Progress in Gynecology and Obstetrics

Progress in Gynecology and Obstetrics

The Proceedings of the
Second European Winter Conference in
Gynecology and Obstetrics held at
Madonna di Campiglio, Italy, March 1989

Edited by
A. R. Genazzani, F. Petraglia and A. Volpe

Department of Obstetrics and Gynecology
University of Modena, Italy

The Parthenon Publishing Group
International Publishers in Science, Technology & Education

Casterton Hall, Carnforth,
Lancs, LA6 2LA, UK

120 Mill Road, Park Ridge,
New Jersey, USA

Published in the UK and Europe by
The Parthenon Publishing Group Ltd.
Casterton Hall
Carnforth, Lancs. LA6 2LA ISBN: 1-85070-299-3

Published in the North America by
The Parthenon Publishing Group Inc.
120 Mill Road
Park Ridge
New Jersey, NJ, USA ISBN: 1-85070-299-3

Typeset by Lasertext Ltd., Stretford, Manchester
Printed in Great Britain by
Dotesios Printers Ltd, Trowbridge, Wiltshire

Contents

Part B Growth factors, puberty and short stature

Part C Dihydroergocriptine and hyperprolactinemia

List of principal contributors

M. Abrate
Dept of Obstetrics and Gynecology
University of Modena
via del Pozzo 71
41100 Modena
Italy

P. Anserini
Clinica Ostetrica e Ginecologica
dell'Universita di Genova
Ospedale San Martino
viale Benedetto XV
16132 Genova
Italy

C. Battaglia
Dept of Obstetrics and Gynecology
University of Modena
via del Pozzo 71
41100 Modena
Italy

C. Belloni
Dept of Obstetrics and Gynecology
University of Milan
Scientific Institute H San Raffaele
via Olgettina 60
20132 Milan
Italy

G. Benagiano
I Institute of Obstetrics and Gynecology
University of Rome "La Sapienza"
Policlinico Umberto 1°
00161 Rome
Italy

C. Benedetto
Institute of Obstetrics and Gynecology
Chair A
University of Torino
via Ventimiglia 3
10126 Torino
Italy

P. Benedetti Panici
Insitute of Obstetrics, Gynecology and
Pathology
Catholic University of Sacred Hearts
Rome
Italy

P. Bergsjo
Dept of Obstetrics and Gynecology
University of Bergen
Kvinneklinikken
N-5021 Bergen
Norway

N. Billestrup
Magedorm Research Laboratory
Niels Steensensvej 6
DK-2820 Gentofte
Denmark

P. Bilotta
Medical Dept
Organon
via Ostilia 15
00184 Rome
Italy

P.F. Bolis
Chair of Semeiotica Ostetrica
University of Pavia
I.R.C.C.S. Policlinico San Matteo
Pavia
Italy

B. Brambati
1st Institute of Obstetrics and Gynecology
University of Milan
via Commenda 12
20122 Milan
Italy

M. Breckwoldt
Division of Clinical Endocrinology
Dept of Obstetrics and Gynecology
University of Freiburg
Hugstetter strasse 55
D-7800 Freiburg i Br
West Germany

H. G. Burger
Prince Henry's Institute of Medical
Research
P.O. Box 118
South Melbourne 3205
Australia

G. Calzolari
Institute of Clinical Medicine
University of Modena
via del Pozzo 71
41100 Modena
Italy

C. Campagnoli
Servizio di Endocrinologia Ginecologica
USL IX Ospedale Sant'Anna
Corso Spezia n 60
10126 Torino
Italy

G.B. Candiani
la Clinica Ostetrica e Ginecologica
Universita di Milano
via Commenda 12
20122 Milan
Italy

G.L. Capitanio
Dept of Obstetrics, Gynecology and Pathology
University of Chieti
Chieti
Italy

E. Cattaneo
Tumor Viruses Laboratory
Infectious Diseases Institute
Pavia
Italy

G. Centini
Dept of Obstetrics and Gynecology
University of Siena
School of Medicine
Siena
Italy

T. Chard
Dept of Reproductive Physiology and Obstetrics and Gynecology
St Bartholomews Hospital Medical College
London EC1A 7BE

T.V. Chervakova
All-Union Research Centre for Maternal and Child Health
Moscow
USSR

A. Cianci
Chair and Obstetrics, Gynecology and Endocrinology
Ospedale S Bambino
via Torre del Vescova
95124 Catania
Italy

N. Colacurci
Dept of Obstetrics and Gynecology
II School of Medicine
University of Naples
Naples
Italy

U.F. Colombo
"L Mangiagalli"
I Clinic of Obstetrics and Gynecology
University of Milan
Milan
Italy

P.F. Conte
Istituto Nazionale per la Ricerca Sul Cancro
Division Oncologia Medica
viale Benedetto XV 10
16132 Genova
Italy

N. Corbino
Istituto do Patologia Ostetrica e Ginecologica
Ospedale di Maternita S Bambino
via Torre del Vescova
95124 Catania
Italy

S. Davolio Marani
Institute of Radiology
University of Modena
C so Adriano 1
41100 Modena
Italy

D. De Aloysio
Dept of Obstetrics and Gynecology
via Massarenti 13
40138 Bologna
Italy

V. De Leo
Dept of Obstetrics and Gynecology
University of Siena
Siena
Italy

G. De Placido
Dept of Obstetrics and Gynecology
II School of Medicine
University of Naples
Naples
Italy

LIST OF PRINCIPAL CONTRIBUTORS

E.C. degli Uberti
Institute of Clinical Medicine
University of Ferrara
44100 Ferrara
Italy

S. Dexeus
Paseo Bonanova, 67
08017 Barcelona
Spain

C. Di Carlo
Istituto di Ginecologica Ostetrica e Fisiopatologia della Riproduzione Umana
II Medical School
University of Naples
via Pansini 5
Naples
Italy

A. Di Lieto
Dept of Pathology
University of Naples
II School of Medicine
Naples
Italy

J. Dor
Dept of Obstetrics and Gynecology
The Sheba Medical Center
Tel Hashomer 52621
Israel

F. Facchinetti
Dept of Obstetrics and Gynecology
University of Modena
via del Pozzo 71
41100 Modena
Italy

J. Falck Larsen
Dept of Obstetrics and Gynecology
Herlev University Hospital
DK-2730 Herlev/Copenhagen
Denmark

L. Falsetti
Via Milziade Tirandi 13
25127 Brescia
Italy

L. Fedele
I Clinica Ostetrica e Ginecologica
University of Milan
via della Commenda 12
20122 Milan
Italy

G. Ferraris
Dept B of Gynecology and Obstetrics Institutes
University of Torino
Torino
Italy

E. Ferrazzi
Clinica Ostetrica e Ginecologica
Universita di Milano
Ospedale San Paolo
via di Rudini 8
20142 Milano
Italy

L. Fioroni
Dept of Obstetrics and Gynecology
University of Modena
via del Pozzo 71
41100 Modena
Italy

R. Forleo
Dept of Obstetrics and Gynecology
Fatebenefratelli S Giovanni
Calibita Area General Hospital
Tiberiria Block
Rome
Italy

G. Forti
Endocrinology Unit
Dept of Clinical Physiopathology
viale Morgagni 85
50134 Florence
Italy

M Franchi
Dept of Obstetrics and Gynecology
Policlinico S Matteo
University of Pavia
27100 Pavia
Italy

P.M. Furneri
Istituto di Microbiologia
University of Catania
via Androne 81
95124 Catania
Italy

G. Garuti
Dept of Obstetrics and Gynecology
University of Modena
via del Pozzo 71
41100 Modena
Italy

A.D. Genazzani
Dept of Obstetrics and Gynecology
University of Modena
via del Pozzo 71
41100 Modena
Italy

A.R. Genazzani
Dept of Obstetrics and Gynecology
University of Modena
via del Pozzo 71
41100 Modena
Italy

C. Gennari
Institute of Medical Semeiotica
University of Siena
Piazza Duome 2
53100 Siena
Italy

G. Giordano
Cattedra di Endocrinologica
ISMI Universita di Genova
viale Benedetto XV 6
16132 Genova
Italy

G. Gragnoli
Servizio di Diabetologia
Piazza Duomo 2
53100 Siena
Italy

A. Groppetti
Dept of Pharmacology
Emilio Trabucchi
University of Milan
Milan
Italy

S. Guaschino
Clinica Ostetrica e Ginecologica
Universita di Pavia
IRCCS Policlinico S. Matteo
P. le Golgi
27100 Pavia
Italy

A. Kauppila
Dept of Obstetrics and Gynecology
University of Oulu
SF-90220 Oulu
Finland

T. Kumasaka
Dept of Obstetrics and Gynecology
Dokkyo University
School of Medicine
Mibu
Tochigi
Japan

V. Kuti
Jozsef Attila 84B
Budapest 1029
Hungary

A. Levi Minzi
Dept of Psychiatry
Fatebenefratelli Hospital
Milan
Italy

V. Locatelli
Dept of Pharmacology
School of Medicine
University of Milan
Milan
Italy

B. Lunenfeld
The Institute of Endocrinology
Chaim Sheba Medical Center
Tel-Hashomer
Israel

S.S. Lynch
Dept of Clinical Endocrinology
Birmingham and Midland Hospital for Women
Showell Green Lane
Sparkhill
Birmingham B11 4HL
UK

R. Maheux
4047, Chemin St-Louis
Cap-rouge, P.Q.
Canada G1Y-IV7

F. Mailland
Dept of Research and Development
Poli Industri Chimica
Milan
Italy

V. Mais
Istituto di Clinica Ostetrica e Ginecologica
Universita degli Studi di Pisa,
56100 Pisa
Italy

S. Mancuso
Dept of Obstetrics and Gynecology
Universita Cattolica del S Cuore
Largo Gemelli 8
00168 Rome
Italy

L.R. Marcellino
Universita di Rome "La Sapienza"
Istituto III Clinica Chirurgia
Cattedra di Metodologia Clinica
Rome
Italy

C. Marcocci
Instituto di Endocrinologia
University of Pisa
viale del Tirreno 64
56018 Tirrenia-Pisa
Italy

P. Martinelli
Dept of Gynecology, Obstetrics and Pathophysiology of Human Reproduction
Faculty of Medicine
University of Naples
Naples
Italy

L. Marzetti
III Dept of Obstetrics and Gynecology Clinic
University of Rome "La Sapienza"
Rome
Italy

G. Masellis
S M I E E – Consultorio Familiare
University of Modena
via Largo del Pozzo 79
41100 Modena
Italy

S. Massobrio
Clinica Ostetrica e Ginecologica
University di Torino
c/o Ospedale Mauriziano
L go Turati 62
10100 Torino
Italy

M. Massobrio
Cattedra "D"-Universitá di Torino
Rep 5-C Ospedale Mauriziano
Largo Turati 62
10128 Torino
Italy

A.M. Mattei
III Dept of Obstetrics and Gynecology
University of Milan
Milan
Italy

S.M. McCann
Dept of Physiology
Neuropeptide Division
The University of Texas South-Western Medical Center at Dallas
5323 Harry Hines Boulevard
Dallas, Texas 75235-9040
USA

H. Meden Vrtovec
Dept of Obstetrics and Gynecology
University Medical Center
Ljubljana
Yugoslavia

G.B. Melis
Istituto di Ginecologica e Ostetrica
Universita degli Studi di Pisa
Ospedale Santa Chiara
via Roma 67
56100 Pisa
Italy

A. Milewicz
Dept of Endocrinology
School of Medicine
University of Wroclaw
ul. Pasteura 4
50-367 Wroclaw
Poland

R.A.V. Milsted
Medical Research Dept
ICI Pharmaceuticals
Alderly Park
Macclesfield
Cheshire SK10 4TG

G. Mollica
Institute of Obstetrics and Gynecology
University of Ferrara
Ferrara
Italy

C. Montoneri
Clinica Ostetrica e Ginecologica dell'Universita
Ospedale Vittorio Emanuele II
via Plebiscito 632
95124 Catania
Italy

T. Motto
I Clinica Ostetrica e Ginecologia
University of Milan
Milan
Italy

C. Nappi
Dept of Obstetrics and Gynecology
University of Naples
via Pansini 5
80131 Naples
Italy

G. Nicoletti
Institute of Microbiology and Chair of Obstetrics and Gynecological Endocrinology
University of Catania
Catania
Italy

C. O'Herlihy
University College of Dublin
National Maternity Hospital
Holles Street
Dublin 2
Ireland

U. Omodei
via Grazie 3
25100 Brescia
Italy

A. Pachi
IV Clinica Ostetrica e Ginecologica
Policlinico Umberto 1
via le Regina Elena 327
00161 Rome
Italy

G. Palumbo
Chairman of Obstetrics, Gynecology and Endocrinology
Ospedale S Bambino
via Torre del Vescovo
95124 Catania
Italy

S. Pecorelli
Dipartimento Materno-Infantile
Spedali Civili di Brescia
p. le Spedali Civili
1-25123 Brescia
Italy

F. Petraglia
Dept of Obstetrics and Gynecology
University of Modena
via del Pozzo 71
41100 Modena
Italy

S. Pinto
Clinica Medica I
viale Morgagni 85
50134 Firenze
Italy

F. Polatti
Istituto di Clinica Ostetrica e Ginecologica
Universita degli Studi di Pavia
Pavia
Italy

A. Porcelli
Institute of Obstetrics and Gynecology
University of Turin
Turin
Italy

N. Principi
Cattedra di Clinici Pediatrica IV
Ospedale L. Sacco
via G.B. Grassi 74
20157 Milan
Italy

P. Pronzato
Instituto Nazionale per la Ricerca sul Cancro e GONO – Gruppo Oncologica del Nord Overt
viale Benedetto XV 10
16132 Genova
Italy

C. Pullé
Istituto di Ginecologica
Policlinico Universitario
98100 Messina
Italy

G. Robustelli della Cuna
Division of Oncology
Fondazione Clinica del Lavaro
via S Boezio 26
27100 Pavia
Italy

C. Romanini
Institute of Obstetrics and Gynecology
University of Ancona
Medical School at Salesi Hospital
Via I. Corridoni II,
60123 Ancona,
Italy

G. Samsioe
Dept of Obstetrics and Gynecology
Goteborgs Universitet
Sahlgrenska Sjukhuset
S-413 45 Goteborg
Sweden

G. Scambia
Dept of Obstetrics and Gynecology
Catholic University of Rome
Largo Agostino Gemelli 8
00168 Rome
Italy

J.G. Schenker
Dept of Obstetrics and Gynecology
Hadassah University Hospital
Jerusalem
Israel

J. Schoemaker
Dept of Obstetrics and Gynecology
Division of Reproductive Endocrinology and Fertility
Free University Hospital
P O Box 7057
1007 MB Amsterdam
The Netherlands

A.E. Semprini
VI Dept of Obstetrics and Gynecology
University of Milan
Ospedale S Paolo
Milan
Italy

G.B. Serra
Istituto di Clinica Ostetrica e Ginecologica
Universita Cattolica del Sacro Cuore
Rome
Italy

R.A. Sherwood
Dept of Clinical Biochemistry
King's College Hospital
Denmark Hill
London SE5 9RS
UK

P. Sismondi
Institute of Obstetrics and Gynecology
University of Torino
via Ventimiglia 3
10126 Torino
Italy

R. Sitruk-Ware
Medical Dept
Ciba-Geigy Ltd
P O Box
4002 Basle
Switzerland

N.O. Sjöberg
Dept of Obstetrics, Gynecology and Orthopaedics
University Hospital
Malmö
Sweden

J. Spona
Division of Molecular Endocrinology
Dept of Obstetrics and Gynecology
University of Vienna
Spitalgasse 23
A-1090 Vienna
Austria

S.S. Stojilković
9000 Rockville Pike
Building 10, Room 8C 407
Bethesda
Maryland 20892
USA

N. Surico
Dept of Obstetrics and Gynecology
Chair B
University of Turin
via Ventimiglia 3
10126 Turin
Italy

M. Szamatowicz
Institute of Obstetrics and Gynecology
Bialystok Medical School
State Teaching Hospital
Bialystock
Poland

G.P. Trentini
Institute of Pathological Anatomy
University of Modena
via del Pozzo 71
41100 Modena
Italy

G.F. Trossarelli
Institute of Obstetrics and Gynecology
University of Turin
AVIS Transfusion Centre
Turin
Italy

P.L. Venturini
Dept of Obstetrics and Gynecology
University of Genova
viale Benedetto XV
16132 Genova
Italy

S. Venturoli
Institute of Reproductive Physiology and Pathology
University of Bologna
Bologna
Italy

P. Vercellini
Ia Clinica Ostetrica e Ginecologica
Universita di Milano
via Commenda 12
20122 Milano
Italy

A. Volpe
Dept of Obstetrics and Gynecology
University of Modena
School of Medicine
via del Pozzo 71
41100 Modena
Italy

A. Zanotti
Dept of Research and Development
Poli Industri Chimica SpA
Milan
Italy

C. Zara
Dept of Obstetrics and Gynecology
University of Pavia
Pavia
Italy

H. Zech
Roemerstrasse 2
A-6900 Bregenz
Austria

Section 1

Gynecological Oncology

Part A

Uterine cancers

1

Epidermal growth factor receptor in gynecological malignancies

G. Scambia, P. Benedetti Panici, F. Battaglia, G. Ferrandina, C. Barletta and S. Mancuso

Peptide growth factors are small molecules which modulate cell proliferation[1]. They have inhibitory or stimulatory effects through an autocrine secretion mechanism in which the same malignant cells and/or, probably, the supporting stromal components are involved[2].

There is much evidence linking growth factors to oncogenes[3]. In particular the *c-sis* proto-oncogene encodes for a homodimer similar to the B chain of platelet-derived growth factor (PDGF)[4,5]; *c-erbB* proto-oncogene and *erbB2-Neu* products are similar to a truncated form of the epidermal growth factor receptor (EGF-R)[6]. On the other hand, growth factors have been shown to positively modulate the transcription of *c-sis* and *c-fos* proto-oncogenes[7]. Moreover, the interaction of peptide growth factors with other growth-modulating substances as steroid hormones, seems to play an important role in cancer cell growth regulation. In fact, estradiol stimulates the production of peptide growth factors[8] and progestins have been found to increase EGF-R expression in breast, endometrial and ovarian cancer cells *in vitro*[9].

EGF and α-transforming growth factor (α-TGF), although different in structure and immunoreactivity, influence the cellular activity with the same mechanisms, interacting with the same membrane receptor, of which they induce autophosphorylation through the activation of the tyrosine-kinase subunit[10–12]. α-TGF activity has been found in the conditioned medium from various transformed and malignant cell lines[11], in solid tumor extracts[13], and in effusions from cancer patients[14]. Increased levels of α-TGF of different molecular weight have also been found in the urine of cancer patients[15,16]. Moreover, EGF was detected in many human tissues[17], and fluids such as urine[18], breast milk and breast cyst fluid[19], homogenates of non-neoplastic mammary tissue and extracts of human breast tumors[17].

EGF-R has been demonstrated to be present in several normal and malignant cell lines, and in most human tumors. In particular, several studies have suggested a biological and clinical significance of EGF and its receptor in gynecological tumors[20,21].

We have recently found EGF-R in many primary breast tumors[22].

Sainsbury *et al.*[23] and Fitzpatrick *et al.*[24] have reported similar results, showing EGF-R expression in about 45% of primary breast cancer. Moreover, these authors reported that EGF-R is negatively related to the estrogen receptors (ER). Our study also demonstrated a negative correlation between EGF-R and ER and progesterone receptors (PR) expression, the last two being a well-known favorable prognostic parameter in breast cancer.

We have also found a positive correlation between EGF-R expression in primary breast tumors and the presence of lymph node metastases, and we hypothesized, in agreement with Macias *et al.*[25], that EGF-R identify more aggressive tumors. In this context the finding that the *Her2-Neu* oncogene is amplified in 30% of primary breast tumors[26] and that this gene amplification is statistically related with the number of metastatic lymph nodes diseased and the disease-free survival, may be relevant.

The inverse relationship between EGF-R and steroid receptors also suggests a possible EGF-R-mediated mechanism of growth control in hormone-independent breast tumors. Much experimental evidence supports this hypothesis. Roos *et al.*[27] have shown significantly higher levels of EGF-R in hormone-independent than in hormone-dependent human breast cancer cells. Moreover, EGF and α-TGF have been demonstrated to decrease the expression of ER and PR in breast cancer cell lines[28] and they may also influence the expression of peptide hormone receptors in mammary tissue.

Table 1 shows the effect of EGF on ER and PR levels in the CG 5 human breast cancer cell line. It appears that the addition of EGF lowers both ER and PR content and that EGF decreases the estrogen-induced stimulation of PR. Therefore it seems to be plausible that the activation of specific EGF-induced intracellular pathways could decrease or modulate those induced by estrogens.

The role of EGF/α-TGF in the processes leading to the neoplastic transformation of human breast epithelium also deserves further attention. Recently we found higher levels of EGF-like substances in the cyst fluid of the apocrine breast cysts than in flattened ones, the former being considered at a higher risk of breast cancer development than the latter[29]. This finding, together with that of detectable levels of EGF/α-TGF activity in the cytosol of primary breast tumors, suggests a possible autocrine regulation of breast cancer cell proliferation through the EGF-R system. In a series of 28 primary breast tumor cytosols analyzed in our laboratory, EGF/α-TGF levels ranging

Table 1 Effects of estradiol (E_2) and EGF on ER and PR levels in the CG 5 cell line

Substance	*ER**	*PR*
None	3566 ± 432	1453 ± 325
E_2 (10 nM)	288 ± 69	2890 ± 415
EGF (5 ng/ml)	1550 ± 320	404 ± 97
E_2 + EGF	821 ± 89	2048 ± 210

*ER and PR were measured according to Taylor *et al.*[33]. Results are expressed as CPM of specific bound. The mean ± SEM of three different experiments performed in triplicate are reported from 0.7 to 22 ng/mg protein have been detected.

Data on EGF-R expression in gynecological malignancies other than breast cancer are more limited. Table 2 shows the levels and expression of EGF-R in a series of 84 female genital tract malignancies collected in our department in the last 2 years. Measurable EGF-R levels were detected in 84.6% of primary ovarian carcinomas and we found a negative correlation between EGF-R and ER expression. Moreover, we demonstrated a measurable EGF/α-TGF activity (ranging from 0.9 to 7.27 ng/mg protein) in all ovarian tumor cytosols. These findings are in agreement with those of Bauchnekt *et al.*[30], who found EGF activity in tumor extracts and related this activity and the EGF-R expression to some prognostic factors of ovarian cancer. These data, together with our recent *in vitro* finding of EGF-R expression and growth regulatory effect of EGF on ovarian cancer cells (manuscript in preparation), seem to indicate a role of EGF-R in the control of ovarian cancer growth. As far as other gynecological malignancies are concerned, we found that 67.8% of endometrial cancer, 73.6% of cervical cancer and 100% of vulvar cancer and uterine sarcomas express EGF-R. In endometrial cancer, in particular, EGF-R were more expressed in less differentiated than in well–moderately differentiated tumors, suggesting that, as in breast cancer, EGF-R may have a negative prognostic significance. Very high EGF-R levels were found in vulvar and cervical tumors with respect to endometrial and ovarian tumors. Therefore in squamous cell tumors that seem to be devoid of a functional estrogen receptor system[31], we can hypothesize that peptide factors, such as EGF or EGF-like substances, may primarily regulate cancer cell growth.

In conclusion, data from our and other laboratories suggest that EGF/α-TGF system is extremely important in the regulation of cancer cell growth by itself and that it may also act as intermediary system through which several mitogens stimulate cell proliferation. Studies on EGF-R system may also provide new insights into the processes leading to cancer development. The modifications of plasma membrane receptor status and the concomitant increase of autocrine growth factor secretion could be important for the development of an independent growth mechanism in neoplastic tissue.

Finally these biological findings may indicate new directions for cancer therapy. It has recently been reported that a monoclonal antibody against EGF-R inhibits the growth of human cancer cells *in vitro* and in nude mice *in vivo*[32].

Table 2 EGF-R expression in 84 gynecological malignancies

		EGF-R (fmol/mg prot.)		*EGF-R* > *1.5*
Tumor type	*No.*	*Median*	*Range*	(%)
Ovarian cancer	26	3.02	0–12.5	84.6
Endometrial cancer	28	6.54	0–20.4	67.8
Cervical cancer	19	9.09	0.4–42.2	73.6
Vulvar cancer	6	12.38	7.9–49.5	100
Uterine sarcomas	5	12.7	7.0–45.3	100

REFERENCES

1. Taketani, Y. and Oka, T. (1983). Biological action of epidermal growth factor and its functional receptors in normal mammary epithelial cells. *Proc. Natl. Acad. Sci., USA*, **80**, 2647–50
2. Sporn, M.B. and Roberts, A.B. (1985). Autocrine growth factors and cancer. *Nature*, **313**, 745–47
3. Heldin, C.H. and Westermark, B. (1984). Growth factors: mechanism of action and relation to oncogenes. *Cell*, **37**, 9–20
4. Waterfield, M.D., Scrace, T. and Whittle, N. (1984). Platelet derived growth factor is structurally related to the putative transforming protein p28-sis of simian sarcoma virus. *Nature*, **304**, 35–9
5. Johnsson, A., Heldin, C.H. and Wasteson, A. (1984). The c-sis gene encodes a precursor of the B chain of platelet derived growth factor. *EMBO J.*, **3**, 921–8
6. Downward, J., Yarden, Y. and Mayes, E. (1984). Close similarity of epidermal growth factor receptor and v-erb-B oncogene protein sequences. *Nature*, **307**, 521–7
7. Kelly, K., Cochran, B.H., Stiles, C.D. and Leder, P. (1983). Cell specific regulation of the c-myc gene by lymphocyte mitogens and platelet derived growth factor. *Cell*, **35**, 603–10
8. Gonzalez, F., Lakshmanan, J., Hoath, S. and Fisher, D.A. (1984). Effect of oestradiol-17β on uterine epidermal growth factor concentration in immature mice. *Acta Endocrinol. (Copenh.)*, **105**, 425–8
9. Imai, Y., Leung, C.K.H., Friesen, H.G. and Shiu, R.P.C. (1982). Epidermal growth factor receptors and effect of epidermal growth factor on growth of human breast cancer cells in long-term tissue culture. *Cancer Res.*, **42**, 4394–8
10. Massague, J. (1983). Epidermal growth factor-like transforming growth factor: II. Interaction with Epidermal growth factor receptor in human placenta membranes and A 431 cells. *J. Biol. Chem.*, **258**, 13614–20
11. Todaro, G.J., Fryling, C. and Delarco, J.E. (1980). Transforming growth factors produced by certain human tumor cells: polypeptides that interact with epidermal growth factor receptors. *Proc. Natl. Acad. Sci., USA*, **77**, 5258–62
12. Reynolds, F.H., Todaro, G.J., Fryling, C. and Stephenson, J.R. (1981). Human transforming growth factors induce tyrosine phosphorilation of EGF receptors. *Nature*, **292**, 259–62
13. Nickell, K.A., Halper, J. and Moses, H. (1983). Transforming growth factors in solid human malignant neoplasms. *Cancer Res.*, **43**, 1966–71
14. Hanauske, A.R., Arteaga, C.L., Clarck, G.M., Buchok, J., Marshall, M., Hazarika, P., Pardue, R.L. and Von Hoff, D.D. (1988). Determination of transforming growth factor activity in effusions from cancer patients. *Cancer*, **61**, 1832–7
15. Twardzik, D.R., Sherwin, S.A., Ranchalis, J. and Todaro, G.J. (1982). Transforming growth factors in the urine of normal, pregnant and tumor bearing patients. *J. Natl. Cancer Inst.*, **69**, 793–8
16. Uchihashi, M., Hirata, Y., Nakjima, H., Fujita, T. and Matsukura, J. (1983). Urinary excretion of human epidermal growth (hEGF) in patients with malignant tumors. *Horm. Metabol. Res.*, **15**, 261–3
17. Kasselberg, A.G., Orth, D.N., Gray, M.E. and Stahlman, M.T. (1985). Immunocytochemical localisation of human epidermal growth factor/urogastrone in several human tissues. *J. Histochem. Cytochem.*, **33**, 315–22
18. Starkey, R.H., Cohen, S. and Orth, D.N. (1975). Epidermal growth factor: identification of a new hormone in human urine. *Science*, **189**, 800–2
19. Jaspar, J.M. and Franchimont, P. (1980). Radioimmunoassay of human epidermal growth factor in human breast cyst fluid. *J. Cancer Clin. Oncol.*, **21**, 1343–8
20. Battaglia, F., Scambia, G., Benedetti Panici, P., Baiocchi, G., Perrone, L., Iacobelli, S. and Mancuso, S. (1989). Epidermal growth factor receptor expression in gynecological malignancies. *Gynecol. Obstet. Invest.*, **27**, 42–4
21. Bauchnekt, T., Rau, B., Meerpohl, H.G. and Pfeiderer, A. (1984). The prognostic value of the presence of EGF receptors in ovarian carcinomas. *Tumor Diagnostik*, **5**, 62–6
22. Battaglia, F., Scambia, G., Rossi, S., Benedetti Panici, P., Bellantone, R., Polizzi, G., Querzoli, P., Negrini, R., Iacobelli, S., Crucitti, F. and Mancuso, S. (1988). Epidermal growth factor receptor in human breast cancer: correlation with steroid hormone receptors and axillary lymph node involvement. *Eur. J. Cancer Clin. Oncol.*, **24**, 1685–90

23. Sainsbury, J.R.C., Farndon, J.R., Needham, G.K., Malcolm, A.J. and Harris, A.L. (1987). Epidermal growth factor receptor status as predictor of early recurrence of and death from breast cancer. *Lancet*, **i**, 1398–402
24. Fitzpatrick, S.L.D., Brightwell, J., Wittliff, J.L., Barrows, G.H. and Schultze, G.S. (1984). Epidermal growth factor binding by breast tumor biopsies and relationship to estrogen receptor and progesterone receptor levels. *Cancer Res.*, **44**, 3448–53
25. Macias, A., Azavedo, E., Perez, R., Rutqvist, L.R. and Skoog, L. (1986). Receptors for epidermal growth factor in human mammary carcinomas and their metastases. *Anticancer Res.*, **6**, 849–52
26. Slamon, D.J., Clarck, G.M., Wong, S.G., Levin, W.J., Ullrich, A. and McGuire, W.L. (1987). Human breast cancer: correlation of relapse and survival with amplification of the HER-2 neu oncogene. *Science*, **235**, 177–82
27. Roos, W., Fabbro, D., Kung, W., Costa, S.D. and Eppenberger, U. (1986). Correlation between hormone dependency and the regulation of epidermal growth factor receptor by tumor promoters in human mammary carcinoma cells. *Proc. Natl. Acad. Sci., USA*, **88**, 991–5
28. Dickson, R.B. and Lippman, M.E. (1987). Estrogenic regulation of growth and polypeptide growth factor secretion in human breast carcinoma. *Endocr. Rev.*, **8**, 29–43
29. Battaglia, F., Rossi, S., Scambia, G., Lanzone, A., Benedetti Panici, P., Ferrandina, G., Lombardi, C.P., Crucitti, F. and Mancuso, S. (1990). Growth factor levels in human breast cysts. *Anticancer Res.* (in press)
30. Bauchneckt, T., Kiechle, M., Bauer, G. and Siebers, J.W. (1986). Characterization of growth factors in human ovarian carcinomas. *Cancer Res.*, **46**, 2614–18
31. Grenman, S., Shapire, A. and Carey, T.E. (1988). *In vitro* regulation of cervical cancer cell line Caski, Hela and ME180 to the antiestrogen Tamoxifen. *Gynecol., Oncol.*, **30**, 228–38
32. Masui, H., Kawamoto, T., Sato, J.D., Wolf, B., Sato, G. and Mendelsohn, J. (1984). Growth inhibition of human tumor cells in athymic mice by antiepidermal growth factor receptor monoclonal antibodies. *Cancer Res.*, **44**, 1002–7
33. Taylor, G.H., Blanchard and Zava, T.D. (1984). A simple method to determine all whole cells uptake of radiolabelled estrogen and progesterone and their subcellular localization in breast cancer cell lines in monolayer culture *J. Steroid Biochem.*, **20**, 1083–8

2

Detection and physical state of human papillomavirus DNAs associated with genital cancers in North-Italian women

G. Garuti, F. Boselli and A.R. Genazzani

INTRODUCTION

Among the known types of human papillomavirus (HPV) infecting the human genital tract[1], some viral strains have been extensively investigated because of their high association rate with cervical and vulvar cancers[2,3] and of the demonstrated *in vitro* transforming activity[4]. In particular, HPV 16 appears the best candidate to play an important role in the natural history of the cervical and vulvar squamous cancers. In fact, percentages of HPV 16 association with genital cancers superior to 60% were detected in all previous studies[5,6]. Moreover, HPV 16 DNA sequences integrated within the host-cell genome characterize the cervical and vulvar malignancies in respect to the benign lesions, carrying episomal forms of viral DNA only[7,8]. Interestingly, interferences between HPV DNA integrations and keratinocyte differentiation were ascertained by the demonstration of viral DNA recombinations sites occurring near activated human cellular oncogenes[9].

In order to define, in our country, the association rate of HPV infection with malignant lesions of the lower genital tract, we studied 50 biopsies collected from patients affected by severe cervical dysplasias, invasive cervical cancers and vulvar carcinomas. The study was performed by restriction endonuclease analysis of the extracted DNA and Southern blot hybridization using genomic radiolabeled probes specific for HPV 6, 11, 16 and 18.

MATERIALS AND METHODS

Fifty women, affected by cervical and vulvar carcinomas were considered as group-study. The patients were referred to Colposcopic division of our Clinic and the diagnosis was performed by histological examination of the haematoxylin-eosin stained sections obtained from colposcopically directed bioptic punches. All the 17 vulvar lesions were invasive squamous carcinomas; among the cervical tumors, we selected 12 grade III Intraepithelial Cervical Neoplasias (CIN III), 16 invasive squamous carcinomas and five well differentiated adenocarcinomas.

Tissue samples suitable for DNA extraction were obtained from surgical or colposcopic collection of the primary neoplastic lesions. The biopsies were immediately frozen and stored in liquid nitrogen until DNA extraction. The genomic DNA was obtained by lysis of the tissue in 10 mM Tris–HCl (pH 7.8), 150 mM NaCl, 10 mM EDTA, 0.6% SDS, 100 μg/ml Proteinase K, followed by one extraction with phenol, two with phenol–chloroform and a final one with chloroform–isoamylalcohol (24/1). The extracted DNA was then digested with RNase and subsequently with Pronase. Then, a further extraction with phenol–chloroform and chloroform–isoamylalcohol was performed. The DNA was ethanol precipitated and resuspended in TE buffer. Various amounts of DNA were digested with *Bam*HI (single cut enzyme for HPV 6, 11, 16 and double cut for HPV 18 DNAs), and *Pst*I (multicut enzyme on the genome of all known HPV 'genital' types) according to manufacturer's instructions (Boehringer). The amounts of the extracted DNA permitted additional restriction analysis in some specimens; *Ava*II, *Eco*RI and *Hin*dIII were other enzymes employed in this study. Four aliquots of digested DNA (10 μg each) obtained from the same tissue sample were separately electrophoresed in 1% agarose gel and blotted onto nylon filters[10]. The recombinant viral DNA cloned at the single *Bam*HI (HPV 6, 11 and 16) and *Eco*RI (HPV 18) sites in pBR322 vector plasmid was digested with the appropriate endonuclease and the linearized DNAs were purified in agarose gel electrophoresis[11]. The total genome of each virus was α-32dATP labelled with DNA polymerase using the random priming technique[12], purified on Sephadex G-50 columns and used as probes, with a specific activity of 2×10^7–6×10^7 cpm/μg DNA. The filters were prehybridized in $2 \times$ SSC, $10 \times$ Denhardt solution, 0.2% SDS and 0.2 μg/ml sonicated salmon sperm DNA, for 10 h at 65°C. The four filters were separately hybridized at 65°C from 15 to 20 h in a mixture containing $2 \times$ SSC, $10 \times$ Denhardt solution, 0.2% SDS, 0.1 μg/ml sonicated salmon sperm DNA and 10^6 cpm/ml of HPV 6, 11, 16 and 18 labelled DNA probes (stringency conditions calculated to -15°C TM). The filters were then washed twice in $2 \times$ SSC, $1 \times$ SSC, $0.1 \times$ SSC (with addition of 0.5% SDS in each wash), for 30 min at 65°C and exposed to Kodak X-Omat AR ray films with an intensifying screen at -40°C from 12 to 72 h.

Episomal forms of HPV DNA were identified on the resulting autoradiograms as a single 7.9 kbp fragment when a single cut enzyme was employed on the viral genome, coupled with the evidence of the expected subgenomic fragments generated by multicut enzymes, according with the known nucleotide sequence of viral genomes[13–16]. Head to tail rearranged viral DNA oligomers have been suspected when some unexpected homologous DNA fragments, representing the junctional sequences, were identified only by use of multicutting enzymes. Integrated physical forms of HPV DNA were suggested from the evidence of more than a 7.9 kbp specific signal generated from the digestion by a single cut enzyme on the viral genome; additional bands represent the junctional regions between viral DNA and host-cell chromosomal DNA.

RESULTS

In Table 1 we report the histological diagnosis and the virus type associated with the studied samples; the physical state of the viral DNA was also

Table 1 Human papillomavirus DNA sequences detected in cervical and vulvar cancers; the physical state of viral DNA suggested from the restriction endonuclease analysis was also indicated (E = Episomal forms; O = Head to tail oligomeric rearranged episomes; I = Integrated forms)

Invasive vulvar squamous carcinomas	*Invasive cervical squamous carcinomas*
1. negative	30. negative
2. negative	31. negative
3. negative	32. HPV 16 (E + I)
4. negative	33. HPV 16 (E + O)
5. negative	34. negative
6. negative	35. HPV 6a (E)
7. negative	36. HPV 16 (E)
8. negative	37. HPV 16 (E)
9. HPV 11 (E)	38. HPV 16 (E)
10. HPV 16 (E + O)	39. HPV 16 (E + O)
11. negative	40. HPV 6 (E)
12. negative	41. HPV 16 (I)
13. negative	42. HPV 16 (E + I)
14. HPV 16 (E)	43. negative
15. negative	44. HPV 16 (E + O)
16. negative	45. HPV 16 (E)
17. HPV 16 (E)	
Cervical intraepithelial neoplasias	*Invasive cervical adenocarcinomas*
18. HPV 16 (E)	46. negative
19. negative	47. negative
20. HPV 16 (E)	48. negative
21. HPV 16 (E + I)	49. HPV 11 (I)
22. negative	50. negative
23. HPV 16 (E + I)	
24. negative	
25. HPV 16 (E)	
26. HPV 16 (E)	
27. HPV 16 (E)	
28. HPV 16 (E)	
29. HPV 16 (E)	

indicated on the basis of the restriction endonuclease analysis performed in each sample. Four out of 17 vulvar squamous carcinomas (23.6%) carried HPV DNA sequences, all defined as episomes of HPV 11 DNA (one case) and HPV 16 DNA (three cases). The sample 10 showed an associated HPV 16 DNA occurring both as monomeric episomes and as oligomeric rearranged physical forms. The percentage of association with HPV infection rise to 75% in the CIN III lesions; the nine positive cases harbored constantly HPV 16 DNA sequences. Monomeric episomes were associated to all the lesions; however, in two samples integrated specific sequences could be identified in association with extrachromosomal episomes. These specimens (cases 21 and 23 of Table 1) revealed a different pattern of integration; in sample 21 a viral DNA sequence of HPV 16 recombines in a single region of the human genome because of the only one homologous additional fragment generated both by *Bam*HI (6.5 kbp) and *Pst*I (2.5 kbp). On the contrary, sample 23, showing a hybridization in the high molecular weight fractions of DNA after the cut by *Bam*HI, coupled with several unexpected positive fragments by *Pst*I digestion, suggests an integration of HPV genome occurring in multiple sites of chromosomal DNA (Figure 1). Twelve out of 16 invasive cervical carcinomas (75%) contained specific sequences related to HPV 6a (two cases) and HPV 16 DNA (ten cases). In six samples we defined only monomeric episomes, in three other cases a contemporaneous presence of head to tail oligomers was detected. HPV 16 DNA sequences observed in the remaining three positive cervical neoplasias showed restriction endonuclease patterns suggesting viral genome rearrangements within the host-cell DNA, with (cases 32 and 42) or without (case 41) the coexistence of episomal physical forms. As well as described for the CIN III lesions, two different patterns of integration could be observed. In the samples 41 and 42 the resulting autoradiograms were consistent with a recombination of the HPV genome in a defined and single region of human DNA, while in the sample 32 a larger number of HPV 16-host cell DNA recombination sites could be suspected on the basis of the more articulated pattern of hybridization generated both by *Bam*HI and *Pst*I enzymes (Figure 1). Among the five cervical adenocarcinomas examined, only one neoplasia carrying HPV DNA showed HPV 11 sequences. In this sample (case 49 of Table 1 and Figure 1), both by *Bam*HI and *Pst*I digestions we detected a principal hybridization of a genomic homologous fragment of around 3.9 kbp. The lack of a 7.9 kbp HPV 11 linearized entire genome after the cut by *Bam*HI, combined with the absence of the known *Pst*I restriction enzyme pattern[14] suggested a particular HPV 11 genome rearrangement within the host-cell genome. It appears consistent with an integration of a HPV 11 partial sequence in a single region of the chromosomal DNA (Figure 1). Our further studies (unshown data) demonstrated that the 3.9 kbp homologous fragment contains viral DNA sequences strongly related to non-coding region and E_6–E_7 open reading frames of the HPV 11 genome.

DISCUSSION

Our results demonstrated that, even in our country, cervical cancers and HPV infection are frequently associated. DNA sequences homologous to HPV types investigated were detected in 66% of cervical specimens. Among the squamous lesions, the detectability of viral DNA rises to 75% because of the lower association of HPV infection with cervical neoplasias originating from endocervical glands. Nineteen out of 22 positive cancers carried DNA sequences related to HPV 16 genome, confirming the well known predominant association between this HPV type and cervical malignancy[2,3]. Our percentage (75%) of CIN III lesions associated with HPV 16 infection is slightly higher than those previously reported[17,18], conversely, the 62.5% detected in the squamous cervical cancers is in accordance with the majority of the epidemiological studies[1,19,20].

Previous studies demonstrated that in malignant squamous vulvar lesions the coexistence of HPV infection is often observed; HPV 16 DNA was detected with a frequency similar to the cervical neoplasias[21,22], suggesting

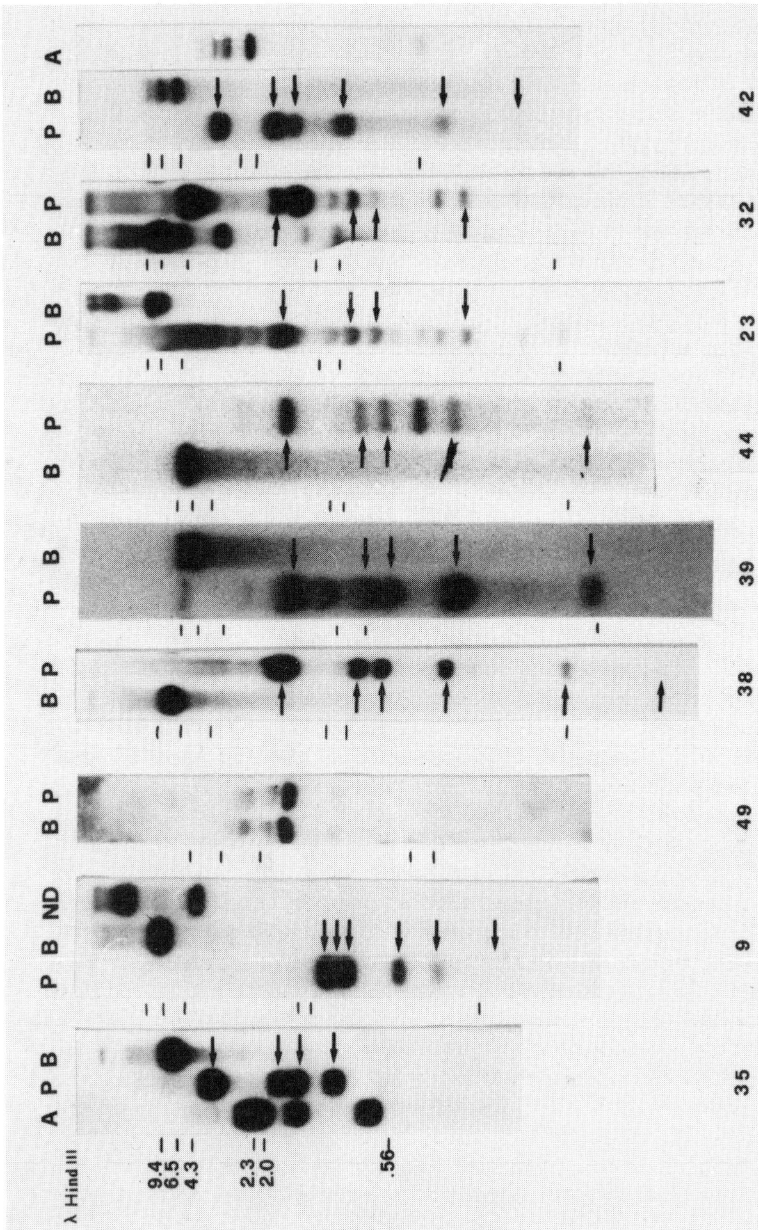

Figure 1 Southern blot hybridizations resulting from some of the studied genital cancers; λ DNA *Hind*III digested was adopted as molecular size marker. At the top of each lane we reported the restriction enzymes employed (B = *Bam*HI, P = *Pst*I, A = *Ava*II, ND = undigested DNA). The numbers indicated below the various autoradiograms correspond to the samples reported in Table 1. The arrows indicate the molecular sizes of the HPV DNA fragments expected after the digestion by *Pst*I on the known nucleotide sequence of HPV 6a (case 35), HPV 11 (case 9) and HPV 16 (cases 38, 39, 44, 23, 32 and 42)

a common etiological role played by this virus in the development of both genital cancers. This observation was not confirmed in the vulvar cancers here investigated where we detected episomal HPV DNA sequences only in four samples (23.5%). Although further confirmations are required, these results suggest the lack of correlation between vulvar cancer and HPV infection. However, adopting only stringent conditions of hybridization, we cannot exclude the association of different HPV types, such as HPV 31, 33, 35, 39 or 42 that, though rarely, are associated with genital neoplasias. A regional prevalence of some of these more recently characterized viral strains within vulvar lesions with respect to HPV 6, 11, 16 and 18 involvement, is not supported from our previous results on the vulvar HPV-related benign lesions, in which the 95.2% of the cases carried HPV 6, 11 or 16 DNA[23]. If the vulvar HPV infection plays a role in the squamous oncogenesis, it is likely that this happens through the more diffuse HPV strains in our geographic areas; thus, we suggest that the failure in HPV detection appears to be the true expression of independence between the vulvar carcinogenesis and the viral infection.

Although the epidemiological studies[1] and biological properties[24] of HPV 16 demonstrated its relationship with genital oncogenesis, it is known that HPV 6 and HPV 11, typically detected in benign lesions, were found in some malignant neoplasias[25,26]. These data were confirmed in our study, in which two squamous cervical carcinomas and one vulvar carcinoma carried HPV 6 and HPV 11 episomal DNA. In addition, a cervical adenocarcinoma contained a rearranged, and most probably integrated, DNA sequence hybridizing to HPV 11 genome.

Among the 19 cervical cancers showing HPV 16-related sequences, the frequency of oligomeric and/or monomeric episomes is greater than the host-cell genome integrated forms. As previously reported[27], episomal HPV 16 DNA coexists with integrated sequences in the majority of the cases investigated. The patterns of integration here observed, indicate that different DNA sequences of the human genome recombine with the viral DNA; this seems to integrate both in a single site of cellular DNA or within various genomic regions, as previously described in other cervical carcinomas.

Although HPV DNA integrations were demonstrated near some activated human cellular oncogenes[9], the role of HPV 16 in the natural history of the cervical carcinoma does not appear to be necessarily related to an integrational event. As shown in previous observations[1] we found that the majority of cervical neoplasias contained HPV 16 episomes only. In these cases, the putative transforming activity of the virus may be due to post-transcriptional and trans-acting events.

REFERENCES

1. Syrjanen, K.J. (1987). Biology of human papillomavirus infection and their role in squamous carcinogenesis. *Med. Biol.*, **65**, 21
2. Durst, M., Gissmann, L., Ikemberg, H. and Zur Hausen, H. (1983). A papillomavirus DNA from a cervical cancer and its prevalence in cancer biopsy samples from different geographic regions. *Proc. Natl Acad. Sci., USA*, **80**, 3812
3. Gupta, J., Pilotti, S., Rilke, F. and Shah, K. (1987). Association of human papillomavirus

type 16 with neoplastic lesions of the vulva and other genital sites by in situ hybridization. *Am. J. Clin. Pathol.*, **127**, 1987

4. Yasumoto, S., Burkhardt, A.C., Doniger, J. and Di Paolo, J. (1986). Human papillomavirus type 16 DNA induced malignant transformation of NIH 3T3 cells. *J. Virol.*, **57**, 572
5. Feinberg, A.P. and Volgestein, G. (1984). A technique for radiolabelling DNA restriction endonuclease fragment to high specific activity. *Anal. Biochem.*, **137**, 266
6. Smotkin, D., Castellano, C., Santos, C., Del Gado, G., Kurman, R.J. and Jenson, A.B. (1986). Human papillomavirus deoxyribonucleic acid in cervical carcinoma from primary and metastatic sites. *Am. J. Obstet. Gynecol.*, **9**, 115
7. Shirasawa, H., Tomita, Y., Kubota, K., Kasai, J., Sekiya, S., Takamizawa, H. and Simizu, B. (1986). Detection of human papillomavirus type 16 DNA and evidence for integration into the cell DNA in cervical dysplasia. *J. Gen. Virol.*, **67**, 2015
8. Durst, M., Kleinheinz, A., Hotz, M. and Gissmann, L. (1985). The physical state of human papillomavirus type 16 DNA in benign and malignant genital tumours. *J. Gen. Virol.*, **66**, 1515
9. Durst, M., Croce, M., Gissmann, L., Schwartz, E. and Huebner, K. (1987). Papillomavirus sequences integrated near cellular oncogenes in some cervical carcinomas. *Proc. Natl Acad. Sci., USA*, **84**, 1070
10. Southern, E.M. (1975). Detection of specific sequences among DNA fragments separated by gel electrophoresis. *J. Mol. Biol.*, **98** 503
11. Maniatis, T., Frisch, E.F. and Sambrook, J. (1983). *Molecular Cloning, a Laboratory Manual.* (Cold Spring Harbor NY: Cold Spring Harbor Laboratory)
12. Smotkin, D., Berek, J.S., Fu, Y.S., Hacker, N.F., Major, F.J. and Wettstein, F.O. (1986). Human papillomavirus deoxyribonucleic acid in adenocarcinoma and adenosquamous carcinoma of the cervix. *Obstet. Gynecol.*, **68**, 241
13. Schwartz, E., Durst, M., Demankowski, C., Lattermann, O., Zech, R., Wolfsperger, E., Suhai, S. and Zur Hausen, H. (1983). DNA sequence and genome organization of genital human papillomavirus type 6b. *EMBO J.*, **2**, 2341
14. Dartmann, K., Schwartz, E., Gissmann, L. and Zur Hausen, H. (1986). The nucleotide sequence and genome organization of human papillomavirus type 11. *Virology*, **151**, 124
15. Seedorf, K., Krammer, G., Durst, M., Suhai, S. and Rovekamp, W.G. (1986). Human papillomavirus type 16 DNA sequence. *Virology*, **145**, 181
16. Cole, S.T. and Danos, O. (1987). Nucleotide sequence and comparative analysis of the human papillomavirus type 18 genome. *J. Mol. Biol.*, **193**, 599
17. Collins, J.E., Jenkis, D. and McCance, D.J. (1988). Detection of human papillomavirus DNA sequences by *in situ* DNA–DNA hybridization in cervical intraepithelial neoplasia and invasive carcinoma: a retrospective study. *J. Clin. Pathol.*, **41**, 289
18. Lehn, H., Villa, I.I., Marizona, F., Hilgarth, M., Hillemans, H.G. and Sauer, G. (1988). Physical state and biological activity of human papillomavirus genomes in precancerous lesions of the female genital tract. *J. Gen. Virol.*, **69**, 187
19. School, S.M., Kingsley, E.M., Robinson, R.E. and Farrel, P.J. (1985). Prevalence of human papillomavirus type 16 in cervical carcinoma samples in east Anglia. *Int. J. Cancer*, **35**, 215
20. Reves, W.C., Caussy, D., Brinton, L.A., Bruns, M.M., Montalvan, P., Gomez, B., Dc Britton, R.C., Morice, E., Gaital, E., DeLao, S.L. and Rawls, W.E. (1987). Case control study of human papillomavirus and cervical cancer in latin America. *Int. J. Cancer*, **40**, 450
21. Sutton, G.P., Stehman, F.B., Ehrlich, C.E. and Roman, A. (1987). Human papillomavirus deoxyribonucleic acid in lesions of the female genital tract: evidence for type 6/11 in squamous carcinomas of the vulva. *Obstet. Gynaecol.*, **70**, 564
22. Karram, M., Tabor, B., Smotkin, D., Wettstein, F., Bhatia, N. and Micha, J. (1988). Detection of human papillomavirus deoxyribonucleic acid from vulvar dystrophies and vulvar intraepithelial neoplastic lesions. *Am. J. Obstet. Gynecol.*, **159**, 22
23. Garuti, G., Boselli, F., Genazzani, A.R., Silvestri, S. and Ratti, G. (1989). Detection and typing of human papillomavirus in histological specimens by *in situ* hybridization with biotinylated DNA probes. *Am. J. Clin. Pathol.* (in press)
24. Giri, I. and Danos, O. (1986). Papillomavirus genome, from sequence data to biological properties. *Trend Genet.*, **2**, 227
25. Rando, R.F., Sedlacek, T.V., Hunt, J., Jenson, A.B., Kurman, R.J. and Lancaster, W.D. (1986). Verrucous carcinoma of the vulva associated with an unusual type 6 human

papillomavirus. *Obstet. Gynecol.*, **78**, 705

26. Gissmann, L., Wolnik, L., Ikemberg, H., Koldvosky, U., Shnurch, H.G. and Zur Hausen, H. (1983). Papillomavirus type 6 and 11 sequences in genital and laringeal papillomas and in some cervical cancers. *Proc. Natl Acad. Sci., USA*, **80**, 560
27. Lehn, H., Krieg, P. and Sauer, G. (1985). Papillomavirus genomes in human cervical tumors. *Proc. Natl Acad. Sci., USA*, **82**, 5540

3

HLA polymorphisms in ovarian and endometrial cancers

P. F. Bolis, M. Martinetti, O. Finco, M. Franchi, A. La Fianza and M. Cuccia

INTRODUCTION

The human leukocyte antigen (HLA) region contains a cluster of genes controlling cell-surface antigens, immune response determinants and complement proteins. HLA markers have also been associated with increased risk for the development of disease[1]. In all these cases an HLA has been found much more often in patients with the disease than in appropriate controls. This indicates either a direct effect of the antigen in question, perhaps on immune response, or a susceptibility control by a gene at a closely linked locus that is in strong gametic association with the allele controlling the associated antigen. There is a long list of HLA specificities and disease associations (Table 1).

In addition certain HLA phenotypes have been shown to be significantly increased in patients with various malignancies[2–6]. Recently, the genes for the tumor α and β necrosis factor have also been shown to be in the HLA region[1]. Relatively few investigations concerning the frequencies of HLA in patients with gynecological malignancies have been undertaken.

Table 1 HLA/disease associations (Bodmer, 1987[1])

Rheumatoid arthritis	80% DR4
Ankylosing spondylitis	~100% B27
Juvenile diabetes	~100% DR3 or DR4
Narcolepsy	100% DR2
Other diseases	
Grave's disease	DR3
Myasthenia gravis	DR3
Multiple sclerosis	DR2
Psoriasis	CW6
Coeliac disease	DR3
Hemochromatosis	A3
Reactive arthritis	B27

Ovarian cancer is the most frequent cause of death for gynecological malignancies and the fifth cause of death for cancer in women in the Western world. Epidemiologic and etiologic studies tried to identify risk factors directly or indirectly related to this cancer, but a review of the literature reveals that currently there is no evidence to incriminate any single etiologic factor for this group of tumors[7]. There is only a growing evidence of familial predisposition in a small group of patients[7]; if current knowledge of the epidemiology of ovarian cancer is to be translated into disease prevention, more attention should be paid to women at risk because of their family history. One of the best ways to investigate hereditary or genetic causes of diseases is the study of HLA polymorphisms.

Endometrial cancer is the most frequent gynecological malignancy in the Western world[8]. Criteria for inclusion in high risk populations have been related more to general clinical correlations such as obesity or infertility than to specifically identifiable laboratory assays.

The present investigation was undertaken in order to define specific HLA profiles in patients affected by ovarian and endometrial cancer. Some authors suggested[9,10] that these neoplasias do not show a strong association with histocompatibility antigens (A, B, C, DR) as it can be noticed in other types of non-malignant disease. From the study of major histocompatibility complex (MHC) supratypes, it is becoming apparent that extended haplotypes rather than individual alleles are the markers for MHC-associated diseases[11].

PATIENTS AND METHODS

Fifty-two women affected by epithelial ovarian carcinoma (mean age 55 ± 10.2 years) (stage I = 11 cases; stage II = six cases; stage III = 31 cases; stage IV = four cases) and 56 patients with endometrial carcinoma (mean age 62 ± 8.7 years) (stage I = 49 cases; stage II = two cases; stage III = five cases) observed at the Clinic of Obstetrics and Gynaecology of Pavia University.

HLA typing was carried out with the microlymphocytotoxicity test. Sera employed were partially standardized during the 10th International Histocompatibility Workshop and partially obtained by international exchanges.

Bf (Properdin factor B) serum samples were subjected to electrophoresis in 1% agarose, as described by Alper *et al.*[12]. Patterns were developed by immunofixation with goat anti-human properdin factor B serum (Atlantic Antibodies Scarborough, ME) and stained.

C4 allotyping was performed on EDTA serum samples treated with neuraminidase according to Awdeh *et al.*[13]. C4 bands were visualized by immunofixation with goat anti-human C4 antiserum (Atlantic Antibodies Scarborough, ME) and stained.

The control group was composed of 388 healthy blood donors attending the AVIS Transfusional Center of Pavia. Their ethnic origin was Northern Italian, the same as the patients.

Double-tailed Fisher's exact test was used to compare the frequencies in the patients and the control population (388 blood donors of the same geographic area, Northern Italy). Strength of the correlation was estimated by relative risk (RR).

RESULTS AND DISCUSSION

The association between HLA and malignant diseases was first suggested by the demonstration of genetic linkage between the MHC of mice (H-2) and certain genes determining resistance to virus-induced leukemia[14]. The relationship between HLA and predisposition of human malignancy is somewhat controversial. As regards ovarian carcinoma there was no difference of the HLA frequencies between patients and healthy controls. Only increased – but not significant – HLA B7, A9, B12 frequencies have been published in the literature[9]. Increased frequency of Aw23, detected in 17.6% of 17 patients with endometrial carcinoma[5], was not confirmed by larger studies. Cw7 and DRw8 increased frequencies in Japanese patients seem to be a new, constitutional previously unreported risk factor involved in endometrial carcinogenesis. No associated antigens of the HLA-A locus or of the B locus were detected[10].

Table 2 shows the altered frequencies of HLA-A, B, C, DR antigens in our ovarian cancer patients ($n = 52$), compared with control ($n = 388$). We noticed statistically significant deviations. The results regarding Bf and C4 allele frequencies are presented in Table 3.

We found three patients with ovarian cancer with following markers: A33, B14, S21, DR1. This HLA supratype is present only in 1% of the general Caucasian population, and in our sample it is present with a frequency of 6%.

The phenotypic and allelic frequencies of HLA class I, II and III markers in patients ($n = 56$) affected by endometrial carcinoma, compared with the control group ($n = 388$) are presented in Tables 4 and 5. HLA supratype A3, B7, S31, DR2 was found in 9% patients affected by endometrial carcinoma, but only in 6% of the Caucasian population.

Our data suggest a correlation between ovarian and endometrial cancers and particular complete HLA supratypes.

The significance of these preliminary findings awaits confirmation by other

Table 2 HLA phenotypic frequencies: a comparison between altered frequencies in patients with ovarian cancer and controls

	Phenotypic frequencies			χ^2		
Allele	*Controls*	*Patients*	χ^2	*with Yate's correction*	*Double-tailed p*	*Relative risk*
A30	2.8351	11.5385	9.3514	7.1550	0.0091	4.4704
A33	2.5773	7.6923	3.8944	2.4110	0.0707	3.1500
B13	5.4124	13.4615	4.9858	3.7265	0.0353	2.7185
B14	5.1546	11.5385	3.3611	2.3109	0.0723	2.4000
CW6	10.5670	26.9231	11.2156	9.7700	0.0020	3.1181
DR3	29.4118	19.2308	2.2729	1.7945	0.0875	0.5714

Table 3 Complement allele frequencies: a comparison between ovarian cancer patients and controls

	Allelic frequencies	
Allele	*Controls*	*Patients*
BfS	80.7692	76.1905
BfF	16.4530	20.2381
BfF1	1.0684	3.5714
BfSO.7	1.7094	0.0000
C4A2	7.1429	6.2500
C4A3	76.8398	85.0000
C4A4	3.6797	1.2500
C4A6	2.5974	5.0000
C4AQ0	8.4416	2.5000*
C4B1	80.5195	76.2500
C4B2	7.5758	12.5000
C4B3	0.4329	0.0000
C4BQ0	9.9567	11.2500

*$\chi^2 = 3.443$, χ^2 with Yate's correction = 2.646, Double tailed $P = 0.0411$, Relative risk = 0.278

Table 4 HLA phenotypic frequencies: a comparison between altered frequencies in endometrial cancer patients and controls

	Phenotypic frequencies			χ^2		*Double*
Allele	*Controls*	*Patients*	χ^2	*with Yate's correction*	*R/R*	*tailed p*
A3	22.6804	28.5714	0.9468	0.6469	1.3636	0.2083
A9	25.5155	39.2857	4.6806	4.0118	1.8889	0.025
B7	11.0825	19.6429	3.3568	2.6034	1.9612	0.059
CW3	9.7938	17.8571	3.2999	2.5166	2.0023	0.0623
DR2	28.0277	41.0714	3.7902	3.1961	1.7897	0.0390
DQW3	30.4498	57.1429	14.7346	13.5813	3.0455	0.0002

Table 5 Complement allele frequencies: a comparison between endometrial cancer patients and controls

	Allelic frequencies			χ^2		*Double*
Allele	*Controls*	*Patients*	χ^2	*with Yate's correction*	*R/R*	*tailed p*
BfS	80.77	70.53				
BfF	16.45	24.10	3.5979	3.0965	1.6130	0.0420
BfS0.7	1.71	0.89				
BfF1	1.07	4.46	6.1508	4.3098	4.3271	0.0273
C4A2	7.14	3.00				
C4A3	76.84	79.00				
C4A4	3.68	6.00				
C4A6	2.60	5.00				
C4AQ0	8.44	7.00				
C4B1	80.51	78.00				
C4B2	7.57	9.00				
C4B5	0.21	1.00				
C4BQ0	9.95	12.00				

investigators. However, these data do suggest that our genetic approach may provide information concerning the predisposition to ovarian and endometrial malignancy which can be used in developing population screening strategies. The association of certain HLA supratypes with a predisposition to the development of malignancy could justify increased screening of the population at risk. This would include increasing frequency of ecographic examination in patients at higher risk of developing ovarian cancer, and the periodic use of endometrial biopsies (hysteroscopy?) in patients at risk of developing endometrial cancer. In addition; studies concerning the association of HLA supratypes with gynecological malignancies could be utilized for the identification of environmental and etiologic factors that are important in the pathogenesis of these diseases.

REFERENCES

1. Bodmer, W.F. (1987). The HLA system: structure and function. *J. Clin. Pathol.*, **40**, 948
2. Rogentine, G.N., Trapani, R.J., Yankee, R.A. and Henderson, E.S. (1973). HLA antigens and acute lymphocytic leukemia. The nature of the HLA-A2 association. *Tissue antigens*, **3**, 470
3. Kissmeyer-Nielsen, F., Kjerbye, K.E. and Lamm, L.U. (1975). HLA and Hodgkin's disease. II. A prospective study. *Transplant. Rev.*, **22**, 168
4. Rogentine, G.N., Dellon, A.L. and Chretien, P.B. (1976). *Prolonged disease-free survival in bronchogenic carcinoma associated with HLA-AW19 and B5. A follow-up, in HLA and disease.* p.234. (Paris: Inserum)
5. Sniecinski, I., Haley, J., Morgan-Byrne, J. and Van Nagell, J. (1981). Histocompatibility antigen distribution in patients with cervical and endometrial carcinomas. *Gynecol. Oncol.*, **11**, 68
6. Dzwonkowski, P., O'Leary, J. and Farid, N.R. (1989). Thyroid papillary carcinoma in HLA identical sibs. *Lancet*, **i**, 971
7. Heintz, A.P.M., Hacker, N.F. and Lagasse, L.D. (1985). Epidemiology and etiology of ovarian cancer: A review. *Obstet. Gynecol.*, **66**, 127
8. Di Saia, P.J. and Creasman, W.T. (1984). Adenocarcinoma of the uterus. In Di Saia, P.J. and Creasman, W.T. (eds). *Clinical Gynecologic Oncology* 2nd ed. p. 146. (St Louis: Mosby)
9. Illeni, M.T., Pasquali, M., La Monica, G., Bohm, S., Rovini, D. and Di Re, E. (1985). HLA antigens in ovarian adenocarcinoma patients. *Eur. J. Gynaecol. Oncol.*, **6**, 121
10. Kanuma, T. and Igarashi, M. (1987). Human leukocyte antigen associated with endometrial carcinoma with a new classification of endometrial carcinoma based on its etiology. *Am. J. Obstet. Gynecol.*, **157**, 427
11. Alper, C.A., Awdeh, Z., Raum, D. and Yunis, E.J. (1985). Complement genes of the Major Histocompatibility Complex (Complotyes), Extended Haplotypes and disease markers. *Biochem. Soc. Symp.*, **51**, 19
12. Alper, C.A., Boenish, T. and Watson, L. (1972). Genetic polymorphism in human-rich beta-glicoprotein. *J. Exp. Med.*, **136**, 68
13. Awdeh, Z.L. and Alper, C.A. (1980). Inherited structural polymorphism of the fourth component of human complement, *Proc. Natl. Acad. Sci., USA*, **77**, 3576
14. Lilly, F. (1966). The histocompatibility-2 locus and susceptibility to tumor induction. *Nat. Cancer Inst. Monogr.*, **22**, 631

4

Amino-terminal propeptide of type III procollagen and CA 125 in ovarian and uterine malignancies

A. Kauppila, J. Penttinen, U. Puistola, J. Risteli, L. Risteli, C. Tomás and J. Vuori

INTRODUCTION

The interaction of carcinoma cells with basement membranes has been intensively studied for many years[1]. Details of the interaction of cancer with the interstitial connective tissue stroma are not known, although the collagen network is an essential structural part of carcinomatous tissue, and different types of collagens and other connective tissue elements participate in the defence of the organism against invasive malignancy by lytic and desmoplastic reactions[2].

Collagen fibers are formed from their precursor procollagen molecules. The development of radioimmunoassays[3] for detecting the amino-terminal propeptide of type III procollagen (PIIINP), present in vascular, interstitial, skin, smooth muscle and uterine tissues, among others, has opened attractive prospects to investigate the significance of collagens in malignant diseases. The PIIINP assay is especially interesting because type III procollagen is one of the most abundant interstitial precursors of collagen, and it is formed in equimolar proportions to collagen.

Using the PIIINP radioimmunoassay, increased serum concentrations of PIIINP have been found in various malignancies[4], including cervical, endometrial and ovarian carcinomas[5], and bone metastases[6]. In ovarian carcinoma, in which the serum PIIINP concentrations directly correlated with the clinical stage of the disease[5], immunohistochemical staining proved that PIIINP is present in different histopathological types of this malignancy[7]. In our preliminary study, the PIIINP radioimmunoassay used was developed against the amino-terminal segment of type III procollagen isolated from fetal calf skin[3,5]. The antibody in our more recent PIIINP radioimmunoassay was raised against the amino-terminal propeptide of human type III procollagen[8]. With this method we have continued to evaluate the clinical significance of PIIINP as a tumor marker in gynecological malignancies, using CA 125, an indicator of epithelial ovarian cancer cell antigeneity, as a reference tumor marker[9–12]. CA 125, however, is not always expressed in ovarian cancer, and during treatment its concentrations do not always correlate with the clinical picture of malignancy[12]. Assay of CA 125 has proved interesting in other gynecological carcinomas[11,13] and in endometriosis[14,15], but complementary methods, such as assay of PIIINP, are also needed.

OVARIAN CANCER

Our recent study[16] involved 30 patients with advanced epithelial ovarian cancer, treated by surgery and cytotoxic chemotherapy. The follow-up time was from 1 to 3 years. Serum concentrations of CA 125 were determined during the treatments, at intervals of 1–2 months. At each visit, blood samples were taken and stored at −20°C until assayed later for PIIINP. The radioimmunoassay of PIIINP has been described elsewhere[16]. In CA 125 determinations we used commercial kits.

Increased concentrations of both CA 125 and PIIINP were found in 26 of the total of 30 cases (87%). CA 125 and PIIINP were each falsely negative four times.

A complete clinical response (CR) was obtained in 18 cases (transient in 11 cases, and still continuing in seven cases). A partial clinical response (PR) was observed in four cases, and stabilization of the disease in eight patients. In the seven cases with a continuing CR, both indicators ($n = 3$) or PIIINP alone ($n = 3$) correlated with the clinical behavior of the disease. In one case, both indicators were initially normal, thus being clinically useless for treatment monitoring.

In cases with a transient response (CR or PR) or stabilization of the disease, the fluctuation in the PIIINP level was less than that of CA 125 (Figure 1). A persistently elevated PIIINP level appeared to be a reliable sign of recurrent cancer after CR (Figure 2), and of progression in patients with PR or stabilization of the disease.

In 16 patients operated upon by non-radical methods, the decrease of CA 125 to normal preceded the CR by 1 to 8 months in eight cases. A normal PIIINP level was reached in two patients 2 and 7 months before CR, and in six patients 2 to 6 months after it. The concentrations of CA 125 and PIIINP were continuously increased in three and six cases, respectively, indicating clinically occult disease.

In the eight second-look laparotomies during CR of five patients (twice in three patients), macroscopic cancer was found in four patients, with elevated CA 125 in three cases and elevated PIIINP in each case. Microscopic cancer was detected three times. Of these CA 125 was increased in two cases, and PIIINP in each case. PIIINP was thus a more precise indicator of malignancy during its regression and, in cases of clinically occult intraperitoneal ovarian cancer, than CA 125 (Figure 2).

In predicting progression after CR in 11 patients, PIIINP and CA 125 were clinically identical. The CA 125 concentration was continuously increased in four patients. In six patients the increase in CA 12 concentration preceded clinical progression by 1 to 13 months, and in one patient it was delayed by

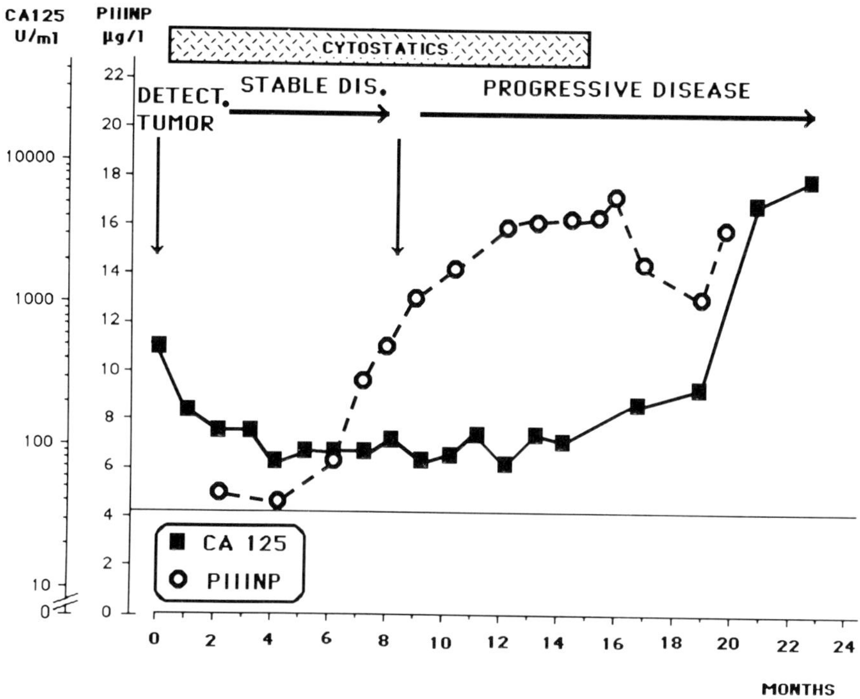

Figure 1 Serum concentrations of CA 125 and PIIINP during cytotoxic chemotherapy following explorative laparotomy of stage III serous ovarian malignancy. Stabilization of the disease for 6 months was followed by progression. PIIINP predicted progression more sensitively than CA 125 in this case

5 months. PIIINP concentrations were continuously increased in six patients; in four patients the PIIINP increase preceded clinical progression by 2 to 19 months, and in one patient the PIIINP concentration was normal all the time.

UTERINE MALIGNANCIES

According to our preliminary results, in endometrial and cervical carcinomas the serum concentrations of PIIINP are increased more often (i.e. in about 40% of the patients) than those of CA 125 (in about 15% of the patients). In clinical stages III and IV, pathological CA 125 and PIIINP recordings were more common than in clinical stages I and II. In the advanced forms of these diseases, CA 125 and PIIINP also appeared to be clinically useful in monitoring the treatment response (Figure 3).

COMMENTS

Serum PIIINP concentrations are commonly increased in advanced ovarian cancer, and changes in PIIINP concentrations are closely correlated with

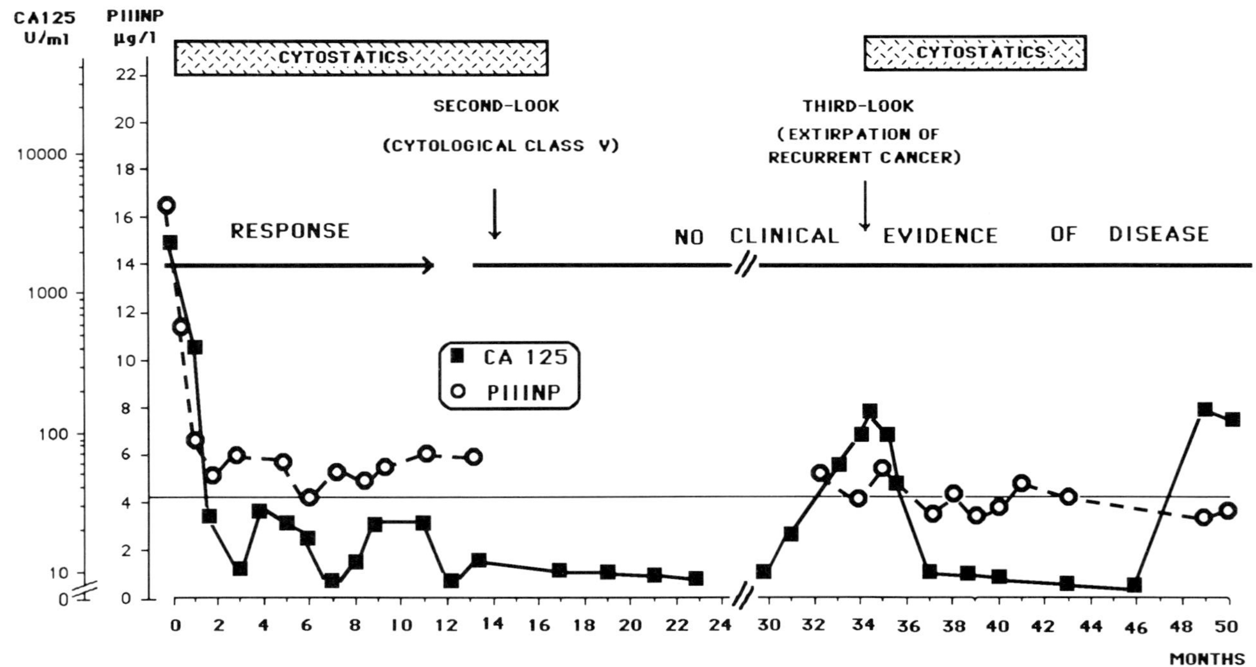

Figure 2 Serum concentrations of CA 125 and PIIINP during different phases of the treatment of patient with an inoperable stage III serous ovarian malignancy. Note that at the time of cessation of cytotoxic chemotherapy at 10 months (complete clinical response) PIIINP level was increased suggesting presence of occult malignancy, which was confirmed at third-look laparotomy at 34 months of follow-up

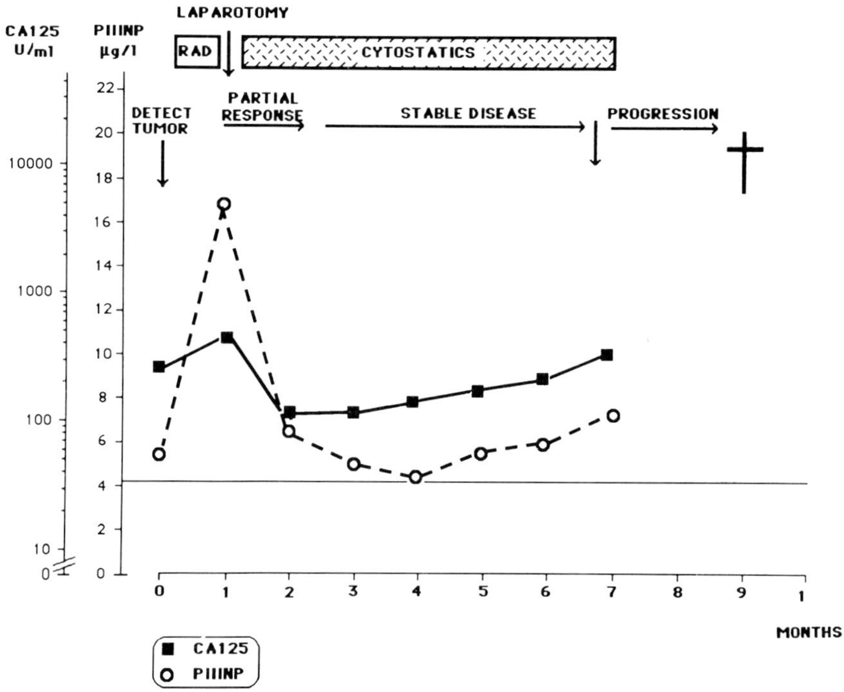

Figure 3 Serum concentrations of CA 125 and PIIINP during cytotoxic chemotherapy of advanced endometrial carcinoma during different phases of the disease

the clinical course of the disease, thus resembling CA 125 in this function[16]. It is worth noticing that in 20% of the cases only one indicator, PIIINP or CA 125, was clinically useful and that the indicators were complementary to each other in 46% of the cases.

Consistent with previous reports, CA 125 antigeneity was expressed in 80% of the cases, and 20% were negative[12]. In addition, CA 125 concentrations commonly decreased to normal many months before clinical CR, and in some cases with residual tumor at second-look laparatomy it was negative. Hence, during the regressive or silent state of ovarian cancer, CA 125 is not an optimal indicator as regards this malignancy. PIIINP was in some cases more informative and more precise. It was always correctly positive at the second-look laparotomies with microscopic or silent macroscopic tumors, and it normalized only twice before clinical CR. On the other hand, as in previous studies, both PIIINP and CA 125 sensitively detected silent progression of ovarian cancer.

In cervical and endometrial carcinomas, there is a general lack of sensitive, specific and precise tumor markers. Our preliminary results suggest that CA 125 and PIIINP separately or together are clinically valuable in monitoring the response of advanced uterine malignancy to chemotherapy.

CA 125 is a membrane antigen of epithelial ovarian cancer cells, whereas PIIINP antigeneity is derived from type III collagen metabolism, thus reflecting different carcinogenic processes. There are two main cellular components in ovarian cancer, epithelial and stromal, the activities of which may possibly be assessed separately by CA 125 and PIIINP measurements. The changes in serum CA 125 and PIIINP concentrations were surprisingly similar in many cases, suggesting that changes in the activities of these tissue elements often run in parallel, especially when they are profound and/or rapid.

REFERENCES

1. Liotta, L.A. (1986). Tumor invasion and metastases – role of extracellular matrix: Rhoads memorial award lecture. *Cancer Res.*, **46**, 1–7
2. van den Hooff, A. (1986). Connective tissue as an active participant in the process of malignant growth. *Anticancer Res.*, **6**, 775–80
3. Risteli, J. and Risteli, L. (1986). Radioimmunoassay for monitoring connective tissue metabolism. *Rheumatology*, **10**, 216–45
4. Hatahara, T., Igarashi, S. and Funaki, N. (1984). High concentrations of N-terminal peptide of type III procollagen in the sera of patients with various cancers, with special reference to liver cancer. *Gann*, **75**, 130–5
5. Risteli, L., Kauppila, A., Mäkilä, U.-M. and Risteli, J. (1988). Aminoterminal propeptide of type III procollagen – an indicator of intraperitoneal invasion in ovarian carcinoma? *Int. J. Cancer*, **41**, 409–14
6. Blomqvist, C., Elomaa, I., Virkkunen, P., Porkka, L., Karonen, S.-L., Risteli, L. and Risteli, J. (1987). Response evaluation of bone metastases in mammary carcinoma. The value of radiology, scintigraphy and biochemical markers of bone metabolism. *Cancer*, **60**, 2907–12
7. Stenbäck, F. (1988). Collagen type III in ovarian tumors. Histological, immunohistochemical and ultrastructural findings. *Eur. J. Obstet. Gynecol. Reprod. Biol.*, **30**, 73–88
8. Risteli, J., Niemi, S., Trivedi, P., Mäentausta, O., Mowat, A.P. and Risteli, L. (1988). Rapid equilibrium assay for the aminoterminal propeptide of human type III procollagen. *Clin. Chem.*, **34**, 715–18
9. Bast, R.C., Jr, Freeney, M., Lazarus, H., Nadler, L.M., Colvin, R.B. and Knapp, R.C. (1981). Reactivity of monoclonal antibody with human ovarian carcinoma. *J. Clin. Invest.*, **8**, 1331–7
10. Kivinen, S., Kuoppala, T., Leppilampi, M., Vuori, J. and Kauppila, A. (1986). Tumor-associated antigen CA 125 before and during the treatment of ovarian carcinoma. *Obstet. Gynecol.*, **67**, 468–72
11. Halila, H., Stenman, U.-H. and Seppälä, M. (1986). Ovarian cancer antigen CA 125 levels in pelvic inflammatory disease and pregnancy *Cancer*, **57**, 1327–9
12. Bast, R.C., Hunter, V. and Knapp, R.C. (1987). Pros and cons of gynecological tumor markers. *Cancer*, **60**, 1984–92
13. Duk, J.M., Aalders, J.G., Fleuren, G.J. and de Bruijn, H.W.A. (1986). Ca 125: a useful marker in endometrial carcinoma. *Am. J. Obstet. Gynecol.*, **155**, 1097–102
14. Pittaway, D.E. and Fayez, J.A. (1986). The use of CA-125 in the diagnosis and management of endometriosis. *Fertil. Steril.*, **46**, 790–5
15. Kauppila, A., Telimaa, S., Rönnberg, L. and Vuori, J. (1988). Placebo-controlled study on serum concentrations of CA-125 before and after treatment of endometriosis with danazol or high-dose medroxyprogesterone acetate alone or after surgery. *Fertil. Steril.*, **49**, 37–41
16. Kauppila, A., Puistola, U., Risteli, J. and Risteli, L. (1989). Aminoterminal propeptide of type III procollagen – a new indicator of ovarian cancer. *Cancer Res.*, **49**, 1885–9

5

Laminin distribution in human endometrial carcinoma

N. Surico, M.R. Amedeo, M. Amedeo, T. Crivello and G. Ferraris

During embryogenesis the first extracellular matrix to appear is the basal membrane, and the first identifiable protein of this matrix is laminin[1]. Laminin is believed to be a multifunctional protein involved in multiple biological processes such as cellular adhesiveness, growth, migration and differentiation[2].

The molecule isolated from cellular cultures, has a molecular weight of 850 000, and consists of four arms (three short, one long) arranged perpendicularly (cruciform shaped) and is composed of three distinct polypeptide chains designated as A_1, B_1, B_2[3] joined by inter- and intramolecular disulfide bonds (Figure 1).

Affinity chromatography has demonstrated the existence of cellular surface receptors for laminin (molecular weight 67 000) characterized by a strong affinity for the glycoprotein ($K_d \simeq 2\,mM$).

These receptors distributed in an orderly fashion, have been visualized on the basal membrane of epithelial cells, and a less orderly distribution has been observed in malignant tumor cells[4]. Laminin has the capability of stimulating 'cellular migration'[5] and thus may be considered a chemotaxic molecule when in solution, and autotaxic when present on the surface. Both forms are capable of 'guiding' cellular movement.

It has been shown that exposing metastatic tumor cells to laminin induces them to become more invasive and produce greater quantities of collagenase IV, an enzyme required for the degradation of the collagen IV reticulum, present in basal membranes. In addition, laminin retains the capability of activating tumor cell migration by auto- and chemotaxic mechanisms.

Research on normal and abnormal human endometrium, has revealed that normal endometrium displays a hormone dependent reactivity for laminin. In fact laminin positivity at the intra- and pericellular level in stromal cells, may be observed only during the endometrial secretory phase[6,7].

Staining by immunological methods may be observed as early as days 14–17 of the menstrual cycle, i.e. before it is possible to evaluate the morphological

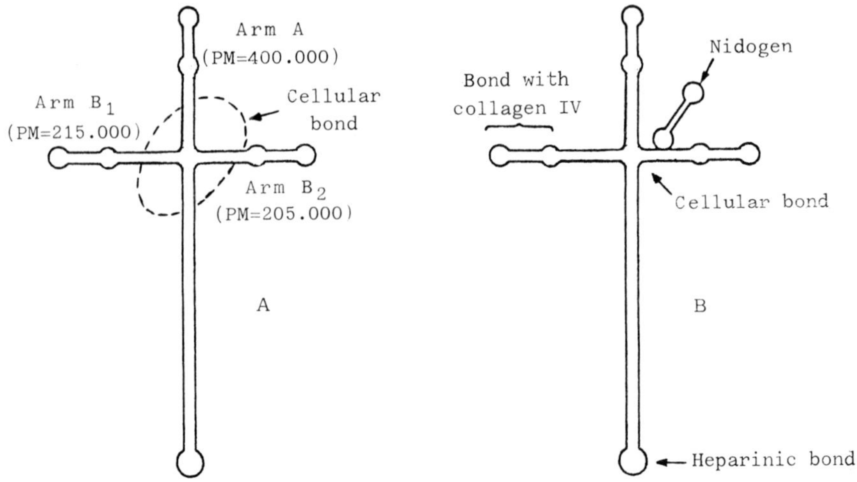

Figure 1 (*a*) Configuration of arms A, B_1 and B_2 of the laminin molecular model; (*b*) interaction complexes of several components found in the basal membrane

changes of the endometrium upon histological examination. A variable number of laminin-positive stromal cells may be identified, and the chromatic intensity gradually increases during the secretory phase. In fact, during the late secretory phase approximately 90% of the stromal cells are immunocolorized at the intracytoplasmic and perivasal levels, and in a discontinuous manner in the pericellular matrix.

During the proliferative phase endometrial stromal cells do not show laminin immunoreactivity[8]. This confirms a correlation between the expression of the protein and hormonal activity, and thus distinguishes proliferative phase stromal cells, from those of the secretory phase.

The precise time period when laminin expression begins in stromal cells is still unknown, but is under research by means of *in situ* hybridization using 'cDNA cloning' for laminin and its receptors.

Endometrial laminin receptors are found in the basal region of the glands, and in the basement membrane during the secretory phase, but are absent during the proliferative phase.

Observed immunohistochemical variations in hyperplastic and carcinomatous endometrial samples have shown a dishomogeneous laminin distribution proportional to the degree of pathological change.

In a study conducted by Faber *et al.*[8], endometrial cystic and endometrial adenomatous hyperplasia with and without atypia were evaluated. In all of the histological types under study, densely crowded fusiform stromal cells, morphologically indistinguishable from proliferative phase stromal cells, were observed[9,10]; yet, immunohistochemical staining for laminin revealed a striking difference between the three hyperplastic variants under study. In 69% of the cystic hyperplasia samples, laminin-positive material was identified in both the cytoplasm and extracellular matrix of the stromal cells, while only 30% of the adenomatous hyperplasia without atypia samples, and none of the atypical adenomatous hyperplasia samples showed laminin immunoreactive material.

In an additional confirming study, a more meticulous ultrastructural examination revealed laminin positivity, in basal membranes, endometrial glands, blood vessels, and smooth muscle fibers[11].

In cystic and adenomatous hyperplasia the basal membrane is visualized due to the laminin reaction, as a continuous band surrounding the glands, whereas in atypcal adenomatous hyperplasia, the basal membrane is often stained in a discontinuous manner.

The localization of laminin in neoplastic endometrium is similar in distribution to that of the hyperplastic type but the carcinomatous preparations show a much greater discontinuous 'pattern' for laminin.

The sites of laminin positivity in well differentiated and moderately differentiated endometrial carcinoma appear as discontinuous staining of the basement membranes, while poorly differentiated carcinoma show a markedly greater staining for laminin within the cytoplasm.

MATERIALS AND METHODS

Human endometrial tissue samples were taken from surgically removed uteri, in endometrial cancer patients, diagnosed previously by D & C.

The endometrial specimens were fixed in Carnoy solution at 0°C for 24 h and set in paraffin blocks. Sections 5 μm thick were cut, and mixed with 0.05% collagenase at 37°C for 40 min with 0.05% calcium chloride ($CaCl_2$).

The preparations were stained by histochemical and immunostaining methods using polyclonal antilaminin antibodies, purified by the authors, from rabbit antiserum, in rabbits previously immunized with purified laminin.

The antiserum was purified using affinity chromatography and covalent bonding of laminin with sepharous and immunoadsorbing antibodies. Antibody dilution was carried out with high strength ionic salt.

Human neuroblastoma samples, from multiple patients were used as positive immunocoloration controls.

RESULTS

The antilaminin antibodies purified by the authors were found to be highly specific for the laminin of the neuroblastoma samples used as controls.

The sites stained immunohistochemically showed a net pattern of coloration, specific for the basal membranes and blood vessels (Figure 2).

Three well differentiated endometrial adenocarcinoma samples and three poorly differentiated endometrial adenocarcinoma samples were evaluated (Table 1).

In the samples stained with the antibody prepared by the authors, laminin was identified, and differed from the neuroblastoma controls in that laminin

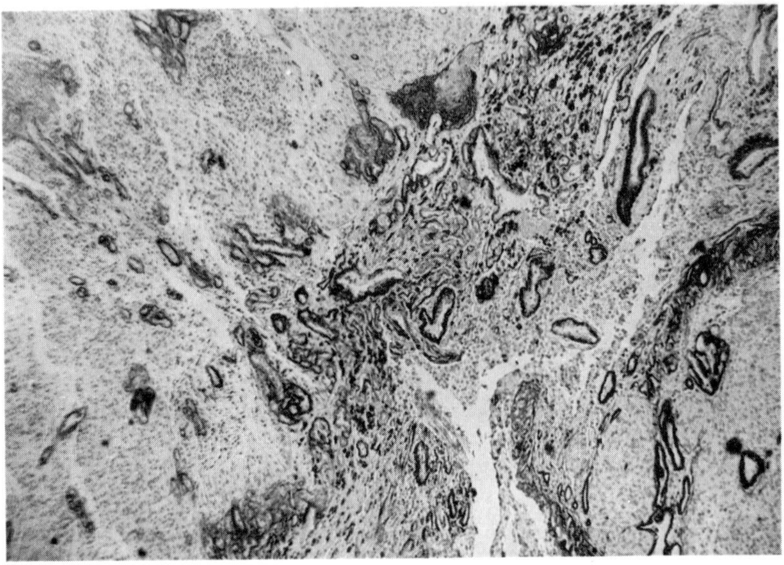

Figure 2 Laminin distribution in human neuroblastoma: immunohistochemical study. All of the basal membranes of the cellular population show pronounced laminin positivity

Table 1 Visualization of laminin presence by immunocoloration

Histological diagnosis	*Number of cases*	*Grading*	*Laminin in stromal cells*
Well differentiated endometrial carcinoma	3	G_1	Present
Poorly differentiated endometrial carcinoma	3	G_3	Present

was not present in the entire cell population.

The antilaminin antibody identifies the glycoprotein in the basal membrane, the cytoplasm and in the pericellular matrix (above all around blood vessels) and is visualized as a discontinuous band.

The results indicate different chromatic intensities for the two types of adenocarcinoma examined, in fact, coloration appears more marked in the poorly differentiated carcinoma (Figure 3) than in the well differentiated type (Figure 4).

DISCUSSION

The neuroblastoma samples used as controls, were well typed immunohistochemically using antilaminin-specific antibodies purified by the authors. All of the examined endometrial carcinoma specimens, resulted laminin positive.

The qualitative and quantitative laminin distribution in endometrial neoplasia reveals a discontinuous staining pattern of the basal membrane,

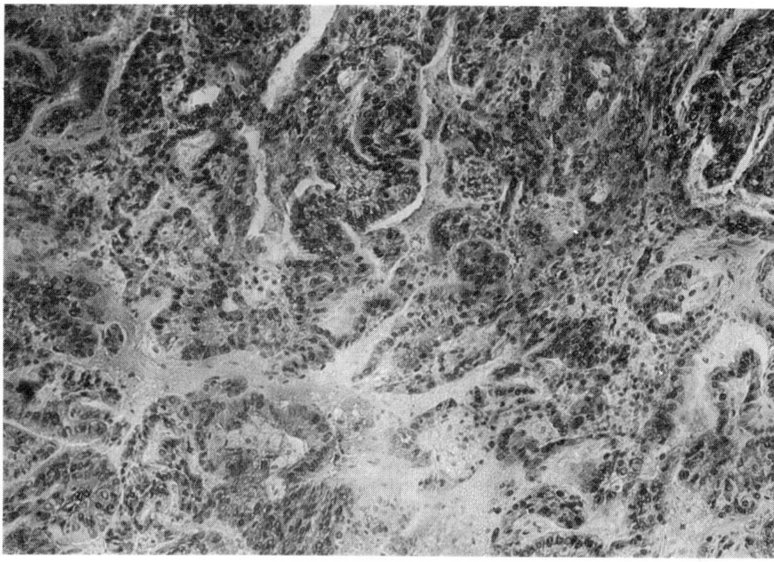

Figure 3 Laminin distribution in poorly differentiated cancer of the endometrium: immunohistochemical study. The neoplastic cells show intense staining of the basal membrane, cytoplasm, and pericellular matrix (and perivasal) in a discontinuous pattern. Not all endometrial stromal cells display laminin positivity

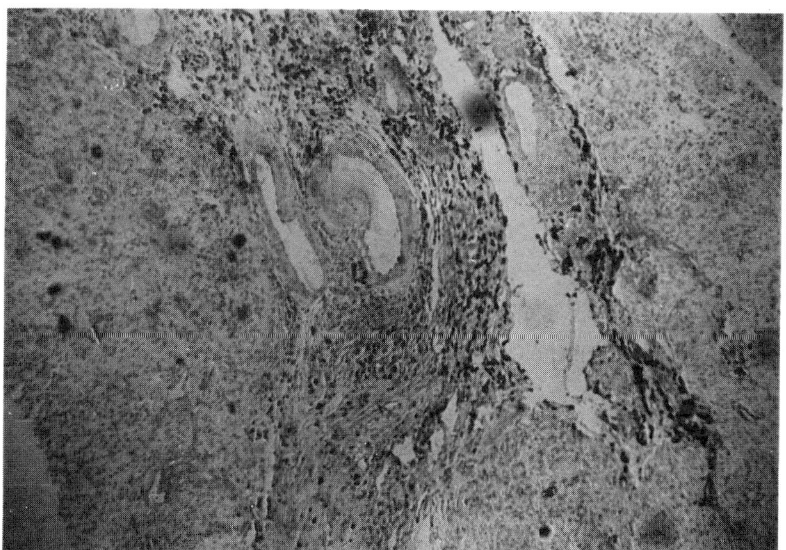

Figure 4 Laminin distribution in well differentiated carcinoma of the endometrium: immunohistochemical study. The neoplastic cells clearly show a staining of the basal membrane and cytoplasm, frequently in a discontinuous pattern. Not all endometrial stromal cells display laminin positivity

particularly in poorly differentiated carcinoma. These data are consistent with other data found in the literature[8] as well as the observation that the disorganization of the basal membrane is related to the level of differentiation of the carcinomatous cells[12–14].

Intracytoplasmic immunocoloration for laminin proved to be more intense in the poorly differentiated carcinomas than the well differentiated forms.

The greater intracytoplasmic laminin positivity in the poorly differentiated forms may be related to a more abundant laminin synthesis, but the more discontinuous and more disorganized immunohistochemical pattern seen in the same poorly differentiated type, points more to an altered capability in assembly of the cytoskeleton.

The above results, in agreement with previous studies conducted on extraendometrial neoplasias[12,15–17] allow us to hypothesize that the greater intracytoplasmatic laminin positivity of cancerous cells may be related to a greater synthesis of receptors for laminin in oncogenic cells, than in normal endometrial tissue.

The correlation between the laminin distribution and the 'grading' of the neoplasia, observed by us, may suggest a diagnostic and/or prognostic application.

With this in mind, we intend to continue this study, thereby increasing the available data and comparing our technique to a similar antibody available commercially as well as to a monoclonal antibody.

REFERENCES

1. Martin, G.R. and Timpl, R. (1987). Laminin and other basement membrane components. *Ann. Rev. Cell. Biol.*, **3**, 57–85
2. Kleinman, H.K., Cannon, F.B., Laurie, G.W., Hassel, J.R., Aumailley, M., Terranova, V.P., Martin, G.R. and Dubois-Dalcq, M. (1985). Biological activities of laminin. *J. Cell. Biochem.*, **27**, 317–25
3. Cooper, A.R., Kurkinen, H., Taylor, A. and Hogan, B.L. (1981). Studies on the biosynthesis of laminin by murine parietal endoderm cells. *Eur. J. Biochem.*, **119**, 189–97
4. Liotta, L.A., Hand, P.H., Rao, C.N., Bryant, G., Darsky, S.H. and Schlom, J. (1985). Monoclonal antibodies to the human laminin receptor recognize structurally distinct sites. *Exp. Cell. Res.*, **156**, 117–26
5. McCarthy, J.B., Palm, S.L. and Furcht, L.T. (1983). Migration by haptotaxis of a Schwann cell tumor line to the basement membrane glycoprotein laminin. *J. Cell. Biol.*, **97**, 772–7
6. Dallenbach-Hellweg, G. (1971). *Histopathology of the Endometrium.* (New York: Springer Verlag)
7. Dallenbach-Hellweg, G. (1985). *Endometrial Histopathology.* (Copenhagen: Hunksgaard)
8. Faber, M., Wewer, U.M., Berthelsen, J.G., Liotta, L.A. and Albrechtsen, R. (1986). Laminin production by human endometrial stromal cells relates to the cyclic and pathologic state of the endometrium. *Am. J. Pathol.*, **124**, 384–98
9. Welch, W.R. and Scully, R.E. (1977). Precancerous lesions of the endometrium. *Human Pathol.*, **8**, 503–12
10. Fenoglio, C.M., Crum, C.P. and Ferenczy, A. (1982). Endometrial hyperplasia and carcinoma: Are ultrastructural, biochemical and immunocytochemical studies useful in distinguishing between them? *Pathol. Res. Pract.*, **174**, 257–84
11. Martinez-Hernandez, A. and Amenta, P.S. (1983). The basement membrane in pathology. *Lab. Invest.*, **47**, 247–57
12. Albrechtsen, R., Wewer, U.M. and Liotta, L.A. (1986). Basement membranes in human cancer. *Pathol. Ann.*, **2**, 251–76

13. Barsky, S.H., Siegal, G.P., Jannotta, F. and Liotta, L.A. (1983). Loss of basement membrane components by invasive tumors but not their benign counterparts. *Lab. Invest.*, **49**, 140–7
14. Gusterson, B.A., Warburton, M.J., Hitchell, D., Ellison, H., Munroe Neville, A. and Rudland, P.S. (1982). Distribution of myoepithelial cells basement membrane proteins in the normal breast and in benign and malignant breast diseases. *Cancer Res.*, **42**, 4763–70
15. Albrechtsen, R., Nielsen, M., Wewer, U., Engvall, E. and Ruoslatc, E. (1981). Basement membrane changes in breast cancer detected by immunochemical staining for laminin. *Cancer Res.*, **41**, 5076–81
16. Haglund, C., Nordling, S., Roberts, P.J. and Ekblom, P. (1984). Expression of laminin in pancreatic neoplasma and in chronic pancreatitis. *Am. J. Surg. Pathol.*, **8**, 669–76
17. McArdle, J.P., Müller, H.K., Raff, B.T. and Murphy, W.H. (1984). Basal laminina redevelopment in tumours metastatic to brain: An immunoperoxidase study using an antibody to type IV collagen. *Int. J. Cancer*, **34**, 633–8

6

Human papillomavirus and cervical cancer

G. Ferraris, G.P. Pescarmona, F. Altruda, R. Bellino, A. Re, G. Gordini, M. Tessarolo and A. Lanza

INTRODUCTION

Initially, numerous studies strongly suggested a significant association of human papillomavirus (HPV) with human neoplasia, especially with dysplasia and carcinoma of uterine cervix[1–10]. That evidence was provided by reports about the association of HPV lesions with cervical dysplasia[9–11]. Furthermore, epidemiological studies supported those data revealing common risk factors[6,12]. The introduction of molecular biology as HPV diagnostic tool allowed the identification of four HPV types (16, 18, 31 and 33) among more than 40, integrated into the cellular genome of cervical dysplasic cells and/or cancer cells[3,4,13–15]. There is increasing evidence that HPV types 16[4,16,17] and 18[17,18] are involved in the dysplasic process, because they have been found associated with up to 30–100% of cervical intraepithelial neoplasias and invasive cancer of the cervix[19]. Furthermore, each of these two types has been found integrated into the cellular genome[17,18] of cell line cultures derived from cervical cancers.

SUBJECTS

In a retrospective study of 45 patients with cervical cancer, we studied the presence of HPV 16 in the primitive site of the neoplasia, in the para-aortic and pelvic nodes and in the cervix adjacent tissues (corpus uteri, parametrium, vagina and bladder).

The patients were divided into two main groups: 20 cases with carcinoma limited to the cervix and 25 cases with invasive carcinoma beyond the cervix.

The first group was further divided into four subgroups:

(1) Five cases without nodal metastases and without recurrences;
(2) Three cases without nodal metastases but with recurrences;
(3) Eight cases with nodal metastases but without recurrences; and
(4) Four cases with nodal metastases and with recurrences.

The second group was divided into the same four subgroups:

(1) Five cases without nodal metastases and without recurrences;
(2) Four cases without nodal metastases but with recurrences;
(3) Seven cases with nodal metastases but without recurrences; and
(4) Nine cases with nodal metastases and with recurrences.

METHODS

The study was performed on a paraffin-embedded specimen to allow retrospective analysis of the cases. The specimens were dewaxed with xylene washing, cut and digested with protease K for 12 h at 37°C. After organic extraction with phenol DNA was obtained with ethanol precipitation[20].

Dot-blot on nylon membranes was performed with purified cellular DNA and samples were tested with ^{32}P-labelled HPV 16 DNA probe for 36 h at 42°C. Labelling was obtained by random-priming reaction, using [^{32}P]nucleotides, on HPV 16 DNA isolated from the vector.

This procedure allowed short exposure of the autoradiograph and increased the sensitivity of the analysis. After hybridization and washing, autoradiography was performed and compared with positive and negative controls.

RESULTS AND DISCUSSION

Results of hybridization on the first and second groups are shown in Tables 1 and 2 respectively.

Table 1 Carcinoma limited to the cervix and HPV 16

	No. cases	*HPV positivity*
Cervical carcinoma	20	17 (85%) 2 borderline
Non-metastatic nodes	13	5 (38.5%) 1 borderline
Metastatic nodes	12	6 (50%) 2 borderline
Neoplasia-free parametrium	1	1 (100%)

Table 2 Carcinoma beyond the cervix and HPV 16

	No. cases	*HPV positivity*
Cervical carcinoma	25	18 (72%) 1 borderline
Non-metastatic nodes	18	8 (44%) 2 borderline
Metastatic nodes	14	10 (72%)
Metastatic parametrium	9	7 (78%)
Vagina	2	2 (100%)
Isthmus	1	1 (100%)
Corpus uteri	1	1 (100%)
Bladder	1	1 (100%)

In the 45 cervical tested specimens, HPV 16 was found in 78%; in the 31 non-metastatic nodes it was present in 48% and in the 26 metastatic nodes, in 62% of the cases. Our results confirm the important association of HPV 16 with human cervical cancer.

We found HPV 16 not only in the primary site of the tumor (78% of the cases) but also in lymph nodes and in the adjacent metastatic and non-metastatic tissues (parametrium, vagina, isthmus, corpus uteri and bladder).

It is well known that lymphovascular invasion is a prognostic factor and it is related to lymph node metastases: it is probable that HPV 16 reaches para-aortic and pelvic nodes not only by cancer cells but through capillary-like spaces too. We in fact found HPV 16 in nine non-metastatic nodes sampled from nine patients with metastatic nodes in other sites: these nine patients had involvement of capillary-like spaces. The histological re-examination of these non-metastatic nodes confirmed the absence of neoplastic cells.

As shown in Table 3 we detected HPV 16 in 48% of non-metastatic nodes. We examined 16 non-metastatic nodes sampled from 16 patients without other metastatic nodes: HPV 16 was found in 25% of the cases. We also studied 15 non-metastatic nodes in 15 patients with nodal metastases in other sites: HPV 16 was found in 60% of the cases. HPV 16 was present in higher percentage in non-metastatic nodes when other nodes were involved by cancer cells.

We also related HPV 16 to recurrent disease. The only significant relation found between HPV 16 and relapses was the following. We examined 11 metastatic nodes sampled from 11 patients who had had a relapse: in these nodes HPV 16 was found in 91% of the cases (including some borderline cases). Then we examined 15 metastatic nodes sampled from 15 patients without relapse (after 5-year follow-up): HPV 16 was found in the 53% of the cases. We did not find a significant relationship between HPV 16 and relapse in non-metastatic nodes. Finally we studied nine patients who had undergone radiotherapy before surgery with a partial or complete local response. We found HPV 16 in seven of these cervical specimens: although radiotherapy has an antineoplastic action it seems that it has no effect on the viruses. Studies on HPV and cervical dysplasia and cancer are needed in order to clarify value of medical adjuvant therapy in the management of cervical cancer.

Table 3 Comprehensive data on cervical carcinoma

	No. cases	*HPV positivity*
Cervical carcinoma	45	35 (78%) 3 borderline
Non-metastatic nodes	31	13 (48%) 3 borderline
Metastatic nodes	26	16 (62%) 2 borderline

REFERENCES

1. Syrjänen, K., Väyrynen, M., Saarikoski, S., Mäntyjärvi, R., Parkkinen, S., Hippeläinen, M. and Castren, O. (1985). Natural history of cervical human papillomavirus (HPV) infections based on prospective follow-up. *Br. J. Obstet. Gynaecol.*, **92**, 1086–92
2. Crawford, L. (1984). Papilloma viruses and cervical tumours. *Nature*, **310**, 16
3. Crum, C.P., Ikenberg, H., Richart, R.M. and Gissmann, L. (1984). Human papillomavirus type 16 and early cervical neoplasia. *N. Engl. J. Med.*, **310**, 880–3
4. Dürst, M., Gissman, L., Ikenberg, H. and zur Hausen, H. (1983). A papillomavirus DNA from a cervical carcinoma and its prevalence in cancer biopsy samples from different geographic regions. *Proc. Natl. Acad. Sci., USA*, **80**, 3812–4
5. Fletcher, S. and Norval, M. (1983). On the nature of the deep cellular disturbances in human papillomavirus infection of the sqamous cervical epithelium. *Lancet*, **ii**, 546–8
6. Franceschi, S., Doll, R., Gallwey, J., La Vecchia, C., Peto, R. and Spriggs, A.I. (1983). Genital warts and cervical neoplasia: an epidemiological study. *Br. J. Cancer*, **48**, 621–8
7. McCance, D.J., Walker, P.G., Dyson, J.L., Coleman, D.V. and Singer, A. (1983). Presence of human papillomavirus DNA sequences in cervical intraepithelial neoplasia. *Br. Med. J.*, **287**, 784–8
8. Okagaki, T., Twiggs, L.B., Zachow, K.R., Clark, B.A., Ostrow, R.S. and Faras, A.J. (1983). Identification of human papillomavirus DNA in cervical and vaginal intraepithelial neoplasia with molecularly cloned virus-specific DNA probes. *Int. J. Gynecol. Pathol.*, **2**, 153–9
9. Syrjänen, K.J. (1984). Current concepts of human papillomavirus infections in the genital tract and their relationship to intraepithelial neoplasia and squamous cell carcinoma. *Obstet. Gynecol. Surv.*, **39**, 252–65
10. Syrjänen, K., Väyrynen, M., Castrén, O., Mäntyjärvi, R., Pyrhönen, S. and Yliskoski, M. (1983). Morphological and immunohistochemical evidence of human papillomavirus (HPV) involvement in the dysplastic lesions of the uterine cervix. *Int. J. Gynecol. Obstet.*, **21**, 261–9
11. De Brux, J., Orth, G., Croissant, O., Cochard, B. and Ionesco, M. (1983). Lesions condylomateuses du coll uterin: evolution chez 2466 patientes. *Bull. Cancer*, **70**, 410–22
12. Sadeghi, S.B., Hsieh, E.W. and Gunn, S.W. (1984). Prevalence of cervical intraepithelial neoplasia in sexually active teenagers and young adults. Results of data analysis of mass Papanicolaou screening of 796,337 women in the United States in 1981. *Am. J. Obstet. Gynecol.*, **148**, 726–9
13. Attila, T. and Lörincz, P.D. (1987). Detection of human papillomavirus infection by nucleic acid hybridization. *Obstet. Gynecol. Clin. N. Am.*, **14**, 451–69
14. Beaudenon, S., Kremsdorf, D., Croissant, O. *et al.* (1986). A novel type of human papillomavirus associated with genital neoplasias. *Nature*, **321**, 246
15. Tsunokawa, Y., Takebe, N., Kasamatsu, T., Terada, M. and Sugimura, T. (1986). Transforming activity of human papillomavirus type 16 DNA sequences in a cervical cancer. *Proc. Natl. Acad. Sci., USA*, **83**, 2200–3
16. Ostrow, R.S. and Faras, A.J. (1987). The molecular biology of human papillomaviruses and the pathogenesis of genital papillomas and neoplasms. *Cancer and Metastasis Rev.*, **6**, 383–95
17. Pater, M. and Pater, A. (1985). Human papillomavirus types 16 and 18 in carcinoma cell lines of the cervix. *Virology*, **145**, 313–8
18. Schwarz, E., Freese, U., Gissmann, L., Mayer, W., Roggenbuck, B., Stremlau, A. and zur Hausen, H. (1985). Structure and transcription of human papillomavirus sequences in cervical carcinoma cells. *Nature*, **314**, 111–4
19. Ostrow, R. and Faras, A. (1986). Human papillomaviruses. *Clin. Microbiol.* Newsletter, **8**, 53–6
20. Lancaster, W.D., Kurman, R.J., Sanz, L.E. *et al.* (1983). Human papillomavirus: detection of viral DNA sequences and evidence for molecular heterogeneity in metaplasias and dysplasias of the cervix. *Intervirology*, **20**, 202

7

The role of hysteroscopy in endometrial carcinoma staging

M. Abrate, P.A. Galli, M. Amidei and G. Covi

INTRODUCTION

The main problem in attempting a therapeutic management of endometrial carcinoma, is the difficulty of an adequate presurgical staging. The FIGO classification is inadequate. Life expectancy for stage I neoplasms varies in relation to factors such as histological differentiation, myometrial infiltration and mostly, the presence of lymphnodal metastases[1].

In stage I, the lymph nodes are involved in about 10%[1-3] of cases, whereas in stage II the percentage is much higher (nearly 23%)[2,4]. Nevertheless, in each stage, the lymph node involvement varies in relation to the histological grade and myometrial infiltration[1,2], with significant differences in recurrences and prognosis[5].

In stage I cases with a low probability of extrauterine involvement, a simple hysterectomy with a bilateral salpingo-oophorectomy is sufficient; in some cases even transvaginally. In stage II, and in high-risk cases, radical surgery is indicated.

With the traditional approach (fractional curettage, cystoscopic and rectoscopic examinations, urography and barium enema) presurgical diagnosis is not higher than 50%[6].

One of the most useful techniques for diagnosis and staging of endometrial carcinoma is hysteroscopy[7]. Signs of endometrial neoplasia include the presence of irregular proliferations, areas of necrosis or hemorrhage, areas of increased vascularization with varicosities, and variations in the vascular design. Hysterocopy can precisely define the borders of the lesion, specifying endocervical involvement[8].

We briefly report our experiences and results of hysteroscopy in the diagnosis and staging of endometrial carcinoma.

MATERIAL AND METHODS

We studied 73 cases of endometrial carcinoma in the Obstetrics and Gynecological Department of the University of Modena. The patients were between the ages of 46 and 79 years old. In each patient, at least one presurgical hysteroscopy was performed.

In 30 days or less after the endoscopic examination, all of the patients underwent transabdominal surgery (17 hysterectomies according to Wertheim and 56 total abdominal hysterectomies with bilateral salpingo-oophorectomy). None of the patients had undergone presurgical therapy.

Using the microcolpohysteroscopy of Hamou, the examination evaluated eventual neoplastic involvement to the endocervix.

Hysteroscopic staging was compared with the pathological surgical specimen. We also took into consideration the validity of the method in the histological diagnosis of the lesion during the first hysteroscopy, which was done on all of the patients.

RESULTS

In eight of the 73 patients, the histological examination demonstrated neoplastic spread to the cervical canal. Hysteroscopy was accurate in staging 67 cases, with five false positives and only one false negative. Therefore, the sensitivity of the test was 87.5% and the specificity was 92.8%. The prognostic value of the positive test was 58.3% and the prognostic value of the negative test was 98.5%).

The hysteroscopic diagnosis of the type of lesion is reported in Table 1, during the first examinations. In 58 cases, the evaluation was correct (79.9% sensitivity). In seven cases, the diagnosis was atypical hyperplasia, in seven patients the lesion was underestimated, and in one it was inconclusive (presence of pyometra).

COMMENT

In evaluating the diagnosis of neoplasia, hysteroscopy has proven to be reliable (79.9% sensitivity). If adenocarcinoma and atypical hyperplasia (histologically very similar lesions) are considered, the percentage rises to 89.7%. In considering our false negatives, we must report that in the diagnosis of dysfunctional endometrium and in one case of atypical hyperplasia, the

Table 1 Hysteroscopic diagnoses in 73 women with endometrial carcinoma

Hysteroscopic diagnosis	*Number of cases*
Inconclusive	1
Regular endometrium	0
Atrophic endometrium	0
Dysfunctional endometrium	1
Polyposis	3
Typical hyperplasia	3
Atypical hyperplasia	7
Carcinoma	58
Total	73

patients were still in their fertile years, a fact which influenced the surgeon's judgement, with a diagnosis of well differentiated adenocarcinoma and coexisting areas of hyperplasia. In two cases of polyps, the neoplastic lesion was in fact of a focal type.

Nevertheless, although hysteroscopy has proven to be highly specific and sensitive with a prediction for negative values near 100%[7], a biopsy is always necessary, since hysteroscopy can be used only for the macroscopic evaluation of the lesion. Hysteroscopy is of utmost importance in differentiating stage I and II of endometrial neoplasia, therefore allowing the accurate definition of neoplasia limits.

It has proven to be undoubtedly reliable, not only from our studies, but also from others[13,14], demonstrating a low percentage of false negatives. These at least in part can be attributed to microscopic lesions of the endocervix, submucosa or limited to the glandular recess and, therefore with a low risk of lymphatic metastases[4,13].

False positives are more numerous: opening isthmic neoplasms with abundant proliferation and heavy bleeding, can be the cause of an erroneous evaluation of the cervical–isthmic region.

The reliability and value of hysteroscopy is appreciated also because there are few alternative diagnostic methods. As we have already mentioned, fractional curettage has a high percentage of false negatives[6,14] and false positives[6,15,16], therefore valuable in diagnosing neoplasms, but not in staging them. Computed axial tomography (CAT) is also unable to differentiate between stage I and stage II: studies that we took into consideration showed a high percentage of false negatives (10–20%)[9], or else were completely unreliable[11–13]. CAT has proven to be a reliable diagnostic tool in the evaluation of myometrial infiltration[10], whereas this is the only serious limitation of hysteroscopy.

The hysteroscopic evaluation is only an indication, even though it has been demonstrated that the histological grading is related to the size of the lesion and the extent of the myometrial involvement[13].

Hysteroscopy should not be used alone in presurgical staging, but it should be used in conjunction with methods that evaluate the risk of myometrial and lymphnodal involvement: CAT has contrasting results[9–11], but after our initial experience, nuclear magnetic resonance (NMR) proved to be most reliable.

Other advantages of the hysteroscopy include: low cost, the possibility of performing it on an outpatient basis with few problems for the patient, and low risk even in neoplasia: peritoneal lavage of the peritoneal cavity during hysterectomy done immediately after the examination in patients with endometrial carcinoma did not show neoplastic dissemination[17].

REFERENCES

1. Boronow, R.C. and Morrow, C.P. (1984). Surgical staging in endometrial cancer: Clinical-pathological findings of a prospective study. *Obstet. Gynecol.*, **63**, 852
2. Lewis, B.W. and Stallworthy, (1970). Adenocarcinoma of the body of the uterus. *J. Obstet. Gynaecol. Br. Cwlth*, **77**, 343

3. Lin, W. and Meigs, J.V. (1955). Radical hysterectomy and pelvic lymphadenectomy. *Am. J. Obstet. Gynecol.*, **69**, 1
4. Homesley, H.D. and Boronow, R.C. (1977). Stage II endometrial adenocarcinoma. *Obstet. Gynecol.*, **49**, 604
5. Di Saia, P.J. and Creasman, T.W. (1985). Risk factors and recurrent patterns in stage I endometrial cancer. *Am. J. Obstet. Gynecol.*, **151**, 1009
6. Cowles, T.A. and Magrine, F.J. (1985). Comparison of Clinical and Surgical Staging in patients with Endometrial Carcinoma. *Obstet. Gynecol.*, **66**, 413
7. Scarselli, G. and Colafranceschi, M. (1988). Rischio oncogeno endometriale e menopausa: utilità dell' isteroscopia diagnostica. *Il climaterio femminile: esperienze di un decennio*, p. 431 (Monduzzi)
8. Scarselli, G. and Mencaglia, C. (1985). L'isteroscopia nelle lesioni precancerose e cancerose dell'endometrio. *Boll. Assoc. Ital. l'endoscop. ginecol.*, **11**, 115
9. Hasumi, K. (1982). Computed tomography in the evaluation and treatment of endometrial carcinoma. *Cancer*, **50**, 904
10. Dore, R. and More, G. (1987). CT Evaluation of Myometrium invasion in Endometrial Carcinoma. *J. Comput. Assist. Tomogr.*, **2**, 282
11. Legrand, I. and Masselot, J. (1984). Tomodensitometrie des cancers du corps uterin (Stades I et II). Confrontations anatomo-pathologiques. *J. Radiol.*, **65**, 767
12. Walsh, J.W. and Goplerud, D.R. (1982). Computer tomography of primary, persistent and recurrent endometrial malignancy. *Am. J. Radiol.*, **139**, 1149
13. Guerra, B. and Mirra, P. (1985). Utilità e limiti dell'isteroscopia nella stadiazione del carcinoma endometriale. In *Isteroscopia Operativa e laser chirurgia in Ginecologia.* pp. 221. (CIC)
14. Scarselli, G. (1986). Problematica della stadiazione del carcinoma endometriale e utilità dell'isteroscopia. *Oncologia Ginecologia*, **5**, 23
15. Berman, L.L. (1982). Risk factors and prognosis in stage II endometrial cancer. *Gynecol. Oncol.*, **14**, 49
16. Wallin, T.E. (1984). Stage II cancer of endometrium: a pathologic and clinical study. *Gynecol. Oncol.*, **18**, 1
17. Parent, B.B. (1985). *Hysteroscopie panoramique.* p. 57. (Paris: Masson)

8

Cisplatin, bleomycin and methotrexate neoadjuvant chemotherapy and radical surgery in locally advanced cervical carcinoma

P. Benedetti Panici, S. Greggi, G. Scambia, G. Ragusa, C. Rabitti and S. Mancuso

INTRODUCTION

Survival of patients with locally advanced inoperable cervical cancer (FIGO stages Ib–III, tumor volume > 4 cm) has not significantly altered during the last decade despite some improvements that have been achieved in radiotherapeutic techniques. The 2-year disease-free survival ranges from 10% to 50% and the 5-year from 30% to 40%[1–6]. Treatment failures may result from the suboptimal treatment of pelvic disease and existence of extrapelvic metastases. Neoadjuvant (primary) chemotherapy offers potential for reducing a bulky pelvic tumor to minimal macroscopic or microscopic curable disease and for controlling micrometastases. Cisplatin-containing regimens have been proved to be the most effective combinations in recurrent cervical carcinoma[7,8]. In the present paper the authors present the preliminary results of a pilot study on patients with locally advanced primary cervical carcinoma treated with cisplatin (P) bleomycin (B) methotrexate (M) (PBM) neoadjuvant chemotherapy followed by radical surgery.

PATIENTS AND METHODS

From January 1986 to October 1988 70 previously untreated patients with locally advanced inoperable (FIGO stages Ib–III, tumor volume > 4 cm) cervical carcinoma were entered in this study. Further eligibility criteria were: histologically proven cervical carcinoma; WHO performance status < 3; age < 70 years; informed patient consent. Patients were excluded in cases of: pulmonary, renal, hepatic or cardiac impairment; white blood cell count < 3500/l; platelet count < 100 000/l; second primary tumor other than basal cell carcinoma of skin. Pretreatment evaluation consisted of: GE, cervical Papanicolaou smear, colposcopy, cervical and vaginal biopsies, chest X-ray, bone scan, abdomino–pelvic ultrasound scan, gynecological examination under general anesthesia, endocervical and endocavitary curettage, cystoscopy, sigmoidoscopy, intravenous pyelogram, and mammography if over 50 years old. All these procedures (except curettage if negative) were repeated 2–3 weeks after the end of chemotherapy. Chemotherapy-induced toxicity was carefully monitored: electrocardiogram, pulmonary, renal and hepatic function tests; complete blood count; audiometry and neurological examination were performed before and after each cycle. The drugs P, B and M were administered according to the following schedule: P, 100 mg/m^2 i.v. on day 1, B, 15 mg i.v. bolus on days 1 and 8 and M, 300 mg/m^2 on day 8 (followed by leucovorin rescue) for three courses every 21 days. Patients underwent radical surgery (Piver's III–V radical hysterectomy, plus systematic para-aortic and pelvic lymphadenectomy) only if a tumor volume < 4 cm had been achieved, and if vaginal and parametrial lesions were judged radically resectable. Patient characteristics are detailed in Table 1. WHO response and toxicity evaluation criteria were adopted. To date a median follow-up of 18 months (range 4–37) from diagnosis has been achieved.

RESULTS

Sixty-eight of the 70 eligible patients were evaluable for response and chemotherapy toxicity. Two patients (with Ib and IIIb tumors) refused further treatment after the first course and were excluded from the study. A total of 201 courses were administered (P, 98%; B, 96%; M, 91.5%). The overall clinical response rate was 80.9% (Table 2). All the 55 responding patients underwent radical surgery and, of the remaining 13, 11 patients received 50 Gy external pelvic irradiation (nine were stable, two had progres-

Table 1 Patients' characteristics

Patients admitted	70
Median age (years)	55 (34–69)
FIGO stage	
Ib–IIa	7 (10.3%)
IIb	32 (47%)
III	29 (42.7%)
Type of surgery	
Type III radical hysterectomy	34 (61.9%)
Type IV radical hysterectomy	20 (36.3%)
Type V radical hysterectomy	1 (1.8%)
Histology	
Squamous cells	55 (80.9%)
Adenocarcinoma	13 (19.1%)
Grade of differentiation	
Good	6 (8.9%)
Moderate	38 (55.9%)
Poor	24 (35.2%)

Table 2 Clinical response according to stage of disease

FIGO stage	*No. of patients*	*Complete response*	*Partial response*	*No change*
Ib–IIa	7	1	5	1
IIb	32	4	25	4
III	29	3	16	8
Total	68	8 (11.8%)	47 (69.1%)	13 (19.1%)

sive disease) and two died respectively 1 and 2 months after the discontinuation of chemotherapy because of early progression. Of the 11 irradiated patients, five died respectively 4, 8, 14, 17 and 18 months after the end of radiotherapy. A mean number of 56 (range 37–128) lymph nodes per patient was removed; the mean duration of radical surgery was 360 min with an average blood loss of 600 ml (range 300–3000). Four intraoperative complications occurred (7.3%); one hemorrhage (blood loss about 3000 ml) because of a lesion of the left common iliac vein, one lesion of the lower tract of the left ureter, and two lesions of the rectum, all intraoperatively repaired and with a good outcome. Non-lethal postoperative complications occurred in 26 patients (47.2%): 12 lymphocystis; three pulmonary microembolisms; six deep venous thromboses; six laparoceles; three temporary ureteral ectasia; two ureteral fistulas; two urinary incontinence; one stress ulcer; one sepsis. Histological evaluation confirmed a response in 63.3%: seven complete response (10.3%), 38 partial response (53%) and no change in 10 patients (17.7%) (Table 3). Pathological response was detected in 87%, 88.4% and 84.5% of parametrial, vaginal and cervical lesions, respectively. Lymph node mestastases were detected in 13 out of 55 cases (23.6%) and of these three had para-aortic and pelvic involvement and 10 had only pelvic involvement. To date a median follow-up of 15 months (range 2–34) from radical surgery has been achieved. Six out 55 operated patients (11%) have so far relapsed (two, IIb; four, IIIb) (median time to relapse 7.5 months, range 3–14). Local recurrences were detected in all cases while one patient showed a concurrent distant relapse (lung). Chemotherapy-induced toxicity was not substantial: all patients experienced nausea and vomiting; grades II and III myelotoxicity were observed in six (8.8%) and five (7.3%) patients respectively; one patient (1.5%) showed grade II neurotoxicity after the third course; no respiratory or severe renal toxicities were observed.

Table 3 Pathological response according to stage of disease

FIGO stage	*No. of patients*	*Complete response*	*Partial response*	*No change*
Ib–IIa	6	1	5	—
IIb	29	3	22*	4
III	20	3	11	6
Total	55	7 (10.3%)	38 (55.9%)	10 (14.7%)

*One patient had complete response on cervical specimen, but was node positive

DISCUSSION

Our results indicate that PBM combination is an active regimen in cervical carcinoma, making radical surgery feasible in over 80% of patients previously considered not amenable to surgery. From our preliminary results on 33 cases[9] vaginal lesions seemed to respond significantly better than parametrial lesions (80% vs 63%) according to Sardi *et al.*[10]. Based on the present data, response rate appears to be approximately the same in the different sites. Age, histological type and grading did not seem to influence the response (Tables 2 and 3). Only in 23.6% of patients (13/55) lymph node metastases were detected, compared with an expected incidence up to 80%[11-13] in such advanced cases thus, it seems reasonable that chemotherapy may have a therapeutic role on lymph node metastases. This hypothesis is supported by Kirsten *et al.*[14] (15 patients, FIGO stages Ib–IV, bulky disease) and Sardi *et al.*[15] (11 patients, FIGO stages IIb, bulky disease) who reported 26.7% and 18.1% positive nodes after PVB neoadjuvant chemotherapy, respectively. Only six patients (11%) have so far relapsed and all had negative lymph nodes. Our results indicate that PBM neoadjuvant chemotherapy plus radical surgery is a feasible combined treatment. Chemotherapy-induced toxicity was acceptable with only 7% of patients having severe side-effects (myelosuppression) and over 90% of dose administered. Radical surgery did not seem to be complicated by previous chemotherapy. Perioperative complications occurred in about 50% of cases but it has to be considered that aggressive surgery was performed. Our results seem to be encouraging, and suggest a positive role of neoadjuvant chemotherapy in improving the cure rates of locally advanced cervical carcinoma. A randomized trial comparing PBM neoadjuvant chemotherapy followed by radical surgery and conventional radical surgery on FIGO stages IIb–IIIb is going to be started in a multicenter setting.

REFERENCES

1. Ballon, S.C., Berman, M.L., La Gasse, L.D. *et al.* (1981). Survival after extraperitoneal pelvic and paraaortic lymphadenectomy and radiation therapy in cervical carcinoma. *Obstet. Gynecol.*, **57**, 90
2. Durrance, F.Y., Fletcher, G.H. and Rutledge, F.N. (1969). Analysis of central recurrent disease in stage I and II squamous cell carcinomas of cervix on intact uterus. *Am. J. Res.*, **106**, 831
3. Jolles, B. (1980). Long term results of treatment of carcinoma of cervix. *Br. J. Obstet. Gynaecol.*, **87**, 315
4. Kottmeier, H.L. (1979). *Annual report of the results of treatment in gynecological cancer.* (Stockholm: International Federation of Obstetricians and Gynecologists, Pogo Print)
5. Nori, D., Valentine, E. and Hilaris, B.S. (1985). The role of para-aortic node irradiation in the treatment of cancer of the cervix. *Int. J. Radiat. Oncol. Biol. Phys.*, **11**, 1469
6. Dargent, D., Frobert, J.L. and Bean, G. (1985). V Factor (tumor volume) and T Factor (FIGO classification) in the assessment of cervix cancer prognosis: The risk of lymph node spread. *Gynecol. Oncol.*, **22**, 15
7. Friedlander, M.L., Keie, S.B., Sullivan, A. *et al.* (1983). Cervical carcinoma: A drug responsive tumor experience with combined cisplatin, vinblastine and bleomycin therapy. *Gynecol. Oncol.*, **16**, 275
8. Vermorken, J.B., Mangioni, C., van Osterom, A.T. *et al.* (1983). Vincristine, bleomycin,

mytomicin C and cisplatin (VMBP) in squamous cell carcinoma of the uterine cervix (SCCUC). *Proceedings of the 2nd European Conference on Clinical Oncology*, **2**, 50 (Oxford: Pergamon Press)
9. Benedetti Panici, P., Scambia, G., Greggi, S., Di Roberto, P. *et al.* (1988). Neoadjuvant chemotherapy and radical surgery in locally advanced cervical carcinoma: a pilot study. *Obstet. Gynecol.*, **71**, 344
10. Sardi, J.E., Di Paola, G.R., Cahan, A. *et al.* (1986). A possible new trend in the management of the carcinoma of the cervix utery. *Gynecol. Oncol.*, **25**, 139
11. Chung, C.K., Nahhas, W.A., Strykew, V.A. *et al.* (1980). Analysis of factors contributing to treatment failures in stage Ib and IIa carcinoma of the cervix. *Am. J. Obstet. Gynecol.*, **138**, 550
12. Benedetti Panici, P., Di Roberto, P., Greggi, S. *et al.* (1987). Squamous cervical cancer at stage Ib and II: A ten years experience, analysis of 231 cases. *Eur. J. Gynecol. Oncol.*, **2**, 76
13. Van Bommel, P.F.J., van Lindert, A.C.M., Kock, H.C.L.V. *et al.* (1987). A review of prognostic factors in early-stage carcinoma of the cervix (FIGO Ib and IIa) and implications for treatment strategy. *Eur. J. Obstet. Gynecol. Reprod. Biol.*, **26**, 69–84
14. Kirsten, F., Atkinsons, K.H., Coppleson, J.V.M., Elliot, P.M. *et al.* (1987). Combination chemotherapy followed by surgery or radiotherapy in patients with locally advanced cervical cancer. *Br. J. Obstet. Gynaecol.*, **94**, 583
15. Sardi, J.E., Di Paola, G.R., Giaroli, A., Sananes, C. *et al.* (1988). Results of a phase II trial with neoadjuvant chemotherapy in carcinoma of the cervix utery. *Gynecol. Oncol.*, **31**, 256

Section 1 continued

Part B

Ovarian cancers

9

Oncogenes and growth factors in ovarian epithelial tumors

G.P. Trentini, C. de Gaetani and L. Losi

INTRODUCTION

An increasing body of evidence suggests that deregulation of cellular proto-oncogenes (*c-oncs*) may play a part in malignant transformation in a variety of human tumors. *c-oncs* are highly conserved regions of the normal genome, which play a part in the transmission and transduction of growth regulatory signals. A change in the coding or controlling regions of these genes, i.e. gene amplification, mutation, rearrangement or increased production of transcript by promoter insertion, is thought to be an important event in tumor initiation, promotion and progression.

The role of *c-onc* in the development of ovarian neoplasia has received relatively scant attention, so far. Recently, attempts have been made to examine the role of *c-onc* activation in ovarian tumors, and possible prognostic implications of such expression have been considered. In particular, amplification of *c-myc* has been shown in three out of 11 ovarian cancers[1] and in ovarian tumor cell lines, which also presented elevation of its transcript[2].

In previous studies[3–6], a good correlation between *c-onc* or specific RNA transcript copy number and antigens encoded by activated *c-onc*, called oncoproteins (OPs), has been demonstrated, an observation which validates the use of OP immunohistochemistry to assess gene activity and provides a new avenue for clinical investigation.

By using specific antibodies raised against such proteins, we have investigated OP distribution and quantity in common epithelial tumors of the ovary with the purpose of beginning to dissect the possible role of *c-onc* in the development of these neoplasias and harness the OPs as tools for diagnosis, prognosis and future therapy.

MATERIALS AND METHODS

A representative series of common epithelial tumors of the ovary, together with samples of normal ovaries, Fallopian tubes and uterine tissues, endometrial glandular hyperplasia and adenocarcinoma were subjected to immuno-

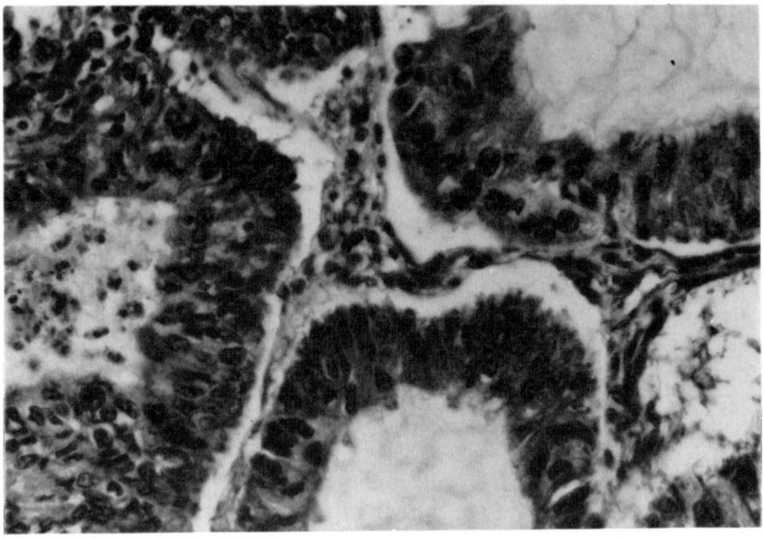

Figure 1 Mucinous cystadenocarcinoma showing diffuse nuclear staining for *c-fos* oncoprotein. A certain reaction is also present in the cytoplasm (ABC immunoperoxidase, ×480)

histochemistry for the search of nine different oncogene-encoded antigens. The following primary monoclonal (MAb) and polyclonal (PAb) antibodies were used: anti-*c-myc* OP (MAb oM-11-905); anti-*N-myc* OP (PAb 0A-11-803 and 0A-11-806); anti-*c-myb* OP (PAb 0A-11-843); anti-*c-fos* OP (PAb 0A-11-825); anti-*ras* p21 (MAb RAP-5); anti-*c-mos* OP (PAb 0A-11-861); anti-*c-fms* OP (PAb 0A-11-815); anti-epidermal growth factor (EGF) receptor (MAb EGFR1 and PAb 0A-11-857). Immunohistochemical staining was performed using the avidin–biotin–peroxidase complex (ABC)–immunoperoxidase method[7] on 5 μm sections of formalin-fixed paraffin-embedded tissues. Each reaction was also controlled on cryostat sections of similar fresh-frozen cases stored at −90°C. Control for the specificity of the immunological reaction was done by incubating sections with primary antibodies absorbed with complementary peptides used to raise antibodies. Antibodies and complementary peptides were purchased from Cambridge Research Biochemicals, U.K., except RAP-5 kindly donated by Dr J. Schlom (NCI, Bethesda) and EGFR1 purchased from Amersham International, U.K.

RESULTS

myc OPs

Concerning *myc* family genes, either *c-myc* or *N-myc*-encoded OPs were investigated (Table 1). *N-myc* OPs were studied by using antibodies directed against two different amino acid sequences, one against the synthetic peptide sequence of human *N-myc*, which does not recognize antigenic determinants present in cells expressing *c-myc* (*N-myc* A), the second against the peptide

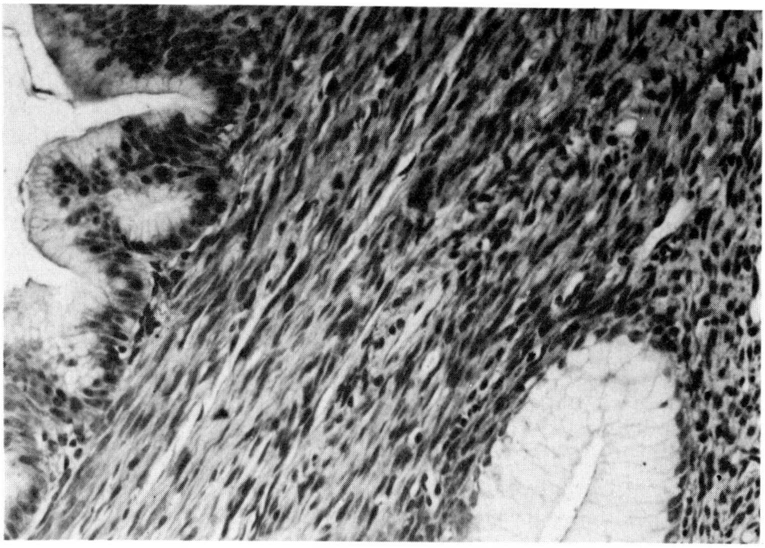

Figure 2 Cytoplasmic staining for *ras* p21 is almost only demonstrated by the borderline component of the mucinous cystadenoma. (ABC immunoperoxidase, ×240)

Table 1 Immunohistochemical staining in common epithelial tumors of the ovary with anti-*c-myc* oncoprotein MAb (microscopic analysis)

Materials	*% of stained nuclei*	*Ab dilution and staining intensity* 1:500	*1:1000*	*1:2000*
Celomic epithelium, mesothelium, inclusion cyst	70	+ +	+ ±	+
Tubal epithelium	30	+	±	±
Serous c-adenoma and adenofibroma	70	+ +	+ ±	+ ±
Serous c-adenoma borderline	80	+ +	+ ±	+ ±
Serous c-adenocarcinoma	*	*	*	*
Mucinous c-adenoma	40	+ +	+	±
Mucinous c-adenoma borderline	80	+ +	+ +	+ ±
Mucinous c-adenocarcinoma	*	*	*	*
Endometrial epithelium	30	+	±	±
Endometrial glandular hyperplasia and adenocarcinoma	50	+	+	±
Endometrioid c-adenoma and adenocarcinoma	50	+	+	±
Brenner tumor	30	+	+	±
Undifferentiated carcinoma	10	+	±	±

*Similar to borderline when well-differentiated; similar to undifferentiated carcinoma when poorly differentiated sequence selected from exon 3 of human *N-myc* OP, which possesses high homology with exon 3 of *c-myc* gene (*N-myc* B). Whereas no reaction was detected with anti-*N-myc* A either on cryostat or paraffin sections, *N-myc* B at the dilution of 1:25, 1:50 and 1:100 showed a staining reaction similar to that of *c-myc* OP, though of minor intensity. This observation appears to suggest that only *c-myc* is expressed in tissues of celomic derivation. The staining reaction for *c-myc* OP was predominantly nuclear, except for tubal and endometrial epithelium, which showed a more uniform and intense cytoplasmic staining. Maximal staining was demonstrated by ovarian surface epithelium, epithelial inclusion cysts and mesothelium with 70% of positive cells. Among ovarian epithelial tumors, serous neoplasms showed a pattern of staining similar to that of celomic epithelium, but with a certain increase in staining intensity and number of positive nuclei in borderline neoplasms, particularly those with a higher grade of dysplasia. In comparison with celomic epithelium, a significantly smaller number of stained nuclei was observed in benign mucinous, endometrioid or Brenner tumors, with a staining similar to that of normal tubal, endometrial or cervical epithelium, suggesting that the gene modification leading to the metaplastic change of celomic epithelium should precede the onset of neoplasia. However, like serous tumors, mucinous borderline cystadenomas were characterized by enhanced levels of *c-myc* OP.

A similar increase was also detectable in endometrioid neoplasms, either benign or malignant, in comparison with normal endometrial epithelium. On the other hand, frankly invasive carcinomas, either serous or mucinous, presented variable degrees of staining in relation to the grade of tumor differentiation, the least staining being shown by the poorly differentiated tumors, as demonstrated also by Polacarz *et al.*[8]

myb OP

A strong reaction was always present, even in spite of progressive antibody dilution from 1:100 to 1:400. The staining reaction was mainly nuclear, except for tubal epithelium, endometrial and endometrioid tissues, or Brenner tumor, which showed an almost exclusive cytoplasmic staining, mainly localized at the gland luminal border. The least staining was shown by undifferentiated carcinoma, presenting, however, numerous cells characterized by an intense dot-like paranuclear reaction. Something similar was detected at cytoplasmic luminal border of tubal and endometrial epithelium. A marked increase in *c-myb* OP was observed particularly in mucinous tumors, in which the percentage of stained nuclei increased from about 10% in benign cystadenoma to approximately 100% in high-grade dysplastic borderline tumor and well-differentiated cystadenocarcinoma. No clear differences were found between celomic epithelium and serous neoplasms.

fos OP

Among normal tissues, celomic epithelium and mesothelium presented a prevalent nuclear staining, whereas tubal and endometrial epithelium showed an almost exclusive and less intense cytoplasmic reaction (Table 2). Benign serous cystadenoma did not appear to differ significantly from celomic epithelium, but a clear increase in the number of stained nuclei was detected in borderline tumors and well-differentiated cystadenocarcinoma. A similar increase was shown by mucinous tumors (Figure 1). On the contrary, endometrial and endometrioid neoplasms did not appear to change in comparison with normal endometrium, a certain increase in percentage of stained nuclei only being observed in endometrial glandular hyperplasia. Like undifferentiated carcinoma, poorly differentiated tumors, either serous or mucinous, only demonstrated a slight cytoplasmic staining. A similar staining was detected in Brenner tumor.

ras p21

As previously reported[9], the search for *ras* oncogene protein p21 failed to discriminate between normal and neoplastic ovarian tissue. However, a tendency to enhanced cytoplasmic staining for p21 was shown by serous tumors, particularly borderline and well-differentiated carcinomas, when compared with normal celomic epithelium (Table 3). A similar increase in comparison with corresponding benign cystadenoma was demonstrated also by mucinous well-differentiated carcinomas and borderline tumors, in the last with a significant correlation to the grade of epithelial dysplasia (Figure 2). No such increase was instead detected in endometrioid or Brenner

Table 2 Immunohistochemical staining in common epithelial tumors of the ovary with anti-*c-fos* OP PAb (microscopic analysis)

Materials	*% of stained nuclei*	*Ab dilution and staining intensity*		
		1:50	*1:100*	*1:300*
Celomic epithelium, mesothelium, inclusion cyst	50	+++	++±	++
Tubal epithelium	2	++	++	+
Serous c-adenoma and adenofibroma	40	+++	++±	++
Serous c-adenoma borderline	70	+++	++±	++
Serous c-adenocarcinoma	*	*	*	*
Mucinous c-adenoma	5	++	+±	+
Mucinous c-adenoma borderline	80†	+++	++±	++
Mucinous c-adenocarcinoma	*	*	*	*
Endometrial epithelium	2	++	+±	+
Endometrial glandular hyperplasia	20	++	++	+
Endometrial adenocarcinoma and endometrioid c-adenoma and adenocarcinoma	2	++	+±	+
Brenner tumor	1	+	±	–
Undifferentiated carcinoma	1	+	±	–

* Similar to borderline when well-differentiated; similar to undifferentiated carcinoma when poorly differentiated

† % of stained nuclei increases together with the grade of dysplasia

Table 3 Immunohistochemical staining in common epithelial tumors of the ovary with anti-*ras* p21 MAb (microscopic analysis)

Materials	*% of stained cells*	*Ab dilution and staining intensity* 1:20 000	1:40 000	1:60 000
Celomic and tubal epithelium, mesothelium, inclusion cyst	70	++	+	−
Serous c-adenoma and adenofibroma	70	+++	++	±
Serous c-adenoma borderline	90	+++	++	±
Serous c-adenocarcinoma	*	*	*	*
Mucinous c-adenoma	30	++	+	−
Mucinous c-adenoma borderline	70†	++	+	−
Mucinous c-adenocarcinoma	*	*	*	*
Endometrial epithelium, glandular hyperplasia, adenocarcinoma	70	++	−	−
Endometrioid c-adenoma	70	++	±	−
Endometrioid c-adenocarcinoma	80	++	±	−
Brenner tumor	100	++	±	−
Undifferentiated carcinoma	100	+	±	−

* Similar to borderline when well-differentiated; similar to undifferentiated carcinoma when poorly differentiated

† % and intensity of staining increases with the grade of dysplasia

tumors. Like undifferentiated carcinoma, poorly differentiated carcinomas demonstrated a tendency to reduced staining.

mos (p37/p43) OP

The cellular distribution of *c-mos* oncogene product was almost exclusively cytoplasmic. No changes were detected in the staining intensity of benign tumors in comparison with correspondent normal tissues, whereas an increase was observed in borderline and malignant tumors, particularly in mucinous and endometrioid (and endometrial) carcinomas (Table 4). In mucinous malignant tumors, the number of positive cells increased to 90%, with a clear correlation to the grade of dysplasia in borderline cystadenoma, and the cellular staining tended to become diffuse, contrary to the basal location presented by cystadenoma. A marked decrease in stainability was observed in poorly differentiated carcinomas, and particularly in undifferentiated carcinoma.

fms OP

The discrete cytoplasmic reaction detected on cryostat sections was markedly reduced, but still detectable, on paraffin sections. No significant differences were presented by different normal tissues and neoplastic lesions, the slight reaction presented with 1:10 antibody dilution being abolished with 1:50 dilution.

Table 4 Immunohistochemical staining in common epithelial tumors of the ovary with anti-*mos* (p37/p43) OP PAb (microscopic analysis)

Materials	*Ab dilution and staining intensity*		
	1:25	*1:50*	*1:100*
Celomic epithelium, mesothelium and inclusion cyst	++	+	±
Tubal epithelium	+	+	−
Serous c-adenoma	++	+	±
Serous c-adenoma borderline	++	++	+
Serous c-adenocarcinoma	*	*	*
Mucinous c-adenoma	++†	+	±
Mucinous c-adenoma borderline and c-adenocarcinoma	++†	++	+
Endometrial epithelium, glandular hyperplasia, endometrioid c-adenoma	±	±	−
Endometrial adenocarcinoma and endometrioid c-adenocarcinoma	++	++	+
Brenner tumor	+	+	±
Undifferentiated carcinoma	±	±	−

*Similar to borderline when well-differentiated; similar to undifferentiated carcinoma when poorly differentiated.
† % of positive cells increases from 5–10 in c-adenoma to 90 in carcinoma, in correlation to the grade of dysplasia in borderline tumors

EGF receptor

Using MAb, a weak and heterogeneous pattern of cytoplasmic staining was only detected on cryosections, paraffin sections giving negative results, and this confirms previous results[10] suggesting EGF receptors are probably expressed in ovarian epithelial tumors (Table 5). A stronger staining was obtained with PAb, even on paraffin sections. Using PAb, a marked increase in staining reaction was observed in all borderline and malignant tumors, in comparison with normal tissues and benign neoplasms. No real difference in staining intensity was observed between gland-like and acanthomatous components in endometrioid carcinomas. In mucinous tumors, the number of positive cells increased together with the progression of neoplasia, all cells being positive in well-differentiated carcinoma, with a pattern of staining analogous to that of *mos* OP. Once again, less differentiated carcinomas were the least stained, though the staining decrease appeared less pronounced than that observed with previous antibodies. The cellular location of staining was mostly cytoplasmic, a certain number of stained nuclei being observed both in benign and malignant tissues.

CONCLUSIONS

The present data underline the existence of over-expression of several *c-oncs* in common ovarian epithelial tumors. Except for *N-myc*, all investigated OPs appeared to be expressed, without discriminating between normal and

Table 5 Immunohistochemical staining in common epithelial tumors of the ovary with anti-human EGF receptor PAb (microscopic analysis)

	Ab dilution and staining intensity		
Materials	*1:50*	*1:100*	*1:200*
Celomic epithelium, mesothelium and inclusion cyst	++	+±	+±
Tubal epithelium	++	+±	+±
Serous c-adenoma	++	++	++
Serous c-adenoma borderline	+++	+++	++±
Serous c-adenocarcinoma	*	*	*
Mucinous c-adenoma	++†	+±	+±
Mucinous c-adenoma borderline	+++†	+++	++±
Mucinous c-adenocarcinoma	*	*	*
Endometrial epithelium	++	+±	+±
Endometrial glandular hyperplasia and adenocarcinoma	+++	++±	++±
Endometrioid c-adenoma and c-adenocarcinoma	+++	++±	++±
Brenner tumor	++	++	+±
Undifferentiated carcinoma	++	+±	+±

* Similar to borderline when well-differentiated; similar to undifferentiated carcinoma when poorly differentiated

† % of positive cells increases from 30 in c-adenoma to 90 in carcinoma, in correlation to the grade of dysplasia in borderline tumors

neoplastic tissues. Among benign tumors, serous neoplasms appeared to reproduce *c-onc* expression shown by celomic epithelium. Mucinous, endometrioid and Brenner tumors showed staining characters analogous to those of equivalent normal tissues of celomic origin. Except for *c-fms*, *c-onc* expression appeared to change in relation with malignant transformation: increased in borderline and well-differentiated carcinomas (particularly mucinous tumors); decreased in poorly differentiated and undifferentiated tumors. The lower absolute levels of OPs in poorly differentiated, therefore clinically aggressive, tumors may reflect an increased protein turnover, or indicate that continuous *onc* expression is not necessary to maintain malignant transformation. A further possibility is that an alteration or partial occlusion of OP epitope may occur in more malignant tumors and thereby decrease the number of cells stained for expression by antibodies.

The detection of *c-onc* expression in ovarian tumors may be useful in predicting tumor prognosis, and in determining genetic relationships between histologically similar but clinically dissimilar tumor types.

ACKNOWLEDGEMENTS

We would like to thank Dr A. M. Martinelli and Mrs Romana Iotti and Milena Tediosi for technical assistance and Gabriella Carpi for typing the manuscript. This work was partially funded by Ministero della Pubblica Istruzione quota 40%.

REFERENCES

1. Serova, O.M. (1987). Amplification of *c-myc* proto-oncogene in primary tumours, metastasis and blood leukocytes of patients with ovarian cancer. *Eksper. Onkol. (Kiev)*, **9**, 25–7
2. Yasue, H., Takeda, A. and Ishibashi, M. (1987). Amplification of the *c-myc* gene and the elevation of its transcripts in ovarian tumour lines. *Cell. Struct. Funct.*, **12**, 121–5
3. Evan, G., Lewis, G.K., Ramsay, G. and Bishop, J.M. (1985). Isolation of monoclonal antibodies specific for human and mouse proto-oncogene products. *Mol. Cell. Biol.*, **5**, 3610–16
4. Hann, S.R., Thompson, C.B. and Eisenman, R.N. (1985). *c-myc* oncogene protein is independent of the cell cycle in human and avian cells. *Nature*, **314**, 366–9
5. Rabbitts, P.H., Watson, J.V., Lamond, A., Fischer, W., Forester, A., Stinton, M.A., Evan, G.I., Atherton, E., Sheppard, R.C. and Rabbitts, T.H. (1985). Metabolism of *c-myc* gene products: *c-myc* mRNA and protein expression in the cell cycle. *EMBO J.*, **4**, 2009–15
6. Sikora, K., Chan, G., Evan, G., Gabra, H., Markham, N., Stewart, J. and Watson, J. (1987). *c-myc* oncogene expression in colorectal cancer. *Cancer*, **59**, 1289–95
7. Hseu, S., Raive, M. and Fauger, H. (1981). Use of avidin-biotin peroxidase complex (ABC) on immunoperoxidase techniques; a comparison of ABC and unlabeled antibody (PAP) procedures. *J. Histochem. Cytochem.*, **29**, 577–80
8. Polacarz, S.V., Hey, N.A., Stephenson, T.J. and Hill, A.S. (1989). *c-myc* oncogene product p62 *c-myc* in ovarian mucinous neoplasms: immunohistochemical study correlated with malignancy. *J. Clin. Pathol.*, **42**, 148–52
9. Rodenburg, C.J., Koelma, I.A., Nap, M. and Fleuren, G.J. (1988). Immunohistochemical detection of the *ras* oncogene product p21 in advanced ovarian cancer. *Arch. Pathol. Lab. Med.*, **112**, 151–4
10. Gullick, W.J., Marsden, J.J., Whittle, N., Ward, B., Bobrow, L. and Waterfield, M.D. (1986). Expression of Epidermal Growth Factor receptors on human cervical, ovarian and vulval carcinomas. *Cancer Res.*, **46**, 285–92

10

Conservative therapeutic approach in sex cord stromal tumors of the ovary

S. Pecorelli, E. Sartori, G. Favalli, F. Rampinelli, C. Bonazzi, S. Chiari and A. Lissoni

Sex cord stromal tumors (SCST) account for approximately 6% of ovarian tumors and for most functioning tumors that have clinical manifestations. The various tumors in this category contain sex cord and stromal elements in varying combinations and with varying degrees of cytologic atypia and mitotic activity. The World Health Organization classification is generally utilized[1], with the addition of several recently recognized types that deserve specific attention[2]. The most important sub-types of these neoplasias are granulosa cell tumors (GCT), juvenile granulosa cell tumors (JGCT) and Sertoli–Leydig cell tumors (SLCT).

GRANULOSA CELL TUMORS

These account for approximately 1.5% of all ovarian tumors and for 6% of ovarian cancers. Approximately 75% of them are estrogenic, but rare examples are androgenic. Two-thirds of the tumors occur in postmenopausal women; the median age is similar in the different reported series, varying from 42 to 53 years while the age range is extremely wide: stillborn infant to 88 years; 2–4% of the cases are prepubertal and 15–20% occur in patients younger than 30 years.

About 80% of GCTs present as stage I and stage IV is exceptional (less than 1%). Bilaterality of the tumor is relatively rare with data varying from 2.1% to 8.2% and an average of 4.1% from the cumulative analysis of 910 cases reported in the literature. At any age GCT is prone to rupture, with hemoperitoneum and acute or subacute abdominal symptoms. Examination of the endometrium in women with functioning GCTs shows a variety of changes ranging from cystic hyperplasia to invasive adenocarcinoma. The latter, which is almost always of low grade, develops in approximately 5% of all women with GCT and is twice as common after the menopause as it is in younger women. Histological grading is now recognized as being of little prognostic value[3,4].

GCTs have a relatively low malignant potential and a propensity for late recurrences and are associated with long-term patient survival (approximately 80% 10 year and 65% 20 year overall survival). Stenwig and colleagues reported a relative 10 year survival of 86% in stage I versus 49% in stage II–IV carcinomas[5]; in another series (Bjorkholm and Silfersward) the relative 10 year survival was 96% for stage I and 26% for stage II to IV[6]. Recurrences are associated with high mortality, the tumor being lethal in 75% of cases. The treatment of GCT depends on its stage and the age of the patient. The basic surgical approach in perimenopausal and postmenopausal women is hysterectomy with bilateral salpingo-oophorectomy. However the majority of authors agree that stage IA tumor, in a young patient in whom the preservation of fertility is desired, can be treated by unilateral salpingo-oophorectomy[7]. Radiotherapy could play some role in advanced or recurrent disease with minimal residual tumor after operative debulking. Chemotherapy appears advisable in patients with large residual disease, inoperable recurrences, or metastases. The few available reports suggest that multidrug regimens, including actinomycin D, 5-fluorouracil, vincristine and cyclophosphamide may be more effective than single alkylating agents. More recently, on the basis of the good results in ovarian germ cell tumors, combination chemotherapy, using cisplatin, vinca alkaloids and bleomycin, was tested with satisfactory preliminary results[8].

About 85% of GCTs that occur before the age of normal puberty have distinctive microscopic features that differ from those of the well-known forms of GCT encountered in older patients and that has led to their designation as 'juvenile granulosa cell tumors'. In Scully's series of 125 cases 44% occurred in the first decade, 34% in the second decade, 19% in the third decade and only 3% beyond the age of 30 years[5].

Although the JGCT usually appears less well differentiated than the typical GCT occurring in older patients the follow-up in the series reported in the literature[9–12] indicates a high cure rate: eight cases with clinically malignant behavior out of 164 patients. However, these few cases have been associated with rapid growth and have spread throughout the abdomen.

Conservative treatment is adequate for most stage IA tumors.

SERTOLI–LEYDIG CELL TUMORS

These account for less than 0.2% of ovarian neoplasms. Their peak occurrence is during the early reproductive years with an average age of 25 years. Approximately half the patients present with hirsutism or virilization. On microscopic examination SLCTs have been divided in four categories: well differentiated, of intermediated differentiation, poorly differentiated and with heterologous elements[13–15].

Ninety-eight per cent of the tumors present as stage I; bilaterality is about 1%. In Scully's series the clinical behavior is related to stage of the tumor (two thirds of recurrences within one year for stage II and III), poor differentiation, presence of mesenchymal heterologous elements and a prominent retiform component[5].

The treatment of these tumors depends on the age of the patient, the stage of the tumor and its degree of differentiation with chance of conservative approach for young stage I patients.

From 1982 to 1988 72 patients suffering from malignant sex cord stromal tumors were treated in our Institutions: the distribution of cases by stage was: stage I = 46; stage II = 3; stage III = 8; stage IV = 2; and relapses = 13. The overall incidence of nodal metastases was 7%.

In this series 65 cases were GCT (53 adult histotype and 12 juvenile type) and seven were SLCT. Twenty-six out of 72 patients (36%) were younger than 36 years at the time of referral to our Institutions and most of them (22/26) were treated conservatively: 17/18 stage I and 5/6 stage IIB–IV (Table 1).

Six out of these 22 patients were treated postoperatively with adjuvant chemotherapy: one of seventeen stage I (undifferentiated GCT stage IC) and all five stage IIB–IV cases. The chemotherapeutic regimen was PVB (cisplatin, 20 mg/m^2 i.v. day 1 to 5; vinblastine, 0.15 mg/kg i.v. day 1 and 2; bleomycin, 30 mg i.v. day 2 (24 h infusion) and 15 mg i.v. bolus day 15; repeated every 28 days).

There was no recurrence in stage I SCSTs, neither after conservative treatment (17 cases) nor after complete surgery (29 cases). Three of the five stage IIB–IV patients treated conservatively had progression/recurrence after PVB chemotherapy (Table 2).

Of the patients treated by chemotherapy after demolitive surgery (seven cases) four are with no evidence of disease at 77, 71, 67, 48 months and three are dead of disease at 11, 20 and 21 months respectively. One of the six patients treated with chemotherapy after conservative surgery is prepubertal while of the remaining five, four suffered from amenorrhea during treatment, with return to regular menstrual function 2–4 months after treatment.

Table 1 Conservative treatment (CT) of SCST (in < 36-year-old patients)

Stage	*CT/Total*
IA	9/10
IC	8/8
IIB–IV	5/6
Relapse*	0/2
Total	22/26

*Previous demolitive surgery

Table 2 Response to primary chemotherapy in SCST after conservative treatment

Stage	*Histology*	*Residual tumor*	*Response**	*Recurrence*	*Status†*
IIB	Juvenile	Micro	CR	–	NED 26 months
IIB	Adult	Micro	CR	–	NED 26 months
III	Adult	< 2 cm	CR	+	DOD 48 months
III	Juvenile	< 2 cm	P		DOD 7 months
IV	Adult	> 10 cm	P		DOD 7 months

* CR, complete regression; P, partial

† NED, no evidence of disease; DOD, dead of disease

Three patients of the 16 submitted to conservative surgery alone and one of the six treated with adjuvant chemotherapy had normal pregnancies and delivered four healthy babies.

From our preliminary results and from data of the literature we can conclude that indication for conservative treatment in SCST is: definite in stage IA; probable in stage I with unfavorable prognostic factors (the role of adjuvant chemotherapy must be established); possible in stage II–IV in some selected cases.

REFERENCES

1. Serov, S.F., Scully, R.E. and Sabin, L.H. (1973). *International Histological Classification of tumors No 9: Histological Typing of Ovarian Tumors.* (Geneva: World Health Organization)
2. Young, R.H. and Scully, R.E. (1983). Ovarian sex cord stromal and steroid cell tumors. In Roth, L.M. and Czernobilsky, B. (eds) *Tumors and Tumors Like Conditions of the Ovary,*
3. Evans, A.T. *et al.* (1980). Clinicopathological review of 118 granulosa and 82 theca cell tumors. *Obstet. Gynecol.*, **55**, 231–8
4. Norris, H.J. *et al.* (1968). Prognosis of granulosa-theca tumors of the ovary. *Cancer*, **21**, 255–63
5. Stenwig, J.T. *et al.* (1979). Granulosa cell tumors of the ovary. A clinicopathological study of 118 cases with long term follow up. *Gynecol. Oncol.*, **7**, 136–52
6. Björkholm, E. and Silfersward, C. (1981). Prognostic factors in granulosa cell tumors. *Gynecol. Oncol.*, **11**, 261–74
7. Scully, R.E. (1977). Ovarian tumors: a review. *Am. J. Pathol.*, **87**, 686–720
8. Colombo, M., Sessa, C. *et al.* (1986). Cisplatin, Vinblastine and Bleomycin combination chemotherapy in metastatic granulosa cell tumors of the ovary. *Obstet. Gynecol.*, **67**, 265
9. Roth, L.M., Nicholas, T.R. and Ehrlich, C.E. (1979). Juvenile granulosa cell tumor. A clinicopathologic study of three cases with ultra-structural observations. *Cancer*, **44**, 2194–205
10. Lack, E.E. *et al.* (1981). Granulosa theca cell tumors in premenarchal girls. A clinical and pathologic study of ten cases. *Cancer*, **48**, 1846–54
11. Zalovdek, C. and Norris, H.J. (1982). Granulosa tumors of the ovary in children. A clinical pathologic study of 32 cases. *Am. J. Surg. Pathol.*, **6**, 503–12
12. Young, R.H. and Scully, R.E. (1984). Ovarian Sex Cord–Stromal Tumours: recent advances and current status. *Clin. Obstet. Gynecol.*, **11**, 93–134
13. Prat, J. *et al.* (1982). Ovarian Sertoli-Leydig cell tumors with heterologous elements (ii). Cartilage and skeletal muscle. *Cancer*, **50**, 2465–75
14. Scully, R.E. (1953). An unusual ovarian tumor containing Leydig cells but associated with endometrial hyperplasia in a postmenopausal woman. *J. Clin. Endocrinol. Metab.*, **13**, 1254–63
15. Young, R.H. *et al.* (1983). A distinctive ovarian sex cord stromal tumor causing sexual precocity in the Peutz Jeghers syndrome. *Am. J. Surg. Pathol.*, **7**, 233–43

11

Study on the possibilities of an early diagnosis of ovarian cancer by pelvic ultrasound scanning

G. Masellis, C. Capodieci, M.R. Bagni, M. Bergamaschi, F. Martinez, M.G. Lucchi and U. Citti

INTRODUCTION

In spite of the progress in the early detection of gynecological cancers of recent years, ovarian cancers continue to show a high mortality rate, owing largely to the difficulty of making an early diagnosis.

It is now clear that if we are to succeed in early detection, we must further define the epidemiological characteristics of cancers of this type and identify sufficiently sensitive, specific instruments which can be used repeatedly on a large scale.

As a contribution to this process, we decided to analyze the advantages and limitations of pelvic ultrasonography and its large-scale use in early detection of ovarian cancers, as other researchers have done in the past.

METHODS AND MATERIAL

We examined 2400 women between 40 and 70 years of age selected at random from the resident population of Modena. The sample was divided into two groups of 1200 individuals; one group contained users of the Modena Family Planning Clinics cytology service, who were invited to take part in the experiment by the service's midwives when they attended for cervical smears, while the other group consisted of women resident in Modena selected at random from the electoral rolls and invited by letter to take part in the experiment after an interview at which they were given further information. The sample was divided into these two groups in order to provide an estimate of the respective percentages agreeing to take part.

A coded card for collection of the following data was filled in at each examination:

(1) main personal, anamnestic and clinical data;

(2) data regarding the risk factors for ovarian cancer (as defined in the literature);
(3) the results of the ultrasound scan; and
(4) information about hospitalization, surgery and histological examination for women who underwent surgery.

These data did not influence the clinical procedures applied, which were decided on the basis of ultrasound findings alone.

The pelvic ultrasound scan was carried out with full bladder using an Aloka SS D 630 machine with sectorial, convex probe 3.5 MHz. Three ovary diameters were measured (longitudinal, anteroposterior and transverse), and the ovary volume was calculated using the ellipse formula. The morphology of the ovary and uterus were described together with any formations in surrounding areas or in the pouch of Douglas.

Ovary volume standards were established on the basis of Campbell's well-known study and the research carried out at the Obstetrics and Gynecology Department of the University of Genoa, which we also bore in mind in deciding our suggested clinical procedures as illustrated in Figures 1, 2 and 3.

Since our sample included pre- and postmenopausal women, we established three different procedures depending on the date of the last menstruation.

The procedure indicated was later modified in relation to simple cysts of diameter not exceeding 3 cm in the two postmenopausal groups. In these cases surgery was recommended only if the cyst was found to have increased in size at later ultrasound checks. Otherwise regular ultrasound scans were recommended.

RESULTS

The results indicated refer to the first examination of the sample group and cover ovary abnormalities found during the ultrasound scan. We are currently processing the overall data referring to the relationship between the ovarian pathologies found and the risk factors, and the numerical distribution of individuals amongst the three groups (premenopause, postmenopause for less than 2 years and postmenopause for over 2 years): these data are important for defining the exact incidence of ovarian pathologies in the three groups. The percentage of those accepting the invitation to undergo the ultrasound examination was 80% in the group of women contacted through the smear test organization, and 15% in the other group. At the first examination, out of 2400 women we found 126 with ovaries of abnormal morphology or volume (8.29%). These abnormalities were also found at further checks in only 73 (3%). Thirty-five women (1.4%) underwent surgery and histological and surgical examination revealed ovarian pathologies in 28 (1.16%): six women presented uterine pathologies (five myomas and one adenomyosis). The results relating to the ovarian pathologies are given in Table 1, broken down according to histological type. Amongst the women operated, we found one *papillary serous carcinoma* (FIGO Stage 1B) which

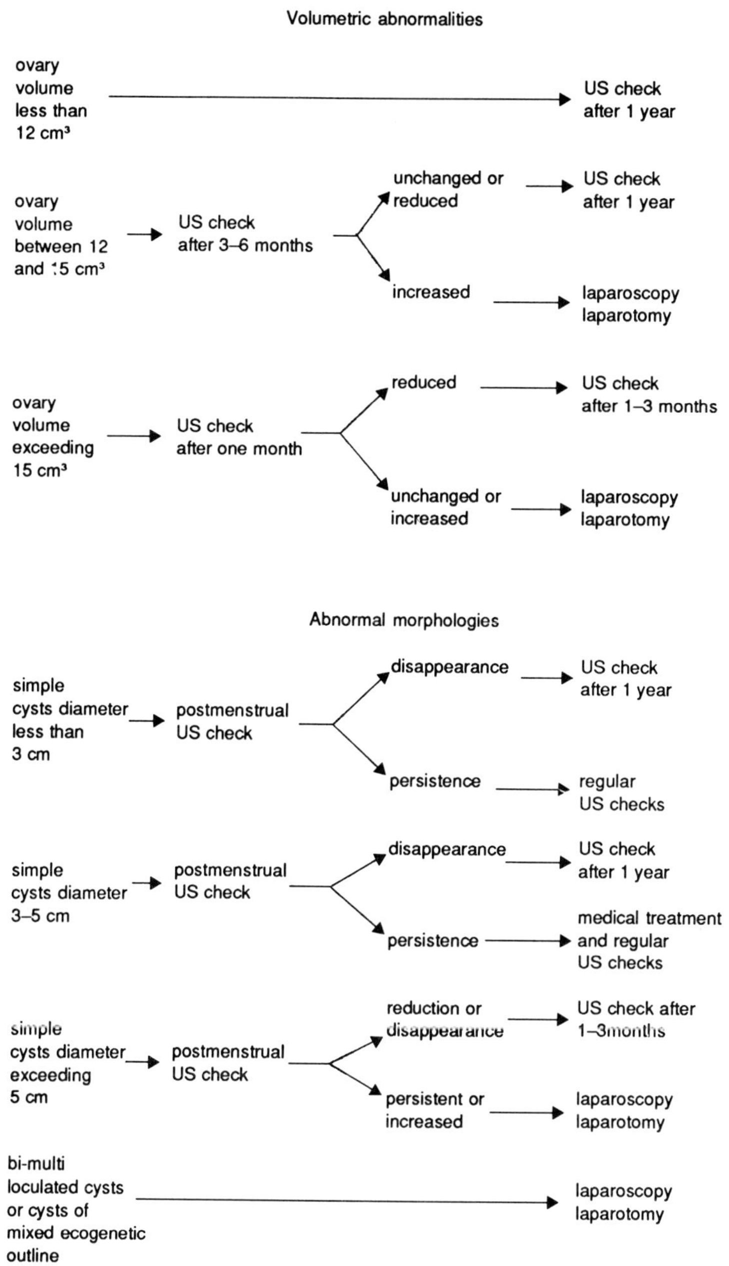

Figure 1 Clinical procedures used for premenopausal women

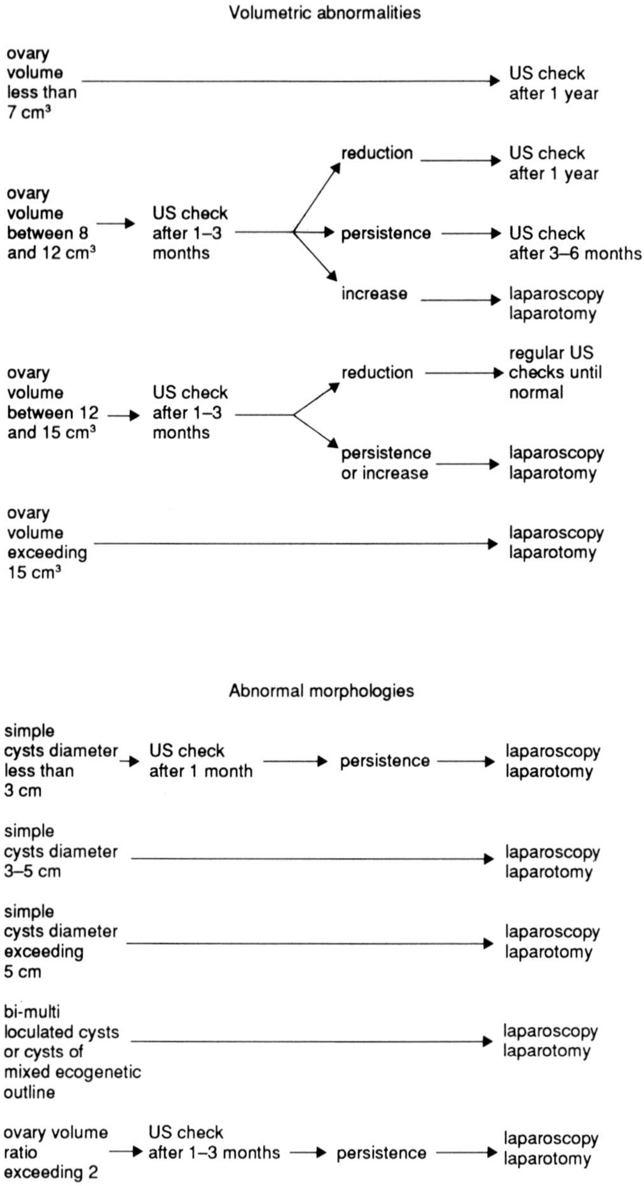

Figure 2 Clinical procedures used for women in menopause for less than 2 years

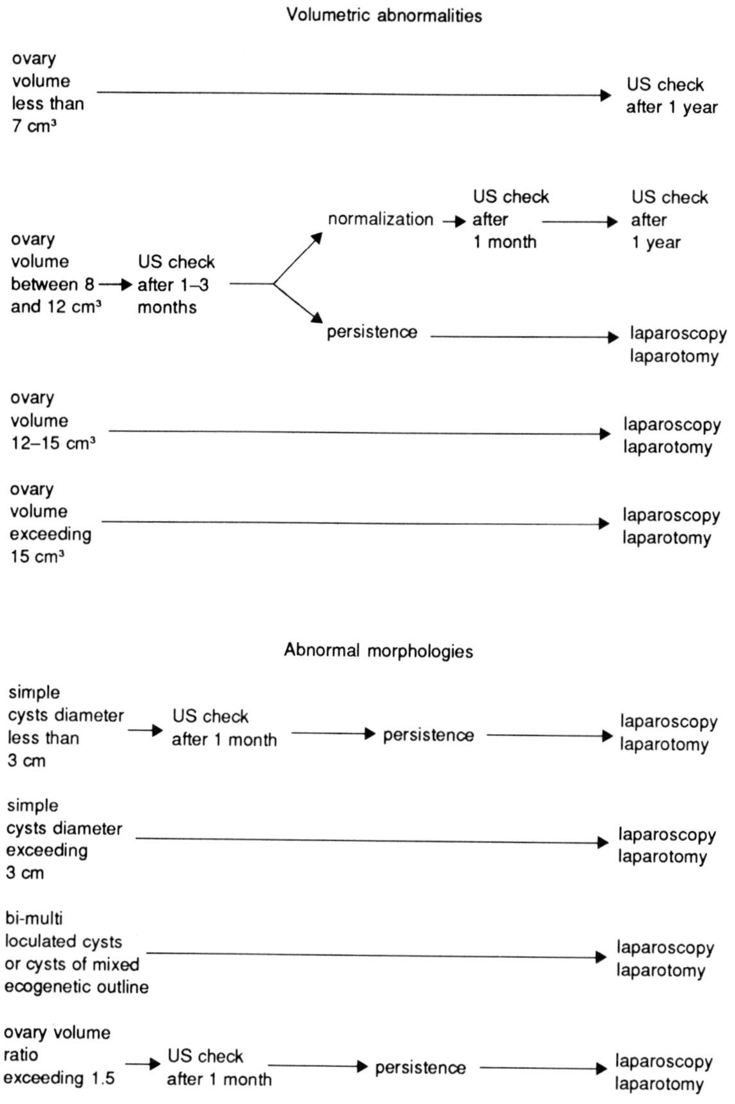

Figure 3 Clinical procedures used for women in menopause for more than 2 years

during the ultrasound scan resembled a regularly shaped liquid-filled ovarian cyst with small solid areas inside, found in both ovaries (the larger of the two growths was on the left and measured 5.4 × 4.9 × 4.7 cm). The patient was 61 years of age, secundipara and obese, and had no symptoms when the examination was carried out. As we expected, epithelial tumors were the most common of the benign neoplasias found. The group of women who

Table 1 Histological breakdown of ovarian pathologies found in women who underwent surgery

	Number	*% of total*	*% of those operated*
Cysts			
Simple	10		
Serous	7		
Mucinous	1		
Total	18	0.75	64.2
Benign epithelial tumor			
Serous cystadenoma	2		
Mucinous cystadenoma	2		
Endometrioma	3		
Total	7	0.29	25
Benign germinal tumor			
Dermoid cysts	1	0.04	3.5
Benign stromal tumor			
Thecoma	1	0.04	3.5
Malignant epithelial tumor			
Papillary serous carcinoma	1	0.04	3.5

had been in menopause for over 2 years had the highest percentage of pathologies, especially of neoplasial type.

As stated previously, we do not yet know the distribution of women between the three groups and thus the exact incidence of the pathology found, meaning that this datum may be modified.

In a woman of 68 years of age who underwent total hysterectomy and bilateral removal of uterine appendages because of an ovarian cyst 6.9 × 4.6 cm in diameter, the postoperative histological examination revealed an adenocarcinoma of the endometrium which was starting to infiltrate the myometrium. One false positive result was obtained in a patient of 50 years of age who had been in menopause for 6 years: both the ultrasound scan and nuclear magnetic resonance (carried out after ultrasonography) revealed a liquid-filled oval mass 4.6 × 3.2 cm in diameter; however laparoscopy gave negative results.

DISCUSSION

We realize that the basic question posed by our research is that of the cost–benefit ratio. In our view, a number of factors must be considered in this way. All the women who underwent surgery except one (who had a techoma 15 cm in diameter) were without symptoms when examined and some of them attended regular gynecological check-ups. Some of them would probably have incurred the most common complications associated with ovarian neoplasias (rupture or torsion) and a few may have risked more dubiously connected phenomena such as malignant change. As we are all aware, the major problem with ovarian cancers is the difficulty of early detection. If a malignant ovarian cancer is detected in Stage 1, instead of in Stage 3 or 4, the 5-year survival rate increases from 20% to 60–80%, which apart from the obvious gain in terms of human suffering may also represent a reduction in the costs sustained by the community for the provision of hospital care, chemotherapy and instrument examinations. Currently, pelvic ultrasonography is the only non-invasive technique which enables us to identify initial modifications in the morphology and volume of the ovaries, so there is no doubt that at the moment it plays an important role in our possibilities of early diagnosis of ovarian tumors. In our opinion, research must be carried out to discover other means of distinguishing which of the growths detected under ultrasonography are benign and which malignant before surgery is carried out. Small ovarian cysts are far from uncommon in postmenopausal women; the frequency with which they were detected and the fact that they did not alter over time led us to consider them a less alarming sign than we had originally believed. We consider that the addition of tumor markers to endocystic fluid collected by aspiration may be a useful additional technique. Moreover, in order to establish the cost–benefit ratio we must also establish the frequency at which pelvic ultrasound scans should be carried out in the various age ranges in order to monitor better the population at greatest risk.

ACKNOWLEDGEMENTS

The research was made possible thanks to the cooperation of the National Association for the Study and Treatment of Solid Cancers, Local Health Authority n. 16 – Modena (Family Planning Clinic Division) and the Obstetrics and Gynecology Department of the University of Modena.

BIBLIOGRAPHY

1. Andolf, E., Svalenius, E. and Astedt, B. (1986). Ultrasonography for early detection of ovarian carcinoma. *Br. J. Obstet. Gynaecol.*, **98**, 1286–9
2. Campbell, S., Goswamy, R., Goessens, L. and Whitehead, M. (1982). Real-Time ultrasonography for determination of ovarian morphology and volume. *The Lancet*, **ii**, 425
3. Costantini, S. and Valenzano, M. (1987). Ruolo dell'ecografia nello screening e nella diagnosi del tumore ovarico. *Presented at Gynaecological Oncology Congress, Turin, 5–7 May*
4. Cramer, D.W., Hutchinson, G.B., Welch, W.R. *et al.* (1983). Determinants of ovarian cancer risk. Reproductive experience and family history. *J. Nat. Cancer Inst.*, **71**, 711
5. Donaldson, E.S., Van Nagell, J.R., Pursell, S. *et al.* (1980). Multiple bio-chemical markers in patients with gynaecologic malignancies. *Cancer*, **45**, 948–53
6. Franceschi, S., La Vecchia, C., Helmrich, S.P. *et al.* (1982). Risk factors for epithelial ovarian cancer in Italy. *Am. J. Epidemiol.*, **115**, 716
7. Goswamy, R., Campbell, S. and Whitehead, M. (1983). Screening of ovarian cancer. *Clin. Obstet. Gynaecol.*, **10**, 3
8. Heintz, A.P.M., Hacker, N.F. and Lagasse, L.D. (1985). Epidemiology and etiology of ovarian cancer: a review. *Obstet. Gynecol.*, **66**, 127
9. Kolstad, P. and Beecham, J.C. (1974). Epidemiology of ovarian neoplasia. In *Proceedings of the American–European Conference on the ovary, Montreux, Switzerland, Excerpta Medica Int. Congress.* Series 364, 56
10. Niloff, J.A., Knapp, R.C., Schaetzl, E. *et al.* (1984). CA 125 antigenal levels in obstetric and gynecologic patients. *Obstet. Gynecol.*, **64**, 703–7

11. Silverberg, E. and Urbera, J.A. (1983). A review of American CANCER society estimates of cancer cases and deaths. *CA-A Cancer J. Clin.*, **33**, 3
12. Van Nagell, J.R., Donaldson, E.S., Hanson, M.B. *et al.* (1981). Biochemical markers in the plasma and tumors of patients with gynecological malignancies. *Cancer*, **48**, 495–503
13. Walsh, J., Taylor, K.J.W., Wasson, J.F., Schwartz, P.E. and Rosenfield, A.T. (1979. Gray scale ultrasound in 204 proved gynecological pelvic masses: accuracy and specific diagnostic criteria. *Radiology*, **130**, 391
14. Young, J.L., Percy, C.L. and Asire, A.J. (1981). Surveillance, epidemiology and end results: incidence and mortality data, 1973–1977. *National Cancer Institute Monograph* 57. (Bethesda: MD, United States Department of Health and Human Services)

12

Ovarian carcinoma treatment with buserelin

L.R. Marcellino, L. Stellato and G. Valducci

INTRODUCTION

It is useless denying that, in the last 8 years, chemotherapy for advanced ovarian carcinoma has given always more encouraging results, with a prolonged average survival, according to the improved and better knowledge of the different protocols used so far.

It is also true that, thanks to Professor Mathe's school, we were among the first to use such therapeutic protocols and it must be said that we were the first to observe the unbinding of the neoplastic cell from the pharmacological action.

Therefore, once obtaining these results and also confirming the need to look at other possibilities, on the basis of a study carried out by S. Kullander[1], we thought it was worthwhile, in cases no longer responding to chemotherapy, to use the luteinizing hormone (LH)-releasing hormone (RH) analogs and antagonists. Much has already been said about their action; hence, we recall Professor Schally's papers and all the other bibliographical references here reported, useful, in our opinion, for a better knowledge of the pharmacological action and each therapeutic effect[2-5].

MATERIALS AND METHODS

The present study includes six cases of ovarian carcinoma. Patients underwent a simple laparotomy or partial removal of the neoplastic mass; their age ranged from 45 to 55 years, hence, in pre- and post-menopausal period.

Two patients received no chemotherapy: in one case due to cardiac reasons and hypertension, and in the other case because of a clear refusal by the patient and her family, who considered such treatment to be physically and psychologically devastating.

The remaining four patients were treated with cyclophosphamide, cisplatinum and pharmorubicyn, each month for at least 6 months, which resulted in partial or total regression of the disease. Two of these patients underwent a second look operation after 1 year, which confirmed, from a histological point of view, the total regression of the disease.

The four cases aforementioned presented a rather marked myelodepression to the point that the white cell count was under 2000 per mm^3. The two cases receiving no chemotherapy were immediately treated with buserelin, one phial intramuscularly per day, for 8 days, followed by 12 inhalations per day.

The four cases receiving chemotherapy were subsequently treated with buserelin, at the same dosage used in the previous cases, as soon as a progression of the disease was registered.

All patients were thoroughly followed-up by means of hematochemical tests, immunological monitoring and other necessary ascertainments according to a specific protocol in which end-points were established at 1 month for laboratory tests and at 3 months for immunological studies or other investigations.

RESULTS

The two cases receiving no chemotherapy, had satisfactory results from the course of treatment. In fact, there was no apparent progression of the neoplastic mass for 2 years in one case, and for 18 months in the other. Such results are also in agreement with S. Kullander's report[1]. No side-effect was registered using LHRH therapy.

Not so encouraging, though, are the results from those patients first treated with chemotherapy. In such cases, perhaps for some weeks or months, a stop in neoplastic mass proliferation was obtained, but it soon ended in ascites and massive metastases, in all cases, within a maximum of 5 months. We are able to say that no side-effects were registered during buserelin treatment even in those patients previously submitted to chemotherapy.

DISCUSSION

It seems evident, even though our series includes only two cases, that hormone therapy with LHRH antagonists is much more effective if neoplastic cells are 'hormone-dependent'. Like prostate cancer, in this type of tumor also, radio- or chemotherapy treatment alters the neoplastic cell, unbinding it from steroid action.

Clear positive results of regression, although partial, have been obtained, in fact, only in those cases not previously treated. Such assertion is confirmed by the other four cases, in which chemotherapy gave some positive results, but there was a progression of the disease clearly before starting buserelin therapy. Unfortunately, as we well know, the number of cells, although minimal, not responding to chemotherapy or hormone therapy, is difficult to control.

So, today, it appears that the simple reduction in proliferation of the cells not hormone-dependent is successful. Chemotherapy was no more effective in those cases, either because of the constant and ineluctable appearance of severe side-effect phenomena, among the first, those due to immunological depression. Buserelin action has also been demonstrated on cells severely altered in their neoplastic biology.

Furthermore, LHRH antagonists have been used in a very advanced phase of the disease, characterized by extensive metastases. For this reason, we cannot illude ourselves about the slightest minimum positive action given by such hormone therapy. In other words, we are not able to hope for any kind of effect by LHRH agonists and antagonists on strongly undifferentiated cells, which do not recognize the hormonal affinity of their original cellular clonus.

The authors hopes for the future are to be able to use a relatively new protocol such as hormone therapy plus immunotherapy.

REFERENCES

1. Kullander, S. (1986). LHRH agonist treatment in ovarian cancer. *Abst. Int. Symp. Hormonal Manipulation of Cancer, Rotterdam*
2. Schally, A.V., Comaru Schally, A.M. and Redding, T.W. (1984). Antitumor effects of analogues of hypothalamic hormones in endocrine-dependent cancer. *Proc. Soc. Exp. Biol. Med.*, **175**, 259
3. Labrie, F., Belanger, A., Cusan, L. *et al.* (1980). Antifertility effects of LH-RH agonists in the male. *J. Androl.*, **1**, 209
4. Tolis, G., Ackman, D., Stellos, A., Mehta, A., Labrie, F., Fazekas, A.T.A., Comaru Schally, A.M. and Schally, A.V. (1982). Tumor growth inhibition in patients with prostatic carcinoma treated with luteinizing hormone-releasing hormone agonists. *Proc. Natl. Acad. Sci., USA*, **79**, 1658
5. Schally, A.V., Coy, D.H. and Arimura, A. (1980). LH-RH agonists and antagonists. *Int. J. Gynaecol. Obstet.*, **18**, 318

Section 1 continued

Part C

Breast cancers

13

Endogenous estrogens in malignant, fatty and normal breast tissues

A. Milewicz, J.H.H. Thijssen, J. Daroszewski and M.A. Blankenstein

INTRODUCTION

Estrogens are involved in the etiology of breast cancer. It has been hypothesized that hormonal hyperstimulation of target cells which are normally under hormonal control may initiate the development of the neoplasm[1]. Several studies on the production rate and plasma levels of estrogens in patients with breast cancer[2,3] do not support this hypothesis. The observation that the unoccupied estrogen receptor is permanently localized in the nucleus of the target cell[4] has led to the suggestion that the intratissue concentration of steroids, i.e. the concentration at their site of action, is more closely related to their biological effects. Previous studies in women living in countries with a high incidence of breast cancer have shown that the concentration of estradiol in the tumor is higher than that in normal breast tissue, whereas for estrone such differences are less manifest[5,6]. The absence of a relationship between tissue and plasma levels of estradiol implies that local factors must be involved in the accumulation of estradiol in breast tumors. The present report extends our observations to samples obtained from a population with a much lower breast cancer incidence, and includes also the estrogen sulfates which may contribute significantly to the intratissue estrogen concentration.

MATERIALS AND METHODS

Patients

Malignant breast tissue was obtained from 39 Polish patients who underwent a mastectomy. Seventeen patients were premenopausal and 21 were postmenopausal. From one patient the menopausal status was unknown. In most patients, plasma, fatty tissue and histologically normal breast tissue were also obtained. Specimens were immediately placed on ice, trimmed free of fat and connective tissue by a pathologist and stored at −80°C until analysis.

The results are compared to those obtained with samples from Dutch breast cancer patients collected under the same conditions, which have been reported earlier[5].

Hormone assays

The concentrations of estrone and estradiol were assessed essentially as described previously[7]. Briefly, 1 g of tissue was pulverized with a Mikrodismembrator (Braun, Melsungen, F.R.G.); the powder was homogenized in 8 volumes phosphate buffer, pH = 7.4 and the homogenate was extracted with 5 volumes ethanol:acetone 1:1 (v/v). The extract was concentrated as far as possible under a gentle stream of nitrogen, delipidated with 70% methanol, concentrated under nitrogen, diluted with 5 ml 0.1 M acetate buffer and extracted twice with 2 volumes of ether. Unconjugated estrogens were assayed in the ether layer by radioimmunoassay. The water phase was subjected to solvolysis by 1500 IU Suc d'Helix Pommatia in acetate buffer for 16 h at 37°C. The solvolyzed samples were extracted with ether and estrone and estradiol were assayed as a measure for their respective sulfates. As extraction recoveries were over 80% and showed little variation, no corrections were made. When the assay result did not exceed the limit of the detection of the assay, a value of 10 fmol/g tissue was arbitrarily assigned to the sample.

Statistical procedures

The distribution of the data was not normal. Therefore non-parametric tests were used. Differences between groups, i.e. pre- and postmenopausal patients were evaluated with Wilcoxon's rank sum test and those within groups, with Wilcoxon's matched pairs signed rank test. The existence of relationships between parameters was tested by calculation of Spearman's rank correlation coefficient. In all cases, p values less than 0.05 were considered to reflect statistical significance.

RESULTS

Table 1 shows the estrogen levels measured in malignant and normal breast tissue as well as in fatty breast tissue from premenopausal Polish women. The same data for postmenopausal women are summarized in Table 2. As expected, estrone concentrations in all tissues dropped significantly with menopause. Strikingly, estradiol concentrations dropped in fatty and normal tissue, but *not* in malignant breast tissue. The concentrations of estrogen sulfates were less than those of the unconjugated estrogens and were less sensitive to the effects of menopause. Only for estrone sulfate significantly lower values were found after menopause. In premenopausal women (Table 1), the concentration of all estrogens measured (except estrone) was significantly higher in tumor than in fatty tissue. Again, with the exception of estrone,

Table 1 Estrogen levels in breast tissues from premenopausal Polish women with breast cancer

Hormone	*Tumor tissue* (n = *17*)	*Fatty tissue* (n = *17*)	*Normal tissue* (n = *8*)
Estrone			
Range	76–1365	405–2000	240–2195
Median	450	1135***	1135
Mean ± SEM	767 ± 20	1181 ± 23	1107 ± 195
Estradiol			
Range	100–3060	10–1005	85–1080
Median	570	375*	480
Mean ± SEM	722 ± 26	409 ± 18	549 ± 105
Estrone sulfate			
Range	30–820	10–1975	70–1820
Median	350	76**	440
Mean ± SEM	415 ± 16	263 ± 21	570 ± 110
Estradiol sulfate			
Range	30–165	10–120	35–275
Median	76	40***	65
Mean ± SEM	88 ± 6	41 ± 5	84 ± 26

All steroid levels are expressed as fmol/g tissue
*$p < 0.05$ vs. tumor
**$p < 0.02$ vs. tumor
***$p < 0.01$ vs. tumor

Table 2 Estrogen levels in breast tissues from postmenopausal Polish women with breast cancer

Hormone	*Tumor tissue* (n = *21*)	*Fatty tissue* (n = *21*)	*Normal tissue* (n = *8*)
Estrone			
Range	32–11 200	141–10 000	215–750
Median	290†††	500†††	380†††‡
Mean ± SEM	886 ± 48	971 ± 45	460 ± 65
Estradiol			
Range	10–1665	10–406	105–295
Median	597	180††****	188††*‡
Mean ± SEM	651 ± 22	148 ± 11	174 ± 20
Estrone sulfate			
Range	10–3630	10–830	45–310
Median	174†††	45***	137
Mean ± SEM	330 ± 27	105 ± 13	154 ± 32
Estradiol sulfate			
Range	10–225	10–148	215–750
Median	60	45	40
Mean ± SEM	80 ± 7	58 ± 6	51 ± 11

All steroid levels are expressed as fmol/g tissue
*$p < 0.05$ vs. tumor
***$p < 0.01$ vs. tumor
****$p < 0.001$ vs. tumor
‡$p < 0.05$ vs. fat
††$p < 0.02$ vs. premenopausal
†††$p < 0.01$ vs. premenopausal

this was also true for tissues from postmenopausal women (Table 2). The concentration of estrogens in normal tissue from premenopausal women did not differ significantly from that in the other types of tissue, but this observation is premature since only eight normal tissues have been analyzed so far. For postmenopausal women, the concentration of estradiol was found to be significantly higher in normal tissue than in fatty tissue. In these patients the estradiol concentration was significantly higher in tumor than in normal tissue (Table 2). In postmenopausal women, a highly significant correlation was found between the estrone concentrations in normal and fatty tissue (Rs = 0.904; $p < 0.01$; $n = 8$). A relationship also existed between the concentrations of estradiol sulfate in tumor tissue and fatty tissue in these women (Rs = 0.561; $p < 0.02$; $n = 21$). In postmenopausal women a correlation was found between the basal body mass index (BMI) and the estrone sulfate concentration in the fatty tissue (Rs = 0.521; $p < 0.02$; $n = 21$). The BMI was not related to any of the other estrogen concentrations tested.

In Table 3 estrone and estradiol concentrations measured in tumor and normal breast tissues from Dutch pre- and postmenopausal patients[5] are given. Again, no difference was found between the estradiol concentrations in tumor tissue from pre- and postmenopausal patients. Estrone concentrations showed the expected decrease with menopause, although the level of significance was not reached ($p < 0.1$). Hormone levels in normal breast tissue were comparable between the Polish and Dutch patients, as was the estradiol concentration in tumor tissue. The estrone concentration in malignant breast tissue from Polish women, by contrast, was approximately 50% lower than in the Dutch women of the corresponding menopausal status.

Table 3 Estrogen levels in breast tissues from pre- and postmenopausal Dutch women with breast cancer

Hormone	*Tumor tissue*	*Normal tissue*
Premenopausal levels		
Estrone		
Range	74–3190	213–> 4000
Median	1040	1028
Mean ± SEM (*n*)	1310 ± 215 (19)	1455 ± 230 (22)
Estradiol		
Range	240–74 000	167–1648
Median	670	435
Mean ± SEM (*n*)	1158 ± 236 (21)	514 ± 71 (22)
Postmenopausal levels		
Estrone		
Range	19–74 000	296–537
Median	610	380
Mean ± SEM (*n*)	859 ± 129 (33)	401 ± 44 (6)
Estradiol		
Range	150–4000	222–444
Median	770	324
Mean ± SEM (*n*)	986 ± 152 (34)	330 ± 37 (6)

All steroid levels are expressed as fmol/g tissue

DISCUSSION

The results described in the present paper confirm and extend our observations[5,6] on the apparent autonomy of human breast cancer to maintain the endogenous estradiol concentration in the tumor tissue irrespective of the existing plasma level. Based on the biochemical pathways for the formation and degradation of estradiol, a number of factors has been identified which might play a role in this respect. On the biosynthetic side these are the endogenous concentrations of estrone, androgens (testosterone and androstenedione) and estrogen sulfates which can be converted to the biologically active estradiol by 17-hydroxysteroid dehydrogenase, aromatase and sulfatase activities respectively. On the catabolic side there are the enzymes which participate in the degradation of estradiol, i.e. the 2-, 4-, and 16-α-hydroxylases[8]. The available data do not allow conclusions yet as to which (combination of) factor(s) is most important in maintaining the intratumor estradiol. The recent finding that breast fibroblasts secrete a polypeptide which is capable of stimulating the conversion of estrone to estradiol in breast epithelial cells[9] indicates that other, as yet unidentified, factors are also important.

Whether the autonomous regulation of intratumor estradiol levels is equally important in pre- and in postmenopausal women can not be derived with certainty yet. In premenopausal women, a statistically significant correlation was found between estrone and estradiol levels in tumor ($Rs = 0.562$; $p < 0.05$; $n = 17$) as well as in fatty tissue ($Rs = 0.793$; $p < 0.01$). In postmenopausal women, by contrast, such a relationship existed only in fatty tissue ($Rs = 0.730$; $p < 0.01$; $n = 21$) but not in tumor tissue ($Rs = 0.161$; NS). From this finding and the fact that the intratumor estradiol concentration does not drop after menopause, we tentatively conclude that in postmenopausal women the autonomy of the tumor with respect to maintenance of estradiol levels is more important than in premenopausal women.

The concentration of estrogen sulfates was lower in fat than in normal and malignant breast tissues (Tables 1 and 2). This is not remarkable in view of the polar nature of the sulfates, but appears to be in contrast with the observed correlation between the BMI and the estrone sulfate level in fatty tissue, especially in view of the absence of further relationships with the BMI.

Preliminary observations indicate that no differences exist between estrogen plasma levels in Polish and Dutch breast cancer patients. Yet, estrone levels are approximately 50% lower in tumors from the Polish women which belong to a population with a relatively low breast cancer incidence. This suggests that breast cancer incidence may be related to the endogenous estrone level. Further investigation is needed in other populations with low, intermediate and high breast cancer incidences.

ACKNOWLEDGEMENTS

The authors gratefully acknowledge the dedication and excellent technical assistance of Mrs M. Haenen-Nabuurs and Mrs I. Maitimu-Smeele.

REFERENCES

1. Henderson, B.E., Ross, R. and Bernstein, L. (1988). Estrogens as a cause of human cancer. *Cancer Res.*, **48**, 246–53
2. Dao, T. (1979). Metabolism of estrogens in breast cancer. *Biochim. Biophys. Acta*, **560**, 397–426
3. Moore, J.W., Clark, C.M.G., Bulbrook, R.D., Hayward, J.L., Murai, J.T., Hammond, G.L. and Siiteri, P.K. (1982). Serum concentrations of total and non-protein bound oestradiol in patients with breast cancer and in normal controls. *Int. J. Cancer*, **29**, 17–21
4. King, W.J. and Greene, G.L. (1984). Monoclonal antibodies localize estrogen receptor in the nuclei of target cells. *Nature*, **307**, 745–7
5. Van Landeghem, A.A.J., Poortman, J., Nabuurs, M. and Thijssen, J.H.H. (1985). Endogenous concentration and subcellular distribution of estrogens in normal and malignant human breast tissues. *Cancer Res.*, **45**, 2900–6
6. Thijssen, J.H.H., Blankenstein, M.A., Miller, W.R. and Milewicz, A. (1987). Estrogens in tissues: Uptake from the peripheral circulation or local production. *Steroids*, **50**, 297–306
7. Van Landeghem, A.A.J., Poortman, J., Helmond-Agema, A. and Thijssen, J.H.H. (1984). Measurement of endogenous subcellular concentrations of steroids in tissue. *J. Steroid Biochem.*, **20**, 639–44
8. Abul Hajj, Y.J., Thijssen, J.H.H. and Blankenstein, M.A. (1988). Metabolism of estradiol by human breast cancer. *Eur. J. Cancer Clin. Oncol.*, **24**, 1171–8
9. Adams, E.F., Newton, C.J., Tait, G.H., Braunsberg, H., Reed, M.J. and James, V.H.T. (1988). Paracrine influence of human breast stromal fibroblasts on breast epithelial cells: secretion of a polypeptide which stimulates reductive 17B-estradiol dehydrogenase. *Int. J. Cancer*, **42**, 119–22

14

Correlation between HER-2 amplification, steroid receptors and epidermal growth factor receptor in primary breast cancer

F. Kury, R. Zeillinger, K. Czerwenka, E. Kubista, G. Sliutz, W. Knogler, J. Huber, C. Zielinski, G. Reiner, R. Jakesz, A. Staffen, A. Reiner, F. Wrba and J. Spona

INTRODUCTION

The management of breast cancer depends on an understanding of the prognostic factors indicating which patients may be at increased risk of relapse and death. Steroid receptors, specifically estrogen receptors and progesterone receptors, predict response to hormonal therapy, disease-free survival, overall survival and site of relapse[1–7]. Receptor-negative patients are at increased risk of relapse and shorter overall survival[8,9]. Similarly, patients with HER-2 amplification were shown to have shorter disease-free survival times and overall survival times when compared to patients with no amplification[10]. In addition, a correlation between epidermal growth factor receptor (EGFR) and relapse-free and overall survival was reported[11]. The aim of the present investigation was to study the association of HER-2 amplification, EGFR and steroid hormone receptor status in mammary carcinoma patients in more detail.

MATERIALS AND METHODS

Tissue samples of 291 patients suffering from primary mammary carcinoma who underwent mastectomy were obtained from 22 different hospitals (see Acknowledgements). Tissue samples were immediately frozen in liquid nitrogen after surgery.

Preparation of cytosol, nuclei and membrane fractions

Tissue samples were homogenized by Ultra-Turrax in 50 mM phosphate buffer pH 7.5. All procedures were carried out at 4°C. The homogenate was centrifuged at 50 000 × *g* for 1 h. The supernatant containing the cytosol fraction was used for the assay of estrogen receptor, progesterone receptor and androgen receptor. The pellet was resuspended in 20 mmol/l 4-(2-hydroxyethyl)-1-piperazine ethane sulfonic acid (HEPES) buffer containing 1 mmol/l phenylmethylsulfonyl fluoride (PMSF), pH 7.2. This suspension was centrifuged at 1000 × *g* for 10 min. The supernatant containing the membrane fraction was used for the determination of EGFR levels and the pellet containing the nuclear fraction was used for the extraction of high molecular weight DNA.

Steroid receptor assays

Estrogen receptor and progesterone receptor levels were determined by a dextrane-coated charcoal method by simultaneous incubation with ^{125}I-labeled estradiol and ^{3}H-labeled R5020 as ligands. Androgen receptor levels were determined by using ^{3}H-labeled R1881 as ligand. Data were evaluated by Scatchard plot analysis. Cut-off points for estrogen receptor, progesterone receptor and androgen receptor levels were at 10 fmol/mg protein.

EGFR assay

EGFR levels were determined by a 12-point displacement assay using ^{125}I-labeled EGF (specific activity 150–200 μCi/μg, NEN, Boston, MA, USA). Cut-off point of EGFR levels was at 15 fmol/mg membrane protein.

Determination of HER-2 copy numbers

DNA extraction and Southern analysis was carried out as described elsewhere[12]. In brief, the nuclear fraction which was obtained after the 1000 × *g* centrifugation of the homogenate was treated with a proteinase-K containing buffer. The incubation mixture was extracted with a phenol:chloroform mixture 1:1 three times followed by two chloroform extractions. High molecular weight DNA was precipitated with 2.5 volumes of ethanol, spooled and dissolved in 10 mM Tris, 1 mM EDTA, pH 7.4 (TE). Ten μg DNA was digested with *Eco*RI, electrophoresed through a 0.7% agarose gel and nicked by exposure to UV light at 302 nm for 20 min. Alkaline blotting and hybridization with a ^{32}P-labeled HER-2 probe were carried out as described[12]. Quantification of autoradiographic signals was carried out by densitometry.

Protein and DNA determination

Protein was determined with Coomassie brilliant blue G-250 using materials obtained from Bio-Rad Laboratories, Munich, West Germany. DNA was determined by fluorometry on a Höfer TKO-100 (Höfer, San Francisco, CA, USA) using Hoechst 33256 as dye.

Statistical analysis

Statistical analysis of data was performed by χ^2 test and Wilcoxon test as indicated in legends of figures and table.

RESULTS

DNA from 291 primary human mammary carcinomas was isolated and analyzed for amplification of HER-2. Amplification of the HER-2 gene was observed in 52/291 (18%), and a single copy was noted in 239/291 (82%) of primary breast tumors. The results obtained with 12 of the 291 tumor DNAs is shown in Figure 1. The amplification was moderate (two- to fivefold) in 36 cases (12%). Examples are shown in lanes 11 and 13 of Figure 1. Higher amplification (five- to 10-fold) was observed in 16 cases (6%). Three tumor samples were noted to contain more than 10 copies of the HER-2 gene. All further data evaluations were done by classifying the degree of amplification as two- to fivefold and greater than fivefold. An example of more than five

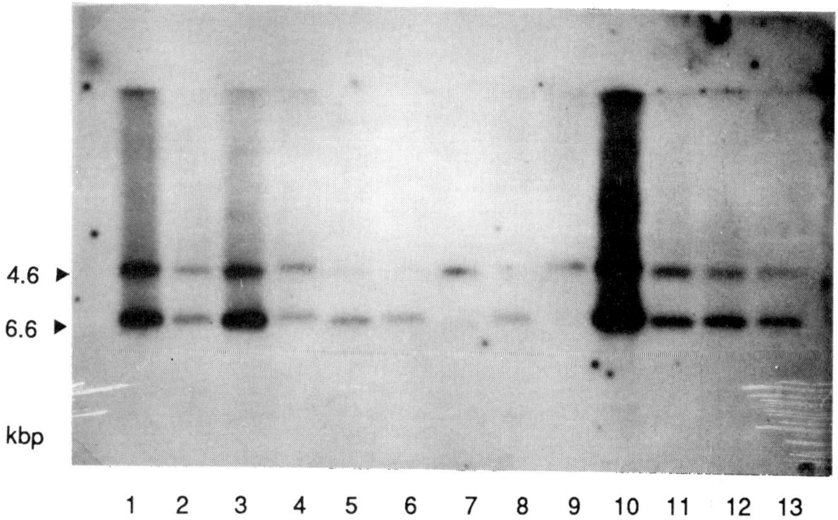

Figure 1 Analysis of HER-2 gene in DNA of primary human breast carcinoma. DNA was digested with *Eco*RI, electrophoresed through 0.7% agarose gels, blotted onto nylon membranes and hybridized to a ^{32}P-labeled RNA derived from a HER-2 cDNA clone. Hybridization was at 52°C for 12 to 18 h. After washing the membranes were exposed to Amersham-MP films. *Hin*dIII-digested λ-DNA was used as a molecular weight marker and the size of the hybridizing fragments was indicated. Copy number was determined by densitometry. Details are given in Materials and Methods. Lane 7, placenta DNA; lanes 11 and 13, two to five copies; lane 4, more than five copies; other lanes, single copy

copies of HER-2 is shown in lane 4 of Figure 1. Single copies were found for DNAs in lanes 1, 2, 3, 5, 6, 8, 9, 10, 12 of Figure 1.

On each filter a control DNA which did not contain amplified HER-2 gene was run. This control DNA was placenta DNA (lane 7, Figure 1). After hybridization with the HER-2 probe the filters were washed and hybridized with an arginase probe which did not detect amplified gene copies in these breast tumor samples. This rehybridization was used to control for the amount of DNA loaded in each lane. Amplification of HER-2 and levels of estrogen receptor as well as of progesterone receptor could be determined in 253/291 tumor samples. The association between HER-2 gene amplification and estrogen receptor is shown in Figure 2. A single copy of HER-2 was found in 86% of estrogen receptor positive patients and amplification was noted in 14% of estrogen receptor positive patients, respectively. But, in estrogen receptor negative patients 72% did not show an amplification of the oncogene whereas 28% of estrogen receptor negative patients were noted to have increased copy numbers (Figure 2). This difference was noted to be

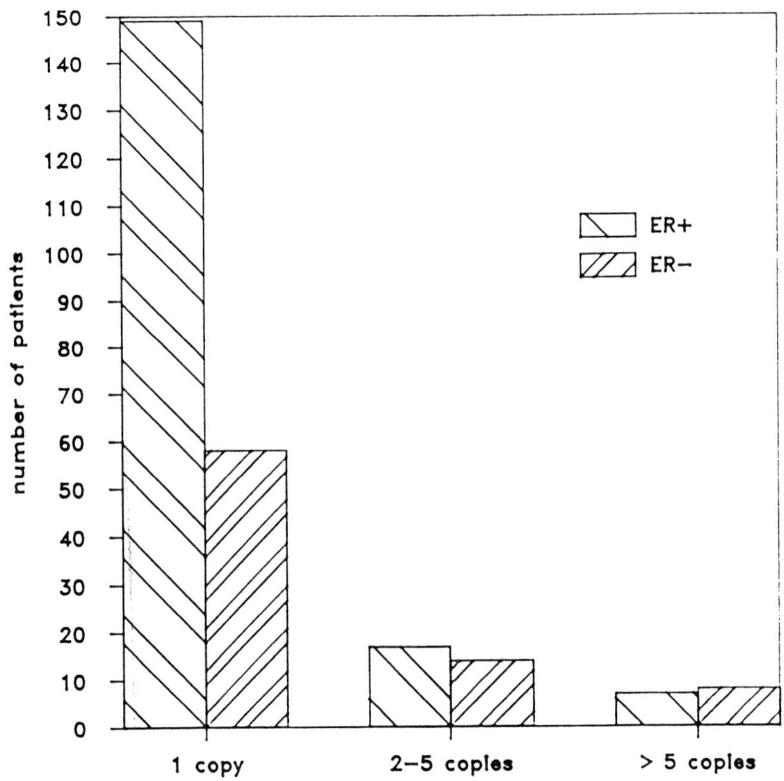

Figure 2 Association of HER-2 amplification and estrogen receptor levels in 253 primary human breast carcinoma. Estrogen receptor levels and HER-2 gene amplification was determined as described in detail in Materials and Methods. Data were calculated for estrogen receptor positive (ER +) and estrogen receptor negative (ER −) patients, respectively, containing a single copy, two to five copies and more than five copies of the HER-2 gene

statistically significant ($p = 0.02$). Similarly 16% of progesterone positive primary breast cancers exhibited an amplification of the HER-2 gene, whereas 22% of progesterone receptor negative tissue samples were found to have increased copy numbers of the HER-2 gene. This difference again was noted to be statistically significant ($p = 0.01$). In addition, the association between HER-2 gene amplification and steroid receptor levels was studied. Although the average number of estrogen as well as progesterone receptor sites was smaller in the amplified groups than in the single copy groups, no statistically significant differences were found.

The association of HER-2 gene amplification and the combination of estrogen receptor plus progesterone receptor was evaluated (Table 1). No significant differences in the degree of HER-2 gene amplification between receptor positive and receptor negative tumors were registered (Table 1). Similar results were obtained when two groups were compared in which only one receptor was positive whereas the second receptor was negative. This data is also shown in Table 1.

The size of tumor samples allowed the simultaneous determination of HER-2 gene amplification, androgen receptor and EGFR in 70 and 50 of 291 primary mammary carcinomas, respectively. It was noted that there was no association between HER-2 gene amplification, androgen receptor and EGFR (Table 1).

In another group of 254 mammary carcinomas, the EGFR content was investigated. Nineteen per cent of the tumors were shown to be EGFR positive (> 15 fmol/mg membrane protein). Seventy per cent of the EGFR negative samples were noted to be ER positive but only 38% of the EGFR positive samples were estrogen receptor positive (Figure 3). Similarly, 60% of EGFR negative patients showed to be progesterone receptor positive but only 33% of the EGFR positive patients were progesterone receptor negative (Figure 3). No association was observed between EGFR and androgen receptor status (Figure 3).

Table 1 Association of HER-2 gene amplification and receptors*

Receptor	*Single copy*	*2 to 5 Copies*	*> 5 Copies*	*p*
EGFR+	6	1	1	0.75
EGFR−	36	3	3	
AR+	47	3	1	0.43
AR−	20	0	1	
ER− PgR−	49	8	6	0.09
ER+ PgR+	118	12	4	
ER+ PgR−	39	5	3	0.11
ER− Pgr+	11	6	2	

Androgen receptor (AR), estrogen receptor (ER), progesterone receptor (PgR) and EGF receptor (EGFR) were determined by methods described in detail in the section Materials and Methods. DNA from primary human breast tumors was isolated and analyzed with a HER-2 probe by methods described in Figure 1. When the amount of tumor material permitted, receptor levels were also estimated. Probabilities were based on χ^2 tests

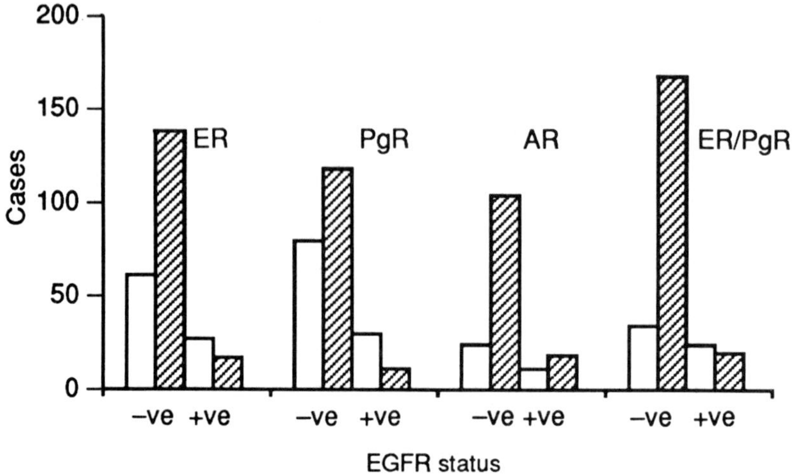

Figure 3 Association of EGFR-levels and steroid hormone receptor status in 254 human breast carcinomas. Steroid receptor status and EGFR was determined as described in Material and Methods. Cut-off levels were 15 fmol/mg membrane-protein for EGFR and 10 fmol/mg protein for steroid receptors, respectively

DISCUSSION

Good correlation was noted between amplification of HER-2 oncogene and the hormone receptor status. HER-2 gene amplification was found more frequently in estrogen receptor negative and progesterone receptor negative breast tumors than in receptor positive cases. This observation is in agreement with a recent study[13]. But, no correlation between HER-2 amplification and estrogen receptor content was observed in previous studies[10,14]. The discrepancy between the results obtained in this investigation and previous studies[10,15] can be explained at least in part by the larger patient numbers of the present investigation. The present observation corroborates the notion that HER-2 amplification may be an independent prognostic factor in primary breast cancer[10,13,14].

It was intriguing to note that steroid receptor negative patients showed HER-2 gene amplification more frequently than steroid receptor positive patients. It seems feasible to speculate that tumor progression is under a more stringent control by the oncogene when hormone dependency is lost[16]. This theory is supported by the present data showing that the steroid receptor levels of patients with an amplified HER-2 gene are, on average, lower than those with a single copy of the oncogene.

Additionally, the good correlation between EGFR and steroid hormone receptor status suggests that EGFR may be an independent prognostic factor. EGFR may be useful to define estrogen receptor positive patients who are at increased risk. Furthermore, EGFR may classify patients who do not respond to endocrine therapy.

The management of breast cancer depends on an understanding of the prognostic factors indicating which patients may be at increased risk of relapse and death. Prognostic factors can identify those breast cancer patients who are at higher risk of recurrence and who could benefit from additional therapy. At present, staging of breast cancer by conventional clinical and histologic techniques and the analysis of estrogen receptors provide the major prognostic guidelines for adjuvant therapy. Present data combine to suggest that the analysis of HER-2 copy number and EGFR status may add to a better understanding of the prognosis of primary breast cancer patients and to define a specific subset of women to whom adjuvant therapy should be directed.

ACKNOWLEDGEMENTS

Tissue samples of primary mammary carcinoma were obtained from various Austrian hospitals other than from the Departments with which the authors are affiliated. We greatly appreciate the provision of the tumor material by: Krankenhaus der Stadt Wien Lainz; A.ö. Nö. Landeskrankenanstalt Tulln; A.ö. Krankenhaus Mistelbach; Krankenhaus der Barmherzigen Schwestern, Wien; Wilhelminenspital der Stadt Wien; A.ö. Krankenhaus Allentsteig; Pathologisches Labor Dr. Kosak, Wien; Krankenanstalt der Stadt Wien Rudolfstiftung; Hanusch-Krankenhaus Wien; A.ö. Krankenhaus Wiener Neustadt; Krankenhaus St. Elisabeth Wien; A.ö. Krankenhaus Baden; Unfallkrankenhaus Meidling, Wien; A.ö. Krankenhaus Melk; A.ö. Krankenhaus Neunkirchen; A.ö. Krankenhaus Stockerau; Kaiser-Franz-Josef-Spital der Stadt Wien; Krankenhaus der Barmherzigen Brüder Wien; A.ö. Nö. Landeskrankenhaus Mödling. In addition, we greatly appreciate a cDNA clone of the human arginase gene from Stephen D. Cederbaum, Department of Pediatrics, University of California Los Angeles, Los Angeles, CA, USA.

REFERENCES

1. Knight, W.A., Livingston, R.B., Gregory, E.J. and McGuire, W.L. (1977). Estrogen receptor as an independent prognostic factor for early recurrence in breast cancer. *Cancer Res.*, **37**, 4669–71
2. Spona, J., Kolb, R., Reiner, G., Jakesz, R., Moser, K. and Rainer, H. (1983). Clinical and Experimental Aspects of Hormone Receptors in Breast Carcinoma Patients. *Cancer Detect. Prev.*, **6**, 227–34
3. Jakesz, R., Bettelheim, P., Bieglmayer, Ch., Chaput, F., Kolb, R., Miksche, M., Moser, K., Rainer, H., Reiner, G. and Spona, J. (1979). Estrogen receptor values in metastatic breast cancer and cytotoxic chemotherapy. *Cancer Treat. Rep.*, **63/7**, 1191–8
4. Jakesz, R., Kolb, R., Moser, K., Rainer, H., Reiner, G. and Spona, J. (1981). Prognostic role of steroid receptor status and its value for adjuvant chemotherapy in early breast-cancer and uncontrolled trial. *Proceedings of the Annual Meeting of the American Society of Clinical Oncology*, **22**, 150 (Baltimore: Waverley Press Inc.)
5. Reiner, G., Jakesz, R., Kolb, R., Kühnl-Brady, K., Reiner, A., Schemper, M. and Spona, J. (1988). Androgenrezeptoren beim primären Mammakarzinom. *Dtsch. Med. Wschr.*, **113**, 892–7
6. Stuller, I., Zielinski, C.C., Aiginger, P., Rausch, P., Pötzi, P., Kubista, E., Salzer, H., Sevelda, O., Langer, M., Staffen, A. and Spona, J. (1987). Der Einfluβ von Hormonrezeptoren auf

die Metaphasenlokalisation beim Mammakarzinom. *Onkologie*, **10**, 302–3
7. Reiner, A., Spona, J., Reiner, G., Schemper, M., Kolb, R., Kwasny, W., Függer, R., Jakesz, R. and Holzner, J.H. (1986). Estrogen Receptor Analysis on Biopsies and Fine-Needle Aspirates from Human Breast Carcinoma. *Am. J. Path.*, **125/3**, 443–9
8. Reiner, A., Kolb, R., Reiner, G., Jakesz, R., Schemper, M. and Spona, J. (1987). Prognostic significance of steroid hormone receptors and histopathological characterization of human breast cancer. *J. Cancer Res. Clin. Oncol.*, **113**, 285–290
9. Zielinski, C.C., Kubista, E., Salzer, H., Sevelda, P., Langer, M., Staffen, A. and Spona, J. (1986). Adjuvant chemotherapy combined with Tamoxifen by postmenopausal patients with stage-III breast cancer. *Lancet*, **i**, 1164–72
10. Clark, G.M., McGuire, W.L., Hubay, C.A., Pearson, O.H. and Marshall, J.S. (1983). Progesterone receptors as a prognostic factor in stage II breast cancer. *Science*, **309**, 1343–6
11. Slamon, D.J., Clark, G.M., Wong, S.G., Levin, W.J., Ullrich, A. and McGuire, W.L. (1987). Human breast cancer: correlation of relapse and survival with amplification of the HER-2/neu oncogene. *Science*, **235**, 177–82
12. Van de Vijver, M., Mooi, W.J., Peterse, J.L. and Nusse, R. (1988). Amplification and over-expression of the neu oncogene in human breast carcinomas. *Eur J. Surg. Oncol.*, **14**, 111–4
13. Sainsbury, J.R., Farndon, J., Needham, G., Malcolm, A. and Harris, A. (1987). Epidermal-growth-factor receptor status as predictor of early recurrence of and death from breast cancer. *Lancet*, **i**, 1398–405
14. Berger, M.S., Locher, G.W., Saurer, S., Gullick, W.J., Waterfield, M.D., Groner, B. and Hynes, N.E. (1988). Correlation of c-erb-2 gene amplification and protein expression in human breast carcinoma with nodal status and nuclear grading. *Cancer Res.*, **48**, 1238–43
15. Van de Vijver, M., Van de Bersselaar, R., Devilee, P., Cornelisse, C., Peterse, J. and Nusse, R. (1987). Amplification of the neu (erbB-2) Oncogene in Human Mammary Tumors Is Relatively Frequent and Is Often Accompanied by Amplification of the Linked c-erbA Oncogene. *Mol. Cell. Biol.*, **7**, 2019–23
16. Zeillinger, R., Kury, F., Czerwenka, K., Kubista, E., Sliutz, G., Knogler, W., Huber, J., Zielinski, C., Reiner,G., Jakesz, R., Staffen, A., Reiner, A., Wrba, F. and Spona, J. (1989). HER-2 amplification, steroid receptors and epidermal growth factor receptor in primary breast cancer. *Oncogene*, **4**, 109–14

15

Neoadjuvant chemotherapy in breast cancer: first results after surgical treatment

L. Marzetti, M.L. Framarino dei Malatesta, G. Galati, M.G. Piccioni, C. Midulla and D. Eleuteri Serpieri

INTRODUCTION

Neoadjuvant chemotherapy is a term chosen from E. Frei[1] and indicates a systemic therapy which is applied after tissue diagnosis of cancer is obtained and before local–regional treatment (surgery or radiotherapy) is started.

This type of chemotherapy aims at several objectives:

(1) To become useful in treating patients with large tumors with the intent of decreasing the extent of surgery;

(2) To provide an *in vivo* assay system for chemosensitivity; and

(3) To destroy the clones responsible for the spreading.

Experimental studies indicate therefore a high correlation between responsiveness of primary tumor and micrometastatic disease.

The high number of failure cases after conventional adjuvant therapy allows clinicians only to improve scheduling of old drugs.

Neoadjuvant chemotherapy is an example of such improvement[2,3].

MATERIALS AND METHODS

Our survey began on 30 March 1985 and it is still underway; 20 women with breast cancer were included. The age ranged between 39 and 74 years (13 were premenopausal and seven postmenopausal). Diagnosis was made by aspiration cytology or needle biopsy. All patients underwent an initial staging work-up that included clinical examination, mammography, liver ultrasonography, bone scintigraphy and chest X-ray.

Criteria for inclusion in this study were: tumor size greater than 2 cm; normal blood counts; liver and kidney functionality and informed consent.

No evidence of metastatic disease was seen in any of the patients. The clinical stages of the patients at the beginning of treatment were as follows: one T2, N0; 16 T2, N1; one T3, N1 and two T3, N2. The patients were subdivided into two groups according to each kind of treatment. The first group (Group I, 9 patients) was subjected to three cycles of preoperative chemotherapy and the second group (Group II, 11 patients) underwent three cycles of preoperative chemotherapy + 30 mg/day tamoxifen. Chemotherapy included the intravenous administration of three drugs every 28 days: 5-fluorouracile 500 mg/m^2, adramycin 50 mg/m^2 and cyclophosphamide 500 mg/m^2 the first day.

On the eighth day another intravenous administration of 5-fluorouracile 500 mg/m^2 followed.

The patients in Group I were in stage T2 or T3 and N0, N1(a-b) or N2.

When the diameter of the lesion was reduced down to category T1, a quadrantectomy with axillary lymphoadenectomy was performed and followed by radiotherapy and three cycles of postoperative chemotherapy + 30 mg/day tamoxifen for 2 years.

When the lesion was restricted or remained at stage T2, the patient was subjected to radical modified mastectomy according to Patey with axillary lymphoadenectomy and three postoperative chemotherapy cycles + 30 mg/day tamoxifen.

The patients in the second group were in stage T2, N1(a-b).

The surgical treatment applied was the same as that given to Group I.

The preoperative evaluation of the local–regional response to therapy was made through clinical examination and ultrasonography after each cycle, the mammography was performed at the beginning and after three treatment cycles.

The objective response was defined as:

(1) Complete (CR) when the lesion had completely disappeared at mammography; or

(2) Partial (PR) when at least two diameters of the lesion were reduced from 25 to 75%.

Responders were defined as women whose tumors decreased in diameter by at least 25%[3]. Since tumor volume is proportional to the cube of the diameter, this implies approximately 60% reduction in tumor volume.

The lesion was considered stationary when at least two diameters of the lesion were reduced by less than 25%; but in progression when at least two diameters increased by 25%.

FINDINGS

A partial response was obtained in 16 patients (eight from Group I and eight from Group II).

In Group II, the response was complete in one patient, no change was observed in two patients and progression occurred in another patient.

The global response (CR + PR) was 85%.

Eighty per cent of the patients in the first group underwent radical Patey mastectomy with axillary lymphoadenectomy and 20% of the patients underwent quadrantectomy and axillary emptying.

In the second group 90% of the patients underwent quadrantectomy + lymphoadenectomy and 10% underwent radical Patey modified mastectomy + lymphoadenectomy.

Pathological findings of neoplasia after chemotherapy showed an increase in reactive regressive phenomena.

With regard to the first phenomenon, large lymphomonocyte cell infiltration can be seen in neoplasia (inflammatory reaction).

With regard to regressive phenomena we found intense necrobiosis with hyaline interstitial degeneration. Atypical polyploid mitosis is prevalent and causes an increase of neoplastic 'terminal' cells (giant cells) and a reduction of stem cells.

Three patients from Group I were N1(a-b) preoperatively and had negative lymph nodes postoperatively.

Two patients in Group I, who were N2 preoperatively, did not show invasion of the lymph nodes at histological examination.

Five patients of Group II, who were classified as N1(a-b) resulted free from metastasis in the axillary lymph nodes.

No local–regional relapse was observed in any of the two groups. The diameter reduction of the lesion in Group II (preoperative chemotherapy + tamoxifen) was greater in premenopausal patients when compared with those in postmenopause.

DISCUSSION

Our data are not comparable to those appearing in the literature due to the less advanced stage of the patients treated (T2 and T3 versus T3 and T4), the type and schedule of antiblastic drug administration, and the type of surgery performed which, especially in Group I, allowed us to adopt a conservative procedure.

In patients both in premenopause and postmenopause in Group II, the association with tamoxifen allowed us to potentiate the cytostatic effect, especially in premenopausal patients.

On the other hand, *in vitro* studies[4] demonstrated that antiestrogens such as tamoxifen, determine the arrest in G1 of mammary carcinoma cells MCF-7. This type of association was thus used together with antiblastic drugs in order to increase the sensitivity of the cells to cytostatic action.

Lippman *et al.*[5] demonstrated that there is a better local and regional response in patients treated with 5-fluorouracil + doxorubicin + methotrexate cyclophosphamide, associated with the administration of conjugated estrogens + tamoxifen, when compared to patients treated with no hormonal synchronization.

Up to now, the short follow-up (maximum of 3 years) has not allowed us to check the impact on the survival rate or the illness-free stage in these patients, when compared to the historical group.

The new concepts on the biology of mammary neoplasia and, in particular, the recognition of similarities to systemic disease from its very onset, as well as the high sensitivity of micrometastasis as regards the metastatic disease, provide convincing evidence for the application of neoaduvant chemotherapy in treating mammary carcinoma.

Moreover, the reduction of the lesion diameter allows us to perform a conservative type of surgery thus improving the quality of the patient's life, whereas the local and regional preoperative sterilization can reduce the incidence of *in situ* relapse.

This type of treatment deserves further verification concerning survival rates; before starting the treatment, accurate information on the biological characteristics of the neoplasia (receptorial stage, grading) should be collected in order to standardize the patient's selection criteria and optimize the schedule of the drugs to be administered.

REFERENCES

1. Frei, E., III (1982). Clinical Cancer research: an embattled species. *Cancer*, **50**, 1979–92
2. Ragaz, J. (1986). Preoperative neoadjuvant chemotherapy for breast cancer: outline of the British Columbia Trial. *Rec. Res. Cancer. Res.*, **103**, 84–93
3. Schwartz, G.F., Cantar, R.I. and Biermann, W.A. (1987). Neoadjuvant chemotherapy before definitive treatment for stage III carcinoma of the breast. *Arch. Surg.*, **122**, 1430–4
4. Green, M.M., Whybourne, A.M., Taylor, I.W. and Sutherland, R.L. (1981). Effects of antiestrogens on the growth and cell cycle kinetics of cultured human mammary carcinoma cells. In Sutherland, R.L. and Jordon, V.C. (eds). *Non-steroidal Antiestrogens*, p. 397. (New York: Academic Press)
5. Lippman, M.E., Cassidy, J., Wesley, M. and Young, R.C. (1984). A randomized attempt to increase the efficacy of cytotoxic chemotherapy in metastatic breast cancer by hormonal synchronization. *J. Clin. Oncol.*, **2**, 28

16

The epithelial–stromal junction of the human breast. Observations about its ultrastructure and physiopathology

A. Di Lieto, G. De Rosa, G. Albano, A.M. Pagnano, M. Campanile, L. Terracciano, R. Ferrara and A. Paladini

INTRODUCTION

Although research has been recently carried out, the etiology of the many clinical, radiological and pathological entities known as benign breast disease (BBD) is still uncertain.

Some authors have blamed it on an anomalous hormonal milieu[1,2], others have cited intrinsic features of the target tissue, which may react abnormally to the cyclical physiological changes of the hormone levels[1–5], because a hormonal abnormality common to the various histological forms of BBD as well as a uniform and symmetrical distribution of the lesions is still undemonstrated[3,5].

For a long time the use of danazol in the symptomatic therapy of BBD has been widely accepted due to the high rate of clinical improvement and the low incidence of side-effects[6–9]. This synthetic steroid, derived from 17α-ethinyltestosterone has various effects on the hypothalamic–pituitary axis[10–12]: inhibition of the ovarian steroidogenesis; modification of the sex hormone-binding globulin plasma level[7] leading to a pseudomenopausal endocrine status responsible for a reduced hormonal stimulation on the target tissues.

Recent studies showed the induction of steroid hormone receptor in the breast suffering from BBD[13], after prolonged administration of danazol, thus justifying the observed favorable clinical response. This finding, if corroborated by further investigations, could disclose new, interesting perspectives for the pharmacological management of benign and malignant breast diseases.

According to Ozzello[14], the epithelial–stromal junction (ESJ) is the portion of the human breast in which epithelium and stroma come in contact with each other. It includes the basal region of the plasma membranes of the epithelial and myoepithelial cells, the intercellular spaces, the lamina lucida, the basal membrane, the fibrillar connective tissue, the ground substance and a layer of 'delimiting fibroblasts'.

The ESJ is a 'morphofunctional unit' which actively mediates the transfer of substances from the bloodstream to the mammary epthelium and vice versa[14,15].

The aim of this study is to explain the modifications of the ESJ of the human breast after prolonged danazol administration in women affected by BBD.

MATERIALS AND METHODS

Our study population consisted of seven healthy volunteers considered as controls and 48 patients affected by BBD and divided into four groups (Table 1): group A, nine patients affected by fibroadenoma, aged from 20 to 35 years (mean $\pm$ SD = 27.2 $\pm$ 5.2); group B, 20 patients with a histological pattern of prevailing cystic disease [age 35–42 (38.7 $\pm$ 2.4) years]; group C, 11 patients affected by prevailing adenosis [age 20–38 (27.6 $\pm$ 6.2) years]; and group D, eight patients affected by prevailing fibrosis [age 25–41 (31.1 $\pm$ 5.1) years].

Patients in group A needed surgical treatment. Patients in the groups B, C and D were treated with danazol 300 mg/day divided into three doses, considering the half-life of the product, for 4 months. They underwent a needle breast biopsy (Rotex H.S.) before and after danazol treatment.

A needle breast biopsy was also performed in the control volunteers.

Two samples were obtained from each specimen. They were fixed, embedded in paraffin, stained and sliced for light microscopy observation.

For electron microscopy observation they were fixed in glutaraldehyde 3% in cacodylate buffer, postfixed in osmic acid 1.5%, stepwise dehydrated in ethanol, transferred in ethylene oxide and then embedded in Epon.

RESULTS

Controls

Electron microscopy observation of biopsy specimens from control women showed the normal architecture of the human mammary ductule. The ESJ was well discernible and structurally undamaged. The ductular basement

Table 1 The different groups of women considered in the study

	No.	*Age*	*Mean $\pm$ SD*
Fibroadenoma (A)	9	20–35	27.2 $\pm$ 5.2
Cystic disease (B)	20	35–42	38.7 $\pm$ 2.4
Adenosis (C)	11	20–38	27.6 $\pm$ 6.2
Fibrosis (D)	8	25–41	31.1 $\pm$ 5.1
Controls	7	20–42	29.3 $\pm$ 7.7

membrane thickness was lower than 120 nm (range = 50–113 nm; mean ± SD = 79.4 ± 20.3) (Table 2).

Fibroadenoma

The most frequently observed ultrastructural aspect in this group was represented by epithelial cells lacking in hemidesmosomes and tight junctions, but provided with imbricated club-shaped projections of the plasma membranes. Myoepithelial cells, on the contrary, showed a reduction in number and size of the aforesaid projections.

A remarkable multilayering with an increase in thickness of the basement membrane (110–800 nm), a disarray of the delimiting fibroblasts and a rarefaction of the stroma were also observed.

The multilayering of the basal lamina in fibroadenomas appeared to be a fairly constant feature.

BBD before danazol administration

The ultrastructural features of the epithelial and myoepithelial cells in these specimens varied according to the histological form of BBD characteristic of each patient.

The ESJ showed remarkable changes. Occasionally, a dispersion of the hemidesmosomes in the basal region of the epithelial and myoepithelial cells' plasma membranes that became flattened, was observed.

The basement membrane appeared to be thickened in all the sections observed [110–800 nm (458 ± 219)] (Table 2) while the delimiting fibroblasts, constantly devoid of the characteristic fence-like aspect, scattered their cytoplasmic processes into the collagen and the elastic fibers of the stroma.

BBD after danazol treatment

A strong epithelial stromal involution was the characteristic feature at the ultrastructural evaluation.

The epithelial cells seemed to be almost lacking in microvilli, so that the luminal surfaces tended to be flattened. The cytoplasm was poor in mitochondria and in rough endoplasmic reticulum. A small Golgi apparatus was often evident. The flattening of the basal region of the myoepithelial

Table 2 Thickness of the basement membrane (nm) in the normal breast, in the breast affected by BBD and after danazol treatment

	Range	*Mean ± SD*
Normal breast	50–113	79.4 ± 20.3
BBD	110–800	458.9 ± 219
After danazol treatment	560–1600	1040.3 ± 339.8

cells plasmalemmas went with a rarefaction of the hemidesmosomes.

The basement membrane was markedly thickened and sometimes distorted [560–1600 nm (1040 ± 339.8), showing a threadlike or a microgranular appearance] (Table 2).

The 'delimiting fibroblasts' were randomly dispersed in a stroma made up of large but disconnected collagen fibers. It was impossible to distinguish the vascular zone from the avascular.

Noteworthy was the finding of intracytoplasmic lumens in the cells from some specimens.

DISCUSSION

These results pointed out that the prolonged danazol administration was able to induce a widespread epithelial–stromal involution of the human mammary gland, with various degrees of thickening of the ductular basement membrane[16,17].

The physiopathological mechanism responsible for that process is still unknown; particularly it will be necessary to clarify if the thickening is due to a further laying down of the basement membrane components and what is the primary damaged structure, able to influence the well-being of the contiguous areas[15].

Considering the basement membrane as a product of an undamaged mammary epithelium it is evident that the harmful stimulus should primarily hit the epithelial cells. It is likewise unanswerable as to whether the basement membrane behaves as physical support or as a selective filter, so that damage should involve the overhanging epithelium[15].

The mechanisms responsible for this multilayering are not known but it may represent new formation of basal lamina, compression of the ductules or possible contraction of the myoepithelial cells. Carstens[18] has stated that the multilayering of basal lamina was never observed in the absence of hemidesmosomes, which are only present at the myoepithelial basal plasma membrane; he also noted that the greatest degree of multilayering of the basal lamina in fibroadenomas was present in old or atrophic fibroadenomas and has suggested that this may interfere with the interchange of oxygen and nutrients between the blood vessels and the epithelial elements; this would account for the tendency of fibroadenomas to undergo atrophy and hyalinization.

The little or ample, localized or widespread thickening of the basement membranes are all found in BBD and after prolonged danazol treatment as well as in other diseases of different organs[15,19]. For instance, in diabetes mellitus a thickening of the endothelial, muscular and glomerular basement membranes resembling the mammary basement membrane damage, can sometimes be shown.

In an attempt to clarify the diabetic thickening of the basement membranes, Vracko and Benditt[20] suggested an interesting hypothesis. Observing that an undamaged basement membrane persisted after the cellular death they hypothesized that the basement membrane acts as a scaffold for tissue remodeling and repair, so that the thickening was due to the new cellular generation that produced further layers.

Recent immunofluorescence studies, done with anti-laminin and anti-type IV collagen antibodies, reliably demonstrated that basement membrane was destroyed and removed from tissues after cellular death[15,21].

The immunohistochemical and ultrastructural study of the ESJ of the human breast, and particularly of the basement membrane is the most recent guide line for the research in several metabolic and degenerative diseases, as well as for comprehension of the mechanism of invasion and metastases of malignant tumors[17,19,22,23].

The data allowed foresight into the probable future uses of danazol in the management of benign and malignant breast diseases[13,24].

Particularly, the ability of danazol to induce steroid hormone receptors in the normal and pathological breast might give, according to Panahy *et al.*[13], a long term protection towards the development of a carcinoma of the breast.

REFERENCES

1. Sitruk-Ware, L.R., Sterkers, N., Mowszowicz, I. and Mauvais-Jarvis, P. (1977). Inadequate corpus luteum function in women with benign breast disease. *J. Clin. Endocrinol. Metab.*, **44**, 771
2. Vorherr, H. (1986). Fibrocystic breast disease: Pathophysiology, pathomorphology, clinical picture and management. *Am. J. Obstet. Gynecol.*, **154**, 161
3. Rannevik, G. (1987). Endocrinological aspects of benign breast disease. In Wood, C. (ed.) *Benign Breast Disease: Is It Worth Treating?* (London: The Royal Society of Medicine Services)
4. Berkowitz, G.S., Kelsey, J.L., Holford, T.R., Livolsi, V.A., Merino, M.J., Beck, G.J., Ort, S., O'Connor, T.Z. and White, C. (1985). Estrogen replacement therapy and fibrocystic breast disease in postmenopausal women. *Am. J. Epidemiol.*, **121**, 238
5. Walsh, P.V., Bulbrook, R.D., Stell, P.M., Wang, D.Y., McDicken, I.W. and George, W.D. (1984). Serum progesterone concentration during the luteal phase in women with benign breast disease. *Eur. J. Cancer Clin. Oncol.*, **20**, 1339
6. Pye, J.K. and Mansel, R.E. (1985). Clinical experience of drug treatments for mastalgia. *Lancet*, **ii**, 373
7. Tobiassen, T., Rasmussen, T., Doberl, A. and Rannevik, G. (1984). Danazol treatment of severely symptomatic fibrocystic breast disease and long-term follow-up – The Hjørring Project. *Acta Obstet. Gynecol. Scand.*, (s)**123**, 159
8. Gorins, A., Perret, F., Tournant, B. and Rogier, C. (1984). Double blind cross-over study of danazol versus placebo in the treatment of severe fibrocystic breast disease. In Baum, M., George, W.D. and Hughes, L.E. (eds.) *Benign Breast Disease*. The Royal Society of Medicine. Distributed by Oxford University Press, Oxford
9. Di Lieto, A., Negri, R., Campanile, M., Albano, G., Magliulo, R. and Paladini, A. (1988). Clinical, morphological and ultrastructural evaluation of benign breast disease (BBD) after danazol treatment. *XII World Congress of Gynecology and Obstetrics*, **22**,
10. Schmidt, C.L. (1985). Endometriosis: a reappraisal of pathogenesis and treatment. *Fertil. Steril.*, **44**, 157
11. Potts, G.O. (1984). Pharmacology of danazol. In Baum, M., George, W.D. and Hughes, L.E. (eds.) *Benign Breast Disease*. The Royal Society of Medicine. Distributed by Oxford University Press, Oxford
12. Rannevik, G. (1987). Hormonal effects of danazol. In Wood, C. (ed.) *Benign Breast Disease: Is It Worth Treating?* (London: The Royal Society of Medicine Services)
13. Panahy, C., Puddefoot, J.R., Anderson, E., Vinson, G.P., Berry, C.L., Turner, M.J., Brown,

C.L. and Goode, A.W. (1987). Effects of danazol on incidence of progesterone and oestrogen receptors in benign breast disease. *Br. Med. J.*, **295**, 464

14. Ozzello, L. (1970). Epithelial–stromal junction of normal and dysplastic mammary glands. *Cancer*, **25**, 586
15. Martinez-Hernandez, A. and Amenta, P.S. (1983). The basement membrane in pathology. *Lab. Invest.*, **48**, 656
16. Martinez-Hernandez, A., Fink, L.M. and Pierce, G.B. (1976). Removal of basement membrane in the involuting breast. *Lab. Invest.*, **34**, 455
17. Bulletti, C., Galassi, A., Jasonni, V.M., Martinelli, G., Tabanelli, S. and Flamigni, C. (1986). Basement membrane components in normal hyperplastic and neoplastic endometrium. *Cancer*, **62**, 142
18. Carstens (1974). Ultrastructure of human fibroadenoma. *Arch. Pathol.*, **98**, 23
19. Liotta, L.A. (1984). Tumor Invasion and metastases: Role of the basement membrane. *Warner-Lambert Parke-Davis Award Lecture. Am. J. Pathol.*, **117**, 339
20. Vracko, R. and Benditt, E.P. (1972). Basal lamina: the scaffold for orderly cell replacement: observations on regeneration of injured skeletal muscle fibres and capillaries. *J. Cell. Biol.*, **55**, 406
21. Gulati, A.K. and Zalewski, A.A. (1982). Renewal of the basement membrane during skeletal muscle regeneration. *J. Cell. Biol.*, **95**, 365
22. Faber, M., Wewer, U.M., Berthelsen, J.G., Liotta, L.A. and Albrechtsen, R. (1986). Laminin production by human endometrial stromal cells relates to the cyclic and pathologic state of the endometrium. *Am. J. Pathol.*, **124**, 384
23. Barsky, S.H., Togo, S., Garbisa, Liotta, L.A. and Albrechtsen, R. (1983). Type IV collagen immunoreactive in invasive breast carcinoma. *Lancet*, **i**, 296
24. Pronzato, P., Amoroso, D., Ardizzoni, A., Bertelli, G., Conte, P.F., Michelotti, A. and Rosso, R. (1987). A phase II study with danazol in metastatic breast cancer. *Am. J. Clin. Oncol.*, **10**, 407

17

Tamoxifen vs. chemotherapy vs. chemotherapy plus tamoxifen in patients with node positive and receptor positive breast cancer: 4-year results of an Italian multicenter trial (GROCTA)

P. Sismondi, F. Boccardo, P. Bruzzi, M. Cappellini, C. De Sanctis, F. Genta, G. Isola, I. Nenci, A. Piffanelli, A. Rubagotti, L. Santi, A. Scanni and other members of GROCTA Group

INTRODUCTION

Only some breast cancer patients have been shown to be cured with both radical or conservative surgery. Actually, about 25% and 50% of patients with negative and positive axillary nodes respectively have local and/or distant recurrences after mastectomy[1]. Most recurrences occur in the first 3 years and after 20 years mortality becomes similar to that of the general population[2]. The number of positive axillary nodes and the hormone receptor status in primary tumors are the most important prognostic factors. The risk of recurrences is higher in patients with four or more positive nodes and estrogen receptor (ER) negative[1,3].

Most investigators now believe that in many cases of breast cancer, micrometastasis are present since diagnosis. The development of remaining micrometastasis after removal of the primary tumor would be responsible for local and distant recurrences. In this respect, the presence of positive axillary nodes should be regarded as the result of distant microdissemination, rather than the cause[4]. In the last few years, many attempts were made to eradicate micrometastasis present at the time of mastectomy, by associating adjuvant treatments with surgery. A recent overview confirmed that although postoperative radiotherapy can decrease the incidence of local recurrences, it cannot increase patient survival[5].

A marked interest in adjuvant medical treatment has grown over the last

15 years. A number of controlled studies have shown that chemotherapy was able to increase the disease-free interval and in some cases also the survival of premenopausal patients. Recently, the Oxford Group carried out a meta-analysis of randomized adjuvant chemotherapy studies on about 15 000 patients. Polychemotherapy, particularly cyclophosphamide methotrexate fluorouracil (CMF), in patients aged less than 50 years, was shown to be able to decrease the risk by 25%. The benefit is less in patients aged more than 50 years, whose mortality risk is reduced by 10–12%[6].

In the last 10 years, many studies faced the problem of the possible role of endocrine therapy as a complementary treatment to mastectomy, due to high toxicity and apparent lack of efficacy of chemotherapy in postmenopausal patients[7–13]. As observed in studies on chemotherapy, adjuvant hormone therapy, particularly with tamoxifen (TAM), was shown to increase disease free interval and in some cases, as in the NATO study, to increase patient survival, independently from main prognostic factors, as for example menopausal and nodal status[11].

More recently, the meta-analysis of endocrine therapy studies showed that endocrine treatment with TAM can reduce by about 20% the 5-year mortality risk in postmenopausal patients and in patients aged over 50 years independently from their menopausal status.

The effect of TAM in premenopausal patients is less clear. However, many data are in favor of a possible positive role of hormone therapy also in premenopausal women; the analysis of nine studies on oophorectomy showed a 29% decrease of mortality risk in women aged less than 50 years. The result is similar to the decrease observed with chemotherapy in the same overview[14–18].

Optimal treatment duration is a key problem. Actually, TAM administration did not exceed 2 years in most studies. The action of TAM is mainly peripheral; TAM is a 17-β-estradiol antagonist at receptor level, however, it cannot inhibit estrogen synthesis and peripheral conversion[11]. Thus, TAM should be administered indefinitely to counteract the effect of estrogen produced by ovaries or via peripheral aromatization of androgens.

Finally, some trials investigated the potential usefulness of the association of chemotherapy with hormone therapy, particularly with antiestrogens, also in the light of the synergism shown in advanced disease. Preliminary results available at the beginning of this study, showed that the association was more effective in postmenopausal patients and in patients with high ER levels[9,10].

RATIONALE AND AIM OF THE STUDY

This study was designed in 1982 based on the following considerations:

(1) Following the introduction of hormonal receptor assay in clinics, the probability of response to hormone therapy could be reliably assessed *a prior*[19]; the efficacy of hormonal therapy was similar to chemotherapy in patients with advanced disease and positive hormonal receptors.

(2) Therapeutic efficacy being equal, hormone therapy should be preferred, due to its lower incidence of side-effects.

(3) Additive TAM therapy proved to be effective, especially in postmenopausal patients. However, some investigators showed that TAM is also effective in premenopausal patients[20]. Responsive premenopausal patients generally experienced amenorrhea; at recurrence, they responded to oophorectomy[20,21].

(4) Some studies showed that chemotherapy–TAM association was more effective than chemotherapy or TAM alone in metastatic breast cancer[22–24]. The therapeutic benefit was mainly due to a higher proportion of objective responses, whilst its effect on response duration and patients' survival was controversial.

In the light of these considerations, the comparison of adjuvant cytotoxic chemotherapy versus adjuvant hormonal therapy with TAM, in patients with positive axillary nodes and ER +, seemed rational, as well as the assessment of the potential usefulness of their association.

Tamoxifen is likely to be at least as active as chemotherapy in this group of patients, and possibly less toxic. Moreover, this association could prove synergistic.

CHOICE OF THERAPEUTIC REGIMEN

Chemotherapy

The impossibility, at present, of controlling metastatic disease with chemotherapy and the relative lack of efficacy of chemotherapy in adjuvant treatment could be explained with the appearance of chemoresistant clones, which results in a neoplastic cell population no longer sensitive to these drugs. According to kinetics, Goldie *et al.*[25] suggested that the alternated sequential use of non cross-resistant regimens could potentially overcome induced chemo-resistance. Moreover, the alternated use of different therapies has the advantage of postponing the onset of cumulative toxic effects relevant to each drug association.

According to these premises, a therapeutic regimen was used, based on sequential administration of two definitely non cross-resistant regimens: CMF (six courses) and 4-epi-doxorubicine (four courses). CMF was administered intravenously, in order to increase patients' compliance and feasibility, even in the light of preliminary results of some feasibility[26] and comparison studies, showing that 1-day intravenously administered CMF efficacy is similar to traditional CMF.

The introduction of 4-epi-doxorubicine, (an analogue of adriamycin with a probable lower cardiotoxicity at equal therapeutic effectiveness) is justified by the fact that adriamycin, when used alone, is as effective as polychemotherapy and certainly non-CMF cross-resistant. Besides, it can be re-employed as a salvage therapy in case of relapse after treatment with adriamycin, with identical possibilities of being successful[27].

As only four courses were administered, a maximal dosage of 300 mg/m^2, which is greatly lower than cardiotoxic dose, is reached.

Hormone therapy

Tamoxifen is a triphenyl-ethylene derivative, provided with estrogenic action, which was shown to be effective in advanced breast cancer with negligible toxicity[28]. Interference with 17-β-estradiol at receptor level seems to be the main mechanism of action; this ultimately results in a delay in cytosolic receptors replacement[29]. However, the drug could also act through different mechanisms, and this could partly explain its partial activity even in ER negative patients. The choice of TAM as adjuvant therapy was also justified by the possibility of a long-term administration with mild side-effects and acceptable costs. Based on physiological premises, TAM is administered for 5 years or until disease progression.

STUDY DESIGN

Selection of patients

The eligibility criteria used for patient selection were:
Operated breast cancer with positive axillary lymphnodes (pT1 a,b; pT2 a,b; pT3 a,b; pN1 according TNM UICC 1982) with at least 10 axillary nodes examined; ER + in primary tumor or its node metastasis > 10 fmol/mg protein; age range 35 to 65 years; performance status (UICC) 0 or 1; creatinine 1.2 mg/dl, bilirubin 1.2 mg/dl, white blood cell count, 4 000, platelets 120 000 and lack of severe ECG alterations.

Exclusion criteria were previous or concomitant malignant neoplasm (contralateral breast included), skin or *in situ* cervical squamous cancer excluded; previous chemotherapy or antiestrogen treatment; presence of diseases which contraindicate chemotherapy or antiestrogens; patients at risk of thromboembolisms; geographical inaccessibility or difficulties for follow-up; mental retardation or psychiatric disorders that could prevent the required compliance to therapy or follow-up program.

Stratification

Stratification per participating center was only performed before randomization, in order to minimize any possible bias linked to operative features of single centers. An *a posteriori* stratification is foreseen, based on: menopausal status, lymphnode status: N +, 1–3, N + 4 +, ER level, or positive progesterone receptors (PR).

Randomization

The randomization process was centralized by telephone. Patients with pN1 and positive estrogen receptors were then randomly assigned to treatment with tamoxifen for 5 years (T); or six courses of CMF and four courses of epi-adriamycin (CT); or the combination of both of the above treatments, tamoxifen, CMF and epi-adriamycin (CTT).

Hormonal receptors

Receptor assay should be performed with a standard technique employing a radiometric method involving dextran-coated charcoal (DCC)[30].

Definition of menopausal status

Patients who had been amenorrheic for the last 2 or more years are regarded as postmenopausal. Hysterectomized patients with no concomitant bilateral oophorectomy are regarded as premenopausal until 54 years old and postmenopausal after 55 years old or when their basal follicle stimulating hormone (FSH) levels are < 60 ng/100 ml.

Postsurgical adjuvant treatment

Tamoxifen treatment (30 mg/day in three doses) should be started within 6 weeks after mastectomy. The drug should be administered continuously for 5 years or until recurrence.

Chemotherapy should be started within 6 weeks after mastectomy. Six CMF courses are administered, followed by four courses of epi-adriamycin, one every 3 weeks. Doses are as follows: cyclophosphamide 500 mg/m^2, i.v., day 1, methotrexate 40 mg/m^2, i.v., day 1, 5-fluorouracil 600 mg/m^2, i.v., day 1, 4-epi-doxorubicine 75 mg/m^2, i.v., day 1.

In cases where white blood cell counts were 4 000 and/or platelets 120 000 at day 21, the treatment should be postponed 1–2 weeks.

Radiotherapy, when indicated, starts together with the first course of adjuvant chemotherapy.

Baseline and follow-up analysis

The baseline and follow-up analyses were performed as shown in Table 1.

Table 1 Baseline and follow-up analysis timing

Timing	*Start*	*Every 3 m*	*Every 6 m*	*Every year*
Physical examination	+	+		
Hematology	+	+		
Chest X-ray	+		+	
Electrocardiograph	+*			
Liver sonography	+†			
Bone scan or X-ray	+			+

*Before each epi-adriamycin course; †if required

RESULTS

Five hundred and four evaluable patients were recruited from November 1983 to June 1987. Table 2 shows the patients' characteristics in the three treatment groups. Table 3 shows the toxicity of different treatments. Survival and disease-free survival, overall and according to menopausal and nodal status are shown in graphs (Figures 1–6).

Table 2 Patient characteristics for treatment types

Treatment	*T*	*CT*	*CTT*
Evaluable patients	168	165	171
Menopausal status			
Premenopause	79	81	77
Postmenopause	89	84	94
Tumor size			
pT1	60	61	63
pT2	97	92	101
pT3	8	9	6
pT4	3	2	1
Unknown		—	1
Nodal status			
1–3	96	88	106
4– +	72	77	65
Estrogen receptors			
< 30 fmol/mg	49	49	47
30–100 fmol/mg	73	57	69
> 100 fmol/mg	46	59	55
Progesterone receptors			
< 10 fmol/mg	19	33	22
> 9 fmol/mg	138	122	134
Unknown	11	10	15

T = tamoxifen (for 5 years), CT = CMF (six courses) and epi-adriamycin (four courses), CTT = tamoxifen plus CMF (six courses) and epi-adriamycin (four courses)

Table 3 Toxicity of treatment types

	Toxicity		
Treatment	*T%*	*CT%*	*CTT%*
Nausea/vomiting	6.7	94.5	97.7
Stomatitis		24.5	21.6
Diarrhea	1.8	12.7	7.6
Infection	0.6	2.4	1.7
Cardiotoxicity	0.6	3.6	4.1
Alopecia	3.6	81.8	86.0
Liver enzymes alteration	5.3	7.9	9.3
Cystitis	4.8	18.8	20.5
Leucopenia	1.8	49.5	39.8
Thrombocytopenia		0.6	0.6
Spotting	17.8	2.4	15.2
Hot flushes	28.6	16.4	39.8
Amenorrhea	27.8	37.1	41.5

T = tamoxifen (for 5 years), CT = CMF (six courses) and epi-adriamycin (four courses), CTT = tamoxifen plus CMF (six courses) and epi-adriamycin (four courses)

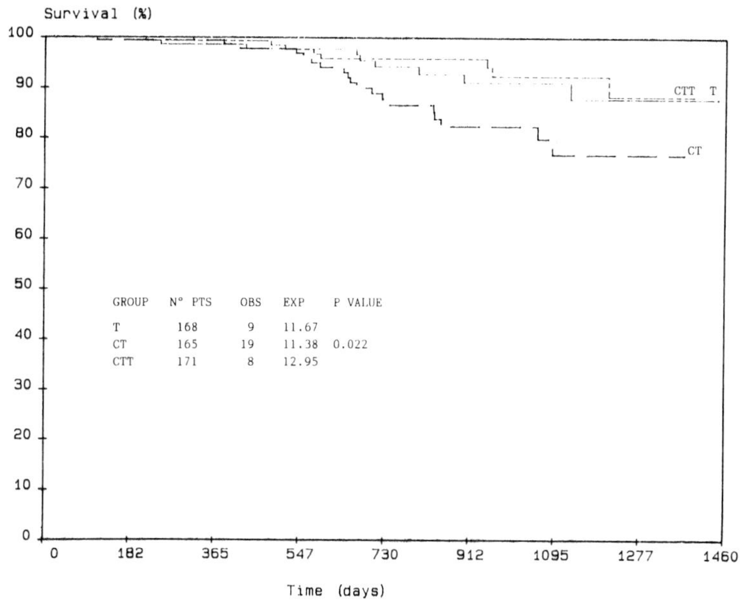

Figure 1 Survival rate for groups overall

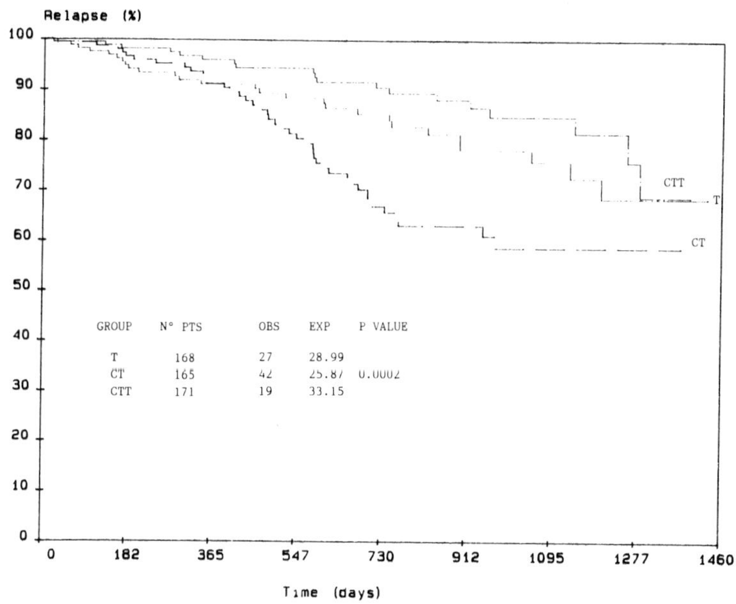

Figure 2 Relapse rate for groups overall

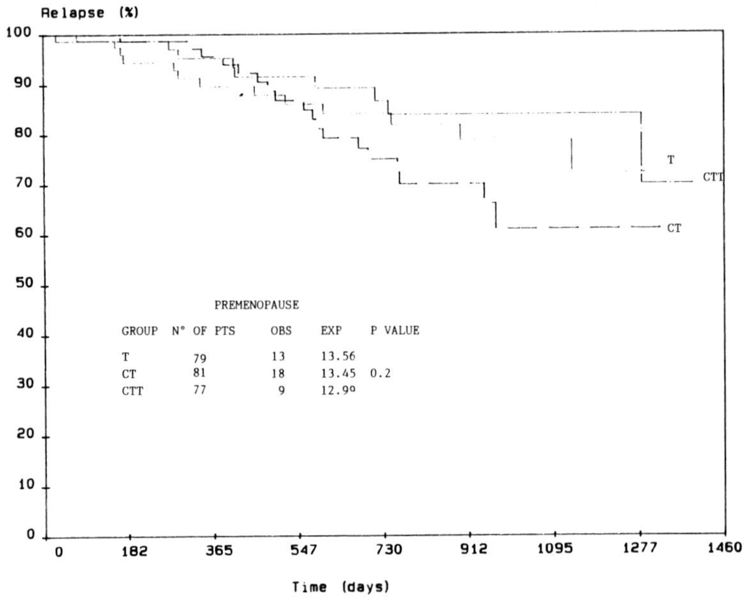

Figure 3 Relapse rate for premenopausal groups

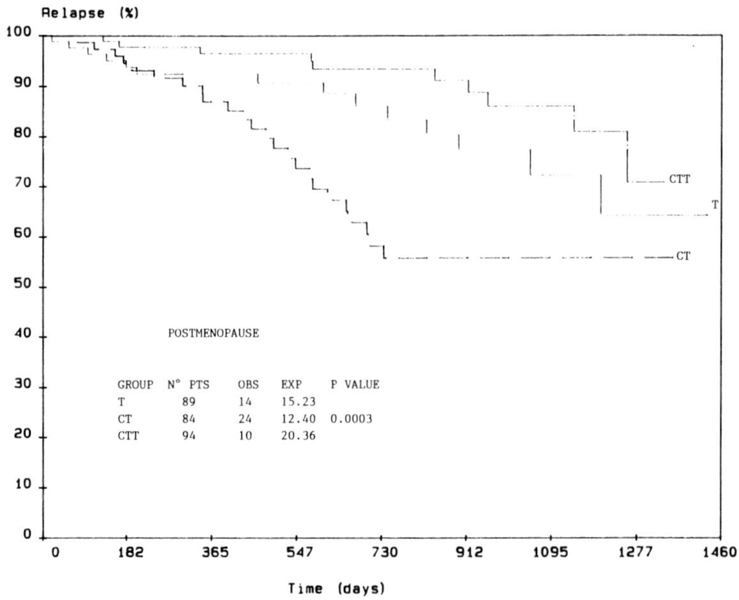

Figure 4 Relapse rate for postmenopausal groups

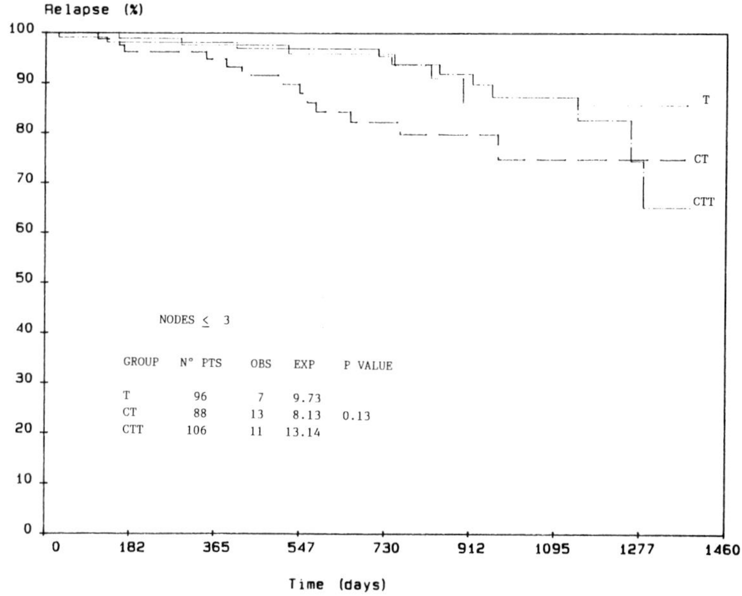

Figure 5 Relapse rate for groups with three or less nodes

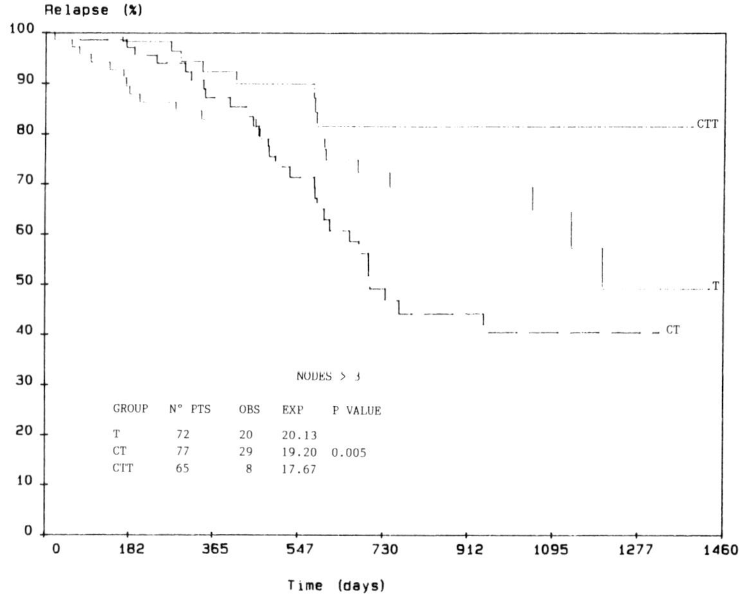

Figure 6 Relapse rate for groups with more than three nodes

CONCLUSIONS

Our results with hormone adjuvant therapy with TAM confirm positive findings reported in the literature in postmenopausal patients. Moreover, our results are at least superimposable on the results obtained with chemotherapy in premenopausal patients with positive nodes and estradiol receptors. The comparison of our results with those obtained in other studies is rather difficult, due to different chemotherapy regimens employed. Our regimen produces slightly lower disease-free survival rates compared with the rates obtained in the first Milan CMF study. However they are comparable to rates obtained in other studies, like ECOG and Ludwig II, where CMF or cyclophosphamide methotrexate fluorouracil prednisone (CMFP) regimens were employed[31,32]. Furthermore, the regimen we employed resulted in an appreciably lower rate of amenorrhea than CMF regimen employed in Milan: this is likely to be linked to the use of a lower dose of alkylating agent.

In the light of these findings, the association of chemotherapy with hormone therapy seems logical, aimed to obtain an additive or synergistic effect. Actually, as already shown in other studies[33–37], association therapy showed no significant advantages compared to TAM or chemotherapy alone, both in pre- and postmenopause.

These data are preliminary, as median follow-up time is still short (2 years) and the number of observed events is small, especially where survival analysis is concerned. When data are analyzed in relation to main prognostic factors, the number of patients in the study and the number of observed events are even smaller. All patients in the TAM group and chemotherapy–TAM group are still under treatment, while in most patients in the chemotherapy group adjuvant treatment is already finished. Nevertheless, some conclusions may already be drawn. Tamoxifen is as effective as chemotherapy in premenopausal women. Association therapy gives no significant advantages to this group of patients. In postmenopausal women, TAM produces better results than chemotherapy. Results of the association therapy are not statistically better than TAM alone. No significant differences between treatment group are seen in low-risk patients; in high-risk patients (more than three positive nodes) association therapy produces a significant amelioration of disease-free interval, but not of survival. Long-term toxicity due to long-term TAM treatment is not yet known, especially in young women. These findings seem stimulating, even if a longer follow-up is needed before definitive conclusions can be drawn.

REFERENCES

1. Valagussa, P., Bonadonna, G. and Veronesi, U. (1978). Patterns of relapse and survival following radical mastectomy. Analysis of 716 consecutive patients. *Cancer*, **41**, 1170
2. Gore, S., Langlands, A., Pocock, S. and Kerr, G. (1982). Natural history of breast cancer. *Rec. Res. Cancer Res.*, **80**, 134
3. Hahnel, R. and Roberts, A.N. (1981). Oestrogen receptor assay and morphology of breast cancer. *Pathology*, **13**, 317

4. Wolmark, N. and Fisher, B. (1981). Surgery in the primary treatment of breast cancer. *Breast Cancer Res. Treat.*, **1**, 339
5. Tubiana, M. and Koscielny, S. (1987). The natural history of human breast cancer: implications for patient management. *Dev. Oncol.*, **51**, 333
6. Henderson, C. (1987). Adjuvant systemic therapy for early breast cancer. *Current problems in cancer*. Vol. XI, 3, p. 125
7. Palshof, T. Carstensen, B., Mouridsen, H.T. and Dombernowsky, P. (1985). Adjuvant endocrine therapy in pre- and postmenopausal women with operable breast cancer. *Rev. Endocr. Rel. Cancer*, **17**, 43
8. Rose, C., Mouridsen, H.T., Thorpe, S.M. *et al.* (1985). For the Danish Breast Cancer Cooperative Group: Antiestrogen-treatment of postmenopausal women with primary high risk breast cancer. 72 months of life table analysis. *Rev. Endocr. Rel. Cancer*, **17**, 117
9. Walgren, A., Baral, E., Nordenskjold, B. *et al.* (1984). Should adjuvant therapy be given for several years in breast cancer? In Jones, S.E. and Salmon, S.E. (eds). *Adjuvant Therapy of Cancer* **IV** p. 331 (Orlando: Grune & Stratton)
10. Ribeiro, G. and Swindell, R. (1985). The Christie Hospital tamoxifen "Nolvadex" adjuvant trial for operable breast carcinoma-seven year results. *Eur. J. Cancer Clin. Oncol.*, **21**, 897
11. *Nolvadex Adjuvant Trial Organization* (1985). Controlled trial of tamoxifen as single adjuvant agent in management of early breast cancer: analysis at 6 years. *Lancet*, **i**, 836
12. Pritchard, K.I., Meakin, J.W., Boyd, N.F. *et al.* (1984). A prospective randomized controlled trial of adjuvant tamoxifen in postmenopausal women with axillary node-positive breast cancer. In Jones, S.E. and Salmon, S.E. (eds). *Adjuvant Therapy of Cancer* **IV.** p. 339 (Orlando: Grune & Stratton)
13. Gelber, R.D. (1984). Adjuvant therapy for postmenopausal women with operable breast cancer: Part II- randomized trials comparing endocrine therapy with surgery alone. In Jones, S.E. and Salmon, S.E. (eds). *Adjuvant Therapy of Cancer* **IV**, p. 393 (Orlando: Grune & Stratton)
14. Lippman, M.E. and Chabner, B.A. (1986). National Institutes of Health Consensus Development Conference on Adjuvant Chemotherapy and Endocrine Therapy for Breast Cancer. Editorial overview. *NIC Monogr.*, **1**, 5
15. Cole, M.P. and Todd, I.D.J. (1975). Tamoxifen (ICI 46, 474) Clinical experience in 129 patients with advanced breast cancer. In Namer, M. and Lalanne, C.M. (eds). *Hormones and Breast Cancer*, p. 245. (Paris: INSERM)
16. Meakin, J.W. *et al.* (1983). Ovarian irradiation and prednisone folowing surgery and radiotherapy for carcinoma of the breast. *Breast Cancer Res. Treat.*, **3**, 45
17. Bryant, A.J. and Weir, J.A. (1981). Prophylactic oophorectomy in operable instances of carcinoma of the breast. *Surg. Gynecol. Obstet.*, **153**, 660
18. Ludwig Breast Cancer Study Group (1985). Chemotherapy with or without oophorectomy in high-risk premenopausal patients with operable breast cancer. *J. Clin. Oncol.*, **3**, 1059
19. Vollenweider-Zeragui, L. *et al.* (1986). The predictive value of estrogen and progesterone receptors' concentrations on the clinical behavior of breast cancer in women. *Cancer*, **57**, 1171
20. Pritchard, K.I. *et al.* (1980). Tamoxifen therapy in premenopausal patients with metastatic breast cancer. *Cancer Treat. Rep.*, **64**, 787
21. Manni, A. and Pearson, O.H. (1980). Antiestrogen-induced remissions in premenopausal women with stage IV breast cancer: effects on ovarian function. *Cancer Treat. Rep.*, **64**, 779
22. Engelsmann, E. *et al.* (1981). CMF versus CMF plus tamoxifen in advanced breast cancer, in postmenopausal women. An EORTC study. *Reviews on Endocrine-Related Cancer* (suppl) **9**, 427
23. Boccardo, F. *et al.* (1982). Chemohormonal therapy of advanced breast cancer: rationale and preliminary results of a randomized study. In Iacobelli, S., Lippman, M. and Robustelli della Cuna, G. (eds). *The Role of Tamoxifen in Breast Cancer*, p. 73. (New York: Raven Press)
24. Cocconi, G. *et al.* (1982). Tamoxifen in combination with or following chemotherapy in advanced breast cancer: results of a randomized prospective study. In Iacobelli, S., Lippman, M. and Robustelli della Cuna, G. (eds). *The Role of Tamoxifen in Breast Cancer*, p. 35 (New York: Raven Press)
25. Goldie, J.H. *et al.* (1982). Rationale for the use of alternating non-cross-resistant chemo-

therapy. *Cancer Treat. Rep.*, **66**, 439
26. Boccardo, F. *et al.* (1982). Kinetic scheduled combination of cyclophosphamide methotrexate and 5-fluorouracil with calcium methyl-tetrahydrofolate in advanced breast cancer: a pilot study. *Chemioterapia*, **6**, 416
27. Buzdar, A.V. *et al.* (1981). Management of breast cancer patients failing adjuvant chemotherapy with adriamycin-containing regimens. *Cancer*, **47**, 2798
28. Heel, R.C. *et al.* (1978). Tamoxifen: a review of its pharmacological properties and therapeutic use in the treatment of breast cancer. *Drugs*, **16**, 1
29. Patterson, *et al.* (1982). The biology and physiology of "Nolvadex" tamoxifen in the treatment of breast cancer. *Breast Cancer Res. and Treat.*, **2**, 363
30. Piffaneli, *et al.* (1982). Protocollo del metodo con charcoal-destrano (D.C.C.) per il dosaggio dei recettori dell'estradiolo e del progresterone nel tessuto neoplastico. *Laboratory*, **9**, 1
31. Goldhirsh, A. and Gelber, R. (1986). Adjuvant treatment of early breast cancer: the Ludwig Breast Cancer Studies. *NCI Monogr.*, **1**, 55
32. Tormey, D.C. *et al.* (1986) Adjuvant systemic therapy in premenopausal (CMF, CMFP, CMFPT) and postmenopausal women with mode positive breast cancer. *NCI Monogr.*, **1**, 75
33. Boccardo, F. (1986). Tamoxifen (TMX) as adjuvant treatment of breast cancer. In Baulieu, E.E., Iacobelli, S. and McGuire, W.L. (eds.) *Endocrinology and Malignancy* p. 489. (Carnforth: Parthenon Publishing)
34. Taylor, IV,S.G. *et al.* (1985). Observation compared to adjuvant chemohormonotherapy in postmenopausal breast cancer: the ECOG trial. *Proc. Am. Soc. Clin. Oncol.*, **4**, 61
35. Tormey, D.C. (1984). In Senn, H. (ed.) *Recent Results in Cancer Research Adjuvant Chemotherapy of Breast Cancer*. p. 155 (Heidelberg: Springer Verlag)
36. Fisher, B. *et al.* (1986). Adjuvant chemotherapy with and without tamoxifen in the treatment of primary breast cancer: 5-year results from the National Surgical Adjuvant Breast and Bowel Project Trial. *J. Clin. Oncol.*, **4**, 459
37. Hubay, C.A. *et al.* (1981). Adjuvant therapy of stage II breast cancer. *Breast Cancer Res. Treat.*, **1**, 77

Section 1 continued

Part D

Nuclear magnetic resonance in gynecology

18

Magnetic resonance imaging (MRI) in the evaluation of adnexal masses

S. Davolio Marani, A. Casolo, G. Nasi, A. Burani, P. Oltramari, F. Martinez, V. Mazza, G. Allessandrini and A.R. Genazzani

INTRODUCTION

At present ultrasonography (US) is the screening method in the evaluation of adnexal lesions; in association with fine needle aspiration under US control, a high percentage of correct diagnosis is gained[1]. However US lacks specificity[2], the field of view is very reduced and it is highly dependable on the operator's skill in certain clinical situations (obesity, abdominal meteorism).

Computerized tomography (CT) is also used when studying this type of pathology especially in the staging of the ovarian carcinomas[3]. The purpose of our study was to verify if at present it is possible to substitute CT with magnetic resonance (MR) in these patients where US is inconclusive. From the early studies of the female pelvis[4,5] it was clear that MR could have more advantageous contrast resolution compared to CT. These studies were however carried out on low to medium field units (0.35–0.6T); as the aspect of various tissues may vary at higher field intensity (due to the increase of T1 and the more pronounced magnetic susceptibility effect of various hemoglobin breakdown products) we wanted to confirm in our unit at 1.5T the past results because better spatial resolution is obtainable at high field strength.

MATERIALS AND METHODS

We examined with MR, 37 patients with a mean age of 48 years presenting an adnexal pathology. The results were controlled by surgery (21 cases), with fine needle aspiration under US guidance or during laparoscopy (10 cases). In the other cases we used the long-term clinical-instrumental control (included US and eventually CT).

In Table 1 our case study is listed. All of the examinations were carried

Table 1 Verified types of adnexal lesions

Diagnosis	*No. of patients*	*No. of adnexal lesions*
Simple cyst	16	16
Hemorrhagic cyst	3	3
Polycystic ovarian disease (PCOD)	1	2
Endometriosis	2	3
Teratoma	2	2
Cystadenoma	3	3
Ovarian carcinoma	3	4
Recurrence of ovarian carcinoma	2	2
Pelvic inflammatory disease (PID)	4	4
Tubal extrauterine pregnancy	1	1
Total	37	40

out on a superconductive unit at 1.5T (Signa, General Electric, Milwaukee, USA). The most useful scans are the coronal and axial ones, occasionally we also obtained sagittal scans. It is essential to have both the T1- and T2-weighted image of the same pathology for the possible presence of hemorrhagic collections. As a localizer we used an SE coronal T1-weighted series at short TR/TE followed by an axial one with asymmetrical SE at long TR (at least 2 s) and two echoes at 20 and 80 ms; spin-density and T2 weighted images are respectively achieved. The field of view was 32–40 cm with a thickness of 5–10 mm and a skip of 1.5 mm. The matrix was 128 × 256 with two excitations. We did not use any specific preparation of the patients but we believe that a certain level of bladder filling may be advantageous.

RESULTS AND DISCUSSION

At present the presurgical evaluation of these patients includes the clinical examination with the sample of certain tumor markers such as CA125, US with fine needle aspiration, and the laparoscopy with eventual needle biopsy. The role of CT was reserved for the staging and follow-up of ovarian carcinomas. In reality the therapeutic strategy depends upon the US reports: small simple cysts are considered as functional and receive only medical treatment; simple anechoic cysts with a diameter less than 5–6 cm are aspirated under US guidance and eventually surgically removed if they should form again; large simple cysts (with a diameter of more than 5–6 cm) and complex lesions are surgically treated. These therapeutic decisions are made considering the fact that US is not so specific. It is also sometimes difficult to distinguish the origin between very large adnexal or uterine masses of the pelvis. Lastly the presurgical staging and control of eventual recurrence of the adnexal carcinomas are not so reliable even with CT. In all of these situations we found that the MR examination was useful as it added important information to the clinical chart. Regarding the specificity, certain images seem completely reliable as in the case of dermoid cysts (Fig. 1a, b) where both the adipose component (fat and/or sebum) with high signal

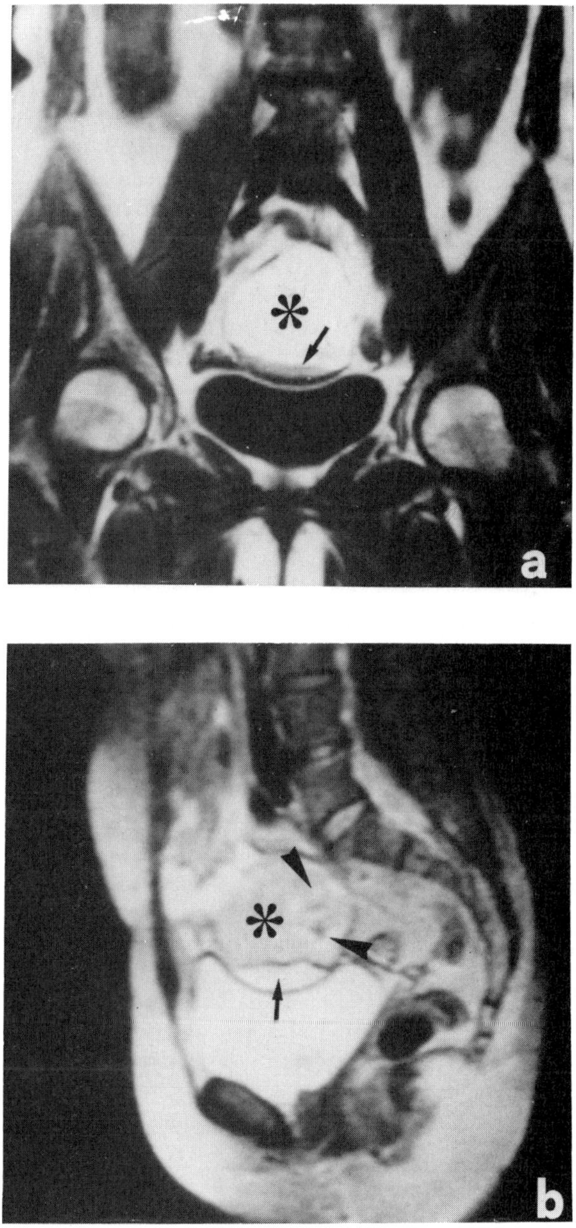

Figure 1 Coronal T1 image (a), sagittal T2 (b) dermoid cyst. Both on T1 and T2 weighted images the predominant fatty tissue (asterisk) shows the same signal as subcutaneous fat. Inferiorly there is a thin band (arrow) with medium signal on T1 and high on T2 images referrable to solid or liquid component. The debris (arrowheads) on the sagittal T2 image on right, show a chemical shift artifact

on T1-weighted scans, and the solid–liquid component, with low signal on T1-weighted image and high on T2-weighted image, are in evidence. There may be debris or protrusions with low signal on every sequence and it is noticeable that the chemical shift artifact corresponds to the liquid–fat interface, a fact already studied by other authors[6]. Simple cysts are shown as round lesions with low signal on T1 images, medium on spin-density and very high on T2 images. When the content is hemorrhagic the signal is generally high on all the sequences due to the presence of extracellular methemoglobin (Fig. 2 a,b). There was an exception with an endometrial cyst in a patient with a tubal extrauterine pregnancy, which showed very low signal even on T2-weighted images; this could be due to the superparamagnetic effects of the other two hematic breakdown products (deoxihemoglobin and hemosiderin) present in other stages of temporal evolution of the hemorrhagic collection. Whilst hematic zones are quite frequent in all the adnexal masses, it seems that the development of a regular cyst with high signal on T1 and T2 images, may be a characteristic of a hematic or endometrial cyst. In endometriosis the adnexal cysts are very easy to identify due also to the contemporary presence of a thick fibrous capsule with low signal[7]; on the other hand it is not possible to say the same of the small pelvic spreading for which at the moment the MR examination is not helpful.

We had one case of a polycystic ovarian disease (PCOD) with an aspect well described in the literature[8] of a crown of small hyperintense cysts on T2 images around a central zone always hypointense probably referring to the cellular stroma. All the masses associated with pelvic inflammatory disease (PID) showed low signal on T1 images with certain hemorrhagic areas and high signal on T2-weighted scans.

The only hematoma associated with a tubal pregnancy had low, heterogeneous signal on T1 and T2 images. In differential diagnosis between very large ovarian cystomas and the adnexal carcinomas (Fig. 3 a, b) MR is not specific: both forms appear as large masses with more or less homogeneous signal, usually low on T1, medium on spin-density and very high on T2-weighted images. Possible fibrous septa are always hypointense, whilst there may be a difference in the various loculi in the case of pluriseptated forms. The staging of adnexal carcinomas is made easier compared to CT due to the excellent contrast between the nearby organs (bladder, rectum, uterus). The large subserosal leiomyoma almost always have a hypointense aspect especially on T2 images and they therefore do not create diagnostic problems.

In the follow-up of carcinomas MR can compete with CT for its wide field of view and the possibility to include in the same slab of axial locations the pelvis and the superior abdomen reducing a great deal the examination time.

The overall diagnostic accuracy was very good, on 40 mass lesions MR correctly identified the final diagnosis in 33 cases, that is 82%. MR proved to be unreliable only in the cases of PID and in extrauterine pregnancy; these cases presented the false negatives.

In conclusion we believe that MR can supply information that neither CT nor US can give.

The specificity also seems good in certain clinical situations (dermoid,

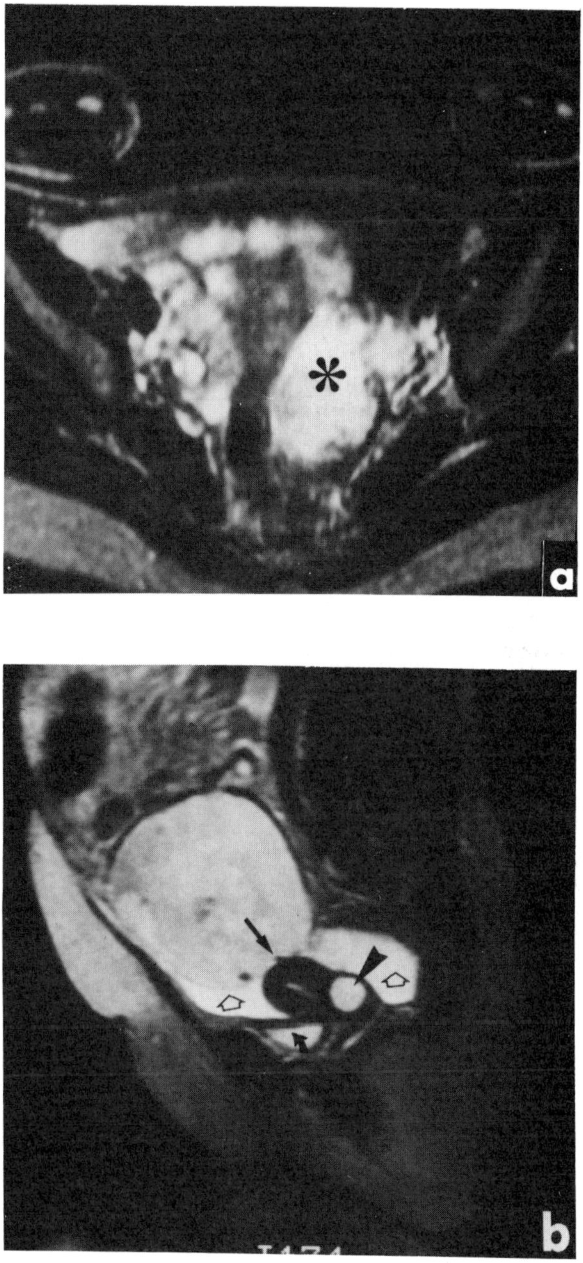

Figure 2 Coronal T1-image (a), axial T2 image (b) left adnexal cyst with hemorrhagic content. The cyst has a high signal (asterisk) both on T1 and T2 images due to the presence of methemoglobin

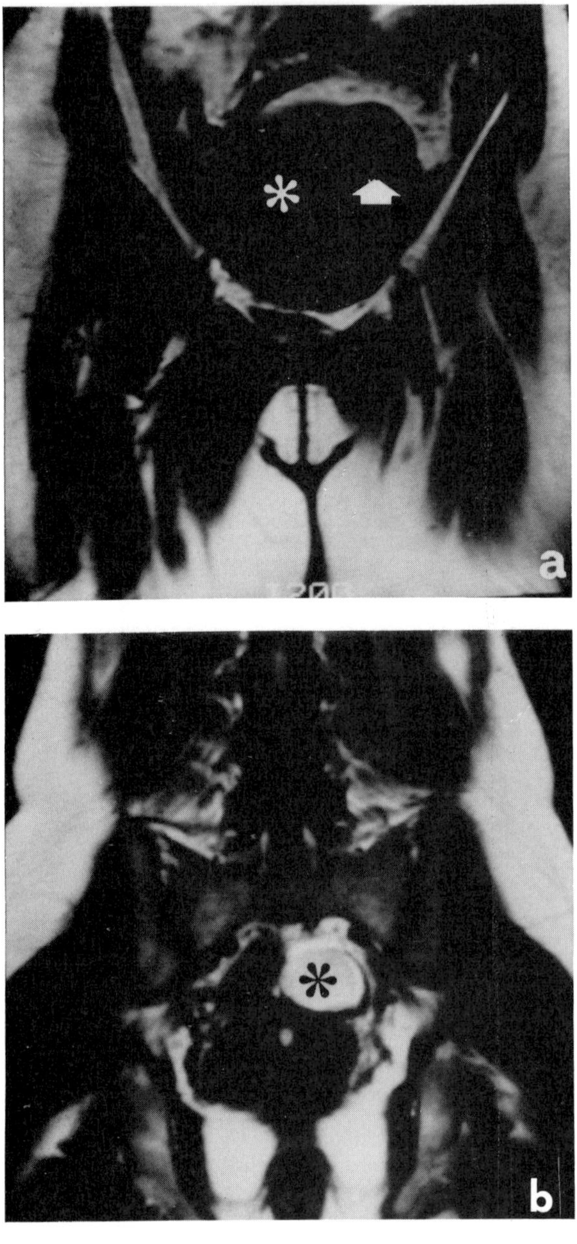

Figure 3 Coronal T1 image (a), sagittal T2 image (b) mucinous ovarian carcinoma. On the coronal T1-weighted image the lesions shows two components with different signal, medium on left (asterisk), low on right (white arrow). On sagittal T2-weighted image the whole lesion has high signal with certain heterogeneities. The uterus is pushed down (arrow) with a cervical Naboth cyst with high signal (arrowhead). There is a liquid collection in the Douglas and vesico-uterine pouch (open arrow). Small bladder with high signal (curved arrow).

endometrial cyst). In the remaining cases where it is not possible to make a differential diagnosis it seems that the excellent soft tissue contrast, the wide field of view and the good spatial resolution favor MR compared to CT as a more thorough examination following US. The capability to visualise the vessels and the bladder without contrast media and the absence of ionizing radiations are also important advantages of this technique.

REFERENCES

1. Kratochwil, A. (1982). Ultrasonography in gynecology. In Kurjak, A. (ed.) *Progress in medical ultrasound*, pp. 123–8. (Amsterdam: Excerpta Medica)
2. Walsh, J.W., Taylor, K.J.W. and McWasson, J.F. (1979). Gray-scale ultrasound in 204 proved gynecologic masses: accuracy and specific diagnostic criteria. *Radiology*, **130**, 391–7
3. Amendola, M.A., Walsh, J.W. and Amendola, B.E. (1981). Computed tomography in the evaluation of carcinoma of the ovary. *J. Comput. Assist. Tomogr.*, **5**, 179–86
4. Butler, H., Bryan, P.J. and Lipuma, J.P. (1986). Magnetic Resonance Imaging of the abnormal female pelvis. *AJR*, **143**, 1259–66
5. Dooms, G.C., Hricak, H. and Tscholakoff, D. (1986). Adnexal structures: MR imaging. *Radiology*, **158**, 639–46
6. Tagashi, K., Kazumasa, N., Kyo, I., Fujisawa, I., Sago, T., Minami, S., Nakano, Y., Harumi, I., Torizuka, K. and Ozasa, H. (1987). Ovarian cystic teratomas: MR imaging. *Radiology*, **162**, 669–73
7. Nishimura, K., Togashi, K., Itoh, K., Fujisawa, I., Noma, S., Kawamura, Y., Nakano, Y., Itoh, H., Torizuka, K. and Ozasa, H. (1987). Endometrial cysts of the ovary: MR imaging. *Radiology*, **162**, 315–8
8. Mitchell, D.G., Gefter, W.R., Spritzer, C.E., Blasco, L., Nulson, J., Livolsi, V., Axel, L., Arger, P.H. and Kressel, H.Y. (1986). Polycystic ovaries: MR imaging. *Radiology*, **160**, 425–9

19

Myometrial infiltration in endometrial carcinoma and preoperative magnetic resonance accuracy

C. Belloni, R. Viganò, G. Colombo, A. Del Maschio, S. Sironi, G.L. Taccagni and M. Vignali

Magnetic resonance (MR) has been recently introduced in medical diagnostic techniques. Due to the new information obtained by this method, it has been possible to perform studies of encephalon, medulla, thorax and liver that are more complete than those obtained by traditional, radiological, ultrasonographic or radioisotopic methods[1,2]. From 1984 MR has been also employed to study the pelvis[3–5], in particular to look for the presence of ovarian masses and/or uterine tumors. Furthermore, its application to the evaluation of the extension of cervical and/or endometrial cancer has already given satisfactory results. The definition of groups at risk for endometrial cancer is essential to make a prognosis and choose a correct therapeutic approach. Clinical staging, according to FIGO parameters, is inadequate for this purpose. All the authors agree to consider three fundamental factors: histological degree, myometrial invasion and presence of lymphnode metastases[6]. The histological degree is always determined on the specimen obtained from the uterine cavity for bioptic purposes. In contrast, the state of lymphnodes and the myometrial invasion are parameters that are not easily studied before surgery by instrumental methods such as echography, computerized axial tomography (CAT) and lymphography[7,8]. Hence, lymphadenectomy should be proposed only for the patients who are reasonably considered 'at risk'. This is the case when a tumor with a low degree of differentiation infiltrates all the myometrium and through the lymphatic vessels may spread into the pelvic and/or para-aortic nodes.

The aim of this study is to evaluate the accuracy of MR examination in determining the presence of myometrial invasion by endometrial cancer before any surgical treatment.

MATERIALS AND METHODS

The clinical staff of the Department of Obstetrics and Gynecology of the University of Milan, Scientific Institute San Raffaele, has followed, by MR, 30 consecutive cases of endometrial carcinoma, aged between 50 and 87 years. For this study, we have utilized the MR equipment which is available at the Radiology Department of the San Raffaele Hospital: a Magnetom Siemens unity which works at a magnetic flux of 1.5 Tesla. In all the patients the MR examination was performed as follows: at the level of the pelvis, both in the axial and sagittal planes, adjacent sections 5–10 mm thick were analyzed. We applied the SPIN-ECHO technique with the following data: Tr 1.5/2.1 s, TE 28/100 ms. These techniques concerning the MR pulse are already used for studying neoplastic pathology of uterus, as reported in the literature[9,10]. Within 10 days from the MR examination, all the 30 patients underwent surgery which included the removal of uterus, uterine adnexa and a vaginal neck of at least 2 cm. In 18 cases we also performed pelvic lymphadenectomy. In 12 cases this kind of surgery was not possible due to the patient's conditions, such as obesity, age. An histological test was performed on the surgical specimens, using the same criteria for all cases, in order to evaluate both macroscopically and microscopically the levels of extent and infiltration of the endometrial tumor. This was done to compare the histological degree (FIGO) of the tumor, its spread and infiltration of myometrium. The myometrial layer was divided into three; we indicated as M1 the invasion of inner third, M2 of that middle third and M3 of that outer third. M0 is the neoplastic growth in the absence of any invasion of myometrium.

RESULTS AND DISCUSSION

Serial histological examination of the surgical specimens indicated that in six cases there was only surface tumor growth (M0); in eight cases the infiltration of the myometrium was limited to the inner third (M1); in nine cases it was extended to the middle third (M2) and in seven cases the infiltration of the tumor was observed in all the myometrial layer (M3). The table compares these results with those obtained by MR examination. The results of this study indicate that magnetic resonance, employed to detect extent of endometrial cancer to myometrial infiltration, has a sensitivity of

Table 1 Invasion of corporeal myometrium: comparison between MR and histological report

Histological evaluation	*MR evaluation*			
	M0	*M1*	*M2*	*M3*
M0 (6)	6	—	—	—
M1 (8)	—	5	3	—
M2 (9)	—	—	8	1
M3 (7)	1	—	2	4
Total (30)	7	5	13	5

93%, a specificity of 78% and an accuracy of 86%. These data are the result of a single and limited study derived from a collaboration between the Pathological Anatomy, the Radiology and the Gynecology Departments of the Institution. However, it is important to note that the results presented confirm those of previous studies performed on a smaller number of patients. Our data are even more interesting if we consider that we classify myometrial infiltration in four stages: M0, M1, M2 and M3 as it is done in the pathological staging. In contrast with the classification proposed by Hricak *et al.*[9] that indicates only three stages (E = extension to the endometrium; I = superficial infiltration and D = deep infiltration). In one case, the instrumental evaluation and the histological test gave opposite results. MR indicated a lack of myometrial infiltration (M0), in contrast the histological test demonstrated that the myometrium was completely infiltrated by the tumor (M3). We believe that this was due to an error in the performance of the test and should not question the validity of the method. In conclusion, we feel that, as already indicated by other studies, our data also strongly suggest that MR might represent an important step in the preoperative staging of endometrial cancer.

REFERENCES

1. Smith, F.W., Mallard, J.R., Hutchinson, J.M.S. *et al.* (1981). Clinical application of nuclear magnetic resonance. *Lancet*, **1**, 78–9
2. Bradley, W.G., Waluch, V., Yadley, R.A. and Wycoff, R.R. (1984). Comparison of LT and MR in 400 patients with suspected disease of the brain and cervical cord. *Radiology*, **152**, 695–702
3. Thickman, D., Kressel, H., Gussman, D. *et al.* (1984). Nuclear magnetic resonance in Gynecology. *J. Obstet. Gynecol.*, **149**, 835
4. Wortmington, J.L., Balfe, D.M. and Lee, J.K.T. (1984). MR imaging of gynecology neoplasm. *Radiology*, **153** (P), 32
5. Hricak, H., Lacey, C., Schriock, E. *et al.* (1985). Gynecologic masses: value of magnetic resonance imaging. *Am. J. Obstet. Gynecol.*, **153**, 31–7
6. Di Saia, P.J., Creasman, W.T., Borrow, R.C. *et al.* (1985). Risk factors and recurrent patterns in stage I endometrial cancer. *Am. J. Obstet. Gynecol.*, **151**, 1009–15
7. Brascho, D.J. and Shawker, T.H. (1980). *Abdominal ultrasound in the cancer patient*, pp. 209. (New York: John Wiley and Sons Inc.)
8. Walsh, J.W. and Goplerud, D.R. (1982). Computed tomography of primary, persistent and recurrent endometrial malignancy. *AJR*, **139**, 1149–54
9. Hricak, H., Stern, J.L., Fisher, M. *et al.* (1987). Endometrial carcinoma staging by MR imaging. *Radiology*, **162**, 297–305
10. Worthington, J., Blafe, D.M., Lee, J.K.T. *et al.* (1986). Uterine neoplasm: MR imaging. *Radiology*, **159**, 725–30

20

MRI in the diagnosis of gynecological diseases in the adolescent

L. Fedele, M. Dorta, D. Brioschi, C. Massari, M. N. Giudici and L. Villa

MATERIALS AND METHODS

Magnetic resonance imaging (MRI), ultrasonography (US), and subsequently laparoscopy were performed on nine girls aged 13–18 years (mean 16.3) with chronic pelvic pain or primary amenorrhea and abnormal pelvic examination, consecutively referred to the outpatient clinic for adolescent diseases at the First Department of Obstetrics and Gynecology, Milan University. Eight girls had pelvic pain (severe dysmenorrhea in two, intermenstrual pain in four, both symptoms in two) and one had primary amenorrhea.

Rectal exploration revealed a retroverted uterus with marked pelvic tenderness in one patient, an adnexal uni- or bilateral mass in three, a pelvic mass in two, an anteverted uterus with marked tenderness of the uterus-sacral ligaments in two, and no palpable uterine structures in one.

Magnetic resonance imaging was performed in another institution by radiologists who were unaware of the patient's medical history, physical findings, or results of US and only knew that the pelvic examination was abnormal. Six girls were in the second phase of the cycle when MRI was done, and two in the proliferative phase, and the other was in amenorrhea. The investigation was performed with a Philips S5 Gyroscan MRI system, with a superconductive 0.5 Tesla upgraded magnet and the standard RF coil (resonance frequency 21 MHz) supplied for total body studies. The spin-echo multislice technique was always employed, with repetition times (TR) varying according to the number of simultaneously acquired slices. In all cases the examination started with some median or paramedian sagittal T_2-weighted slices to show the uterine orientation. For this sequence TR were of the order of 1000 ms with echo times (TE) of 50 and 100 ms (double echo sequence). Once the orientation of the uterus was established, the organ was examined with sets of oblique slices as parallel as possible to the anatomical plane containing the tubal ostia and internal uterine os. These spin-echo T_2-weighted images were always obtained with multislice, double echo technique using TE of 50 and 100 ms, TR ranging from 1500 to 2000 ms, with 256×256

matrix and 2 free induction decay. Slice thickness varied from 6 to 10 mm according to uterine size. For particular conditions, mainly to obtain morphological images, coronal and/or sagittal T_1-weighted (TR of 500 ms, TE of 20 ms) thin slices were acquired.

Ultrasonography was performed with a real-time Ansaldo 920 sector scanner and a 3.5 or 5 MHz transducer. The pelvis was scanned in longitudinal, transverse and oblique planes with the bladder half full and full.

Bicornuate and didelphic uteri were differentiated from partial and complete septate uteri according to the presence in MR and US images of a fundal indentation more than 10 mm deep associated with an angle of at least 60° between the medial margins of the hemicavities. These parameters are arbitrary but were found to be reliable in our previous US study[1]. The level of the lower apex of the myometrial septum was used to differentiate didelphic from bicornuate uteri and complete from partial septate uteri.

All the patients then underwent laparoscopy to assess diagnosis, and four were subsequently operated on to correct the underlying pathology.

MRI data were compared with the US, laparoscopic and surgical findings.

RESULTS

Table 1 shows MRI, US, laparoscopic and surgical findings. The presence or absence of a uterus was demonstrated by MRI and also the orientation and overall size of the organ. It was more or less anteverted in seven patients, retroverted in one, and absent in one. Uterine malformation was observed in three cases: unicornuate uterus with rudimentary horn in one, septate in one, and didelphic in one (respectively classes II, V and III according to Buttram and Gibbons[2]).

Ultrasonography visualized the uterine fundal profile in the girl with uterus didelphys, but could not define the other 'double' uterus as septate or didelphic due to its retroversion. The unicornuate uterus and cavitation of its rudimentary horn were correctly diagnosed by US.

In the case of didelphic uterus with imperforate hemivagina laparoscopy demonstrated only the presence of a bicornuate uterus with asymmetry of the two horns (the hemiuterus corresponding to the imperforate hemivagina was about twice the size of the controlateral hemiuterus).

DISCUSSION

In this preliminary study MRI was generally found to be a valid means of diagnosis of benign organic gynecologic pathology in the adolescent, particularly considering that it is a non-invasive method and ionizing radiations are not used.

However, the efficiency of MRI differed for the various pathologies examined. It was excellent for uterine malformations. It correctly identified the absence of the uterus in one case, the unicornuate structure and cavitation of its rudimentary horn in another, a 'double' uterus in two girls (and the respective subclasses), and a normal uterus in five. This success was facilitated

Table 1 MRI, US, laparoscopic and surgical findings

Patient no.	*Age*	*MRI*	*US*	*Laparoscopy*	*Surgery*
1	18	retroverted uterus, septum	retroverted 'double' uterus	retroverted uterus, stage I endometriosis	—
2	13	didelphic uterus, imperforate vagina	didelphic uterus, imperforate vagina	asymmetric bicornuate uterus	asymmetric bicornuate uterus
3	14	unicornuate uterus, cavitary rudimentary horn	unicornuate uterus, cavitary rudimentary horn	unicornuate uterus, rudimentary horn	unicorunate uterus, cavitary rudimentary horn
4	15	serous ovarian cyst	'uniloculata' ovarian cyst	mesosalpingeal cyst	mesosalpingeal cyst
5	17	polycystic ovaries	polycystic ovaries	polycystic ovaries	—
6	18	ovarian cyst	hydrosalpinx	pelvic inflammatory disease	—
7	18	hemorrhagic ovarian cyst	ovarian cyst with mixed content	hemorrhagic corpus luteum	—
8	17	Rokitansky's syndrome	Rokitansky's syndrome	Rokitansky's syndrome	Rokitansky's syndrome
9	17	no abnormal findings	no abnormal findings	stage II endometriosis	—

by exploring the uterus in frontal and transverse scans, oriented as closely as possible to the plane containing the tubal ostia and internal uterine os so as to visualize the peritoneal fundal contour and any indentation. Unlike US, MRI can also be used successfully to examine retroverted uteri and those with marked displacement when it is difficult to perform a correct fundal scan. Magnetic resonance imaging was more useful than laparoscopy in the case of uterus didelphys with imperforate hemivagina since it was possible to demonstrate simultaneously the presence of the vaginal sac not visible at intraperitoneal exploration.

Our only case of pelvic inflammatory disease (PID) was not diagnosed by MRI although it is reported in the literature that in these cases T_1-weighted images show regions of low intensity along the uterine surface and within pelvic peritoneal recesses due to inflammatory fluid[3]. In our patient MRI detected only a cystic formation of the ovary which at laparoscopic examination was revealed to be a periovarian serocele; the sonographer found only an enlargement of the left salpinx. Only with laparoscopy was it possible to obtain a precise picture of the extent of the disease, a sample of endoperitoneal exudate (on which to base treatment), and a prognosis.

Magnetic resonance imaging was reliable in identifying the nature of ovarian masses. Functional cysts in the patient with polycystic ovaries were correctly diagnosed as was the hematic content in the case of corpus luteum cyst. In the third patient with an ovarian mass, a cyst of the mesosalpinx was incorrectly diagnosed by MRI as a serous ovarian cyst. These usually generate low signal intensity on T_1- and high signal intensity on T_2-weighted images but are similar to cysts of the mesosalpinges and to the sequelae of PID[4].

In our study MRI failed to diagnose both minimal and mild endometriosis. It is reported in the literature that MRI is sufficiently precise in identifying the endometriotic nature of ovarian cysts[4] which present a homogeneous high signal intensity on T_1- and T_2-weighted scans. However, since such findings resemble those obtained for other hemorrhagic ovarian cysts, in our opinion endoscopy is still the best diagnostic tool in these cases.

In conclusion, we consider that MRI may have a role in differential diagnosis of benign organic gynecological pathology of the adolescent, especially of malformations. It does not require hospitalization or narcosis and thus is less costly than laparoscopy. It is non-invasive, allows a complete and detailed exploration of the subperitoneal structures, and can be performed even in patients in whom laparoscopic examination is risky or not desired.

REFERENCES

1. Fedele, L., Ferrazzi, E., Dorta, M., Vercellini, P. and Candiani, G.B. (1988). Ultrasonography in the differential diagnosis of 'double' uteri. *Fertil. Steril.*, **50**, 361–5
2. Buttram, V.C., Jr and Gibbons, W.E. (1979). Müllerian anomalies: a proposed classification (an analysis of 144 cases). *Fertil. Steril.*, **32**, 361–70
3. Hricak, H., Lany, C. and Schriock, E. (1985). Gynecologic masses: value of magnetic resonance imaging. *Am. J. Obstet. Gynecol.*, **153**, 31–7
4. Dooms, G.C., Hricak, H. and Tscholakoff, D. (1986). Adnexal structures: MR imaging. *Radiology*, **158**, 639–46

Section 1 continued

Part E

LHRH analogs: biochemical and clinical aspects

21

Growth factors as modulators of ovarian and endometrial function

G. Forti and M. Serio

INTRODUCTION

The menstrual cycle can be considered as the repetitive expression of the hypothalamic–pituitary–ovarian axis which induces structural and functional changes in the target tissues of the female reproductive tract (uterus, endometrium, vagina and oviduct). The primary regulators of ovarian activity are the two gonadotropins, follicle-stimulating hormone (FSH) and luteinizing hormone (LH): however several recent studies have focused on the potential role of local paracrine or autocrine signalling systems in the modulation of the ovarian activity induced by gonadotropins. The synergistic relationship between FSH and estradiol produced by granulosa cells represents a well known intraovarian positive autoregulatory feedback mechanism responsible for stimulating the rapid division of granulosa cells thus promoting follicular growth[1,2]. Recently many authors have reported that several growth factors can be produced and act at the ovarian level[3]. Moreover there is increasing evidence that growth factors can modulate the effects of ovarian steroids at the level of the uterus.

In this paper we will discuss some data concerning: the modulation of ovarian activity by insulin-like growth factor-I (IGF-I); and the modulation of the effects of gonadal steroids on uterine tissue by epidermal growth factor (EGF), IGF-I and other growth factors.

IGF-I, IGF-II AND OVARY

In vitro experiments have demonstrated that immunoreactive and bioactive ovarian IGF-I is present in granulosa cells of the rat. Its production is controlled by gonadotropins and growth hormone (GH)[4]. Moreover the IGF-I gene expression has been observed in rat ovary by determination of the specific mRNA levels[3].

In humans, gonadotropins are able to stimulate accumulation of IGF-II mRNA in granulosa cells, but GH is not[5]. However, in other experiments human granulosa cells stimulated with LH and FSH were able to produce considerable amounts of immunoassayable IGF-II in the culture medium, but also high doses of GH had the same effect[6]. Therefore the effect of GH on IGF-II production by granulosa cells *in vitro* remains questionable.

Concerning the effects of IGF-I on granulosa cells it has been demonstrated that this growth factor is able to stimulate the FSH-induced steroidogenesis and FSH-induced synthesis of LH receptors. These effects seem to be mediated throughout the type I IGF-I receptor[7].

Studies *in vivo* suggest that the major site of IGF-I production in the human is the liver. Moreover the circulating levels of IGF-I are clearly correlated with GH secretion[8].

We measured IGF-I by radioimmunoassay in the follicular fluid of eight women undergoing ovarian hyperstimulation for *in vitro* fertilization and we did not find any significant gradient in comparison to circulating levels (follicular fluid: 1.94 ± 1.1 mU/ml; serum 2.45 ± 1.1 mU/ml; mean $\pm$ SD). Similar results were obtained by Adashi *et al.*[7] Even if these data do not rule out the possibility of intraovarian IGF-I production, as *in situ* hybridization histochemistry experiments are not available at the moment, we can reasonably hypothesize that the majority of IGF-I reaches the follicle through the systemic circulation.

In addition, in collaboration with some colleagues from the Department of Anatomy of our University, we tried to localize the presence of IGF-I type I receptors in the human ovary by histoimmunochemical techniques using a very specific monoclonal antibody (α-IR3), which was kindly provided by Dr S. Jacobs (The Wellcome Research Laboratories, Research Triangle Park, NC, USA). The results of this study suggest that the amount of these receptors in granulosa cells and oocytes of the human ovary are not equal during the different phases of follicular growth. In particular the highest positivity for type I IGF-I receptor in the oocyte was found during the preantral phase of follicular development, whereas the granulosa cells were more positive during the antral phase[9].

These data suggest that the type I IGF-I receptor seems to be involved in the modulation of oocyte growth during the preantral phase and of granulosa cell differentiation during the antral phase.

GROWTH FACTORS AND UTERUS

EGF

EGF was detected by radioimmunoassay in uteri of 16-day-old mice and increased fivefold after estradiol administration[10]. EGF mRNA was also detected in uteri of immature mice and a twofold increase was observed after estrogen treatment[11]. Specific EGF receptors have been demonstrated in the rat uterus[12] and a threefold increase of these receptors has been reported in immature[13] and mature[14] female rats treated with pharmacological doses of estradiol. Taken together these data suggest estrogen modulation of EGF and its receptor. Autoradiographic studies in rat uterus have shown specific EGF binding to epithelial cells, stroma and myometrium[15]. In the human uterus specific binding sites for EGF have been demonstrated in myometrium, endometrium and leiomyomas[16]. Autoradiographic studies reported EGF binding in all major uterine cell types in the human[17]. It has also been reported that the proliferation of mouse uterine epithelial cells *in vitro* is enhanced by EGF[18].

Insulin-like growth factors

It has recently been reported that, liver apart, uterine expression of IGF-I mRNA was higher than in any other tissue tested[19]. In ovariectomized hypophysectomized rats acute estradiol administration has been reported to increase the uterine IGF-I gene expression 20-fold without affecting hepatic IGF-I gene expression[20]. Chronic estradiol administration is less effective, increasing uterine IGF-I gene expression only about fivefold[20]. These data suggest that estradiol is the physiological stimulator of IGF-I gene expression in uterine tissue whereas GH is the physiological stimulator of IGF-I gene expression in the liver.

Concerning the human, it has been recently reported that membrane preparations of human endometrium possess IGF-I receptors with the same size, affinity and specificity of those found in tissues regarded as targets for IGF-I action[21]. The number of these receptors does not change in the different phases of the cycle, however the human secretory endometrium in the luteal phase secretes a specific binding protein (which is identical to placental protein 12) which competes with membrane receptors for IGF-I binding[21,22]. According to these data it has been suggested:

(1) As a possible role for IGF-I in the proliferation and in the differentiation of the human endometrium;
(2) The specific binding protein could act as an autocrine–paracrine inhibitor of IGF-I action in the human endometrium.

Concerning the myometrium, Hoppener *et al.*[23] have recently reported the presence of IGF-I and IGF-II mRNAs in benign and malignant tumors from smooth muscle origin whereas in normal smooth muscle tissue of the uterus only IGF-I mRNA was present. Moreover the IGF-I mRNA content of tumors from smooth muscle origin was higher than in normal myometrium[23].

Transforming growth factor α (TGFα)

TGFα is a polypeptide with a 30% homology to EGF which shares the same receptor. Recently TGFα mRNA expression was reported in decidua[24].

Colony stimulating factor-1 (CSF-1)

CSF-1 is a glycosylated homodimeric polypeptide required for the survival, proliferation and differentiation of cells of the mononuclear phagocyte lineage[24]. CSF-1 (which would be better considered as a cytokine, i.e. a non-enzymic peptide involved in immunoinflammatory responses) was detected by radioimmunoassay in mouse uterus and its levels increased during pregnancy[25]. CSF-1 mRNA was also detected in mouse uterus and increased during pregnancy[26].

Other growth factors

Several other growth factors such as so called 'estromedins' and uterus-derived growth factors with similarities to the acidic and basic fibroblast growth factors have been described, but not yet fully characterized[27].

CONCLUSION

The reported ability of IGF-I to potentiate several FSH driven ovarian functions may account, at least in part, for the well known association between delayed puberty and isolated growth hormone deficiency and for the normal pubertal maturation observed during GH replacement therapy. According to this hypothesis it has been recently reported that GH treatment may facilitate ovarian maturation in postmenarchial monkeys[28].

Concerning the uterus the preliminary available data seem to suggest that endometrial and myometrial growth are probably modulated by EGF, IGF-I (and probably other growth factors and cytokines) which could mediate, at least in part, the *in vivo* mitogenic action of ovarian gonadal steroids.

We suggest also the possibility that peptide growth factors and cytokines could be involved in the pathogenesis of some uterine diseases, such as, respectively, endometriosis and fibroleiomyomata.

ACKNOWLEDGEMENT

This paper was supported by a grant from the University of Florence.

REFERENCES

1. Hsueh, A.J.W., Jones, P.B.C., Adashi, E.Y., Wang, C., Zhuang, L.Z. and Welsh, T.H. (1983). Intraovarian mechanisms in the hormonal control of granulosa cell differentiation in rats. *J. Reprod. Fertil.*, **69**, 325–31
2. Adashi, E.Y.G. and Hsueh, A.J.W. (1982). Estrogens augment the stimulation of ovarian aromatase activity by follicle-stimulating hormone in cultured rat granulosa cells. *J. Biol. Chem.*, **257**, 6077–82
3. Fauser, B.C.J.M., Golwzy, B. and Hsueh, A.J.W. (1988). Differentiation of ovarian and testicular cells: intragonadal regulation by growth factors. In Cooke, B.A. and Sharpe, R.M. (eds). *Molecular and Cellular Endocrinology of the Testis*, pp. 281–95 (New York: Raven Press)
4. Hsueh, A.J.W. (1986). Paracrine mechanisms involved in granulosa cell differentiation. *Clin. Endocrinol. Metab.*, **15**, 117–25
5. Voutilainen, R. and Miller, W. (1987). Coordinate tropic hormone regulation of mRNAs for insulin-like growth factor II and the cholestrol side chain cleavage enzyme, p 450 scc, in human steroidogenetic tissues. *Proc. Natl. Acad. Sci., USA*, **84**, 1590–5

6. Ramasharma, K. and Li, C.H. (1987). Human pituitary and placental hormones control human insulin-like growth factor II secretion in human granulosa cells. *Proc. Natl. Acad. Sci., USA*, **84**, 2643–51
7. Adashi, E.Y., Resnick, C.E., D'Ercole, A.J., Svoboda, M.E. and Van Wik, J.J. (1985). Insulin-like growth factors as intraovarian regulators of granulosa cell growth and function. *Endocr. Rev.*, **6**, 400–21
8. Wallis, M. (1988). Mechanism of action of growth hormone. In Cooke, R.J.B. and Van Der Molen, H.J. (eds). *Hormones and their Action*, part II, pp. 265–73. (Amsterdam: Elsevier)
9. Balboni, G.C., Vannelli, G.B., Barni, T., Orlando, C. and Serio, M. (1987). Transferrin and somatomedin C receptors in the human ovarian follicles. *Fertil. Steril.*, **48**, 796–801
10. Gonzalez, F., Lakshmanan, J., Hoath, S. and Fisher, D.A. (1984). Effect of oestradiol-17β on uterine epidermal growth factor concentration in immature mice. *Acta Endocrinol. (Kbh)*, **105**, 425–8
11. DiAugustine, R.P., Petrusz, P., Bell, G.I., Brown, C.F., Korach, K.S., McLachlan, J.A. and Teng, C.T. (1988). Influence of estrogens on mouse uterine epidermal growth factor precursor protein and messenger ribonucleic acid. *Endocrinology*, **122**, 2355–63
12. Mukku, R.V. and Stancel, G.M. (1985). Receptors for epidermal growth factor in the rat uterus. *Endocrinology*, **117**, 149–54
13. Mukku, R.V. and Stancel, G.M. (1985). Regulation of epidermal growth factor receptor by estrogen. *J. Biol. Chem.*, **260**, 9820–4
14. Gardner, R.M., Verner, G., Kirkland, J.L. and Stancel, G.M. (1989). Regulation of uterine epidermal growth factor (EGF) receptors by estrogen in the mature rat and during the estrous cycle. *J. Steroid Biochem.*, **32**, 339–43
15. Lin, T.H., Mukku, V.R., Verner, G., Kirkland, J.L. and Stancel, G.M. (1988). Autoradiographic localization of epidermal growth factor receptors to all major uterine cell types. *Biol. Reprod.*, **38**, 403–11
16. Hofmann, G.E., Rao, C.V., Barrows, G.H., Schultz, G.S. and Sanfilippo, J.S. (1984). *J. Clin. Endocrinol. Metab.*, **58**, 880–4
17. Chegini, N., Rao, C.V., Wakim, N. and Sanfilippo, J. (1986). Binding of ^{125}I-epidermal growth factor in human uterus. *Cell Tissue Res.*, **246**, 543–8
18. Tomooka, Y., DiAugustine, R.P. and McLachlan, J.A. (1986). Proliferation of mouse uterine epithelial cells *in vitro*. *Endocrinology*, **118**, 1011–18
19. Murphy, L.J., Bell, G.I. and Friesen, H.G. (1987). Tissue distribution of insulin-like growth factor-1 and 2 messenger ribonucleic acid in the adult rat. *Endocrinology*, **120**, 1279–82
20. Murphy, L.J. and Friesen, H.G. (1988). Differential effects of estrogen and growth hormone on uterine and hepatic insulin-like growth factor-I gene expression in the ovariectomized hypophysectomized rat. *Endocrinology*, **122**, 325–32
21. Rutanen, E.M., Pekonen, F. and Makinen, T. (1988). Soluble 34K binding protein inhibits the binding of insulin-like growth factor-I to its cell receptors in human secretory phase endometrium: evidence for autocrine/paracrine regulation of growth factor action. *J. Clin. Endocrinol. Metab.*, **66**, 173–80
22. Bell, S.C. (1988). Endometrial IGF-binding protein: a paracrine role in controlling endometrial or trophoblast growth. *Res. Reprod.*, **20**, 3
23. Hoppener, J.W.M., Mosselman, S., Roholl, P.J.M., Lambrechts, C., Slebos, R.J.C., de Pagter-Holthuizen, P., Lips, C.J.M., Jansz, H.S. and Sussenbach, J.S. (1988). Expression of insulin-like growth factor-I and -II genes in human smooth muscle tumors. *EMBO J.*, **5**, 1379–85
24. Han, V.K.M., Hunter, E.S., Pratt, R.M., Zendegui, J.G. and Lee, D.C. (1987). Expression of rat transforming growth factor alpha mRNA during development occurs predominantly in maternal decidua. *Mol. Cell. Biol.*, **7**, 2335–43
25. Bartocci, A., Pollard, J.W. and Stanley, E.R. (1986). Regulation of colony-stimulating factor 1 during pregnancy. *J. Exp. Med.*, **164**, 956–61
26. Pollard, J.W., Bartocci, A., Arceci, R., Orlofsky, A., Ladner, M.B. and Stanley, E.R. (1987). Apparent role of the macrophage growth factor, CSF-1, in placental development. *Nature*, **330**, 484–6
27. Brigstock, D.R., Heap, R.B. and Brown, K.D. (1989). Polypeptide growth factors in uterine tissues and secretions. *J. Reprod. Fertil.*, **85**, 747–58
28. Wilson, M.E., Gordon, T.P., Rudman, C.G. and Tanner, J.M. (1989). Effects of growth hormone on the tempo of sexual maturation in female rhesus monkeys. *J. Clin. Endocrinol. Metab.*, **68**, 29–38

22

Pharmacology of the luteinizing hormone-releasing hormone analog, Zoladex*

R. A. V. Milsted and B. J. A. Furr

INTRODUCTION

It is well established that androgens stimulate the growth of a majority of prostate cancers and estrogens enhance the growth of about one-third of all breast cancers. A variety of approaches have been adopted to induce androgen and estrogen withdrawal from the tumor cell in order to prevent prostate and breast tumor progression. Antiestrogens, like Nolvadex*[1] and antiandrogens such as cyproterone acetate[2], flutamide[3], nilutamide[4] and Casodex*[5] compete with the relevant stimulatory hormone for binding to a cytosolic receptor protein, but have little or no intrinsic activity as estrogens or androgens respectively.

A knowledge of the processes which regulate gonadal steroid synthesis has led to further approaches to tumor therapy. Administration of estrogens to men with prostate cancer inhibits gonadotropin secretion from the pituitary gland, which leads to a form of medical castration[6]. However, clinical remissions seen in prostate cancer patients were offset by increased serious cardiovascular complications[7].

Recently, the availability of potent analogs of luteinizing hormone-releasing hormone (LHRH) has led to a selective effect on pituitary gonadotropin release which has caused, in turn, a form of medical castration: the side-effect profile is greatly superior to that associated with the administration of estrogens and, indeed, the only side-effects reported are those predicted from a medical castration. Zoladex* (ICI 118,630: D-Ser(Bu^t)^6,Azgly^{10}-LHRH; Figure 1), is a novel, potent LHRH analog which can be used for the treatment of hormone-responsive diseases[8]. This paper describes pharmacological studies with Zoladex, attempts to explain its mode of action and reports on an exciting and innovative depot formulation which allows the drug to be released continuously over at least 28 days.

*Zoladex, Nolvadex and Casodex are trade marks, the property of Imperial Chemical Industries PLC

Pyro - Glu - His - Trp - Ser - Tyr - Gly - Leu - Arg - Pro - Gly - NH_2

LH - RH

Pyro - Glu - His - Trp - Ser - Tyr - D - Ser (Bu^t) - Leu - Arg - Pro - Azgly NH_2

ZOLADEX (ICI 118,630 D - SER (Bu^t)^6 $AzGly^{10}$ - LH - RH)

Figure 1 Structures of LHRH and Zoladex

PHARMACOLOGICAL STUDIES WITH AQUEOUS SOLUTIONS OF ZOLADEX

Zoladex is an LHRH agonist and when given acutely will induce follicle-stimulating hormone (FSH) and luteinizing hormone (LH) secretion (Figure 2). In the rat, a single intramuscular injection of 5 μg Zoladex elicits a supraphysiological release of LH (Figure 2). In this respect it is at least 100 times as potent as LHRH[9].

Zoladex will also initiate LH release and ovulation in androgen-sterilized constant estrus rats (Table 1). When given by the intramuscular (i.m.), subcutaneous (s.c.) or intravenous (i.v.) routes Zoladex is at least 100 times as potent as LHRH. It should be emphasized, however, that it is far less effective when given intravaginally, orally (p.o.) or intranasally and in the latter case absorption was noted to both low and variable.

The high potency of Zoladex is due in part to an enhanced affinity for the pituitary LHRH receptor (Figure 3), which leads to around a 10-fold increase in potency compared with LHRH at releasing LH from pituitary cells in culture (Figure 4). The high potency *in vivo* is also due to a longer elimination halflife; in man, the halflife of Zoladex is more than 4 h compared with values of less than 10 min for LHRH[10].

When given chronically, Zoladex induces an inhibition of gonadal steroid secretion which produces a castration-like state in rats, dogs and primates[8,11,12]. Superficially, this is unexpected and has frequently, but inappropriately, been described as the paradoxical effect of LHRH agonists. An explanation for this observation is clearly required.

MODE OF ACTION OF ZOLADEX

Figure 5*a* illustrates the release of gonadotropin from the pituitary gland in response to endogenous LHRH. Normally, LHRH is released from the hypothalamus as a series of small pulses at approximately 90 min intervals[13,14]. The LHRH travels via the hypothalamic–pituitary portal system to the pituitary gland where it binds to LHRH receptors present on the cell surface. Receptors occupied by LHRH aggregate into clumps, 'coated pits' are formed and the receptor–ligand complex is internalized thus disappearing from the cell surface. There is usually an excess of LHRH receptors present on the pituitary cell and receptor resynthesis occurs at a rate which allows replenishment before the next LHRH pulse occurs. This process allows an

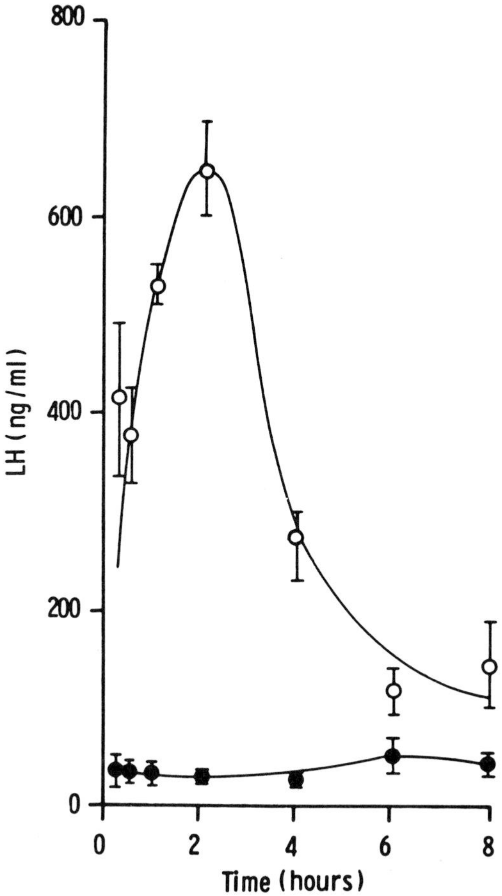

Figure 2 Plasma LH concentrations in mature virgin female rats given a single intramuscular injection of 5 μg Zoladex at time 0 (open circles). The closed circles are the values for saline-treated controls. The points indicated are the mean values for five animals with the standard error of the mean

orderly and systematic secretion of LH. When Zoladex is first given at relatively high dosage, the majority of the receptors are occupied (Figure 5*b*) and subsequently internalized. This leads to supraphysiological LH secretion and an initial stimulation of gonadal function. However, the marked loss of LH receptors and the failure of receptor replenishment due to the continuing presence of Zoladex leads to a pituitary cell which has few receptors and which is, therefore, unable to respond to Zoladex (Figure 5*c*). Consequently LH secretion is markedly reduced which results in gonadal atrophy, a reduction in steroid secretion and the regression of hormone-responsive tissues including mammary and prostate tumors. This phenomenon has long been recognized and termed either tachyphylaxis or tissue desensitization but is perhaps more appropriately now described as receptor down-regulation. It

Table 1 Induction of ovulation in androgen-sterilized, constant estrus rats by Zoladex

Route	*Dose* (μg)	*Number ovulating/ number treated*	*% response*
Intravenous	0.005	9/9	100
	0.0031	10/18	55.6
	0.0016	5/21	23.8
	0.0008	0/12	0
Per os	25	3/3	100
	10	5/6	83.3
	5	5/12	41.7
	2.5	2/6	33
Intravaginal	25	2/3	67
	10	0/3	0
Intranasal	1	2/5	40

is, therefore, clearly a predictable, not paradoxical, effect of chronic therapy with LHRH agonists. Usually tachyphylaxis is regarded as a serious disadvantage in a drug therapy. Here, for the first time, advantage is taken of this phenomenon to produce an effective therapy.

DEVELOPMENT AND PROPERTIES OF A DEPOT FORMULATION OF ZOLADEX

Although early preclinical studies clearly demonstrated the effectiveness of daily s.c. injections of Zoladex in inducing regression of sex hormone-responsive tumors[11], it was felt that this would limit clinical acceptability and reduce patient compliance with therapy. Several formulations were considered but the majority were rejected because of concerns about reliability of drug delivery or convenience. Administration of Zoladex by vaginal pessaries limited treatment to women and there was low and variable absorption. Similarly, in our experience, absorption of the drug after nasal administration was also low and unacceptably variable. Furthermore, nasal application had to be made several times daily to achieve the desired biological effect which again raised concerns about the likelihood of compliance. Others have found nasal spray formulations to be acceptable but compliance is recognized as a problem[15].

A very ambitious target was selected for a drug delivery system for Zoladex namely the development of a biodegradable, sustained release formulation which would deliver the drug over a period of at least 28 days. Efforts were concentrated on poly (d, l-lactide) and poly (d, l-lactide-*co*-glycolide) since these have been used for the sustained delivery of low molecular weight compounds such as steroids[16], narcotic antagonists[17] and antimalarial drugs[18]. Moreover, since these polymers have been evaluated as biodegradable surgical sutures and prostheses it is known that they are both pharmaceutically and toxicologically acceptable. This work culminated in the development of a depot based on a 50:50 poly (d, l-lactide-*co*-glycolide) polymer throughout which the drug is homogeneously dispersed. The depot

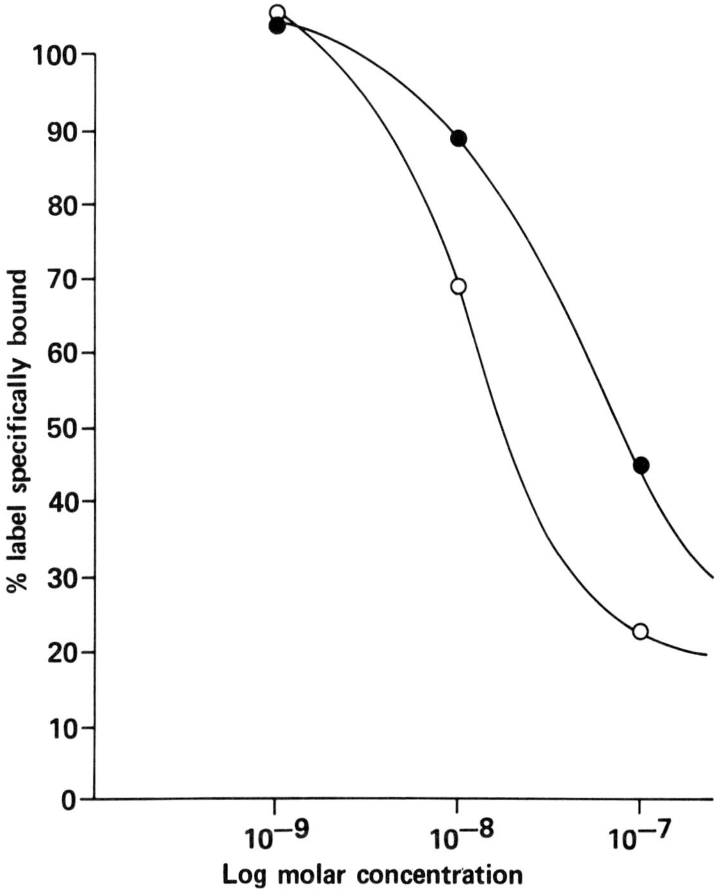

Figure 3 Relative potencies of Zoladex (open circles) and LHRH (closed circles) in causing displacement of $[I^{125}]$D-Leu^6-proethylamide^9-LHRH from a rat pituitary membrane receptor preparation

is in the form of a rod approximately 1 mm in diameter and 3–6 mm length containing 500–1000 μg Zoladex and will suppress ovarian function in rats for a period of 33 days. Figure 6 shows the suppression of estrogen secretion in adult female rats, assessed by vaginal smear inspection, following a single depot containing 500 μg Zoladex.

Although the primary objective was to produce a formulation of the drug which was more convenient to administer and which would secure improved compliance, the depot formulation also appears to have improved efficacy. This was demonstrated in rats which were given a single subcutaneous bolus dose of 50 μg Zoladex after either pretreatment with daily subcutaneous injections of saline or 50 μg Zoladex for 6 weeks or, alternatively, at the start of the experiment and at 4 weeks, a single subcutaneous depot, calculated to release a dose of Zoladex equivalent to 50 μg daily. Rats were killed at various times after the final treatment and serum LH was determined by

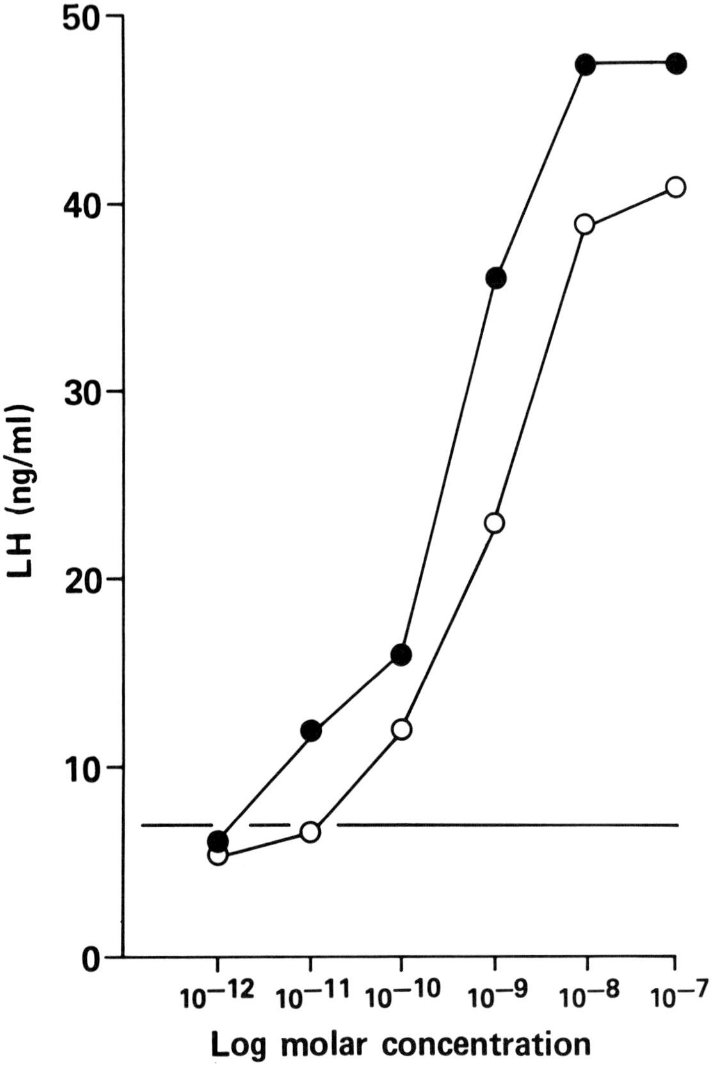

Figure 4 Release of LH from dispersed rat pituitary cells into the culture medium after 4 h incubation in response to increasing concentration of Zoladex (closed circles) and LHRH (open circles). Control values shown by the horizontal line indicate the release rate in the absence of LHRH or LHRH agonist

radioimmunoassay in blood collected from the dorsal aorta. The results are shown in Figure 7.

As expected, the bolus dose of Zoladex elicited a massive secretion of LH in the rats pretreated with saline. In spite of pretreatment for 6 weeks with 50 μg Zoladex daily, the bolus dose of the drug still caused a substantial release of LH, although a clear degree of desensitization of the pituitary

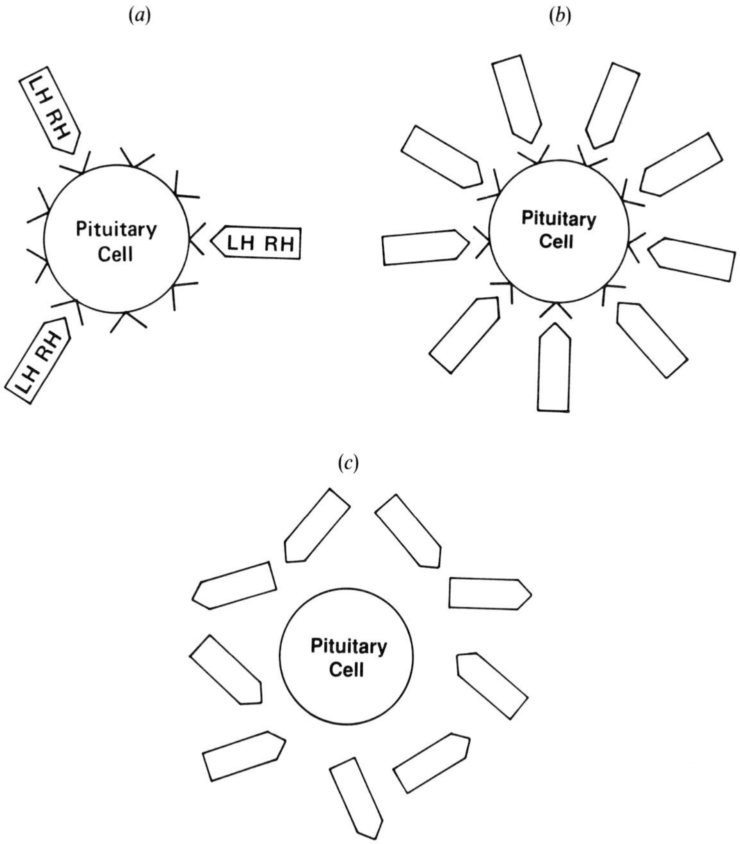

Figure 5 Diagrammatic representation of pituitary gland response to (*a*) an endogenous pulse of LHRH; (*b*) an acute bolus of Zoladex; (*c*) chronic presence of Zoladex

gland occurred. In contrast, there was negligible LH secretion in response to the bolus injection in rats pretreated with the Zoladex depot, indicating an improved level of pituitary desensitization by this formulation. Similarly, in the male monkey, *Macacca nemestrina*, the depot formulation of Zoladex induces a fall in plasma testosterone into the castrate range whereas daily s.c. injections are relatively ineffective. It should be noted that recovery of testis function occurred around 40 days after the final depot was administered. This advantage of depot Zoladex has also been observed in the clinic where incomplete pituitary desensitization is seen in some patients given daily s.c. injections of the drug in contrast to complete pituitary desensitization in those given Zoladex depot[19].

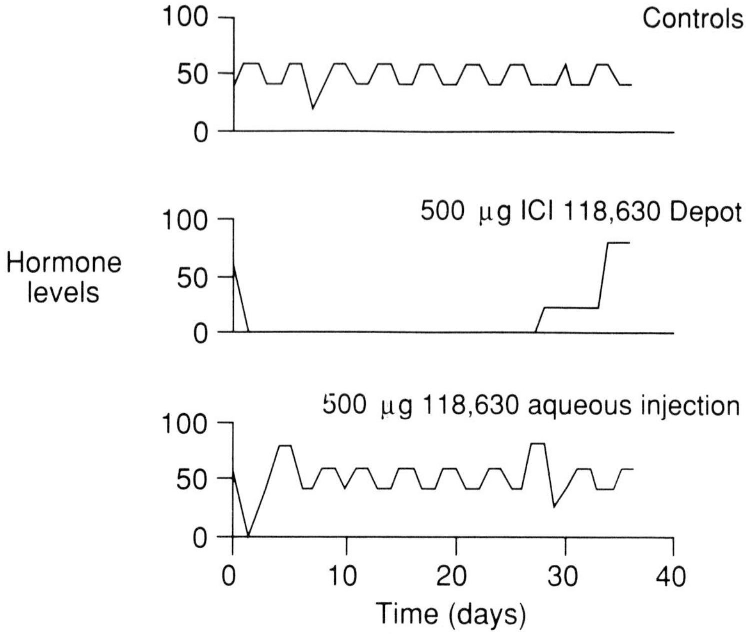

Figure 6 Effect of a single s.c. injection of 500 μg Zoladex (ICI 118,630) either as a depot formulation or as an aqueous injection on 1% hydroxmethyl cellulose on ovarian activity in adult female rats. Control data are shown in the upper panel for comparison

EFFECTS OF DEPOT ZOLADEX IN ANIMALS BEARING SEX HORMONE-RESPONSIVE TUMORS

The androgen-responsive, Dunning R3327H, transplantable rat prostate, tumor[20] was used in several studies to determine the efficacy of Zoladex depot administration.

Single subcutaneous depots containing 1 mg Zoladex given every 28 days to rats bearing Dunning R3327H prostate tumors implanted on each flank, caused a marked inhibition of tumor growth to values indistinguishable from those in surgically castrated rats (Figure 8). Twenty-one days after the eighth depot was given the rats were killed and the weights of the sex organs assessed and serum hormone concentrations measured by radioimmuno-assay.

Testes weights were about 10% those of control rats of a similar age and weight and showed atrophic histological changes; ventral prostate gland and seminal vesicle weights were identical to those in the surgically castrated group and, histologically, were also completely atrophic. Serum LH and testosterone were undetectable in the group given Zoladex depot and serum FSH was decreased by 60–70%.

A comparison of the efficacy of surgical castration, depot Zoladex, a novel peripherally-selective antiandrogen[5] and the combination, in the treatment of Dunning R3327H tumors is shown in Figure 9. All of the treatments cause a significant reduction in tumor growth compared to values found for control

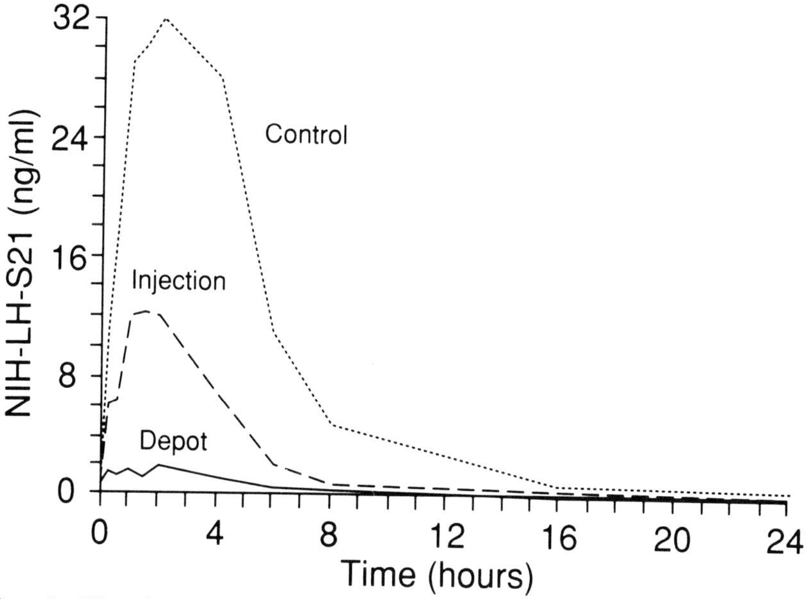

Figure 7 Effect of a 50 μg s.c. bolus dose of Zoladex on LH release in mature male rats given either saline (......) or 50 μg Zoladex (– – –) daily for 6 weeks or a single s.c. depot containing Zoladex calculated to release approximately 50 μg daily (———) at the start of the experiment and at day 28. The bolus dose of 50 μg Zoladex was injected 6 weeks after the start of the experiment and serum LH was measured by radioimmunoassay at the times shown

animals but none of the treatments is more effective than any other. Since the rat does not secrete significant quantities of adrenal androgens these data, while interesting, should not be taken to disprove the total androgen withdrawal hypothesis advanced by Labrie and co-workers[21].

Zoladex depot has also proved to be highly effective against dimethylbenz-anthracene-induced rat mammary tumors. Administration of single subcutaneous depots containing 500 μg Zoladex every 28 days caused an inhibition of estrogen secretion, the disappearance of cornified cells from vaginal smears and frequently complete tumor regression[11]. When given at days 30, 58 and 86 after administration of the carcinogen, single depots containing 500 μg Zoladex delayed the appearance of tumors for a period of around 100 days, i.e. the expected duration of action of such a treatment regimen[11].

When given at 28 day intervals, starting on day 30 after administration of the carcinogen, single s.c. depots of Zoladex caused a more profound inhibition of tumor appearance and only nine out of 21 rats had mammary tumors at the end of the study on day 450[11]. Those tumors which were found did not regress following ovariectomy and so were classified as non-hormone responsive. It is concluded from this study, which approximates the adjuvant therapy setting, that Zoladex may be of benefit as a treatment for primary breast cancer postmastectomy in premenopausal women.

In none of these studies were side-effects observed and there was no lesion at any injection site.

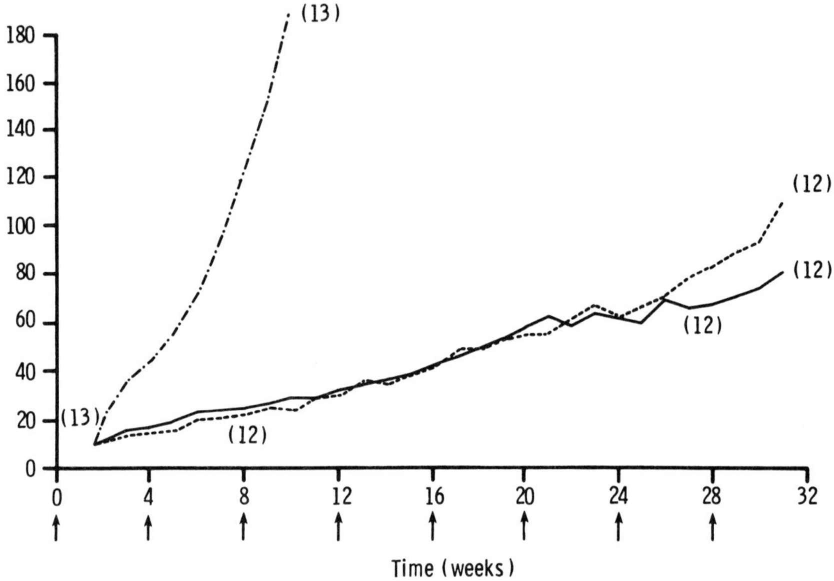

Figure 8 Growth of Dunning R3327H androgen-responsive prostate tumors in male rats which were either surgically castrated (——) or given a single s.c. depot without Zoladex (–·–) or containing 1 mg Zoladex (- - - -) at 28 day intervals on eight occasions as shown by the arrows. The values are expressed as % increase in mean tumor area

CONCLUSIONS

Zoladex is a potent LHRH agonist which, when given chronically at relatively high doses, causes a predictable pituitary desensitization and consequently an inhibition of pituitary gonadotropin secretion: this in turn leads to gonadal and accessory sex organ atrophy. The biodegradable, biocompatible Zoladex depot, which releases the drug continuously over at least 28 days, is both more convenient to administer and more efficacious in a number of test systems than daily s.c. injections. Particularly, it is highly effective at inducing regression of sex hormone-responsive prostate and mammary tumors.

The pharmacological profile of Zoladex depot, its excellent tolerance and its convenience to administer make it a genuine alternative to surgery for treatment of sex hormone-responsive tumors in men and women.

ACKNOWLEDGEMENT

NIAMDD, Professor L. E. Reichert and G. D. Niswender for reagents for FSH, LH and prolactin radioimmunoassays. The US National Prostate Cancer Agency for supplies of rats bearing Dunning R3327H tumors. The many colleagues in ICI Pharmaceuticals Division Research Department who have made this development possible, particularly A. S. Dutta, F. G. Hutchinson and B. E. Valcaccia.

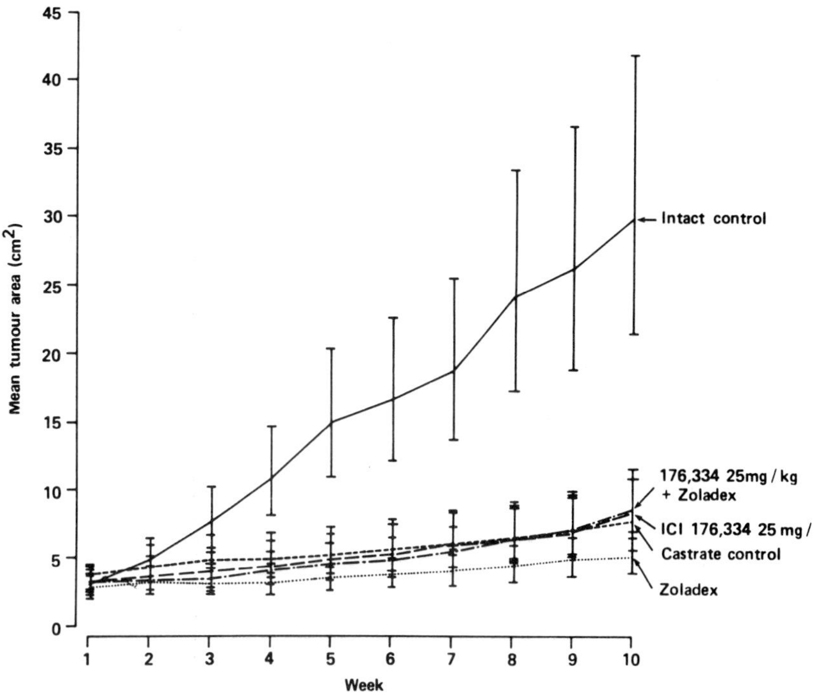

Figure 9 Effect of surgical castration, depot Zoladex given s.c. every 28 days, ICI 176,334 (novel peripherally selective antiandrogen) given p.o. daily and the combination of the two drugs on growth of the Dunning R3327H prostate tumor. Data from intact control animals are shown by comparison. The results show the mean tumor area ± SEM

REFERENCES

1. Furr, B.J.A. and Jordan, V.C. (1984). The pharmacology and clinical uses of tamoxifen. *Pharmacol. Ther.*, **25**, 127–205
2. Neumann, F. (1987). Pharmacology and clinical uses of cyproterone acetate. In Furr, B.J.A. and Wakeling, A. E. (eds). *Pharmacology and Clinical Uses of Inhibitors of Hormone Secretion and Action.* pp. 132–59. (London: Bailliere Tindall)
3. Neri, R. and Kassem, N. (1987). Pharmacology and clinical uses of flutamide. In Furr, B.J.A. and Wakeling, A.E. (eds). *Pharmacology and Clinical Uses of Inhibitors of Hormone Secretion and Action*, pp. 160–9 (London: Bailliere Tindall)
4. Moguilewsky, M., Fiet, J., Tournemine, C. and Raynaud, J-P. (1986). Pharmacology of an antiandrogen, Anandron, used as an adjuvant therapy in the treatment of prostate cancer. *J. Steroid Biochem.*, **24**, 139–46
5. Furr, B.J.A., Valcaccia, B., Curry, B., Woodburn, J.R., Chesterson, G. and Tucker, H. (1987). A novel non-steroidal, peripherally selective antiandrogen. *J. Endocrinol.*, **113**, R7–R9
6. Robinson, M.R.G. (1982). Carcinoma of the prostate: hormonal therapy. In Furr, B.J.A. (ed). *Clinics in Oncology*, *Volume* 1, pp. 233–43 (London: W.B. Saunders)
7. Veterans Administration Cooperative Urological Research Group. (1967). Treatment and survival of patients with cancer of the prostate. *Surg. Gynecol. Obstet.*, **124**, 1011–17
8. Furr, B.J.A. (1981). Treatment of hormone-responsive rat mammary and prostate tumors with Zoladex depot. In Klijn, J.G.M., Paridaens, R. and Foekens, J.A. (eds). *Hormonal Manipulation of Cancer: Peptides, Growth Factors and New (anti) Steroidal Agents.* pp. 213–23 (New York: Raven Press)
9. Maynard, P.V. and Nicholson, R.I. (1979). Biological effects of high dose levels of a series

of new LH-RH analogues in intact female rats. *Br. J. Cancer*, **39**, 274–9
10. Swaisland, A.J., Adam, H.K., Barker, Y., Holmes, B. and Hutchinson, F.G. (1988). Tailored release profiles for Zoladex using biodegradable polymers. *Pharm. Weekblad.*, **10**, 57
11. Furr, B.J.A. and Nicholson, R.I. (1982). Use of analogues of luteinizing hormone-releasing hormone for the treatment of cancer. *J. Reprod. Fertil.*, **64**, 529–39
12. Furr, B.J.A. and Hutchinson, F.G. (1985). Biodegradable sustained release formulation of the LH-RH analogue Zoladex for the treatment of hormone-responsive tumors. In Schroeder, F.H. and Richards, B. (eds.) *EORTC genitourinary group monograph* 2, *Part A. therapeutic principles in metastatic prostatic cancer.* pp. 143–53 (New York: Liss)
13. Nankin, H.R. and Troen, P. (1971). Repetitive luteinizing hormone elevations in serum of normal men. *J. Clin. Endocrinol. Metab.*, **33**, 558–60
14. Santen, R.J. and Bardin, C.W. (1973). Episodic luteinizing hormone secretion in man. *J. Clin. Invest.*, **52**, 2617–28
15. Rajfer, J., Handelsman, D.J., Crum, A., Steiner, B., Peterson, M. and Swerdloff, R.S. (1986). Comparison of the efficacy of subcutaneous and nasal spray Buserelin treatment in suppression of testicular steroidogenesis in men with prostate cancer. *Fertil. Steril.*, **46**, 104–10
16. Beck, L.R., Cowsar, D.R., Lewis, D.H. *et al.* (1979). A new long-acting injectable microcapsule system for the administration of progesterone. *Fertil Steril.*, **31**, 545–51
17. Schwope, A.D., Wise, D.L. and Howed, J.F. (1975). Lactic/glycolic acid polymers as narcotic antagonist delivery systems. *Life Sci.*, **17**, 1877–85
18. Wise, D.L., McCormick, G.J., Willet, G.P. and Anderson, L.C. (1976). Sustained release of an antimalarial drug using a copolymer of glycolic/lactic acid. *Life Sci.*, **19**, 867–73
19. Grant, J.B.F., Ahmed, S.R., Shalet, S.M., Costello, C.B., Howell, A. and Blacklock, N.J. (1986). Testosterone and gonadotropin profiles in patients on daily or monthly LH-RH analogue (Zoladex) compared with orchidectomy. *Br. J. Urol.*, **58**, 539–44
20. Smolev, J.K., Heston, W.D.W., Scott, W.W. and Coffey, D.S. (1977). Characterisation of the Dunning R3327H prostatic adenocarcinoma: an appropriate animal model for prostatic cancer. *Cancer Treat. Rep.*, **61**, 273–87
21. Labrie, F., Dupont, A. and Belanger, A. (1985). Complete androgen blockade for the treatment of prostate cancer. In DeVita, V.T., Hellman, S. and Rosenberg, S.A. (eds). *Important Advances in Oncology*, pp. 193–217 (Philadelphia: Lipincott)

23

Endometriosis: past, present and future

G. Benagiano, C. Napolitano and R. Marziani

INTRODUCTION

It is commonly believed that the first mention of endometriosis was that made by Sampson[1] in March 1921 when he described 'perforating hemorrhagic (chocolate) cysts of the ovary' and pointed out their importance and especially their relation to 'pelvic adenomas of endometrial type (adenomyoma of the uterus, rectovaginal septum, sigmoid, etc.)'. In his original work Sampson reported that 'the cyst on the ovary is found adherent, and in freeing-in the chocolate contents escape because of a previous perforation. The histological study of these hematomas shows that periodic hemorrhage similar to that of menstruation, occurs'. He concludes: 'we have come to the conclusion that these ovarian hematomas are of endometrial type'.

In his second major paper on the subject, published in 1927[2], Sampson describes endometriosis as: 'The presence of ectopic tissue which possesses the histological structure and function of the uterine mucosa', and states 'it also includes the abnormal conditions which may result not only from the invasion of organs and other structures by this tissue, but also from its relation to menstruation'.

Notwithstanding the major contribution by Sampson, a review of the literature on endometriosis reveals extensive investigation of this subject by several authors prior to him, since Cullen[3] in March 1895 reported at a meeting of the Johns Hopkins Hospital Medical Society the first case ever described of ectopic uterine mucosa, that of an 'adenomyoma' of the uterus; this tumor consisted of non-striped muscle with islands of uterine mucosa. The following year Cullen[4] reported a case of 'adenomyoma' of the round ligament; he states: 'on the histological examination, they are found to be made up of non-striped muscle, fibrous tissue, and the characteristic uterine glands'.

In 1898, Russel[5] reported a case of a strange tumor in which he found endometrial tissue within an ovary. He states 'on microscopic study we were astonished to find areas which were an exact prototype of the uterine glands and interglandular connective tissue'. In spite of this early report, none of the studies published in subsequent years on 'ovarian haematomas'[6-10] mentioned the possibility that they may originate as a consequence of the presence of endometrial tissue, until Lockyer[11] in 1918 reported 'a bloody cyst in the ovary' and named it 'extrauterine adenomyoma'.

Continuing his work on 'adenomyomas', Cullen[13] reported a series of cases collected between 1913 and 1919 where endometriotic implants were found in the rectovaginal septum and elsewhere in the pelvis. Additional cases of ovarian endometriosis were published before Sampson's first description: in 1919 Casler[14] detailed a case of 'menstruation after complete hysterectomy due to uterine mucosa in remaining ovary'; the following year Mahle and MacCarty[15] reported 10 cases of 'adenomyoma' of uterine type where 'tarry' cysts were found in both ovaries and Norris[16] described 'a case of a well developed and apparently functioning endometrium within the ovary'. It was however, the publication of the first of Samspon's classic articles, read before the American Gynecologic Society in 1921[1] that intensified the investigation of endometriosis, particularly of its histogenesis.

ETIOPATHOGENESIS

Various hypotheses have been formulated to explain the pathogenesis and histogenesis of endometriosis. The first, and probably – until recently – the most widely accepted, dates back to Sampson's[2] classic paper of 1927: 'endometriosis is due to menstrual dissemination and implantation of endometrial tissue into the peritoneal cavity'. The simple implantation theory was followed by a more complex one proposed by Novak[17]: according to his theory, menstrual debris acts by causing mesothelial metaplasia.

Several experimental data support Sampson's theory: Blumenkrantz *et al.*[18] reported in 1981 that nine of 11 menstruating women, undergoing peritoneal dialysis, had blood present regularly in the dialysate during the time of their period. Furthermore, Halme *et al.*[19] reported in 1982 that, of 80 peritoneal fluid samples, four obtained during menses were bloody and in 1984[20] that blood was found at laparoscopy or laparotomy in the peritoneal fluid in 90% of 331 women with patent tubes during the perimenstruum.

The second theory, advanced by Iwanoff and Meyer[21,22] in 1930 suggests that 'endometriosis is the result of metaplasia of the celomic epithelium'. This theory is based on known embryological facts. It offers a logical explanation for the development of endometriosis in males and explains its growth in all known locations. Nevertheless, the irritative or hormonal stimuli which cause the celomic epithelium to develop into endometrial-like tissue are still unknown. This theory was further elaborated by Meigs[23] who believes that 'endometriosis is the result of activation of the celomic epithelium by an unusual number of uninterrupted menstrual cycles'. There is good experimental support also for the Iwanoff and Meyer theory. Indeed, endometriosis has been observed in: males on hormonal therapy[24]; the urinary bladder of a man with prostatic carcinoma[25]; a case of Turner's syndrome treated with cyclical estrogen–progestogen combinations[26] and a woman with Rokitanski–Kuster–Hauser syndrome[27]. Finally, the observation by Vasquez *et al.*[28] of the existence of microscopic metaplastic endometriotic lesions, not covered by mesothelium but in direct sequence with it, lends credibility to the existence of 'continuous' metaplastic processes in the peritoneum.

Additional theories suggest that endometriosis may be due to the diffusion of endometrial cells through the vascular and lymphatic systems[29] and could be facilitated by the presence of genetic[30,31], immunological and hormonal[32] factors.

DIAGNOSIS

In the early days clinical diagnosis of endometriosis was considered difficult and in many cases impossible. Indeed, before laparoscopy became commonly utilized, the existence of additional pelvic pathology, which in many cases accompanies endometriosis, obscured its presence thereby clouding the diagnostic picture[33]. It is generally agreed that it is difficult to estimate accurately the extent of pelvic endometriosis by bimanual examination[34]. This is why clinical diagnosis of endometriosis remains difficult and suspicion must be confirmed by direct visualization of endometriotic lesions at laparoscopy or laparotomy.

The symptoms of endometriosis are variable and may not be directly related to the extent and severity of the disease. They are: pelvic pain, dysmenorrhea, infertility, dyspareunia, rectal pain and tenesmus.

More recently some limited hope for a non-invasive technique for the diagnosis of endometriosis has been provided by the observation that cells deriving from celomic embryonic epithelium possess the surface antigen Ca-125, which can then be measured in peripheral blood[35-6]. Unfortunately this technique lacks specificity and it is unlikely that it will contribute to the accuracy of diagnosis.

ENDOMETRIOSIS AND INFERTILITY

Sampson[1,2] was the first to report that the 'association of infertility with endometriosis has been repeatedly found in the analysis of case histories of the lesions'. A definite decrement in fertility even in patients with mild endometriosis, has been demonstrated[37,38]. In fact, between 30% and 40% of women with endometriosis are infertile, twice the general population rate[39,40].

Whereas it is easy to understand the many possible reasons why severe endometriosis and the ensuing adhesions can cause infertility, the relationship is more dubious in patients with mild endometriosis where the oviducts are usually patent and cycles are usually ovulatory. Mettler and Semm[41] have listed several factors which may be involved in infertility associated with mild endometriosis. They are: interference with spermatozoal or ovum transport because of mechanical factors within the Fallopian tubes; disturbance of the ovum pick-up mechanisms by blood secretion in the pouch of Douglas, with fimbriae touching; presence of cross-reactivity between zona pellucida antibodies and those in sera of patients with endometriosis; disturbance of implantation because of the presence of intrauterine endometriomas.

Recent investigations have identified several interesting but disparate hypotheses by which mild endometriosis could lead to infertility; they include ovarian dysfunction (luteal phase defects; luteinized unruptured follicle)[42]; increased prostaglandin secretion[43,44]; presence of autoimmune disorders[45–47]; action of genetic factors[30,31].

CLASSIFICATION

According to Candiani[48], a satisfactory classification of endometriosis must take into account the following criteria: be based on endoscopic or laparotomic findings; have not only good descriptive potential but also be simple and practical to use; allow a reliable prognosis for probabilities of conception; indicate probabilities of recurrence; allow a precise follow-up and; facilitate a comparison of results. The idea of staging endometriosis is not a new one; indeed, the first classification of the disease was made by Sampson[2] in his classic paper. In 1949 Wick and Larsen[49] presented a classification based on the histological characteristics of the lesions, and proposed a system to correlate symptomatology and objective findings with disease grading. A variety of additional systems for classifying endometriosis was published in the 1950s and 1960s[50–60]. The principal methods to evaluate endometriosis published to date are listed in Table 1.

The first classification specifically based on laparoscopic/laparotomic findings was published in 1973 by Acosta *et al.*[37]. Although it allowed a more exact staging of actual lesions, it had its drawbacks because of the insufficient definition of pelvic pathology, which occasionally may result in doubts in staging. In addition, the lack of discrimination between unilateral and bilateral adnexal lesion groups, classified together cases with evident different prognosis. Finally, it did not consider subperitoneal lesions, such as those in the rectovaginal septum.

In view of the need for a widely accepted scoring system, the American Fertility Society[57] published in 1979 its first official classification, devised to

Table 1 Classifications of endometriosis

Sampson[2]	1927	*Am. J. Obstet. Gynecol.* **14**, 422
Wick and Larsen[49]	1949	*Northwest. Med. J.* **48**, 611
Huffman[34]	1951	*Am. J. Obstet. Gynecol.* **62**, 1243
Riva *et al.*[50]	1962	*Obstet. Gynecol.* **19**, 111
Beecham[62]	1966	*Obstet. Gynecol.* **28**, 437
Acosta *et al.*[37]	1973	*Obstet. Gynecol.* **42**, 19
Mitchell and Faber[52]	1974	In *Controversies in Ob-Gyn.* 631
Dmowski and Cohen[33]	1975	*Obstet. Gynecol.* **46**, 147
Kistner *et al.*[54]	1977	*Fertil. Steril.* **28**, 1008
Buttram[56]	1978	*Fertil. Steril.* **30**, 240
AFS[57]	1979	*Fertil. Steril.* **32**, 633
Revised AFS[59]	1985	*Fertil. Steril.* **43**, 347

be used in connection with laparoscopy or laparotomy; it is based on the attribution of a score varying according to the location and extent of lesions. A series of obvious defects soon became apparent in the AFS scoring method system and in 1984 the AFS committee was convened again to revise it; the result was the 'Revised AFS classification of endometriosis'[59] published in 1985, in which determination of the stage or degree of endometrial involvement is based on a weighted point system. To ensure complete evaluation, inspection of the pelvis in a clockwise or counterclockwise fashion is encouraged. Number, size and location of endometrial implants, plaques, endometriomas and/or adhesions must be noted.

Buttram *et al.*[60] compared the capacity of Acosta's, AFS 1979, and AFS 1985 classifications to predict future pregnancy and found that the AFS 1985 new system gave better results than the other two in correlating severity of endometriosis with pregnancy outcome following treatment, although differences were minimal and not statistically significant. Nonetheless the AFS 1985 classification should be utilized as widely as possible because it enables all those who treat endometriosis to speak the same language.

TREATMENT

In the early days treatment of endometriosis was achieved exclusively through surgery. Radical or conservative management was decided in relation to the patient's age, the severity of symptoms and the removability of the major lesions[61–65]. Irradiation therapy at castration or subcastration levels has never been popular; only a select group of patients was ever submitted to this therapy; those with major surgical risks, and those with recurrence after surgery[34].

The first major advance in the medical treatment of the disease was made possible by hormonal therapy: high doses of diethylstilbestrol (DES)[66] or methyltestosterone (MT)[67,68] both achieved moderate degrees of success in providing relief from the symptoms of endometriosis. However, the high percentage of disturbing side-effects produced by these hormonal regimens precluded their widespread application.

The introduction in the late 1950s of 'progestin only' and 'pseudopregnancy regimens'[69–71] resulted in a marked improvement in the medical management of endometriosis. They provided symptomatic relief in 50 to 80% of patients with a much smaller percentage of disturbing side-effects when compared to DES or MT therapy.

The next step in improving treatment was the introduction by Greenblat *et al.* of danazol[72]. This drug has a complex mechanism of action: it abolishes midcycle incretion peaks of follicle-stimulating hormone (FSH) and luteinizing hormone (LH)[73,75] while not affecting their basal levels[73,76]; it does not impair pituitary response to gonadotropin-releasing hormone (GnRH) stimulus[77,78]; it lowers estradiol production but does not abolish it[79,80] and decreases sex hormone-binding globulin (SHBG)[81]. In addition, the drug binds to receptors in the myometrium[82] and may have a direct action on the ovary[79,83].

Danazol possesses a complex metabolism, leading to approximately 60 molecules, some of which have independent pharmacological effects[84] and androgenic activity; it binds to androgen receptors and the danazol–androgen receptor translocates into the nucleus with initiation of androgen-specific RNA synthesis[83]. Although the very high testosterone plasma concentrations observed after danazol administration are, at least in part, due to artifacts, androgenic side-effects are common[85]. It has also progestational and antiprogestational activity: it binds to progesterone receptors but the danazol–progesterone receptor translocates poorly[83]. The drug affects liver function by causing a significant increase in serum glutamic-pyruvic transaminase and glutamic-oxalic transaminase; it also modifies lipid metabolism by increasing low density lipoprotein cholesterol (LDL-C) and decreasing high density lipoprotein cholesterol (HDL-C) (specifically the subunits HDL-C_2 and HDL-C_3); total cholesterol is not altered[86,87]. Side-effects to be expected from danazol include: weight gain, edema, muscle cramps (myalgia), acne, oily skin and/or hair, depression, decreased breast size, headache, hot flushes, changes in libido, nausea, hirsutism, arthralgia, voice change, skin rashes[88].

The most recent development in the medical therapy of endometriosis is the introduction over the past few years of GnRH superagonist analogs[89–92]. The analogs induce a 'medical oophorectomy' and allow temporary suppression of ovarian function, without measurable peripheral effects; unfortunately they cause 'menopausal-like' side-effects: hot flushes, sweating, depression, insomnia, headache, vaginal dryness, changes in libido. A comparison of the side-effects observed during therapy with a buserelin GnRH analog, danazol and in normal menopausal women is presented in Figure 1.

A role still to be fully evaluated in the management of endometriosis is that of gestrinone (R2323), a drug with antiestrogenic and antiprogestogenic properties. The remarkable effect of this compound on endometriosis results not only from its antigonadotropic action, but also from its antiestrogenic effect. Unfortunately, the drug has androgenic activity and can cause annoying side-effects[93].

In the field of invasive techniques, the recent availability of bipolar diathermy[94,95] for the laparoscopic coagulation of endometriotic implants in women with mild endometriosis, seems to offer the advantage of a decreased risk of adhesions. Finally laser techniques[96] (CO_2; KTP/532 nm) represent a further improvement in the laparoscopic coagulation of endometriotic implants, the excision of endometrioma capsules and the lysis of adnexal adhesions.

CONCLUSIONS

This brief summary of the work carried out to investigate endometriosis clearly shows that, in spite of a large body of clinical and experimental data, the pathogenesis of this disease is still unclear. Therefore further animal work will be necessary in order to elucidate the respective roles of metaplasia and retrograde menstruation. A fascinating hypothesis, supported by the finding

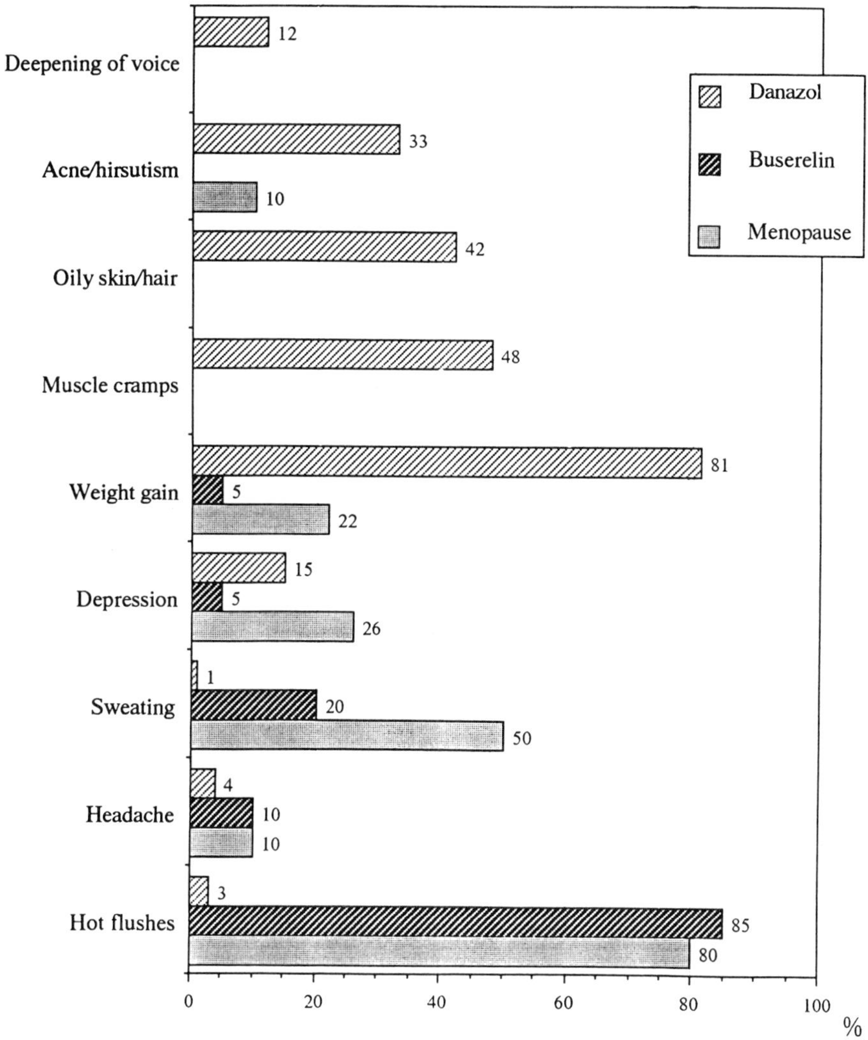

Figure 1 Incidence of side-effects in subjects treated with danazol or buserelin and in healthy menopausal women

of microscopic 'endometrial-like' foci in otherwise normal peritoneum[28] is that peritoneal mesothelium metaplasia may be a 'paraphysiological' process of widespread occurrence.

The situation is at least as confused when it comes to therapy. Recent data have proven that, a variety of pharmacological agents are equally effective in relieving pain, and improving the AFS score, although they act with very different mechanisms. In contradistinction to this, all comparative trials have failed to observe any statistically significant difference in the occurrence of pregnancy when comparing danazol, progestins and expectant management or danazol and GnRH analogs[97].

This seems to indicate that treatment, whereas markedly affecting actual lesions by inactivating endometriotic implants, has a less profound action on the still incompletely understood relationship between mild endometriosis and infertility.

REFERENCES

1. Sampson, J.A. (1921). Perforating hemorrhagic (chocolate) cysts of the ovary. Their importance and especially their relation to pelvic adenomas of endometrial type ('adenomyoma' of the uterus, rectovaginal septum, sigmoid, etc.). *Arch. Surg.*, **3**, 245
2. Sampson, J.A. (1927). Peritoneal endometriosis due to the menstrual dissemination of endometrial tissue into the peritoneal cavity. *Am. J. Obstet. Gynecol.*, **14**, 422
3. Cullen, T.S. (1986). Adenomyoma uteri diffusum benignum. *Johns Hopkins Hosp. Bull.*, **6**, 133
4. Cullen, T.S. (1896). Adenomyoma of the round ligament. *Johns Hopkins Hosp. Bull.*, **7**, 112
5. Russel, W.W. (1898). Aberrant portions of the Mullerian duct found in an ovary. *Johns Hopkins Hosp. Bull.*, **10**, 8
6. Savage, S. (1906). Haematoma of the ovary and its pathological connection with the ripening and the retrogression of the graffian follicle. *Br. Gynaecol. J.*, **21**, 285
7. Wolf, E.H. (1908). Ueber haematoma ovarii. *Arkiv. Gynäkol*, **84**, 211
8. Hedley, J.P. (1910). Haematoma of the ovary, with reports of 18 cases. *J. Obstet. Gynaecol. Br. Emp.*, **18**, 21
9. Novak, E. (1917). Abdominal hemorrhage of ovarian origin. *J. Am. Med. Assoc.*, **68**, 1160
10. Novak, E. (1917). Hematomata of the ovary, including corpus luteum cysts. *Johns Hopkins Hosp. Bull.*, **28**, 349
11. Lockyer, C. (1918). Fibroids and allied tumors (myoma and adenomyoma). Their pathology, clinical features and surgical treatment. pp. 324–8 (London: MacMillan)
12. Cullen, T.S. (1917). Adenomyoma of the recto-vaginal septum. *Johns Hopkins Hosp. Bull.*, **28**, 343
13. Cullen, T. (1920). The distribution of adenomyomas containing uterine mucosa. *Arch. Surg.*, **1**, 215
14. Casler, W.B. (1919). A unique, diffuse uterine tumor, really an adenomyoma, with stroma, but no glands. Menstruation after complete hysterectomy due to uterine mucosa in remaining ovary. *Trans. Am. Gynecol. Soc.*, **44**, 69
15. Mahle, A.E. and MacCarty, W.C. (1920). Ectopic adenomyoma of uterine type (a report of ten cases). *J. Lab. Clin. Med.*, **5**, 218
16. Norris, C. (1921). Ovary containing endometrium. *Am. J. Obstet. Gynecol.*, **1**, 831
17. Novak, E. (1926). The significance of uterine mucosa in the Fallopian tubes with a discussion of the origin of aberrant endometrium. *Am. J. Obstet. Gynecol.*, **12**, 484
18. Blumenkrantz, M.J., Gallagher, R.N., Bashore, R.A. and Tenckhoff, H. (1981). Retrograde menstruation in women undergoing chronic peritoneal dialysis. *Obstet. Gynecol.*, **57**, 667
19. Halme, J., Becker, S., Hammond, M.G. and Ray, S. (1982). Pelvic macrophages in normal and infertile women: the role of patent tubes. *Am. J. Obstet. Gynecol.*, **142**, 890
20. Halme, J., Hammond, M.G.G., Hulka, J.F., Ray, S.G. and Talbert, L.M. (1984). Retrograde menstruation in healthy women and in patients with endometriosis. *Obstet. Gynecol.*, **64**, 151
21. Iwanoff, N.S. (1898). Drusiges cystenhaltiges uterusfibromyom complicirt durch sarcom und carcinom. (Adenofibromyoma cysticum sarcomatodes carcinomatosum). *Monat. Geburst. Gynecol.*, **7**, 295
22. Meyer, R. (1930). Adenomyosis, adenofibrosis und adenomyome. In Stockel, V. (ed.) *Handbuch der Gynakol.*, (Munich: J.F. Bergmann)

23. Meigs, J.V. (1953). Endometriosis: etiologic role of marriage, age and parity: conservative treatment. *Obstet. Gynecol.*, **2**, 46
24. Oliver, A.J. and Harris, A.E. (1971). Endometriosis of the bladder in a male patient. *J. Urol.*, **106**, 858
25. Pinkert, T.C., Catlow, C.E. and Straus, R. (1979). Endometriosis of the urinary bladder in a man with prostatic carcinoma. *Cancer*, **43**, 1562
26. Binns, B.A.O. and Banerjee, R. (1983). Endometriosis with Turner's syndrome treated with cyclical estrogen/progestogen. Case report. *Br. J. Obstet. Gynaecol.*, **90**, 581
27. Rosenfeld, D.L. and Lecher, B.D. (1981). Endometriosis in a patient with Rokitanski–Kuster–Hauser syndrome. *Am. J. Obstet. Gynecol.*, **139**, 105
28. Vasquex, G., Corneillie, F. and Brosens, I.A. (1984). Peritoneal endometriosis: scanning electron microscopy and histology of minimal pelvic endometriotic lesions. *Fertil. Steril.*, **42**, 696
29. Halban, J. (1924). Hysteroadenosis metastatica. *Wien. Klin. Wochenschr.*, **37**, 1205
30. Simpson, J.L. (1982). Genetic aspect of gynecologic disorders occurring in 46, XX individuals. *Clin. Obstet. Gynecol.*, **15**, 157
31. Simpson, J.L., Elias, S., Malinak, L.R. and Buttram, V.C. (1980). Heritable aspects of endometriosis. *Am. J. Obstet. Gynecol.*, **137**, 327
32. Muse, K.N. and Wilson, E.A. (1982). How does mild endometriosis cause infertility? *Fertil. Steril.*, **38**, 145
33. Payne, F.L. (1940). The clinical aspects of pelvic endometriosis. *Am. J. Obstet. Gynecol.*, **39**, 373
34. Huffman, J.W. (1951). External endometriosis. *Am. J. Obstet. Gynecol.*, **62**, 1243
35. Barbieri, R.L. (1986). Ca-125 in patients with endometriosis. *Fertil. Steril.*, **45**, 767
36. Barbieri, R.L., Niloff, J.M., Bast, R.C. Jr., Schaetzl, E., Kistner, R.W. and Knapp, R.C. (1986). Elevated serum concentrations of Ca-125 in patients with advanced endometriosis. *Fertil. Steril.*, **45**, 630
37. Acosta, A.A., Buttram, V.C., Besch, P.K., Malinak, L.R., Franklin, R.R. and Vanderheyden, J.D. (1973). A proposed classification of pelvic endometriosis. *Obstet. Gynecol.*, **42**, 19
38. Strathy, J.H., Molgaard, C.A., Coulam, C.B. and Melton, L.J. (1982). Endometriosis and infertility: a laparoscopic study of endometriosis among fertile and infertile women. *Fertil. Steril.*, **38**, 667
39. Kistner, R.W. (1962). Infertility with endometriosis: a plan of therapy. *Fertil. Steril.*, **13**, 237
40. Kistner, R.W. (1979). Endometriosis and infertility. *Clin. Obstet. Gynecol.*, **22**, 101
41. Mettler, L. and Semm, K. (1984). Three-step therapy of genital endometriosis in cases of human infertility with Lystrenol, Danazol or Gestrinone administration in the second step. Raynaud, J.P. *et al.* (ed.) *Medical Management of Endometriosis* (New York: Raven Press)
42. Pittaway, D.E., Maxson, W., Daniell, J., Herbert, C. and Wentz, A.C. (1983). Luteal phase defects in infertility patients with endometriosis. *Fertil. Steril.*, **39**, 712
43. DeLeon, F.D., Vijayakumar, R., Brown, M., Rao, C.V., Yussman, M.A. and Schultz, G. (1986). Peritoneal fluid volume, estrogen, progesterone, prostaglandin, and epidermal growth factor concentrations in patients with and without endometriosis. *Obstet. Gynecol.*, **68**, 189
44. Sgarlata, C.S., Hertelendy, F. and Mikhail, G. (1983). The prostanoid concentration in peritoneal fluid and plasma of women with endometriosis. *Am. J. Obstet. Gynecol.*, **147**, 563
45. Weed, J.C. and Arquembourg, P.C. (1980). Endometriosis: can it produce an autoimmune response resulting in infertility? *Clin. Obstet. Gynecol.*, **23**, 885
46. Dmowski, W.P., Steele, R.W. and Baker, G.F. (1981). Deficient cellular immunity in endometriosis. *Am. J. Obstet. Gynecol.*, **141**, 377
47. Halme, J., Becker, S. and Haskill, S. (1987). Altered maturation and function of peritoneal macrophages: Possible role in pathogenesis of endometriosis. *Am. J. Obstet. Gynecol.*, **156**, 783
48. Candiani, G.B. (1986). The classification of endometriosis: historical evolution, critical review, and present state of the art. *Acta Europ. Fertil.*, **17**, 85
49. Wick, M.J. and Larsen, C.D. (1949). Histologic criteria for evaluating endometriosis. *Northwest. Med. J.*, **48**, 611
50. Riva, H.L., Kawasaki, D.M. and Messinger, A.J. (1962). Further experience with Norethynodrel in treatment of endometriosis. *Obstet. Gynecol.*, **19**, 111
51. Beecham, C.T. (1966). Classification of endometriosis. *Obstet. Gynecol.*, **28**, 437

52. Mitchell, G.W. and Faber, M. (1974). Medical versus surgical management of endometriosis. In Reed, D. and Christian, D. (eds). *Controversies in Ob-Gyn, II*, p. 631 (Philadelphia: W.B. Saunders)
53. Dmowski, W.P. and Cohen, M.R. (1975). Treatment of endometriosis with an antigonadotropin, Danazol. *Obstet. Gynecol.*, **46**, 147
54. Kistner, R.W., Siegler, A.M. and Behrman, S.J. (1977). Suggested classification for endometriosis: relationship to infertility. *Fertil. Steril.*, **28**, 1008
55. Adamson, G.D., Frison, L. and Lamb, E.J. (1982). Endometriosis: studies of a method for the design of a surgical staging system. *Fertil. Steril.*, **38**, 659
56. Buttram, V.C. (1978). An expanded classification of endometriosis. *Fertil. Steril.*, **30**, 240
57. The American Fertility Society (1979). Classification of endometriosis. *Fertil. Steril.*, **32**, 633
58. Guzic, D.S., Bross, D.S. and Rock, J.A. (1982). Assessing the efficacy of the American Fertility Society's classification of endometriosis: application of a dose-response methodology. *Fertil. Steril.*, **38**, 171
59. The American Fertility Society (1985). Revised American Fertility Society Classification of Endometriosis. *Fertil Steril.*, **43**, 351
60. Buttram, V.C. (1985). Evolution of the revised American Fertility Society Classification of Endometriosis. *Fertil. Steril.*, **43**, 347
61. Schmitz, H.E. and Towne, J. E. (1948). The treatment of pelvic endometriosis. *Am. J. Obstet. Gynecol.*, **55**, 583
62. Beecham, C.T. (1949). Surgical treatment of endometriosis. *J. Am. Med. Assoc.*, **139**, 971
63. Brosens, I.A., Boeckx, W. and Gordts, S. (1987). Conservative surgery of ovarian endometriosis in infertility. *Eur. J. Obstet. Gynecol. Reprod. Biol.*, **8**, 277
64. Buttram, V.C. (1979). Surgical treatment of endometriosis in the infertile female: a modified approach. *Fertil. Steril.*, **32**, 635
65. Schenken, R.S. and Malinak, L.R. (1982). Conservative surgery versus expectant management for the infertile patient with mild endometriosis. *Fertil. Steril.*, **37**, 183
66. Karnaky, K.J. (1948). The use of stilbestrol for endometriosis. *South. Med. J.*, **41**, 1109
67. Hirst, J.C. (1943). Favorable response of advanced endometriosis to testosterone therapy. *Am. J. Obstet. Gynecol.*, **46**, 97
68. Miller, J.R. (1944). Preoperative use of testosterone propionate as aid to surgical treatment of endometriosis. *J. Am. Med. Assoc.*, **125**, 207
69. Kistner, R.W. (1958). The use of newer progestins in the treatment of endometriosis. *Am. J. Obstet. Gynecol.*, **75**, 264
70. Andrews, M.C., Andrews, W.W. and Strauss, A.F. (1959). Effects of progestin-induced pseudopregnancy on endometriosis: Clinical and microscopic studies. *Am. J. Obstet. Gynecol.*, **78**, 776
71. Thomas, H.H. (1960). Conservative treatment of endometriosis: use of the long-acting ovarian steriod hormones. *Obstet. Gynecol.*, **15**, 498
72. Greenblatt, R.B., Dmowski, W.P., Mahesh, V.B. and Scholer, H.F.L. (1971). Clinical studies with an antigonadotropin-danazol. *Fertil. Steril.*, **22**, 102
73. Colle, M.L. and Greenblatt, R.B. (1976). Contraceptive properties of danazol. *J. Reprod. Med.*, **17**, 98
74. Lauersen, N.H. and Wilson K.H. (1977). Evaluation of danazol as an oral contraceptive. *Obstet. Gynecol.*, **50**, 91
75. Ward, G.D. (1977). Dosage aspects of danazol therapy in endometriosis. *J. Int. Med. Res.*, **5**, 95
76. Scott, J.Z., Kletzky, O.A., Brenner, P.F. and Mishell, D. (1978). Comparison of the effects of contraceptive steroid formulations containing two doses of estrogen on pituitary function. *Fertil. Steril.*, **30**, 141
77. Shane, J.M., Kates, R., Barbieri, R.L., Todd, R.B. and Davies, I.J. (1978). Pituitary gonadotropin responsiveness with danazol. *Fertil. Steril.*, **29**, 637
78. Franchimont, P. and Cramilion, C. (1977). The effect of danazol on anterior pituitary function. *Fertil. Steril.*, **28**, 814
79. Barbieri, R.L., Canick, J.A., Makris, A., Todd, R.B., Davies, I.J. and Ryan, K.J. (1977). Danazol inhibits steroidogenesis. *Fertil. Steril.*, **28**, 809
80. Asch, R.H., Fernandez, E.O., Siler-Khodr, T.M., Bartke, A. and Pauerstein, C.J. (1980). Mechanism of induction of luteal phase defects by danazol. *Am. J. Obstet. Gynecol.*, **136**,

932
81. McGinley, R. and Casey, J.H. (1979). Analysis of progesterone in unextracted serum: A method using danazol–a blocker of steroid binding to proteins. *Steroids*, **33**, 127
82. Chamness, G.C., Asch, R.H. and Pauerstein, C.J. (1980). Danazol binding and translocation of steroid receptors. *Am. J. Obstet. Gynecol.*, **136**, 246
83. Tamaya, T., Furuta, N., Motoyama, T., Boku, S., Ohono, Y. and Okada, H. (1978). Mechanisms of antiprogestational action of synthetic steroids. *Acta Endocrinol.*, **88**, 190
84. Dmowski, W.P., Scholer, H.F.L., Mahesh, V.B. and Greenblatt, R.B. (1971). Danazol–a synthetic steroid derivative with interesting physiologic properties. *Fertil. Steril.*, **22**, 9
85. Davison, C., Banks, W. and Fritz, A. (1976). The absorption, distribution and metabolic fate of danazol in rats, monkeys and human volunteers. *Arch. Int. Pharmacodyn.*, **221**, 294
86. Allen, J.K. and Fraser, I.S. (1981). Cholesterol, high density lipoprotein and danazol. *J. Clin. Endocrinol. Metab.*, **53**, 149
87. Fahraeus, L., Larsson-Cohn, V., Ljungberg, S. and Wallentin, L. (1984). Profound alterations of the lipoprotein metabolism during danazol treatment in premenopausal women. *Fertil. Steril.*, **42**, 52
88. Barbieri, R.L., Evans, S. and Kistner, R.W. (1982). Danazol in the treatment of endometriosis: analysis of 100 cases with a 4-year follow-up. *Fertil. Steril.*, **37**, 737
89. Lemay, A. and Quesnel, G. (1982). Potential new treatment of endometriosis: reversible inhibition of pituitary–ovarian luteinizing hormone by chronic intranasal administration of a luteinizing hormone-releasing hormone (LH-RH) agonist. *Fertil. Steril.*, **38**, 376
90. Cortes-Prieto, J., Lledo, A., Avila, C., Cortes-Garcia, L.C., D'Acunto, A., Luini, M., Comaru-Schally, A.M. and Schally A.V. (1987). Long-acting agonist of LH-RH in the treatment of large ovarian endometriosis. *Int. J. Fertil.*, **32**, 290
91. Steiregold, K.A., Cedars, M., Lu, J.K.H., Randle, D., Judd, H.L. and Meldrum, D.R. (1987). Treatment of endometriosis with a long-acting gonadotropin releasing hormone agonist. *Obstet. Gynecol.*, **69**, 403
92. Lemay, A., Maheux, R., Huot, C., Blanchet, J. and Faure, N. (1988). Efficacy of intranasal or subcutaneous luteinizing hormone-releasing hormone agonist inhibition of ovarian function in the treatment of endometriosis. *Am. J. Obstet. Gynecol.*, **158**, 233
93. Coutinho, E.M., Husson, J.M. and Azadian-Boulanger, G. (1984). Treatment of endometriosis with gestrinone – Five years experience. In Raynaud, J.P. *et al.* (eds). *Medical Management of Endometriosis*, (New York: Raven Press)
94. Hasson, H.M. (1979). Electrocoagulation of pelvic endometriosis lesions with laparoscopic control. *Am. J. Obstet. Gynecol.*, **135**, 115
95. Nowroozi, K., Chase, J.S., Check, J.H. and Wu, C.H. (1987). The importance of laparoscopic coagulation of mild endometriosis in infertile women. *Int. J. Fertil.*, **32**, 442
96. Nezhat, C., Crowgey, S.R. and Garrison, G.P. (1986). Surgical treatment of endometriosis via laser laparoscopy. *Fertil. Steril.*, **45**, 778
97. Henzl, M.R., Corson, S.L., Moghissi, K., Buttram, V.C., Berqvist, C. and Jacobson, J. (1988). Administration of nasal nafarelin as compared with oral danazol for endometriosis. A multicenter double-blind comparative clinical trial. *N. Engl. J. Med.*, **318**, 485

24

Endometriosis therapy with Zoladex

V. Mais, G.B. Melis, A.M. Paoletti, M. Gambacciani, A. Spinetti, F.D. Petacchi, G.A. Mauro and P. Fioretti

INTRODUCTION

Over the last 30 years a variety of non-surgical methods has been suggested for curing or controlling endometriosis. First, Kistner[1] proposed the concept of producing a 'pseudopregnancy' state by the simultaneous prolonged use of estrogen and progestogen, as an alternative to pregnancy-induced improvement in endometriosis. Then, 'pseudomenopause' therapy utilizing danazol has been proposed after Greenblatt *et al.*[2] published the first results of clinical use of this 'antigonadotropic' drug. Recently, 'medical oophorectomy' therapy using gonadotropin-releasing hormone (GnRH) agonists has been shown to be a promising approach to medical treatment of endometriosis[3]. However, GnRH agonists so far used in clinical studies have been administered in multiple daily doses[3].

Zoladex (Goserelin, ICI Pharmaceuticals, Macclesfield, UK) is a potent GnRH agonist that has recently become available in a biodegradable, sustained-release depot preparation[4,5]. The drug may be administered as a monthly subcutaneous implant, thus improving patient compliance[4,5].

The aim of the present study was to evaluate clinical, endocrine and metabolic effects of Zoladex depot in patients with symptomatic endometriosis treated for 6 months.

MATERIALS AND METHODS

Five women, 25 to 38 years of age, were included in the study. All of the patients had symptomatic endometriosis (pelvic pain and/or progressive dysmenorrhea) and underwent a laparoscopy before beginning the treatment. Pelvic endometriosis was scored according to the revised American Fertility Society classification: 1985[6].

Zoladex depot (3.6 mg) was administered subcutaneously every 4 weeks into the anterior abdominal wall using a prepacked syringe. Therapy was continued for 6 months. In all of the patients the first depot was given during the early follicular phase (day 2–7 of the cycle).

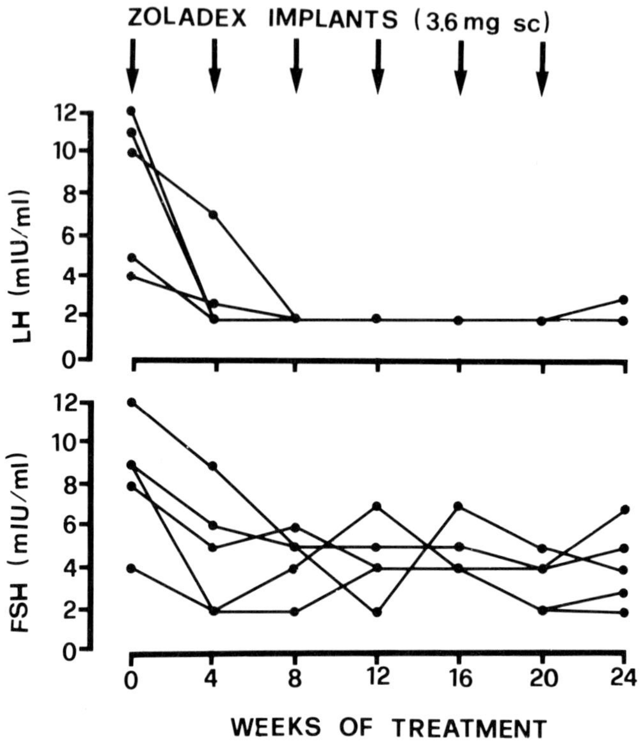

Figure 1 Plasma levels of LH and FSH measured in the five subjects (at 4-week intervals) before, during and at the end of treatment with Zoladex depot (3.6 mg s.c. every 4 weeks)

Clinical, endocrine and metabolic evaluations were performed at 4-week intervals before, during and at the end of treatment. At each visit, the patients were asked about timing and occurrence of vaginal bleeding, pelvic pain and side-effects attributable to therapy. Blood was taken at each visit for immunoradiometric (IRMA) assay of luteinizing hormone (LH) and follicle-stimulating hormone (FSH), for radioimmunoassay (RIA) of estradiol (E_2) and progesterone (P), and for enzymic analyses of high density lipoprotein cholesterol (HDL-C) and HDL_3-C fraction. The IRMA assay method for LH and FSH was based on the use of mouse monoclonal antibodies.

Bone density was measured in the distal radius before and after treatment by dual photon absorptiometry (sources, ^{125}I and ^{241}Am).

RESULTS

The grade of endometriosis was II in three patients, III in one patient and IV in one patient. All of the patients completed 6 months of therapy.

One patient became amenorrheic after the first Zoladex implant, all patients were amenorrheic after the second. Dysmenorrhea and pelvic pain were relieved in three patients after the first implant and in all patients after the second.

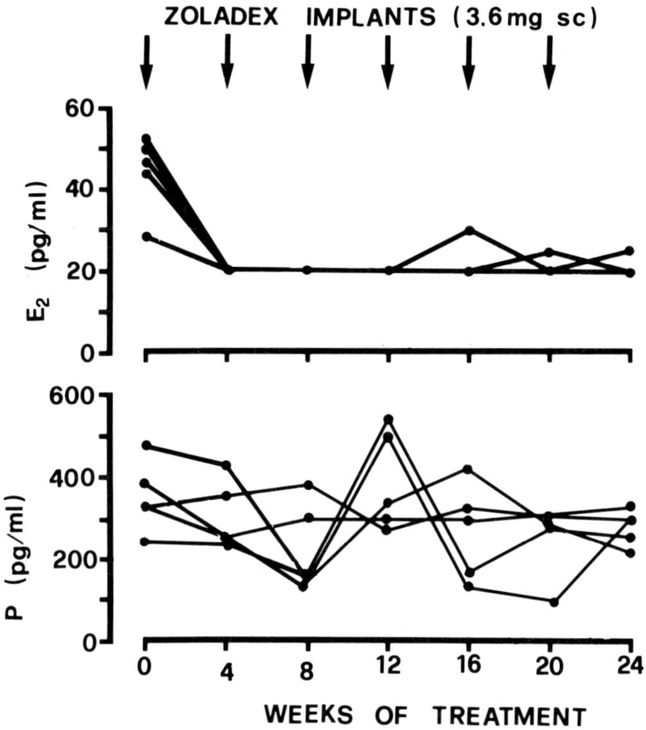

Figure 2 Plasma levels of E_2 and P measured in the five subjects (at 4-week intervals) before, during and at the end of treatment with Zoladex depot

Two patients reported hot flushes after the first implant, one patient after the second, one patient after the third and one patient after the fourth. Two patients reported headache at the second and at the third visit, respectively.

As for endocrine evaluation, plasma LH was reduced to the limit of sensitivity of the assay in all of the patients, while no reduction of plasma FSH was evident (Figure 1). Similarly, plasma E_2 was reduced to the limit of sensitivity of the assay, while P fluctuated in the early follicular phase range (Figure 2).

No major modifications of HDL-C or HDL-C fractions (HDL_2-C and HDL_3-C) were detected (Figure 3). Similarly, bone density measured in the distal radius did not seem to be modified by 6 months of ovarian suppression with Zoladex implants (Figure 4).

DISCUSSION

The present study confirmed that GnRH agonist-induced 'medical oophorectomy' is an effective approach to medical management of endometriosis[3]. The therapy was well tolerated and the only symptoms associated

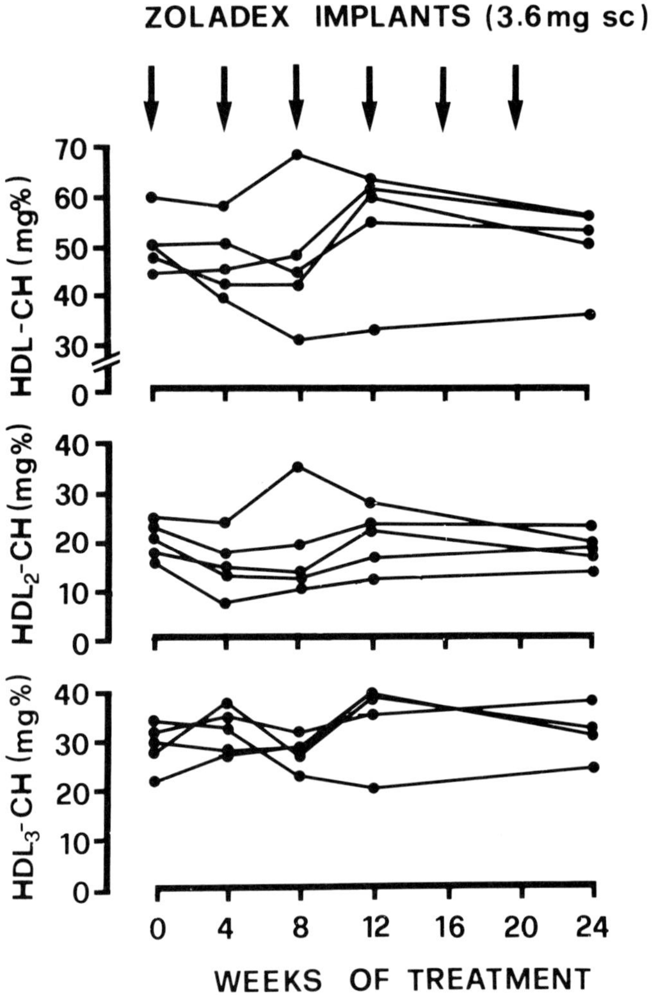

Figure 3 High density lipoprotein cholesterol (HDL-C) and HDL-C fractions measured in the five subjects before, during and at the end of treatment with Zoladex depot

with estrogen deficiency were hot flushes. Moreover, the possibility of administering Zoladex as a monthly subcutaneous implant actually improved patient's compliance, as previously reported by West *et al.*[7] in premenopausal women receiving Zoladex depot as medical approach to the management of uterine fibroids.

As for objective markers of estrogen action (bone and lipid metabolism), the present study confirmed the observations of Steingold *et al.*[8] showing that HDL-C remain unchanged in women with endometriosis treated with a potent GnRH agonist for 6 months. By contrast, Steingold *et al.*[8] also reported an increase in the fasting urinary calcium/creatinine and hydroxyproline/creatinine ratios to the range of women who underwent

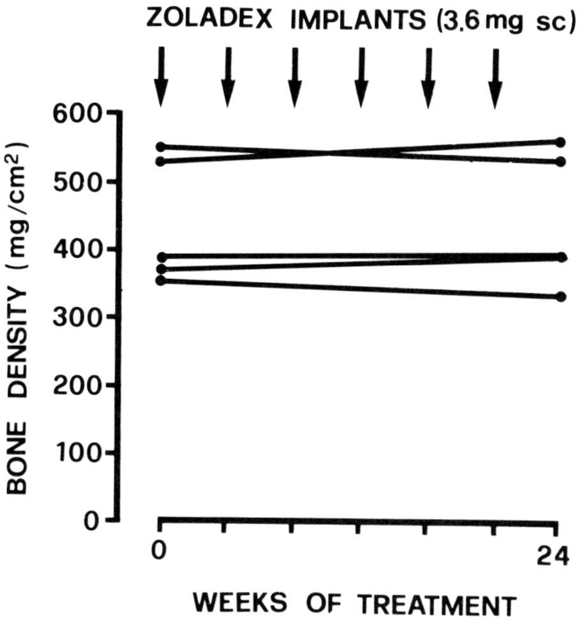

Figure 4 Bone density measured in the five subjects in the distal radius before and after treatment with Zoladex depot (3.6 mg s.c. every 4 weeks)

bilateral oophorectomy. However, from the results of the present study, treatment with Zoladex depot (3.6 mg every 4 weeks) does not seem to induce significant changes in bone density measured in the distal radius.

REFERENCES

1. Kistner, R.W. (1958). The use of newer progestins in the treatment of endometriosis. *Am. J. Obstet. Gynecol.*, **75**, 264–78
2. Greenblatt, R.B., Dmowski, L.P., Mahesh, U. and Scholer, H.F.C. (1971). Clinical studies with an antigonadotrophin-danazol. *Fertil. Steril.*, **22**, 102–13
3. Lemay, A., Maheux, R., Faure, N., Jean, C. and Fazekas, A.T.A. (1984). Reversible hypogonadism induced by a luteinizing hormone-releasing hormone (LH-RH) agonist (Buserelin) as a new therapeutic approach for endometriosis. *Fertil. Steril.*, **41**, 863–71
4. Dowsett, M., Cantwell, B., Lal, A., Jeffcoate, S.L. and Harris, A.L. (1988). Suppression of postmenopausal ovarian steroidogenesis with the luteinizing hormone-releasing hormone against Goserelin. *J. Clin. Endocrinol. Metab.*, **66**, 672–7
5. Matta, W.H.M., Shaw, W.R. and Burford, G.D. (1988). Endocrinologic and clinical evaluation following a single administration of gonadotropin-releasing hormone agonist (Zoladex), in a depot formulation, to premenopausal women. *Fertil. Steril.*, **49**, 163–5
6. The American Fertility Society (1985). Revised American Fertility Society classification of endometriosis: 1985. *Fertil. Steril.*, **43**, 351–2
7. West, C.P., Lumsden, M.A., Lawson, S., Williamson, J. and Baird, D.T. (1987). Shrinkage of uterine fibroids during therapy with goserelin (Zoladex*): a luteinizing hormone releasing hormone agonist administered as a monthly subcutaneous depot. *Fertil. Steril.*, **48**, 45–51
8. Steingold, K.A., Cedars, M., Lu, J.K.H., Randle, D., Judd, H.L. and Meldrum, D.R. (1987). Treatment of endometriosis with a long-acting gonadotropin-releasing hormone agonist. *Obstet. Gynecol.*, **69**, 403–11

25

Treatment of uterine leiomyomata: past, present and future

R. Maheux

INTRODUCTION

The objective of this chapter is to review the management of uterine leiomyomata from the situation in the 19th century and before, to the present time with particular emphasis on medical treatment and its future development.

THE 19TH CENTURY AND BEFORE

In 1853, Washington Hatley won the annual prize essay award of the American Medical Association for his report on successful abdominal myomectomy[1]. Among the 15 patients reported, 10 survived. He is probably the one who, with his brother John, performed the first successful abdominal operation for uterine leiomyoma in 1844[2]. The 19th century was a time of pioneers. In 1846, John Collins Warren (1778–1856) removed under anesthesia a tumor from the jaw of a young man in a room at the Massachusetts General Hospital known henceforth as the Ether Dome. Ephraim McDowell in 1809, in Kentucky, 1000 miles from the nearest hospital, performed the first successful ovariectomy whereas Robert Lawson Tait from England performed in 1883 the first successful salpingectomy for extrauterine pregnancy.

Before the introduction of modern surgery with suture, anesthesia and asepsis, hysterectomy had a bleak record. In 1880, C.D. Palmer reviewing the 119 cases collected by Pozzi up to 1875 reported a mortality of 64%[3]. Symptomatic women harboring fibroids had to rely on often bizarre and strange therapeutic regimens. Canadian Indians used decoctions of bloodroot or of blue cohosh, also called squaw root, for menorragia and infusions of Labrador tea for dysmenorrhea; this infusion was also utilized for labor pain. Probably influenced by the experiments of Galvani, a lot of women utilized Perkin's tractors at the beginning of the nineteenth century. The idea was that metal stroked across the body was able to draw off noxious electrical fluids. George Washington purchased a pair for his family. The most popular remedy for female diseases at the beginning of this century was Pinkham's vegetable compound which has been produced in American for more than a century. This brown, bitter brew of herbs and alcohol (18%), was strongly recommended for 'female weakness including leukorrhea, irregular and painful menstruation, inflammation and ulceration of the womb, etc . . .' Although the Federal Trade Commission had forbidden advertising of this compound in 1941 and the original factory in Lynn, Massachusetts has been closed since 1972, it was still possible until recently to find this most famous American remedy for woman's diseases on the shelves of some drugstores.

There was a dramatic improvement in the mortality rate reported following hysterectomy during the last quarter of the 19th century. As gynecologists feared the abdominal cavity less and less, more and more hysterectomies were performed. At the 19th annual meeting of the American Gynecological Society, in 1894, William T. Lusk[3] in his presidential address said: 'Not many years ago we preached to a patient with a myomatous growth the virtues of fortitude and resignation; we comforted her with figures showing the statistical frequency of the disease, and with the assurance that it was not malignant; and we held out the hope that the progress of the tumor would be arrested by the occurrence of the climacteric . . . Perhaps no achievement in surgery has ever borne witness so completely to the triumph of human ingeniosity over anatomical difficulties as the safe extirpation of an enlarged uterus'.

Still other forms of treatment for uterine leiomyoma persisted at the end of the 19th century. Electricity which was condemned by some such as E. Stansbury Sutton as 'an absolute piece of rot'; was promoted by others such as William H. Baker who insisted that 'electricity for fibroids has, in my hands, proved a success. I am well satisfied with this treatment in certainly 19 cases out of 20'[3]. However, enthusiasm for Faradism and Galvanism apparently waned with the 20th century. The same happened to the treatment of uterine leiomyomata by means of thyroid and mammary gland extracts such as advocated by Malcolm McLean. It is interesting to note that as early as the 1900 meeting of the American Gynecological Society, George Engelmann[3] reviewing the progress made in gynecological surgery, noted in his presidential address that 'along the lines of extirpation we can no longer advance; we must look to preservation, to the conserving of the function and this must be the guiding star for the surgery of the 20th century'. Advice, as we will see, which has not been well followed.

HYSTERECTOMY

Hysterectomy is the most frequently performed major operation in the United States[4]. The hysterectomy rate increased between 1971 and 1975 and plateaued thereafter (Table 1). A total of 649 000 hysterectomies were performed in United States in 1980 (a rate of 563 per 100 000 women). An estimated 3 536 000 women between the ages of 15 and 44 years underwent hysterectomy (excluding radical procedures) during the 9-year period of 1970 to 1978[5]. If the actual rate continues in the future, this would result in loss of the uterus by more than half the female population by the age of 65 years[6].

Table 1 Numbers* and rates of hysterectomy by year, in the United States, 1971–1980

Year	*Number (in thousands)*	*Rate (per 100 000 women)*
1971	570	544
1972	649	614
1973	690	648
1974	695	648
1975	725	670
1976	678	622
1977	705	642
1978	644	582
1979	639	572
1980	649	563

Hysterectomy is one of the most controversial operations of our times, widely discussed and criticized by the general public. The risk of death from hysterectomy is low. Large multicenter studies indicate a death-to-case rate of one to two deaths per 1000 operations[7]. However, with the actual number of hysterectomies performed per year, the Committee on Gynecologic Practice of the American College of Obstetricians and Gynecologists[8] has estimated hysterectomy-related deaths at over 600 per year in United States. This operation is also associated with a substantial complication rate and Dicker *et al.*[7] reported that one-quarter to one-half of women who undergo hysterectomy will sustain complications. Most often this will be only transient hyperthermia but hemorrhage, pelvic infection, septicemia and injuries to the urinary tract may occur. Also some late complications of hysterectomy are now recognized. The rate of depression within 3 years after hysterectomy in a 1973 English study was nearly five times that observed in a set of unoperated female control patients[9]. This difference persisted when patients with pre-existing depression were excluded from the analysis. The 'residual ovary syndrome' consists of development of pain, dyspareunia and pelvic mass after hysterectomy when the ovaries are retained. Most series reported an incidence of 1% to 4%[10]. Vascular diseases may also develop following this operation, even when the ovaries are not removed. Reports[11] indicate that premenopausal hysterectomy is associated with a threefold increase in the risk of coronary heart disease during the remaining premenopausal years. Finally, significant psychological and emotional sequelae may follow this operation: sexual dysfunction, loss of self-esteem, alteration in the perception of femininity. The costs associated with this operation are also extremely important. Over 1.7 billion dollars are spent for hysterectomy each year in the United States alone[8].

Uterine leiomyoma is essentially benign (0.7% sarcomatous degeneration) but still represent the most common indication for hysterectomy[12] (Figure 1). For example, at St-François d'Assise Hospital in Quebec City, 1047 hysterectomies have been performed during the last 3-year period. In 310 cases, uterine leiomyoma was the main surgical indication. More hysterectomies have been performed in our hospital for uterine leiomyoma than for the second and third indications together.

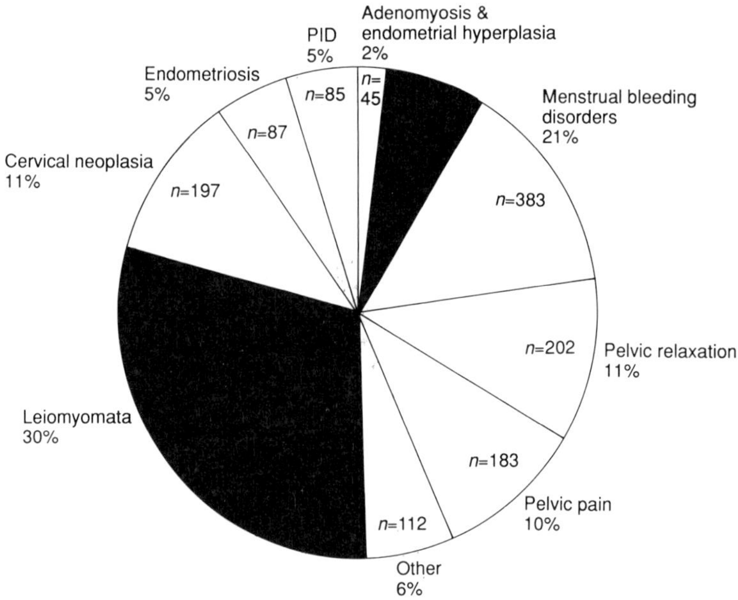

Figure 1 Indication for hysterectomy according to Lee *et al.*[1]. Over 1/3 of hysterectomies performed in USA are for leiomyomata or for menstrual bleeding related to leiomyomata

MYOMECTOMY

Uterine leiomyoma may cause infertility especially during the late reproductive years and in the black population. It may also seriously complicate a pregnancy. A review in 1981 of 1941 cases of myomectomy revealed a 41% preoperative abortion rate[13]. Pain, hemorrhage, abnormal presentation or placentation, premature labor or rupture of the membranes, fetal death, infection or degeneration of leiomyoma are other potential complications of this tumor during pregnancy. The occurrence of one of these complications in a prior pregnancy may be an indication for surgical myomectomy. Also, until now the classical approach for a young woman harboring a symptomatic uterine leiomyoma but desiring to preserve her fertility was to perform selective surgical myomectomy.

This operation is, however, not an easy procedure because often leiomyomata are multiple and those with which we are more concerned are deep in the myometrium. Significant blood loss is reported with postoperative formation of adhesions. Furthermore, we have to consider the anesthetic risk and the possible need, if the operation is successful, for Caesarean section. The pregnancy rate following surgical myomectomy is approximately only 40%[13].

Fifteen per cent of the patients having had a surgical myomectomy will present a recurrence, two-thirds of them necessitating second surgery[13].

The technique of surgical myomectomy has been extensively reviewed by Buttram and Reitter[13]. As stressed in their article, we also think that anterior middle incision is preferable to minimize adhesions. However, to reduce the subsequent rate of Caesarean section and the risk of subsequent intrauterine adhesions, we avoid, when possible, entering the endometrial cavity and the proximal third of the myometrium. Therefore, we almost never attempt 'transcavity enucleation' as described by Bonney[14]. We have found it preferable, for posterior tumors of the lower uterine segment, to remove the leiomyoma by a posterior vertical incision. The leiomyoma is sectioned in two and then enucleated. Normal myometrium should be spared even if it looks in excess; the stretched myometrium covering a leiomyoma will retract postoperatively, strengthening the incision. Careful surgical techniques using 0-Vicryl interrupted suture on the myometrium and a 4-0-Vicryl running 'in-and-out' suture on the serosa effectively reduce the raw surface and the subsequent risk of adhesions. When we perform posterior or fundal incisions, we routinely suspend the uterus and place 100 cc of dextran 70 (Hyscon*) in the pelvic cavity at the time of peritoneal closure. We never use clamps or tourniquet to occlude uterine vessels. Moreover, in our hands, the utilization of CO_2, YAG or Argon lasers has been found unhelpful during myomectomy by laparotomy and the injection of vasopressives around the tumor unnecessary. The only adjuvant that we use to minimize blood loss is preoperative luteinizing hormone-releasing hormone agonist (LHRH-A) therapy. Matta *et al.*[15] have shown in patients with uterine fibroids a significant reduction in uterine arterial blood flow, as assessed by Doppler ultrasound, following treatment with LHRH-A. Pregnancy rates following surgical myomectomy approximate only 40%. As the success of this operation seems inversely related to the size of the myoma at the time of surgery[13], it is logical to think that preoperative shrinkage of the myoma with LHRH-A will yield a better prognosis. We recommend routine preoperative utilization of LHRH-A in all patients who are candidates for surgical myomectomy. This therapy may also prove helpful before hysterectomy to facilitate surgery technically when the tumor is large or to allow vaginal instead of abdominal hysterectomy. In fact, 28% of the hysterectomies performed in the United States are vaginal hysterectomies[5]. As preoperative adjunctive therapy, LHRH-A should be used for a short-term period; 8 to 12 weeks of treatment is usually enough for maximum volume reduction of the fibroid.

Myomectomy by laparoscopy with or without CO_2 laser vaporization has been described by us[16] and others[17]. Although still experimental, this technique is an outpatient procedure and may allow the removal of some subserosal or pedunculate leiomyoma. If we can develop in the near future a tool able to predict which fibroid will grow, laser endoscopic vaporization combined with preoperative LHRH-A may allow us to remove those myomata before they begin to give problems.

A vaginal approach is usually preferable to remove submucous leiomyomata provided they are not associated with other myomata necessitating a laparotomy and are not already too large technically for removal by this approach. Here again, preoperative LHRH-A treatment is recommended. If the fibroid has prolapsed in the vagina or if a submucous leiomyoma has a thin stalk, it can usually be removed by twisting the pedicle[18]. Submucous leiomyomata with large and thick pedicules are better removed by hysteroscopy with electrical resectoscopes[19–20]. If the tumor is large, it may be necessary to use laminaria the night before surgery to facilitate the removal of the fibroid transcervically[21].

MEDICAL TREATMENT

Progestins

The concept of a medical treatment for uterine leiomyoma is not new. As early as 1946, the utilization of progesterone in six cases of uterine leiomyoma was reported by Goodman[22]. Although Goldzieher[23] has reported intense degenerative change in myomata following large doses of progestogens, small doses seem to have no effect. Segaloff[24] has not observed evidence to indicate involution of uterine leiomyomata in his study. This poor response of uterine leiomyomata to progestogens may be explained by the fact that progesterone receptors do not increase in uterine leiomyomata as they normally do in the myometrium during the menstrual cycle[25]. It is also possible that progesterone acts differently in the myometrium from the way it does in the endometrium. Boulet and Fortier[26] have reported in cultured cells of rabbit myometrium that progesterone does not have an antiestrogenic effect in these tissues as it does when observed in the endometrium. It potentiates the stimulatory effects of estradiol on protein content and on the ratio of protein/DNA. Increased mitotic activity has also been reported in myomata following prehysterectomy utilization of progestins[27].

Danazol

The first medication that we used (in 1981) for uterine leiomyoma was danazol. As danazol was effective in endometriosis, an estrogen dependent pathology, we presumed that it would be useful for uterine leiomyomata. At the 1983 annual meeting of the American Fertility Society in San Francisco, we presented the results of a study conducted at Yale University on the use of danazol in eight patients harboring uterine leiomyomata[28]. Although we obtained a good hormonal response following the use of 800 mg of danazol per day for 6 months in those patients, the reduction observed in the volume of the uterine leiomyomata was only 20–25%. At the same period, Basel Ho Yuen[29] from Vancouver reported the development of small myomata, in a patient receiving treatment for endometriosis with danazol for 6 months. These had been absent at the laparoscopy performed before treatment. The poor results obtained following the utilization of danazol is probably explained by the fact that this synthetic steroid has androgenic properties. Androgen receptors are present in uterine leiomyomas[30] with an increased 5α-reductase activity when compared to the endometrium and myometrium[31].

Yamamoto *et al.*[32] have demonstrated that, unlike normal myometrium, leiomyomata have a high aromatase activity and were able to synthesize estrogens from androgens.

Gestrinone

Gestrinone (Roussel-Uclaf, Paris, France) is a synthetic trienic 19-non-steroid, also known as R-2323, which shares many properties with danazol: it is effective in endometriosis and induces prolonged amenorrhea in women through ovulation-inhibition and endometrial atrophy[33]. As for danazol, its exact antiestrogenic effect is still not completely understood but it is probably multifactorial. Its side-effects are similar: acne, seborrhea, hirsutism, hoarseness, muscular pain, edema of the legs, weight gain, etc . . . The efficacy and the occurrence of side-effects seem proportional to the dosage used. However, unlike danazol, it has a longer duration and can be administered orally weekly or twice weekly. Silastic implants containing gestrinone have also been tested as a contraceptive measure[34].

In 1981 Coutinho[35] reported a significant volume reduction of a pelvic leiomyoma and subsequent pregnancy in an 18-year-old infertile patient treated for 14 months with gestrinone 5 mg *per os* every 2 days for 2 months then twice a week for the rest of the treatment period. A more extensive study[36] was published by the same group in 1986; 97 women were studied. 34 patients (group A) received 5 mg of gestrinone twice a week whereas 36 (group B) took half that dosage at the same interval. The other 27 women (group C) were instructed to insert tablets containing 2.5 mg of gestrinone in the vagina three times weekly. The duration of therapy was variable. Some took the medication for 4 months, others up to 13 months. Most patients discontinued therapy because they considered themself cured, others because of side-effects or because the treatment failed to alleviate symptoms. Data on all the patients are therefore only available after 4 months of treatment with gestrinone. At that time, uterine volume decreased by 18% and 27% respectively in groups A and B and increased by 5% in group C. Thirty-two patients were observed after 10 months; uterine volume changes were respectively −26%, −15% and +10% in groups A, B and C. Forty patients completed 13 months of treatment, respective uterine volume change being −21%, −37%, −2% in the three groups. Overall the mean reduction in uterine volume has not been impressive; the volume of the leiomyoma was, in fact, increased or unchanged in 26 women. Those results are in accordance with what has been observed during treatment with danazol. Although blood levels of gestrinone in group C were sufficient to inhibit ovulation and prevent menstruation, the authors claim that the poor results observed in the group treated vaginally are probably related to levels inadequate 'to saturate myometrial receptors and inhibit tumor growth'[36]. This hypothesis is hard to verify as no blood levels of gonadotropins or sex steroid hormones were reported before, during or after treatment in these three groups of patients. Also, although more than 50% of patients had more than 1 year of follow-up at the time of the report, no data was reported on the volume of the fibroids after the treatment stopped. Almost half of patients (47%) reported side-effects, mostly androgenic. No blood safety data are reported.

In summary, the efficacy of gestrinone in reducing uterine volume in women harboring leiomyomata is not very impressive at the present time and seems comparable to the poor results obtained with danazol. Gestrinone should be recommended in this pathology when a good clinical trial has been completed with hormonal blood levels measured and safety laboratory data assessed.

Chinese approach

Meiling[37], in 1980, reported in the Acta Academial Medicinal Sinical the use of gossypol in 30 women with menopausal functional bleeding, myoma of uterus or endometriosis. Estrogen levels were lowered and in 70% endometrial sampling showed highly atrophied endometrium. In 62.5%, there was a reduction in the volume of leiomyoma. Although it is said that 'no or little side-effect could be observed under adequate dosage', my main concern with this approach is the possible side-effects. Fatigue and non-reversible hypokalemia has been reported in clinical trials using gossypol for male contraception. Direct permanent effect on the gonad is also possible.

For many years, acupuncture has been used successfully to treat various menstrual disorders including menorrhagia and dysmenorrhea[38]. It seems particularly effective for dysmenorrhea. A recent prospective randomized study from California[39] has demonstrated its effectiveness in primary dysmenorrhea. As reliable acupuncture is increasingly available in Western countries, it may be worth a trial if the symptomatology is mild and the patient wants to avoid standard treatment regimens.

Antiprostaglandins

Prostaglandin synthesis inhibitors reduce excessive menstrual blood loss in women with essential menorrhagia[40] or menorrhagia associated with an intrauterine contraceptive device[41]. Therefore, it was reasonable to think that they may also be effective for myoma-induced menorrhagia. However, a recent prospective placebo controlled study from Finland[42] has recently shown the opposite. The utilization of naproxen, 500–1000 mg daily for 5 days, although it has reduced by 35.7% menstrual blood loss in women with idiopathic menorrhagia, had no consistent effect on myoma-induced menorrhagia.

LHRH agonist

Mechanism of action

Roger Guillemin and Andrew Schally received the Nobel Prize for medicine in 1971 for their work on peptide hormones secreted by the brain. They

Table 2 LHRH agonists

Molecular changes		*Company*	*Potent*	*Half life*
6	10			
D-Trp	Net	Salk, Ferring	144	30 min
D-Ser(But)	Net	Hoechst	20–40	75–80 min
D-Leu	Net	Abbott	20–30	1.3 h
D-Na12	Net	Syntex		120 min
D-His(Imbzl)	Net	Ortho	140	
D-Ser(But)	Azgly	ICI	50–100	4.5 h
Long-acting LHRH agonists				
Zoladex	ICI	3.6 mg	lactide–glycolide polymer	
Decapeptyl-Cr	Ferring	4.0 mg	poly(dl)lactide–glycolide microcapsules	

had isolated and defined the decapeptide LHRH which, secreted by the hypothalamus, controls the hypophyseal secretion of gonadotropins. Slight structural modifications of the original molecule have allowed development of superactive agonists (LHRH-A). It was believed initially that LHRH-A would enhance fertility but instead it has been shown that they exercise a paradoxical effect. To obtain physiological secretion of gonadotropins, *pulsatile* hypothalmic secretion of LHRH is necessary. On the contrary, *continuous* occupation of hypophyseal LHRH receptors by natural LHRH or one of its long-acting agonists provokes a *down-regulation*, i.e. inhibition of hypophyseal production and secretion of gonadotropins with resulting hypogonadism and hypoestrogenism. This is why this treatment has often been called ‘pseudomenopause’. LHRH-A are not active *per os*, they are therefore administered by nasal insufflation or by subcutaneous injection; new monthly depot forms have recently been developed. LHRH-A are very effective in hormone-dependent pathologies. They have been used with success in prostatic carcinoma, precocious puberty, uterine leiomyoma and endometriosis. Table 2 illustrates the LHRH-A currently used.

Short-term administration of LHRH-A in uterine leiomyoma

In August 1985, we reported the first pilot study on the utilization of LHRH-A in uterine leiomyoma[43]. Ten women with 12 uterine leiomyomata ranging from 7.5 to 420 cc (mean 112.6 ± 39.4) were treated with subcutaneous injections of buserelin, $200\,\mu g$ three times daily for 1 week and then $500\,\mu g$ daily for the rest of the 6-month treatment period. Following initial stimulation the pituitary–ovarian axis was suppressed after 3 weeks of treatment with mean serum estradiol ranging between 17 and 36 pg/ml. Seven uterine leiomyomata have shown a marked regression in size following treatment with LHRH-A; two were undetectable and the volume of the other five diminished by an average of 80%. One tumor did not respond to treatment, two regressed by 25%, and two, following an initial reduction of 65% and 50%, re-enlarged during the last 2 months of treatment to 75% and 100% respectively of their initial volume. Three case reports have been published before. The first was by Filicori[44] in November 1983 who treated a symptomatic patient harboring a myoma for 15 weeks with subcutaneous injections of 8 μg/kg of D-Trp^6-Pro^9-NET-LHRH. An 88% reduction in the 151 cc initial volume of the fibroid was observed. In October 1984, we reported[45] on three patients harboring four myomata treated once daily with subcutaneous buserelin for 6 months. The reduction in size of the leiomyomata was 91.2% for patient 1, 80.8% for patient 2 and 61.5% and 100% respectively for the two leiomyomata that patient 3 was harboring. In November 1984, Healy[46] observed in a patient treated for 16 weeks with pulsatile subcutaneous administration of buserelin 6 μg every 45 min, an 85% reduction of her myoma. These results have been corroborated by many other studies. Table 3 summarizes the results obtained up to now by different groups of investigators in 201 cases. Significant reduction of the volume of the uterus or the leiomyoma has been reported (39% to 71%, mean 46%). An average 10% of the leiomyomata have not responded or have responded poorly to the LHRH-A treatment. This could be related to the histological nature of some myomata which after a while are mostly composed of fibrous tissue and are not hormonally active. Seven patients treated with intranasal leuprolide as reported by the Boston group[55] did not respond to treatment, four dropping out of the study after 3 months. The lack of response observed in this subgroup is probably related to insufficient dosage or frequency of administration (nasal leuprolide 800 μg bid) as estradiol levels were not properly suppressed (50–156 pg/ml) during the treatment period.

The most common side-effects reported during LHRH-A treatment are hot flushes. They usually start 3 to 4 weeks after initiating therapy and most patients are affected. Fortunately, they are usually not severe and are tolerated by the patients. Few women have reported dryness of the vagina or decreased libido. Scanty results concerning bone density have been published during LHRH-A treatment for myoma[54,55,59]. A short-term treatment up to 6 months does not seem to exert a deleterious effect. High density lipoprotein (HDL)-cholesterol does not change or is slightly but significantly increased during LHRH-A treatment[52,59]. This beneficial effect may be explained by an alteration of the androgen/estrogen ratio or by the fact that when low dosage of LHRH-A is used[52,59], some estrogen stimulation is preserved whereas progesterone production is blocked. No other significant effect has been reported in the safety data.

It is clear at the present time, that shrinkage of fibroids during LHRH-A treatment is only transitory and if no surgery is performed at the end of the treatment period, rapid regrowth of the myomas is the rule for most of the patients. Therefore, short-term LHRH-A treatment should not be clinically recommended other than as an adjunctive therapy before surgery.

Long-term treatment

Overall the hysterectomy rate among women of reproductive age averaged 8.5 per 1000 women[5]. This rate more than doubled with increasing age (18.4/1000 women aged 35 to 44 years). Uterine leiomyoma is the most common indication for hysterectomy[12] and as most of these tumors will become asymptomatic during the climacteric period, if it is possible to control

Table 3 Utilization of LHRH-A in uterine leiomyoma

Authors	Year	Patient n	LHRH-A	Dosages	Duration	Reduction %
Maheux[43]	1985	10	buserelin	500 μg s.c. daily	24	−55
Matta[47]	1986	10	buserelin	300–400 μg i.n. tid	24	−52–58
Healy[48]	1986	5	buserelin	6 μg s.c. q45min	20	−60
Leusden[49]	1987	6	D-Trp6–LHRH	4 mg s.c. monthly	16	−50
Goddington[50]	1986	6	histrelin	4 μg/kg s.c. daily	24	−56
Leusden[51]	1987	13	zoladex	3.6 mg s.c. monthly	12	−40
Maheux[52]	1987	9	buserelin	400 μg i.n. tid	24	−71
West[53]	1987	13	zoladex	3.6 μg s.c. monthly	24	−55
Perl[54]	1987	10	D-Trp6-LHRH	100 μ s.c. daily	12	−39
Friedman[55]	1987	7	leuprolid	800 μg i.n. bid	24	+9
		7	leuprolid	500 μg s.c. daily	24	−54
Benagiano[56]	1988	10	buserelin	1.5 mg s.c. daily	24	−82
Eckstein[57]	1988	7	decapeptyl-cr	3.2 mg s.c. monthly	24	−45–75
		5	decapeptyl	500 μg s.c monthly	24	−70–90
		5	buserelin	600 μg i.n. tid	24	−35–60
Oltramari[58]	1988	17	buserelin	i.n. tid	24	−33
Maheux[59]	1988	10	buserelin	350 μg s.c. tid	24	−58
		10	buserelin	200 μg s.c. tid	24	−53
Kessel[60]	1988	9	histrelin	20–50 μg s.c. daily	24	−40
		6	D-Trp6–LHRH	20–50 μg s.c. daily	24	−40
Friedman[61]	1988	7	leuprolide	500 μg s.c. daily	24	−51
		9	leuprolide and provera	500 μg s.c. daily 20 mg	24	−14
Andreyko[62]	1988	10	nafarelin	400 μg i.n. bid		−46
TOTAL		201		Mean reduction		−48.2%

the symptomatology associated with these tumors during the years before the menopause with LHRH-A, some hysterectomies may be avoided. Hysterectomy was often recommended in the 1960s as prophylaxis against future cancer, this was especially true if the patient was harboring a leiomyoma. However, as prophylaxis against future cancer, hysterectomy can be expected to increase life expectancy by approximately 2 months, at a considerable cost in dollars and morbidity[6]; only 0.1% to 0.5% of uterine leiomyomata are believed to degenerate into cancer[13]. The true incidence of sarcomatous degeneration is probably lower. Recently, most of the pathological slides of sarcomatous degeneration of uterine myomata which have been reported in the Quebec area have been reviewed by Dr J. Bonenfant, a senior pathologist in Canada. In many instances, the diagnosis of cancer was made during the 1950s and 1960s not on the number of mitoses per high power field but on the presence of bizarre hyperchromatic, polymorphous nuclei. These atypical nuclei are not diagnostic of cancer and may be only secondary to degenerative changes. The true incidence of sarcomatous degeneration in a leiomyoma is therefore probably extremely rare. So rare, that the probability of finding a cancer will probably be greater if instead of a hysterectomy, the surgeon removed the breasts of the patient harboring a uterine leiomyoma, as one of 11 women will have a breast cancer during her life. Elective prophylactic hysterectomy for an asymptomatic patient is therefore to be condemned. As the incidence of sarcomatous degeneration in a uterine leiomyoma is lower than the incidence of breast carcinoma, prophylatic hysterectomy does not make any more sense than prophylactic bilateral mammectomy.

Severe hypoestrogenism is associated with an increased risk of atherosclerosis and osteoporosis. If to control the symptomatology associated with uterine leiomyomata, we have to induce in a patient severe hypoestrogenism with LHRH-A, the cure of her disease may be worse than the initial problem she presented. Fortunately this does not seem the case. Figure 2 illustrates the mean estradiol levels and myoma volume reduction that we have observed in the four groups of patients that we have treated up to now with four different dosages of buserelin. Patients in groups A, C and D received respectively 500, 350 and 200 μg s.c. daily whereas women in group B received 400 μg t.i.d. by nasal insufflation. From this graph, we can see that, once we remove the high fluctuations of estradiol encountered in the ovulation cycle, it does not make any difference whether some basal estradiol is conserved or not; the reduction observed in the volume of uterine leiomyoma being statistically the same among these four groups although basal estradiol is different (group A > group B, $p < 0.05$). In terms of side-effects, however, the preservation of some estrogen stimulation makes a great difference, fewer hot flushes[52], bone preservation[59] and increased HDL cholesterol[52-59]. Therefore it seems possible to control uterine leiomyomata while preserving some blood estrogens.

We have treated with LHRH-A during the last 3 years a premenopausal woman harboring symptomatic uterine leiomyoma (Figure 3). With the LHRH-A given subcutaneously at a dose of 500 μg daily, we have induced severe hypoestrogenism with amenorrhea and significant hot flushes. A

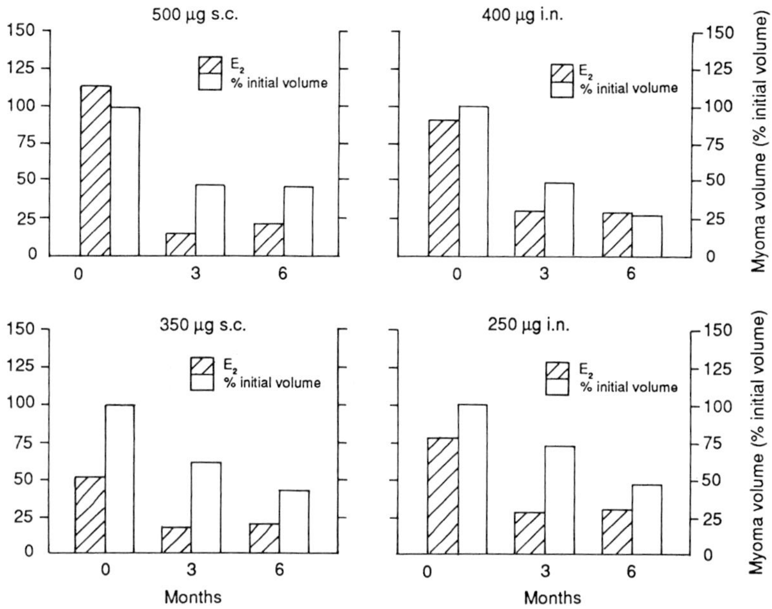

Figure 2 Serum estradiol and volume of uterine leiomyoma in four groups of patients treated with different dosages of buserelin

91.2% reduction in the volume of the uterine leiomyoma was observed during this first period. The leiomyoma re-enlarged to 66% of its initial volume during the next 6-month period without medication. As symptoms recurred, the patient was placed a second time on LHRH-A treatment, this time with intranasal insufflation of 400 μg three times a day. Serum estradiol levels were not well controlled during this second episode of treatment with minimal hot flushes and regular bleeding. Interestingly, a reduction, although less pronounced, in the volume of her leiomyoma was observed. This indicates that, in some patients at least, severe hypoestrogenism, with all the resulting side-effects, may not be necessary to control uterine leiomyomata. During the next year and a half, we tried to adjust the dosage of the LHRH-A so that the patient conserved some estrogen stimulation with uterine bleeding and minimal hot flushes. To prevent possible hyperplasia of the endometrium, medroxyprogestereone acetate 10 mg *per os* daily for 10 days has been added to the treatment regimen. In April 1986, more than 3 years after first administration of LHRH-A, dual photon bone densitometry has shown no sign of osteoporosis with bone mineral content of respectively 0.93 gHA/cm^2 (69th percentile) and 0.71 gHA/cm^2 (50th percentile) for the lumbar spine and the femoral neck. Here also, HDL-cholesterol increased during treatment, from a value of 47 up to 70 mg/100ml. The fact that we have been able to control the volume of the leiomyoma in this patient and the associated symptomatology with mild hypoestrogenism is encouraging, however dose adjustment of LHRH-A has been shown to be impractical and the patient

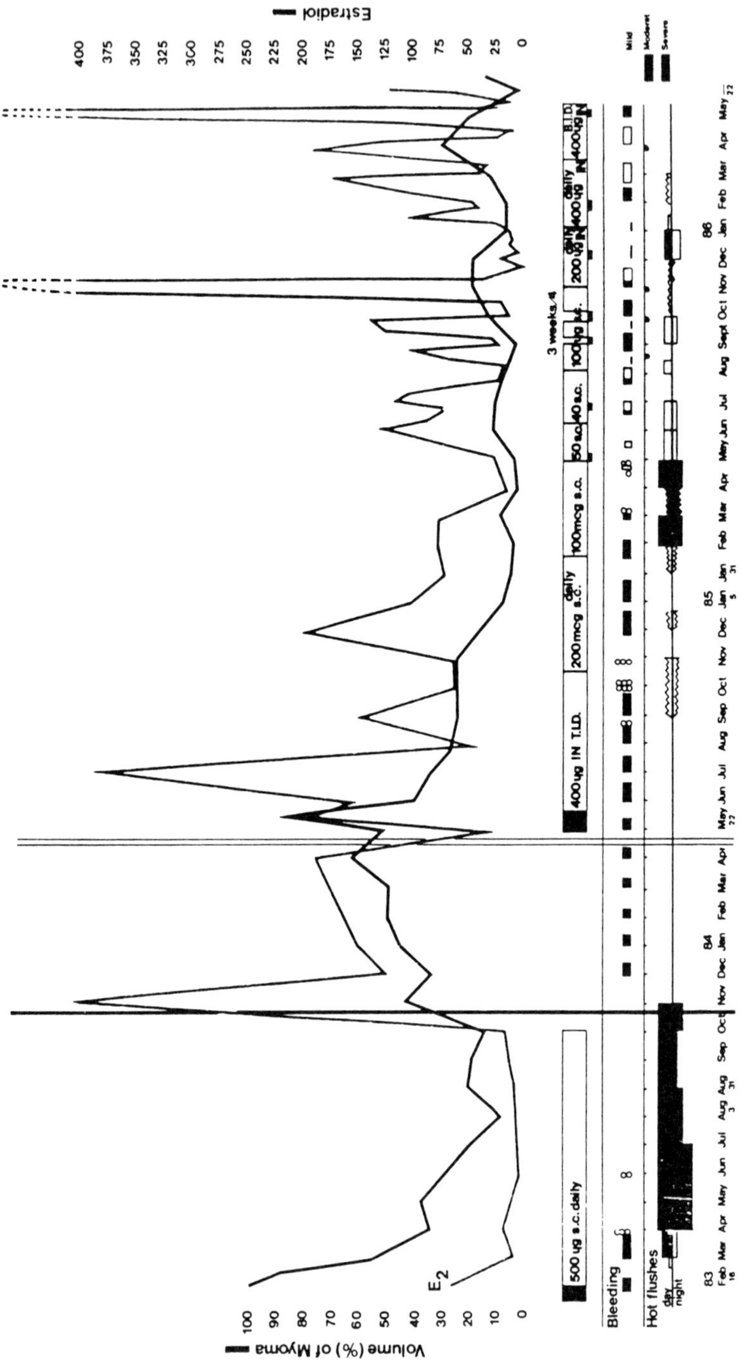

Figure 3 Serum estradiol, volume of uterine leiomyoma, bleeding pattern and hot flushes observed in a premenopausal patient treated between February 83 and May 86 with buserelin

had to undergo hysterectomy.

We have recently tried a new approach which is discussed in this chapter; the combined utilization of LHRH-A with low-dose hormonal replacement therapy. The study was conducted in ten premenopausal women harboring symptomatic myomata. Zoladex (3.6 mg; ICI Canada) was administered monthly for 1 year. After the initial 3 months, maximum regression of myomata was obtained (mean 65.4%). During the remaining 9 months, Premarin 0.3 mg (Ayerst Canada) from day 1 to 25 and Provera 5 mg (Upjohn Canada) from day 16 to 25 have been added to the treatment regimen. No significant regrowth of the myomata was observed so far, hot flushes were minimal and the bleeding pattern was predictable. The safety laboratory data including HDL-cholesterol and dual photon bone densitometry stayed in the normal range during the treatment period. We concluded that in selected cases, this approach may be a valid alternative to hysterectomy in premenopausal women harboring symptomatic uterine leiomyomata.

CONCLUSION

Treatment of uterine leiomyoma has changed drastically during recent centuries. With the introduction of modern surgery with suture, anesthesia and asepsis, hysterectomy can now be considered a safe procedure. Effective medical treatment is now available. The preoperative LHRH-A administration greatly facilitates surgical procedure, allowing myomectomy in some women desiring to preserve their fertility potential who otherwise would have needed hysterectomies. In selected cases, especially by the end of the reproductive period, LHRH-A may become a valid alternative to hysterectomy as most of the uterine leiomyomata are going to be asymptomatic after menopause. However, a great deal of research should be done not only on treatment but also on the etiology of this disease. However, as this pathology seems to attract the attention of the scientific community more and more, the future is looking brighter.

REFERENCES

1. Atlee, W.L. (1853). The surgical treatment of certain fibrous tumours of the uterus, heretofore considered beyond the resources of art. *Trans. Am. Med. Assoc.*, **6**, 547–643
2. Atlee, W.L. (1845). Case of a successful extirpation of a fibrous tumor of the peritoneal surface of the uterus by the large peritoneal section. *Am. J. Med. Sci.*, **9**, 309–35
3. Speert, H. (ed.) (1980). *The Nineteenth Century: a Specialty Evolves. Obstetrics and Gynecology in America: A History*, vol. 4, pp. 37–71. (Baltimore: Waverley Press)
4. National Center for Health Statistics. (1982). Utilization of shortstay hospitals, Annual Summary for the United-States, 1980. *Vital and Health Statistics, Series 13* **64**
5. Dicker, R.C., Scally, M.J., Greenspan, J.R., Layde, P.M., Ory, H.W., Maze, J.M. and Smith, J.C. (1982). Hysterectomy among women of reproductive age. Trends in the United States, 1970–1978. *J. Am. Med. Assoc.*, **248**, 323–7
6. Bunker, J.P., Donahue, V.C., Cole, P., Notman, M.T. and Bunker, J.P. (1976). Public-health rounds at the Harvard School of public health. *N. Engl. J. Med.*, **295**, 264–8
7. Dicker, R.C., Greenspan, J.R., Strauss, L.T. *et al.* (1982). Complications of abdominal and

vaginal hysterectomy among women of reproductive age in the United States. *Am. J. Obstet. Gynecol.*, **144**, 841–8
8. Easterday, C.L., Grimes, D.A. and Riggs, J.A. (1983). Hysterectomy in the United States. *Obstet. Gynecol.*, **62**, 203–12
9. Richards, D.H. (1973). Depression after hysterectomy. *Lancet*, **ii**, 430–3
10. Christ, J.E. and Lotze, E.C. (1975). The residual ovary syndrome. *Obstet. Gynecol.*, **46**, 551–6
11. Centerwall, B.S. (1981). Premenopausal hysterectomy and cardiovascular disease. *Am. J. Obstet. Gynecol.*, **139**, 58–61
12. Lee, N.C., Dicker, R.C., Rubin, G.L. and Ory, H.W. (1984). Confirmation of the preoperative diagnoses for hysterectomy. *Am. J. Obstet. Gynecol.*, **150**, 283–7
13. Buttram, V.C. and Reiter, R.C. (1981). Uterine leiomyomata: etiology, symptomatology, and management. *Fertil. Steril.*, **36**, 433–45
14. Dolmey, V. (1931). The technique and results of myomectomy. *Lancet*, **i**, 171
15. Matta, W.H.M., Stabile, I., Shaw, R.W. and Campbell, S. (1988). Doppler assessment of uterine blood flow changes in patients with fibroids receiving the gonadotropin-releasing hormone agonist Buserelin. *Fertil. Steril.*, **49**, 1083–5
16. Maheux, R. (1986). LH-RH agonist – How useful against uterine leiomyomas? *Contemp. Obstet. Gynecol.*, **28**, 66–77
17. Murphy, A.A. (1987). Operative laparoscopy. *Fertil. Steril.*, **47**, 1–18
18. Dicker, D., Feldberg, D., Dekel, A., Yeshaya, A., Samuel, N. and Goldman, J.A. (1986). The management of prolapsed submucous fibroids. *Aust. N.Z. J. Obstet. Gynaecol.*, **26**, 308–11
19. Fried, F.A. and Hulka, J.F. (1987). Transuterine resection of fibroids: a new approach to the management of submucous fibroids in selected patients. *J. Urol.* **138**, 1256–7
20. Hallez, J.P., Netter, A. and Cartier, R. (1987). Methodical intrauterine resection. *Am. J. Obstet. Gynecol.*, **156**, 1080–4
21. Goldrath, M.H. (1987). Vaginal removal of the pendunculated submucous myoma: the use of laminaria. *Obstet. Gynecol.*, **70**, 670–2
22. Goodman, A.L. (1946). Progesterone therapy in uterine fibromyoma. *J. Clin. Endocrinol. Metab.*, **6**, 402–8
23. Goldzieher, J.W., Maqueo, M., Ricaud, L., Aguilar, J.A. and Canales, E. (1966). Induction of degenerative changes in uterine myomas by high-dose progestin therapy. *Am. J. Obstet. Gynecol.*, **96**, 1078–87
24. Segaloff, A., Weed, J.C., Sternberg, W.H. and Parson, W. (1949). The progesterone therapy of human uterine leiomyomas. *J. Clin. Endocrinol.*, **9**, 1273–91
25. Pollow, K., Geilfuss, J., Boquoi, E. and Pollow, B. (1978). Estrogen and progesterone binding proteins in normal human myometrium and leiomyoma tissue. *J. Clin. Chem. Clin. Biochem.*, **16**, 503–11
26. Boulet, A.P. and Fortier, M.A. (1987). Preparation and characterization of rabbit myometrial cells in primary culture: influence of estradiol and progesterone treatment. In Vitro *Cell. Dev. Biol.*, **23**, 93–9
27. Tiltman, A.J. (1985). The effect of progestins on the mitotic activity of uterine fibromyomas. *Int. J. Gynecol. Pathol.*, **4**, 89–96
28. Maheux, R., DeCherney, A. and Polan, M.L. (1983). Use of danazol in treatment of myomata uteri. Presented at the 1983 *Annual Meeting of the American Fertility Society*
29. Yuen, B.H. (1981). Danazol and uterine leiomyomas. *Can. Med. J. Assoc.*, **124**, 963–4
30. Tamaya, T., Motoyama, T., Ohono, Y., Ide, N., Tsurusaki, T. and Okada, H. (1979). Estradiol 17B, progesterone and 5 alpha-dihydro-testosterone receptors of uterine myometrium and myoma in the human subject. *J. Steroid Biochem.*, **10**, 615–22
31. Reddy, V.V. and Rose, L.I. (1979). Delta-4-3-ketosteroid 5 alpha-oxidoreductase in human uterine leiomyoma. *Am. J. Obstet. Gynecol.*, **135**, 415–18
32. Yamamoto, T., Takamori, K. and Okada, H. (1984). Estrogen biosynthesis in leiomyoma and myometrium of the uterus. *Horm. Metabol. Res.*, **16**, 678–9
33. Sakiz, E., Azadian-Boulanger, G., Laraque, F., Raynaud, J.P. (1974). A new approach to estrogen-free contraception based on progesterone receptor blockage by mid-cycle administration of ethyl norgestrienone (R-2323). *Contraception*, **10**, 467–74
34. Coutinho, E.M., Da Silva, A.R., Carreira, C.M., Chaves, M.C. and Filho, J.A. (1975). Contraceptive effectiveness of Silastic implants containing the progestin R-2323. *Contracep-*

tion, **11**, 625–35

35. Coutinho, E.M. (1981). Conservative treatment of uterine leiomyoma with the antiestrogen antiprogesterone R-2323. *Int. J. Obstet. Gynecol.*, **19**, 357–60
36. Coutinho, E.M., Azadian Boulanger, G. and Gonçalves, M.T. (1986). Regression of uterine leiomyomas after treatment with gestrinone, an antiestrogen, antiprogesterone. *Am. J. Obstet. Gynecol.*, **155**, 761–7
37. Meiling, H. (1980). Gossypol treatment for menopausal functional bleeding, myoma of uterus and endometriosis: Preliminary report. *Acta Acad. Med. Sin.*, **2**, 170
38. Chamfrault, A. (1964). *Traité de Médecine Chinoise*. pp. 928–47 (Angoulême: Coquemard)
39. Helms, J.M. (1987). Acupuncture for the management of primary dysmenorrhea. *Obstet. Gynecol.*, **69**, 51–6
40. Fraser, I.S., Pearse, C., Shearman, R.P., Elliot, P.M., McIlveen, J. and Markham, R. (1981). Efficacy of mefenamic acid in patients with a complaint of menorrhagia. *Obstet. Gynecol.*, **58**, 543–51
41. Guillebaud, J., Anderson, A.B.M. and Turnbull, A.C. (1978). Reduction by mefenamic acid of increased menstrual blood loss in association with intrauterine contraception. *Br. J. Obstet. Gynaecol.*, **85**, 53–62
42. Ylikorkala, O. and Pekonen, F. (1986). Naproxen reduces idiopathic but not fibromyoma-induced menorrhagia. *Obstet. Gynecol.*, **68**, 10–12
43. Maheux, R., Guilloteau, C., Lemay, A., Bastide, A. and Fazekas, A.T.A. (1985). Luteinizing hormone-releasing hormone agonist and uterine leiomyoma: A pilot study. *Am. J. Obstet. Gynecol.*, **152**, 1034–8
44. Filicori, M., Hall, D.A., Loughlin, J.S., Rivier, J., Vale, W. and Crowley, W.F. (1983). A conservative approach to the management of uterine leiomyoma: pituitary desensitization by a luteinizing hormone-releasing hormone analogue. *Am. J. Obstet. Gynecol.*, **147**, 726–7
45. Maheux, R., Guilloteau, C., Lemay, A., Bastide, A. and Fazekas, A.T.A. (1984). Regression of leiomyomata uteri following hypoestrogenism induced by repetitive LHRH agonist treatment: preliminary report. *Fertil. Steril.*, **42**, 644–6
46. Healy, D.L., Fraser, H.M. and Lawson, S.L. (1984). Shrinkage of a uterine fibroid after subcutaneous infusion of a LHRH agonist. *Br. Med. J.*, **289**, 1267–8
47. Matta, W., Shaw, R.W. and Nye, M. (1986). Blair bell research society. Papers presented at the meeting in May 1986 at the Royal College of Obstetricians and Gynaecologists. *Br. J. Obstet. Gynaecol.*, **93**, 1194–7
48. Healy, D.L., Lawson, S.R., Abbott, M., Baird, D.T. and Fraser, H.M. (1986). Toward removing uterine fibroids without surgery: subcutaneous infusion of a luteinizing hormone-releasing hormone agonist commencing in the luteal phase. *J. Clin. Endocrinol. Metab.*, **63**, 619–25
49. VanLeusden, H.A.I.M. (1986). Rapid reduction of uterine myomas after short-term treatment with microencapsulated D-Trp^{6}–LHRH. *Lancet*, **ii**, 1213
50. Goddington, C.C., Collins, R.L., Shawker, P.H., Anderson, R., Loriaux, D.L. and Winkle, C.A. (1986). Long-acting gonadotropin hormone-releasing hormone analog used to treat uteri. *Fertil. Steril.*, **45**, 624–9
51. Lumsden, M.A., West, C.P. and Baird, D.T. (1987). Goserelin therapy before surgery for uterine fibroids. *Lancet*, **i**, 36
52. Maheux, R., Lemay, A. and Mérat, P. (1987). Use of intranasal luteinizing hormone-releasing hormone agonist in uterine leiomyomas. *Fertil. Steril.*, **47**, 229–33
53. West, C.P., Lumsden, M.A., Lawson, S., Williamson, J. and Baird, D.T. (1987). Shrinkage of uterine fibroids during therapy with goserelin (Zoladex): a luteinizing hormone-releasing hormone agonist administered as a monthly subcutaneous depot. *Fertil. Steril.*, **48**, 45–51
54. Perl, V., Marquez, J., Schally, A.V., Comaru-Schally, A.M., Leal, G., Zacharias, S. and Gomez-Lira, C. (1987). Treatment of leiomyomata uteri with D-Trp^{6}-luteinizing hormone-releasing hormone. *Fertil. Steril.* **48**, 383–9
55. Friedman, A.J., Barbieri, R.L., Benacerraf, B.R. and Schiff, I. (1987). Treatment of leiomyomata with intranasal or subcutaneous leuprolide, a gonadotropin-releasing hormone agonist. *Fertil. Steril.*, **48**, 560–4
56. Benagiano, G., Primiero, F., Morini, A., Isidori, C., Addi, G. and Tunnera, G. (1988). Multimodal pharmacological approach to the treatment of leiomyomata uteri. Presented at the *First Congress of the International Society of Gynecological Endocrinology*, Crans

Montana, March 6–12. *Gynecol. Endocrinol.*, **2**, 50

57. Eckstein, N., Wagman, I., Eshel, A., Mann, A. and Ayalon, D. (1988). Results of long term treatment of patients with uterine leiomyoma with GnRH agonists. Presented at the *First Congress of the International Society of Gynecological Endocrinology*, Crans Montana, March 6–12. *Gynecol. Endocrinol.*, **2**, 199
58. Oltramari, P., Volpe, A., Petraglia, F., La Marca, S., Adama, R., La Torre, L. and Genazzani, A.R. (1988). LH-RH analogous in the treatment of endometriosis and leiomyomatosi uteri: clinical and endocrinal aspects. Presented at the *First Congress of the International Society of Gynecological Endocrinology*, Crans Monana, March 6–12. *Gynecol. Endocrinol.*, **2**, 200
59. Maheux, R., Lemay, A. and Mérat, P. (1988). A prospective randomized study comparing 2 subcutaneous dosages of the luteinizing hormone-releasing hormone agonist (LHRH-A) buserelin in the treatment of uterine leiomyoma. Presented at the 44*th Annual Meeting of the American Fertility Society*, Atlanta, Georgia, October 8–13
60. Kessel, B., Liu, J., Mortola, J., Berga, S. and Yen, S.S.C. (1988). Treatment of uterine fibroids with agonist analogs of gonadotropin-releasing hormone. *Fertil. Steril.*, **49**, 538–41
61. Friedman, A.J., Barbieri, R.L., Doubilet, P.M., Fine, C. and Schiff, I. (1988). A randomized, double-blind trial of a gonadotropin releasing-hormone agonist (leuprolide) with or without medroxyprogesterone acetate in the treatment of leiomyomata uteri. *Fertil. Steril.*, **49**, 404–9
62. Andreyko, J.L., Blumenfeld, Z., Marshall, L.A., Monroe, S.E., Hricak, H. and Jaffe, R.B. (1988). Use of an agonistic analog of gonadotropin-releasing hormone (naferelin) to treat leiomyomas: Assessment by magnetic resonance imaging. *Am J. Obstet. Gynecol.*, **158**, 903–10

26

Treatment of leiomyomata uteri and menorrhagia with goserelin depot

P. Vercellini, L. Fedele, L. Arcaini, S. Bianchi, M. Sideri and G. Battista Candiani

INTRODUCTION

Leiomyomata uteri are the commonest pelvic mass, being present in 20–25% of women over 35[1]. Sarcomatous degeneration probably occurs in under 0.03–0.7% of cases[2]. In the United States the most frequent surgical operation, after Caesarean section, is hysterectomy, which was performed on 673 000 women in 1983[3]. Uterine myomata constitute the main indication for this operation[4], and according to some authors are the reason for 60% of gynecological laparotomies[1]. Each year 1.7 billion dollars are spent on hysterectomies in the United States[4]. The possibility of alternative treatments for symptomatic uterine leiomyomata would have important social and health-care effects. Recently various gonadotropin-releasing hormone agonists (GnRH-A) have been used to induce transient hypoestrogenism with volume reduction of leiomyomata[5,6]. We administered a GnRH-A, goserelin, in a depot formulation to 14 premenopausal women with symptomatic fibroids with the aim of evaluating the safety, ovarian suppression potential and efficacy of this treatment in reducing uterine volume and in resolving symptoms.

MATERIAL AND METHODS

Fourteen women of mean age 46 years (range 33–53) with symptomatic fibroids participated in the study after giving informed consent. Mean parity was 1.9 (range 0–4). The main disturbance was severe menometrorrhagia in eight women and pressure symptoms in six. The inclusion criteria were:

(1) Non-pregnant women not wanting children;
(2) Uterine body of at least twice normal volume;
(3) Menometrorrhagia with hemoglobin (Hb) under 11 g/dl;
(4) Negative Pap smear and endometrial biopsy in the month preceding the start of treatment;

(5) No adnexal disease at pelvic exploration and ultrasound scanning; and
(6) Follicle stimulating hormone (FSH) under 30 mIU/ml.

Goserelin depot 3.6 mg (Zoladex, ICI Pharma-Italia, Milano, Italy), a decapeptide LHRH agonist incorporated in a biodegradable lactide–glycolide copolymer vehicle from which the drug is released at a constant rate of 120 μg/day, was injected subcutaneously into the anterior abdominal wall using a prepacked syringe every 28 days for 6 months. Eight patients started the treatment between days 22 and 24 of the menstrual cycle, and six between days 1 and 3. In no case was local anesthesia used.

Evaluation of the patients before treatment and at monthly intervals during the 6-month study included a complete medical history, physical examination with blood pressure measurement, and a battery of laboratory tests (serum estradiol (E_2), progesterone (P), prolactin (PRL), FSH, luteinizing hormone (LH), triiodothyronine (T_3), thyroxin (T_4), free unbound T_4 (FT_4) index, thyrotropin (TSH), complete blood count, serum iron, total iron binding capacity (TIBC), serum glucose, blood urea nitrogen (BUN), serum creatinine, aspartate aminotransferase, alanine aminotransferase, bilirubin, alkaline phosphatase, γ-glutamyl transferase, prothrombin time, partial prothrombin time, electrophoresis of serum proteins, triglycerides, total and high density lipoprotein (HDL)-cholesterol, electrolytes, complete urine analysis). Specific radioimmunoassays (Biodata, Milan, Italy) were used to perform quantitative determinations of serum LH and FSH over the range of 1.5–200 mIU/ml (2nd International reference preparation of human menopausal gonadotropin). With the E_2 ^{125}I radioimmunoassay (RIA) kit (Biodata, Milan, Italy) direct quantitative determinations of E_2 were obtained with a standard curve between 25 to 2000 pg/ml.

Overall uterine volume excluding the cervix was calculated at sonography according to the formula for a prolate ellipsoid (length $\times$ width $\times$ depth $\times$ 0.5233). All ultrasound measurements were performed by one of two observers using a real time Ansaldo 440 scanner with a 3.5 MHz convex transducer. Uterine volume was determined in each patient before treatment and at monthly intervals during the study. All patients were instructed to use a barrier method of contraception during the study period.

Statistical analysis of the laboratory data was performed with analysis of variance for repeated measures. Analysis of ultrasound data before, during and at the end of treatment was performed with the Wilcoxon rank test for matched pairs. All data are expressed as means $\pm$ SEM.

RESULTS

All the patients completed the study. The subcutaneous injections of goserelin depot were always well tolerated although a 16 gauge needle was used with no local anesthesia. No subject reported disturbances at the injection site, which was always normal at the monthly examinations.

In the eight patients who started treatment in the midluteal phase of the cycle, the next menstrual flow was slightly earlier, lighter, and of longer duration (mean 13 days, range 8–16) than expected. The next menstruation in the six women who started the treatment at the beginning of the cycle was at the expected time, more abundant, and slightly longer (mean 7 days, range 5–11). Five weeks from the start of treatment 12 women were amenorrheic whereas two had spotting for 10 weeks. All the women reported hot flushes starting after the second injection, but in no case was the disturbance so severe as to require treatment suspension. For four patients night sweats were uncomfortable, slightly disturbing sleep, and three others reported transient headache. Six subjects had vaginal dryness, but application of a lubricating gel resolved discomfort during intercourse. Two patients reported reduced libido, and five noted a decrease in breast size. Pressure symptoms were relieved by 3 months of treatment. Ovulation was inhibited in all the subjects during treatment, with serum P levels never exceeding 1 mg/ml. Pretreatment E_2 concentrations obtained in the midluteal phase were 142 pg/ml ± 37. Four weeks after the start of treatment gonadal suppression was profound and uniform in all patients except two who began treatment while menstruating (Table 1). At 2 months E_2 levels fell to < 20 pg/ml, with only one subsequent flare-up in two women at 3 and 4 months respectively. Serum LH values ranged from 14.8 to 24.4 mIU/ml, and FSH values were between 7.8 and 10.7 mIU/ml. Neither of the two gonadotropins altered significantly during the treatment period (Table 1). PRL, T_3, T_4, FT_4 index and TSH remained in the normal range.

The mean pretreatment uterine volume of the 14 patients was 519 cm^3 ± 68.

Table 1 Serum LH, FSH and estradiol concentrations in 14 women with uterine leiomyomas before and during goserelin depot treatment (mean ± SEM)

Month	E_2 (pg/ml)	*LH* (mIU/ml)	*FSH* (mIU/ml)
Pretreatment	142.0 ± 37	18.3 ± 1.2	10.2 ± 1.5
1	29.6 ± 4.2	24.1 ± 1.6	7.8 ± 1.0
2	< 20	25.4 ± 1.8	10.1 ± 1.8
3	23.7 ± 3.1	28.4 ± 2.6	9.6 ± 1.2
4	31.5 ± 9.5	19.6 ± 1.4	10.7 ± 1.2
5	< 20	14.8 ± 1.1	9.7 ± 1.7
6	< 20	20.2 ± 1.6	8.4 ± 0.7

Table 2 Uterine volume by ultrasound scan in 14 women with uterine leiomyomas before and during goserelin depot treatment

Month	*Volume* (cm^3) *mean ± SEM*	*Reduction/cycle* (%)	*Pretreatment volume* (%)
Pretreatment	519 ± 68	—	100.0
1	396 ± 57	23.7	76.3
2	324 ± 49	18.2	62.4
3	273 ± 46	15.7	52.6
4	284 ± 51	−4.0	54.7
5	269 ± 47	5.3	51.8
6	263 ± 44	2.3	50.7

$p < 0.01$ 3 months *vs* pretreatment; *p*, NS 3 months *vs* 6 months

All the women responded to treatment with a mean volume reduction of 49.3% at 6 months (Table 2), the individual reductions being between 32 and 67% independently of the initial size. The greatest mean percentage reduction was observed after 1 month of treatment (23.7%) with a progressive good response over the next 2 months to reach a mean uterine volume of $273\,cm^3 \pm 46$, that is a 47.4% reduction ($p < 0.01$ versus baseline). The response over the last 3 months was limited, and at the end of the study the mean volume was $263\,cm^3 \pm 44$ (p = NS). Significant differences were not found between the patients who started treatment in the midluteal phase and those who started in the early follicular phase at any of the time-points. No increase in uterus size was observed in the two women with a rise in E_2 levels at 3 and 4 months.

Eight patients with severe menometrorrhagia started treatment with a mean hemoglobin (Hb) level of 7.7 g/dl corresponding to a mean hematocrit (Hct) of 26.3% (Table 3). After 3 months of treatment the values normalized (Hb, 13.1 g/dl; Hct, 40.2%) ($p < 0.01$). In the same period we observed a significant rise in serum iron from 37.3 to 72.6 μg/dl ($p < 0.01$) and a significant fall in TIBC from 396.2 to 334.1 mg/dl ($p < 0.01$). The further modification of Hb, Hct, serum iron and TIBC that occurred in the second 3 months of the study did not reach statistical significance.

No alterations were seen in the monthly blood pressure measurements. Routine blood tests remained in the normal range in all the women during the treatment period. In particular, total cholesterol, HDL-cholesterol, triglycerides and the total/HDL-cholesterol ratio did not vary significantly.

DISCUSSION

Treatment of leiomyomata uteri has always been surgical. Clinical and experimental data have demonstrated the sensitivity of fibroids to estrogens[7]. We used monthly goserelin depot injections to induce transient hypoestrogenism in 14 women with symptomatic fibroids. The injections were practical and did not require local anesthesia, nor did they provoke local reactions. Gonadal suppression was prompt and uniform. Only on two occasions did serum E_2 levels exceed the postmenopausal threshold. FSH and LH levels did not present significant modification. It is known that during treatment with GnRH-A there is a marked decrease in the bioactive LH/immunoreactive LH ratio (the B/I ratio), especially using the conventional polyclonal antibody

Table 3 Hemoglobin, hematocrit, serum iron, and total iron binding capacity (TIBC) in eight patients with uterine leiomyomata and severe menometrorrhagia before and during goserelin depot treatment (mean ± SEM)

	Pretreatment	*3 months (% variation)*	*6 months (% variation)*
Hemoglobin (g/dl)	7.7 ± 0.3	13.1 ± 0.2* (+70)	13.8 ± 0.2† (+ 79)
Hematocrit (%)	26.3 ± 0.7	40.2 ± 0.9* (+53)	41.6 ± 0.6† (+ 58)
Serum iron (μg/dl)	37.3 ± 6.1	72.6 ± 3.6* (+94)	82.5 ± 7.5† (+121)
TIBC (μg/dl)	396.2 ± 23.7	334.1 ± 18.9* (−15)	327.2 ± 15.4† (− 17)

$p < 0.01$ *vs* pretreatment; †p, NS *vs* 3 months treatment radioimmunoassay[5,8]. Women treated with a GnRH analog synthesize non-glycosylated α and β protein chains of FSH[9]. Non-glycosylated FSH is not biologically active, but it binds to FSH receptors more avidly than glycosylated bioactive hormone. GnRH-A could act not only by determining a reduction in the number of LHRH receptors in the anterior pituitary (down-regulation) but also by inducing the synthesis of iso-LH and iso-FSH non-glycosylated forms. When *in vitro* bioassays and monoclonal immunoradiometric assay for LH and FSH are not available, endocrine monitoring by FSH and LH measurements during GnRH-A treatments may not reflect the real state of gonadal supression[10,11]. The side-effects of hypoestrogenism were fairly well tolerated by our patients and treatment never had to be suspended.

At the end of the treatment the mean uterine volume was reduced by about 50%. In the first 3 months there was a rapid and constant fall in the mean size ($p < 0.01$ versus baseline) followed by only minor changes over the next 3 months (p = NS). The individual variability in fibroid response did not relate either to the initial overall uterine volume or, as suggested by others[6,10], to the degree of hypoestrogenism reached, since from 2 months onwards all the serum E_2 measurements except two were under 20 pg/ml. Moreover, an excellent reduction of myoma size has also been reported in the presence of incomplete ovarian suppression[12,13]. The difference in response could depend on the ratio between the muscular and fibrous components. A fall of E_2 may induce a reduction in size of the smooth muscle cells but it has a scanty effect on the fibrous connective tissue. The greatest percentage reduction was obtained, as reported by others[11], in the first months. Estrogens have a vasodilating effect on uterine arteries of sheep[14]. Cytoplasmic and nuclear estrogen receptors have been identified in human uterine arteries[15,16].

During buserelin treatment an increase of vascular resistances of uterine arteries and of arteries supplying fibroids has been demonstrated using a pulsed wave Doppler system[17]. The rapid reduction of uterine volume after only 1 month of treatment may be partially due to a marked decrease of blood flow. Lumsden *et al.*[18] have reported a reduction in the binding of epidermal growth factor (EGF) to fibroid tissue and not to myometrium during goserelin depot treatment. Their results suggest that the fibroid shrinkage associated with hypoestrogenism may be partly mediated by EGF.

The increase of Hb (+ 79%) and Hct (+58%) in our patients with menometrorrhagia was impressive, and emergency hysterectomy with blood transfusions was avoided. The most marked improvement was obtained in the first trimester, the subsequent increase not being statistically significant. Farrer-Brown *et al.*[19,20] have demonstrated radiologically that menometrorrhagia associated with myomas may derive from pressure on venous plexuses of the adjacent myometrium and endometrium. Fibroids may obstruct the return of venous blood from the internal myometrium, or impair the radial or arcuate veins in the intramural and subserous myometrium. A volume reduction of fibroids, associated with a decreased blood flow in the uterine vascular bed due to increased arterial resistances, may result in resolution of the venous ectasias probably responsible for excessive bleeding.

Routine blood tests did not present any modifications. In particular the blood lipid profile was not influenced by transient hypoestrogenism. The administration of goserelin for 6 months was found to be practical, acceptable and safe. The continuous availability of the drug ensured by the depot formulation results in a constant plasma concentration and avoids unpredictable fluctuation of the ovarian steroids[21,22]. According to our data, continuation of the treatment for longer than 3 months does not improve the results in terms of uterine volume and blood tests. The prolonged use of GnRH-A raises the question of a possible effect on bone metabolism[21]. It is known that the effects of GnRH-A are rapidly reversible at suspension, with the return of the uterus and fibroids to pretreatment size[11].

When hysterectomy is indicated, preoperative treatment for 3 months with goserelin depot would correct iron deficiency anemia and thus avoid transfusions, reducing the risks of parenteral infections and the costs of care. A decrease in intraoperative blood loss and postoperative febrile morbidity has been reported in patients hysterectomized after treatment with goserelin depot compared with a control group[23]. It is probable that excessive bleeding, frequency of blood transfusions, and risk of infections and the formation of adhesions, may be even more reduced by an accurate surgical technique. According to various authors[12,24,25], the administration of GnRH-A before a myomectomy facilitates the operation by reducing the myometrial thickness and vascularization of the uterus and fibroids, shrinking the latter and thus assisting their enucleation; it would also minimize blood loss and the risk of a hysterectomy, and the postoperative course and the probability of subsequent pregnancy would be improved. That the degree of vascularization is a decisive factor in the favorable outcome of myomectomy is not proven: the variables are multiple[2,7]. Preoperative administration of GnRH-A may increase the risk of missing small intramural fibroids at surgery, increasing the frequency of recurrence in the short term[24].

Treatment of symptomatic leiomyomata uteri with GnRH-A for a limited period may be appropriate for premenopausal women until they reach the physiological climacteric. The treatment period could possibly be prolonged by adding low-dose estrogen–progestogen combinations or by inducing moderate ovarian suppression and administering a progestogen at regular intervals. Either of these modalities would avoid the undesired effects of premature hypoestrogenism.

REFERENCES

1. Merril, J.A. and Creasman, W.T. (1986). Lesions of the corpus uteri. In Darforth, D.N. and Scott, J.R. (eds). *Obstetrics and Gynecology*, 5th Ed, pp. 1068–96 (Philadelphia: J.B. Lippincott)
2. Mattingly, R.F. and Thompson, J.D. (1985). Leiomyomata uteri and abdominal hysterectomy for benign disease. In Te Linde, S. (ed.) *Operative Gynecology*. 6th edn, pp. 203–55 (Philadelphia: J.B. Lippincott)
3. Rutkow, I.M. (1986). Obstetric and Gynecologic operations in the United States 1979 to 1984. *Obstet. Gynecol.*, **67**, 755–9
4. Easterday, C.L., Grimes, D.A. and Riggs, J.A. (1983). Hysterectomy in the United States. *Obstet. Gynecol.*, **62**, 203–12

5. Perl, V., Marquez, J., Schally, A.V., Comaru-Schally, A.M., Leal, G., Zacharias, S. and Gomez-Lira, C. (1987). Treatment of leiomyomata uteri with D-Trp^6 luteinizing hormone-releasing hormone. *Fertil. Steril.*, **48**, 383–8
6. Friedman, A., Barbieri, R.L., Benacerraf, B.R. and Schiff, I. (1987). Treatment of leiomyomata with intranasal or subcutaneous leuprolide, a gonadotropin releasing hormone agonist. *Fertil. Steril.*, **48**, 560–4
7. Buttram, V.C. and Reiter, R.C. (1985). Uterine leiomyomata. In Brown, C.L. (ed.) *Surgical Treatment of the Infertile Female*, pp. 201–28 (Baltimore: Williams and Wilkins)
8. Bischof, P. and Herrmann, W.L. (1988). Absence of immunoreactive luteinizing hormone following gonadotropin-releasing hormone against therapy in women with endometriosis. *Gynecol. Obstet. Invest.*, **25**, 130–4
9. Dahl, K.D., Bicsak, T.A. and Hsveh, A.J.W. (1988). Naturally occurring antihormones: secretion of FSH antagonists by women treated with a GnRH analog. *Science*, **239**, 72–4
10. Friedman, A.J., Barbieri, R.L., Doubilet, P.M., Fine, C. and Schiff, I. (1988). A randomized double-blind trial of a gonadotropin releasing-hormone agonist (leuprolide) with or without medroxyprogesterone acetate in the treatment of leiomyomata uteri. *Fertil. Steril.*, **49**, 404–9
11. West, C.P., Lumsden, M.A., Lawson, S., Williamson, J. and Baird, D.T. (1987). Shrinkage of uterine fibroids during therapy with goserelin (Zoladex): a luteinizing hormone-releasing hormone agonist administered as a monthly subcutaneous depot. *Fertil. Steril.*, **48**, 45–51
12. Maheux, R., Lemay, A. and Merat, P. (1987). Use of intranasal luteinizing hormone releasing hormone agonist in uterine leiomyomas. *Fertil. Steril.*, **47**, 229–33
13. Maheux, R., Lemay, A. and Turcot Lemay, L. (1988). Dose-related inhibition of acute luteinizing hormone response during luteinizing hormone-releasing hormone agonist treatment for uterine leiomyoma. *Am. J. Obstet. Gynecol.*, **158**, 361–4
14. Resnik, R., Killam, A.P., Battaglia, F.C., Makowski, E.L. and Meschia, G. (1974). The stimulation of uterine blood flow by various estrogens. *Endocrinology*, **94**, 1192–6
15. Lantta, M., Karkkainem, J. and Lehtovirta, P. (1983). Progesterone and estradiol receptors in the cytosol of the human uterine artery. *Am. J. Obstet. Gynecol.*, **147**, 627–33
16. Batra, S. and Iosif, S. (1987). Nuclear estrogen receptors in human uterine arteries. *Gynecol. Obstet. Invest.*, **24**, 250–5
17. Matta, W.H.M., Stabile, I., Shaw, R.W. and Campbell, S. (1988). Doppler assessment of uterine blood flow changes in patients with fibroids receiving the gonadotropin releasing hormone agonist Buserelin. *Fertil. Steril.*, **49**, 1083–5
18. Lumsden, M.A., West, C.P., Bramley, T., Rumgay, L. and Baird, D.T. (1988). The binding of epidermal growth factor to the human uterus and leiomyomata in women rendered hypoestrogenic by continuous administration of an LHRH agonist. *Br. J. Obstet. Gynaecol.*, **95**, 1299–1304
19. Farrer-Brown, G., Beilby, J.O.W. and Tarbit, M.H. (1970). The vascular patterns in myomatous uteri. *J. Obstet. Gynaecol. Br. Cwlth.*, **77**, 967
20. Farrer-Brown, G., Beilby, J.O.W. and Tarbit, M.H. (1971). Venous changes in the endometrium of the myomatous uteri. *Obstet. Gynecol.*, **38**, 743
21. Matta, W.H., Shaw, R.W., Hesp, R. and Katz, D. (1987). Hypogonadism induced by luteinizing hormone-releasing hormone agonist analogues: effect on bone density in premenopausal women. *Br. Med. J.*, **294**, 1523–4
22. Matta, W.H.M., Shaw, R.W. and Burdford, G.D. (1988). Endocrinologic and clinical evaluation following a single administration of a gonadotropin-releasing hormone agonist (Zoladex), in a depot formulation to premenopausal women. *Fertil. Steril.*, **49**, 163–5
23. Lumsden, M.A., West, C.P. and Baird, D.T. (1987). Goserelin therapy before surgery for uterine fibroids. *Lancet*, **i**, 36–7
24. Kessel, B., Liv, J., Mortola, J., Berga, S. and Yen, S.S.C. (1988). Treatment of uterine fibroids with agonist analogs of gonadotropin-releasing hormone. *Fertil. Steril.*, **49**, 538–41
25. Andreiko, J.L., Blumenfeld, Z., Marshall, L.A., Monroe, S.E., Hricak, H. and Jaffe, R.B. (1988). Use of an agonistic analog of gonadotropin-releasing hormone (nafarelin) to treat leiomyomas: Assessment by magnetic resonance imaging. *Am. J. Obstet. Gynecol.*, **158**, 903–10

Section 1 continued

Part F

Epirubicin in gynecological tumors

27

Epirubicin: a new anthracyclin analog

G. Robustelli della Cuna

Besides the discovery of new active drugs, the search for analogs with improved activity has become an increasingly important part of drug development programs, particularly when the parent compound has its therapeutic indications limited by undue acute and/or chronic toxicity. However, the major difficulty in developing effective analogs is that a superior therapeutic index, and not just a therapeutic activity is required. Epirubicin (EPI) is a new anthracycline analog resulting from epimerization of the 4′-hydroxyl of doxorubicin. In the last decade EPI has been one of the few new compounds proven effective in the management of hematological malignancies and solid tumors[1].

Starting from July 1977 (when it was first introduced into clinical use), EPI has been evaluated as a single agent in a series of conventional and disease-oriented phase II clinical trials. Those first generation trials, including more than 1600 evaluable patients, defined doses and schedules of the drug: namely 75 to 90 mg/m^2 i.v., daily for 3 weeks, as single agent or 60 to 75 mg/m^2 i.v. in combination with other cytotoxic agents[2]. Some single-institution trials also suggested the therapeutic value of the analog administered in weekly doses (20 mg or 20 mg/m^2 i.v.) mainly in aged women, or pretreated cases with advanced breast carcinoma[3].

Randomized comparisons of EPI versus the parent compound doxorubicin showed comparable therapeutic activity both as a single agent, and as a component of combination regimens, again in disseminated breast cancer[4]. However, these results notwithstanding, a clear dose-equivalence between epirubicin and doxorubicin cannot, by now, be clearly stated.

As compared to parent compound, EPI appears less toxic both in terms of myelotoxicity, cardiac toxicity and alopecia. At dosages of 75 to 90 mg/m^2 i.v. the leukocyte nadir occurs between days 8 and 14; recovery is usually completed by day 21. Even if the median cumulative dose to produce $> 10\%$ decrease in the left ventricular ejection fraction was reported to be 850 mg/m^2, congestive heart failure (CHF) is rare at cumulative epirubicin dosages below 1000 mg/m^2. Complete alopecia, qualitatively similar to that of doxorubicin, is somewhat lower ($< 65\%$) and mild at equal doses[5].

Studies designed to assess the therapeutic efficacy of EPI included neoplasms known as sensitive to parent compound (i.e. breast and ovarian cancer, gastric and small cell lung cancer, soft tissue sarcomas, nodular histiocytic lymphomas, liver and pancreatic carcinoma), as well as tumors believed to be sensitive to EPI, even if scarcely or not at all sensitive to parent compound (i.e. cervical, endometrial, prostatic, head and neck cancer)[6].

Epirubicin possesses a wide spectrum of activity both as a single agent and as a component of effective combinations with other drugs. The major efficacy (objective response in the range of 60–70%) is reported in malignant lymphoma, breast cancer and ovarian carcinoma. Consistent therapeutic activity (in the range of 30–40% objective response) has been observed in small cell lung cancer, soft tissue sarcomas, pediatric acute leukemias, and bladder cancer. The analog has been proven of moderate activity (20% objective response) in non-small cell lung cancer, gastric and pancreatic carcinoma, and cervical cancer. It failed to show any consistent activity in renal cell carcinoma, malignant melanoma, and colon carcinoma. In the frame-work of gynecological malignancies ovarian cancer seems the most sensitive tumor to the antiproliferative effect of EPI. As a consequence of early favorable clinical evaluations, more than 250 women with advanced ovarian carcinoma are currently on treatment with EPI-containing regimens. Platinum plus epirubicin regimens seem to be as effective as platinum plus doxorubicin combination for the management of advanced ovarian cancer[6].

The results obtained so far in advanced endometrial cancer are quite disappointing. Response rate ranging between 17 and 20% has been reported on a small series of patients. More than 100 women with advanced cervical carcinoma are currently on study in ongoing phase II clinical trials in South-East Asia and Latin America. Preliminary results on a limited number of fully evaluable cases show a response rate around 20%.

In conclusion, by including 1600 cases of phase II trials, a total of 4000 patients with advanced solid tumors and hematological malignancies has now received epirubicin treatment at various dosages and schedules. More than 2000 patients are now under evaluation in ongoing disease-oriented clinical trials involving more than 100 qualified institutions around the world[8]. The most important points we are expecting to be clarified in a larger number of evaluable patients are first, the certainty of achieving superimposable results by substituting the analog for parent compound in effective doxorubicin-containing regimens, and second, the therapeutic efficacy of epirubicin in solid tumors, known to be scarcely sensitive to parent compound doxorubicin.

REFERENCES

1. Bonadonna, G. (1984). *Advances in Anthracycline Chemotherapy: epirubicin.* (Milano: Masson Italia Editor)
2. Nagel, G.A. and Robustelli della Cuna, G. (1986). *Fortschritte in der Chemotherapie.* (Munchen, Bern, Berlin: W. Zuckschwerdt, Verlag)
3. Cersosimo, R.J. and Hong, W.K. (1986). Epirubicin: A review of pharmacology, clinical activity and adverse effect on an Adriamycin analogue. *J. Clin. Oncol.*, **4**, 425–39
4. Robustelli della Cuna, G., Da Prada, G.A., Preti, P., Pavesi, L. and Fiore, G. (1988). Nuove antracicline: risultati clinic. *Progr. Oncol. Clin.*, **4**, 153–64

5. Young, C.W. (1988). Epirubicin. In Droz, J.P., Cvitkovic, E., Armand, J.P., and Khoury, S. (eds). *Handbook of Chemotherapy in Clinical Oncology*, pp. 130–132. (Paris: FIIS Publisher)
6. Robustelli della Cuna, G., Pavesi, L., Preti, P., Ganzina, F. and Da Prada, G.A. (1985). Review of clinical trial with epirubicin: updated October 1984. *Akt. Onkol.*, **15**, 162–75
7. Robustelli della Cuna, G., Pavesi, L., Preti, P., Da Prada, G.A. and Intini, G. (1986). Ubersicht uber laufende klinische studien mit Epirubicin. *Akt. Onkol.*, **29**, 25–35
8. Confidential Report on Epirubicin (1988). (Milano: Farmitalia Carlo Erba)

28

Hormonal modulation of sensitivity to anthracyclines in breast cancer

P.F. Conte, L. Repetto, G. Gardin and A. Alama

INTRODUCTION

Tumor growth is controlled by specific mitogenic signals. Hormone-dependent tumors represent a model of choice to study kinetic manipulation in cancer treatment.

Estrogens play a critical role in the etiology of breast cancer inducing normal breast cell growth and development. Breast cancer retains the hormone-dependent phenotype in approximately one-third of advanced disease, thus it is the most widely studied neoplasm. This paper concerns the stimulatory effects of low-dose estrogen studied by recruiting G0 cells into the cell cycle to increase the tumor growth fraction and to enhance the cell killing of sequentially administered chemotherapy.

Hormonal manipulation of breast cancer has employed the cytostatic effect of the antiestrogen Tamoxifen to arrest hormone-dependent cancer cells in G0–early G1 phases; after synchronization, estrogens are given to induce cancer cell proliferation before chemotherapy treatment[1]. We report the North West Oncological Group experience using diethylstilbestrol (DES) as recruiting agent in locally advanced breast cancer.

CLINICAL RESULTS

Locally advanced breast cancer (LABC) was selected as a tumor model because sequential Tru-cut biopsies are easily obtained. Cell cycle recruitment was monitored by thymidine labelling index (TLI) and primer-dependent αDNA polymerase (PDP) in patients suitable and willing to receive multiple tumor biopsies[2]. The first kinetically designed study was started in 1983. Aims of the study were: to verify whether tumor proliferative activity is associated with other prognostic parameters; to evaluate the impact of basal proliferative activity on objective response rate, disease-free survival and survival; to analyze the effect of induction chemotherapy on the kinetics of residual tumor mass.

Stage IIIA or IIIB LABC patients received treatment with DES 1 mg/day for 3 days followed by CAF (cyclophosphamide 600 mg/m^2; adriamycin 50 mg/m^2 and fluorouracil 600 mg/m^2) on day 4. After three courses, responding patients underwent radical surgery or radiotherapy followed by six courses of alternating CAF with CMF (cyclophosphamide 600 mg/m^2; methotrexate 50 mg/m^2; fluorouracil 600 mg/m^2) regimens: 39 patients were treated. Median age was 56 years (range 38–76) and performance status (PS) 0 (0–2), 14 patients had clinical and/or histological findings of inflammatory carcinoma; 20 patients had negative estrogen receptors, 13 patients had positive estrogen receptors and in six patients their status was unknown. The objective response rate was 71.8% with 15.4% complete remission. After induction chemotherapy and local treatment 36 of 39 patients (92.3%) were free of disease.

Results of this trial have already been published[3]. Because of encouraging results achieved in this pilot study a randomized trial was started in which patients received the CAF regimen with or without 3 days of prior treatment with DES. In this ongoing study 56 patients entered and 46 were clinically evaluable (26 CAF, 20 DES–CAF).

Characteristics of patients are comparable in the two groups. No differences in objective response rate after induction chemotherapy (53% versus 55%) and in disease-free survival after chemotherapy and local treatment (75% versus 70.4%) were noted in the conventional versus the kinetic chemotherapy respectively. No survival and relapse data are presently available.

KINETIC RESULTS

Results evaluations were performed in 111 tumor specimens. TLI and PDP were measured before and after DES, 24 h after chemotherapy and at surgery as shown in Table 1.

After DES exposure a kinetic recruitment (> 50% increase in TLI and/or PDP value) was noted in 76.2% of cases and a kinetic inhibition (> 50% decrease in TLI and/or PDP value) was evident in 56.3% of the patients after the first course of CAF and in 76% at mastectomy. Kinetic parameters were not significantly correlated with prognostic variables such as age, receptor status, stage of disease and diagnosis of inflammatory breast cancer; moreover no correlation was shown among pretreatment kinetic data, objective response rate and relapse rate (Table 2). Overall 5-year survival was 41.1% and 71.9% in patients with low and high TLI and 56.4% and 66.3% in patients with low and high PDP respectively. These differences were not significant.

Table 1 Tumor proliferative activity in locally advanced breast cancer during treatment, median with range in parentheses

Time	*No. of patients*	*TLI*	*PDP*
Diagnosis	49	1.7 (0.1–19.4)	5.5 (0.4–41.2)
After DES	21	2.2 (0.17–18.5)	7.6 (0.4–20.7)
After 1st chemotherapy	16	0.9 (0.2–23.5)	2.8 (0.9–8.8)
Mastectomy	25	0.7 (0.1–6.2)	2.2 (0.4–13.7)

Table 2 Tumor proliferative activity in locally advanced breast cancer: patterns of response and relapse according to basal proliferative activity

	*OR** (%)	*Relapse* (%)
Low TLI	17/24 (70.8)	11/25 (44)
High TLI	17/23 (73.9)	8/24 (33.3)
Low PDP	11/17 (64.7)	7/17 (41.2)
High PDP	12/15 (80.0)	6/16 (37.5)
Total	34/47 (72.4)	19/49 (38.8)

* OR, objective response

CONCLUSIONS

No definitive data are available, nevertheless preliminary analysis of DES chemotherapy showed that low-dose estrogens induce *in vivo* tumor cell recruitment even in hormone receptor negative tumors, moreover kinetically designed chemotherapy is feasible and allows high objective response rate, overall 5-year survival and disease-free survival[4–6]. These results encourage further investigation to optimize the potential advantage of kinetic chemotherapy a high-dose intensity DES regimen is starting in our institute. Patients will receive full doses of cyclophosphamide and fluorouracil on days 4 to 21, DES on days 1–3, 8–10, 15–17 and fractionated doses of epirubicin on days 4, 11 and 18.

Recently, specific factors, i.e. growth factors (GFs) able to stimulate tumor cell proliferation have been identified. At present there are few clinical applications due to the unavailability of sufficient amounts of purified GFs. The administration of growth hormone can induce an increase in the production of insulin-like growth factor 1 (IGF-1) which has been demonstrated to be an important GF for breast cancer. We are now evaluating the efficacy of growth hormone as a recruiting agent in breast cancer patients.

Seven patients with advanced breast cancer were treated with growth hormone followed by chemotherapy. TLI, serum and tumor IGF-1 were evaluated before and after treatment. Median TLI values before and after growth hormone exposure were 0.7 (*r* 0.4–8.1) and 2.7 (*r* 0.16–11.5).

Serum IGF-1 values in two patients were 38 and 50 ng/ml before and 197 and 214 ng/ml after growth hormone. Finally, in one patient tumor IGF-1 was 1.31 ng/g before and 1.39 ng/g after growth hormone administration.

The identification of new active cytotoxic agents is warranted to overcome genetic drug resistance, nevertheless tumor growth manipulations designed around hormonal recruitment or targeted to expression of growth factors represent future prospects for clinical trials.

ACKNOWLEDGEMENTS

This work was supported by CNR contract no. 88.00601.44 and AIRC.

REFER

1. Lippma
S. (1987
carcino
of Canc
2. Conte,
Drewin
fraction
3. Conte,
and sur
40, 490-
4. Conte,
results
cancer.
Cancer,
5. Conte,
polyche
random
6. Conte,
sequent
cancer.

While node-positive premenopausal patients should take combination chemotherapy, node-positive postmenopausal women should take tamoxifen ± chemotherapy, if estrogen receptor positive, or chemotherapy ± tamoxifen, if estrogen receptor negative[5].

Node-negative patients should be considered in relation to prognostic factors (tumor size, estrogen receptor, nuclear grade, tumor proliferative activity) in order to define the relative risk. High-risk patients should be treated with chemotherapy (in addition with tamoxifen, if postmenopausal), low-risk patients should be treated with tamoxifen.

ANTHRACYCLINES IN THE ADJUVANT TREATMENT OF BREAST CANCER

The role of anthracyclines in the adjuvant treatment of breast cancer is not well established. Their introduction in several trials has been suggested by the high activity of doxorubicin in advanced breast cancer; nevertheless, the effectiveness of doxorubicin-containing regimens may be defined only by prospective randomized trials, since eventual cardiotoxic effects could negatively influence the survival of the group as a whole.

In some institutions large series of patients have been treated with doxorubicin containing regimens. At M.D. Anderson, Houston, the FAC regimen (5-fluorouracil, adriamycin and cyclophosphamide) yielded a better survival compared to a historical control both in premenopause (68% versus 48%) and postmenopause (67% versus 50%)[6]. Postmenopausal patients with one to three positive nodes, treated at NCI of Milan with CMF (cyclophosphamide, methotrexate and 5-fluorouracil) followed by AV (adriamycin and vincristine) did better than patients treated with adjuvant CMF (survival: 84% versus 67%)[3]. In a randomized trial carried out by the NSABP group the addition of doxorubicin to PF (L-Pam + 5-FU) in premenopause and to PFT (PF + tamoxifen) in postmenopause resulted in a relapse-free survival and overall survival advantage[6].

The final results of other randomized trials on the utility of doxorubicin are needed: for example, CMF versus CMF alternated with doxorubicin in patients with one to three positive nodes, performed at Tumor Institute of Milan.

EPIDOXORUBICIN AND DOXORUBICIN IN BREAST CANCER

Epidoxorubicin is a new analog of doxorubicin extensively studied in breast cancer. Two large multicenter randomized trials have been carried out in Italy and France on the comparison of the two anthracyclines in advanced breast cancer[7,8]. In both trials doxorubicin has been compared to epidoxorubicin at the same dosage (50 mg/m^2) and in combination with the same anticancer drugs (cyclophosphamide and 5-fluorouracil). The two regimens (FAC and FEC) yielded the same response rate: in the Italian study 53% objective response rate (complete responses in 10%) for FEC and 56%

objective response rate (complete responses in 15%) for FAC; in the French study 50% objective response rate (complete responses in 12%) for FEC and 52% objective response rate (complete responses in 8%) for FAC. These and other trials show that the acute toxicity determined by epidoxorubicin or epidoxorubicin-containing regimens is lower compared to that of the parent compound: in fact, alopecia, nausea/vomiting and marrow toxicity are less frequent. For the cardiotoxicity the cumulative data of the two above mentioned trials show that seven cases of congestive heart failure occurred among 239 patients treated with doxorubicin against one case among 248 patients treated with epidoxorubicin. In the Italian trial a significant difference for ECG changes and PEP/LVET ratio in favor of FEC has been observed.

In conclusion, the available data indicate that epidoxorubicin seems to be equiactive, but less toxic than doxorubicin.

EPIDOXORUBICIN IN THE ADJUVANT SETTING

There are several reasons why epidoxorubicin seems to be more suitable than the parent compound in the adjuvant setting. In fact about 50% of patients treated with surgery and conventional adjuvant treatment are cured; therefore for the introduction of a new agent in this setting it must be remembered that all the patients undergo the toxic effects, while only a minority will benefit from the procedure. So it is very important to choose drugs that have no long-term toxic effects, able to influence negatively vital organ outcome and, consequently, shorten survival for non-cancer reasons; moreover, drugs inducing heavy acute toxicity should be avoided mainly so as not to worsen the quality of life of these apparently healthy patients.

At present, epidoxorubicin seems to be less cardiotoxic than doxorubicin, even if the differences in cardiac damage are clearly quantitative and not qualitative in nature. We can consider that the incidence of congestive heart failure is 5% at a cumulative dose of 550 mg/m^2 and 800–900 mg/m^2 of doxorubicin and epidoxorubicin respectively. Therefore, with the new anthracycline we can almost double the anthracycline total dose. Nevertheless, in the adjuvant setting, conventional dose schedules do not require the administration of threatening total dose. The opportunity of utilizing epidoxorubicin should exist mainly for those patients who have recurrences in spite of the anthracycline adjuvant treatment. In fact for most of them, the best choice for the treatment of metastases is anthracycline again and this choice can be limited by the drug used in the adjuvant setting. For example, if we have treated a patient with 10 cycles of doxorubicin at the dose of 50 mg/m^2, a total dose of 500 mg/m^2 has been reached and the treatment of recurrence with doxorubicin is not recommendable because of the cardiac risk. On the contrary, with 500 mg/m^2 of epidoxorubicin (10 cycles at the same dose) we are far from the threatening cumulative dose and the new anthracycline can be applied for a second time. However, the most important aspect for introducing epidoxorubicin in the place of doxorubicin in the adjuvant setting is probably the lower acute toxicity (alopecia, gastrointestinal toxicity). A lower acute toxicity, in fact, could assure a better quality of life and a better patient compliance to chemotherapy.

Epidoxorubicin has been employed in several adjuvant trials. At Royal Marsden Hospital, London, premenopausal patients are randomized to six cycles of classic CMF or eight cycles of FEC and postmenopausal patients are randomized to tamoxifen or eight cycles of FEC + tamoxifen.

A large multicenter study (GROCTA trial) has been performed in Italy about the comparison between tamoxifen, chemotherapy and chemotherapy + tamoxifen in estrogen receptor positive patients. Chemotherapy consisted of six cycles of i.v. CMF followed by four cycles of epidoxorubicin (75 mg/m^2). In this trial, a survival advantage in favour of the chemohormonal treatment has been observed in a preliminary report[8].

Finally at our Institution a randomized trial is ongoing with the perioperative FEC.

PERIOPERATIVE CHEMOTHERAPY

The first course of adjuvant chemotherapy is conventionally administered 3–4 weeks after the tumor removal to allow the healing of the surgical wound.

The effect of the delay of chemotherapy beginning is theoretically negative because of the increasing number of cells in micrometastases. Since the number of genetically chemoresistant cells is related to the total number, the delay is expected to determine a reduction of chemotherapy curability. Ragaz and colleagues applying their mathematical model to this situation, have calculated that, for a doubling time of 40 days, the micrometastatic cells nearly double in an interval time of a month, but the increase is much more if the doubling time shrinks as a result of primary tumor removal. Consequently, the probabilities of cure may be reduced from 70% to 45%[9].

The tumor kinetics changes after primary tumor removal have been demonstrated in experimental models[10,11]. The tumor proliferative activity measured by means of the thymidine labelling index (TLI) of metastases increases about 48–72 h after the primary tumor removal in C3H/HeJ mammary adenocarcinoma in mice.

If the kinetics changes occur also in human micrometastases, we can expect that the total number of cells and the number of genetically chemoresistant cells rapidly increase; moreover, since most anticancer drugs act mainly on cycling cells, the administration of drugs at the time of cell recruitment into the cycle should result in a higher kill rate.

More than 25 years ago several trials of perioperative chemotherapy had been carried out with the aim to kill the cells released in the circulation at the time of mastectomy. The rationale of these trials was later demonstrated to be wrong, but the results are surprisingly positive to a certain degree. The NSABP tested perioperative Thiotepa demonstrating an increased survival for premenopausal patients with four or more positive axillary nodes[7]. The Scandinavian Adjuvant Chemotherapy Group randomized patients to receive perioperative cyclophosphamide or nothing; after more than two decades of follow-up, there is an advantage in favor of treatment in all subsets of patients (premenopause and postmenopause; node-positive and node-negative). The benefit was not present among patients of one Center in which chemotherapy was delayed after chest irradiation. Similar results have been obtained by a Cancer Research Campaign study, in which the same regimen of perioperative cyclophosphamide has been employed[12].

Furthermore, an improved Relapse Free Survival was observed among patients receiving adjuvant AC during the first postoperative 4 weeks compared to patients in whom treatment was delayed[13] and among patients beginning CMF within 35 days after surgery compared to patients in whom treatment started after 35 days[14].

Based on these data, some groups have started a new series of perioperative adjuvant trials. The Ludwig Breast Cancer Study Group has carried out a trial in which node-negative patients have been randomized to observation or perioperative CMF and node-positive patients are randomized to conventional chemotherapy or perioperative CMF or both[15]. The EORTC is performing trials in which patients are randomized to observation or perioperative CAF then only premenopausal/node-positive patients are given six cycles of CMF.

At the Cancer Institute in Genoa more than 400 patients have so far entered a randomized trial of perioperative FEC. Stage I–II patients are randomized at the time of surgery to a cycle of perioperative FEC (cyclophosphamide 600 mg/m^2, epidoxorubicin 60 mg/m^2, 5-fluorouracil 600 mg/m^2) or no therapy; then, node-negative patients receive no further treatment, while node-positive patients receive further cycles of chemotherapy (12 for patients who had not the perioperative cycle and 11 for patient having had the perioperative cycle). This study is ongoing and data on the chemotherapy effectiveness on relapse-free survival and overall survival are not available until now.

Toxicity results related to the perioperative FEC are of some interest. Vomiting is present in more than 50% of patients, hair loss in 55%; stomatitis and infections are rare. Interestingly, the perioperative FEC did not produce any negative effect on healing of the surgical wound as demonstrated by an analysis on 180 patients. For 92 patients given perioperative FEC the mean duration of recovery was 7 days (range 5–13); the mean drainage was 431 cm^3; fever occurred in two cases; the mean number of dressings was 4 (range 1–8); a healing delay was observed in four patients and lymphocele occurred in about 25% of patients. These results are superimposable on those of patients who had not the perioperative cycle.

ACKNOWLEDGEMENT

Supported in part by CNR, Rome: contracts 86.00645.44, 87.01516.44.

REFERENCES

1. (1986). Introduction and Conclusions. National Institutes of Health Consensus Development Panel on Adjuvant Chemotherapy and Endocrine Therapy for Breast Cancer. *NCI Monographs*, **1**, 1–4

2. (1988). NCI alert on node negative breast cancer. *Breast Cancer Res. Treat*, **12**, 3–5
3. Bonadonna, G., Valagussa, P., Tancini, G., Rossi, A., Brambilla, C., Zambetti, M., Bignami, P., Di Fronzo, G. and Silvestrini, R. (1986). Current status of Milan Adjuvant Chemotherapy Trials for node-positive and node-negative breast cancer. *NCI Monographs*, **1**, 45–9
4. Baum, M., Brinkley, D.M. and Dossett, J.A. (1985). Controlled trial of tamoxifen as single adjuvant agent in management of early breast cancer. *Lancet*, **i**, 836–40
5. Glick, J.H. (1988). Meeting highlights: adjuvant therapy for breast cancer. *NCI Journal*, **80**, 471–5
6. Buzdar, A.U., Hortobagyi, G.N., Marcus, C.E., Smith, T.L., Martin, R. and Gehan, E.A. (1986). Results of adjuvant chemotherapy trials in breast cancer at M.D. Anderson Hospital and Tumor Institute. *NCI Monographs*, **1**, 81–5
7. Fisher, B., Redmond, C., Fisher, E.R. and Wolmark, N. (1986). Systemic adjuvant therapy in treatment of primary operable breast cancer: National Surgical Adjuvant Breast and Bowel Project Experience. *NCI Monographs*, **1**, 35–43
8. Boccardo, F., Bruzzi, P. and Cappellini, M. (1988). Tamoxifen versus chemotherapy versus chemotherapy plus tamoxifen in stage II ER+ breast cancer patients: 4 years results of a multicentric Italian study. *Proc. ASCO*, **7**, 11
9. Ragaz, J., Baird, R., Rebbeck, P., Goldie, J., Coldman, A., Spinelli, J. and Simpson-Herren, L. (1984). Preoperative adjuvant chemotherapy (neoadjuvant) for cancer of the breast: rationale and safety report. *Rev. Endocr. Rel. Cancer*, Suppl. 14, 233–7
10. Fisher, B., Gunduz, N. and Saffer, E.A. (1983). Influence of the interval between primary tumor removal and chemotherapy and growth of metastases. *Cancer Res.*, **43**, 1488–92
11. Braunschweiger, P.G., Schiffer, L.M. and Betancourt, S. (1982). Tumor cell proliferation and sequential chemotherapy after partial tumor resection in C3H/HEJ mammary tumors. *Breast Cancer Res. Treat.*, **2**, 323–9
12. Nissen-Meyer, R., Host, H., Kjellgren, K., Mansson, B. and North, T. (1986). Treatment of node-negative breast cancer patients with short course of chemotherapy immediately after surgery. *NCI Monographs*, **1**, 125–8
13. Brooks, R., Jones, S.E. and Salmon, S.E. (1983). Improved outcome with early treatment in an adjuvant breast cancer program. *Proc. ASCO*, **2**, 431
14. Pronzato, P., Campora, E., Amoroso, D., Bertelli, G., Botto, F., Conte, P.F., Sertoli, M.R. and Rosso, R. (1989). *Am. J. Clin. Oncol.*, **6**, 481–5

Section 2

Infective Diseases in Gynecology and Obstetrics

Part A

Infections in the female reproductive tract

30

Inactivation of HIV-1 by Euclorina

E. Cattaneo, M. Danesino, G. Achilli, P. Ferrante and E.G. Rondanelli

INTRODUCTION

One of the most up-to-date aspects of infectious pathology is the outbreak of the infection by exogenous human retroviruses, among which the lentiviridae subfamily is the most important from a pathogenetic point of view as it includes the viral etiological agents of a wide range of syndromes, namely lymphadenopathy syndrome (LAS), acquired immune deficiency syndrome (AIDS), AIDS-related complex (ARC). Human immunodeficiency virus (HIV-1) formerly called HTLV-III, LAV or ARV, was isolated for the first time in 1983 from AIDS patients[1-3] and spread epidemically in USA, in Europe and to date AIDS cases are reported almost all over the world.

The main route of spreading of the infection is the blood stream because the main target cells of this virus are OK T4 phenotyped T lymphocytes carrying the CD4 receptor molecule specific for HIV-1 on their surface[4].

MATERIALS AND METHODS

The study of Euclorina's disinfecting activity was performed using a continuous line of human lymphocytes persistently infected with HIV and testing several dilutions at different exposure periods to check their *in vitro* ability to counteract the viral action.

We took into account the effect of lymphocytes on the specific antigens of the persistently infected cells, and also evaluated the possible presence of free viral particles in the surnatants of lymphocyte cultures as indicated by the presence of reverse transcriptase (RT) activity.

We used the uninfected lymphocyte cell-line H9 as a control and the persistently infected cell-line H9/HTLV-III (a kind gift from Dr R.C. Gallo, National Cancer Institute, Bethesda, MD, USA)[5]. Euclorina powder, whose active principle is sodium toluen-p-sulfonchloramide, was provided by Zambeletti firm in the same trade envelopes weighing 2.5 g.

RESULTS

H9 and H9/HTLV-III lymphocytes at the concentration of 1 x 10 cells/ml were incubated at room temperature in Euclorina at the concentrations of 0.1%, 0.25%, 1%, 2.5% in RPMI-1640 culture medium. After 30 s, 60 s, 2 min, 5 min, 10 min, 5 ml of fetal bovine serum (FBS) were added to the cultures to block the activity of Euclorina, which was instantly removed by means of three washings in RPMI-1640.

After this treatment the lymphocytes were cultivated at 37°C in 5% CO_2 atmosphere with a mixture of RPMI-1640, FBS 10%, L-glutamine 2 mM, 100 U/ml of penicillin, 50 ug/ml of streptomycin.

On the 2nd, 5th and 8th days, the cell cultures were monitored to evaluate the presence of reverse transcriptase[6] in the culture medium and to demonstrate the expression of viral antigens in the lymphocytes by indirect immunofluorescence using monoclonal antibodies versus the main core protein (p 24) of HIV[7].

The survival percentage of the lymphocytes treated with Euclorina at the concentrations of 2.5%, 1% and 0.25% and at the different exposure times turned out to be 0%.

At the concentration of 0.1% the survival percentage of the lymphocytes progressively decreased from 85% after a 30 s exposure to 0% after 5 min (Table 1).

The day after no lymphocytes were found was vital in all cultures. The expression of p 24 protein, tested the day after by indirect immunofluorescence (IFA), turned out to be negative for Euclorina concentrations from 2.5% to 0.25% right after a 30 s exposure to the disinfectant. At the concentration of 0.1% a progressive decrease of fluorescent lymphocyte percentage was noticed from 80% for the 30 s exposure time down to 20% for the 2 min exposure time (Table 2).

No reverse transcriptase (RT) activity was detected from the 2nd day in all cultures at all the tested Euclorina dilutions.

DISCUSSION

Our results indicate that the virucidal activity of the active principle of Euclorina is total at the 2.5%, 1%, 0.25% dilutions, which represent the recommended usage dilutions while at the dilution of 0.1% vital cells persist

Table 1 Percentages of vital H9/HTLV-III lymphocytes after exposure to Euclorina

Euclorina concentrations (%)	*Exposure times*				
	30 s	*60 s*	*2 min*	*5 min*	*10 min*
2.5	0	0	0	0	0
1	0	0	0	0	0
0.25	0	0	0	0	0
0.1	85	60	40	0	0

Table 2 Expression of p 24 protein in H9/HTLV-III lymphocytes after exposure to Euclorina

Euclorina concentrations (%)	*Exposure times*				
	30 s	*60 s*	*2 min*	*5 min*	*10 min*
2.5	0	0	0	0	0
1	0	0	0	0	0
0.25	0	0	0	0	0
0.1	80	50	20	0	0

during the first 24 hours after exposure to the disinfectant. Viral antigens were detected up to 2 min exposure times while at longer exposure periods no specific antigens were in evidence. No reverse transcriptase (RT) activity was found and, as a consequence, the survival of infectious viral particles is considered unlikely.

The Euclorina concentrations recommended as disinfectant prove to be effective on intra- and extracellular HIV-1 virus.

REFERENCES

1. Barre Sinoussi, F., Chermann, J.C., Rey, F. *et al.* (1983). Isolation of T-lymphotropic retroviruses from a patient at risk for AIDS. *Science*, **220**, 869
2. Popovic, M., Sarngadharan, M.G., Read, E. and Gallo, R.C. (1984). Detection, isolation and continuous production of cytopathic retroviruses (HTLV-III) from patients with AIDS and pre-AIDS. *Science*, **224**, 497
3. Levy, J.A., Hoffman, A.D., Kramer, S.M. *et al.* (1984). Isolation of lymphocytopathic retroviruses from San Francisco patients with AIDS. *Science*, **225**, 840
4. Fauci, A.S. (1988). The human immunodeficiency virus: infectivity and mechanism of pathogenesis. *Science*, **239**, 617
5. Gallo, R.C., Salahuddin, S.Z., Popovic, M. *et al.* (1984). Frequent detection and isolation of cytopathic retroviruses (HTLV-III) from patients with AIDS and at risk for AIDS. *Science*, **224**, 500
6. Rabson, A.B. (1988). In Levy J.A. (ed.), *AIDS: Pathogenesis and Treatment.* (Dekker: New York)
7. Di Marzo Veronese, F., Sarngadharan, M.G., Rahman, R. *et al.* (1985). Monoclonal antibodies specific for p 24, the major core protein of human T-cell leukemia virus type III. *Proc. Natl. Acad. Sci., USA*, **82**, 5199

31

Mycoses during pregnancy: results of a wide screening and treatment

U.F. Colombo, L. Ghisoni, T. Viezzoli, M. Orlandella and G. Zuliani

INTRODUCTION

Mycetes, *Candida albicans* in particular, are the pathogens which are met most often in the vaginal secretion microbiological screening of pregnant women. The glycogen increase in the vaginal epithelium and the cellular immunity depression which occur during pregnancy favor the growth of *C. albicans* and justify the high prevalence of vulvovaginites from candida (VVC) at that period.

In fact, symptomatic VVCs develop in about 10% of pregnant women during the first trimester, with a constant increase in the second and third trimesters[1,2]. In addition, if the woman was already a carrier of *C. albicans* before becoming pregnant, the occurrence of vaginitis during pregnancy itself is more frequent (from 61 to 90% according to some studies). It must also be kept in mind that therapeutic failures and reinfections are more frequent during pregnancy.

The presence of VVC during pregnancy is also important for the fetus and the newborn. Serious intrauterine cerebral candidiasis[3,4] has been observed. On the other hand, there is a significant increase (from two to 35 times) in the risk of oral cavity colonization by *C. albicans* in the newborns of *C. albicans*-infected women compared to the newborns of non-infected women[5,6].

We have performed a cultural screening in *C. albicans*-infected pregnant women with the scope of evaluating the efficiency and tolerability, as well as its results on newborns, of a local therapy with capsules of cyclopiroxolamin (Dafnegyn–Poli).

MATERIALS AND METHODS

During the April 1987–October 1988 period, 598 pregnant patients from 8 to 38 weeks of pregnancy, admitted at the Pregnancy pathology ward of the

'L. Mangiagalli' I Obstetrical and Gynecological clinic of the University of Milan, were subjected to vaginocervical screenings of the main sexually transmitted pathogens. The isolation percentage of each pathogen found was: *Chlamydia trachomatis* (7.3%); *Mycoplasma hominis* (15.6%); *Ureaplasma urealiticum* (11.4%); *Trichomonas vaginalis* (2.1%); *Gardnerella vaginalis* (7.8%); Group B *Streptococcus* β hemolitic (5.5%); and *Candida albicans* (19.7%).

The main indications at the time of admission of the patients in our ward were the following (with number of patients per group in parentheses): Diabetes (58); gestoses, underdevelopment, arterial hypertension (80); Rh isoimmunization (42); threatened miscarriage (12); threatened premature birth (24); cervical incompetence (38); polyabortivity (19); therapeutic abortion (61); prenatal diagnosis (37); missed abortions (35); intrauterine death (7); hazardous pregnancy check (151); fetal malformation (19); and premature membrane rupture (15).

RESULTS

C. albicans was isolated from 118 patients (19.7%). Table 1 indicates the prevalence of *C. albicans* isolation distributed in age groups; Table 2 shows its prevalence as the main indication for admission.

We recorded the objective clinical signs and the subjective symptomatology reported by 94 *C. albicans* isolation cases (Table 3). We excluded from the study 24 patients whose pregnancy did not proceed (19 cases of therapeutic abortion, four of missed abortion, one of fetal intrauterine death). The remaining 94 patients were treated with capsules of cyclopiroxolamin for 6 days.

Within a week of the end of the treatment, a second vaginal tampon was applied to determine its efficiency. Objective clinical signs were also re-evaluated, as well as the subjective symptomatology reported by the patient (Table 3). Out of 94 treated patients, 61 (65%) were negative for *C. albicans*, whereas the remaining 33 still showed the presence of pathogens.

A second 12-day treatment with the same pharmaceutical was performed in 25 of the still-infected patients. It was not possible to repeat the treatment in eight patients as they had delivered in the meantime. For this last group

Table 1 Prevalence of *C. albicans* infection in relation to the age of the patient

Age (yr)	*Total no.*	*No. with* C. albicans	%
< 20	48	14	29.2
21–25	92	18	19.6
26–30	181	32	17.7
31–35	164	31	18.9
36–40	92	17	18.5
> 40	21	6	28.6
Total	598	118	

Table 2 Prevalence of *C. albicans* in relation to pathological conditions

Pathology	*Total no.*	*No. with C. albicans*	*%*
Diabetes	58	11	19.0
Intrauterine growth retardation EPH gestosis	80	15	13.8
Rh immunization	42	12	28.6
Threatened abortion	12	0	0
Preterm labor	24	6	25.0
Cervical incompetence	38	4	10.5
Polyabortivity	19	7	36.8
Therapeutic abortion	61	19	31.1
Prenatal diagnosis	37	4	10.8
Missed abortion	35	4	11.4
Intrauterine death	7	1	14.3
Fetal malformations	19	3	15.8
Premature membrane rupture	15	2	13.3
Other	151	30	19.9
Total	598	118	

Table 3 Clinical signs and symptoms before and after the first treatment (94 patients) and the second treatment (25 patients); number with % in parentheses

	Signs		*Symptoms*	
	Vulvar edema	*Discharge*	*Itching*	*Burning*
Before 1st treatment	54 (57)	79 (84)	57 (61)	31 (33)
After 1st treatment	12 (13)	19 (20)	19 (20)	5 (5)
Before 2nd treatment	10 (40)	7 (28)	9 (36)	4 (16)
After 2nd treatment	2 (8)	5 (20)	3 (12)	2 (8)

objective clinical signs and subjective symptomatology, before and after treatment are also indicated in Table 3. Eleven out of 25 patients were negative to the pathogen after the second course of treatment.

To summarize the results obtained with both treatments: 61/94 were negative after the first treatment and 11/25 after the second; recovery was achieved in 72 cases out of 94 (76.6%).

DISCUSSION

Our screening, performed over a wide population of pregnant women, shows the high prevalence of *C. albicans* (approx. 20%). The distribution by age of *C. albicans* isolation indicates a higher prevalence in the youngest group (< 20 years old) and in the over 40 years old group. These data, contradictory only in appearance, are explained by the high prevalence of sexually-transmitted pathogens in younger women and the high frequency of diabetic patients in the older women.

Harder to explain is the correlation between *C. albicans* isolation and type of obstetric pathology. Polyabortivity, Rh isoimmunization, threatened premature delivery seem to correlate to a higher pathogen prevalence. Comments can be made on the relatively low prevalence of *C. albicans* in

Table 4 Cultural results after treatment

	First treatment	*Second treatment*	*Total clinical results*
No. of patients	94	25	94
C. albicans −ve culture	61 (65%)	11 (44%)	61 + 11 = 72 (76.6%)
C. albicans +ve culture	33 (35%)	14 (56%)	14 + 8* = 22 (24.4%)

* Eight patients delivered before 2nd treatment

diabetic women, which can be explained by the fact that in most cases it concerns women with gestational diabetes well compensated with insulin therapy.

Objective clinical signs of the presence of the pathogen do not always show and, in almost one-half of the patients no typical symptomatology was present (Table 3). The decrease in clinical signs and subjective symptomatology after local treatment with cyclopiroxolamin is significant (Table 4). Of the 14 patients who did not respond after the second treatment, three cases were kidney transplant patients under immunosuppressant therapy, four cases were non-compensated diabetic patients, and two were cases of premature membrane rupture (<27th week) being treated with antibiotics.

As for pharmaceutical tolerability, some patients reported vaginal burning during the first and second days of therapy, although they all completed the treatment. One single case of neonatal oral cavity colonization was observed after premature membrane rupture in a 34th week of pregnancy newborn.

CONCLUSIONS

It is our opinion that screening and treatment for *C. albicans* infections during pregnancy are justified both by the patient's subjective symptomatology remission and the feto–neonatal repercussions which that pathogen can produce.

Cyclopiroxolamin treatment can be considered safe, well tolerated and efficient. The effect of *C. albicans* on the fetus is not yet totally clear and thus requires further in-depth study.

REFERENCES

1. Morton, R.S. and Rashid, S. (1977). Candidal vaginitis: natural history, predisposing factors and prevention. *Proc. R. Soc. Med.*, **70**, (suppl. 4), 1
2. Carroll, C.J., Hurley, R. and Stanley, V.C. (1973). Criteria for diagnosis of candida vulvovaginitis in pregnant women. *J. Obstet. Gynaecol. Br. Cwlth.*, **80**, 258
3. Hopsu-Havu, V.K., Gronroos, M. and Punnoren, R. (1980). Vaginal yeasts in parturients and infestation of the newborns. *Acta Obstet. Gynecol. Scand.*, **59**, 73
4. Levin, S., Zaidel, L. and Bernstein, B. (1978). Intrauterine infection of fetal brain by candida. *Am. J. Obstet. Gynecol.*, **130**, 597
5. Kozinn, P.J., Tashdjian, C.L. and Wiener, H. (1958). Incidence and pathogenesis of neonatal candidiasis. *Pediatrics*, **21**, 421
6. Drake, T.E. and Maibach, H.I. (1973). Candida and candidiasis: cultural conditions, epidemiology and pathogenesis. *Postgrad. Med.*, **53**, 83

32

Enoxacin in the treatment of *Chlamydia trachomatis* genital infection

N. Colacurci, G. De Placido, F. Zullo, G. d'Agostino, I. Strina and M. Galasso

INTRODUCTION

Chlamydia trachomatis infections are the most common sexually transmitted disease. *C. trachomatis* is the main pathogenic agent of non-gonococcal urethritis (about 50%) and of epididimitis in young men; in women the infection usually has few symptoms but it is of great importance for the possible long-term damage it can cause to Fallopian tubes[1]. Up to now the first choice treatment in uncomplicated *C. trachomatis* infections has been a monochemotherapy using tetracycline or a macrolide[2,3]; the success rate with this treatment is generally good but to get optimal results it is necessary to continue treatment for not less than 2 weeks; furthermore, there is a significant percentage of recurrence[4]. Our aim has been to evaluate the effectiveness of enoxacin, a new compound of the quinolonic group, in the treatment of *C. trachomatis* infections.

The quinolonics are a group of antibacterial agents which inhibit DNA replication[5] by means of a specific cessation of DNA girase inhibition, which is an important component of the bacterial DNA replicative system[6]. Until now they have been used in urinary tract infections because of the high concentrations they reach in the urine[7]. The latest generation compounds, as a result of the introduction of a carboxylic group in 4th position, show a wider spectrum than first and second generation precursors and their possible therapeutic use is in other fields than urinary tract infections[8-10].

MATERIALS AND METHODS

We studied a population of 45 infertile couples affected by an asymptomatic or paucisymptomatic *C. trachomatis* infection not associated with other microbial agents, screened during the initial diagnostic approach. Each couple was fully informed and signed a consent form. In 17 couples both partners were affected; in 17 couples only the female partner was positive and in the remaining 11 couples only the male was affected, so we had a total number of 62 positive patients and 28 negative patients.

The diagnosis of *C. trachomatis* infection was made by means of an indirect immunofluorescence technique using cervical, urethral and rectal samples in women, urethral and rectal specimens in men (T0). A complete infective screening including a cervicovaginal culture and a sperm culture with specific research of *Gonococcus*, *Pseudomonas* and anaerobic flora was performed 2–4 days after treatment (T1), after 15 days (T2), and 45 days (T3). Enoxacin was administered to both partners at a dosage of 300 mg/12 hours for 10 days starting on day 1 of the menstrual cycle of the female partner. Exclusion criteria were; severe liver or kidney disease, pregnancy, breastfeeding, known hypersensitivity to chinolonics, other antibiotic therapies.

RESULTS

The results are shown in Table 1; in which is shown the success rate of 88.7% of positive cases rendered negative with an eradication in 88.9% of couples. The infection was eradicated in 15/17 males and females (88.3%) and in 25/28 males or females (89.3%) giving 40/45 (88.9%) of couples free from infection. In no one case was a recurrence noticed by 45 days of treatment. In 26 cases a control has been carried out after 3 months and it has not shown any recurrence. In nine patients of the 90 treated, a development of enoxacin-resistant microbiological flora was noticed, after treatment with chinolonics. In 70 cases (85%) there were no side-effects; in the remaining cases the side-effects were always mild (Table 2), except for one in which a severe urticarial reaction with vulvovaginal skin rash was observed on the last day of treatment. The hematochemical parameters did not show any significant modifications during therapy.

Table 1 Microbial response to enoxacin treatment

	T_0	T_1	T_2	T_3
Positive culture	62	8	7	7
Negative culture	0	54	55	55 (88.7%)

Table 2 Side-effects to enoxacin treatment ($n = 90$)

Skin rash	4
Itching	4
Diarrhea	2
Nausea/vomiting	7
Stomach ache	9
Headache	1

DISCUSSION

This study has shown that enoxacin can be used successfully in uncomplicated *C. trachomatis* infections. Data indicating the possible use of this drug as a first choice treatment are:

(1) A very good percentage of eradication of the infection;
(2) No recurrence after 45 days nor after 3 months;
(3) Duration of treatment significantly less than previous treatments; and,
(4) High sensitivity of *Gonococcus* to enoxacin, avoiding polychemotherapy in urethritis caused by both micro-organisms.

In our study we have not discovered any severe side-effects, which have been described sometimes in literature during 4-quinolonic use; this fact is probably determined by the low dosage we have used.

In conclusion, enoxacin appears a very good drug for the treatment of *C. trachomatis* infections even where they are associated with *Gonococcus*.

REFERENCES

1. Centers for disease control. (1985). *Chlamydia trachomatis* infections: policy guidelines for prevention and control. *MMWR*, **34** (suppl.3), 53S
2. Orfila, J. (1984). Action des antibiotiques sur les chlamydiae. *Med. Hyg.*, **42**, 1057
3. Sanders, L.L. *et al.* (1986). Treatment of sexually transmitted chlamydial infections. *J. Am. Med. Assoc.*, **255**, 1750
4. Wise, R. *et al.* (1986). The comparaive pharmacokinetics and tissue penetration of four quinolones including intravenously administered enoxacin. *Infection*, **14** (suppl. 3), 196
5. Dubois, J. *et al.* (1986). *In vitro* activities of Enoxacin and CI-934 against urinary tract and gastrointestinal tract pathogens. *Curr. Ther. Res.*, **40**, 6 1084
6. Fernandes, C.J. *et al.* (1986). *In vitro* antibacterial activity of Enoxacin (CI-919). *Pathology*, **18**, 240
7. Thomas, M.G. *et al.* (1985). Enoxacin treatment of urinary tract infections. *J. Antimicrob. Chemother.*, **15**, 759
8. Naber, K.G. *et al.* (1985). *In vitro* activity, pharmacokinetics, clinical safety and therapeutic efficacy of Enoxacin in the treatment of patients with complicated urinary tract infections. *Infection*, **13**, 5 219
9. Notowicz, A. *et al.* (1984). A double blind study comparing two dosages of Enoxacin for the treatment of uncomplicated urogenital gonorrhoea. *J. Antimicrob. Chemother.*, **14** (suppl. C), 91–4
10. Storz, B. *et al.* (1986). Quinolones in the treatment of gonorrhoea and *Chlamydia trachomatis* infections. *Pharmaceutisch Weekblad Scientific Edition*, **8**, 60

33

Rationale of the use of cefotetan in the treatment of gynecological surgical infections

G. Nicoletti, P.M. Furneri, A. Cianci, L. Roccasalva and G. Palumbo

The incidence of infections in the gynecology and obstetrics departments have been evaluated at about 10%, all these cases following surgery, delivery or abortion[1]. The incidence of surgical infections is closely related to the 'risk class'. In the obstetric and gynecological fields, in which operations belong to the 'clean–contaminated' and 'contaminated' classes, it is now recognized that infections of the upper genital tract are polymicrobic in nature and due to synergism between aerobic and anaerobic bacteria[2]. Because of these findings the use of a broad spectrum antibiotic drug is becoming indispensable.

Because of the increasing use of cephalosporins there has been a rise in the incidence of bacterial strains producing cephalosporinases that render many of this class of antibiotic therapeutically useless[3]. Attempts to overcome this problem resulted in the discovery of the cephamycin class of antibiotic; the presence of a 7α-methoxy substituent confers a high degree of stability to β-lactamases[4].

Cefotetan[5] is a well known cephamycin with a broad spectrum, stable to both the transferable β-lactamases of Gram negative bacteria and the chromosomal β-lactamase of *Bacteroides* species[6]. It exhibits a high degree of activity against a wide spectrum of Gram positive and Gram negative bacteria. The 90% of strains of *Escherichia coli*, *Klebsiella* species and *Proteus mirabilis* are inhibited at concentrations of less than 1 ml/l. Moreover Cefotetan is active against *Bacteroides fragilis*[1,6]. Its pharmacokinetic behavior evidenced a long halflife, which ensures therapeutically effective plasma levels for more than 12 hours[1]. Tissue concentrations of cefotetan likely to be effective are achieved in the genitourinary tract, female genital tissue and many others[1].

Clinical studies indicated an impressive clinical efficacy, particularly in obstetric–gynecological infections including salpingitis and endometritis[1]. Moreover the preoperative administration of one dose of Cefotetan has been shown to reduce the incidence of postoperative infections in patients undergoing surgical procedure.

EVALUATION OF THERAPEUTIC EFFICACY

Fifty patients who developed infections after gynecological and obstetrical surgery (Table 1) were studied. Thirty-two of these were suffering from *in situ* infections (Table 2), whereas postsurgical urinary tract infections and respiratory tract infections were found respectively in 14 and two patients (Table 2).

Whenever possible pathological specimens were collected (43/50) and assayed for micro-organism content. The microbial results are shown in Table 3: mixed infections occurred in 22 of 43 cases (51.16%) with an incidence of 66.66% (18/27 cases) in wound infections, 14.28% (2/14 cases) in urinary tract infections and 100% (2/2 cases) in endometritis; single infections were observed in 21 of 43 cases (48.83%) with an incidence of 33.33% (9/27 cases) in wound infections and 85.71% (12/14 cases) in urinary tract infections.

Seventy micro-organisms were isolated from 43 patients: 70% were aerobic bacteria and 30% anaerobic. Among the aerobic bacteria *E. coli* and *Klebsiella pneumoniae* were the more frequently isolated; *B. fragilis* was the more frequently isolated among the anaerobes.

Therapy with Cefotetan started at the clinical evidence of infection; in all the patients Cefotetan was administered 2 g every 12 hours for 7 days. Moreover, in four cases of severe infection, Cefotetan was used in association with netilmicin (150 mg/day). In two patients the combined therapy started from the beginning, while in two others netilmicin was administered when the clinical symptoms were still present at the 4th day of therapy with

Table 1 Type of surgery on 50 patients

Abdominal surgery	9
Vaginal hysterectomy	12
Wertheim hysterectomy	3
Myomectomy	3
Caesarean section	23

Table 2 Postoperative infections following obstetric and gynecological surgery

In situ infections (32/50)	
Wound infections	27
Endometritis	2
Parametritis	1
Pelvic sepsis	2
Other infections (18/50)	
Pyrexia of unknown origin	2
Lower respiratory tract infections	2
Urinary tract infections	14

Table 3 Microbiological results

Wound infections (27)	
4	*Bacteroides* spp.
3	*E. coli*
2	*K. pneumoniae*
1	*Peptostreptococcus* spp. + *P. aeruginosa* + *S. epidermidis*
4	*Peptococcus* spp + *E. coli*
4	*Bacteroides* spp + *K. pneumoniae*
1	*Bacteroides* spp. + *E. faecalis* + *K. pneumoniae*
2	*C. freundii* + *E. coli*
1	*Peptostreptococcus* spp. + *E. coli*
1	*Peptostreptococcus* spp. + *E. faecalis*
1	*Clostridium* spp. + *K. pneumoniae*
2	*E. agglomerans* + *Bacteroides* spp. + *E. coli*
1	*E. coli* + *E. faecalis*
Urinary tract infections (14)	
9	*E. coli*
3	*K. pneumoniae*
1	*E. coli* + *E. agglomerans*
1	*E. coli* + *S. marcescens*
Endometritis (2)	
1	*P. aeruginosa* + *Peptococcus* spp. + *S. epidermidis*
1	*Peptococcus* spp. + *E. coli*

Cefotetan. In these cases *Pseudomonas* was isolated.

Clinical evaluation indicated that Cefotetan alone was effective in 46 of 50 patients; moreover, the association of Cefotetan with netilmicin, in four cases, was very successful.

Side-effects were mild and few transient changes in laboratory parameters were found.

Our results showed that Cefotetan is an effective and safe therapeutical agent in the therapy of severe polymicrobial infections.

REFERENCES

1. Bertelli, A. and Cocuzza, G. (1986). Cefotetan. *Drugs Expt. Clin. Res.*, **XII**, (Suppl. 2), 1–82
2. Nicoletti, G., Cianci, A., Nicolosi, V.M., Tempera, G. and Palumbo, G. (1988). Epidemiologia ed eziologia delle infezioni in chirurgia ginecologica ed ostetrica: attuali criteri classificativi. *Farmaci Terapia*, **V**, 206–16
3. Neu, H.C., Fu, K.P., Aswapokee, P. and Kung, K. (1979). Comparative activity and β-lactamase stability of cefoperazone, a piperazine cephalosporin. *Antimicrob. Agents Chemother.*, **16**, 150–7
4. Ishiyama, S., Akeida, Y., Kawaguchi, H. and Nakayama, I. (1981). A clinical study of cefotetan (YM 09330) in aerobic and anaerobic surgical infections. Presented at *12th International Congress of Chemotherapy*, Florence, Italy. Abstract 187.
5. Ayers, L.W., Jones, R.N., Barry, A.L., Thornsberry, C., Fuchs, P.C., Gavan, T.L., Gerlach, E.H. and Sommers, H.M. (1982). Cefotetan, a new cephamycin: comparison of *in vitro* antimicrobial activity with other cephems, β-lactamase stability, and preliminary recommendations for disk diffusion testing. *Antimicrob. Agents Chemother.*, **22**, 859–77
6. Watt, B. and Brown, F.V. (1985). Anaerobes in clinical practice: significance and treatment. In Lode, H., Periti, P. and Strachan, C.J.L. (eds). *Cefotetan – A Long Acting Antibiotic for Polymicrobial Infections*, pp. 8–13. (Edinburgh, London and New York: Churchill Livingstone)

34

Prevalence and treatment of Chlamydial infections in pregnancy

P. Martinelli, C. Nappi, G. Ribera, E. Grandone, A. Nicotra and D. Paladini

Chlamydial infections are among the most common sexually transmitted diseases (STD). In the USA and Scandinavia, the role played by *Chlamydia trachomatis* infections in the recent increase of STD is well known and established, *C trachomatis* being the most widespread pathogen in the world[1-4].

In detail, the Center for Disease Control (CDC) of Atlanta claims that during 1986 in the USA 5 million people, mostly young heterosexuals, were infected by *C. trachomatis* which is responsible, on its own, for 500 000 of the million pelvic inflammatory disease (PID) cases occurring yearly in the USA, with a cost of some $1.3 billion[1,3-5].

The incidence of *C. trachomatis* infections in the male subject with STD has been calculated to be around 14% if heterosexual and 5% if homosexual; in women, the incidence is 3–7% in the general population, 20–30% in patient with STD and 37% among pregnant women[2,6-8]; finally, it can be cultured from 60–70% of the partners of chlamydial non-gonococcal urethritis (NGU) affected males.

C. trachomatis infections are asymptomatic in most cases, especially in women.

The key reservoir for transmission (to the partner, to the vaginally delivered neonate and to the female genitourinary tract itself) is Chlamydial cervicitis. The occurrence of carrier status has been well documented among women, persisting, in some cases, even after the menopause[2,5,9,10].

Several reports on *C. trachomatis* prevalence agree that there is an increase among teenagers and young individuals (13 to 27 years), the age group for which the highest incidence of STD has been demonstrated, with a peak in the 20–24-year-old group followed by the 25–29 and 15–19 age groups, though with a high variability according to the social, moral, and religious background of the sample population[3,11-17].

Among women, prevalence has also been found to increase with the number of sexual partners[1,12,18,20].

Another factor responsible for the current rise in *C. trachomatis* infections is the increasing use of oral contraceptives: in fact, the estroprogestins bring about both a decrease in the use of the barrier methods (condom, diaphragm), and an increase in the susceptibility of the cervix to *C. trachomatis* infections, via the oral contraceptive-induced ectropion, showing *C. trachomatis*' peculiar predilection for the columnar epithelium[1,2,19,21]. This is also the case for the other conditions in which a cervical ectropion occurs: i.e. adolescence and pregnancy[7,8,19,21].

During pregnancy, *C. trachomatis* has been related to first trimester miscarriage, postabortive infections, extrauterine pregnancies, postpartum endometritis and premature rupture of membranes! An association between *C. trachomatis* and intrauterine growth retardation has also been noted, though not yet confirmed[2,8,18,19,22–24].

These data have led us to assess the incidence of *C. trachomatis* infections among Neapolitan pregnant women, and to evaluate the feasibility of a screening program in terms of costs and benefits.

A screening program on a sample population of 168 women referred to us mainly for delivery was carried out between March and December 1988. The method chosen for the screening was an immunofluorescence (IF) test on cervical smears (Monoclonal Antibody Direct Specimen Test, ORTHO-Diagnostics, USA). Anamnestic behavioral and clinical data of the 168 patients were also recorded.

It has to be underlined that the IF test is, according to several reports[3,4,9,20] a reliable alternative to cell culture, requiring less time (0.5 vs 40 h) with a good sensibility (94.9%) and specificity (97.9%), if properly handled[4,9,13,20].

All the screened patients were from the same geographic area: Naples and its hinterland. Mean age of the sample population was 27.9 (SD 5.7) yr, ranging between 16 and 42 yr.

Of the 168 women screened for *C. trachomatis* near term (36–40 weeks of gestation), 39 (23.2%) showed a positive IF test.

There was no statistically significant difference in age or socioeconomic background between the two groups (age 28 (SD 4.7) vs 27 (SD 5.8); low social status: 75.6% vs 72%).

Ten (25.6%) of the affected patients had used contraception: four of them (10.2%) had used barrier methods, but irregularly; three patients (7.6%) had used oral contraceptives for 1 to 4 years.

As to clinical signs, only three positive patients mentioned itching, soreness and/or signs of cervicovaginitis at pelvic examination. Most women showed leucorrhea of varying intensity. This is so frequent in pregnancy as to appear statistically not significant in comparison to the control group.

As to the neonates at risk from *C. trachomatis* infections, a conjunctival smear for IF testing was performed by the 3rd day after birth.

Four neonates dropped out; of the remaining 35, 12 (34.2%) showed a positive IF test. Two of these (16.6% of the infected babies) showed clinical signs of conjunctivitis, one (8.2%) developed interstitial pneumonia, while no apparent sign of infection could be found in the remaining nine (75%) babies, in agreement with the widely documented self-limiting nature of neonatal infection[2,7,21,23,24].

However, it should be stressed that all the neonates underwent antibiotic prophylaxis for conjunctivitis in the first hours of life with a collirium containing chloramphenicol, colistine, and tetracycline (Colbiocin, SIFI).

The reason prophylaxis failed in 12 cases is probably due to systemic rather than local spread of the infection, as reported by some authors[7,8,23]. Noteworthy is also the fact that one of the infected babies was delivered by Caesarean section, though with ruptured membranes. Some authors commenting on a similar occurrence, hypothesized three mechanisms of infection: prenatal, postnatal and intrapartum,[8,21,22,24]. In the first instance, there would be an ascending infection from the cervix, favored by prematurely ruptured membranes, contaminating the fetus and the placenta; the postnatal mechanism of infection would be through breastfeeding, but this route of infection is still controversial[7,20]; the last mechanism, obviously, depends on the contact between the fetus and an infected birth canal.

Given the high prevalence of *C. trachomatis* infections in the Neapolitan area, which has also been reported by other researchers, we decided to carry out a clinical trial on the effectiveness of an oral antibiotic regimen on a selected group of 27 pregnant women between the 34th and 36th week of gestation, with a positive IF test. The schedule used was: erythromycin ethylsuccinate (Eritrocina, cp 500 mg, Abbot), 500 mg four times daily for 10 days for both the patients and their partners, the patients were also advised not to have sexual intercourse during therapy.

Two weeks after the end of the therapy, a control smear was taken. Twenty-five (92.5%) patients completed the treatment schedule; 22 of them (81.4%) showed a negative IF test. Two patients interrupted the therapy for the occurrence of mild gastrointestinal side-effects (nausea, vomiting, pyrosis, flatulence); nevertheless, one of these two patients resulted negative at the control smear, despite the early withdrawal from therapy (only 4 days of treatment).

None of the cured mothers' neonates showed a positive result to the IF test performed on the conjunctival specimen, while the neonate of the only patient with a positive control test was infected.

In spite of the high percentage of success achieved with erythromycin, further studies are needed to identify the drug of choice for *C. trachomatis* infections in pregnancy, it being very difficult to persuade an asymptomatic woman to take a drug which could cause even mild side-effects. The detection of a suitable drug becomes much more difficult if we consider that tetracyclines are contraindicated during pregnancy; that new trials are needed to test the new quinolones (Ciprofloxacin, Enoxacin, Perfloxacin) in pregnant women; that, finally, serious dose-dependent effects have been reported in experimental models (the rat) with the quinolones of the previous generation (Pipemidic acid): delayed ossification, ureteral dilatation.

The last resort is, therefore, represented by macrolides and, among them, the ones with the longest half-lives (Miocamicin, Iosamicin), which could improve the patient's compliance.

However, multicenter studies are needed to assess the effectiveness of these drugs in gestational *C. trachomatis* infections.

Conclusively, it can be affirmed that a screening program through cervical smears is mandatory, especially in the third trimester of gestation. As Sweet *et al.*[9] calculated, such a screening would be economically feasible even for a population with a prevalence of 4.5%, if followed by the treatment of all the infected women.

REFERENCES

1. Westrom, L. (1980). Incidence, prevalence and trends of acute pelvic inflammatory disease and its consequences in industrialized countries. *Am. J. Obstet. Gynecol.*, **138**, 880
2. Schachter, J. (1978). *Chlamydia* infection. *N. Engl. J. Med.*, **298**, 428, 490, 540
3. (1982). Sexually transmitted disease treatment guidelines. *MMWR*, **31** (suppl 2), 33–60
4. (1985). *Chlamydia trachomatis* infections: Policy guidelines for prevention and control. *MMWR*, **34** (suppl 3) 53S
5. Fraser, J.J., Rettig, P.J. and Kaplan, D.W. (1983). Prevalence of cervical *Chlamydia trachomatis* and *Neisseria gonorrhoeae* in female adolescents. *Pediatrics*, **71**, 333–6
6. Isselbacher, K.J., Adams, R.D., Braunwald, E., Petersdorf, R.G. and Wilson, J.D. (1983). In *Harrison's Principles of Internal Medicine*, 10th edn. (New York: McGraw-Hill)
7. Harrison, H.R. (1983). Cervical *Chlamydia trachomatis* and mycoplasmal infections in pregnancy. *J. Am. Med. Assoc.*, **250**, 1721–9
8. Martin, D. (1982). Prematurity and perinatal mortality in pregnancies complicated by maternal *Chlamydia trachomatis. J. Am. Med. Assoc.*, **247**, 1587–91
9. Hammerschlag, M.R., Anderka, M., Semine, D.Z. *et al.* (1979). Prospective study of maternal and infantile infection with *Chlamydia trachomatis. Pediatrics*, **64**, (2) 142
10. Nagashima, T. (1987). A high prevalence of chlamydial cervicitis in postmenopausal women. *Am. J. Obstet. Gynecol.*, **156**, 31–2
11. Panconesi, E. and Zuccati, G. (1987). Sexually transmitted *Chlamydia trachomatis* infection in adolescence. In *Third European Symposium on Pediatric and Adolescent Gynaecology, Florence*, pp. 619–23 (Rome: CIC Edizioni Internacionali)
12. Bump, R.C., Sachs, L.A. and Buesching, W.J. (1986). Sexually transmissible infectious agents in sexually active and virginal asymptomatic adolescent girls. *Pediatrics*, **77**, 488
13. Shafer, M.A., Sweet, R.I., Ohm-Smith, M.J. *et al.* (1985). Mycrobiology of the lower genital tract in postmenarchal adolescent girls: difference by sexual activity, contraception, and presence of nonspecific vaginitis. *J. Pediatr.*, **107**, 974–81
14. Chacko, M.R. and Lovchik, J.C. (1984). *Chlamydia trachomatis* infection in sexually active adolescents: prevalence and risk factors. *Pediatrics*, **73**, 836–40
15. Brunham, R.C., Paavonen, J., Stevens, C.E. *et al.* (1984). Mucopurulent cervicitis – the ignored counterpart in women of urethritis in men. *N. Engl. J. Med.*, **311**, 1–6
16. Shafer, M.A., Beck, A., Blain, B. *et al.*, (1984). *Chlamydia trachomatis*: Important relationship to race, contraception, lower genital tract infection, and Papanicolau smear. *J. Pediatr.*, **104**, 141–6
17. Harrison, H.R., Costin, M., Medler, J.B. *et al.* Cervical *Chlamydia trachomatis* infection in university women: relationship to history, contraception, ectopy, and cervicitis. *Am. J. Obstet. Gynecol.*, **153**, 244–51
18. Sweet, R.L., Schachter, J. and Landers, D.V. (1983). Chlamydial infections in obstetrics and gynecology. *Clin. Obstet. Gynecol.*, **26**, 143
19. Alexander, E.R. (1979). *Chlamydia T.*: the organism and the neonatal infection. *Hosp. Practice*, 63–9
20. Sweet, R.L. and Mead, P.B. (1986). Le infezioni da *Chlamydia* in ginecologia. *Medico e Paziente*, **3**, 240–8
21. Helin, J. (1982). Maternal–neonatal transmission of *Chlamydia trachomatis* and its consequences. *Scand. J. Infect. Dis.* **32**, (suppl) 135–40
22. Piccaro, M. (1984). Ruolo dell Chlamydie nella patologia genitale e neonatale. *Minerva Ginecol*, **36**, (12) 861–9
23. Khurana, C.M., Deddish, P.A., Delmundo, F. (1985). Prevalence of *Chlamydia trachomatis* in the pregnant cervix: *Obstet. Gynecol.*, **66**, 241–8
24. Heggie, A. (1981). *Chlamydia trachomatis* infections in mothers and infants: a prospective study. *Am. J. Dis. Child.*, **135**, 507–604

35

Cyclopyroxolamin in treating mycotic vulvovaginites

R. Forleo, F. Baiocco, L. Tamassia and P. Forleo

INTRODUCTION

Mycotic vulvovaginites, generally supported by *Candida albicans*, represent today a more and more frequent and constantly increasing pathology[1]. For the gynecologist they constitute a serious problem, in particular in overcoming the infection which can be difficult because of predisposition factors, which must be carefully considered in order to obtain complete recovery[2–7].

A critical part in encouraging infection seems to be played in many cases by iatrogenic factors, for example, the intake of:

(1) Antibiotics, especially those with a wide range of action which are taken over a long period. These favor the development of mycetes because of the decreased presence of normal bacterial flora in the vagina[7].

(2) Antiblastic, chemotherapic or corticosteroid pharmaceuticals which weaken the body defences.

(3) Estroprogestinics, because of the interference occurring with the woman's hormonal balance[5,8,10]

Also significant are certain hygiene habits which involve the indiscriminate and incongruous use of soaps and so-called 'specific' douches[1].

Beside the iatrogenic factors, several pathological factors are important, such as chronic debilitant, dysmetabolic, and/or endocrine diseases and congenital or acquired immune deficits[11–13].

It has also been seen that certain physiological conditions, such as pregnancy, premenstrual phase, periclimacteric period, can also contribute to disease development[14,15]. As yet, many of the mechanisms these various conditions act with are not perfectly clarified: this confronts the gynecologist with further problems concerning the causes of the disease and, in consequence, the medication. In fact, many therapeutic attempts have been made, both using pharmaceuticals, and through systemic and local administration. The most common pharmaceuticals have been imidazole derivatives[16–19].

Cyclopyroxolamin, a brand new pharmaceutical, has been recently introduced. This is characterized by an original chemical structure which does not seem linked to either the imidazole group of pharmaceuticals or any other type of medicine so far used in therapy. Cyclopyroxolamin is in fact an antimycotic product belonging to the hydroxypyridone class, with a remarkable antifungal action (inhibition of amino acid, potassium and phosphate ions intracytoplasm transport and membrane permeability alteration)[20,21]. This pharmaceutical product has proved efficient not only on mycotic forms, but also in various types of bacteria, both Gram negative and Gram positive, the former character being unique and making the difference between cyclopyroxolamin and the antimycotic so far used[22]. In addition, its efficiency on *Gardnerella vaginalis*, so often responsible for aspecific vaginites, has recently been demonstrated[23].

The clinical activity of cyclopyroxolamin has been so far verified on small groups of patients suffering mostly from pure vaginal candidiasis[24–29]. We have therefore performed a prospective epidemiological study whose objects were to:

(1) Evaluate, treating a wider and heterogeneous population of patients suffering from mycotic vulvovaginitis, whether cyclopyroxolamin is able to influence the clinical picture either by making the microbiological results negative or by improving the symptoms, and

(2) Evaluate the tolerance of the pharmaceutical product by identifying possible noxious and unexpected reactions.

PATIENTS AND METHODOLOGY

Experimental design

Each gynecologist was asked to provide outpatient treatment to 12 patients suffering from mycotic vulvovaginitis, which had been ascertained by the examination of either fresh or after staining vaginal secretion. The possible presence of other microbes did not constitute an exclusion criterion from the study. However, patients suffering from ascertained cyclopyroxolamin hypersensitivity were excluded.

Treatment

Each patient was treated with one 100 mg cyclopyroxolamin (Dafnegin®) capsule per day for 3 days. In cases of persistent symptoms and/or lack of negative microbiological results, the cycle was repeated with the same posology. All patients were asked to abstain from sexual intercourse during the treatment period.

Procedure

The investigation included an admission examination followed by another at the end of the study.

At the admission examination, after verification of the patients admissibility, the experimenter proceeded to the evaluation of the following parameters: presence of various micro-organisms in the vaginal secretion, vulvovaginal erythema, vulvovaginal edema, leucorrhea, itch, burn and dysuria. These were all evaluated by a semiquantitative estimate through pre-established scores.

At the final examination, the clinical picture was evaluated and the vaginal secretion microbiological examination was repeated. From these the experimenter assessed the treatment efficiency; excellent (fully negative microbiological results and symptomatological picture resolution), good (still positive microbiological results but absent-to-light symptomatology), acceptable (still positive microbiological results with light-to-moderate symptomatology), none (unvaried microbiological and clinical pictures).

Tolerance

In order to evaluate correctly the side-effects at the end of the study, the experimenter had to fill in a report card of possible undesired effects, spontaneously indicated by the patient or evidenced by the gynecologist, their intensity, duration and the possible pharmaceutical intervention adopted to solve them.

Characteristics of the study population

Two hundred and eighty hospital/university gynecologists participated during the 1987–8 period. Patients (3368) from all over Italy (44.9% from northern Italy, 21.3% from central Italy and 33.8% from southern and insular Italy) suffering from mycotic vulvovaginitis have been admitted to the study.

As can be noted from Table 1, the age range of the treated patients was between 18 and 70 ($\bar{x} \pm$ SEM: 32.0 ± 0.18). The most represented age group (73.3%) was that between 21 and 40, that is the one corresponding to the highest sexual and reproductive period. The majority (97.0%) showed *C. albicans*, 3.2% showed *Trichomonas vaginalis* and 19.4% showed mixed bacterial flora. Moreover, it can be seen that 66.5% of the patients showed in their medical history predisposition to the development of a vaginal infection and/or, specifically, mycosis (Table 1).

Almost half of the patients (1559 equal to 46.3%) had had previously at least one episode of vulvovaginitis; out of these 1483 (95.1%) had already received treatment (Table 1).

At the time of the study 1370 patients (40.6%) suffered from a concomitant pathology which, in some cases, could have some connection with the vulvovaginitis: 223 showed colpites–cervicites; 177, urinary passage infection; 65, adnexites; 38, vulvovaginal dystrophy; 37, cutaneous mycosis; 34, condylomatosis; 10, genital herpes.

During the study period, 57.8% of the patients took cyclopyroxolamin only, 1.2% took other specific pharmaceuticals and 41.0% followed a therapy

Table 1 Characteristics of patients admitted to the study

	n	%
Patients	3368	
Age (years)		
$\bar{x} \pm$ SEM	32.0 ± 0.18	
Range	18–70	
Classes ≤20	316	9.4
21–40	2469	73.3
41–60	514	15.3
>60	69	2.0
Geographical distribution		
North	1512	44.9
Center	718	21.3
South and islands	1138	33.8
Type of bacteriological ascertainment		
Fresh	1851	55.0
After staining	1513	44.9
Pathology type		
1st episode patients	1809	53.7
Previous vulvovaginitis patients	1559	46.3
Previous treatments		
Medical history information		
Oral contraceptives	892	26.5
Pregnancies	384	11.4
Antibiotic therapy	293	8.7
IUD	156	4.6
Ectropion. exocervix erosion, DTC	130	3.8
Diabetes	113	3.4
Physiological menopause	83	2.5
Menopause + diabetes	48	1.4
Surgical menopause	46	1.4
Confinement	42	1.2
Pregnancy + diabetes	13	0.4
Bartholinitis	10	0.3
Drug addiction	4	0.1

for the concomitant afflictions. For 753 (22.3%) patients only was it considered necessary to go through a second treatment cycle.

RESULTS

Out of the 3368 patients, 38 (1.3%) did not complete the study with cyclopyroxolamin for reasons indicated in Table 2. Of the 3330 patients who completed the experimentation, the pharmaceutical action was studied both in regard to the microbiological picture and the clinical symptomatology.

Microbiological picture

The bacteriological ascertainment performed on vaginal secretion was carried out in 'fresh' conditions in 1851 cases (55%) and after coloration in 1513

Table 2 Patients who did not complete the study

Motivation	*Number of cases* *1st cycle*	*2nd cycle*	*% of total admitted patients*
Intolerance	12	—	0.3
Did not show up	17	1	0.6
Scarce compliance	6	2	0.4
Total	35	3	1.3

Table 3 Etiological and symptomatological characteristics of the treated and controlled cases

Series of cases	*Basic* *n*	*%*	*Before 2nd treatment* n	%
Number of patients under treatment	3368		753	22.3
Microbiological results				
C. albicans	3268	97.0	693	92.0
T. vaginalis	109	3.2	43	5.7
Mixed bacterial flora	654	19.4	182	24.1
Clinical symptomatology				
Vulvovaginal erythema	2381	70.6	425	56.4
Vulvovaginal edema	1790	53.1	283	37.5
Leucorrhea	3259	96.8	664	88.1
Itch	3144	93.3	583	77.4
Burn	2636	78.3	451	59.8
Dysuria	1318	39.1	193	25.6

cases (44.9%) (Table 1); in four cases the method has not been indicated.

Table 3 shows the composition of the cases treated. Out of 3268 ascertained mycosis cases, *C. albicans* was found alone in 80.5% of the cases, associated with *T. vaginalis* in 2.5%, with mixed bacterial flora in 16.4% and with both in 0.6% of the cases.

Table 4 shows how at the end of the first treatment cycle *C. albicans* had disappeared in 2377 cases out of 3268 (72.8%), *T. vaginalis*, in 57 cases out of 109 (52.3%), and mixed bacterial flora, in 378 cases out of 654 initial cases (57.8%).

Of the 753 patients who, because of the absence of negative microbiological results or of the persistence of some symptom, received the second cycle of treatment, 693 (92%) showed a mycosis (*C. albicans*) which, at the end of that cycle, had become negative in 83.3% of the cases, and had improved in 10.8% of the cases.

Together, these two 3-day cycles of treatment have registered complete eradication of *C. albicans*, *T. vaginalis* and mixed bacterial flora in 90.4%, 75.2% and 75.7% of the cases respectively (Figure 1).

Clinical symptomatology

At the end of the first cycle of treatment with cyclopyroxolamin, we noticed the disappearance of erythema and vulvovaginal edema in 1706 (71.6%) and

Table 4 Evaluation of the microbiological picture after the 1st and 2nd treatment cycles

Micro-organisms	*Microbiological picture*	*1st cycle end* *n*	*1st cycle end* %	*2nd cycle end* *n*	*2nd cycle end* %
C. albicans	Negativity	2377	72.8	577	83.5
(3268 cases)	Improvement	801	24.5	74	10.8
	Unchanged	55	1.6	32	4.6
	Worsened	—	—	1	—
	Missing	35	1.1	9	1.3
T. vaginalis	Negativity	57	52.3	25	58.1
(109 cases)	Improvement	42	28.5	4	9.3
	Unchanged	6	5.5	6	14.0
	Worsened	—	—	—	—
	Missing	4	3.7	8	18.6
Mixed bacteriological flora					
	Negativity	378	57.8	117	64.3
(654 cases)	Improvement	231	35.4	15	8.2
	Unchanged	39	5.9	40	22.0
	Worsened	—	—	—	—
	Missing	6	0.9	10	5.5

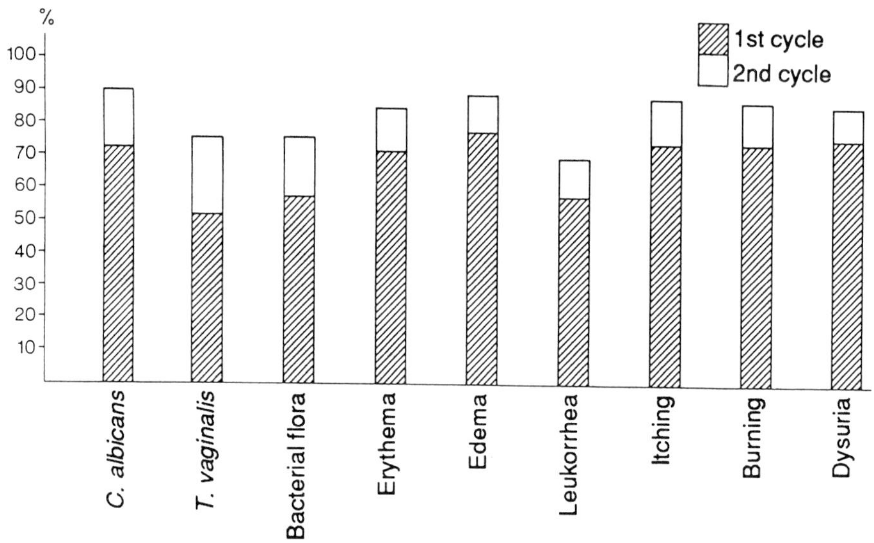

Figure 1 Eradication of micro-organisms and disappearance of symptomatology per cent at the end of the treatment (1st and 2nd cycle)

1383 (77.3%) of patients respectively who had shown the symptoms in basal conditions, leucorrhea had ceased in 1865 (57.2%) cases whereas itch, burn and dysuria were no longer mentioned in 2303 (73.2%), 1953 (74.1%) and 994 (75.4%) of patients respectively.

At the end of the second treatment cycle, the vulvovaginal erythema had disappeared in 319 out of the 425 women (75.0%) who still showed signs of it at the time of the treatment repeat. Edema had disappeared in 407 out of 664 cases (61.3%), itching had ceased in 461 women out of 583 (79.1%), burning had completely regressed in 347 out of 451 (76.9%) and, finally, dysuria had disappeared in 139 cases out of 193 (72.0%).

The symptomatology disappearance ratio was therefore further increased by the second cycle of treatment, stabilizing itself on 85.0% for the vulvovaginal erythema, 89.6% for edema, 69.7% for leucorrhea, 87.9% for itch, 87.2% for burn and 85.9% for dysuria (Figure 1).

Therapeutical efficiency

The efficiency statement expressed by the experimenting physician at the end of the treatment was excellent in 61.8% of the cases, good in 29.2%, acceptable in 6.8% and none in 1.1% (Table 5).

The therapeutic efficiency of cyclopyroxolamin did not show significant links with the geographic origin or the age of the patients, whereas it confirmed itself of different degree according to the etiological agent.

The least satisfying results were obtained in treating vulvovaginites caused by *T. vaginalis* or by the association of *C. albicans* with *T. vaginalis* and mixed bacterial flora. In *C. albicans* only vulvovaginites cases, the cyclopyroxolamin treatment efficiency was judged excellent in 65.2% of the cases, good in 27.4% and acceptable in 6.3%. In the case of mixed bacterial flora only, therapeutic efficiency was judged excellent in 57.6% of the cases, good in 31.5% and acceptable in 8.7%. The treatment of conditions caused by mycetes and bacteria gave excellent results in 51% of the cases, good in 40.1% and acceptable in 7.9%.

TOLERANCE

Cyclopyroxolamin was extremely well tolerated, having caused no side-effects in 99.1% of the women (Table 6). Only 30 patients reported the

Table 5 Statement on cyclopyroxolamin treatment efficiency

	Frequency	%
Excellent	2087	61.8
Good	985	29.2
Acceptable	228	6.8
None	36	1.1
Missing	38	1.1

Table 6 Incidence of side-effects

Side-effects	*Number of episodes*	*Drop-outs*
Vulvovaginal burn/reddening	12	6
Erythema	11	
Pelvicalgia	1	3
Urine retention	1	1
Nausea	3	
Gastralgia	1	
Malaise	1	1
Cutaneous rash	1	1
Edema	2	
Total number of episodes	33	12

appearance of side-effects; among those, the most frequent were vulvar burning and reddening (12 cases), erythema (10 cases) and nausea (three cases). In addition one case of each of the following symptoms has been observed: pelvicalgia, gastralgia, malaise, urine retention and cutaneous rash. In three cases patients experienced two side-effects (Table 6).

Incidence and type of side-effect have shown no statistically significant difference in the various diagnostic groups.

Side-effects were responsible for 12 drop-outs, six for burning, three for erythema, three for urine retention, cutaneous rash and malaise respectively.

CONCLUSIONS

The results of this multicenter study performed on a wide number of ambulatory cases (3330 patients), and aimed at verifying the efficiency of the cyclopyroxolamin treatment (Dafnegin®) in its actual operational conditions, confirmed its efficiency which had been already largely demonstrated in previous studies.

In patients suffering from mycotic vulvovaginites (pure or mixed) a complete *C. albicans* eradication ratio has been registered in 90.4% of the cases at the end of the treatment.

The data are linked to the improvement of both the subjective symptomatology (with disappearance of itches, burns and dysuria in over 86% of the cases) and the objective clinical signs (erythema, edema and leucorrhea) no longer showed in more than 85% of the cases.

The cyclopyroxolamin treatment efficiency has been judged positive (excellent + good) in 92.6% of the *C. albicans* vulvovaginitis cases. This pharmaceutical has, besides, confirmed its efficiency, not only against pure mycotic forms but also against conditions caused by mycetes and bacteria (with 89% of the results judged as excellent or good).

Where there is relapse, it is always good practice to extend the treatment for at least 3 days since our results have shown that the administration of six capsules was enough to turn the vaginal mycetes negative in over 90% of the cases.

As regards tolerance, no unexpected or unacceptable side-effect has been noticed and those which were reported were similar to those indicated in previous studies with cyclopyroxolamin.

This drug therefore appears effective in most vaginal candidiasis cases, and is very well tolerated, to the point that we consider it could be administered in the case of relapses which are frequent in this type of pathology.

REFERENCES

1. Difonzo, E.M., Vannini, P., Palleschi, G.M. and Panconesi, E. (1986). Vulvovaginiti micetiche: aspetti epidemiologici. Presented at *Le infezioni in Ostetricia e Ginecologia*, II Congresso Interdisciplinare; Pavia 4–7, May
2. Senft, H.H. and Karte, W. (1982). Epidemiology, pathology and clinical features of genital mycoses – 1981 status. *Chemotherapy*, **28** (suppl. 1), 3
3. Venturini, P.L. (1988). Le vulvovaginiti da Candida. *Doctor*, **14**, 50–2
4. Sobel, J.D. (1985). Epidemiology and pathogenesis of recurrent vulvovaginal candidosis. *Am. J. Obstet. Gynecol.*, **152**, 924
5. Miles, M. *et al.* (1987). Recurrent vaginal candidiasis. *J. Am. Med. Assoc.*, **238** (1), 836
6. Cassone, A. (1985). Candida e candidosi. *Fed. Med.*, **38**, 1018
7. Cassaro, N., Caschetto, S. and Abbadessa, M.G. (1986). Micosi vulvovaginale: fattori predisponenti. Note preliminari. Presented at *Le infezioni in Ostetricia e Ginecologia*, II Congresso Interdisciplinare, Pavia 4–7 May
8. Costa, S. *et al.* (1983). Sui rapporti tra ambiente vaginale e portio uterina nei processi flogistici locali. *Min. Ginecol.*, **35**, 549
9. Conti, M. *et al.* (1986). Contraccezione e malattie sessualmente trasmesse. Presented at *Le infezioni in Ostetricia e Ginecologia*, II Congresso Interdisciplinare, Pavia 4–7 May
10. Powell, B.L., Frey, C.L. and Drutz, D.J. (1983). Estrogen receptor in *Candida albicans*. A possible explanation for hormonal influences in vaginal candidiasis. Presented at the *Twenty-third Interscience Conference on Antimicrobial Agents and Chemotherapy*, Las Vegas
11. Finucci, R. and Marcozzi, A. (1988). Le vulvovaginiti da *Candida albicans*. *Dermatologia*, **3** (1), 28
12. Morton, R.D. and Rashid, S. (1977). Candidal vaginitis: natural history, predisposing factors and prevention. *Proc. R. Soc. Med.*, **70** (suppl. 4), 3
13. Odds, F.C. (1982). Genital candidosis. *Clin. Exp. Dermatol.*, **7**, 345
14. Conti, M. (1983). La gravidanza predispone alle forme vaginali. *Le Micosi, Quaderni del Corriere Medico*, **9**, 20
15. Meloni, G.A. (1986). Ecologia microbica dell'apparato genitale femminile. Presented at *Le infezioni in Ostetricia e Ginecologia*, II Congresso Interdisciplinare, Pavia 4–7 May
16. Borges, M. (1980). Mechanism of action of antifungal drugs, with special reference to the imidazole derivates. *Rev. Infect. Dis.*, **4**, 520
17. Pasetto, N., Baschieri, L. and Piccione, E. (1986). Le vulvovaginiti candidosiche recidivanti: orientamenti terapeutici. Presented at *Le infezioni Ostetricia e Ginecologia*. II Congresso Interdisciplinare, Pavia 4–7 May
18. Dennerstein, G.J. and Langley, R. (1982). Vulvovaginal candidiasis: treatment and recurrence. *Aust. N.Z. J. Obstet. Gynecol.*, **22**, 231
19. Gargani, G. (1985). Le malattie micotiche. *Terapia Oggi*, **4**, 50
20. Sakurai, K. *et al.* (1978). Mode of action of 6-cyclohexyl-1-hydroxy-4-methyl-2-(1H)-pyridone ethanolamine salt (Hoe 296). *Chemotherapy*, 24–28
21. Koch, H. (1982). Cyclopiroxolamin: antifungal agent. *Pharm. Int.*, **2**, 46
22. Dittmar, W. *et al.* (1981). Microbiological laboratory studies with cyclopiroxolamine. *Arzneim. Forsch/Drug Res.*, **31**(II) 8a, 1317
23. Riganti, A. and Martinetto, P. (1988). Gardnerella vaginalis e vaginiti non specifiche. *Medical News*, **21**, 1
24. Nencioni, T., Pamparana, F. and Jacobellis, M. (1988). Vulvovaginiti micotiche e ciclopirox-olamina per via topica. *Min. Ginecol.*, **40**, 719

25. Salvadoti, B., Cavalli, C. and Bonini, R. (1988). Efficacia e tollerabilità di un nuovo antimicotico per uso topico: la ciclopiroxolamina. *G. Ital. Ostet. Ginecol.*, **5**, 813
26. Russo, I., Oliveri, S., Greco, A.M., Sardo, S., Cammarata, E., Cosentina, R. and Palumbo, G. (1987). Valutazione clinica e microbiologica di ciclopiroxolamina nel trattamento di candidosi vaginali. *G. Ital. Ostet. Ginecol.*, **11**, 895
27. Rustichelli, S., Coppola, C., Tumiati, L., Giacardi, M., Carbone, G. and Cosentina, R. (1987). Ciclopiroxolamina: considerazioni preliminari sull'impiego di un nuovo antimicotico non imidazolico nella patologia infettiva genitale. *Min. Ginecol.*, **39**, 793
28. Mezzatesta, M., Maneschi, F. and Garofalo, C. (1984). Terapia della candidosi vulvovaginale con Ciclopiroxolamina. *Medical Praxis*, **5**, 221

36

Genital herpes simplex virus infection: current epidemiological, serological and therapeutic problems

N. Corbino, G. Calvo, L. Ciravolo, G. Boemi and A. Castro

One of the most relevant consequences of the cultural revolution that, during the 1960s, spread to the western countries, has been a dramatic increase in sexually transmitted diseases. Particularly, between 1966 and 1979, the incidence of genital herpes simplex virus (HSV) infection, has increased about tenfold. Current reports indicate that in the United States the number of patients consulting per year, for this disease, has increased from 30 000 to 300 000[1].

Based on these numbers and on an estimated 30 to 70% recurrent rate for genital HSV lesions, it can be calculated that each year, there are 5 to 9 million cases of clinically overt genital HSV infections[1]. These findings have caused a renewed interest among biologists and clinicians that has improved our current knowledge. However, genital HSV infection shows some critical points that are still poorly understood. Among these are the relationship between infection and clinical symptoms as well as some peculiarity about the spread of infection.

Most physicians see a relatively small number of patients with clinically evident HSV lesions and direct patient questioning suggests that primary infection often occurs following exposure to an asymptomatic partner[2]. Furthermore, the diffusion of the disease that has spread to the entire society, probably has changed the classic epidemiological patterns, mainly collected in the early 1970s. These data indicated that the risk of infection was related to social class and professional activity with a rate of specific seropositivity about 80 to 90% among sexually active, young males of lower social classes[3] as well as among prostitutes[4] but of about 50% among males of middle and higher classes[5] and about 25 to 30% among medical doctors[6]. There was also the evidence that less than 0.5% of women undergoing routine cytopathological examination[7] as well as women university students[8] shed infectious virus.

On the other hand, the rates of virus shedding among women attending sexually transmitted disease clinics were considerably higher and ranged from 1.6 to 6.9%[9]. Indeed, one of the most significant pieces of epidemiological evidence acquired in the last years has been the demonstration that HSV infection of the genital tract may be subclinical but, nevertheless, it remains associated with viral shedding[10]. The fundamental importance of detecting these subclinically infected spreaders of disease has become imperative, during early 1980, when a new drug, able to effectively stop viral replication, without any relevant side-effect or toxicity has become available: Acyclovir[11].

The search for the spreaders calls for a suitable screening method of risk subjects as well as for a virological assessment of suspected patients. On the other hand, normal serological diagnosis cannot be used, because of the latency and the great diffusion of infection among population. Now, because genitourinary tracts in humans are covered by mucosal epithelia, we measured, together with complement fixing immunoglobulin (Ig) serum levels also the serological patterns of HSV IgA response. We also used detection by monoclonal antibodies of viral antigens expressed on cervicovaginal exfoliated cells as well as viral culture isolation and typing.

In order to ascertain if epidemiological parameters, collected during the early 1970s were still reliable, particularly in our population, we studied 421 subjects, 184 men and 237 women (aged between 20 and 47 years), sexually active, free of any symptoms, among doctors and nurses in our hospital staff as well as among medical students.

A direct individual questioning about previous history of sexually transmitted diseases was positive only in 39 out of 421 subjects (9.26%). Of them, 21 men and six women reported experience of genital herpes (6.41%), six men and two women of genital warts, two men of gonorrhea and finally two men of genital herpes associated with warts. Serology was negative in 60 out of 184 men (32.6%) and 94 out of 237 women (39.6%). When this population was distributed according to age-classes (Table 1), it became evident that actual prevalence of seropositivity is certainly higher than in the past, even in a low-risk population.

It is important to notice that the males' seropositivity curve is progressively increasing from younger to older age-classes whereas in females after an initial age-related increase, the curve reaches the plateau level at about 30 to 34 years of age. This is presumably related to a different behavior among the sexes in reaching and maintaining a stable and exclusive sexual partnership.

Table 1 Age distribution of men and women showing seropositivity

Age-class	*Men*	%	*Women*	%
20–24	17/32	53.1	20/39	51.2
25–29	26/42	61.9	29/53	54.7
30–34	19/28	67.8	28/43	65.1
35–39	21/29	72.4	26/40	65.0
40–44	19/25	76.0	22/35	62.8
45–49	22/28	78.5	18/27	66.6
All	124/184	67.4	143/237	60.3

In seropositive subjects (124/184 men and 143/237 women) serum levels of specific complement fixing Ig showed a monomodal (normal) distribution curve with a peak for men and women, respectively, at the dilutions of 1/32 and 1/64 (Table 2).

On the other hand, the distribution of IgA serum levels showed a bimodal curve with two peaks, respectively at the dilution of 1/32 and 1/256 for men and 1/64 and 1/256 for women (Table 3). Indeed, in both sexes, the dilution of 1/128 may be considered as a threshold level that discriminates between two different subpopulations. Of them, the first, constituted by subjects with IgA levels between 1/8 and 1/128, includes 95 out of 124 men and 107 out of 143 women, that means 75% of studied subjects.

In order to ascertain if these two subpopulations were somehow related to active virus replication, a population of 256 clinically unaffected, sexually active women, undergoing routine Pap-test examination in our Department, was studied. A blind virus isolation/identification and determination of complement fixing antibodies and fluorescent assayed IgA were done, together with routine cytology and colposcopy (Table 4). Surprisingly, virus identification was positive in 34 out of 256 cervical swabs (13.28%). HSV2 was identified in 27, HSV1 in five and HSV2 together with HSV1 in two.

In this population, seropositivity rates in different age-classes were similar to those shown by the hospital staff population with a seronegativity percentage of 34.3%. However, the seropositivity distribution closely resembles masculine rather than feminine hospital staff population (Table

Table 2 Serum levels of HSV-cf-Ig in seropositive men and women

Dilution	*1/8*	*1/16*	*1/32*	*1/64*	*1/128*	*1/256*	*1/ 512*	*Total*
No. of men	9	23	36	24	18	9	5	124
Per cent	7.25	18.54	29.03	19.35	14.51	7.25	4.03	99.96
No. of women	13	25	26	33	25	11	10	143
Per cent	9.09	17.48	18.18	23.07	17.48	7.69	6.99	99.98

Table 3 Distribution of HSV-IgA serum levels in seropositive men and women

Dilution	*1/8*	*1/16*	*1/32*	*1/64*	*1/128*	*1/256*	*1/ 512*	*Total*
No. of men	11	19	25	22	18	23	6	124
Per cent	8.87	15.32	20.16	17.74	14.51	18.54	4.83	99.97
No. of women	11	19	26	32	19	27	9	143
Per cent	7.69	13.28	18.18	22.37	13.28	18.88	6.29	99.97

Table 4 Virus identification in Departmental population

Virus isolates	*HSV 2*	*HSV 1*	*HSV 1 + HSV 2*
No. of patients	27	5	2
Per cent	79.41	14.70	5.88

Table 5 Distribution of seropositivity in women undergoing routing Papanicolaou tests and coposcopy

Age-class	*Women*	*%*
20–24	19/37	51.3
25–29	37/63	58.7
30–34	32/48	66.6
35–39	29/41	70.7
40–44	27/36	75.0
45–49	24/31	77.4
All	168/256	65.6

5). For this, we do not have, at the moment, any explanation.

In the seropositive population, distribution curves of specific Ig serum levels were similar to those shown by hospital staff population with a monomodal (normal) distribution for complement fixing Ig, and bimodal distribution as far as IgA is concerned (Table 6).

However this particular point must be considered: In the virus-positive population 33 out of 34 patients showed IgA titers equal or higher than 1/128 whereas in the virus-negative population only 34 out of 222 patients had these titers. Furthermore, the serum dilution geometrical mean was 88.16 in virus-negative and 322.81 in virus-positive individuals with a significant difference (Table 7).

Finally, when virus-positive patients were excluded from the seropositive population, IgA distribution curves of remainders became monomodal (Table 8).

It is now clear that the two subpopulations distinguished by HSV-IgA are indeed constituted by subjects either with or without active virus replication. Data collected in overtly infected patients confirm this interpretation.

Table 6 Distribution of HSV-cf-Ig and HSV-IgA levels in seropositive patients

Dilution	*1/8*	*1/16*	*1/32*	*1/64*	*1/128*	*1/256*	*1/ 512*	*Total*
Cf-Ig	14	29	31	40	31	16	7	168
Per cent	8.33	17.26	18.45	23.80	18.45	9.52	4.16	99.97
IgA	11	22	31	37	26	31	10	168
Per cent	6.54	13.09	18.45	22.02	15.47	18.45	5.95	99.97

Table 7 HSV-IgA levels in virus-positive and virus-negative patients

Dilution	*Neg*	*1/8*	*1/16*	*1/32*	*1/64*	*1/128*	*1/256*	*1/512*	*Total*
Positive	—	—	—	—	1	4	21	8	34
Per cent	—	—	—	—	2.94	11.76	61.76	23.52	99.98
Negative	88	11	22	31	36	22	10	2	222
Per cent	39.63	4.95	9.90	13.96	16.21	9.90	4.50	0.90	99.95

Table 8 Distribution of HSV-IgA levels in seropositive patients

Dilution	*1/8*	*1/16*	*1/32*	*1/64*	*1/128*	*1/256*	*1/512*
No. of patients	11	22	31	36	22	10	02
Per cent	8.20	16.41	23.13	26.86	16.41	7.46	1.49

Between July 1984 and December 1988, we studied 192 women affected with clinically overt genital HSV infection. HSV2 was identified in 161 patients, HSV1 in 23, HSV2 together with HSV1 in eight (Table 9).

In this population, the IgA distribution curve was monomodal (normal) with a single peak at the dilution of 1/256 (Table 10).

We also studied 187 sexual partners of previously reported patients, measuring complement fixing HSV-Ig as well as HSV-IgA serum levels.

Also in this population, complement fixing Ig showed a monomodal (normal) distribution whereas IgA distributed bimodally (Table 11).

Among partners 62 out of 187 agreed to undergo urological examination, urinalysis, bacterial culture and bladder washing with cytological assessment of recovered cells. Surprisingly, although the inspection of external genitalia was completely negative, a prostate enlargement was detected in 37 out of 62 subjects (59.67%). Furthermore 34 out of 62 patients had a white blood cell blood count higher than 20 cells per microscopical field whereas a

Table 9 Virus identification in women with clinically overt genital HSV infection

Virus isolates	*HSV 2*	*HSV 1*	*HSV 1 + HSV 2*
No. of patients	161	23	8
Per cent	83.85	11.97	4.16

Table 10 Distribution of HSV-IgA in women with clinically overt genital HSV infection

Dilution	*1/64*	*1/128*	*1/256*	*1/512*	*Total*
No. of patients	6	31	106	49	192
Per cent	3.12	16.14	55.20	25.52	99.98

Table 11 Distribution of HSV-cf-Ig and HSV-IgA levels in sexual partners of infected patients

Dilution	*1/8*	*1/16*	*1/32*	*1/64*	*1/128*	*1/256*	*1/ 512*	*Total*
Cf-Ig	17	32	43	35	33	19	8	187
Per cent	9.09	17.11	22.99	18.71	17.64	9.64	4.27	99.97
IgA	13	24	37	32	26	32	23	187
Per cent	6.95	12.83	19.78	17.11	13.90	17.11	12.29	99.97

significant bacterial growth was evident only in nine specimens. Papillary hyperplasia of bladder urothelium was present in 46.77% (29 out of 62).

As far as therapy is concerned, 128 women underwent specific antiviral treatment together with 27 partners. Acyclovir was administered by intravenous injection on a daily basis (15 mg/kg) in three refracted doses of 5 mg/kg each for 5–7 consecutive days. Courses were repeated 1–3 times at 3–9 day intervals. Twenty-four controls were placebo-treated receiving normal saline. The effectiveness of Acyclovir therapy was assessed by controlling morphological evolution of mucocutaneous lesions, until crusting (healing time) as well as by checking for viral presence during the 3rd, 6th, 9th and 12th days after starting the treatment. HSV-IgA serum levels were measured before and at the 21st and 42nd days post-treatment. In treated patients at the 3rd and at the 6th day, the virus was present, respectively, in 29 out of 128 and in five out of 128 swabs or scrapings, whereas in untreated controls corresponding figures were 21 out of 24 and 15 out of 24. During the 9th day all treated patients were virus-free whereas eight out of 24 untreated controls were positive (Table 12).

Also the healing time of mucocutaneous lesions, when they were present before therapy, was significantly shortened in treated patients (average of 5 ± 2 days) when compared to controls (average of 9 ± 5 days). As far as IgA serum levels on day 21 post-therapy are concerned, three different groups of women were identified:

The first (74 out of 128) in which post-treatment titers were lower than pretreatment ones;

The second (46 out of 128) in which pre- and post-treatment titers were similar;

The third (eight out of 128) in which post-treatment titers were higher than pretreatment ones.

During the 42nd day, 121 out of 128 patients had stable titers equal to those on the 21st day. Only seven patients showed decreasing titers. It is important to stress that these seven patients include six of the eight subjects with increasing titers on the 21st day.

Furthermore, when the threshold value of one of 128 is considered, it is clear that before therapy only 23 out of 128 patients had normal values whereas on the 21st and 42nd day after treatment, the corresponding figures were 86 out of 128 and 93 out of 128 respectively (Table 13).

The same was evident in partners (Table 14).

Table 12 Effectiveness of Acyclovir therapy

		Day after starting treatment			
		3rd	*6th*	*9th*	*12th*
Symptomatic treated	(104)	25	4	—	—
	Per cent	24.03	3.84	—	—
Asymptomatic treated	(24)	4	1	—	—
	Per cent	16.66	4.16	—	—
Controls	(24)	21	15	8	4
	Per cent	87.50	62.50	33.33	16.66

Table 13 Response of IgA levels to therapy

Dilution		*1/32*	*1/64*	*1/128*	*1/256*	*1/512*
Pretreatment		—	4	19	63	42
	Per cent	—	3.12	14.84	49.21	32.81
21st day		19	36	31	23	19
	Per cent	14.84	28.12	24.21	17.96	14.84
42nd day		22	40	31	22	13
	Per cent	18.75	43.75	15.62	11.71	10.05

Table 14 Response of IgA levels to therapy in partners

Dilution		*1/32*	*1/64*	*1/128*	*1/256*	*1/512*
Pretreatment		—	—	4	16	7
	Per cent	—	—	14.81	59.25	25.92
21st day		4	5	9	7	2
	Per cent	14.81	18.51	33.33	25.92	7.40
42nd day		4	7	8	6	2
	Per cent	14.81	25.92	29.62	22.22	7.40

CONCLUSIONS

The salient features of this study are the following observations. Current seropositivity rate is certainly higher than in the past and among individuals in the medium–high social classes, seropositivity generally does not differ from that of lower classes. There is a relevant proportion of genital infections due to HSV1 that relates to major changes in sexual behavior of younger subjects. Asymptomatic subjects can shed infectious virus (HSV2 or HSV1 or both). There is a good correlation between virus shedding and increased titers of HSV-specific serum IgA antibodies. This particular Ig class may indeed be considered as a marker of active virus replication in the genital tract[12] and therefore, it can be useful in detecting asymptomatic shedders, in confirming clinical diagnosis as well as in monitoring the effectiveness of treatment. Sexual partners of infected women are generally infected with a surprisingly high rate of urogenital subclinical colonization. Accordingly, we recommend a policy of routine 'couple-treatment' instead of single-patient treatment in order to avoid reinfection by an asymptomatic, infected and untreated sexual partner[13,14]. Intravenous Acyclovir therapy reduces virus shedding in both symptomatic and asymptomatic individuals with a relevant shortening of healing time and with a decrease in severity of disease, without any significant side-effects or toxicity.

ACKNOWLEDGMENT

It is a pleasure for the authors to acknowledge the fundamental importance of the support received from Sigma-Tau Pharmaceutical Co., during the preparation of this study.

REFERENCES

1. Genital Herpes Infection – United States, 1966–1979. *Morbidity and Mortality Weekly Report* 1982, **31**, 137–9
2. Rawls, W.E. and Gardner, H.L. (1972). Herpes genitalis: venereal aspects. *Clin. Obstet. Gynecol.*, **15**, 912–18
3. Nahmias, A.J., Josey, W.E. and Naib, Z.H. (1970). Antibodies to herpesvirus hominis types 1 and 2 in humans. *Am. J. Epidemiol.*, **91**, 539–46
4. Duenas, A., Adam, E. and Melnick, J.L. (1972). Herpesvirus type 2 in a prostitute population. *Am. J. Epidemiol.*, **95**, 583–90
5. Rawls, W.E., Gardner, H.L. and Flunders, R.W. (1971). Genital herpes in two social groups. *Am. J. Obstet. Gynecol.*, **110**, 682–7
6. Brooks, S.L., Rowe, N.H. and Drach, J.C. (1981). Prevalence of herpes simplex virus in a professional population. *J. Am. Dent. Assoc.*, **102**, 31–6
7. Kleger, B. and Prier, J.E. (1969). Herpes simplex infection of the female genital tract. II. Association of cytopathic effect in cell culture with site of infection. *J. Infect. Dis.*, **120**, 376–8
8. Mccaughtry, M.G., Fleagle, G.S. and Docherty, J.J. (1982). Inapparent genital herpes simplex virus infection in college women. *J. Med. Virol.*, **10**, 283–90
9. Josey, W.E., Nahmias, A.J. and Naib, Z.M. (1972). The epidemiology of type 2 (genital) herpes simplex infections. *Obstet. Gynecol. Surv.*, **27**, 295–302
10. Aurelian, L. and Kessler, I.I. (1985). Subclinical herpesvirus infections of the genital tract are commonly associated with viral shedding. *The Cervix & l.f.g.t.*, **3**, 235–48
11. Corey, L. and Holmes, H.K. (1983). Genital herpes simplex virus infection: current concepts in diagnosis, therapy and prevention. *Ann. Intern. Med.*, **98**, 973–82
12. Corbino, N., Guglielmino, S., Moschetti, P., Cianci, A. and Garozzo, A. (1986). Le IgA sieriche come possible marker di infezione herpetica. In Danesino, V. and Rondanelli, G. (eds). *Le Infezioni in Ostetricia e Ginecologia* pp. 38–41. (Roma: Monduzzi Editore)
13. Corbino, N. and Guglielmino, S. (1986). L'Acyclovir per via intravenosa nel trattamento di coppia dell'herpes genitalis. *Quad. Clin. Ostet. Ginecol.*, **41**, 93–106
14. Corbino, N., Guglielmino, S., Ciravolo, L. and Tempera, G. (1987). Therapeutical effects of intravenous Acyclovir administration in patients affected with genital herpes. *Chemioterapia*, **6**, suppl. 2, 667–70

37

Colposcopic and microcolpohysteroscopic diagnosis of viriasis

S. Dexeus, M. Montesinos, D. Jakob and R. Rubio

GENERAL CHARACTERISTICS OF HUMAN PAPILLOMA-VIRUS (HPV)

Papillomavirus belongs to the *papovaviridae* family in which polio virus is included and to which it is closely related.

Human papillomavirus is a specific DNA virus. The biology and behavior of HPV is not well-known. It induces epithelial proliferation, characterized by hyperkeratosis and hyperplasia. HPV replication is related to maturation of the squamous eptihelium. The virus requires mature cells for duplication which makes culture studies difficult.

CANCER RELATIONSHIP

There is a large variety of HPVs. During the last years, 20 new types have been described and more than 48 HPVs had been discovered up to October. Approximately 12 of these affect the genital tract (types 6, 11, 16, 18, 31, 35, 39 and 44).

In Table 1, the viruses of known clinical manifestations are specified. Their relationship to cancer was suspected years ago. Therefore, it was no surprise that Dürst *et al.*[1] found HPV DNA in different female genital tract neoplasms. Up to date, types 16, 18, 31 and 33 accounted for 85% of HPV found in cervical carcinomas[2]. Other authors[3] believe that types 35, 39 and 42 also have oncogenic capacity.

Zurhausen[4] believes that the HPV carcinogenic action is provoked by the production of cellular clones capable of initiating the process under the action of other carcinogens or mutants. At a molecular level, the HPV oncogenic action develops due to the failure of the proliferative host cells to control the presence of viral genomes producing an imbalance in the viral transcription.

In summary, all these theories point to a multifactorial etiology of the low genital tract neoplasm (GTN). The HPV infection could be a cervical intraepithelial neoplasm (CIN) and cancer precursor. However, both are

Table 1 HPV types and associated clinical presentation

Type	*Clinical presentation*
1	Plantar and palmar warts
2	Common warts
3	Juvenile flat warts
4	Plantar and common warts
5	EV
6	Genital condyloma, laryngeal papilloma (GTN)
7	Butcher's wart
8,9	EV
10	Juvenile flat wart, EV
11	Genital condyloma, laryngeal papilloma (GTN)
12	EV
13	Oral focal epithelial hyperplasia (Heck's disease)
14,15	EV
16	GTN, Bowenoid papulosis (genital condyloma)
17	EV
18	GTN (Genital condyloma)
19–25	EV
26–29	Immunosuppressed host, EV
30	Immunosuppressed host, laryngeal carcinoma+
31	GTN
32	Oral focal epithelial hyperplasia (Heck's disease)
33	GTN, bowenoid papulosis
34	Premalignant squamous lesions of skin (actinic keratosis Bowen's disease), Bowenoid papulosis
35	GTN
36	EV, premalignant squamous lesions of skin (actinic keratosis, Bowen's disease, keratoacanthoma)
37	Keratoacanthoma
38	Malignant melanoma+
39	Cutaneous squamous lesions (GTN)
40	Laryngeal carcinoma
41	Juvenile flat wart
42	GTN

EV, epidermodysplasia verruciformis; GTN, genital tract neoplasms

known to coexist and quite frequently a colposcopist detects HPV lesions close to CIN-type lesions.

Taking into account that not all gynecological services are capable of diagnosing HPV infection and identification of the type through hybridization techniques, it is important that the colpo- and microcolpohysteroscopists know how to individualize the images compatible with HPV.

CLINIC

Usually, HPV infection does not show any clinical manifestation. However, some patients complain of vulvodynia and/or dyspareunia in some vulvar and vaginal locations. Smelly leucorrhea and burning sensation, signs of overinfection depending on the type of vaginitis, may appear in condylomatosis.

DIAGNOSIS

The most common indication for colposcopic exploration is alteration compatible with HPV in cytological smears. Seventy to 75% of abnormal cytologies show only HPV[5]. Forty per cent of CIN are associated with HPV.

COLPOSCOPY

Two forms of HPV can be diagnosed through colposcopy: exophitic form; flat form.

Among the exophitic forms, we must consider the folowing: (a) acuminate condyloma, sometimes called macropapillar; (b) spiked or papillar condyloma, and (c) extended condylomatous forms or micropapillar.

Acuminate or macropapillar condylomas appear as a necrotic white formation with digitations. Vascularization is difficult to observe when there is an important keratinization. In general, they are multiple and easy to detect by the naked eye (Figure 1). Spiked papillar forms show irregularities and asperities in the surface of lesion whitened with acetic acid (acidophilic). The end of a capillary can be observed in papillas. Micropapillar condyloma or condylomatosed cervicovaginitis[6] is characterized by extensive lesions on the irregular surface, showing spikes or asperites on a surface without other pathology. It is usually associated to other HPV manifestations but sometimes it is the only lesion. Flat forms are acidophilic without surface anomalies.

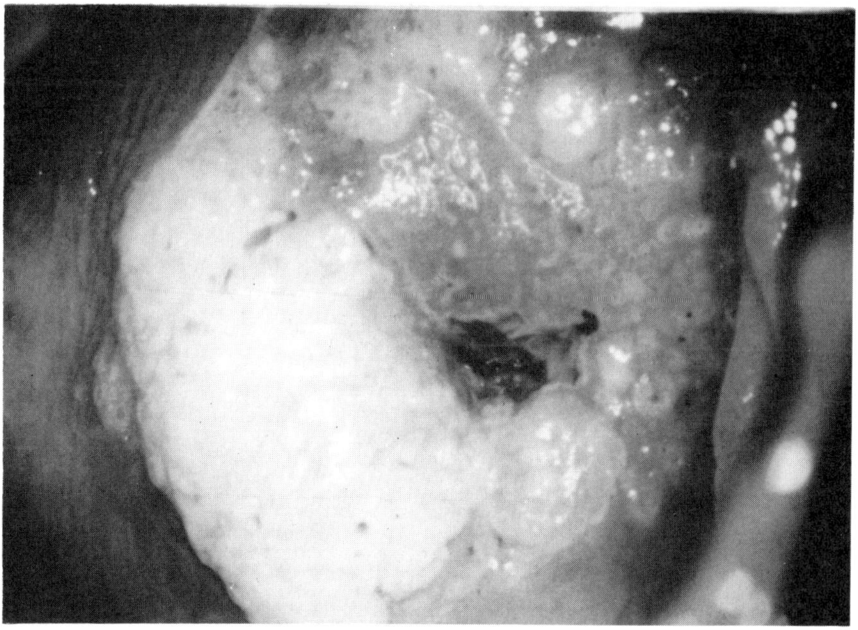

Figure 1

they can show mosaic or base images. When they are located in the transformation zone, they are difficult to distinguish from CIN, therefore guided biopsy is required. If flat forms appear in exocervix outside the transformation zone, they are generally benign. However, flat forms in the vagina usually show severe atypia (intraepithelial vaginal neoplasia).

Other colposcopic signs may be associated with HPV infection. Limited hyperkeratosis which is visible, without preparation, under white spots aspect. They change slightly with acetic acid but Lugol's iodine makes them clear (Figure 2). Cerebroid pattern, according to Bouchard, confirms CIN.

DIFFERENTIAL COLPOSCOPIC DIAGNOSIS

Differential diagnosis of HPV infection should be established with: ectopia; atypical transformation zone without virus infection; invasive neoplasia; polyps; granulomas; and vaginal neoplasic recurrences.

Papillar condyloma and ectopia are clearly distinguished by colposcopy. Pure ectopia is not frequent but it is usually associated with the transformation zone at the metaplastic process, (a not frequently observed coexistence in condyloma). Vascularization of papillar condyloma is different from ectopia. In the former, in each of its papillar elements a capillar which is similar to each papilla runs through. On the other hand, the ectopic spots have no special vascularization. Condylomatose lesions are usually raised, sometimes as a platform, from the rest of the epithelium. However, if ectopia is associated

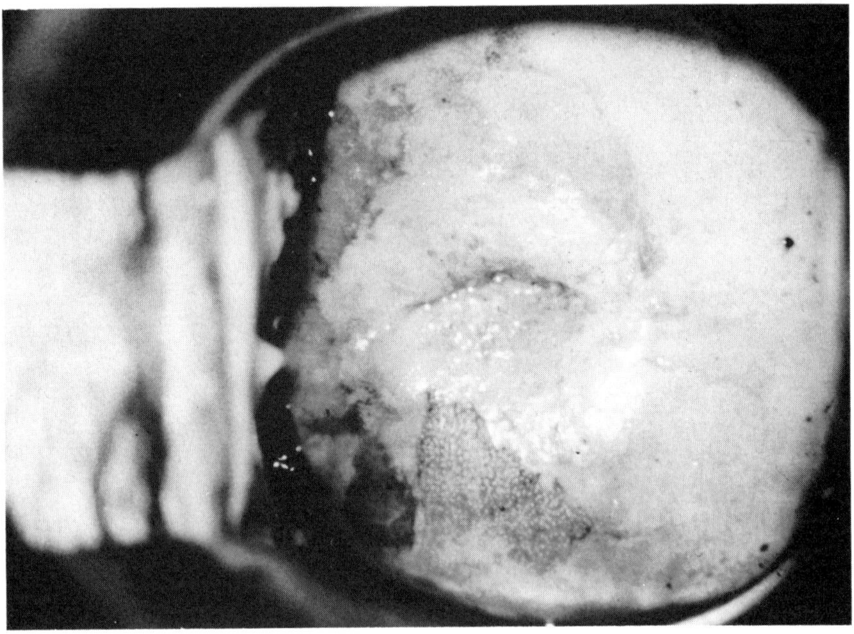

Figure 2

with infection or deciduosis it obtains a greater visual intensity and more diffuse character. To be able to make a good differential diagnosis, the application of Lugol's iodine is very important. Lugol's iodine on condyloma will give a weak fixation and no fixation at all on ectopia.

It is difficult if not impossible to diagnose the viral origin of a concrete atypical transformation zone through colposcopy. Irregularities of mosaic forms, the presence of wide spaces between its brick-shape or early keratosis, very clear in any of the atypical images, can *only* signal a diagnosis of viral etiology. On other occasions, there is an apparent absence of viral signs. After application of Lugol's it is heterogeneously fixed by the suspected atypical transformation zone. Therefore, the colpocopist will be able to consider the possibility of a viral lesion. Incipient metaplasia, due to thin tissue showing the sinuosities of subjacent chorion, can also confuse the diagnosis (Figure 3).

Some exophitic papillar carcinomas look like viral lesions of similar configuration. The atypical vascularization, even though of small significance, is specific enough to allow differential diagnosis: abnormal vessels, weak, tortuous vessels with irregular ramifications, have nothing to do with the vascular uniformity of viral lesions. In this situation, Schiller's test can help to distinguish between the two lesions by showing a negative result when there is cancerous tumoration and a weak positive result for viral papillomatose lesion.

Viral growths, polyps and vaginal granulomas are not difficult to distinguish. The colposcopic vision of polyps shows their epithelialized surface

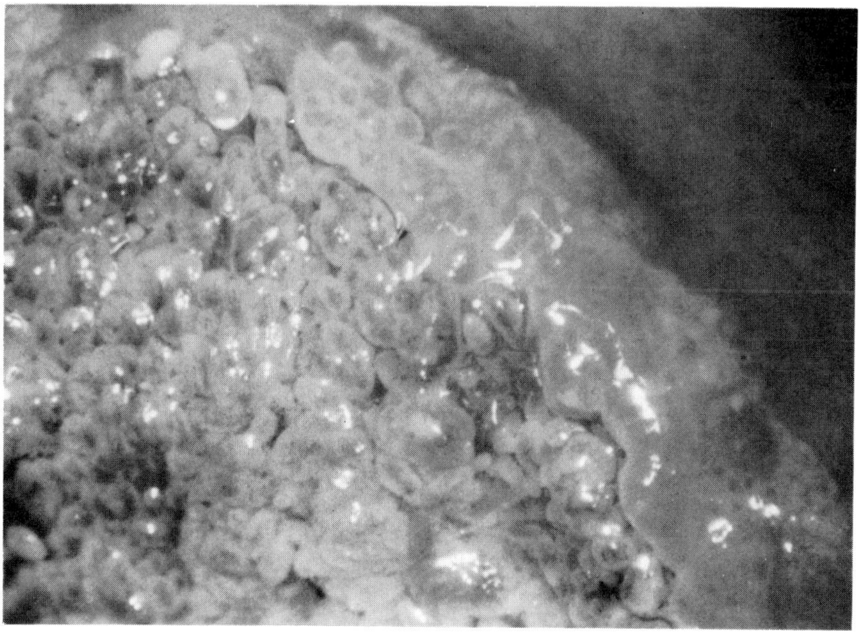

Figure 3

or columnar nature but never characteristics of HPV. Only the polyp's infection, necrosis or deciduosis provoke alterations in its structure thus changing its image and making it much more difficult to recognize.

Vaginal granulomas originating on a hysterectomy scar or episiorraphias are easily recognizable (Figure 4). The granuloma is a fragile formation which bleeds on minimal contact. The bleeding makes proper colposcopic observation difficult, sometimes confusing the untrained explorer. Recurrences of vaginal neoplasia adopt a micropapillar structure similar to viral growth. Vascular irregularities, weakness and wide extension help to establish a correct diagnois.

MCH AND VIRIASIS

Since HPV infection is related to sexual transmission and oncogenic role of CIN appearance[7], HPV detection is necessary to obtain a wide epidemiological knowledge and principally, to prevent cervical carcinoma.

Some authors[8,9] believe that only 12–18% of patients with viral infection by HPV develop CIN. However, MCH study, able to locate nucleocytoplasmatic alterations and direct the biopsy, shows that CIN incidence is higher than expected[10]. Furthermore, some authors[11] think that CIN recurrence and persistence are only due to intraepithelial neoplasias associated with viral infection. The images shown by these lesions in MCH observations are various.

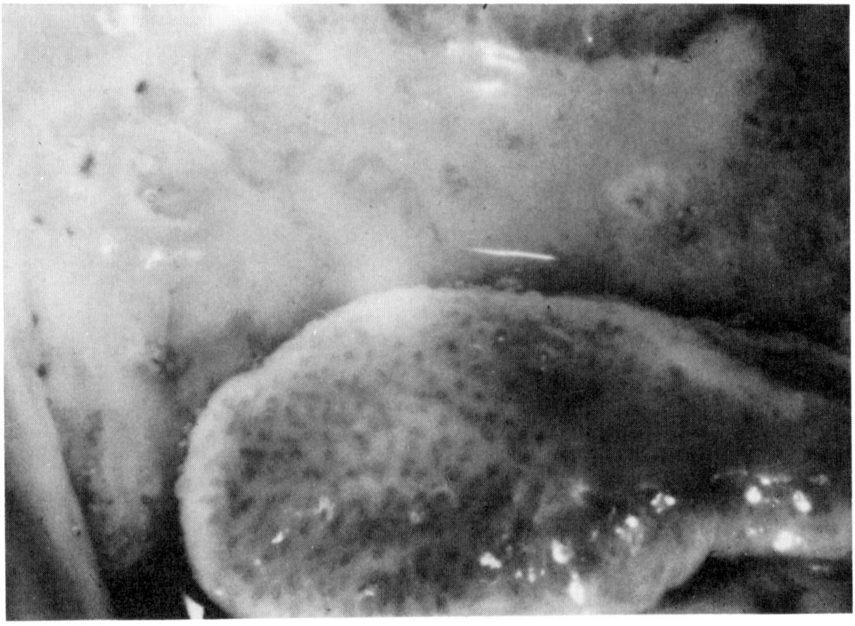

Figure 4

Superficial keratosis

Superficial keratoses are areas which weakly and heterogeneously absorb vital coloring with Lugol's iodine prevalence. In these areas, silent areas or white–yellow color spaces made up of anucleated scales, some detached folded cells or groups of them which absorb intensively Waterman Blue and, more rarely well disposed superficial cells weakly absorbing dye, are observed. All these gives a 'dirty' impression. These areas have a poorly defined limit with surrounding epithelium. Some leucoplasias or hyperkeratosis zones, especially the small ones and ones close to the transformation zone, can hide, in their inferior layers, dysplasic alterations which will be missed on first examination. It is convenient to separate this zone or explore its limits meticulously, restaining the underlying layers.

Koilocytosis

They usually appear in the distal limit of the transformation zone, close to mature epithelium, where they are found in larger concentrations.

Alterations of the cellular cytoplasm in papovavirus infection: perinuclear halo, strengthening of cytoplasmic limit, and vacuolization are better observed in this zone by MCH as this area is made up of superficial cells with enough cytoplasm to allow a correct nucleocytoplasmic contrast.

Nuclear alterations

Some nuclear alterations, especially the bi- or multinucleations, more frequently appear in zones built up of intermediate and deep cells, and they are more clearly seen in zones where there are internuclear spaces.

On the opposite side, the most obvious nuclear alterations are more remarkable in squamocylindrical junctions where the cells are more immature and there is more nuclear concentration allowing better contrast between the different types of nucleus. An obvious nuclear pleomorphism exists, from the big clear nucleus, of irregular limits, and sometimes lobulated to the shrunk and picnotic ones, all with strengthening of the cytoplasmic limit. Comparison between them and especially with the normal adjacent squamous tissue makes the diagnosis easier. Some HPV infections provoke hypertrophic (some giants), hyperchromatic and irregular nuclei. Hamou[12] qualified them as grotesque for being similar to the ones produced in carcinoma *in situ*. Differential diagnosis is established when the lowest nuclear concentration, diameter and regular distribution of these nuclei, and cytoplasmic conservation in the cells, is verified.

Spiral distribution

They probably correspond to the first phase of the papillar condyloma in which superficial cells, preferentially iodine negative, are arranged in a spiral shape, forming the base of future papillas[13] (Figure 5). They are difficult to observe because of the pressure or optical system within these cells, which breaks the spiral configuration. This is the reason for finding them at the beginning of the exploration.

Micropapillar condylomas

They appear as small, spiked digits of a more intense blue color than the surrounding epithelium because they are covered with iodine negative squamous cells. Some of these spikes show a white halo in their base because the dye has not been absorbed in the base. They are mobile, generally multiple and occasionally show the central vascular axis.

Papillar condyloma

They are made up of papillas covered with squamous iodine negative cells with few alterations (rarely associated to atypy) and a tortuous vessel in the center which runs along the papilla.

Vascular alterations

When micropapillar condyloma appear in the thickness of the cylindrical epithelium, very elongated dilated mobile vascular ansas are shown. They

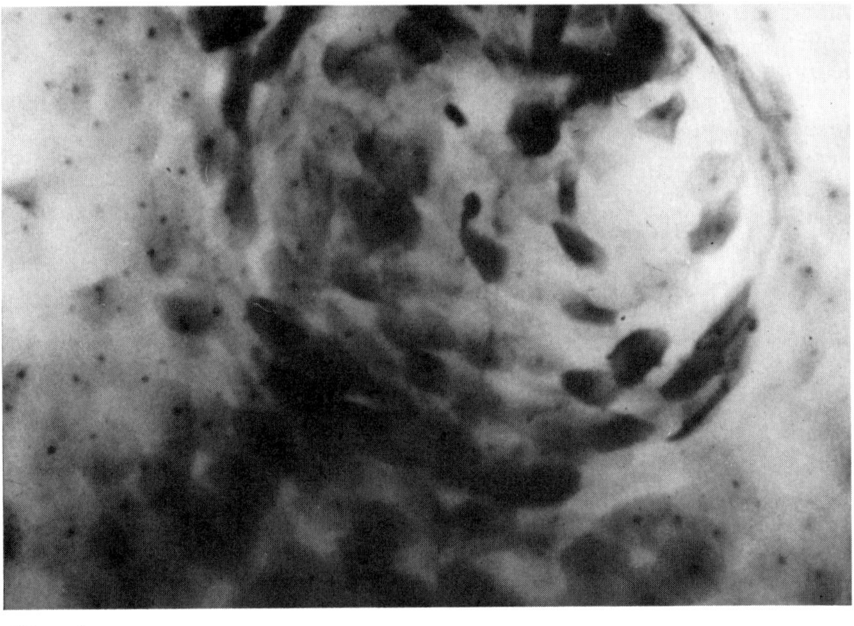

Figure 5

absorb Waterman Blue intensively and in contrast to papillar condyloma originate in metaplastic tissue they have a dilated rounded upper pole with a narrow base, adopting a match-like shape. They are not frequent and are located in specific zones.

Obviously, HPV infection diagnosis generally presents difficulties because, excepting clear lesions, it is possible that its subclinical manifestation is not detected by any of the habitual methods of cervical pathology study.

Out of 19 cervices affected only by ectopia, Toon *et al.*[14] found HPV-specific DNA in 14 cases. Possibly when hybridization techniques of HPV-specific DNA are more routinely performed, then another important diagnostic tecnique will be obtained. This involves the differentiation between HPV of low and high risk, helping to establish a correct treatment of the papillomavirus lesion.

Many characteristics of the HPV infection physiopathology are still unknown. Facing the recently increasing number of published studies in the universal bibliography, describing vulvar and vaginal lesions of HPV, it should be pointed out that HPV infection is a generalized disease and located manifestations may represent the failure in a very limited area of self-defence capacity of the organism towards the virus. Therefore, the existence of subclinical disease is a highly probable hypothesis. That is the reason why Reid[15] pointed out that approximately 10% of cervical lesions without importance carry HPV 16, 18 and 31. In 160 cases the sensitivity of MCH reached 86% and the specificity 42%, giving the positive predictive value of 85% and the negative one of 45%.

CONCLUSIONS

Colpocopy and MCH are not competitive techniques in HPV diagnosis but complementary.

Colposcopy helps to diagnose exophytic condylomas. Flat and endophytic condylomas are better diagnosed by MCH.

MCH is a good method to diagnose HPV in patients previously selected (positive predictive value = 85%).

REFERENCES

1. Durst, M., Gissmann, L., Ikenberg, H. and Zur Hausen, H. (1983). A papillomavirus DNA from cervical carcinoma and its prevalence in cancer biopsy samples from different geographical regions. *Proc. Natl. Acad. Sci., USA*, **80**, 3812
2. Boshart, M., Gissmann, L., Ikenberg, H. *et al.* (1984). A new type of Papillomavirus DNA, its presence in genital cancer biopsies and in cell lines derived from cervical cancer. *EMBO J.*, **3**, 1151
3. Winkler, B. and Richart, R.M. (1987). Human papillomavirus and gynecologic neoplasia. *Cur. Prob. Obstet. Gynecol. Fertil.*, **10**, 51
4. Zur Hausen, H. Intracellular surveillance of persisting viral infections. *Lancet*, **2**, 489
5. Meisels, A., Morin, C. and Casas-Cordero, M. (1984). Lesions of the uterine cervix associated with papillomavirus and their clinical consequences. In Koss, L.G. and Coleman, D.V. (New York: Masson)

6. Roy, M., Fortier, M. and Meisels, A. (1979). Colposcopy of cervical condyloma acuminatum. *Obstet. Gynecol. Survey*, **34**, 853
7. Syrjänen, K.J. (1981). Cytologic evidence of the association of condylomatous lesions with dysplastic and neoplastic changes in the uterine cervix. *Acta Cytol.*, **25**, 17
8. Syrjänen, K.J. and Syrjänen, S.M. (1985). Human papillomavirus infections related to cervical intraepithelial neoplasia and squamous cell carcinoma to the uterine cervix. *Am. Clin. Res.*, **17**, 45
9. Mitchell, H., Drake, M. and Medley, G. (1986). Prospective evaluation of risk of cervical cancer after cytological evidence of human papillomavirus infection. *The Lancet*, **1** 573
10. Labastida, R. and Cararach, M. (1987). Comunicación personal. I Curso Patologia Cervical. Instituto Dexeus. Barcelona
11. Sjöstedt, L. (1987). What is the significance of koilocytosis in cervical intra-epithelial neoplasia? *Acta Obstet. Gynecol. Scand.*, **66**, 41
12. Hamou, J. (1986). De la colposcopie et la microcolpohystéroscopie. *Gyn. Obstét.*, **92**, 1118
13. Montevechi, L. and Vechione, A. (1986). Microcolpohysteroscopic features of cervical condilomatosis and the accuracy in detecting subclinical papillomavirus infection. *The Cervix and L.f.g.t.*, **4**, 225
14. Toon, P.G., Arrand, J.R., Wilson, L.P. *et al.* (1987). Infección del cuello uterino por el papilomavirus humano en mujeres sin signos citológicos de neoplasia. *British M. Journal* (Ed. Espanola), **11**, 38
15. Reid, R. (1987). Understanding HPV infection: The key to rational triage. *Colposcopy and Gynecologic laser surgery*, **3**, 37

Section 2 continued

Part B

Chlamydiae infections

38

Diagnostic problems in *Chlamydia trachomatis* genital infections

A. Cianci, G. Palumbo and G. Nicoletti

Chlamydia trachomatis has recently been recognized as the most common 'sexually transmitted disease' (STD) agent and its increasing incidence in genital infection is becoming a major problem in the reproductive life of the young population.

The rate of *Chlamydia* positivity is highly age-correlated. Thus in younger age groups, up to one-third will experience one or more such infections during their life-time.

The clinical manifestations in women include mucopurulent cervicitis, acute urethral syndrome, pelvic inflammatory disease (PID) (endometritis, salpingitis, tubo-ovarian abcess, perihepatitis), postpartum endometritis, adverse pregnancy outcome (premature rupture of membranes, preterm delivery), tubal pregnancy, tubal infertility and cellular atypia of cervical epithelium.

Pelvic inflammatory disease is the most serious complication of bacterial lower genital tract infections; plasma cell endometritis represents an intermediate stage of infection between cervicitis and frank salpingitis. The increase in the incidence of PID seems to be associated with the epidemic situation of STD, that has prevailed during the last 2 decades.

Most cases are caused by an infection ascending from the cervix, colonized by organisms known to be spread by sexual intercourse.

Actually, low genital tract infections, very common in sexually active young women, represent the first stage of *C.trachomatis* infection. The microorganism can remain in the cervix for some years before infection spreads to the pelvis, leading to a salpingitis, with its inherent risk of permanent sterility.

Apart from that, tubal infection can occur as 'hospital' and 'iathrogenic' infections, after surgery or diagnostic/therapeutic procedures (curettage, insertion of an intrauterine device).

In this 'non-venereal' type of salpingitis, the infection of the Fallopian tubes generally seems to stem from an endogenous infection, caused by bacteria of the indigenous flora of the lower genital tract.

A variety of organisms alone or in combination produce salpingitis, but *Neisserria gonorrhoeae* and *C.trachomatis* are the most common initial invaders. *N.gonorrhoeae* attaches to tubal epithelium and causes a rapid influx of leucocytes and tubal swelling, which commonly results in the acute onset of peritoneal signs.

In contrast, *C.trachomatis* usually produces only symptoms and signs without peritonitis, which is related perhaps to a long replication time of the organism and protection of the organism within tubal cells from immune mechanisms.

Special mention should be made of the two- to fivefold increased risk of salpingitis among women who wear an intrauterine device (IUD). There is evidence that the cervico-vaginal flora ascend along the tail to colonize the lower part of the uterus.

In contrast, lower than expected rates of salpingitis have been found among users of oral contraceptives. These steroids may cause changes in the cervical mucus that prevent bacterial penetration. Thus, oral contraceptives form a particularly attractive choice of contraception among teenagers, who have the highest rate of salpingitis.

The sequelae of these genital infections (tubal pregnancy and infertility) are a rapidly increasing problem in most European countries, reflecting the endemic nature of genital *C.trachomatis* infections. Following an acute episode of salpingitis, 25% of women develop recurrent infection and recurrent salpingitis leads to high rates of infertility[1]. Infertility is one of the most common and dreaded consequences of salpingitis occurring in 10% of women following a single episode and 25% of women following two episodes of infection[1]. Even newer antibiotic regimens have not influenced this infertility rate.

Ectopic pregnancy is seven times more common among women who have had salpingitis than among those who have not.

About 5% of women who become pregnant following an episode of salpingitis will have an ectopic pregnancy. Chronic abdominal pain occurs in about 15% of women following salpingitis[2].

The inability of clinicians to make an accurate diagnosis of salpingitis remains the major obstacle in the treatment of this infection. Frequent false-negative and false-positive errors in clinical diagnosis are made. It is well-known that it is not possible to observe or to culture the Fallopian tubes except by laparoscopy or laparotomy. So, laparoscopy is the best means to establish an accurate diagnosis. However, laparoscopy requires hospitalization and general anesthesia, and is costly. The accuracy of diagnosis using laparoscopy has to be weighed against the disadvantages of a frequent error in the clinical diagnosis.

In a large study of consecutive women laparoscoped because of suspected salpingitis, the clinical diagnosis was confirmed in only 65% of women; 12% of women had other abnormalities that appeared as salpingitis, including ectopic pregnancy, appendicitis, ovarian cysts and endometriosis; and 23% of women had a normal laparoscopic examination[3].

This study demonstrated the difficulty of establishing a diagnosis of salpingitis by clinical criteria, because of the tremendous range of symptoms and physical signs among women and the overlap of symptoms caused by salpingitis and other diseases.

In addition, up to 50% of women with salpingitis have symptoms that are so mild, that they are not diagnosed and treated.

Among women who do present with symptoms, there is a very limited correlation between severity of symptoms and severity of tubal damage. The textbook example of a patient with salpingitis having moderate physical findings, a fever, and leukocytosis occurs in only about 20% of women with laparoscopically verified salpingitis[4]. In fact, only one third of women with salpingitis have a temperature of more than 38°C[3]. Because of the limited accuracy of a clinical diagnosis based on symptoms and physical signs, physicians have often relied heavily on laboratory data to assist in the diagnostic process. Unfortunately, the white blood cell count is abnormal in only 45% of women and the sedimentation rate is elevated in only 75% of women with laparoscopically confirmed salpingitis[3].

Ultrasonographic techniques are at present too insensitive to detect mild tubal infection.

Because the infection ascends through the uterus from cervical source *en route* to the Fallopian tube, the use of endometrial biopsy is being explored to diagnose endometritis.

If all patients with salpingitis have detectable endometritis, endometrial biopsy could be used to diagnose uterine infection in symptomatic women. However, the proportion of symptomatic women with endometritis who have salpingitis will first have to be confirmed by laparoscopy to assess the accuracy of this method.

Until newer diagnostic techniques are further refined, the physicians can utilize a practical method of diagnosis. Women with moderate or severe clinical findings should be treated for presumed salpingitis. Women with mild manifestations, in whom the diagnosis is unclear, should be laparoscoped if there is the possibility of appendicitis or ectopic pregnancy. Patients who fail to have a clinical response to therapy should be laparoscoped.

Finally, laparoscopy should be utilized more widely to establish a diagnosis among women with acute abdominal pain because some of these women, who by clinical criteria are diagnosed as having ovarian cysts and endometriosis, actually have salpingitis.

In conclusion, clinical diagnosis of PID appears very difficult to perform because of a lack of specific symptoms. For this reason we think that clinical diagnosis should be confirmed by celioscopy which reveals tubal occlusion and more or less widespread adherences.

As regards microbiological diagnosis, we must underline that the choice of both microbiological test and pathological sample are very important to avoid false negative results which could cause great problems such as wrong therapy and *C.trachomatis* persistence. Endocervical swab is the correct sampling procedure in cervicitis, but when the infection has already reached the upper genital tract, it is possible to draw directly a pathological sample for microbiological diagnosis without vaginal flora contamination, only by celioscopy.

REFERENCES

1. Westrom, L. (1975). Effect of acute pelvic inflammatory disease on fertility. *Am. J. Obstet. Gynecol.*, **121**, 707–13
2. Westrom, L., Josif, S. and Svensson, L. (1979). Infertility after acute salpingitis: Results of treatment with different antibiotics. *Curr. Ther. Res.*, **26** 752–9
3. Jacobson, L. and Westrom, L. (1969). Objectived diagnosis of acute pelvic inflammatory disease: Diagnostic and prognostic value of routine laparoscopy. *Am. J. Obstet. Gynecol.*, **105**, 1088–98
4. Westrom, L. (1980). Incidence, prevalence and trends of acute pelvic inflammatory disease and its consequences in industrialized countries. *Am. J. Obstet. Gynecol.*, **138**, 880–92

39

Chlamydia trachomatis and infertility

G. De Placido, N. Colacurci, F. Zullo, A. Nazzaro, G. Portella and R. Magliulo

Female genital tract infections are more and more frequent and our data lead us to consider this phenomenon as an epidemic. It is very interesting that, at the same time, there is a decrease, on the whole, of infectious disease. At the moment sexually transmitted diseases (STDs) are exceeded only by respiratory viral infections. During the years we have seen a 'shift' of pathogenic agents of STDs and now the possible agents are over 20. A serious problem, besides the large diffusion, is the modification of the clinical course which is very often completely asymptomatic. We have frequently to treat just the long-term consequences of STDs rather than an acute event. The new generation, greatly at risk of STD, are the most involved in the diffusion of the disease by means of, as it has been said, 'tender loving care'. A terrific prospective evaluation comes from Weström[1] who calculated that in the year 2000 90% of women, which in 1970 were 19, will have developed an STD and 20% of these women will be infertile.

The STD is essentially an infection starting at the uterine cervix and tending to spread with a rising movement to the endometrium, to the tubes and to the pelvic peritoneum. The women who have had one or more events of STD have a real risk of infertility of 20%; likewise the extrauterine pregnancies, likely determined by tubal damage, appear with an incidence which is from 6 to 10 times higher than that of non-affected women[2,3].

The etiological agent which appears as the most important cause of infertility is *Chlamydia trachomatis*, whose incidence is increasing with a positive trend to decreasing age (60% <20 years). The pathology of *C.trachomatis* often shows more serious long-term consequences as its trend to run in an asymptomatic way, leads to a lack of treatment. Since *C.trachomatis* infections are not included among the diseases that have to be reported, its real incidence will always be underestimated. Also the different means of sample collection seem to have a great importance. Mardh and Punnonen[4], found an association between *C.trachomatis* and STD in 67% of cases, while Sweet[5] in the USA found it only in 25–40% of cases. The Swedish authors[6] made multiple biopsies in the involved areas, while the American authors used only a tubal sample picked up by aspiration. The infertility caused by *C.trachomatis* can be caused by a modification of the immune system, of cervical mucus and of endometrium and salpingis. The cellular cycle and the damage caused in the host cells by *C.trachomatis* leads to consideration of the involvement of the host's immune system in the development of a *C.trachomatis* STD. It is well-known that the elemental bodies are able to modify the surface characteristics of infected cells, and the defence mechanism of the host. The humoral immune response, during a *C.trachomatis* infection can appear as a polyclonal expansion of B-lymphocytes with plasmacellular infiltration and local immunoglobulin (Ig) synthesis[7]. To verify the efferent cell-mediated arm of immune response during a *C.trachomatis* infection is more difficult. If the T lymphocyte were present in the lesions, their presence would result in either an advantageous or deleterious effect on the host. The infected epithelial cells could be the target of lymphotoxins. The macrophage migration inhibition and the induction of their proliferation by lymphokines could make macrophages, locally available, possible hosts or victims or 'killers' of parasites.

The activation of macrophages could cause a recovery of the infection by the production of enzymes in the phagolysosomes. In this case, some of the antigenic material, could remain and continue to stimulate the immune system even after all the *C.trachomatis* has been killed[8]. It is possible that an immune response to a *C.trachomatis* infection could both have protective effects and cause damage. Furthermore an immune response could cause massive destruction of infected cells, and at the same time, could show autologous antigens able to prime an autoimmune response[9]. Further activation of the immune response can cause irreparable damage especially when the course of tissue repair results in a fibrous obstruction, that seems to be caused by interleukin 1 (IL-1) production during immune system activation. In our experience the cell mediated response shows several variations in the antigenic surface expression in women affected by *C.trachomatis* with an increase of the positive T lymphocytes (T8) and of activated lymphocytes (Ia positive)[10]. The presence of the Ia positive lymphocytes can cause pathological modifications which may be found both at cervical and seminal side. At seminal side an inflammation caused by *C.trachomatis* appears able to activate an autoimmune anti-nemaspermic response, with the production of anti-spermatozoa antibodies[11]. The mechanisms which show the possible relationship between *C.trachomatis* infection and Ab anti-nemaspermic includes:

(1) The epididimitis with monolateral obstruction;
(2) The appearance of nemasperms to immune cells in the urethra after a course of an acute urethritis;
(3) The *C.trachomatis* can be a marker of another STD, which would be due to production of the antisperm antibodies.

The subclinical epididimitis caused by *C.trachomatis* can bring out a monolateral epididimal obstruction involving an increased phagocytosis of the trapped spermatozoa and production of antisperm antibodies in over 80% of affected patients[11]. The leucocytes in the infection site can be phagocytic to the spermatozoa and take the sperm antigens in to the lymphatic system. The contacts between sperm and blood can bring out an activation of the complement with a following chemotaxis of leucocytes by

C3a[12]: this could increase in turn the production of antisperm antibodies. Some authors have shown a relation between the presence of antisperm antibody and the fertilizing capacity of spermatozoa titer of > 1:32[11]. How the *C.trachomatis* targets different anatomical sites from this biological primary site, (the glandular epithelial cell of the uterine cervix), is still an unsolved problem, even if the spermatozoa seem to be responsible. Hausen and Mardh have shown that *in vitro* at acid pH the *C.trachomatis* are able to bind to the spermatozoa with the possibility of transport along the female genital tract[13]. The most important infection sites for *C.trachomatis* are the uterine cervix and the tubal epithelium. In the uterine cervix the presence of inflammation caused by *C.trachomatis* can result in a quantitative and/or qualitative modification of the rheologic characteristics of the mucus that can become detrimental for a normal fertilizing course. The modification of pH of the molecular structure of the mucus, the presence of an inflammatory infiltrate and the presence of Ig, can inhibit normal gamete transfer. The possibility that the spermatozoa can act as 'preferential' vehicles of *C.trachomatis* has not yet been demonstrated *in vivo* The diagnostic problem regarding cervicitis by *C.trachomatis* is caused by the complete lack of symptoms and the most *frequent* colposcopic picture show an aspecific appearance of pseudopapillar ectropion with possible mucopurulent secretions. The picture of poor cervical mucus, with the production of the cervical mucus considerably reduced with a negative postcoital test (PCT) appears more frequently, even if some authors deny a negative interference between the *C.trachomatis* infection and PCT. The possibility that *C.trachomatis* infections could be misinterpreted necessitates infective screening tests. In the first diagnostic cycle, in both partners researching specifically *C.trachomatis* by immunofluorescence identification (IFI), even in cases which are asymptomatic, with a negative PCT or in presence of the sperm agglutination. When the *C.trachomatis* goes over the cervical filter it can easily spread to the tubes. The relation between *C.trachomatis* infections and infertility was clearly shown by a significant relationship between serum positivity anti-*C.trachomatis* and tubal factor infertility. This relation was also demonstrated by culture tests. Only one in three of these women were positive for pelvic inflammatory disease (PID) anamnesis. In the remaining cases the tubal damage appeared as a long-term consequence of an asymptomatic and non-treated infection.

In our experience 49% of women affected by tubal factor infertility diagnosed laparoscopically were *C.trachomatis* positive at the cervix and the tubal pathology was mainly distal (idrosalpingitis), further complicated by endopelvic large adhesions. In 25% of cases we found perihepatitis[14]. Since an infection caused by *C.trachomatis* can be misunderstood and therefore not treated, necessitates research into more reliable methods for diagnosis.

At the present time we are trying to get suitable samples of tubal fluid by hysteroscopic catheterism for *C.trachomatis* research by IFI. These samples are compared with those obtained by laparoscopy from the Douglas and Fallopian tubes. Furthermore, during hysteroscopy we get bioptic sample from endometrium. All patients in the study were examined for cervical *C.trachomatis.* Our data referred to 57 sterile women with pathological hysterosalpingography and they show a good relationship between endometrial and tubal *C.trachomatis* positivity with an incidence of cervical negative samples of 20% in cases of tubal positivity. Leaving out the variables caused by the technique, the trend of this micro-organism is to spread from the low female genital tract to the high one, with persistent infection also with a cervical negativization. The persistence of the infection at the cervix seems to be the cause of the higher incidence of tubal pregnancies in the *C.trachomatis* positive women. It is very interesting to notice the possibility that *C.trachomatis* infections could interfere with a normal fertilization and implantation by assisted reproductive techniques. The data about it are still few, but it seems that a *C.trachomatis* serum positivity does not reduce significantly the success rate of gamete intrafallopian transfer (GIFT) or an IVF. In a study of Torode[15] in 244 couples who underwent embryo-transfer or GIFT, 34 became pregnant. Forty-one per cent of these 34 couples were serum positive for *C.trachomatis* in comparison with the 38% for women who were not pregnant. Likewise an antibiotic treatment does not seem to interfere with the success rate of IVF-ET/GIFT, independently from *C.trachomatis* positivity or negativity. Also the fertilizing ability of spermatozoa from serum positive men does not appear to be lower than that of those men without antibodies. Yet the presence of anti-*C.trachomatis* antibodies is a sign of a previous exposure to the *C.trachomatis* and does not necessarily indicate the presence of an infection However it is possible that a cervicitis caused by *C.trachomatis* followed by a uterine infection can interfere with implantation thus lowering the pregnancy rate of IVF/GIFT. In these cases we have set up a therapy before using these techniques.

BIBLIOGRAPHY

1. Weström, L. (1980). *Am. J Obstet. Gynecol.*, **138**, 880
2. Svesson, L. *et al.* (1985). *Fertil. Steril.*, **44**, 313
3 Barnes, A.B. *et al.* (1983) *Obstet. Gynecol. Surv.*, **38**, 345
4. Mard, *et al.* (1987). *N. Engl. J. Med.*, **296** 1377–9
5 Sweet, R.L. (1980). *Am J. Obstet. Gynecol.*, **138**, 985
6. Grayston, J.T. *et al.* (1975). *J. Infect. Dis.*, **87**, 132
7. Schachter, J. (1978). *N. Engl. J. Med.*, **298**, 498
8. Wang, S.P. (1973). In Nichols, R.L. (ed.) *Trachoma and related disorders caused by chlamydial agents.* p. 217, (Amsterdam: Excerpta Medica)
9. Wakefield, D. *et al.* (1983). *Clin. Exp. Immunol.*, **51**, 191
10. De Placido, *et al.* In Danesino, V. (ed.) *II Congresso Interdisciplinare sulle Infezioni in Ginecologia.*
11. Close, C.E. *et al.* (1987). *Fertil. Steril.*, **48**, 880
12. Clark, R.A *et al.* (1976). *J. Immunol.*, **117**, 1378
13. Wallmer-Hanssen, P. and Mardh, P.A. (1984). *Fertil. Steril.*, **42**, 102
14. Mercorio, F. *et al.* In Danesino, V. (ed.) *I Congresso Interdisciplinare sulle Infezioni in Ostetricia e Ginecologia.*
15. Torode, H.W. *et al.* (1987). *J. In Vitro Fert. Embryo Transfer*, **4**, 148

40

Modern strategies in diagnosis of *Chlamydia trachomatis* genital infections

A. Cianci and G. Tempera

It is well-known that *Chlamydia trachomatis* genital infections involve many diagnostic problems and in both cervicitis and salpingitis, it is very important to establish etiological diagnosis in order to perform a rapid and specific therapy.

Only in this way is it possible to avoid disappointing sequelae, such as recurrent cervicitis, ectopic pregnancy, tubal occlusions, infertility, chronic abdominal pain, due to the persistence of *C.trachomatis.* Methods for diagnosing chlamydial infections are basically the same as those used for other bacteria and include: isolation of the organism, direct detection of the presence of specific antigen or specific antibodies.

ISOLATION

The most reliable method for detecting chlamydial infection is isolation using cycloheximide-treated McCoy cells.

The sensitivity of this procedure, being a reference test, is unknown, while the specificity is 100%. Nevertheless, cell culture techniques are laborious and therefore limit their use, i.e. it is compulsory to use a special transport medium (2 SP); the specimens must be kept refrigerated after collection and processed within 18 hours or they must be frozen soon after collection; swabs must be proven non-toxic to McCoy cells; negative specimens in the initial isolation attempt are often subjected to a blind passage. Finally, the method is time-consuming and expensive.

NON-CULTURE METHODS OF CHLAMYDIAL INFECTION

Recently two rapid immunological methods have been introduced to detect *C.trachomatis* directly from patient specimens. They are based either on immunofluorescence technique (IF), using fluorescein isothiocyanate conjugated monoclonal antibodies or enzyme immunoassay (EIA).

Immunofluorescent assay

The direct examination of pathological specimens using fluorescent antibodies was the original means of demonstrating typical chlamydial inclusions.

Although IF is a more sensitive procedure than Giemsa stain, it is less sensitive than cell culture because of the non-specificity of polyclonal antibodies.

More recently, fluorescein conjugated, species-specific monoclonal antibodies have become commercially available.

Direct IF test takes less than 1 hour and costs no more than cell culture while culture takes about 72 hours.

The technology is easy, but needs a highly skilled microscopist.

The procedure is approximately 90% as sensitive as cell culture, while the specificity appears to be quite good (98%) only in the hands of experienced microscopists. Especially, for genital specimens, the sensitivity and specificity of direct IF tests depend on the rate of *C.trachomatis* infection prevalence in the population studied.

In conclusion, the direct monoclonal antibody test is a valuable alternative to culture in high prevalence settings, while it is not useful for screening when prevalence of *C.trachomatis* infection is less than 10%.

Enzyme immunoassay

Recently EIA has been used to detect chlamydial antigen in clinical specimens. The test appears to be as sensitive as cell culture using first passage results, but showed a certain number of false-positive results. The latter became more important as the prevalence of infection in the population under study decreases.

Enzyme-immunoassays present different advantages with cell culture: ease of transport of specimens, speed of diagnosis (4 to 5 h), objective photometrical measurement and automation.

However results demonstrated that the sensitivity of EIA is greatly influenced by the population studied. In high risk groups, EIA seems an effective screening both for symptomatic women and others who are contacts of those with the disease. However, asymptomatic women in a low risk group, mainly pregnant women, may not benefit from such a test because sensitivity is too low. Furthermore in cases of PID, a peritoneal specimen is not suitable since sensitivity is very low (50%).

Serological means

The diagnostic value of serological studies for *C. trachomatis* genital infections, is the most important, unsolved problem among microbiologists.

In fact, a wide variety of serological tests are currently available for detection of *C.trachomatis* antibodies. These tests may provide evidence of infection, although considerable confusion abounds concerning the validity, or the predictive accuracy of these tests for diagnosis of individual cases of chlamydial infection.

Treharne[1] says that except on very rare occasions (when both acute and convalescent sera are available, or a rising or falling level of antibodies can be demonstrated, or when significant level of immunoglobulin (Ig) M antibodies are present) chlamydial serology may be best regarded as a confirmatory test, used in tandem with other tests when there are strong suspicions of infection.

Furthermore, Treharne reported that IgM antibodies in humans with genital chlamydial infections persist for 8 to 10 weeks after infection. Other studies[2] suggest that such antibodies persist for a longer period of time. If this were so, the demonstration of IgM antibodies would be of limited value for the establishment of current genital chlamydial infections.

On the contrary, Sarov[3] suggested that this type of antibody can be considered as a marker of active and persistent chlamydial infections, since the half-life of serum IgA is 5 to 6 days.

On this basis he observed a close correlation between high titers of serum IgA and chlamydial salpingitis[3], epididymitis[4] or cervicitis[3]. The finding that chances of conception after *in vitro* fertilization are lower if the candidate has specific IgA and elevated IgG antibody titers to *C.trachomatis* was also suggested by Lunefeld[5]. Therefore serological assays may play an important role in the control of chlamydial infections in certain conditions, but they should be extensively studied in infections in which their predictive value has not been determined yet.

Another important problem in the etiological diagnosis of *C.trachomatis* genital infection is the choice of type of specimens for microbiological tests. In the lower genital tract, cervical and urethral swabs should be examined.

In pelvic inflammatory disease (PID) many attempts have been performed to isolate *C.trachomatis* from peritoneal fluids or from tubal biopsy. In our experiences peritoneal fluids are unsuitable and tubal biopsy too traumatic. We believe that the best pathological sample for microbiological diagnosis (isolation and/or direct antigen detection) is a scraping from tubal cells obtained by using a cytobrush during celioscopy, slightly carried over the fimbriated end. In our experiences this method was very effective and provoked no bleeding or other side-effect in the follow-up. Furthermore specimens collected in this way were suitable for microbiological tests, both in direct IF and in McCoy cells.

However, the choice of microbiological test for *C.trachomatis* diagnosis can be connected with the pathology and/or the type of patient. We suggest a protocol for *C.trachomatis* genital infection diagnosis which uses different strategies in four population groups: (1) women with cervicitis, (2) Women with clinical suspicions of PID, (3) Asymptomatic sterile women and (4) Asymptomatic women exposed to a risk of ST D.

Whenever we found evidence of *C.trachomatis* in endocervical and/or urethral swabs in women with cervicitis and in those asymptomatically exposed to a risk of sexually transmitted disease (STD), we propose celioscopy to control spread of *C.trachomatis* to the upper genital tract. Routine celioscopy and tubal scraping by cytobrush will be performed in the other two groups of women. The isolation of *C.trachomatis* on McCoy cells will be carried out in comparison with direct IF or EIA tests. If *C.trachomatis* cannot be isolated, serological diagnosis based on level of serum IgG, IgA and IgM and secretory IgA may be performed.

All positive patients and their sexual partners will be treated for 15 days with 1800 g/day of Miocamicin.

Clinical and microbiological evaluation will be performed at the end of therapy and 2 months later, on the basis of disappearance of symptoms and *C.trachomatis* eradication. The aim of the protocol was to perform an epidemiological study of the prevalence of *C.trachomatis* infection in a large series of women who were divided into four main groups depending on their clinical manifestations and risk factors of infection. We would also evaluate the foundation of these risk factors and suitability of the diagnostic method proposed to detect the various clinical manifestations the infection can assume.

We would then evaluate the clinical effectiveness and tolerability of antibiotic treatment using Miocamycin.

REFERENCES

1. Treharne, J.D. (1988). Chlamydial serodiagnosis. Luxury or necessity? In Mardh, P.A. and La Placa, M. (eds). *Proceedings of The European Society for Chlamydial Research*, pp. 230–233. (Bologna: Società Editrice Esculapio)
2. Schachter, J. (1978). Chlamydial infections. *N. Engl. J. Med.*, **298**, 428, 490, 540
3. Sarov, I. (1988). The significance of *Chlamydia* specific serum IgA antibodies in *Chlamydia trachomatis* infections. In Mardh, P.A. and La Placa, M. (eds). *Proceedings of The European Society For Chlamydial Research*, pp. 234–8. (Bologna: Società Editrice Esculapio)
4. Kanety, S., Sarov, B. and Sarov, I. (1990). IgG and IgA antibodies specific for *Chlamydia trachomatis* in acute epididymitis. *Eur. Urology* (In press)
5. Lunefeld, E., Shapiro, B., Sarov, I., Sarov, B., Insler, V. and Decherney, A.H. (1990). The effect of Chlamydia on pregnancy outcome in a IVF program (In preparation)

41

Miocamycin in the treatment of *Chlamydia trachomatis* genital infections: microbiological, pharmacokinetic and therapeutic aspects

P.M. Furneri and L. Roccasalva

The macrolides comprise a large group of very similar antibiotics. Although a number of new antibiotics have been discovered in the past several decades, macrolides, and erythromycin especially, have been extensively used on a world-wide basis. In fact, it is generally recognized that macrolides are among the safest and best tolerated of all antimicrobial agents. They are a safe alternative in cases in which patients are known to be allergic to penicillin or other antibiotics, or instead of tetracyclines during pregnancy. To date, not all the newer macrolides which have been investigated have offered a significantly wider antimicrobial spectrum, increased potency or superior pharmacokinetic characteristic. Moreover, if a drug of equal, or more than, erythromycin microbiological and pharmacological properties was discovered, for which increased stability and improved pharmacokinetic characteristics have been established, it might be useful not only as therapeutic agent of respiratory tract infections, but also for other clinical fields, especially gynecology.

Improvement in the macrolide family especially involved the group of 16-membered macrolides. These 16-membered macrolides are claimed to be more active against mycoplasmas than 14-membered macrolides; moreover their *in vitro* activity is frequently higher than that of erythromycin because of the low incidence of cross resistance. Miocamycin, the 10, 3″-di-O-acetyl ester of midecamycin, is a well-known antibiotic belonging to the group of 16-membered macrolides. Its synthesis and chemical properties have been described elsewhere[1] and its metabolic pathway and the chemical structures of its metabolites have been found from studies on its metabolism[2].

MICROBIOLOGY

Its *in vitro* activity has been well viewed and the spectrum is quite similar to that shown by other macrolides[3,4]. A very low incidence of cross resistance or resistance has been reported (Furneri, personal communication). The authors' experience on *in vitro* activity confirmed these findings and also the high activity against erythromycin-resistant *Staphylococcus aureus* and *Ureaplasma urealyticum* was noted[5]; moreover, miocamycin is active against naturally resistant micro-organisms such as *Mycoplasma hominis*[4] (Table 1).

Its activity against sensitive microorganisms is often bactericidal, especially against ureaplasmas and mycoplasmas[4]. Lacey and co-workers showed the same features against beta-haemolytic streptococci, on which its activity is similar to that of penicillin[6]. Miocamycin also interferes with O_2 uptake and with the synthesis of protein P_1 in *Mycoplasma pneumoniae*[4]. Its *in vitro* activity against *Chlamydia trachomatis* is similar to that shown by other macrolides[7] (Table 1).

PHARMACOKINETICS

The pharmacokinetic data collected in the last years indicated miocamycin as a typical drug for the therapy of the respiratory tract infection (pneumonol-

Table 1 *In vitro* activity of miocamycin against gram-positive, gram-negative bacteria, mycoplasmas and chlamydiae[3,4,7] (minimal inhibitory concentration (MIC) in μg/ml)

Gram-positive bacteria		Gram-positive anaerobes	
S. aureus	0.39	*P. asaccharolyticus*	0.26
S. epidermidis	0.78	*P. variabilis*	1.56
S. pyogenes	0.39	*P. constellatus*	1.56
S. pneumoniae	0.05	*P. parvulus*	0.20
E. faecalis	0.78	*P. acnes*	0.78
B. subtilis	0.39	*B. bifidum*	0.20
B. anthracis	0.39	*B. adolescentis*	0.78
C. diphtheriae	0.39	*E. lentum*	0.39
L. monocytogenes	1.56	*C. tetani*	0.20
		C. perfringens	3.12
Gram-negative bacteria		*C. difficile*	0.78
H. influenzae	0.78		
H. parainfluenzae	0.39	Gram-negative anaerobes	
H. paraphrofilus	0.78	*B. fragilis*	1.56
H. aphrophilus	0.39	*B. distansonis*	3.13
C. jejuni	1.56	*F. russii*	0.39
B. pertussis	0.78		
N. gonorrhoeae	0.78	Mycoplasmas	
L. pneumophila	0.50	*M. pneumoniae FH*	0.01
E. coli	>100	*M. pneumoniae FIC*	0.003
S. enteritidis	>100	*M. hominis*	0.05
P. aeruginosa	>100	*M. orale*	0.25
K. pneumoniae	>100	*M. salivarium*	0.25
P. vulgaris	>100	*M. mycoides*	1
S. marcescens	>100	*M. gallisepticum*	0.05
		U. urealyticum	0.25
		Chlamydiae	
		C. trachomatis	0.06

ogical and otorhinolaryngological field)[8,9]. Moreover, many data are available on the concentrations in human secretions as sputum, bronchial secretion, nasal secretion[9]. In our observations[10] miocamycin after oral administration is rapidly absorbed in all the patients studied as T value proved in Table 2: the area under the curve obtained appears to be dose dependent (Table 2) and higher than those obtained in other studies[2,8,11]. $t\frac{1}{2}\beta$ was, also, recorded higher than that obtained in the study of Fraschini and co-workers[8], this difference is partly due to the use of a different pharmacokinetic model; in fact, those authors, unlike us that have described pharmacokinetics through a time limited zero-order absorption model, have studied the pharmacokinetics of miocamycin through first-order kinetics. Unlike Fukaya[2] we did not determine the concentrations of the metabolites, and Qu was recorded as total because of the high antibacterial activity of the urinary metabolites[3]. In any case the determination of the metabolites requires the original standard substances not yet available in Italy.

Nevertheless, miocamycin is poorly eliminated in the urine, like the other macrolides and our results confirm those of Fukaya[2], with a urinary recovery of about 1.2% of the administered doses in 24 h (data not shown). Therefore, miocamycin after 6 h from the last administration showed a urinary excretion rate in the first group of 0.78% (range 0.67%–0.84%), in the second of 1.1% (range 0.67%–1.5%) and in the third of 2.78% (range 1.85%–3.51%). Miocamycin excretion rate is lower than that showed by josamycin but higher than that of erythromycin. Unlike josamycin[12], miocamycin reached higher prostatic levels at a lower dosage, as demonstrated by Furneri and co-workers[10] (Table 3). This is, in our opinion, due to the higher

Table 2 Derived parameters after analysis with zero-order absorption model

Parameters	*First group**	*Second group*** (Average ± SD)	*Third group†*
K (1/h)	0.3667 ± 0.1002	0.38 ± 0.1229	0.295 ± 0.0991
Ko (mg/h)	1100.3567 ± 64.3358	1098.4133 ± 182.7353	2284.69 ± 294.4818
C_{max}-abs (μg/ml)	1.77 ± 0.7662	1.6767 ± 0.9815	4.5 ± 2.9147
C_{max}-est (μg/ml)	2.2913 ± 0.6071	2.1753 ± 0.6846	4.22 ± 4.7141
T_{max} (h)	0.62 ± 0.0173	0.6833 ± 0.0864	0.422 ± 0.2333
$t\frac{1}{2}\beta$(h)	1.99 ± 0.5524	1.94 ± 0.6018	2.525 ± 0.7053
AUC (mg h/l)	7.5767 ± 0.2511	6.7333 ± 0.6058	18.682 ± 15.1555
AVD (l)	228.45 ± 69.9870	248.4933 ± 118.6034	329.965 ± 181.7157
Qu (mg)	4.8867 ± 0.2491	13.4433 ± 5.0461	33.352 ± 8.6235
Clp (l/h)	79.23 ± 2.6709	89.8767 ± 10.2641	100.777 ± 68.9604
Clr (l/h)	0.6467 ± 0.0153	2.0514 ± 0.8715	2.8 ± 2.1907

*First group received a single dose of 600 mg of miocamycin
** Second group received 600 mg twice a day of miocamycin up to 1200 mg
† Third group received 1200 mg of miocamycin in a single administration
K, first order kinetic constant; Ko, zero order kinetic constant; C_{max}-abs, maximal concentration absorbed; C_{max}-est, maximal concentration by the computer assisted fitting program; T_{max} time when is reached the C_{max}; $t\frac{1}{2}\beta$, elimination phase half-life; AUC, area under the curve; AVD, apparent volume of distribution; Qu, quantity of drug eliminated with urine; Clp, plasmatic clearance; Clr, renal clearance.

Table 3 Prostatic concentrations in μg/g[10]

Patients	*Time after administration* (h)	*Relative concentration in* μg/g*
1	2	5 (1)
2	2	4.9 (0.9)
3	2	5 (1)

*The obtained value in the serum at the same time is given in parentheses

hydrophobicity of the molecule and to the better tissue penetration power as shown in other sites.

Recently, Furneri and co-workers[13] described the pharmacokinetic behavior of miocamycin in the female genital tissue (vagina, cervix, endometrium, ovary and tube) and the results are shown in Table 4. The highest levels were obtained in the endometrium the lowest in the vagina. Both in the prostate and in the female genital tissues the levels of the drug were frequently higher than those in the serum at the same time[10,13].

In our studies we did not investigate the possibility of drug accumulation during therapy. Sanders and co-workers[11] demonstrated an increase from day 1 to day 6 of about one-half or the whole of the concentration obtained, especially for area under the curve (AUC). The same authors also evidenced an increase of urinary excretion from 1.8 mg to 3.2 mg after a 6 day duration therapy, and they concluded that this is indicative of some drug accumulation.

THERAPEUTIC ASPECTS

In a recent paper we investigated the therapeutical efficacy of miocamycin, in a 12 day duration therapy with two administrations per day of 600 mg each, against two urogenital disorders (non-gonococcal urethritis and acute urethral syndrome)[5]. Our results carried out a 100% therapeutic efficacy in both syndromes, and the regression of the clinical signs was always followed by the eradication of the causative micro-organisms. Particularly, clinical symptoms in *C.trachomatis*-positive non-specific genital infections (NSGI) were noticed from day 6 of the therapy.

Before us, in 1986 Marziani and co-workers[14] investigated the therapeutical

Table 4 Female genital tissue concentrations (in μg/g) of miocamycin after a 2 day preoperative administration (600 mg three times a day, last administration of 600 mg)[13]; average of two patients

Patient samples	*Time* (h)	
	2	3
Vagina	1.1	0.8
Cervix	1.5	1
Endometrium	2.5	2
Serum	1.2	0.8

efficacy of miocamycin against pelvic inflammatory disease with positive isolation of *C.trachomatis* carrying out a therapeutic efficacy of 94%. Unlike us[5] and Marziani[14], Cianci and co-workers (personal communication), Riillo and co-workers[15] have chosen a different dosage, in which they increased the dosage from 1200 mg to 1800 mg a day. Moreover, in the paper of Cianci and co-workers they left unchanged the 12 days duration therapy, while in the paper of Riillo and co-workers they reduced from 12 to 10 the duration of the therapy. The microbiological results of these two experiences carried out a percentage of success of 89% and 100% respectively. Recently, another two studies have been made about the therapeutic efficacy of miocamycin in same pathological conditions of the female genital tract due to *C.trachomatis*, by Furneri and co-workers[13] and Roccasalva and co-workers[16]. In both cases the eradication of *C.trachomatis* has been achieved, but different durations of therapy have been used, that is, 15 days and 12 days respectively.

REFERENCES

1. Omoto, S., Iwamatsu, K., Inouye, S. and Niida, T. (1976). Modification of a macrolide antibiotic midecamycin (SF837). I. Synthesis and structure of 9,3″-diacetylmidecamycin. *J. Antibiot.*, **XXIX(5)**, 536–48
2. Fukaya, K., Shomura, T., Someye, S., Kitai, S., Murata, S. and Unemura, K. (1981). Absorbtion, metabolism and excretion of 9,3″-di-acetyl-midecamycin (MOM) in human. *Acta Tocxicol. Ther.*, **2**, 45–62
3. Yoshida, T., Watanabe, T., Shomura, T., Someya, S., Okamoto, R., Ishihara, S., Miyauchi, K. and Kazuno, Y. (1982). Bacteriological evaluation of midecamycin acetate and its metabolites. *Jpn. J. Antibiot.*, **35(6)**, 1462–74
4. Furneri, P.M., Tempera, G., Bisignano, G., Cottarelli, F.V. and Nicoletti, G. (1987). Antimycoplasmal activity of a new macrolide: miocamycin. *Chemiotherapia*, **6**, 341–5
5. Furneri, P.M., Roccasalva, L., Fallica, L. and Tempera, G. (1988). Efficacy of miocamycin in the therapy of non-specific genital infections (NSGI): Non gonococcal urethritis (NGU) and acute urethral syndrome (AUS). *Int. J. Clin. Pharm. Res.*, **VIII(2)**, 111–16
6. Lacey, R.W., Lord, V.L. and Howson, G.L. (1984). In vitro evaluation of miocamycin: bactericidal activity against streptococci. *J. Antimicrob. Chemother.*, **13**, 5–13
7. Ridgway, G.L., Mumtaz, G., Gabriel, G. and Oriel, J.D. (1983). The activity of miocamycin (MOM) against *Chlamydia trachomatis* and mycoplasma *in vitro*. *J. Antimicrob. Chemother.*, **12**, 511–14
8. Fraschini, F., Scaglione, F., Cantarella, G., Marchi, E., Scarpazza, P., Falchi, M. and Braga, P.C. (1985). Plasma and tissue concentrations of miocamycin in humans. In Ishigami, J. (ed.) *Recent Advances in Chemotherapy – Antimicrobial section* (*Proceedings of the 14th International Congress of Chemotherapy, Kyoto*, June 23–28, 1985), pp. 1447–9. (Tokyo: University of Tokyo Press)
9. Fioretti, M., Bandera, M. and Rimoldi, R. (1984). Attività terapeutica e comportamento farmacocinetico della miocamicina a livello dell'apparato respiratorio. *G. Ital. Chemioter.*, **31**, 145–8
10. Furneri, P.M., Scalia, G., Garozzo, A. and Tempera, G. (1988). Pharmacokinetic data and therapeutical efficacy of miocamycin: serum, urinary and prostatic levels. *Drugs Exptl. Clin. Res.* (In press)
11. Sanders, S.W., Jaeger, H., Cunci, R., Fujita, M. and Maurette, J.M. (1985). Single and multiple dose pharmacokinetics and tolerance of miocamycin in healthy European volunteers. In Ishigami, J. (ed.) *Recent Advances in Chemotherapy – Antimicrobial section* (*Proceedings of the 14th International Congress of Chemotherapy, Kyoto*, June 23–28, 1985), pp. 1452–3. (Tokyo: University of Tokyo Press)
12. Fagioli, A., Cruciani, E., Riario Sforza, G., Ferrone, G. and Di Silverio, F. (1982). Livelli

tissutali prostatici di josamicina. *G. Ital. Chemioter.*, **29** (Suppl.), 85–7

13. Furneri, P.M., Blandino, G., Roccasalva, L., Cianci, A., Palumbo, G. and Tempera, G. (1988). Some features of miocamycin in gynaecological field: pharmacokinetic data using preoperative administration and therapeutical aspects against gynaecological chlamydial infections. Presented at the *6th Mediterranean Congress of Chemotherapy*, May 22–27. (Taormina-Giardini Naxos)
14. Marziani, R., Buzzi, M., Napolitano, C., Morini, A. and Mogini, C. (1986). Flogosi pelviche da Chlamydia trachomatis: trattamento con eritromicina e miocamicina.In Danesino, V. and Rondanelli, G. (eds). *Le infezioni in ostetricia e ginecologia – Le malattie a trasmissione sessuale negli anni* 80, pp. 637–40. (Bologna: Monduzzi)
15. Riillo, S., Furneri, P.M., Roccasalva, L., Tempera, G. and Cianci, A. (1987). Efficacia di miocamicina nella terapia della infezioni ginecologiche da Chlamydia trachomatis. In Montoneri, C. and Zarbo, G. (eds). *Malattie in Gravidanza* (*Atti del convegno – Malattie in gravidanza. Attuali orientamenti diagnostici e terapeutici*, Catania, 1–3 June, 1987), pp. 195–7. (Bologna: Monduzzi)
16. Roccasalva, L., Vaccaro, F., Sardo, S., Pafumi, C., Cianci, A. and Furneri, P.M. (1988). Impiego razionale di miocamicina quale terapia di scelta nella infezioni genitali da Chlamydia tracomatis. Presented at the *LXV Congresso Nazionale della Società Italiana di Ginecologia e Ostetricia,* 29 May–2 June, Giardini Naxos – Taormina

42

Cost–benefit analysis of screening and therapy of *Chlamydia trachomatis* infections

S. Guaschino, A. Spinillo, I. Prinetti and A. Pistoni

INTRODUCTION

Chlamydia trachomatis infection is considered the most common sexually transmitted disease in western countries[1]. In the last few years there has been an improvement in standards of screening, diagnosis and therapy. Many studies have been carried out to clarify epidemiological factors affecting prevalence; unfortunately, risk factors are not the same in different populations.

The real problems of the *C.trachomatis* epidemics, both for social and economic reasons, are the sequelae of infection such as pelvic inflammatory disease (PID), ectopic pregnancy, infertility and perinatal infections[2].

At present chlamydial infections may be diagnosed, in screening program, by culturing the organism or detecting the antigens with enzyme-linked immunosorbent assay (ELISA) and immunofluorescence tests. Serology is also available, but not recommended in patients at high risk from past infection. Cell culture from both urethral and cervical specimens is probably the most sensitive and specific test (sensitivity 88%; specificity 99.9%), but it is the most expensive. Direct and indirect immunofluorescence and ELISA tests have a range of sensitivity from 60 to 90% and specificity from 65% to 95%. Serological screening may be effective in populations with low rates of serological positivity and in detecting high risk groups[3].

Although screening for *C.trachomatis* infection has been routinely performed in many clinics, the cost-effectiveness of using one of the above tests has not been adequately evaluated.

COST–BENEFIT BALANCE

The factors that affect cost–benefit balance are: prevalence of the disease, cost of test, diagnostic accuracy of the test, and rate, cost and seriousness of untreated infections.

The prevalence of the infection changes in different risk groups and countries. In some risk groups (lower socioeconomic status, prostitutes, homosexuals) prevalence is higher than 25%[1]. Risk groups are defined on historical or clinical findings such as: purulent cervical discharge, cervical ectopy, cervical erythema/friability, positive culture for *N. gonorrhoeae* and clinical diagnosis of PID. Historical risk groups include partners of men with non-gonococcal urethritis (NGU); young, sexually active women with genital symptoms; lower socioeconomic status and multiple sexual partners; past or current history of sexually transmitted diseases (STD); persistent abnormal Pap-smear; pill users[4,5].

Evaluation of the screening

A screening for *C.trachomatis* infection was performed in the Obstetrics and Gynecology Department of University of Pavia on 610 outpatients attending to cytology, colposcopy and STD departments.

Screening was effected by cell culture and direct immunofluorescence test (Micro-Trak) of urethral and cervical specimens. The results of cultures were: positivity or urethra specimen in 7/610 cases (1.15%), of cervix specimen in 15/610 cases (2.5%), and both urethra and cervix in 2.5% of cases for a total of 6.06% positive women. Our population is then at low risk of infection. This is confirmed by the fact that among epidemiological factors only cervical ectopy and pill use were positively correlated to infection (Table 1).

The cost of test is one of the main factors in the evaluation of cost-effectiveness of the screening. The cost of a combined urethral-cervical culture, direct antigen detection tests and serological screening are respectively $25–30, $12 and $8 for each woman tested[6,7].

Sensitivities and specificities of the test used are important factors in determining the cost/effectiveness of the screening. Table 2 reports the

Table 1 Historical and clinical factors in a low-risk population

	Positive	*Negative*	*p*
Pill users	18/30	72/580	<0.01
Cervical ectopy	13/30	126/580	<0.01
Mucopurulent discharge	12/30	168/580	N.S.

Table 2 Accuracy of the test (DFA) in %

	Cervix	*Urethra*
Sensitivity	60	63.6
Specificity	99.5	99.5
Positive predictive value	85.7	85.7
Negative predictive value	98	98

diagnostic accuracy of direct fluorescent antigen detection (DFA) in our population. The specificity and sensitivity are comparable to other studies[8].

The frequency, seriousness and economic costs of the sequelae of an uncured infection are reported in many studies[2,6,9]. The risk of PID following uncured positive cervical culture is estimated to be 10–30%. About 20% of these women will be hospitalized. The rates of ectopic pregnancy and infertility are estimated to be 4% and 20% respectively. The rate of spontaneous cure is estimated to be 10% of infected women, and 25% is the rate of infection in the male sexual partner. The average cost associated with complications of an uncured chlamydial infection is $347 per uncured woman. Now we apply the principles of cost–benefit analysis to our cases. The total cost of the screening was $22.57 ($15.25 for cultures and $7.32 for antigen detection). Table 3 reports the costs of the screening (culture only) and the costs resulting from the unidentified/uncured cases. These costs were subtracted from the costs associated with preventable cases. The same calculations are reported in Table 4 for antigen detection only (DFA). It is clear, from the results, that cultural screening for *C.trachomatis* in a low-moderate risk population is cost-effective.

The diagnostic accuracy of the test is the key of cost-effectiveness. Assuming the use of ELISA test (85% sensitivity and 81% specificity), the costs of the screening are comparable to DFA test, but false negative rates are lower. In order to avoid treating the 19% false positives, the best approach is cultural confirmation of positive cases.

The knowledge of infection prevalence in the population and the relation to known risk factors is another critical point in evaluating the efficacy of the screening. For a prevalence ranging from 5% to about 7% there is not a great difference in cost–effectiveness between cell culture only or targeted culture after antigenic tests. Antigenic detection only, is cost-effective, in low-moderate risk populations, for tests costing less than $12 and with at least 80% sensitivity[6].

In high risk groups (prevalence more than 15%) other suitable approaches are selective screening and empiric ('epidemiological') treatment[10,11]. Nettle-

Table 3 Costs of the consequences

Culture only (88% sensitivity)		
Cost of screening	610	$15.250
Non-preventable cases	4	$1.388
Preventable cases	37	$12.839
Net cost		$3.800

Table 4 Cost of the consequences

Antigen detection only (DFA) (65% sensitivity)		
Cost of screening	610	$7.320
Non-preventable cases	15	$5.205
Preventable cases	24	$8.328
Net cost		$4.200

man *et al.*[7] have demonstrated that empiric treatment in high risk groups (e.g. patients attending STD clinics) and culture based treatment of low-risk women is the best cost-effective strategy.

Therapy

The drugs actually used for treatment of *C.trachomatis* infections are: tetracyclines (doxycycline, mynocycline), macrolides (erithromycin, josamycin, miocamycin) and quinolones (ofloxacin, ciprofloxacin).

The efficacy of these drugs, evaluated as per cent of bacterial eradication, is similar and the range is 85–95%[12].

The rate of adverse reactions is higher for tetracycline therapy (10–12%) than macrolides or quinolones (2–4%)[6,12]. In the evaluation of cost-effectiveness of drugs, in association with the costs of medications, the costs of adverse effects should be considered. The cost of adverse reactions (nausea, vomiting, yeast infections etc.) for tetracycline therapy has been estimated to be $27 per complication[6]. Because of this estimate and of the low compliance of tetracycline therapy, alternative methods of treatment (macrolides, quinolones) can be cost-effective almost in presumptive treatment of high risk groups.

REFERENCES

1. Harrison, H.R. and Alexander, E.R. (1984). In Holmes, K.K., Mardh, P., Sparling, P.F. and Wiesner, P.J. (eds). *Sexually Transmitted Disease*, pp. 270–80. (New York: McGraw-Hill)
2. Washington, A.E., Johnson, R.E. and Sanders, L.L. (1987). *Chlamydia trachomatis* infections in the United States. *J. Am. Med. Assoc.*, **257**, 2070–2
3. Embil, J.A., Thiebaux, H.J. and Manuel, F.R. (1983). Sequential cervical specimens and the isolation of *Chlamydia trachomatis*; factors affecting detection. *Sex Transm. Dis.*, **10**, 62–6
4. Thompson, S.E. and Washington, A.E. (1983). Epidemiology of sexually transmitted *Chlamydia trachomatis* infections. *Epidemiol. Rev.*, **5**, 96–123
5. Harrison, H.R., Costin, M. and Meder, J.B. (1985). Cervical *Chlamydia trachomatis* infection in university women: relationship to history, contraception, ectopy and cervicitis. *Am. J. Obstet. Gynecol.*, **153**, 244–57
6. Nettleman, M.D. and Jones, R.B. (1988). Cost-effectiveness of screening women at moderate risk for genital infections caused by *Chlamydia trachomatis*. *J. Am. Med. Assoc.*, **260**, 207–13
7. Nettleman, M.D., Jones, R.B., Roberts, S.D., Katz, B.P., Washington, A.E., Dittus, R.S. and Quinn, T.S. (1986). *Annals of Internal Medicine*, **105**, 189–96
8. Kent, G.P., Harrison, H.R., Berman, S.M. and Keenlyside, R.A. (1988). Screening for *Chlamydia trachomatis* infection in a sexually transmitted disease clinic: comparison of diagnostic tests with clinical and historical risk factors. *Sex Transm. Dis.*, **15**, 51–7
9. Washington, A.E., Arno, P.S. and Brooks, M.A. (1986). The economic cost of pelvic inflammatory disease. *J. Am. Med. Assoc.*, **255**, 1735–8
10. 1985 STD treatment guidelines. (1986). *J. Am. Acad. Dermatol.*, **14**, 707–26
11. Meriwether, C.D., Evans, M.I. and Sokol, R.J. (1986). *Chlamydia trachomatis*: a practical obstetric/gynecologic management approach. *Int. J. Gynaecol. Obstet.*, **24**, 407–15
12. Watts, D.H. and Eschenbach, D.A. (1988). Treatment of *Chlamydia*, *Micoplasma* and Group B streptococcal infections. *Clin. Obstet. Gynecol.*, **31**, 435–52

43

Chlamydial infections in newborns and infants

N. Principi

Chlamydial infections undoubtedly represent an emerging pathology in pediatrics. Up until a few years ago it was believed that these infectious agents were only responsible for conjunctivitis in neonates and pneumonia in infants in relation to vertical transmission of the infection from mother to child during passage through the birth canal. Today it is known that older children may contract chlamydial infections, especially pharyngotonsillitis and otitis but also lower respiratory tract infections. In addition the more precocious initiation to sexual activity has spread these genital infections to the later pediatric ages. In fact, these infections are readily demonstrable in significant percentages in sexually active adolescents.

The incidence of neonatal infection varies with the variation of the incidence of infection in pregnant women at the time of birth. This figure is very variable in that it may go from a minimum of 2% to a maximum of 40% depending on the prevalence in the sample of women considered (more or less at risk for sexually transmitted diseases) and the number of check-ups and therapeutic interventions carried out during pregnancy.

In any event, neonatal conjunctivitis represents the most precocious pediatric chlamydial pathology to be manifested. It is the most common neonatal eye infection having substituted gonococcal eye infection in both importance and frequency. Its appearance is usually delayed and doesn't arise before the 4th–5th day of life. This, on one hand indicates the necessity for the neonatologist to consider other diagnostic possibilities if the symptoms are more precocious, while on the other hand, alerts us to the fact that the first manifestations of the disease may become evident when the baby has already gone home increasing the risk of permanent eye damage.

If, in fact, the acute clinical presentation is that of any other purulent conjunctivitis, late or insufficient treatment may lead to irreversible alterations such as a corneal pannus. The importance of a swift and effective therapy is therefore obvious. In pediatrics, this means the utilization of macrolides, since the other antibiotics that are theoretically active against *Chlamydiae*, the tetracyclines and quinolones, are not usable in younger children because of the irreversible damage that they may cause. The antibiotics of choice are administered at doses of 50 mg/kg/day in 3–4 doses. Treatment is carried out over 2 weeks. Topical therapy may be associated, but must not represent the only therapeutic solution since it is not sufficient to eradicate the infection.

Pneumonia caused by *Chlamydia* is a clinical entity that is not yet adequately understood even though it has been recognized for approximately 15 years. The reason for the scarce attention given to this form by pediatricians is linked, above all, to the difficulty in making a definitive diagnosis, along with its apparently benign evolution. Clinically, it appears between 3 and 12 weeks after birth and presents with an afebrile state characterized by a dry pertussoid cough and findings of wheezing, hisses and fine rattles on auscultation. Diffuse infiltrations with peribronchial thickening, and at times, focal consolidation are demonstrated radiologically. Useful for making the diagnosis, are eosinophils, typically found in bronchial secretions and in the circulation where elevated levels of immunoglobulin G (IgG) and immunoglobulin M (IgM) are consistently found.

In contrast to other infections of the lower respiratory tract, there seems to be a correlation with the finding of the infectious agent and its antigens in the pharynx, in this way offering the possibility of a ready etiological diagnosis with the use of immunofluorescence or pharyngeal culture. Although often benign, the evolution may take on a protracted course or end in death due to crises of apnea or sovraposition of infections by other germs. Even in this case, treatment is with a macrolide at the same doses recommended for the conjunctivitis. It is interesting to note that approximately one half of the cases of penumonia occur in subjects that had no ocular symptoms. This may delay diagnosis and favor a less favorable outcome. Another important fact is that eventual treatment of the mother does not exclude the possibility of infection in the child. It is therefore only from the clinical pulmonary presentation, hematochemical analysis and cultural exams that the suspicion and then confirmation of the diagnosis can be made. Therapy therefore seems to be more effective if initiated precociously.

In pediatric experience in the Milan area, therapy with miocamycin (50 mg/kg in three doses) was effective in approximately 80% of subjects diagnosed as having a form of *Chlamydia*. Of these subjects, 22 had conjunctivitis, 10 upper respiratory infections, three pneumonia and six were asymptomatic carriers. The efficacy of the drug was almost identical in premature as well as term infants as well as in children of drug abusers that were human immunodeficiency virus positive or negative. For the most part these data were analogous to those found in the literature regarding similar cases treated with other macrolides.

Recent notation that subjects declared healed due to sterilization of the initial infection site, may present a successive localization at another site (anal or vaginal) implies that the percentage of effective healings may be less than those cited. In any case, future research must take into account the possible extension of the infection outside of the commonly considered sites as well as treatment's interference on the long-term evolution of the infection.

BIBLIOGRAPHY

1. Bell, T.A., Stamm, W.E., Küo, C.C. *et al.* (1987). Delayed appearance of *Chlamydia trachomatis* infections acquired at birth. *Ped. Infect. Dis. J.*, **6**, 928–31

2. Brayden, R.M., Paisley, J.W. and Laner, B.A. (1987). Apnea in infants with Chlamydia trachomatis pneumonia. *Ped. Infect. Dis. J.*, **6**, 423–5
3. Numez, R.M., Duque, J. and De Gonzales, B. (1988). Viral and chlamydial etiology of acute infections of the lower respiratory tract in Colombian children. *Ped. Infect. Dis. J.*, **7**, 69–70
4. Paisley, J.W., Laner, B.A., Melinkovich, P. *et al.* (1986). Rapid diagnosis of *Chlamydia trachomatis* pneumonia in infants by direct immunofluorescence microscopy of nasopharyngeal secretions. *J. Pediatr.*, **109**, 653–5
5. Persson, K., Ronnerstam, R., Svanberg, L. *et al.* (1986). Neonatal chlamydial conjunctivitis. *Arch. Dis. Child.*, **61**, 565–8
6. Preece, P.M., Brooks, J.M., Anderson, J.M. *et al.* (1986). The prevalence of Chlamydia trachomatis infection in infants following maternal infections. *Arch. Dis. Child.*, **61**, 627

44

Oral miocamycin in the prophylaxis and treatment of reproductive tract infections in infertile couples

A.R. Genazzani, P.G. Artini, G. Coukos, M. Monaco, F. Boselli and A. Volpe

INTRODUCTION

Asymptomatic or subclinical infection may be an important contributor to female and male infertility[1,2]. Particularly, *Chlamydia trachomatis* seems to be a frequent cause of infertility. In fact, *C. trachomatis* is a possible causal agent of female urethritis, infection of the cervix and less frequently of endometrial and adnexal infections[2,4]. Moreover, the presence of serum antibodies against *C. trachomatis* in women undergoing *in vitro* fertilization (IVF) cycles is associated with failure of the treatment[3]. *C. trachomatis* is also the causal agent of prostatitis as well as of epididymitis in males[1,5].

Subclinical and asymptomatic chlamydial infections may be successfully treated with miocamycin, a recent semisynthetic macrolide[6,7]. The efficacy of miocamycin has been proven not only against Gram positive and negative bacterial infections, but also against infections caused by micro-organisms devoid of a bacterial wall, as *Mycoplasma hominis* and *Ureaplasma urealyticum* and micro-organisms with intracellular growth as *C. trachomatis* and *Lysteria*[6,7]. Moreover, clinical trials have shown an optimal acceptance of this compound[7]. In this study we have evaluated the clinical efficacy and acceptance of miocamycin in infertile couples.

MATERIALS AND METHODS

Female infertility

One hundred and eighty-nine infertile patients have been evaluated for the presence of cervical *C. trachomatis* by means of a micro-immunofluorescent technique[8]. The presence of *C. trachomatis* in the peritoneal fluid has also been tested in 44 infertile patients during a diagnostic laparoscopy, routinely performed in our IVF unit.

Patients proven positive for *C. trachomatis* in the cervix or the peritoneal fluid have been administered oral miocamycin, 600 mg three times a day, for 15 days. An endocervical biopsy and investigation of *C. trachomatis* by employment of an immunofluorescent technique were repeated at the end of treatment in case of chlamydial cervicitis proven before. A second immunofluorescent test of the peritoneal fluid was also performed 4–6 months later, during laparoscopy for follicular aspiration of an IVF/gamete intrafallopian transfer (GIFT) cycle following diagnostic laparoscopy.

Male infertility

In our IVF unit oral antibiotic treatment is usually given, as a general prophylaxis, prior to artificial insemination procedures. The efficacy of oral miocamycin, 600 mg twice a day, for 11–15 days has been evaluated in 60 patients, who presented inflammatory aspects of semen. Sperm count and motility and presence of inflammatory aspects have been compared before and after therapy in these patients. Moreover, the semen of 45 out of these 60 patients has been compared, in terms of oocyte fertilization rate, at the time of insemination of oocytes (2 weeks of treatment), to that of 90 controls at the time of IVF, who had received no treatment in terms of oocyte fertilization rate.

RESULTS

Female infertility

Seventeen patients out of 189 (8.9%) have proven positive for endocervical *C. trachomatis* at immunofluorescent tests, while in four out of 44 patients (9.1%) there was detected a peritoneal fluid positivity for *C. trachomatis*.

Both groups of patients showed a complete negativization of immunofluorescence at the second examination after 15 days of miocamycin 180 mg/day treatment.

Male prophylaxis with oral miocamycin

Semen analysis compared before and after treatment revealed a significantly improved sperm motility and a disappearance of the inflammatory aspects in 52 out of 60 patients treated (Table 1). There was no observed difference

Table 1 Semen analysis before and after miocamycin treatment

	Sperm count (10^6/ml)	*Motility* %	*Leucocytes* 10^6/ml	*Viscosity*	*Agglutination*
Pretreatment	74.5	53.7	>1	+ +	+ −
Post-treatment	65.7	70.1	<0.5	+ −	− −

however in terms of the oocyte fertilization rate between treated patients (78%) and controls (72%).

A very low percentage of patients treated, of both sexes, presented side-effects. In fact, only six out of 119 patients (5%) complained of nausea and epigastric pain. In no case was treatment withdrawn because of these side-effects.

DISCUSSION

Non-specific genital infection is frequently encountered in infertile couples.

In our study, 23 out of 233 infertile women presented an asymptomatic chlamydial infection of the endocervix or the peritoneal fluid. In all of them, treatment with miocamycin for 2 weeks resulted in a negativization of the immunofluorescence for *C. trachomatis*.

The relevance of *C. trachomatis* in seminal fluid to the success rate of IVF is still unknown. Some data indicate the presence of the micro-organism in the seminal plasma being of no importance for the success of this procedure[9]. Cultures of samples of fertilization medium have shown no significant occurrence of bacterial growth[10]. Moreover, in our experience, no infection attributable to organisms present in the semen occurred in women undergoing embryo-transfer (unpublished data). On the other hand, it has been postulated that asymptomatic or subclinical prostatitis is an important contributor to male infertility[1]. Schaeffer *et al.*[11] found that infertile men had increased numbers of leukocytes in expressed prostatic secretion when compared to normal men. Although the risk of infection appears to be small, the microbiological investigations are continuing to determine whether micro-organisms may represent an important cause of failure of *in vitro* fertilization or of subsequent embryo wastage due to some disorder during implantation or pregnancy.

Our data show that the oocyte fertilization rate in couples with the male partner treated with miocamycin does not show any significant difference compared to controls.

We have however observed a significant improvement of sperm motility, which appears an interesting finding especially concerning oligoastheno-spermic patients undergoing artificial insemination.

In comparison to the control group, miocamycin prophylactic treatment improved the inflammatory aspects. This result may be important in view of the fact that inflammatory phagocytic cells may release cytotoxins reactive with the membranes of the oocyte or the spermatozoa[12].

The clinical efficacy of miocamycin in the treatment of chlamydial genital infections as well as in the prophylaxis prior to artificial insemination procedures derives also from its optimal acceptance.

Alternative antibiotic treatments like erythromycin or tetracyclines are often associated with more pronounced side-effects[13] and this makes mioca-mycin a first choice compound for the prophylaxis and treatment of genital aspecific infections in the infertile couple.

REFERENCES

1. Elliasson, R. (1979). Clinical examination of infertile men. In Hafez, E.S.E. (ed.) *Human Semen and Fertility Regulation in Men*. p. 321. (CV Mosby Co: St. Louis)
2. Paavonen, J. and Wolner-Hanssen, P. (1989). *Chlamydia trachomatis*: a major threat to reproduction. *Hum. Reprod.*, **4**, 111
3. Rowland, G.E., Forsey, T., Moss, T.R., Steptoe, P.C., Hewitt, J. and Darougar, S. (1985). Failure of *in vitro* fertilization and embryo replacement following infection with *Chlamydia trachomatis*. *J. Vitro Fertil. Embryo Transf.*, **2**, 151
4. Moore, D.E., Foy, H.M., Daling, J.R., Grayston, J.T., Spadoni, L.R., Wang, S.P., Kuo, C.C. and Eschenbach, D.A. (1982). Increased frequency of serum antibodies to *Chlamydia trachomatis* in infertility due to distal tubal disease. *Lancet*, **ii**, 547
5. Holmes, K.K., Bell, T.A. and Berger, R.E. (1984). Epidemiology of sexually transmitted diseases. *Urol. Cin. N. Am.*, **11**, 3
6. Ridgway, G.L., Mumtaz, G., Gabriel, G. and Oriel, D. (1983). The activity of miokamycin (MOM) against *Chlamydial trachomatis* and mycoplasma *in vitro*. *J. Antimicrob. Chemother.*, **12**, 511
7. Furneri, P.M., Roccasalva, L., Fallica, L. and Tempera, G. (1988). Efficacy of miocamycin in the therapy of non-specific genital infections (NSG): non-gonococcal urethritis (NGU) and acute urethral syndrome (AUS). *Int. J. Pharm. Res.*, **8(2)**, 111
8. Yoder, B.L., Stamm, W.E., Koester, C.M. and Alexander, E.R. (1981). Microtest procedure for isolation of *Chlamydia trachomatis*. *J. Clin. Microbiol.*, **13**, 1036
9. Torode, H.W., McPetrie, R.A., Wheeler, P.A., Medcaif, S.C., Sounders, D.M. and Ackerman, V.P. (1987). The role of chlamydial antibodies in an *in vitro* fertilization program. *Fertil. Steril.*, **48**, 987
10. Edwards, R.G. (1982). Discussion on the fertilization of human oocytes *in vivo* and *in vitro*. In Edwards, R.G. and Purdy, J.M. (eds) *Human Conception in Vitro*, p. 196. (Academic Press: London)
11. Schaeffer, A.J., Wendel, E.F., Dunn, J.K. and Graychack, J.T. (1981). Prevalence and significance of prostatic inflammation. *J. Urol.*, **125**, 215
12. Berger, R.E., Karp, L.E., Williamson, R.A., Koehler, J., Moore, D.E. and Holmes, K.K. (1982). The relationship of pyospermia and seminal fluid bacteriology to sperm function as reflected in the sperm penetration assay. *Fertil. Steril.*, **37**, 557
13. Oriel, J.D. and Ridgway, G.L. (1982). *Genital infection by* Chlamydia trachomatis, (Edward Arnold: London)

Section 3

Obstetrics

Part A

Early pregnancy

45

α-Fetoprotein, chorionic gonadotropin and biopsy of the chorionic villi

C. Pullé, G. Baviera, N. Carlo Stella, F. Corrado, O. Triolo and C. Dugo

INTRODUCTION

The prenatal diagnosis of chromosomal alterations, carried out on couples at risk, permits the individualization of affected subjects but only in a relatively low percentage of cases. Therefore, the need was felt to discover other parameters of screening to support those already ascertained (the mother's age, previous child affected, balanced parental translocation) so as to be able to enlarge the basis of the population at risk that should undergo the study. Among the parameters proposed up to now the dosage of α-fetoprotein (αFP) plays a prominent role. The first author to hypothesize a correlation between maternal serum levels of αFP and eventual fetal autosomal trisomies was Merkatz[1]. The relative observation of a 'case report', later supported by a survey, referred to the possibility that low αFP levels could represent a further prenatal screening method of chromosomal alterations. Later, other authors confirmed such an observation, basing themselves on personal survey[2,3] until combined tables of autosomal trisomy risk with the mother's age and serum α levels were elaborated[4]. Such an observation, verified in the serum obtained from patients between the 14th and 20th weeks of pregnancy whose diagnosis had been carried out by means of amniocentesis, was later reported in earlier pregnancies (9th to 12th weeks) of patients who underwent chorionic villus sampling[5–7] and the correlation was confirmed. An analogous attempt to correlate a variation of serum human chorionic gonadotropin (hCG) levels to the pregnancies with the fetus affected by chromosomal alteration, has not given definite results up to now, even if a correlation with the high levels of the hormone in circulation seems to be present when the determination is carried out from the 18th to 25th weeks of pregnancy[8].

On the basis of such studies and in consideration of the disagreement of data, our prenatal diagnosis center has also undertaken analogous experience in subjects who have undergone a chorionic villus biopsy.

MATERIAL AND METHODS

The study was carried out on 136 women who requested prenatal diagnosis on account of advanced age (>39 years). Those subjects who underwent biopsy for chorionic villi for a different reason were not considered. The period of pregnancy covered between 9 and 12 weeks and the sampling was carried out using a transcervical approach with a Portex catheter and continuous ultrasound guidance. The hCG and the αFP determinations were performed before and after biopsy. A first sample of venous blood (5 ml) was taken 15 min before the biopsy and the serum was separated within an hour and preserved at −20°C until the analytic determination.

In order to evaluate the best time to take the second postbioptic sample to have the highest variation of the secretion of the two substances, another sample of blood was taken at 0.5, 1, 2, 4, 6 and 18 h after the chorionic villus sampling in 19 patients. The αFP secretion in these patients was later evaluated at 16–18 weeks, a period in which the screening for neural tube defects is carried out. So as to be able to interpret the results obtained at various periods of pregnancy, we preferred to transform the units obtained into multiples of median (MoM). This form of expression of the data obtained, proposed for the first time in an English collaborative study[9] permits an interpretation of universally accepted results.

After the results obtained in the first 19 patients, a successive sample of blood was taken in all the others 2–4 h after the villus sampling and the αFP concentration in the serum, preserved at −20°C together with the sample obtained before the intervention, was determined. The αFP responses obtained after the biopsy were classified, in agreement with the work of Brambati[5], into four groups: from 0 to 19%; from 20 to 49%; from 50 to 99%; and ⩾100%. The αFP determination[10] and that of hCG[11] were carried out with the immunofluorescent monoclonal antibody technique.

RESULTS AND DISCUSSION

In 136 examined women five autosomal trisomies have been observed (two Down syndromes, two Edwards syndromes, one Patau syndrome).

On examining the other 131 patients in the various periods of pregnancy (9th–12th weeks) and reporting the results with the MoM, we have met with a distribution of hCG values between 0.25 and 2.5 MoM. In three of the five pregnancies with a fetus with aneuploidies, the hCG levels were 2.5 MoM higher. In a case with trisomy 21 the hCG levels were within 2 MoM, while a in case of trisomy 18 they were under 0.5 MoM (Figure 1). As outside pregnancy dosable αFP levels can be met with so as to be able to evaluate the interference of same during the first trimester of pregnancy we have compared the αFP values encountered in the 131 control subjects at various weeks of pregnancy with those obtained from 64 non-pregnant women between 35 and 45 years old. It can be deduced from Figure 2 that the difference of αFP levels is significant only at the 10th, 11th, and 12th weeks while in the 9th week the results, though different, are not statistically significant compared with those encountered in non-pregnant women.

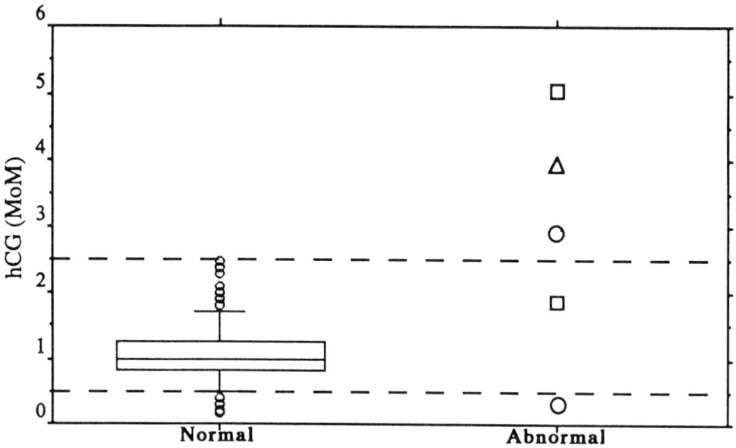

Figure 1 hCG multiples of median (MoM) from normal (131) and chromosomally abnormal pregnancies (trisomy 21 (□), trisomy 18 (○), trisomy 13 (△))

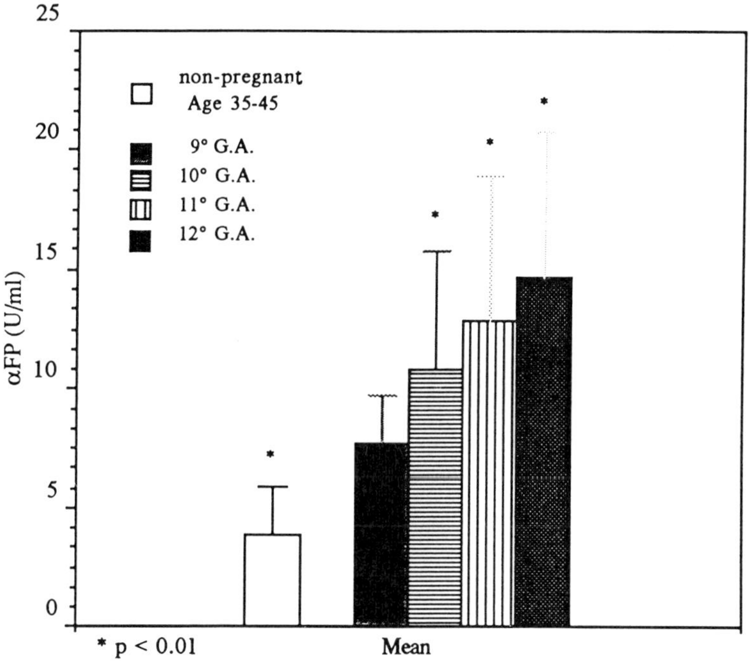

Figure 2 AFP values (U/ml) in non-pregnant women (64) and in women during first trimester of pregnancy (131)

The analysis of αFP data normalized with the determination of median at various weeks of pregnancy shows levels lower than 0.5 MoM in two of the five patients. In one of these cases with trisomy 21 hCG levels within the 2 MoM were present at the same time; in the case with trisomy 13, on the contrary, the hCG levels were higher than 2.5 MoM.

As regards the other three subjects with chromosomal alterations and specifically two with trisomy 18 and one with trisomy 21 levels between 0.5 and 1.5 MoM were encountered (Figure 3). These results have pointed out, analogously to what other authors[3] have shown, low αFP levels only in two of the five subjects with chromosomal aberration.

The high hCG levels (>2.5 MoM) in three of the five subjects with trisomy would point out a higher percentage of subjects affected analogously to what was observed by others in a later period[8]. In our experience the association of the two parameters is positive in four cases out of five, however, in our opinion, it would increase in a limited way the risk of autosomal trisomy to the population at risk.

Besides, we have analyzed the behavior of αFP and of hCG after the chorionic villus biopsy.

From a preliminary study on 19 cases an increase of the αFP levels has been noticed in all the subjects who have undergone biopsy, while the hCG concentration has shown a tendency towards a decrease in most cases. However, the hCG variation was so slight that is was not possible to evaluate a moment of excellent sampling to be able to study this behavior. In the case of αFP, instead (Figure 4) it is deduced that the highest frequency of maximal increase is verified between 2 and 4 h even if the levels are still high at 18 h. In the light of these data the αFP behavior in all other subjects has been studied taking the sample from 2 to 4 h after the villus sampling. From the analysis of the results obtained it is deduced that the chorionic villus biopsy increases the serum αFP level. However, only 27.5% (36/131) of the

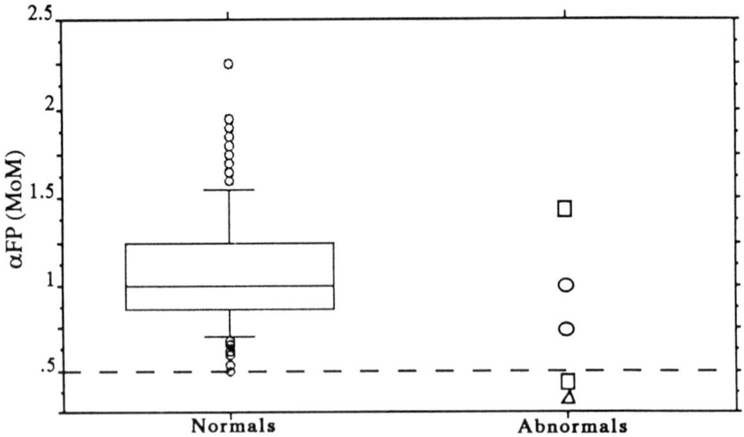

Figure 3 AFP multiples of median (MoM) distribution from normal (131) and chromosomally abnormal pregnancies (trisomy 21 (□), trisomy 18 (○), trisomy 13 (△))

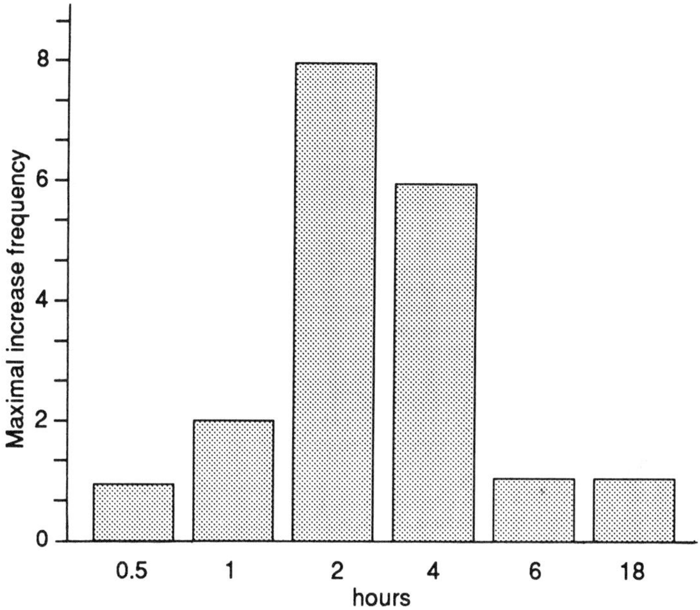

Figure 4 Frequency of maximal increase (hours) in 19 patients after CVS

subjects have shown an increase superior to 100%. With the increase of the percentage to 39.7% (52/131) if we assume as a base a rise of the levels as 50% (Figure 5).

Besides the increase of the αFP levels has been evaluated in respect to the quantity of trophoblast taken and to the number of insertions of the cannula. The αFP increase has been noticed with the number of insertions.

In order to be able to evaluate whether the increase of the αFP levels continues in time or whether it is a transitory event connected with the biopsy we have evaluated the αFP secretion at 16–18 weeks, a period in which the screening for the neural tube defects is carried out. The comparison between the αFP levels in pregnancies that have undergone a CVS and a group of control patients (84) aged between 21 and 44 has not shown any significant differences.

We have also tried to establish whether the elevated increase of αFP (≧100%) encountered in some patients could be correlated with a higher percentage of miscarriages. The absence of correlation in some women (32/36) who presented an increase of αFP ≧100% (Figure 6) makes us believe that such an increase does not influence the outcome of pregnancy.

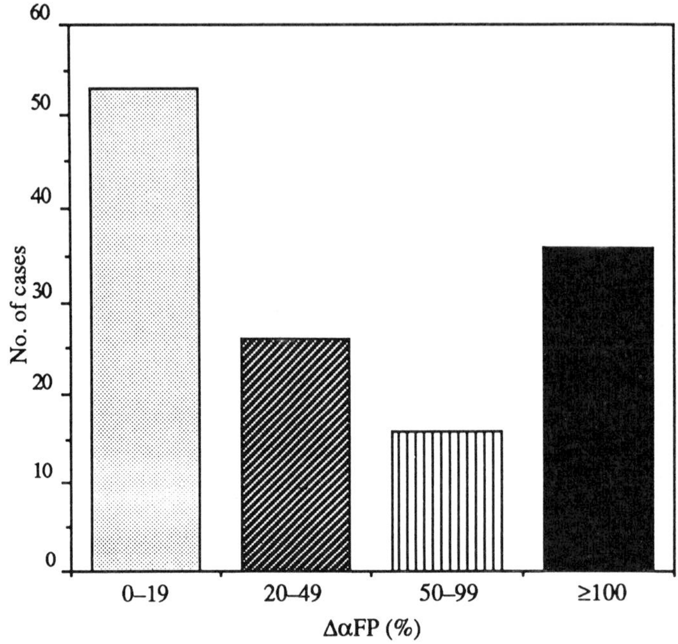

Figure 5 Incidence of increased maternal serum AFP concentration following CVS

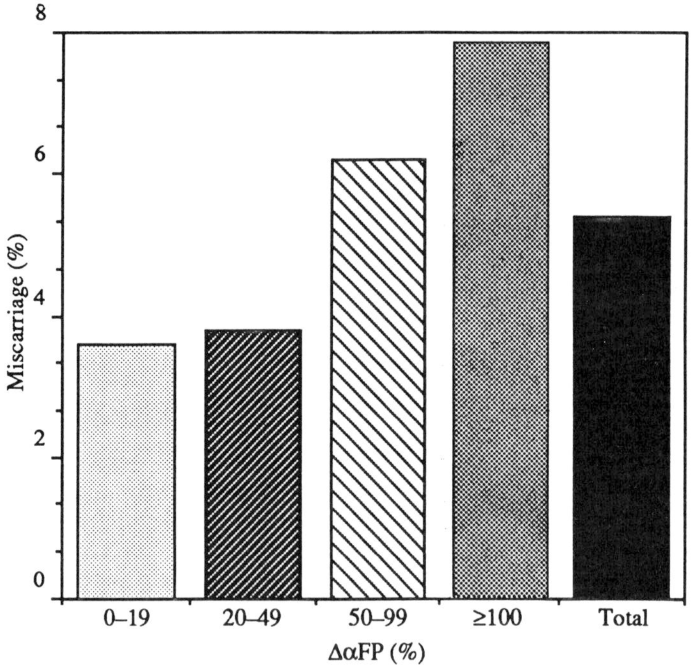

Figure 6 Relationship between increase of maternal serum AFP after CVS and the frequency of miscarriage in 131 cases

CONCLUSIONS

The data in our possession, even if from a rather exiguous survey and not permitting us to draw any definite conclusions, allow us to make some considerations. The hCG and the αFP determinations after chorionic villus sampling point out that marked hCG variations do not exist, while an increase of αFP levels, often significant, always exists. This mentioned increase seems to be in correlation with the quantity of villi taken but does not seem to be in relation to the greater number of miscarriages.

The αFP increase, re-entering the range of normality at 16–18 weeks, makes us presuppose that it is of a transitory nature connected probably to the alteration found in the seat of the sample taking and therefore it does not question the reliability of the determination of the above mentioned parameter at 16–18 weeks of pregnancy, a period in which screening for neural tube defects is carried out.

The determinations of the above mentioned parameters if carried out in the population at risk increase the possibility of the observation of a chromosomal alteration. It would be desirable to enlarge the combined evaluation of such parameters to pregnant women within the first trimester of pregnancy so as to be able to point out the presence of potentially pathological data for selecting these patients to be sent for prenatal diagnosis.

REFERENCES

1. Merkatz, I.R., Nitowsky, H.M., Macri, J.N. and Johnson, W.E. (1984). An association between low maternal serum alpha-fetoprotein and fetal chromosomal abnormality. *Am. J. Obstet. Gynecol.*, **148**, 886
2. Cuckle, H.S., Waldn, J. and Lidenbaum, R.H. (1984). Maternal serum alphafetoprotein measurement: a screening test for Down syndrome. *Lancet*, **i**, 926
3. Doran, T.A., Cadesky, K., Wong, P.Y., Mastrogiacomo, C. and Capello, T. (1986). Maternal serum alphafetoprotein and fetal autosomal trisomies. *Am. J. Obstet. Gynecol.*, **154**, 277
4. Palomaki, G.E. and Haddow, J.E. (1987). Maternal serum alphafetoprotein, age and Down syndrome risk. *Am. J. Obstet. Gynecol.*, **156**, 460
5. Brambati, B., Guercilena, S., Bonacchi, I., Oldrini, A., Lanzani, A. and Piceni, L. (1986). Fetomaternal transfusion after chorionic villus sampling: clinical implications. *Hum. Reprod.*, **1**, 37–40
6. Barkai, G., Shaki, R., Pariente, C. and Goldman, B. (1987). First trimester alpha-fetoprotein in normal and chromosomally abnormal pregnancies. *Lancet*, **ii**, 389
7. Jones, S.R., Evans, S.E., MacKenzie, W.E. and Hodgkins, P. (1988). First trimester alpha-fetoprotein levels and fetal chromosomal aneuploidies. *Lancet*, **i**, 826–7
8. Bogart, M.H., Pandian, M.R. and Jones, O.W. (1987). Abnormal maternal serum chorionic gonadotropin levels in pregnancies with fetal chromosome abnormalities. *Pren. Diagn.*, **7**, 623
9. UK collaborative study on alpha-fetoprotein in relation to neural tube defects. (1977) Maternal serum alpha-fetoprotein measurement in antenatal screening for anencephaly and spina bifida in early pregnancy. *Lancet*, **i**, 1323
10. Suonpaa, M.U., Lavi, J.T., Hemila, J.A. and Lovgren, T. (1985). A new sensitive assay of human alpha-fetoprotein using time-resolved fluorescence and monoclonal antibodies. *Clin. Chim. Acta*, **145**, 341–8
11. Petterson, K., Siitari, H., Hemila, I., Soini, E., Lovgren, T., Hanninen, V., Tanner, P. and Stenman, U.-H. (1983). Time-resolved fluoroimmunoassay of human choriogonadotropin. *Clin Chem.*, **29**, 60–4

46

New trends in prenatal diagnosis and fetal monitoring in the first trimester

B. Brambati, A. Lanzani, I. Bonacchi and L. Tului

INTRODUCTION

First trimester is still considered a black-box where fundamental questions are waiting to be answered and the outcome is frequently known in terms of embryo or fetal death. There is increasing evidence that 10–20% of clinically recognized pregnancies end in abortion, and the rate of loss is strongly related to advancing maternal age[1].

Chromosomal aberrations have been accounted responsible for up to 80% of clinical abortions before the 8th week[2], and are the only ascertained causes, together with severe structural abnormalities (e.g. neural tube defects) found in excess in aborted fetuses[3]. For several other factors, e.g. endocrine and neurological status of the mother, causal relationships with pregnancy failure are not well established.

Chorionic villus sampling (CVS) together with high resolution ultrasound and new biochemical markers, i.e. α-fetoprotein (αFP), pregnancy-associated plasma protein A (PAPP-A), and unconjugated estriol (uE_3) were recently reported[4,5] to be very promising tools for investigating the earliest stages of pregnancy (Table 1).

METHODS

The study was performed on 3968 pregnant women referred to our Prenatal Clinic for fetal diagnosis by CVS. Ultrasound investigation and maternal

Table 1 Possibilities of early detection of embryo-fetal anomalies

Method	*Abnormal conditions*
CVS	Genetic diseases
Ultrasound	Malformations
	Growth retardation
α-Fetoprotein + unconjugated estriol	Screening of aneuploidies
Pregnancy-associated plasma protein A + α-fetoprotein + ultrasound (crown–rump length)	Imminent conceptus death

blood sampling were performed at the same time as genetic counseling and just before CVS.

For sonographic embryo biometry and morphological study a 5 MHz sector scanner (ATL MK300) and a 6.5 MHz transvaginal probe (Ansaldo AU440) have been used.

CVS was obtained by aspiration using either transcervical Portex catheter or transabdominal 20G spinal needle, as previously described[6].

PAPP-A was evaluated by radioimmunoassay in collaboration with Professor J. G. Grudzinskas, The London Hospital, London[4].

RESULTS AND DISCUSSION

Ultrasonography provides fundamental information on the viability of the conceptus by detecting heart activity from the 6th week of gestation. Spontaneous fetal death rate was evaluated by serial ultrasound checks in a series of 2427 cases referred to us between 6 and 8 weeks (Table 2). Missed abortion was diagnosed at the first control in 200 cases (12%) by failure to detect heart activity or any embryo pole in a gestational sac of 5 ml or more. The remaining patients with a viable pregnancy were checked once again between 9 and 11 weeks just before undergoing CVS, and fetal death was recognized in 4.4% of them. Moreover, fetal loss rate showed a significant increase with advancing maternal age (Table 3).

Estimation of fetal wastage due to chromosome abnormalities was attempted by direct karyotyping of the chorionic tissue obtained at the evacuation of the uterine cavity in 35% of cases of retained abortion[7]. The

Table 2 Chromosomal abnormalities in 2427 pregnancies referred for CVS

Population series	*Chromosomal aberrations*
200 missed abortion cases (12%) detected between 6 and 8 weeks	86.5%
106 missed abortion cases (4.4%) detected between 9 and 11 weeks before CVS	78.9%
2027 pregnancies undergoing CVS and still viable at the time of the result	2.9%

Table 3 Spontaneous abortion rate in the first trimester before chorionic villus sampling divided by maternal age

Maternal age (yr)	*Total number of cases*	*Abortion cases*		
≤30	333	18	5.4%	NS
31–35	374	28	8.1%	$p < 0.005$
36–40	1351	178	15.2%	$p < 0.001$
>40	672	145	27.5%	
Total	2730	369	15.8%	

very high percentage of cases in which an abnormal chromosomal constitution was found in the early abortion series is in striking contrast with the low rate found in the population undergoing CVS, and confirms the primary importance of this factor in pregnancy failure (Table 3).

Crown–rump length (CRL) measurement is currently used in the first trimester to estimate gestational age. Therefore in women with menses at regular intervals and thus a reliable date for their last menstrual period CRL should be considered a sensitive tool to detect abnormal intrauterine growth. By this criteria CRL was measured in a series of 92 viable embryos dying days or weeks later, and compared to the normal limits (Table 4 and Figure 1). The sensitivity and specificity of CRL to detect cases at risk of early fetal

Table 4 Value of first trimester crown–rump length (CRL) measurement in predicting first trimester abortion

CRL	*No. of abortions*	*No. of normal pregnancies*	*Total no. of cases*
≤5th centile	60	105	165
>5th centile	32	1995	2027
Total	92	2100	2192
Sensitivity	65.2%		
Specificity	95.0%		
Predictive value of CRL ≤5th centile		36.36%	
Predictive value of CRL >5th centile		98.40%	
Relative risk of CRL ≤5th centile		23	

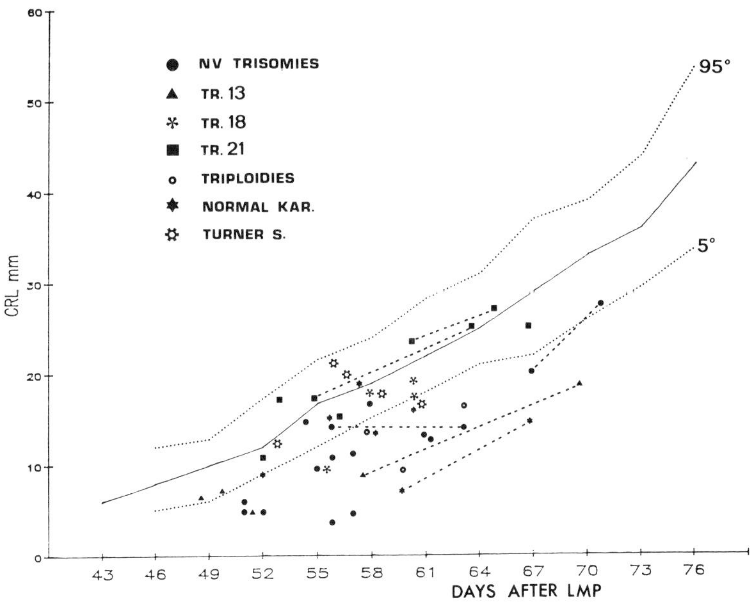

Figure 1 Distribution of crown–rump length (CRL) measurements in cases later ending in spontaneous abortion

death was 65.2% and 95.0%, respectively, and the predictive value of a positive test was 36.3%. Moreover, the percentage of low CRL values increased significantly in respect to the whole series of missed abortion cases (30.3%) when only the aneuploidic embryo group was considered (61%). These findings would suggest that an abnormally low CRL measurement in the first trimester is most likely to predict imminent death of the conceptus, together with a high possibility of chromosomal abnormality.

Several biochemical markers have been used in the past to predict the evolution of early gestation, but with very poor success, mainly because of lack of correlation with fetal heart activity. However, recently PAPP-A, a large glycoprotein produced by the trophoblast, and detectable in the maternal blood after about 30 days post-ovulation, was reported to be of prognostic value in threatened abortion cases. In 167 unthreatened cases PAPP-A was evaluated in maternal blood when embryo heart activity was evident. Levels below 0.6 multiple of the median were found in 81% of the 37 cases in which fetal death was detected days or weeks later (Figure 2).

Although the value of maternal serum PAPP-A levels and CRL measurements to predict early pregnancy failure need to be further defined in large perspective studies, their clinical use is advisable to obtain a rough and quick prognostic estimate of the gestation.

Chorionic tissue can now be sampled after the 6th week of gestation by transcervical catheter or transabdominal fine needle aspiration under direct

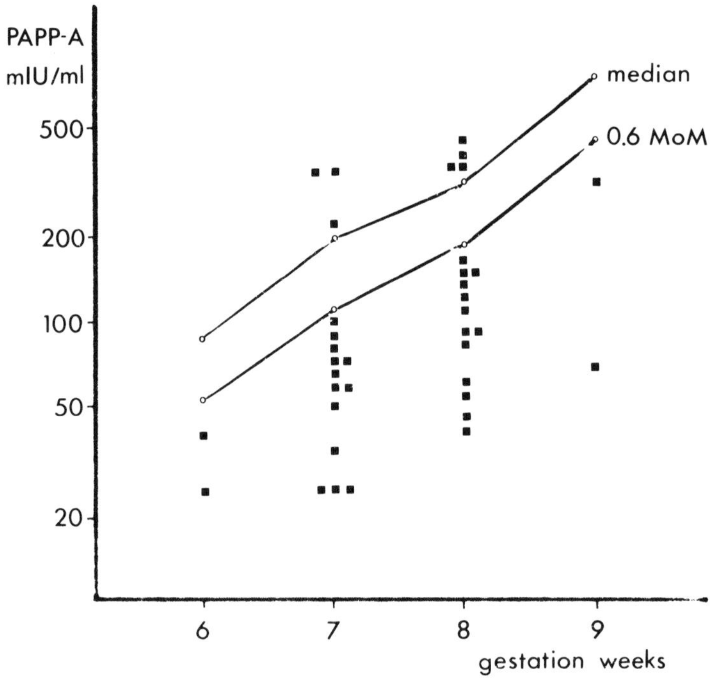

Figure 2 PAPP-A levels in maternal serum in cases later ending in spontaneous abortion

guidance of high resolution ultrasound. Because of its precocity, accuracy and safety first trimester CVS has become the method of choice to diagnose genetic diseases. Since its introduction in clinical routine in 1983, CVS has been performed in more than 100 000 cases by diagnostic centers all over the world. About 14 000 CVS were performed by the European centers in 1987, and the number per year is rapidly increasing. Fetal loss risk has been evaluated comparing CVS and amniocentesis, and no significant differences were demonstrated between methods in both randomized and control case trials, recently concluded in Canada and in USA, respectively[8,9]. Moreover, so far no fetal or neonatal abnormal conditions were reported as causally related to chorionic tissue sample. Although the risk of chromosomal aberrations remains by far the most frequent indication for CVS (Table 5), the number of hereditary diseases diagnosable by direct or indirect DNA analysis is in continuous progress, and by the end of 1988 more than 40 of the most frequent and severe diseases had already been diagnosed. In addition, the recent advances in recombinant DNA technology (e.g. polymerase chain reaction), together with transabdominal fine needle chorionic tissue aspiration allow genetic diagnosis in the very early stages of the pregnancy, and it is expected in the near future to be possible even before blastocyst implantation.

Although first trimester imaging of fetal anatomy can be achieved with a 5 MHz abdominal ultrasound probe, screening for fetal anomalies is usually scheduled to take place after the 16th week. High-frequency transvaginal sonography has been reported as an efficient method to detect some of the gross developmental defects becoming visible in the 2nd and 3rd months of pregnancy (Table 6). Transvaginal scanning in the first trimester should be recommended in cases at risk of specific fetal anomalies, however its wide use for the general population may give the opportunity not only to detect embryo abnormalities but also to make a reliable diagnosis by offering CVS and rapid fetal karyotyping.

Table 5 Diagnostic indications for chorionic villus sampling in 3468 cases from the Mangiagalli Clinic

Chromosomal abnormalities	91.6%
Fetal sexing	2.4%
Inborn errors of metabolism	1.2%
DNA analysis*	4.8%

* for Duchenne and Becker muscular dystrophies, cystic fibrosis, congenital adrenal hyperplasia, thalassemia and hemophilia A and B

Table 6 Fetal abnormalities diagnosable in the first trimester by ultrasound

Anencephaly	Conjoined twins
Spina bifida	Vanishing twins
Encephalocele	Anembryonic sac
Omphalocele	Fetal death
Cystic hygroma	Growth retardation

ACKNOWLEDGEMENT

This work was partially supported by a grant from Associazione Italiana Studio Malformazioni, Milano, Italy.

REFERENCES

1. Miller, J.F., Williamson, E., Glue, J., Gordon, Y.B., Grudzinskas, J.G. and Sykes, A. (1980). Fetal loss after implantation. *Lancet*, **ii**, 554–6
2. Guerneri, S., Bettio, D., Simoni, G., Brambati, B., Lanzani, A. and Fraccaro, M. (1987). Prevalence and distribution of chromosome abnormalities in a sample of first trimester internal abortions. *Hum. Reprod.*, **2**, 735–9
3. Fantel, A.G., Shepard, T.H., Vadheim-Roth, C., Stephens, T.D. and Coleman, C. (1980). Embryonic and fetal phenotypes: prevalence and other associated factors in a large study of spontaneous abortion. In Potter, I.H. and Hook, E.B. (eds), *Human Embryonic and Fetal Death*, pp. 71–88. (London, New York: Academic Press)
4. Westergaard, J.G., Teisner, B., Sinosich, M.J., Madsen, L.T. and Grudzinskas, J.G. (1985). Does ultrasound examination render biochemical tests obsolete in the prediction of early pregnancy failure? *Br. J. Obstet. Gynaecol.*, **92**, 77–83
5. Cuckle, H.S., Wald, N.J., Barkaj, G., Fuhrmann, W., Altland, K., Brambati, B., Knight, G., Palomaki, G., Haddow, J.E. and Canick, J. (1988). First trimester biochemical screening for Down syndrome. *Lancet*, **ii**, 851–2
6. Brambati, B., Oldrini, A., Ferrazzi, E. and Lanzani, A. (1987). Chorionic villus sampling: an analysis of the obstetric experience of 1000 cases. *Prenat. Diagn.*, **7**, 157–69
7. Simoni, G., Brambati, B., Danesino, C., Rossella, A.F., Terzoli, G.L., Ferrari, M. and Fraccaro, M. (1983). Efficient direct chromosome analysis and enzyme determination from chorionic villi samples in the first trimester of pregnancy. *Hum. Genet.*, **63**, 349–57
8. Canadian Collaborative CVS-Amniocentesis Clinical Trial Group (1989). Multicentre randomised clinical trial of chorionic villus sampling and amniocentesis. *Lancet*, **i**, 1–6
9. Rhoads, G.G., Jackson, L.G., Schlesselman, S.E. *et al.* (1989). The safety and efficacy of chorionic villus sampling for early prenatal diagnosis of cytogenetic abnormalities. *N. Engl. J. Med.*, **320**, 609–17

47

Vaginal echoscopy in early pregnancy

G. Centini and F. M. Severi

INTRODUCTION

Endovaginal sonography can be profitably employed in the study of the first trimester of pregnancy thanks to the significant advancement this technique has recently undergone.

The first endovaginal probes were used about 20 years ago but were soon abandoned due to their poor technical features and the discomfort their difficult handling caused patients[1].

These limitations have been overcome in present probes whose dimensions are very small and whose exploration fields range from 60° to 180°[2,3]. Sonography was first applied in gynecology for follicle monitoring and oocyte withdrawal for artificial insemination[4,5], whereas it is presently employed to monitor the growth of a fertilized ovule until the 3rd month of pregnancy[6–9].

Endoscopy introduces the advantage of bringing the ultrasound source into contact with internal genital organs[10]. This removes the interference in ultrasound transmission which obesity and/or anatomical alteration of the expectant mother may cause yielding unreliable results, particularly during earliest pregnancy.

Due to the physical properties of ultrasounds, resolution power of the echograph linearly increases along with the ultrasonic emission frequency, whereas penetration in depth of ultrasounds decreases. As a result, vaginal endoscopes can work at high frequencies allowing clear, high resolution images, but their exploration field is limited to 10 cm depth[10–13]. Therefore, this technique can be fully exploited only during the first trimester of pregnancy, although it may still be useful in the following 6 months to locate the closest edge of the placenta, for example, or to visualize that part of the fetus next to the cervix.

Vaginal probing does not require filling up the bladder in order to remove intestinal ansae, thus, the immediate benefit to the patient who is spared the pelvic discomfort caused by a hyperdilated bladder. Moreover, the ovule is not compressed by outer agents and can be probed in its correct morphology and physiological position.

When patients are properly informed about the advantages of vaginal probing they approve of this technique without fear of possible discomfort;

a favorable atmosphere is a crucial element of this methodology.

And finally, endoscopy supplies gynecologists with images of higher quality[6–11,14] than those taken through transabdominal exploration even when the same ultrasound frequencies are employed.

We conducted a comparison between the two methods in order to verify whether the higher resolution achievable through endoscopy provides more accurate data than transabdominal probing. For this purpose, we monitored the first appearance of the embryo and its annexes (yolk sac, celomatic and amniotic cavities, umbilical cord, etc.) and plotted growth curves for the gestational sac, crown–rump length and the biparietal diameter.

MATERIALS AND METHODS

We employed a Siemens 'Sonoline SL2' echograph with mechanical sector scanning probes; the ultrasound frequencies were 3.5 and 5 MHz in transabdominal probing and ranged from 5 to 7.5 MHz in transvaginal probing. The scanning angle was 100°, the exploration field was 200° wide.

The population we tested consisted of 178 expectant mothers whom we examined on routine check-ups or for suspected pathologies during their first trimester of pregnancy (between the 4th and the 12th week). Out of this group we chose to follow 156 cases with known last menstruation date and no pathology and/or clinical symptomatology.

We performed both transabdominal and transvaginal single session probing for a direct comparison between the data taken by each technique. During endoscopic exploration, the patient assumed the gynecological position for a correct physiology; a condom guaranteed the transducer probe asepsis.

We performed the first 50 endoscopies on a partial bladder filling in order to localize the scanning planes, from then on, our examinations were conducted after a complete emptying of the bladder.

We personally performed all the examinations. The biometric parameters were determined calculating the average values of low scattered data.

The results were compared in terms of visualization, definition and biometry of gravidic structures such as gestational sac, embryo and relative annexes.

RESULTS

Our patients reported that endoscopies performed with either a moderately full or an empty bladder are equally acceptable. The elimination of the waiting time for complete bladder-filling was advantageous to both gynecologist and patient.

The earliest endovaginal observation of a gestational sac was possible after 4 weeks and 2 days of pregnancy. The gestational sac appeared as a highly echogenic ring with a diameter of 2 mm (Figure 1a). It was not aligned with the uterine cavity, presented an anechoic area in the center, a strong signal peak in the rear and was clearly visible against the surrounding myometrium[14]. We could observe the gestational sac in 12 patients out of 15 we examined between their 4th and 5th week of amenorrhea associated with a positive pregnancy test (Table 1). After the 5th week, we were able to identify the yolk sac, the embryo and to sound cardiac activity in almost all cases. From the 6th week on, embryonic vibrations were noticeable, starting with the 3–4 mm crown–rump length. After 7 to 8 weeks, we could visualize adipose tissue, amniotic sac, celomatic cavity and limb buds; we were also able to measure the cephalic pole (in the 8th week). In the 9–10th week, we could discern the movements of the arms and identify ribs and scapulae. After 11 to 12 weeks, cerebral ventricles and pelvic bones became clearly visible while the umbilical cord was still very voluminous for the presence of allantoic residues. Sometimes, at this stage, we could detect the gender of the fetus. This is difficult to do in the 10th week when genital buds are similar to male ones in both genders.

Early observation and accuracy

Endovaginal echoscopy allows for the observation of all the anatomic and functional structures of the embryo about a week earlier than transabdominal echoscopy.

A pregnancy diagnosis between the 4th and the 5th week was possible on 80% of cases (12 out of 15 patients) by means of transvaginal probing versus 20% of cases (three out of 15 patients) by means of transabdominal probing. In the 6th week, the diagnosis was possible on 100% cases by endoscopy versus 80% cases by traditional echoscopy. Likewise, in the 5th week, we detected embryo, cardiac activity, celomatic and amniotic cavities in 90% versus 50% cases. Finally, between the 5th and the 6th week, we visualized celomatic and amniotic cavities in 100% cases versus 50% only (Figure1*b–d*).

Moreover, the higher image definition achievable through endoscopy allowed for a more detailed analysis of the embryonic anatomy. We were thus able to detect malformations better and at an earlier stage than with traditional echoscopy.

Table 1 Time of observation of some anatomical structures by transvaginal echoscopy

Week	*Structure*
4th	Gestational sac
5th	Yolk sac, amniotic cavity, embryo, embryonic cardiac activity
6th	Embryonic vibrations
7th	Cephalic pole, limb buds
7–8th	Embryonic movements
8th	Embryonic adipose tissue, umbilical cord
10th	Cerebral ventricles, choroid plexi, face (orbits, ears, mouth movements), clavicle, limbs, ribs, stomach, perineum
12th	Specific embryo movements, pelvic bones, external genital organs, umbilical cord vessels, bladder, crystalline, spine

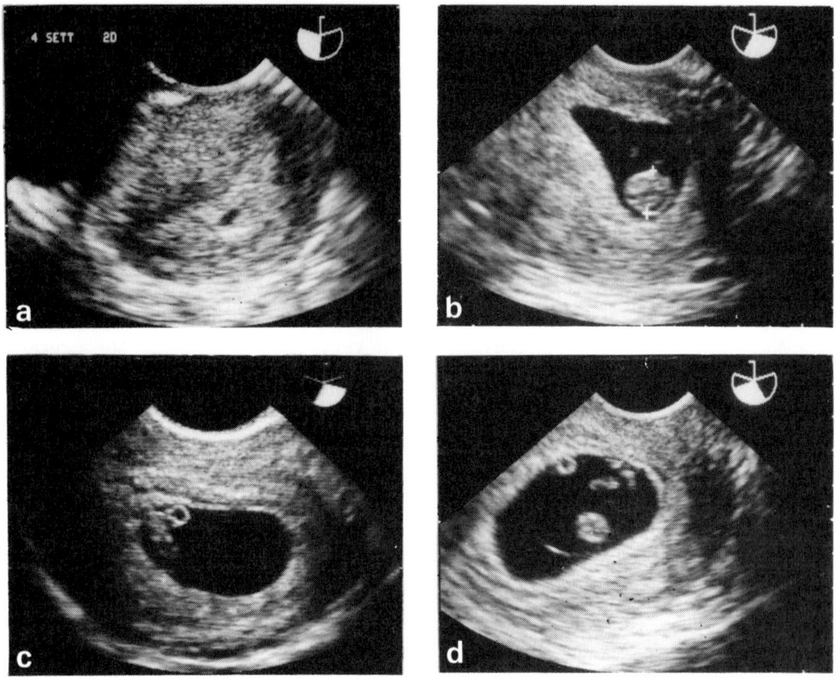

Figure 1 (*a*) The gestational sac in the 4th week: an asymmetrical hyperechogenic area with an anechoic region; (*b*) biparietal diameter in the 8th week; (*c*) yolk sac and embryo in the 6th week; (*d*) embryo yolk sac and amnios in the 7th week

Comparison between curves

Contrary to our expectations, the regression curves from transvaginal and transabdominal probing agree for all the structures we monitored: gestational sac, yolk sac, crown–rump length and biparietal diameter (Figures 2 and 3). Transabdominal measurements slightly overestimate transvaginal ones, still, the curves match almost perfectly.

The only curves which differ noticeably are those for the yolk sac growth: endoscopy shows an acme in the 10th week, followed by a quick and regular dimensional decrease until the 12th week (i.e. when amniotic and chorionic layers usually fuse together thus compressing the yolk sac). Transabdominal echoscopy, instead, shows an acme in the 9th week followed by a plateau, which is probably due to poor resolution.

Miscarriages

Eight of our 178 patients (4.5%) were diagnosed a miscarriage between the 6th and the 9th week. Such early diagnoses were possible by transvaginal sonography. In the 6th week, in four out of eight patients, we could clearly identify yolk sac, amniotic and celomatic cavities and the embryo lacking

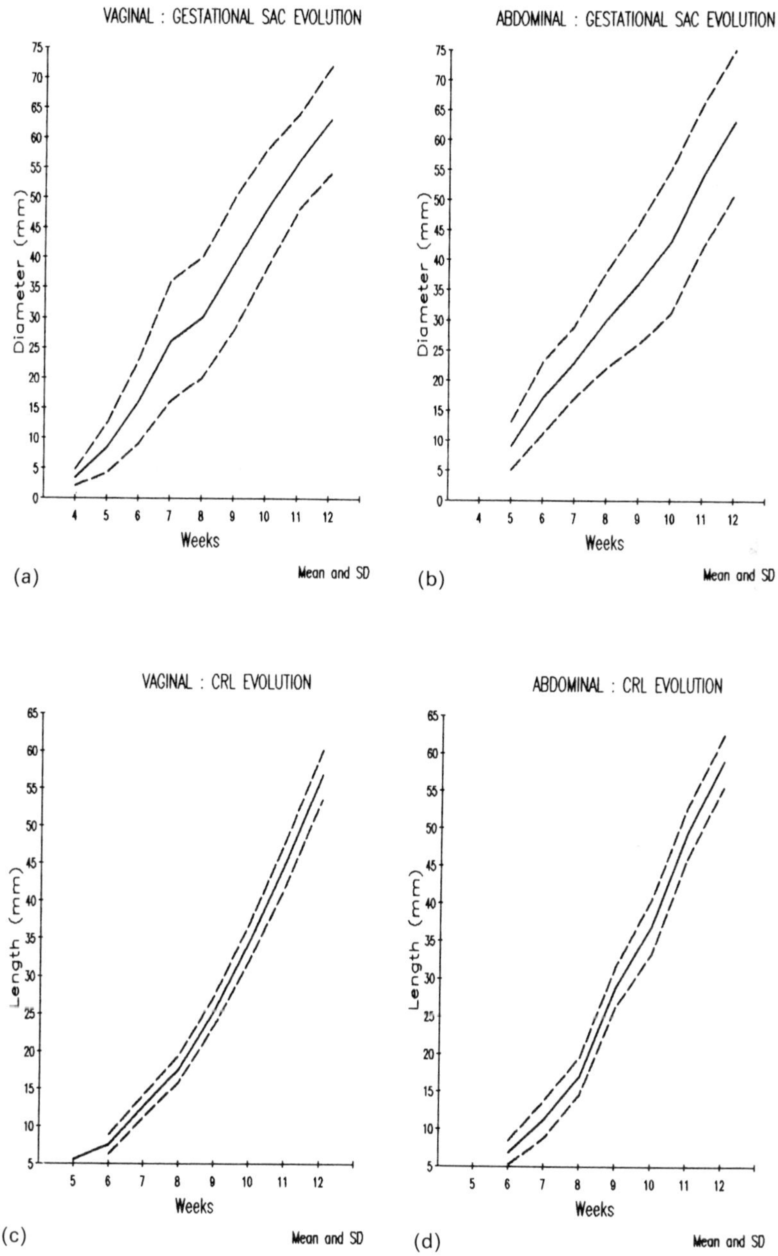

Figure 2 Comparison of mean $\pm$ SD values for gestational sac evolution (*a*, *b*) and crown–rump length (CRL) evolution (*c*, *d*) as measured by transvaginal (*a*, *c*) and transabdominal (*b*, *d*) echoscopy

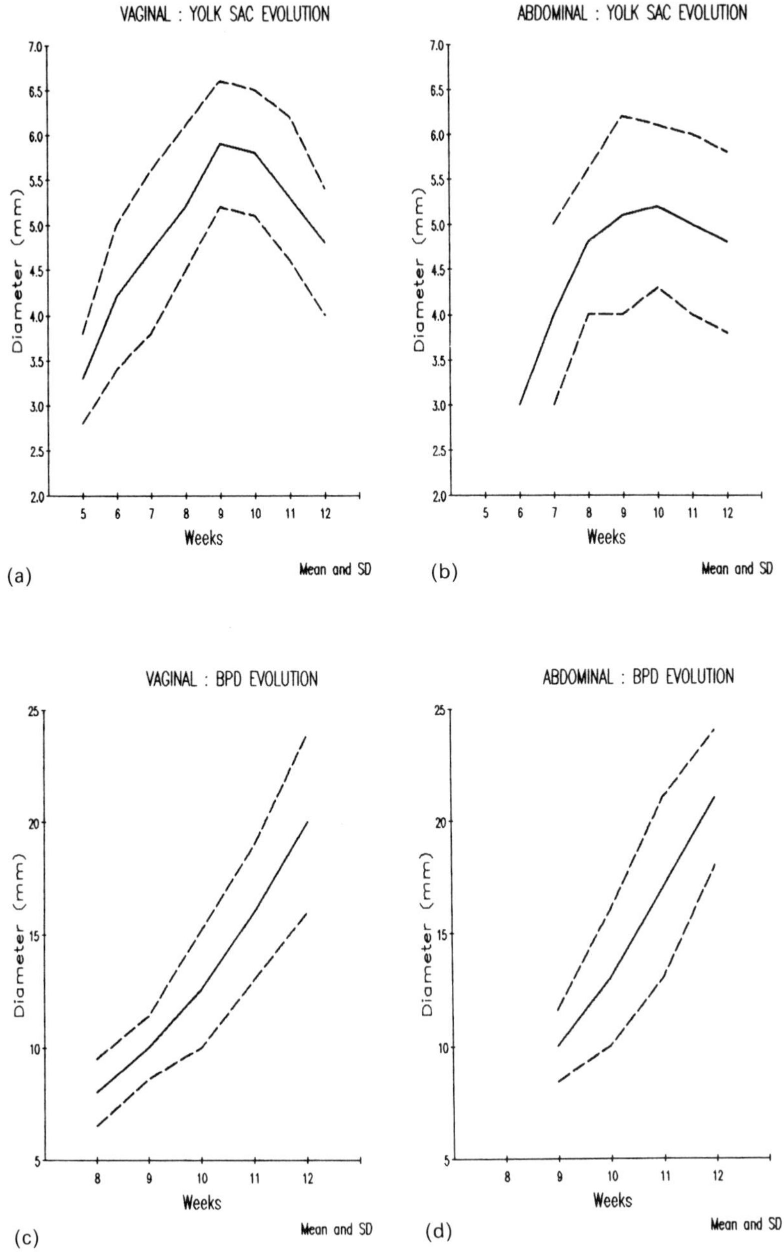

Figure 3 Comparison of mean ± SD values for yolk sac evolution (*a*, *b*) and biparietal diameter (BPD; *c*, *d*) as measured by transvaginal (*a*, *c*) and transabdominal (*b*, *d*) echoscopy

cardiac activity. Transabdominal sonography required further testing to diagnose miscarriage.

CONCLUSIONS

Our results are promising beyond all expectations: we registered an improved precision in all the parameters we analyzed by transvaginal sonography. The ratio of correct diagnoses was an astounding 92%; traditional echography matches the accuracy of endoscopy only in the measurement of biometric quantities.

This study, in line with many others, documents the fundamental improvement introduced by endoscopy: it brings the ultrasound source in proximity to the region of interest, so that higher frequency ultrasounds may be used. The cases in which endoscopy is recommended are shown in Table 2 and the characteristics of the method are listed in Table 3.

Endoscopy causes less discomfort than vaginal exploration and was soon accepted by our patients; we met with no refusals and very little hesitation. The authority and professionality of the gynecologist clearly play an important role with regard to this. Correct information, a favorable atmosphere and images of matchless quality are the crucial elements for the acceptance of endoscopy, which allows expectant mothers the joy of a perfect vision of their embryo.

This study verified that traditional transabdominal echography yields substantially correct information and deserves the importance it has in diagnostics. Still, endoscopy constitutes great progress in this field offering improved quality pictures and the possibility of an earlier observation of embryonic structures. These features are of the greatest importance in all pregnancy-related pathologies including abortions, malformations and extrauterine pregnancies. The use of endoscopy will bring immediate advan-

Table 2 Cases in which endoscopy is recommended

Adipose panniculus thicker than 1 cm
Retroversion of uterus
Early diagnosis of pregnancy
Early diagnosis of abortive pathology
Improved chorion visualization for biopsy
Previous cicatrixes
Pathology relative to the 1st trimester of pregnancy

Table 3 Characteristics of vaginal endoscopy

Gynecological position
Asepsis of transducer probe
Same discomfort as in a vaginal exploration
No dilated bladder
Higher frequency ultrasounds (5–10 MHz)
Exploration field limited to 8–10 cm
No compression of gestational sac

tages such as early diagnosis, reduced psychological and physical stress on women and a substantial reduction of social costs.

REFERENCES

1. Kratochwil, A. (1969). Ein neues vaginales ultraschall-schnittbildverfahren. *Geburtsh. Frauenheilk.*, **29**, 379
2. Mendelson, E.B., Bohm-Velez, M. and Joseph, N. (1988). Endometrial abnormalities: evaluation with transvaginal sonography. *Am. J. Radiol.*, **150**, 139
3. Timor-Tritsch, I.E. and Rottem, S.Y. (1987). Transvaginal ultrasonographic study of the fallopian tube. *Obstet. Gynecol.*, **70**, 424
4. Deutinger, J., Reinthaller, A. and Riss, P. (1987). Comparison of the results of vaginal and abdominal follicle scans. *Arch. Gynecol.*, **241**, 171
5. Kemeter, P. and Feichtinger, W. (1986). Trans-vaginal sector scan probe with an automated puncture device. *Hum. Reprod.*, **1**, 21
6. Bonilla-Musoles, M., Perez-Gil, R., Barron, V., Serra, G. and Pardo, F.J. (1988). Transvaginal ultrasound in the first trimester of pregnancy. *Riv. Ostet. Ginecol.*, **I**, 6, 247
7. Levi, S. (1988). Anatomie de la grossese debutante par echographie endovaginale. In Centini, G. and Severi, F.M. (eds). *Patologia dell'Accrescimento Fetale, Fisiopatologia dell'Ovulazione*, p. 5. (Rome: CIC Ed. Internaz)
8. Nardelli, G.B., Onnis, G.L., Siliotti, F. and Crocco, M. (1988). Impiego delle sonde vaginali in ostetricia. In Centini, G. and Severi, F.M. (eds). *Patologia dell'Accrescimento Fetale, Fisiopatologia dell'Ovulazione*, p. 769. (Rome: CIC Ed. Internaz)
9. Urquharty, D.R. and Fisk, N.M. (1988). Transvaginal ultrasound in suspected ectopic pregnancy. *Br. Med. J.*, **8**, 415
10. Timor-Tritsch, I.E. and Rottem, S. (1988). High-frequency transvaginal sonography: new diagnostic boom. *Contemp. Obstet. Gynecol.*, **31**, 111
11. Bernaschek, G., Rudelstorfer, R. and Csaicsich, P. (1988). Vaginal sonography versus human chorionic gonadotropin in early detection of pregnancy. *Am. J. Obstet. Gynecol.*, **158**, 608
12. Nyberg, D.A., Mack, L.A. and Jeffrey, R.B. Jr, (1987). Endovaginal sonographic evaluation of ectopic pregnancy a prospective study. *Am. J. Radiol.*, **149**, 1181
13. Timor-Tritsch, I.E., Bar-Yam, Y., Elgali, S. and Rottem, S. (1988). The technique of transvaginal sonography with use of a 6.5 MHz probe. *Am. J. Obstet. Gynecol.*, **158**, 1019
14. Yeh, H. and Rabinowitz, J.G. (1988). Amniotic sac development: ultrasound features of early pregnancy the double bleb sign. *Radiology*, **166**, 97

48

Immunological approach to recurrent pregnancy loss

A.E. Semprini, A. Vucetich, S. Garbo, C. Barbieri, A. Zanini, F. Ragusa, M. Costa, R. Sarli, C. Livi, M. Lovotti and S. Norchi

Recurrent miscarriage is defined as the consecutive loss of three pregnancies before the 20th week of gestation. This reproductive failure affects 1% of all fertile women and exceeds what is expected by statistical chance alone, suggesting that a mechanism other than prenatal selection of chromosomally abnormal embryos is involved. Viviparity in an immunocompetent host requires that the pregnant organism does not reject the implanted embryo, which is as a rule semiallogenic, deriving half of the genes from the father and half from the mother. This semi-isogeneity is not an essential prerequisite as is well shown from embryo transfer procedures in animals and man. Different specific etiologies can be found for recurrent pregnancy loss if they are correctly investigated. In our collaborative study (four university departments and one major referral hospital) we have examined 118 women with three early spontaneous abortions and no living child. In 20 patients clinical screening revealed a specific cause generating the reproductive failure: this is shown in Table 1.

The low percentage of patients with a clinical cause is possibly the result of the good quality of prereferral screening of the patients' own doctors. In all these cases a specific therapy has been discussed with the patients and results of treatment will be reported in the future. In our study all patients without a clinical cause underwent a complex immunological screening to evaluate whether there was an autoimmune basis generating the pregnancy loss or if maternal immunomodulation during early pregnancy was inadequate to allow embryo growth and survival. The immunological screening is

Table 1 Results of clinical screening in 118 patients with three or more recurrent pregnancy losses

Patients with a specific cause	20/118 (17%)
Müllerian anomaly	9/20 (45%)
Chromosomal anomaly	1/20 (5%)
Luteal phase deficit	5/20 (25%)
Diabetes	1/20 (5%)
Genital infection	4/20 (20%)

represented in Table 2. Ten women showed an abnormal autoimmune and coagulatory profile: three women had elevated levels of antinuclear antibodies, and seven had an elevated KCT ratio indicating the presence of anticoagulant activity. These women were not further investigated and immunosuppressive and anticoagulant treatment was recommended in the next pregnancy. Eighty-eight couples were screened by histocompatibility locus antigen (HLA) typing (results are not reported here) and modified mixed lymphocyte reaction to evaluate materno–paternal immune response in culture medium and in the woman's serum. Maternal response to unrelated control lymphocytes and specificity of blocking factors were also assessed. A standard National Institutes of Health cross-match was performed in all cases (results are not reported here). Couples with negative clinical and autoimmune screening, showing poor materno–paternal immunoreactivity and defective blocking activity were offered immunostimulation with paternal lymphocytes after careful screening of the husband for blood transmissible diseases. Pregnancy following immunostimulation was carefully followed and results are available in 10 couples who experienced a successful pregnancy and 10 couples who repeatedly aborted (Table 3).

The data presented show that patients with recurrent abortion who respond well to immunostimulation by paternal antigens and obtain a successful pregnancy clearly differentiate from women who repeatedly abort after receiving identical treatment. These preliminary results indicate that in the future there will be a need to define which couples with negative clinical, autoimmune and coagulatory screening will be helped by immunostimulation in correcting their abnormal immune response to the gestational antigenic stimulus and which couples will receive no benefit from this experimental therapeutic approach.

Table 2 Immunological screening in 98 couples with three or more pregnancy losses with a negative clinical screening

A Autoimmune and coagulatory screening of the women
Antinuclear, antimitochondrial, antismooth muscle antibodies, anticardiolipin antibodies IgG and IgM, C3 and C4, protein electrophoresis, IgA–IgM–IgG levels, apTT, KCT
B Immunogenetic screening of the couple
Histocompatibility locus antigen typing of the couple
C Maternal immune response to paternal antigens
Mixed lymphocyte reaction (MLR)
Titration of maternal blocking factors in MLR
Titration of maternal antipaternal lymphocytotoxic antibodies by microlymphotoxicity assay

Table 3 Materno–paternal immune response (as stimulation index) in mixed lymphocyte culture of 20 couples with recurrent miscarriage after maternal immunostimulation with paternal lymphocytes

	Pretreatment	*Post-treatment*	*Pregnant*
Aborted AB serum	11 ± 12	41 ± 38	28 ± 18
Delivered AB serum	46 ± 58	82 ± 81	13 ± 16
Aborted female serum	7 ± 11	17 ± 21	7 ± 7
Delivered female serum	35 ± 41	19 ± 20	3 ± 3

Section 3 continued

Part B

Use of Doppler in reproductive medicine

49

Biophysical profile, Doppler velocimetry and acid–base balance in growth-retarded fetuses

E. Ferrazzi, S. Della Peruta, M. Rodolfi, A. Barbera, G. Bulfoni and G. Pardi

INTRODUCTION

Prenatal assessment of fetal growth and wellbeing relies mainly on biophysical parameters provided by sonography (pattern of fetal growth, amniotic fluid volume, fetal movements) and fetal heart rate recordings. More recently Doppler velocimetric studies and transabdominal cord sampling have been introduced in prenatal diagnosis.

These new techniques are open to many controversies. The physiopathological meaning of Doppler waveform analysis is not yet generally accepted, its relative importance in the definition of fetal risk is still to be quantified. The timing of cordocentesis or even the clinical dropout of intrauterine biochemical information has only recently been addressed.

PATIENTS AND PROCEDURES

We report our experience with a series of 23 growth-retarded fetuses diagnosed *in utero* by sonographic criteria. Cordocentesis was performed in these fetuses under ultrasound guidance. A reinjection of few millilitres of blood into the sampling site allowed verification of the venous site by means of the bubbling effect. This confirmation was established in 17 cases. In spite of the venous goal of the procedure the remaining six showed an arterial sampling site. This occurred among fetuses with oligohydramnios (two cases) and severe growth retardation (three cases below 800 g). Oxygen content (hemoglobin × oxygen saturation × 0.05982), Po_2, pH, Pco_2 and lactate concentration were determined[1].

A coaxial pulsed Doppler equipment was used in this series. Pulsatility Index (PI) was measured on hard copies by means of a computerized map measurer according to the simplified Gosling formula. Fifteen fetuses of this series were delivered before 35 weeks of gestation. Twenty-one fetuses were delivered by Caesarean section. Seventeen fetuses weighed below the 5th percentile. Three neonatal deaths occurred in this series, one fetus of 450 g died *in utero*.

In our clinical approach to this series of growth retarded fetuses, the combination of sonographic and cardiotocographic parameters can identify three groups with different degrees of prenatal risk.

RESULTS AND COMMENTS

Fetal oxygenation *in utero* was described by means of a gestational age independent parameter, i.e. oxygen content[2]. In Figure 1*a* the values of oxygen content are plotted for the three above-mentioned groups. Both venous and arterial samples are reported. Fetuses with abnormal Doppler velocimetric findings on the umbilical arteries are represented by full markers. As expected the O_2 content was consistently abnormal in Group 3 while Groups 1 and 2 were significantly different (Mann–Whitney U test: $p<0.06$). In Group 1 all four umbilical PI were normal. In Group 2, seven fetuses showed abnormal PIs and only one of these had O_2 content value above 6 mmol/l. Unfortunately, venous values decribe oxygenation before fetal oxygen consumption.

The same criteria were used to analyze the observed values of acid–base balance, i.e. $P\text{co}_2$, pH, and lactate concentration (Figure 1 *b–d*). Group 3 shows consistently the worst values for all these acid–base data, all these fetuses had abnormal PI values and non-reactive fetal heart rate tracings. This strong association of non-reactive heart rate tracings and acidosis must be taken into consideration in the timing of delivery of premature growth-retarded fetuses.

Venous findings of Group 1 and Group 2 were significantly different (Mann–Whitney U test: $p<0.006$, $p<0.006$, $p<0.06$). Full dots represent cases with abnormal PI data. Not all abnormal PI values were associated with fetal acidosis. However, acidemic conditions were not found in fetuses with normal PI values on the umbilical artery both in Group 1 and 2.

The most interesting clinical result is that fetuses in Group 2 took advantage from fetal blood sampling before the appearance of ominous signs on the fetal heart rate recordings. The clinical significance of umbilical waveform analysis lies in the fact that acidotic fetuses were found only among those with abnormal PI, whatsoever the other biophysical parameters. As a matter of fact the four acidotic fetuses of Group 2 ($P_{CO_2}>42$ mmHg, pH <7.34, lactate >1.8 mmol/l) had PI values on the umbilical artery above the 3rd standard deviation (about 1.6).

These data suggest that fetuses whose PI exceeds values of 1.5–2.0 could be reasonably and reliably investigated by means of intrauterine cord sampling for the assessment of fetal oxygenation and acid–base balance[3].

The evaluation of the PI of the middle cerebral artery can be of great help in improving the sensitivity of Doppler investigations. The correlation between lactate versus the PI of the middle cerebral artery was possible only in the last 10 fetuses of this series.

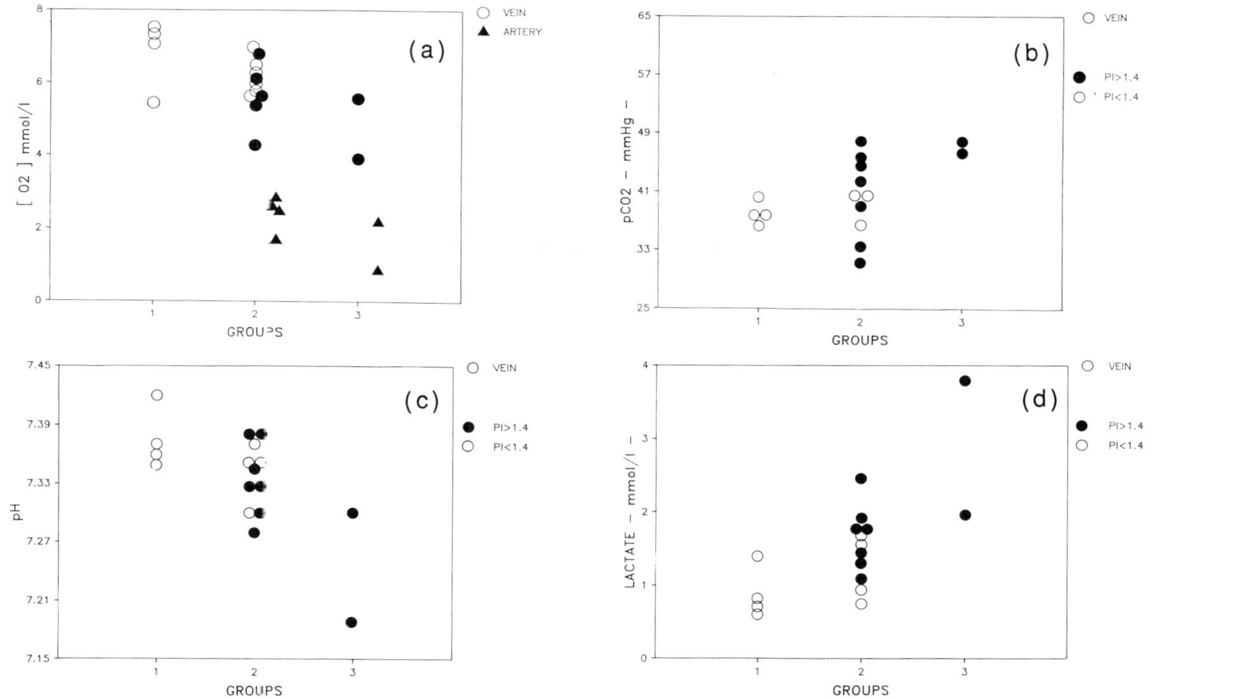

Figure 1 (*a*) Oxygen content values in fetal blood collected at cordocentesis for the three groups of fetuses. Open circles represent venous values, triangles represent arterial values. Solid circles represent fetuses with abnormal velocimetric findings on the umbilical artery. (*b*) P_{CO_2} values in fetal venous blood collected at cordocentesis for the three groups of fetuses. Solid circles represent fetuses with abnormal velocimetric findings on the umbilical artery (PI > 1.4). (*c*) pH values in venous fetal blood collected at cordocentesis for the three groups of fetuses. Solid circles represent fetuses with abnormal velocimetric findings on the umbilical artery (PI > 1.4). (*d*) Lactate concentration values in venous fetal blood collected at cordocentesis for the three groups of fetuses. Solid circles represent fetuses with abnormal velocimetric findings on the umbilical artery (PI > 1.4)

A significant linear regression was observed for lactate concentration ($p < 0.05$).

In conclusion our experience induces us to suggest a cordocentesis in those cases in which there is the coexistence of an abnormal PI with other biophysical parameters which do not clearly indicate whether pregnancy should be allowed to continue or the fetus should be delivered before ominous signs appear on the heart rate tracings.

REFERENCES

1. Pardi, G., Buscaglia, M., Ferrazzi, E., Bozzetti, P., Marconi, A.M., Cetin, I., Battaglia, F.K. and Makowski, E.L. (1987). Cord sampling for the evaluation of oxygenation and acid-base balance in growth-retarded human fetus. *Am. J. Obstet. Gynecol.*, **157**, 1221
2. Bozzetti, B., Buscagli, M., Cetin, I., Marconi, A.M., Nicolini, U., Pardi, G., Makowski, E.L. and Battaglia, F.C. (1987). Respiratory gases, acid base balance and lactate concentration of the mid-term human fetus. *Biol. Neonate*, **51**, 188
3. Ferrazzi, E., Pardi, G., Buscaglia, M., Makowski, E.L. and Battaglia, F.K. (1988). The correlation of biochemical monitoring versus umbilical flow velocity measurements of the human fetus. *Am. J. Obstet. Gynecol.*, **159**, 1059

50

Doppler measurement of uterine blood flow in IVF

C. Battaglia, C. Steere, G. D'Ambrogio, A. Volpe and A.R. Genazzani

INTRODUCTION

There is a high percentage of couples who, after extensive investigations, have a diagnosis of unexplained infertility. Many explanations have been suggested. These include: tubal damage not detectable by the normal patency tests; luteinization of unruptured follicles; failure of fertilization/implantation. A possible further cause of infertility is a reduction of blood flow which prevents successful implantation of the blastocyst[1]. Inducing multiple follicular growth raises serum estrogens and as a consequence might increase uterine blood flow. It is now possible to investigate on this aspect of infertility using Doppler ultrasound which has the ability to study patterns of blood flow and identify functional changes.

Until a few years ago the use of this method for examination of flow in specific deep vessels has been difficult since continuous wave Doppler provided confusing signals from flow occurring anywhere along the length of the ultrasound beam[2]. The availability of the pulsed-Doppler machine has made it possible to sample signals at a chosen depth and thus to detect flow in any selected deep vessel[3]. Furthermore, the so-called Duplex system allows the precise localization of a deep vessel and the positioning of the Doppler sample within it[4]. The most recent development of Doppler ultrasound is the Color Imaging Doppler. With this the direction and the velocity of blood flow are displayed in color superimposed upon a real-time image[5]. The Doppler-shifted frequencies are conventionally represented with different colors. Thus the brighter shades of red represent faster velocities towards the transducer, whilst brighter shades of blue represent faster velocities away from the transducer. The identification of vessel position is not dependent upon ultrasound imaging but on the presence of movement within it. Smaller vessels which are hardly seen by B-mode ultrasound are thus seen in color as long as there is movement of blood within then. These techniques hitherto have been used to detect blood flow in medicine and obstetrics but their application in the study of pelvic blood has not yet been fully explored. The aim of this study is to quantify changes in uterine blood flow throughout the normal menstrual cycle and stimulated IVF cycle, to verify if it is possible to predict by the pulsatility index (PI) in midluteal phase those patients who will become pregnant[6].

PATIENTS AND METHODS

For this study we used: 3.5 MHz convex pulsed transducer (Ansaldo AU 940); 3.5 MHz pulsed color sector imaging (Acuson 128): 4 MHz pulsed color vaginal probe (Diasonic Vingmed CFM 700)[5]. The ascending branch of the uterine artery was visualized just lateral to the cervix by performing an oblique longitudinal abdominal scan. Distension of the bladder was needed so that the uterine fundus could be adequately visualized. Ten multiparous patients with a normal menstrual cycle of 26–30 days had a transabdominal scan on alternate days from the 7th day of the cycle up to the time of the ovulation was evidenced by the collapse of the leading follicle which was measured taking the average of three follicular diameters[7]. They were then scanned in the midluteal phase until the 25th day of the cycle. The second group was represented by 16 patients entered in the IVF program for tubal damage. This group was prescribed a stimulation regimen of clomiphene citrate (Clomid) 100 mg/day from day 3 to day 7 of the cycle of urofollithropin (Metrodin) 150 I.U./day from day 3 to day 5 of the cycle both associated with Pergonal ampoules in a quantity depending on past IVF attempts and reaction to initial stimulation. The Doppler scan was performed on days 7, 10, 12, 13, 18, 20, 25 and 27 of the cycle. On the first 4 days of the scans blood was taken for the measurement of serum estradiol. The analysis of flow velocity waveform (FVW) was performed using the pulsatility index (PI: $a - b/\bar{x}$)[8] which is an expression of impedance and enables the assessment of changes in flow patterns when there is no diastolic component.

RESULTS

In the first group we obtained a decrease of PI from day 7 (PI 4.43 $\pm$ 1.02) up to day 13 (2.34 $\pm$ 0.32) (Figure 1*a*). On day 14 we had a smooth increase of PI (2.77 $\pm$ 0.5) which up to the midluteal phase was stable and after grew up to 4.88 $\pm$ 1.0 in the perimenstrual period. While this is in accordance with the estradiol variation in the follicular phase up to the periovulatory drop, we obtained discordant results from Goswamy[9] because we did not note any decrease of PI in the luteal phase. On the contrary we found a slight progressive decrease of the PI from 5.27 $\pm$ 1.04 on day 7 to 3.4 $\pm$ 0.8 on day 13 of 10 I.U. Profasi administration (Figure 1*b*). The values were proportionally correlated with estradiol increase (Figure 1*c*). In correspondence with the pick up day we had a slight increase of PI (3.72 $\pm$ 0.78) which decreased until the late luteal phase (3.08 $\pm$ 0.94; Figure 1*b*). In two cases (Figure 1*d*) we had high values of PI (respectively of 8.20 $\pm$ 5.31 and 12.58 $\pm$ 4.52) in the follicular period (7th and 12th day) which associated with an estradiol value respectively of 156 and 318 pg/ml on day 12 of the cycle, caused us to suspend the stimulation program. In two other cases (Figure 1*d*), after embryo transfer (ET) we had a steep decrease of PI (respectively 2.53–2.38 and 2.34–2.27 on days 20 and 25 of the cycle). In these patients we had two chemical pregnancies with a positive serum β human chorionic gonadotropin test on the 12th day from ET. During the study we failed to obtain reproducibility of good values. We believed that this was due to the length of vessel imaged by transducer being extremely small and the imaging beam needing to be at a right angle to the vessel to visualize it[3]. These variables can be modified by scanning at different time intervals. Because of this we utilized color flow mapping which has the advantage that a vessel can be visualized at a low angle. Nevertheless the intraobserver error was not decreased but it was possible to note that excessive bladder distension gave consistent rise of PI. Then we performed Doppler analysis of the uterine artery in 10 patients in the late luteal phase comparing the values obtained with full bladder and after emptying of 300 cc of urine in a fractionated container. A significant PI difference of 0.61 ($p < 0.01$) was found in the two groups.

DISCUSSION

These data show that uterine flow response to spontaneous or induced hormonal changes can be assessed using a Doppler machine. Because we ascertained that the full bladder distorting pelvic anatomy is responsible for a higher PI and because it is well known that the closeness of pelvic structures to a scanner improves the image resolution, we are continuing with this study utilizing a color vaginal Doppler[4]. With vaginal color imaging of the uterine artery the vessel can be seen at an angle consistent with a near maximum Doppler frequency shift. It is thus possible to say with confidence which vessel is being studied and with a high color intensity there is no loss of FVW due to scanning at an angle to the vessel approaching the perpendicular. The Doppler signal obtained by placing the gate across the artery is potentially more reproducible than other systems in which the gate is placed blindly across the anatomical site of the vessel. The technique of obtaining the uterine FVW with a vaginal probe is to view the uterus longitudinally and from a view of the right side of the cervix the scanning angle is tilted until the ascending branch of the uterine artery is located as a blue pulsation along the lateral uterine border. A red coloration indicates flow towards the probe in the descending branch of the artery.

CONCLUSION

If the result obtained using the transabdominal approach is confirmed by the transvaginal Doppler analysis we will be able to identify the abnormal group and, by manipulating their hormonal levels, improve the uterine blood flow and thus chances of conception. Furthermore, Doppler ultrasound

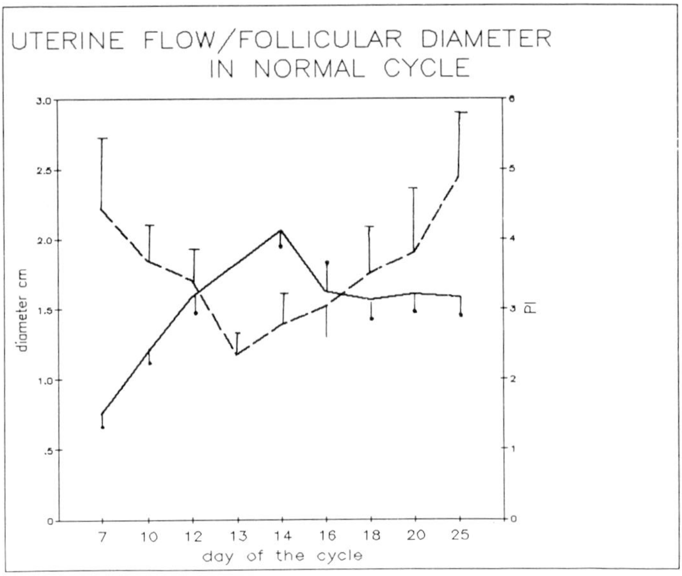

(*a*)

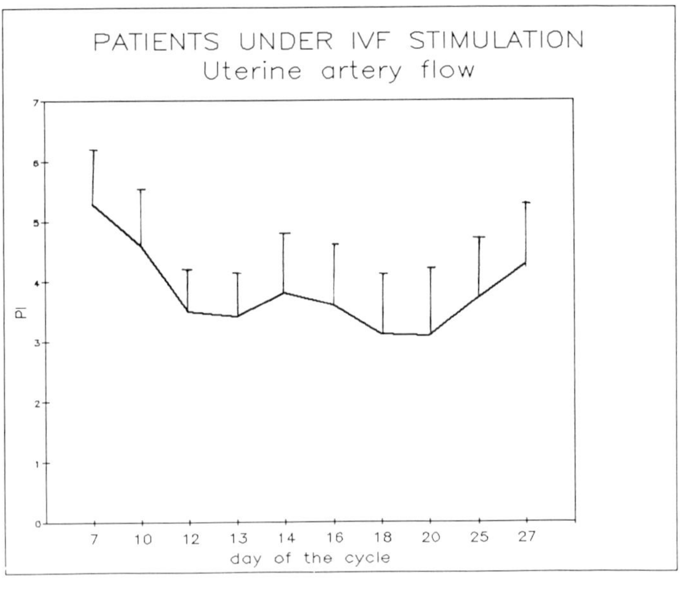

(*b*)

Figure 1 (*a*) Uterine flow (---) and follicular diameter (—) in normal cycle; (*b*) uterine artery flow in patients under IVF stimulation; (*c*) estradiol levels in patients under IVF stimulation;

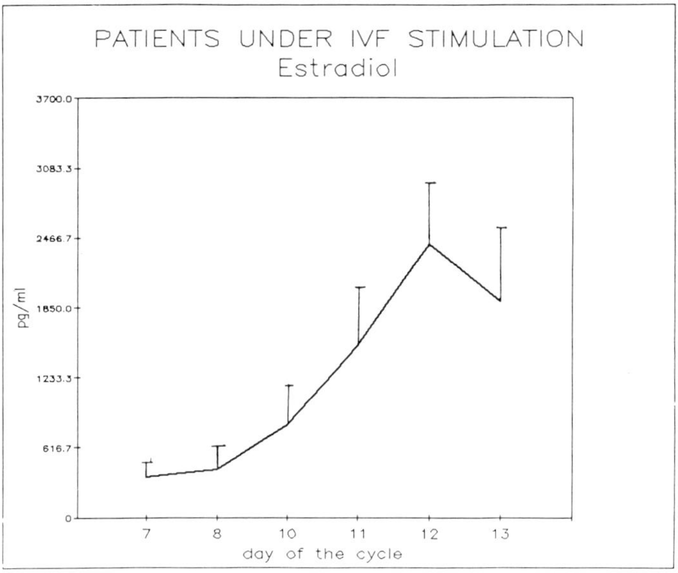

(*c*)

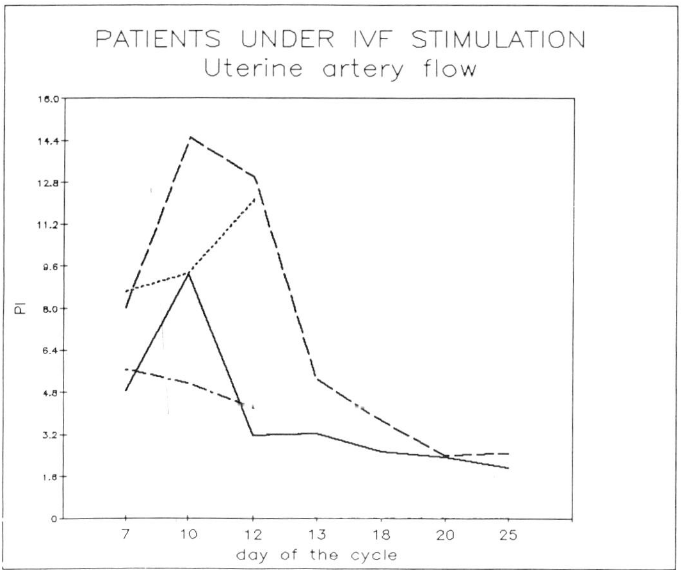

(*d*)

Figure 1 *continued* (*d*) uterine artery flow in patients with chemical pregnancies (– – – ——) and with suspension of IVF program (· · ·, – · –)

investigation may be of prognostic value in predicting pregnancy outcome for patients enrolled in an IVF program.

REFERENCES

1. Goswamy, R.K. and Steptoe, P.C. (1987). Abnormal uterine blood flow patterns – a possible cause for failed implantation in IVF patients? *Hum. Repr.*, **2**, (Suppl. 1), 56
2. Atkinson, P. and Woodcock, J.P. (1982). Doppler ultrasound and its use in clinical measurement, pp. 134–197, (London: Academic Press)
3. Kenneth, J.W., Taylor, M.D., Burns, P.N., Woodcock, J.P. and Wells, P.N.T. (1985). Blood flow in deep abdominal and pelvic vessels: Ultrasonic Pulsed-Doppler Analysis. *Radiology*, **154**, 487–93
4. Taylor, K.J.W., Burns, P.N., Wells, P.N.T., Conway, D.I. and Hull, G.R. (1985). Ultrasound Doppler flow studies of the ovarian and uterine arteries. *Br. J. Obstet. Gynaecol.*, **92**, 240–6
5. Steere, C.V. Transvaginal colour flow Doppler measurement of uterine and ovarian blood flow as related to hormone secretion in the menstrual cycle. (Unpublished data.)
6. McSweeney, M.B., Baber, R.G., Gill, R.W., Kossoff, G., Saunders, D., Porter, R. and Piker, R. (1988). Prediction of IVF and Gift outcome using transvaginal Doppler assessment of ovarian blood flow. *J. Ultrasound Med.*, **7**, S239–S283
7. William, G.M. and Ritchie, M.D. (1985). Ultrasound in the evaluation of normal and induced ovulation. *Fertil. Steril.*, **43**, (2)
8. Gosling, R.K. and King, D.M. (1985). Ultrasound Angiology. In Marcus, A.W. and Adamson, L. (eds). *Arteries and Veins*, pp. 289–310. (Edinburgh: Churchill Livingstone)
9. Goswamy, R.K. and Steptoe, P.C. (1988). Doppler ultrasound studies of the uterine artery in spontaneous ovarian cycles. *Hum. Repr.*, **3**, 721–6

51

Changes of fluximetric indices in pregnancy

C. Montoneri, G. Zarbo, M. Vasta and L. Lupo

INTRODUCTION

Studies on utero–placental, umbilical and fetal blood flow by means of Doppler velocimetry have raised new expectations in obstetric monitoring, since the fluximetric changes should anticipate the appearance of irreversible fetal damage by a number of weeks. So diagnosis should take place early in gestation allowing early, safe action[1–5].

However, a consensus has not been reached yet about the limits and clinical usefulness of this technique although the recently available color-Doppler equipment has increased interest in these studies[6].

The aims of the present report are to evaluate changes of the most usual fluximetric indices during pregnancy, to define the normal limits in the Sicilian population and to test diagnostic accuracy with respect to fetal hypoxia.

MATERIALS AND METHODS

A cross-sectional study was carried out on 179 pregnant women (Table 1): 159 were regarded as normal and 20 as pregnancies at risk (Table 2). Duplex-pulsed Doppler equipment with 3.5 MHz probe was used (Esacord 80 – Ansaldo); the angle of insonation was ≤ 45 grades and the observation time was about 1–2 min on each vessel during the absence of fetal movements (when the measurement was pathological it was repeated in a different projection).

Table 1 Study group characteristics

Number of patients	179
Weeks of pregnancy	15–40
Age (years)	20–37
Parity	0–2
Number of measurements in the same subject	1–3

Table 2 Distribution of pregnancies

Normal pregnancies	159	88.93%
Pregnancies 'at risk'	20	11.17%
Pregnancy-induced hypertension	10	
Systemic lupus erythematosus	1	
Cardiopathy	1	
Diabetes	2	
Tuberculosis	1	
Multiple pregnancy	4	
Toxoplasmosis	1	

Table 3 Fluximetric indices

$$\text{PI (pulsatility index)*} = \frac{A - B}{M}$$

$$\text{RI (resistance index)} = \frac{A - B}{A}$$

*A = peak-systolic flow; B = end-diastolic flow; M = mean flow

As usual, the following vessels were investigated:

(1) uterine arteries: 27 measurements;
(2) umbilical arteries: 201 measurements;
(3) descending aorta: 178 measurements.

The most usual fluximetric indices were considered[7–10] (Table 3).

RESULTS

Results were analyzed statistically. Firstly, data were examined to evaluate the distribution of the measurements relative to each index, to find out the occurrence of incidental outliers and, mainly, to study the behavior of the data according to gestational age.

Distribution of pulsatility index (PI) proved to be symmetrical enough; conversely, resistance index (RI) and A/B ratio distributions were pretty skewed both for the umbilical arteries and descending aorta. Data for the uterine arteries were not analyzed since they were very few.

Only one outlier was found with reference to PI measured at 24th week of pregnancy in the umbilical artery (PI = 0.09); accordingly, this measurement was left out of the subsequent data processing.

Curves of the isopercentiles for each index can be constructed according to the weeks of pregnancy. These indices may be regarded as anthropometric ones concerning a growing organism. Thus, they act as a temporal series of correlated data.

Also, since the pattern of the indices was asymmetrical with a standard deviation changing in some cases with the mean (RI and A/B ratio), a distribution-free method suggested by Healy *et al.*[11] was used. It is based on techniques for smoothing a scatter diagram described by Cleveland[12]. It is very flexible, allowing for every percentile to follow a smooth curve with time.

According to the method, every percentile (dependent variable) can be predicted by a polynomial regression in which time is the independent variable. However, a polinomy in z (standard normal deviate) is fitted to each coefficient. The value of z depends on the selected percentile. This procedure gives a linear model for the whole of the data which can be fitted by least squares.

Results regarding the umbilical arteries showed a decrease of all three indices according to the week of pregnancy and they were used to construct reference charts. The 3rd and 97th percentiles were selected respectively as the lower and upper limit since they are conventionally used in statistics to establish normal values for biological variables.

The fitted regression with time is always significant ($p < 0.05$). Thus, every index changes significantly according to the week of pregnancy. However, the degree of the polynomies both in the independent variable and in z is different for the three indices.

The expressions of these polynomies are listed separately for the three examined indices, as shown in Table 4.

The curves obtained from measurements on the umbilical arteries for the 3rd, 50th and 97th percentiles and for each index according to the weeks of pregnancy are shown in Figures 1, 2 and 3.

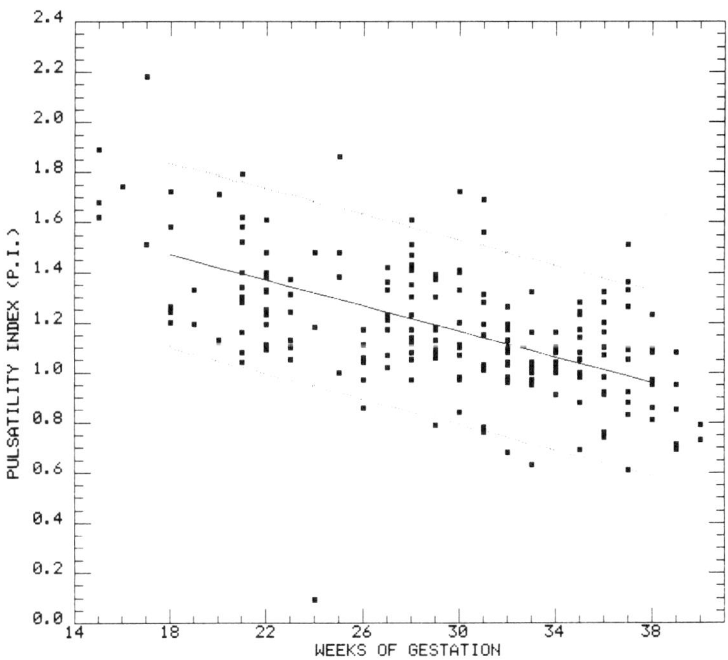

Figure 1 The 3rd, 50th and 97th percentile and the reference range for the pulsatility index (PI) from the umbilical arteries

Table 4 The expression of the polynomies used for the three indices

PI (199 measurements)
$y_i = 1.930 + 0.196\ z_i - 0.025\ t_i$
RI (199 measurements)
$y_i = 9.331 + 0.155\ z_i - 0.0012\ z_i^2 - (0.0082 - 0.0017\ z_i)\ t_i$
A/B ratio (200 measurements)
$y_i = 11.269 - (0.556\text{-}0.096\ z_i)\ t_i + (0.0153 - 0.00217\ z_i)\ t_i^2 - 0.00017\ t_i^3$

y_i = ith percentile; z_i = normal standardized deviate connected with the ith percentile; t_i = ith week of pregnancy

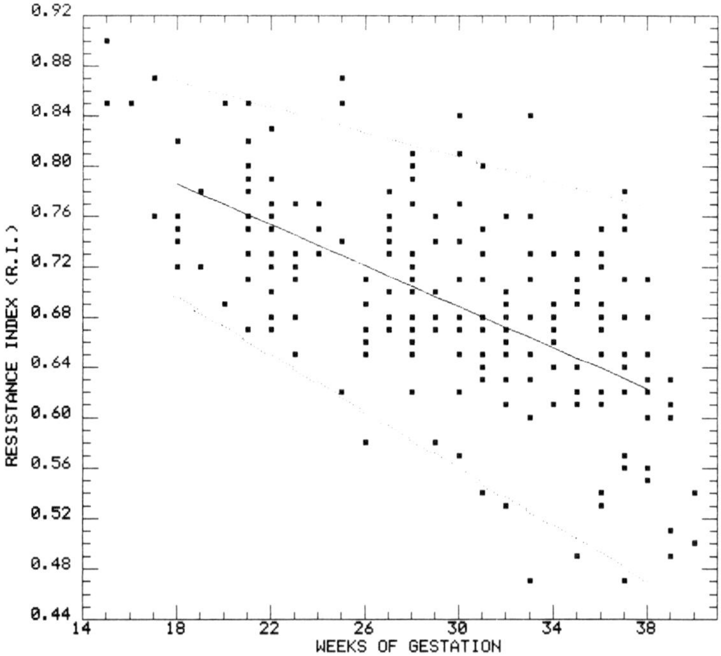

Figure 2 The 3rd, 50th and 97th percentile and the reference range for the resistance index (RI) from the umbilical arteries

Table 5 Normal ranges for the fetal descending aorta

Index	*Median value*	*Normal values*	*Number of measurements*
PI	1.67	1.02–2.32	175
RI	0.79	0.63–0.92	174
A/B ratio	5.04	2.69–11.43	174

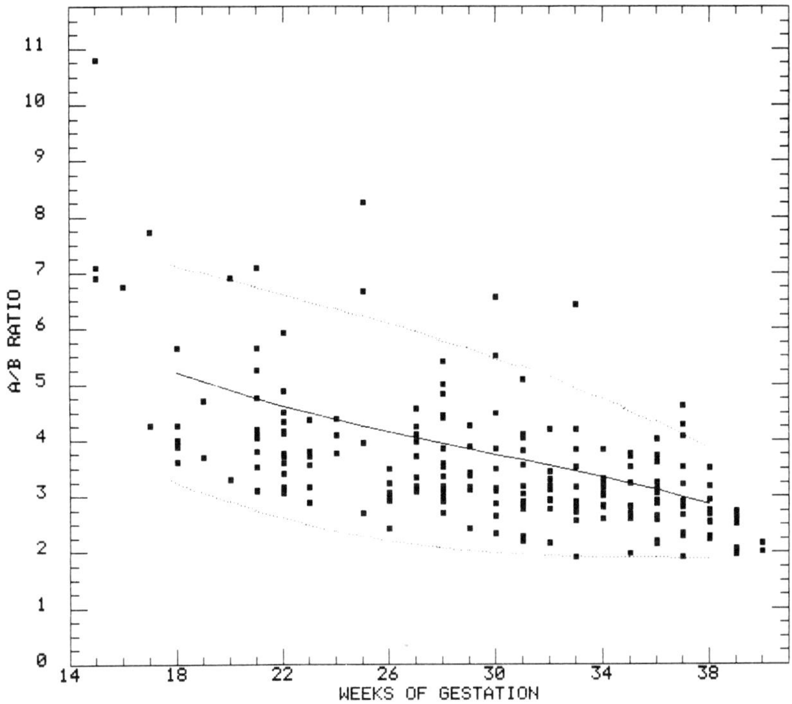

Figure 3 The 3rd, 50th and 97th percentile and the reference range for the A/B ratio from the umbilical arteries

Furthermore, as regards the fetal descending aorta, analysis of the pattern of the three indices showed no significant change according to the week of pregnancy. In other words, measured indices on the descending aorta do not change significantly while the pregnancy progresses. Therefore, the median value (50th percentile) and the normal limits (2.5th and 97.5th percentile) of the three indices were calculated without taking the weeks of pregnancy into account (Table 5).

These normal limits were calculated assuming a normal distribution of the data. However, given the asymmetry of the distribution of the three indices, a family of power transformations based on the first three moments of the distribution, as described by Box and Cox[13], was previously applied to the raw data. The value for the power which minimized the skewness was estimated by maximum likelihood (MLE).

Figures 4, 5 and 6 show graphs of the three indices according to the week of pregnancy. The median curve was overlapped in order to point out that the indices were independent of the age of pregnancy in which they were measured.

Finally, as regards the uterine arteries, unprocessed curves of the three indices are shown in Figure 7. Data were few since these vessels are difficult to locate with certainty without color-Doppler equipment.

Percentages of cases below the lower limit or above the upper limit are

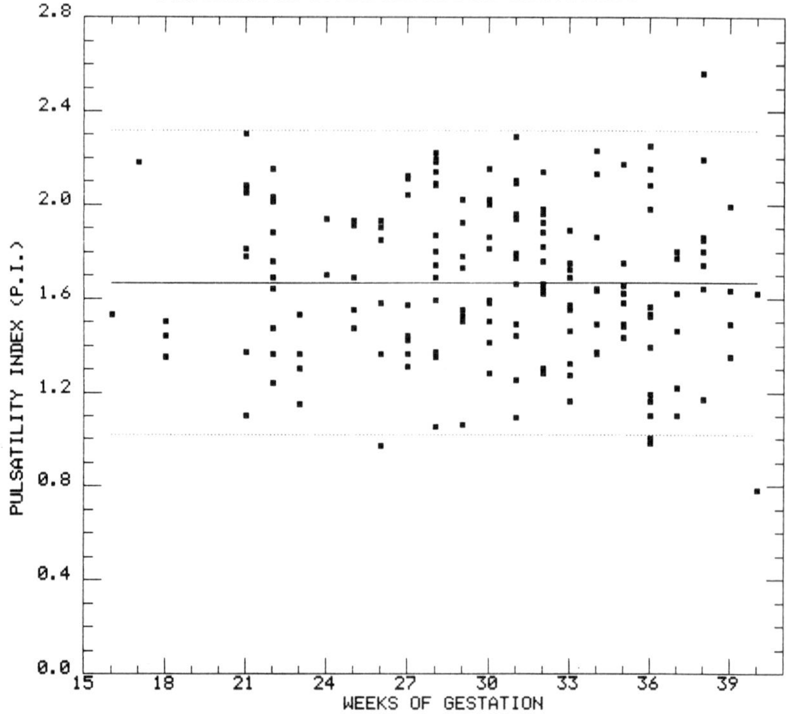

Figure 4 The 2.5th, 50th and 97.5th percentile and the reference range of the PI from the fetal descending aorta

Table 6 Abnormal cases (numbers with % in parentheses)

Index	*Cases below the lower limit*	*Cases above the upper limit*	*Total*
Umbilical arteries (201 *measurements*)			
PI	5 (2.81)	9 (4.48)	14 (6.97)
RI	6 (2.99)	5 (2.49)	11 (5.47)
A/B ratio	1 (0.50)	10 (4.98)	11 (5.47)
Descending aorta (178 *measurements*)			
PI	5 (2.81)	1 (0.50)	6 (3.37)
RI	3 (1.69)	— —	3 (1.69)
A/B ratio	3 (1.69)	4 (2.25)	7 (3.93)

shown in Table 6 according to the normal ranges we obtained for the umbilical arteries and descending aorta.

Tables 7 and 8 show respectively the outcome of pregnancies and the results of the perinatal mortality and morbidity. In spite of the small number of pathological cases, an attempt to evaluate the accuracy of this diagnostic method was carried out.

Sensitivity (% of the affected subjects recognized as affected by the test) and *specificity* (% of the unaffected subjects recognized as healthy by the

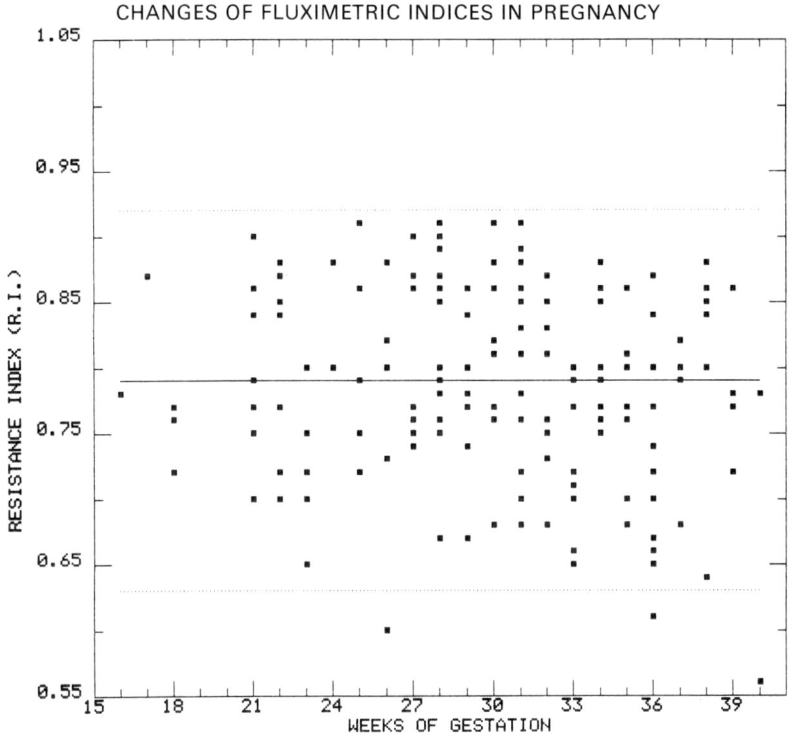

Figure 5 The 2.5th, 50th and 97.5th percentile and the reference range of the RI from the fetal descending aorta

test) were calculated according to the following well known formulae:

$$\text{sensitivity (\%)} = \frac{\text{true positive cases}}{\text{true positive cases + false positive cases}} \times 100$$

$$\text{specificity (\%)} = \frac{\text{true negative cases}}{\text{false positive cases + true negative cases}} \times 100$$

Distribution of the true and false, positive and negative cases in the present study is listed in Table 9.

The following results were obtained: sensitivity = [3/(3 + 7)] × 100 = 30%; specificity = [62/(1 + 62)] × 100 = 98.4%. Thus, specificity was excellent; on the contrary, sensitivity was very inadequate. This could depend on the improper distribution of true and false, positive and negative cases. Indeed, some cases could have been regarded as false negative ones just because of extreme scrupulousness.

However, the predictive value of the positive test is quite adequate (3/4 = 75%), although the relevance of the period between fluximetric measurement and delivery has to be clarified since the predictive value is strongly different when the fluximetric measurement is taken a few days before delivery rather than a number of weeks earlier.

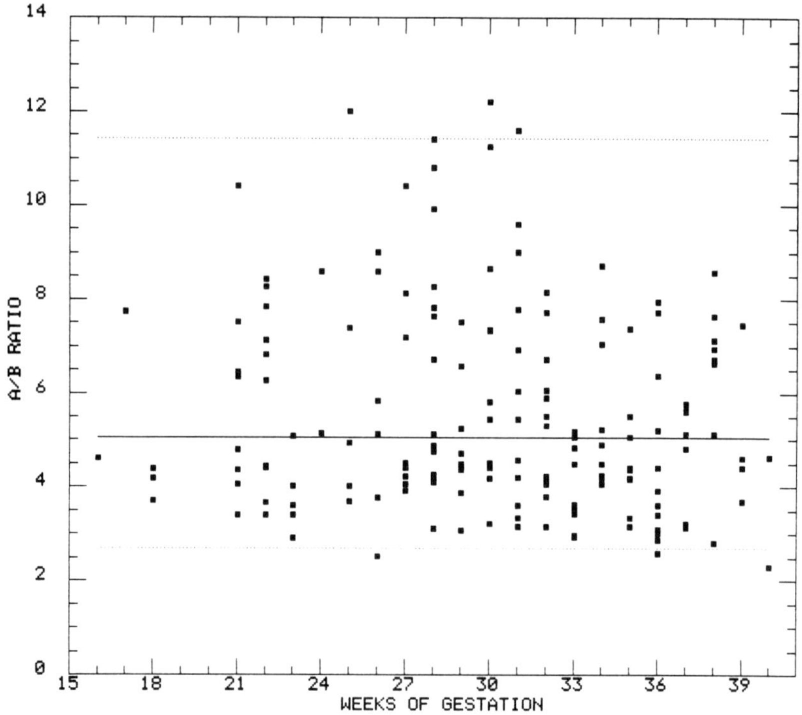

Figure 6 The 2.5th, 50th and 97.5th percentile and the reference range of the A/B ratio from the fetal descending aorta

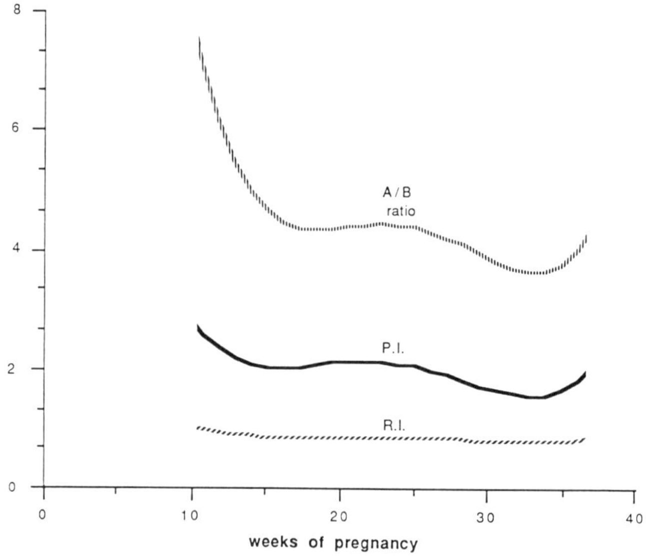

Figure 7 Unprocessed curves of the three indices from the uterine arteries

Table 7 Outcome of the pregnancies

Pregnancies in progress	48				
Deliveries	73	Caesarean section	29	Repeat Caesarean section	8
				Maternal diseases	11
				Fetal hypoxia	1
				Dysfunctional labor	4
				Abnormal presentation	5
		Vacuum extraction	2	Dysfunctional labor	1
				Fetal hypoxia	1
		Spontaneous	42		
Lost to follow up	58				
Total	179				

Table 8 Perinatal outcome

Perinatal mortality 4
- 1 spontaneous delivery at 28th week (lupus and fetal death)
- 1 multiple spontaneous delivery at 26th week (PIH)
- 1 spontaneous delivery at 33rd week (PIH and fetal death)
- 1 spontaneous delivery at 34th week (fetal death)

Apgar score <7 3
- 1 Caesarean section at 37th week (diabetes)
- 1 Caesarean section at 39th week (breech presentation and fetal malformation)
- 1 Caesarean section at 38th week (placental insufficiency and fetal malformation)

Small for gestational age fetuses (<5th perc.) 2
- 1 Caesarean section at 39th week (2300 g)
- 1 spontaneous delivery at 40th week (2750 g)

PIH, pregnancy-induced hypertension

Table 9 Distribution of the true and false, positive and negative cases

Positive cases (4)

True 3	PIH; CS at 39th week; Apgar score 10; PI 1.51
	PIH; spontaneous delivery at 33rd week; fetal death; PI 1.72
	Spontaneous delivery at 34th week; fetal death; PI 1.60
False 1	Spontaneous delivery at 36th week; Apgar score 10; PI 1.69

Negative cases (69)

True 62	
False 7	diabetes; CS at 37th week; Apgar score 5; PI 1.24
	Placental insufficiency; CS at 38th week; Apgar score 5; PI 1.23
	Breech presentation; CS at 39th week; Apgar score 4; PI 1.39
	Spontaneous delivery at 40th week; SGA fetus; Apgar score 10; PI 1.19
	Fetal hypoxia; CS at 39th week; SGA fetus; Apgar score 10; PI 1.13
	Spontaneous delivery at 28th week; fetal death; PI 1.61 and 1.33
	PIH; multiple spontaneous delivery at 26th week; PI 1.58 and 1.20

PIH, pregnancy-induced hypertension; CS, Caesarean section

CONCLUSION

In conclusion, the assessment of the sensitivity of this method has to be examined more carefully. In addition, the real advantage of taking only a single fluximetric measurement as compared with longitudinal repeated measurements (as in hormonal monitoring) on the same subject must be checked. As regards this question, it has to be remembered that most of the data in the present study concerned single measurements taken a number of weeks before delivery, while longitudinal observations could have increased sensitivity.

REFERENCES

1. Campbell, S., Griffin, D.R., Pearce, J.M., Diaz-Recanses, J., Cohen-Overbeek, T.E. and Wilson, K. (1983). New Doppler technique for assessing utero placental blood flow. *Lancet*, **i**, 675–7
2. Griffin, D., Cohen-Overbeek, T.E. and Campbell, S. (1983). Fetal and utero-placental blood flow. *Clin. Obstet. Gynecol.*, **10**, 565–601
3. Trudiger, B.J., Cook, C.M. and Colins, J. (1985). Fetal umbilical arterial velocity waveforms and placental resistance: clinical significance. *Br. J. Obstet. Gynaecol.*, **92**, 23–30
4. Arduini, D., Rizzo, G., Shash, H., Giaquinto, P., Romanini, C. and Mancuso, S. (1986). Valore predittivo della flussimetria fetale nella insorgenza dell'iposviluppo. Presented at the *LXIV Congresso Nazionale SIGO*, Rome
5. Wladimiroff, J.W., Wizngaard, J.A.G.W., Degani, S., Noordan, M.J., Eyck, J.V. and Tonge, H.M. (1987). Cerebral and umbilical arterial blood flow velocity waveforms in normal and growth retarded pregnancies. *Obstet. Gynecol.*, **69**, 705–9
6. Switzer, D.F. and Nanda, N.C. (1985). Doppler color flow mapping. *Ultrasound Med. Biol.*, **11**, 3
7. Goslin, R.C. and King, D.H. (1974). Continuous wave ultrasound as an alternative and complement to X-rays in vascular examinations. In Reneman, R.S. (ed.), *Cardiovascular Applications of Ultrasound*, pp. 266. (New York: Elsevier)
8. Pourcelot, L. (1974). Applications cliniques de l'examen Doppler transcutáne. In Peroneau, P. (ed.). *Velocimetric ultrasonor Doppler. INSERM.*, **34**, 213–40
9. Goslin, R.C. (1976). Extraction of physiological information from spectrum analysed Doppler-shifted continuous wave ultrasound signal obtained non-invasively from the arterial tree. In Hill, D.M. and Watson, B.W. (eds). *IEE Medical Electronic Monographs*, 13–22, p. 73. (London: Peter Perigrinus)
10. Stuart, B., Drumm, J., Fitzgerald, D. and Duignan, N.M. (1980). Fetal blood velocity waveforms in normal pregnancy. *Br. J. Obstet. Gynaecol.*, **87**, 780–5
11. Healy, M.J.R., Rasbash, J. and Young, M. (1988). Distribution free estimation of age-related centiles. *Ann. Hum. Biol.*, **15**, 17–22
12. Cleveland, W.S. (1979). Robust locally weighted regression and smoothings scatterplots. *J. Am. Stat. Assoc.*, **74**, 829–37
13. Box, G.E.P. and Cox, D.R. (1964). An analysis of transformation. *J.R. Stat. Soc. B.*, **26**, 211–25

Section 3 continued

Part C

Intrauterine growth retardation

52

Intrauterine growth retardation – semantics and diagnostics

P. Bergsjø

INTRODUCTION

The term intrauterine growth retardation (IUGR) implies that the fetus does not attain its biological potential. A growth-retarded newborn should be bigger at birth if growth retarding factors did not operate. Fetal growth, and thereby newborn size, is determined partly by genetic and partly by environmental factors. Although this distinction is not clear-cut, it serves to emphasize that one fetus is biologically determined to be small at birth while another is impeded by a pathological condition. The former is normal and can be left to itself, while the other needs help. This chapter will deal with definitions and give examples of how epidemiological research can help us understand the condition better. I shall give my philosophy of the diagnostic approach to detect IUGR but leave the details to other authors. Treatment options are few and largely debatable; the crucial question when the condition is deemed life-threatening concerns the timing and mode of delivery.

DEFINITIONS

By international agreement, low birth weight (LBW) and very low birth weight (VLBW) denote newborns below 2500 g and 1500 g, respectively, without reference to gestational age. Preterm refers to those born before 37 completed weeks, with no reference to birth weight. A premature baby is one which the pediatrician believes to have been born preterm. The expression should not be used in scientific work, being conditioned upon subjective interpretation. Combining weight and age we can define weight-by-gestational-age in percentiles of a given reference birth population. These are divided into three broad groups:

(1) large-for-gestational-age (LGA),
(2) appropriate-for-gestational-age (AGA), and
(3) small-for-gestational-age (SGA).

The limit for SGA is variously drawn at the 10th, 5th, or the 2.5th centiles (or at 2 standard deviations below the mean).

It is important that percentile weight charts are population-based and that they include the whole birth population without undue exclusions. They should also be representative of the population which they are to serve as reference. It is ironic that the 'Lubchenko charts', which for many years served as international standards, were based on a high altitude birth population in Colorado, USA[1], in which the 10th percentile corresponds approximately to the 2.5th percentile in Norway[2]. Computer-derived charts, using information about the dates of the last menstrual period and birth, tend to be erratic in the low birth weight range[2], and may therefore require smoothing (Figure 1). As boys and girls of the same population have different birth weight distributions, they should be defined separately, as should singleton births. Other factors known to influence birth weight, are parity and the mother's height and prepregnancy weight, all of which may be adjusted for in nomograms.

IUGR is lacking in this exposé of definitions. IUGR is a clinical term which eludes strict definition. In the extreme case of malnourishment there is no doubt about the diagnosis, but in others it is pure guesswork, for example in most of the children born to smoking mothers. Many IUGR newborns are in the SGA range, but an AGA baby may also be growth retarded, if biologically destined to weigh more at birth than it actually does. The smaller twin of a discordant set is a perfect example of IUGR (Figure 2).

The body contour of a newborn child is symbolized by the ponderal index (PI), which expresses its weight-for-height, with 'skinny' and 'fat' as the two extremes[3]. The PI varies with gestational age, and its practical use is therefore restricted.

INTERNATIONAL COMPARISONS AND PROGNOSTIC POINTS

It is important to realize that birth weights in populations of different geographical and ethnic origins differ, not only in average values, but also in the shape of their standardized distribution curves. Figure 3 shows that California black and Japanese newborns in 1981 were 400 g lighter than Norwegians, on average, but with different shapes of the distribution curves[4]. The curve for Japan was much narrower than for the two other populations, and that for California blacks more drawn-out toward the lighter weights. Assuming that there is a high share of IUGR babies in the low birthweight range, these observations are relevant. The next point to consider is the hypothesis put forth by Wilcox and Russell, that when the birth weight distribution curve deviates from the Gaussian curve, the 'residual' area of the deviation (mainly in the low birth weight range), expresses the proportion of pathological births in the population[5].

On comparing birth weight specific perinatal mortality rates in the populations just described, we find a correlation between the characteristics of the birth weight distribution curves, and the shifting mortality rates along the weight axis (Figure 4 as compared to Figure 3)[6]. However, the interpretation with regard to IUGR as a risk factor is largely conjectural, in particular as long as the causes of death are lacking.

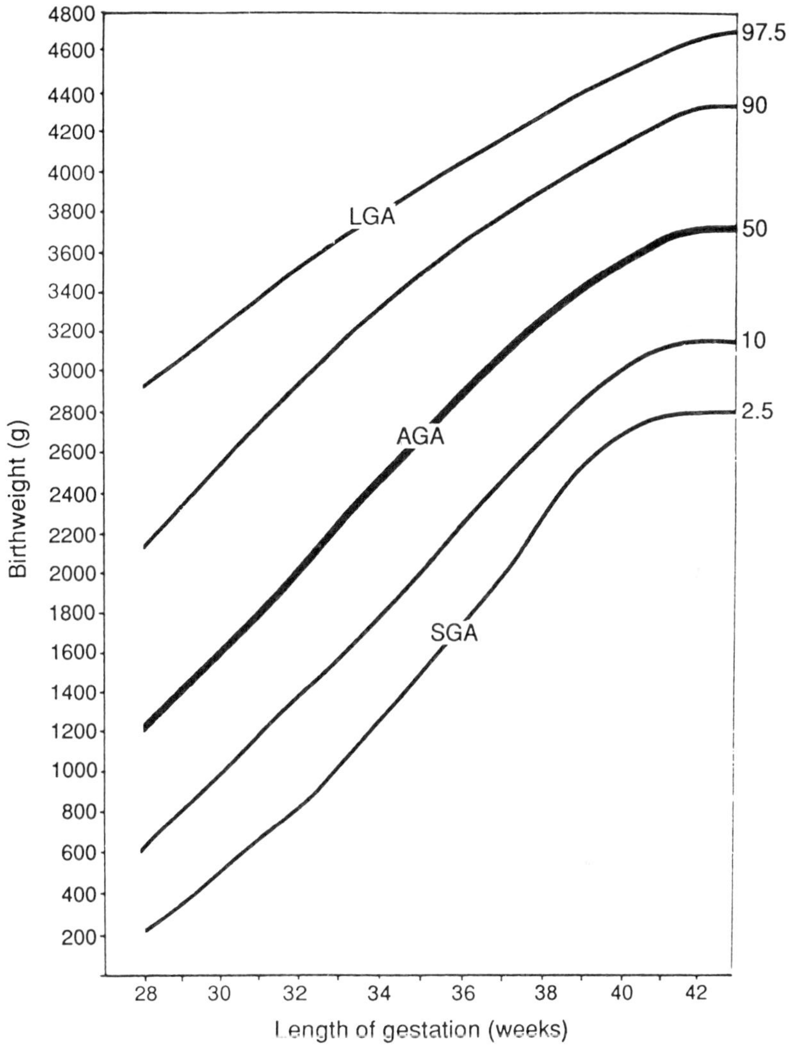

Figure 1 Smoothed weight percentiles of Norwegian firstborn singleton boys 1967–84. Based on data from the Medical Birth Registry of Norway

Another epidemiological observation is of clinical interest. Bakketeig and colleagues, using data from the birth registry of Norway, have demonstrated that mothers have a strong tendency to repeat birth performance in succeeding pregnancies. This is also true of SGA births. Furthermore, on studying perinatal mortality rates, they found that the risk of death was much higher in non-repeater than in repeater SGA births (Table 1)[7]. The clinical lesson is that an apparent SGA fetus in a mother with previous AGA birth(s) is a high risk fetus which needs close monitoring.

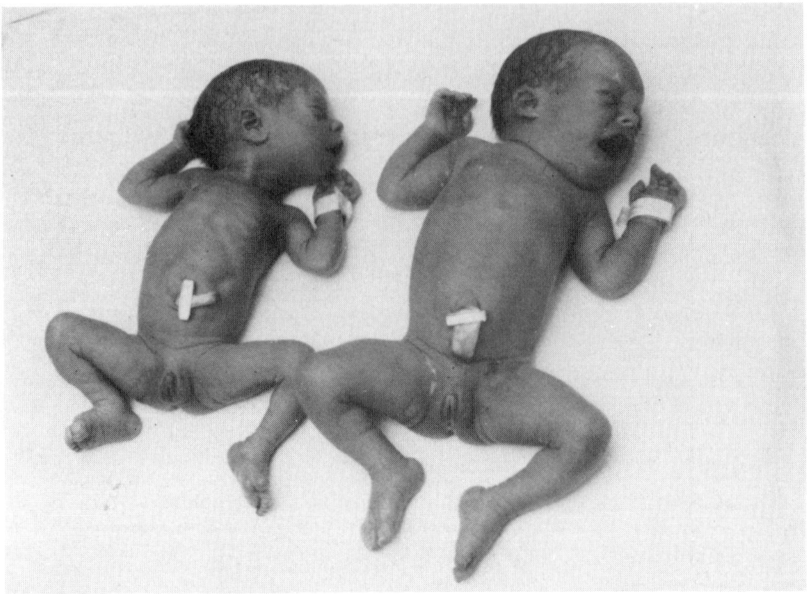

Figure 2 The smaller twin is a perfect illustration of intrauterine growth retardation

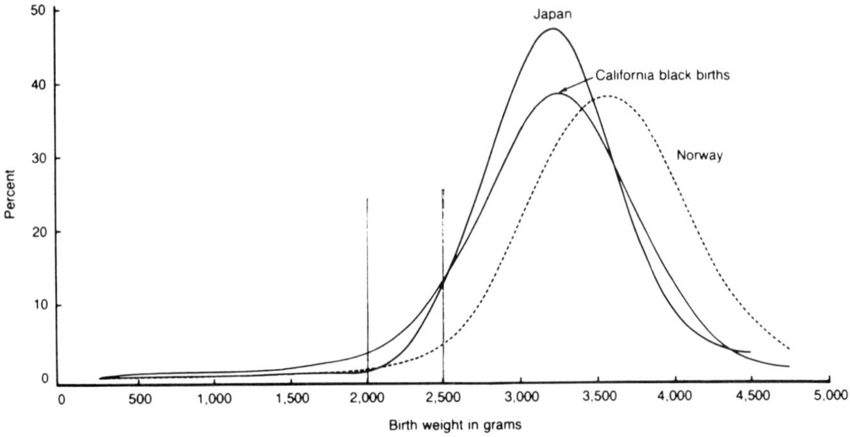

Figure 3 Birth weight distribution of singleton births in populations of California blacks, Japan and Norway, 1981[4]

CAUSES

The single most important cause of IUGR is cigarette smoking. Table 2, taken from a study in Bergen[8], shows that the effect is dose-dependent. The average birth weight when the mothers smoked 10 cigarettes or more per

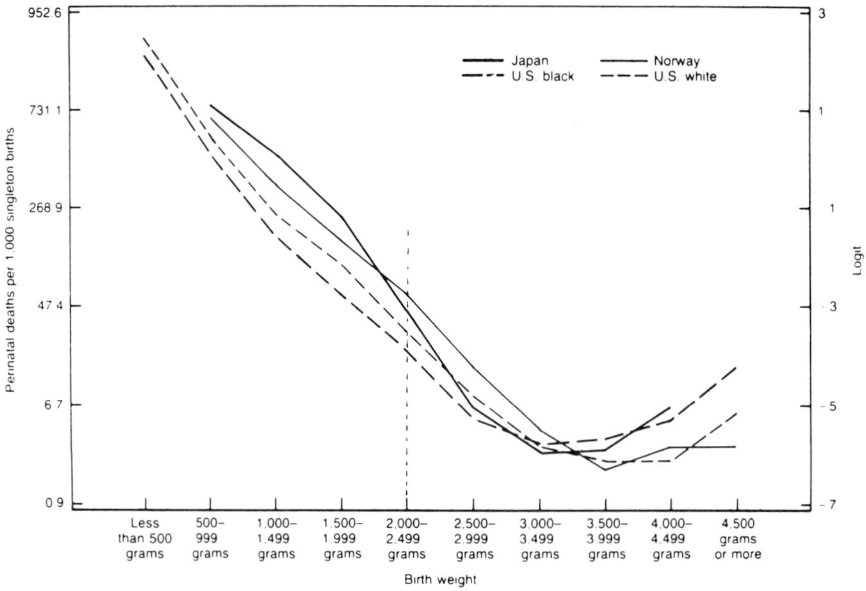

Figure 4 Birth weight-specific perinatal mortality rates of singleton births in Japan, Norway, U.S. blacks and U.S. whites, 1980–82. U.S. rates are based on births occurring in five States[6]

Table 1 The perinatal mortality rate (PMR) per 1000 births for small-for-gestational age (SGA) second births by weight-for-gestation of the elder sibling. Based on 134 629 mothers with their first and second single births in Norway, 1967–76[7]. Data from the Medical Birth Registry of Norway

Weight-for-gestation of elder sibling	*SGA second births*	
	No.	*PMR*
SGA	4578	33.0
AGA	10 070	39.5
LGA	180	100.0
Unknown	466	38.6
Total	15 294	38.6

day was 300 g less than for babies of non-smokers. There is also a correlation between birth weight and maternal weight gain, which to some degree could be linked to cigarette smoking.

It has been established that fetuses and children of smoking mothers run a higher risk of perinatal death than those of non-smokers[9]. Therefore, persuading mothers to stop smoking may be the single most effective way to reduce the incidence of IUGR and improve perinatal survival.

The effect of smoking is mediated through the toxic and vasoconstrictory effects of nicotine, plus the carbon monoxide affinity to hemoglobin. Another basic mechanism which causes IUGR is the lack of trophoblast downgrowth

Table 2 Maternal weight gain and birth weight in 811 singleton normal pregnancies in Bergen, Norway, by the mothers' smoking habits[8]

Smoking status	*Maternal weight gain* (kg ± SD)	*Birth weight* (g ± SD)
Non-smokers	14.2 (3.8)	3589 (492)
1–9 cig./day	14.7 (4.2)	3486 (467)
≥10 cig./day	13.3 (3.5)	3262 (592)

Weight gain difference is significant between light and heavy smokers ($p = 0.01$), and all birth weight differences are highly significant ($p = 0.004$ or less)

along the walls of the decidual spiral arteries, resulting in poor maternal circulation through the intervillous space. This is commonly linked to pre-eclampsia, but has also been demonstrated in normotensive cases with IUGR[10]. The underlying cause remains to be found.

In addition to these, there is a long list of causes, or rather, risk factors of IUGR. Some are merely statistical associations, such as socioeconomic status, level of formal education, living in high altitude, race, ethnicity, and previous birth of an IUGR baby. Mothers with certain specific conditions run a high risk of fetal growth retardation. Foremost among these are pre-eclampsia, hypertension and renal disease. Diabetes is linked to growth retardation as well as to macrosomia. Smoking has been mentioned. Alcohol use is also correlated to birth weight[11], as are addictive drugs.

Fetuses may be affected by maternal infections, with growth retardation resulting. Some fetuses with chromosomal aberrations and some malformed fetuses are small. Erythroblastosis is a risk factor.

In some instances growth retardation is associated with a small placenta due to ill-explained maternal–fetal mismatching, possibly determined by immunological factors.

DIAGNOSTICS

The list of causes, which is not complete, indicates that there are diverse pathogenetic mechanisms of IUGR. However, many instances exhibit vasoconstriction with poor arterial supply to the placental bed as a common feature. Generalized vasoconstriction leads to hemoconcentration, which may occur both in pre-eclamptic and in otherwise normal pregnancies. Consequently, the finding of a high hemoglobin concentration (or a high hematocrit value), is a diagnostic warning sign, which should be followed up by more intensive monitoring. Table 3 shows the correlation between hemoglobin levels and birth weight at term in normal pregnancies. In another study we have demonstrated the value of the hemoglobin concentration as an indicator of adverse outcome[12].

Table 3 Birth weight according to hemoglobin concentration shortly before birth, in 811 singleton normal pregnancies in Bergen, Norway[8]

Hemoglobin concn (g/dl)	*Number*	*Birth weight*	
		Mean	*1 SD*
9.0–11.9	341	3748	426
12.0–12.9	275	3514	458
13.0–15.0	195	3158	457

PHILOSOPHY OF DIAGNOSTIC APPROACH

Antenatal care is prophylactic medicine. The various diagnostic measures are screening tools aimed at discovering threatening conditions at an early stage. Hemoglobin (*vide supra*) is a good example. The tape-measure gives the symphysis-to-fundus distance, indicating the size and, by repeated measurements, the growth of the fetus. The mother's weight gain chart is another useful indicator. Fetal kick counting, with sensible warning rules, appears to be of value[13]. Such simple tools should be used for screening, to be followed by more sophisticated methods in those found to be at risk. In my experience as a peer reviewer of perinatal deaths, physicians are more often to blame for omitting to do the simple examinations, or to fail to react properly when they indicate pathology, than for neglect in performing high technology diagnostics.

The second line approach, of course, includes ultrasound, cardiotocography and biochemical tests of fetoplacental function. Fetal blood stream waveform examination with pulsed Doppler ultrasound is highly complex and still in the experimental stage.

REFERENCES

1. Lubchenko, L.O., Hansman, C., Dressler, M. and Boyd, E. (1963). Intrauterine growth as estimated from liveborn birth-weight data at 24 to 42 weeks of gestation. *Pediatrics*, **34**, 793–800
2. Bjerkedal, T., Bakketeig, L. and Lehmann, E. H. (1973). Percentiles of birth weights of single, live births at different gestation periods. Based on 125 485 births in Norway, 1967 and 1968. *Acta Paediatr. Scand.*, **62**, 449–57
3. Gruenwald, P. (1974). Pathology of the deprived fetus and its supply line. In *Ciba Foundation Symposium 27 (new series): Size at Birth*, pp. 3–19. (Amsterdam: Elsevier)
4. Alberman, E.D. and Evans, S.J.W. (1988). Trends in birth weight distribution: 1970–83. In *Proceedings of the International Collaborative Effort on Perinatal and Infant Mortality*, Vol. II, pp. III-37–III-47. (Hyattsville: Department of Health and Human Services, DHHS Publication No. (PHS)88-1252-1)
5. Wilcox, A. and Russell, I.T. (1983). Birthweight and perinatal mortality: I. On the frequency distribution of birthweight. *Int. J. Epidemiol.*, **12**, 314–25
6. Hoffman, H.J., Bergsjø, P. and Denman, D.W., III (1988). Trends in birth weight-specific perinatal mortality rates: 1970–83. In *Proceedings of the International Collaborative Effort on Perinatal and Infant Mortality*, Vol. II, pp. III-51–III-71 (Hyattsville: Department of Health and Human Services. DHHS Publication No. (PHS)88-1252-1)
7. Bakketeig, L.S., Bjerkedal, T. and Hoffman, H.J. (1986). Small-for-gestational age births in successive pregnancy outcomes: results from a longitudinal study of births in Norway. *Early Human Development*, **14**, 187–200

8. Nilsen, S.T., Sagen, N., Kim, H.C. and Bergsjø, P. (1984). Smoking, hemoglobin levels, and birth weights in normal pregnancies. *Am. J. Obstet. Gynecol.*, **148**, 752–8
9. Cnattingius, S., Haglund, B. and Meirik, O. (1988). Cigarette smoking as risk factor for late fetal and early neonatal death. *Br. Med. J.*, **297**, 258–61
10. Brosens, I., Dixon, H.G. and Robertson, W.B. (1977). Fetal growth retardation and the arteries of the placental bed. *Br. J. Obstet. Gynaecol.*, **84**, 656–64
11. Mills, J.L., Graubard, B.I., Harley, E.E., Rhoads, G.G. and Berendez, H.W. (1984). Maternal alcohol consumption and birth weight. How much drinking during pregnancy is safe? *J. Am. Med. Assoc.*, **252**, 1875–9
12. Sagen, N., Nilsen, S.T., Kim, H.C., Koller, O. and Bergsjø, P. (1984). The predictive value of total estriol; HPL and hb on perinatal outcome in severe pre-eclampsia. *Acta Obstet. Gynecol. Scand.*, **63**, 603–8
13. Neldam, S. (1986). *Fetal Movements as an Indicator of Fetal Well-being.* p. 34 (København: Laegeforeningens forlag)

53

Epidermal growth factor in urine of pregnant women and in amniotic fluid throughout pregnancy

T. Kumasaka, H. Watanabe and M. Tanaka

INTRODUCTION

Epidermal growth factor (EGF) is a single chain 53 amino acid polypeptide mitogen that has been isolated from the male mouse submaxillary gland[1] and from human urine[2]. EGF has been identified in maternal, cord blood and amniotic fluid[3]. It has attracted attention, since it has a striking property to stimulate growth of a variety of tissues. These actions are thought to be mediated by EGF binding to specific high affinity receptors present in human amnion, chorion, decidua and placenta[4]. Therefore, it is presumed to play a role in fetoplacental growth and development through it's mitogenic action. The aim of this work was to investigate the relationships among EGF concentrations in urine, amniotic fluid and fetoplacental development during pregnancy.

SUBJECTS AND METHOD

Thirty urinary samples from non-pregnant women, 85 from normal pregnant women, 21 from women with toxemic pregnancy, 17 from postpartum women (at 3–4 days after delivery), 30 from newborns (at 3–4 days after the birth) and 55 amniotic fluid samples from pregnant women with a variety of conditions necessitating amniotomy and amniocentesis at 25 to 39 weeks of gestation were collected. Non-pregnant women were recruited from those with unexplained infertility asked to collect urine in their follicular phase. All had regular menstrual cycles and no known medical, renal or gynecological disease. Each subjects' collected first morning voided urine and samples were stored frozen until brought to the laboratory for analysis. EGF concentrations were measured by double antibody radioimmunoassay[5]. The sensitivity of this assay was equivalent to 20 pg/ml of EGF. Nerve growth factor, insulin or fibroblast growth factor did not cross-react in the assay. Urinary and amniotic fluid creatinine concentrations were measured by alkali picrin acid method. Urinary EGF concentrations were expressed as ng EGF/mg creatinine. Comparison of data from each subject was performed using Student's *t* test.

Determination of gestational age

Gestational age was determined by the last menstrual period and measurement of fetal weight by ultrasound examination. The criterion of intrauterine growth retardation (IUGR) was based on the definition by Japanese Ministry of Health and Welfare[6].

RESULTS

Urinary EGF

Though urinary EGF concentrations in early pregnancy (< 14 weeks) or at term did not differ significantly from those in non-pregnant women, urinary EGF concentrations during pregnancy reached maximal levels at 20–21 weeks gestation, then they gradually declined toward term (Figure 1). At puerperium, they were similar to those during pregnancy. However, the concentrations in toxemic women and in women carrying IUGR were lower than normal pregnancy (Figure 2). On the other hand, neonates had higher urinary EGF concentration than those in pregnant women.

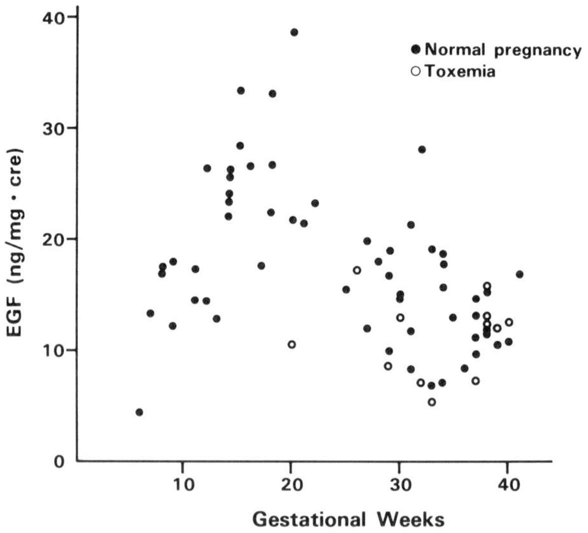

Figure 1 Urinary EGF levels corrected for creatinine through gestation in normal pregnancy and in toxemia

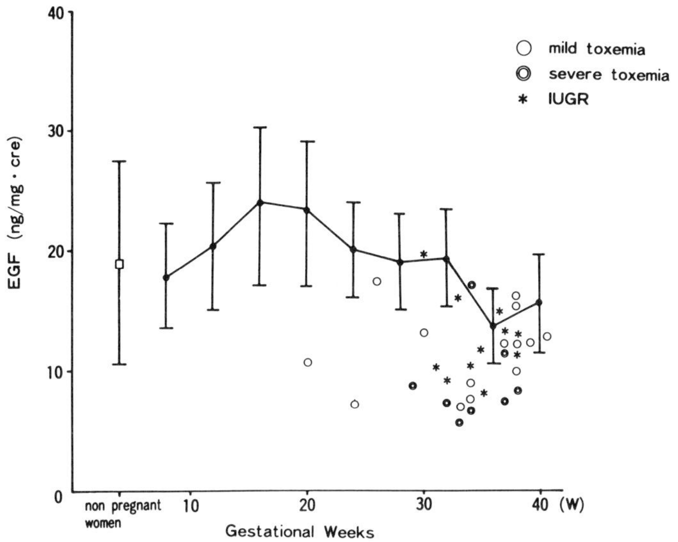

Figure 2 Urinary EGF levels corrected for creatinine during gestation in normal pregnancy, toxemic pregnancies and in those with IUGR

EGF in amniotic fluid

Though EGF concentrations in amniotic fluid were extremely low (24–137 pg/ml), they were detectable with our radioimmunoassay system. As shown in Figure 3, significant correlation between gestational weeks and EGF concentrations in amniotic fluid was recognized. EGF concentrations

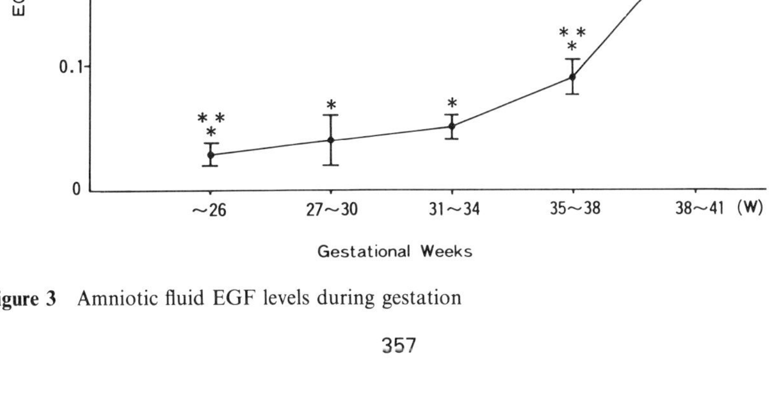

Figure 3 Amniotic fluid EGF levels during gestation

in amniotic fluid and creatinine levels were also correlated significantly (Figure 4). However, when EGF concentrations in amniotic fluid were corrected by the creatinine levels, that is, expressed as ng EGF/mg creatinine, no significant relation between gestational weeks and EGF concentration was observed.

DISCUSSION

Urinary EGF concentrations increased from early pregnancy on, reaching maximal levels at 19–22 weeks gestation, and then declined toward term. This gestational profile is very similar to that of serum EGF concentrations throughout pregnancy[7]. Urinary EGF concentrations are highest when placental EGF receptor density is highest[4]. From these findings it could be speculated that EGF has a role in fetoplacental growth and development. There was no significant difference between urinary EGF concentrations in non-pregnant and normal pregnant women, and also no significant difference according to fetal weight in normal pregnancy. However, women with toxemia and delivering an IUGR infant had significantly lower urinary EGF concentrations than women delivering normal appropriate for gestational age infants (AGF). Especially, there were no identifiable fetal or placental anomalies in women delivering an IUGR infant, therefore the significance

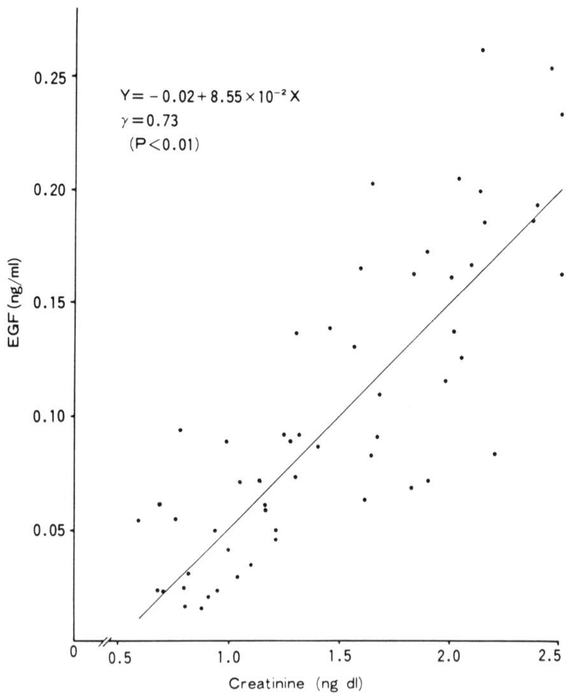

Figure 4 Correlation between amniotic fluid levels of EGF and creatinine

of this result on IUGR is uncertain. In this study, we could detect EGF from amniotic fluid as early as 25 weeks gestation. This work is the first report to demonstrate that EGF concentrations in amniotic fluid are clearly related to gestational weeks and from 36 weeks they rapidly increased toward term. The origin of amniotic fluid EGF has not been certain. Fetal urine was suspected to be a source[3]. Our data also suggest that fetal urine must be the major source of amniotic fluid EGF. The first reason is that EGF concentration in amniotic fluid increased parallel to creatinine, which obviously derived from fetal urine. Second, as urinary excretion of EGF is demonstrated parallel to creatinine excretion, amniotic fluid EGF concentrations corrected by creatinine were also close to adult urine levels. The physiological role of amniotic fluid EGF is not clear. EGF may modulate placental growth, because EGF levels in amniotic fluid and placental weight were significantly related[3]. As EGF receptor has been demonstrated in fetal lung[8], increased amniotic fluid EGF in late pregnancy possibly accelerates fetal lung maturation. But absolute values measured in our study seem to be too low to stimulate fetoplacental organ growth, and the possibility exists that amniotic fluid EGF is only an excretory product. Analysis of amniotic fluid in renal agenesis (Potter syndrome), frequently with hypoplastic lung, must be important to elucidate the origin and role of EGF in amniotic fluid. Apart from the physiological function, measurement of amniotic fluid EGF may become available for the clinical assessment of fetal maturation, such as creatinine and lecithin/sphingomyeline ratio. Furthermore, prospective studies comparing urinary EGF concentration at 19–21 weeks gestation, or amniotic fluid EGF concentration at two different periods during pregnancy and pregnancy outcome might clarify the clinical significance of EGF during pregnancy.

REFERENCES

1. Cohen, S. (1962). Isolation of a mouse submaxillary gland protein accelerating incisor eruption and eyelid opening in the new-born animal. *J. Biol. Chem.*, **237**, 1555–60
2. Starkey, R.H. and Orth, D.N. (1977). Radioimmunoassay of human epidermal growth factor (Urogastrone). *J. Clin. Endocrinol. Metab.*, **45**, 1144–53
3. D'Souza, S.W., Haigh, R., Micklewrighy, L., Donnai, P. and Keys, A. (1985). Amniotic fluid epidermal growth factor and placental weight at term. *Lancet*, **ii**, 272–3
4. Chegini, N. and Rao, C.V. (1985). Epidermal growth factor binding to human amnion, chorion, decidua and placenta from mid- and term pregnancy: Quantitative light microscopic autoradiographic studies. *J. Clin. Endocrinol.*, **61**, 529–35
5. Sasaki, T. (1987). Measurement of urinary EGF by radioimmunoassay. *SRL HOKAN*, **11**, 27–30
6. Nishida, H., Sakagami, M., Kurachi, K., Asada, M., Kubota, S. and Funakawa, H. (1984). Japanese intrauterine fetal development. *Acta Neonatol. Jpn*, **20**, 90–7
7. Ances, I. G. (1973). Serum concentrations of epidermal growth factor in human pregnancy. *Am. J. Obstet. Gynecol.*, **115**, 357–62
8. Adamson, E.D., Deller, M.J. and Warshaw, J.B. (1981). Functional EGF receptors are present on mouse embryo tissues. *Nature*, **291**, 656–9

54

Evaluation of glycemia and C-peptide in maternal and fetal blood

A. Pachi, E. Maggi, A. Ferrero, M. Marceca, S. Balducci and F. Fallucca

INTRODUCTION

Endocrine activity of fetal pancreas starts early during intrauterine life: insulin production might even begin at the 7th week of development. Nevertheless, it seems that human fetal pancreas does not begin its production of insulin as a response to glucose before the 26th week of gestation[1,2]. Hormonal activity of the pancreas, involving not only the production of insulin but also of glucagon and polypeptide hormones such as somatostatin[3], constitutes an important control factor of growth and development of the fetus. Extrapancreatic factors, such as growth hormone, human placental lactogen (hPL) and somatomedins[4,5] also have an important role of this kind. They act according to complex mechanisms that depend on the different concentrations reached by these substances at hematic and histic levels. The pancreatic function of the fetus was studied both on animal experimental models[6,7] and on the human fetus by means of determinations carried out on amniotic fluid[8], on fetal blood sampled at birth[4,9,10], and on cultures obtained from fetal tissues after abortion[5,11].

The recent use of cordocentesis, that can be performed as early as the second trimester of pregnancy, seems to constitute the method of choice for sampling fetal blood directly from the funicle[12].

Furthermore, the possibility of using fetal blood has permitted a more accurate physiopathological evaluation of fetal functions, in particular the endocrinometabolic mechanism regarding the growth processes of the fetus.

MATERIALS AND METHODS

Glycemia and C-peptide were comparatively evaluated in maternal and fetal blood during the performance of various cordocentesis tests carried out according to different conditions. The evaluation was done on 40 fetal blood samples taken between the 18th and the 37th week of gestation. At sampling, the groups were constituted by 19 cases of hemoglobinopathy, 17 cases of malformation of fetus assessed by ultrasound; one sampling was performed for the cytogenetic study of a diabetic patient (White Class D) with a fetus affected by intraventricular defect. Another sampling was performed on a diabetic patient (White Class A) for a hemogasanalytical evaluation. Finally, two samplings were carried out in order to obtain a rapid determination of the fetal karyotype. Five ml of venous blood samples were drawn from fasting mothers, just before cordocentesis.

An Ansaldo AU 440 apparatus with a convex 3.5 MHz probe was used for the ultrasound study. Cordocentesis was performed with the free hand technique, utilizing 20 and 22 Gauge spinal needles. After visualization of the umbilical cord, under local anesthesia, 1.5–2 ml of fetal blood were taken, preferably at the placental insertion of the funicle. The sampling lasted 6–7 min on average. The quality of the sampled blood was verified by a Coulter Counter Analyzer. Thirty minutes after sampling, the fetal heart rate (FHR) was evaluated and the insertion point of the needle observed once more. The blood samples were placed in test tubes with EDTA trasylol, then centrifuged and stored at $-28°C$.

Glycemia was measured on frozen plasma by the enzymatic method, whereas C-peptide was measured on plasma by the radioimmunological method using the Biodata commercial kit.

RESULTS

Taking into account the whole population studied, two well-defined groups emerged. The first included 19 cases at risk for hemoglobinopathy, the second consisted of 17 cases of fetal malformation pathology. Samplings were performed at week 19.9 ± 0.2 for the first group, and at week 22.6 ± 1 for the second.

For the first group, the average values for maternal and fetal glycemia were 82.8 ± 4 mg/100 ml and 41.4 ± 4.5, respectively. For the second, the corresponding values were 94.2 ± 5.5 and 36.7 ± 4.2 ml.

In the group at risk for hemoglobinopathy, the average values for maternal and fetal C-peptide were 677 ± 118 pmol/l and 615 ± 77 pmol/l, respectively; the corresponding values for the malformation pathology group were 365 ± 34 pmol/l and 601 ± 152 pmol/l.

The glycemia and fetal C-peptide values of the two diabetes cases were 160 mg/100 ml and 3102 pmol/l for the patient belonging to White Class D; 56 mg/100 ml and 758 pmol/l for the patient belonging to White Class A.

Finally, the two samplings performed to obtain a rapid determination of the fetal karyotype (that happened to be normal) gave the following results for glycemia and fetal C-peptide: 42 mg/100 ml and 395 pmol/l in the first case, and 60 mg/322 pmol/l in the second.

57

Placental status in pregnant patients with a history of Caesarean section

T. V. Chervakova and Zh. M. Dairbaeva

Considerable rates of Caesarean section have given rise to increased numbers of pregnant patients with a uterine scar after past abdominal delivery. Given a certain percentage of developmental fetal abnormalities in this category of patients, the purpose of this study was to assess fetoplacental activity in 248 pregnant patients with a history of Caesarean section. In order to exclude fetoplacental effects of systemic disease and pregnancy complications, apparently normal women with uncomplicated pregnancy were studied. Indications for Caesarean section included abnormalities of pelvic bones, fetal malpresentations and abnormal fetal head engagement, breech presentation and incompetent uterine scar, which, as a rule, did not affect the fetoplacental system.

The period of time since the previous operation varied from 11 to 75 months, being less than 24 months (2 years) in the vast majority of patients (208, or 83%). Incompetent uterine scar was observed in 103 (45.1%). It was associated with a high incidence of inflammation (28.4%) and induced and spontaneous abortions (49.9%) within 1 to 6 months after surgery. It should be noted that morphofunctional insufficiency of the uterine scar can be with and without clinical manifestations. Where medical history and clinical results in the current pregnancy pointed to a possible incompetent scar in 23.48% of the cases, the intraoperative rate was nearly twice as high, 45.1% (103 patients). The formation of the scar was influenced by placental localization (Table 1).

To assess fetoplacental status, placental lactogen and estriol were measured

Table 1 Placental localization

Placental site	*Number of cases*	*Percentage*
Anterior wall	50	20.2
Lateral wall to anterior wall	67	27.0
Lateral wall to posterior wall	69	27.8
Posterior wall	62	25.0

in the blood of pregnant patients with a history of Caesarean section. Hormonal levels were found to be related to the dates of pregnancy and placental site (Figure 1). For example, before 24–27 weeks of pregnancy, maternal blood placental lactogen was on a higher level, as compared to the respective values in normal pregnant patients. The highest values were associated with posterior localization of the placenta. From 28 to 30 weeks onward, placental lactogen began to fall behind the respective values in normal patients, and was particularly low if the placenta was attached to the anterior uterine wall, especially so in the vicinity of the scar (Figure 2). Blood estriol in uterine scar patients kept on a higher level throughout pregnancy, as compared to the scar-free patients, its values being particularly high if the placenta was attached to the posterior uterine wall.

The only exceptions here were the dates between 13 and 16 weeks when blood estriol of patients with a uterine scar dropped below normal values. As pregnancy progresses, the myometrium grows thin around the scar, which may account for the increased risk of uterine rupture at these dates. Blood placental lactogen dropped by 20–40% by this time, as compared to normal pregnancy. Beginning at 35–36 weeks of pregnancy, estriol in the blood of postcaesarean patients was lowered (1.4-fold at 37–38 weeks, and 2.8-fold at 39–40 weeks) as compared to normal pregnant patients. The level was particularly low where the placenta was located on the anterior wall and near the scar. Apparently, increased hormonal levels, seen in the second and third trimesters of pregnancy, may be due to the mobilization of protective and adaptive placental reactions. These reactions are more marked in postcaesarean patients, obviously due to more considerable circulatory deviations from normal, associated with the uterine scar. Lower estrogen levels at 13–16 weeks of pregnancy may be related to the fact that placental

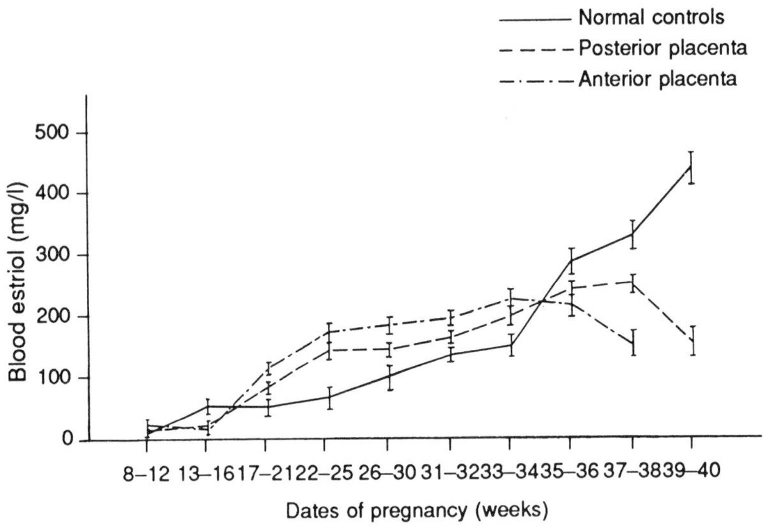

Figure 1 Blood estriol variation in normal controls (——) and in postcaesarean patients with posterior placenta (– – –) or anterior placenta (–·–·–) measured in mg/l

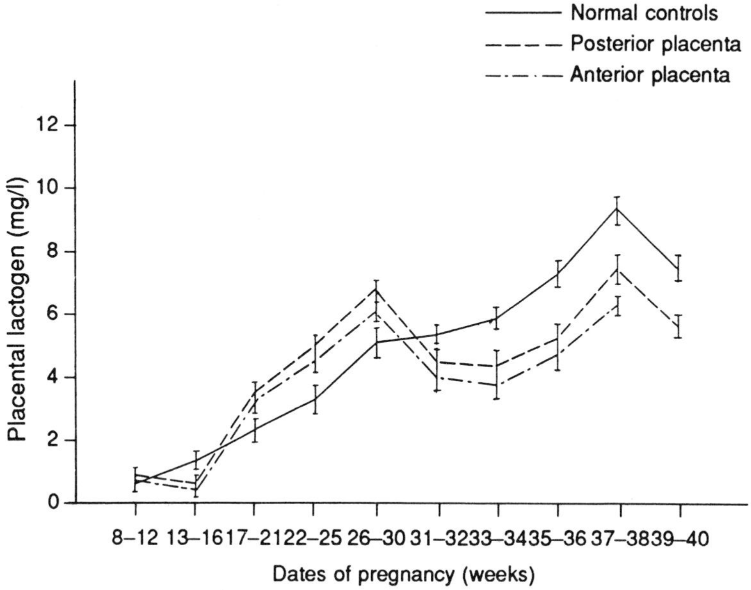

Figure 2 Placental lactogen in normal controls (——) and in postcaesarean patients with posterior placenta (– – –) or anterior placenta (–·–·–) measured in mg/ml

formation is completed by those dates, and the placenta joins the fetoplacental circulatory network. In the presence of a uterine scar, this process is slowed down somewhat as manifested in slower mobilization of protective mechanisms. At 24–26 weeks, the uterus grows rapidly. In the presence of myometrial morphofunctional changes, fetoplacental circulation is disrupted around the scar, and adaptation becomes impaired. Signs of threatened abortion often develop at these dates.

Anterior placental localization is less conducive to the mobilization of these reactions which are soon exhausted. Drops of hormonal levels at 13–16, 26–30 and 34–36 weeks of pregnancy suggest that these dates are critical ones for pregnancy, when placental insufficiency associated with a uterine scar is particularly pronounced.

To assess the activity of placental metabolic compensatory reactions, detect functional placental disorders and make fetal prognosis, the activity of heat-labile and heat-stable alkaline phosphatase was determined in 40 pregnant patients, and the ratio of the heat-labile form to the heat-stable form was estimated as this can reflect the contribution of alkaline phosphatase to blood phosphate activity.

A study by Nasyrov has demonstrated that altered enzyme activity (both the rise and the drop) is an evidence of transformation in the adaptive mechanisms[1,2]. Whereas normally the heat-labile to heat-stable alkaline phosphatase ratio is 1.4 ± 0.2, its drop to 0.69–0.96 is an evidence of a compensated incompetence, and its rise to 2.3–3.1 points to a decompensated incompetence (Table 2). In all cases, changes in blood phosphate activity

Table 2 Heat-stable/heat-labile alkaline phosphatase activity in blood of normal patients and those with uterine scar

Diagnosis	*Dates of pregnancy* (weeks)	*Mean ratios*	*Variability range*
Normal pregnancy	38–40	1.4 ± 0.2	1.0–1.8
Uterine scar (compensated incompetence)	38–40	0.7 ± 0.2	0.3–1.1
Uterine scar (decompensated incompetence)	38–40	2.7 ± 0.2	2.3–3.1

were accompanied by developing signs of fetal hypoxia and growth retardation. This test allows a more accurate assessment of the severity of fetoplacental disorders.

The evaluation of fetoplacental activity on the basis of the heat-labile to heat-stable alkaline phosphatase ratio was verified by clinical data and demonstrated high incidence of fetoplacental insufficiency in uterine scar patients, its severity showing correlation to the placental site and being particularly great in cases of anterior placental attachment (Figure 3). The rate of decompensated fetoplacental insufficiency reached 71%.

Fetoplacental diagnosis and the assessment of fetal condition made use of ultrasonic complex scanning and fetal heart rate monitoring, which are extensively used in current obstetrical practices. Ultrasonography was used to monitor the condition of the scar, placental thickness and site, as well as fetometric measurements, since the first trimester of pregnancy.

Particular attention was paid to the identification of an incompetent scar. A competent uterine scar typically shows a distinct homogeneous echo structure throughout pregnancy. Incompetent scar may be associated with interrupted or deformed structures and echo-negative areas of varying sizes. Using this method, the diagnosis of incompetent uterine scar was made in 87% of the cases.

Placental thickness and reduced fetal biparietal diameter (Table 3) were important indicators of fetoplacental insufficiency. One can see from the table that fetal biparietal diameter and placental thickness were reduced in all cases, pointing to developing signs of placental insufficiency and fetal growth retardation. The accuracy of ultrasonic diagnosis of fetoplacental

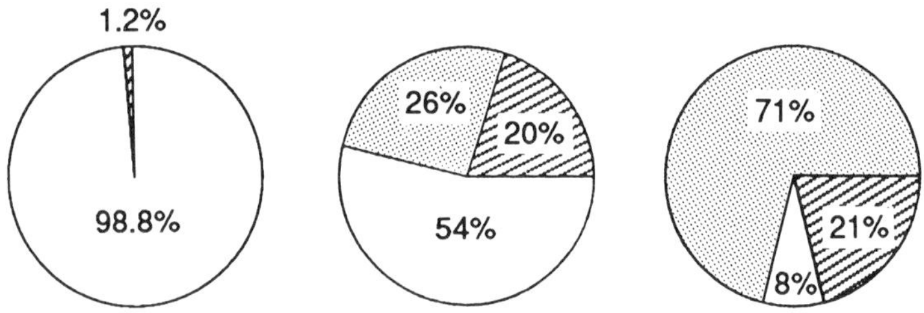

Figure 3 Incidence of compensated and decompensated fetoplacental insufficiency in normal and postcaesarean patients with compensated incompetence (hatched area) or decompensated incompetence (stippled area) as evidenced by heat-labile and heat-stable alkaline phosphatase, normal placenta is shown by open area

Table 3 Fetal biparietal diameter and placental thickness in pregnant patients with and without uterine scar

Dates of pregnancy (weeks)	*Pregnant patients with uterine scar*	*Normal pregnant patients*
Fetal biparietal diameter (mm)		
28–32	73.45 ± 1.54	76.5 ± 1.5
33–36	83.57 ± 0.72	86.8 ± 0.9
37–40	91.19 ± 1.01	93.3 ± 0.8
Placental thickness (mm)		
28–30	26.76 ± 0.82	28.8 ± 3.2
33–36	31.0 ± 0.35	35.2 ± 3.4
37–40	34.04 ± 0.32	35.2 ± 3.4

insufficiency was confirmed at surgery in 68% of cases.

Ultrasonic complex scanning is of particular importance for placental localization. High diagnostic accuracy (97%) allows the recommendation of this method to all postcaesarean pregnant patients. In our series, the placenta was attached to the posterior uterine wall reaching out to other walls in 45%, and to the anterior wall (around or close to the scar) in 55%.

Fetal heart rate monitoring using non-invasive tests helped to detect developmental disorders due to developing placental insufficiency and related to the site of the uterine scar. A correlation has been established between placental localization and fetal heart rate disorders. The latter was particularly pronounced in cases of anterior placental attachment (Figure 4). The demonstrated fetoplacental disorders and fetal cardiodynamic changes suggest that the fetus is suffering from hypoxia in the presence of a uterine scar, its severity being largely related to the placental site. After-effects of chronic intrauterine hypoxia were seen in 37% of the infants, delivered by postcaesarean mothers.

Placental morphological studies have demonstrated that placental localization has a considerable impact on the markedness of arising morphological changes. The changes were particularly marked in cases of anterior placental localization. For example, macroscopic changes (additional lobules, lipid degeneration, calcification and hemorrhage sites, etc.) were seen in 16% of normal pregnant patients, 39% of pregnant patients with posterior placenta and in 88% of patients with anterior placenta. Microscopic studies demonstrated intact structures with marked adaptive reactions on the part of villous

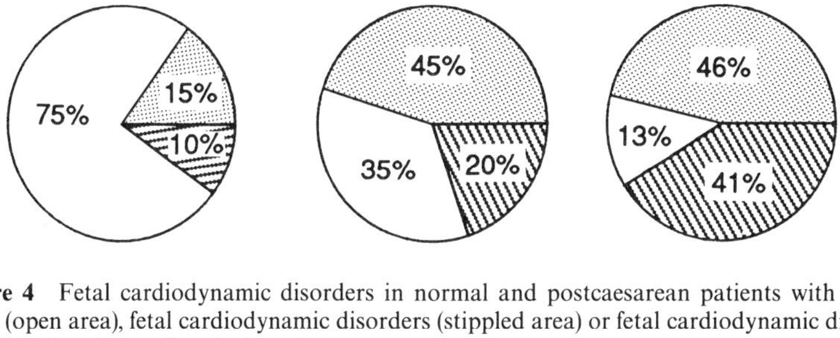

Figure 4 Fetal cardiodynamic disorders in normal and postcaesarean patients with normal heart (open area), fetal cardiodynamic disorders (stippled area) or fetal cardiodynamic disorders after functional tests (hatched area)

syncytium and the absence of dystrophic changes in patients undergoing Caesarean section for the first time.

The placentas of patients with a history of Caesarean sections showed more marked compensatory reactions, increased numbers of capillaries in terminal villi, syncytial nodes, from which new villi developed, and syncytioendothelial membranes. At the same time, degenerative changes were revealed: hemorrhages into intervillous space, excessive fibrinoid deposition (villous necrosis?). The changes were particularly marked in the placenta attached to the anterior uterine wall, especially in the vicinity of the scar. The type of change was determined by the state of the scar. Quantitative correlations of individual structural elements in the placenta, visualized stereomorphometrically, are presented in Table 4. This shows structural changes distinctly prevailing in numbers in the placenta located on the anterior uterine wall.

In all cases of repeated Caesarean section, the myometrium shows expanded growth of connective tissue with manifestations of hyalinosis, tissue defibration and edema, circulatory disturbances, massive hemorrhages and dystrophic changes of muscle fibers. These changes were combined with signs of acute inflammation in 22%, and with signs of chronic inflammation of myometrial tissues in 17.5%.

Histological studies of myometrial walls demonstrated, in addition to changes, typical for pregnancy, some changes related to the site of the scar and the placenta. Where the placenta is located in the area of the scar, there is deep invasion of trophoblastic elements into the myometrial and endometrial tissue in 50% of the cases. Placenta adherens was detected in seven cases.

In cases where the placenta was located on the anterior wall somewhat off the scar, trophoblastic elements could be seen in the myometrium in 25% of the patients, and decidual in-growth in 40% of the patients. Apparently, those changes were a factor leading to a disturbance of uterine contractility.

Placental studies demonstrated that the placentas attached to the anterior wall or around the scar showed greater dystrophic changes in their compensa-

Table 4 Major quantitative manifestations of placental structural change in relation to placental location as evidenced by stereomorphometric methods

	Controls	*Patients with placenta on posterior wall*	*Patients with placenta on anterior wall*
Terminal villous stroma	12.2 ± 0.02	16.6 ± 0.08	18.5 ± 0.04
Terminal villous capillaries	13.5 ± 0.05	13.5 ± 0.05	18.1 ± 0.05
Syncytiotrophoblastoma nuclei	6.3 ± 0.01	8.1 ± 0.01	7.75 ± 0.01
Syncytiotrophoblastoma cytoplasm	4.7 ± 0.05	5.8 ± 0.06	5.8 ± 0.05
Syncytiella node	1.0 ± 0.01	1.2 ± 0.01	2.7 ± 0.02
Syncytioendothelial membranes	3.0 ± 0.03	4.6 ± 0.03	4.9 ± 0.04
Intervillous spaces	31.2 ± 0.04	33.6 ± 0.03	30.4 ± 0.04
Fibrins	3.0 ± 0.01	5.6 ± 0.06	4.05 ± 0.04

tory and adaptive mechanisms. The great strain of placental compensatory and adaptive mechanisms was a factor that promoted normal gas exchange in infants and contributed essentially to normal births.

Marked fetoplacental changes had an impact on fetal and neonatal condition. Among the causes of perinatal morbidity fetal growth retardation came first (22%), and was followed by asphyxia (10%) and pneumonia (6%).

Studies of neonatal condition (Table 5) have demonstrated considerable influence of the placental site on birth weight and Apgar score at birth as well as the course of the early neonatal life and the development of the infant through the first years of life.

The follow-up of infants in the first year of life demonstrated differences between infants born at first and repeat Caesarean section. There was a significant physical retardation within the first 3 months of life in infants whose mothers had exhibited signs of fetoplacental insufficiency.

It can be concluded, on the basis of our results, that postcaesarean pregnant patients with a uterine scar are a high-risk group for fetoplacental insufficiency.

Placental localization on the anterior wall and, particularly, in the vicinity of the scar, increased the risk of fetoplacental insufficiency considerably.

To prevent the development of fetal abnormalities, a combination of therapeutic and preventive factors was prescribed with regard to fetoplacental status, as determined at least once every 7–10 days.

All pregnant patients underwent outpatient preventive treatment for fetoplacental insufficiency at critical dates of pregnancy (13–16 weeks, 24–26 weeks, 34–36 weeks) with regard to fetoplacental status, as assessed every 7 or 10 days. It included drugs, improving uteroplacental circulation (tonicol), fetal energy metabolism and cardiac activity and tissue metabolism (glucose, vitamin C, co-carboxylase).

All patients were treated with vitamins and spasmolytic agents. The preventive course takes 2 to 3 weeks. To detect fetoplacental insufficiency, patients were admitted to hospital for a comprehensive clinical and laboratory monitoring, including weekly measurement of blood hormones and urinary estriol, heat-stable alkaline phosphatase (measured twice a week) and functional tests (weekly or twice weekly where necessary).

Where signs of placental insufficiency were demonstrated, intravenous drip infusion of 2% sigetin (6.0–10.0 ml per 200 ml hemodez) or 400 ml rheopolyglucin solution, were added to the therapeutic complex in order to improve placental microcirculation and fetal nutrition.

To prevent and control fetal growth retardation, we used: pholic acid, 0.02 g three times daily; vitamin B_{12}, 200 μg every second day, i.m.; galascorbin, 0.5 g three times a day; intramuscular co-carboxylase, 100 mg once daily and ATP, 1.0 ml per 20 ml of 40% glucose solution.

β-mimetics are also given to improve uteroplacental circulation (1.0 ml alupent, diluted with 300.0–400.0 ml physiological saline, or 10 ml partusisten per 500 ml 5% glucose solution). In addition, dexamethazone (four tablets four times daily for 2 days, or a total of 16 mg per course of treatment) was administered to prevent fetal distress syndrome where preterm delivery was indicated. Dexamethazone was given at any dates of pregnancy beginning

Table 5 Neonatal condition in relation to placental location

Placental location	*Birth weight* (g)	*Apgar score*	*Course of early neonatal period*	*Infant development*
Control group	3621 ± 58.82	8.5 ± 0.4	Normal	Normal
Placenta on posterior-to-lateral uterine wall	3223 ± 68.76	8.1 ± 0.3	After-effects of hypoxia in 19%	Increased morbidity in 12%
Placenta on anterior-to-lateral uterine wall	2852 ± 49.43	7.6 ± 0.4	After-effects of hypoxia in 27%	Increased morbidity in 19% Retarded physical development in 10%
Placenta near the scar	2637 ± 51.32	6.8 ± 0.3	After-effects of hypoxia in 44%, retarded physical development	Increased morbidity in 35%, retarded physical development

at 27–28 weeks, yet not later than 2 days in advance of the elective section.

Fetal monitoring allowed fetal condition and treatment efficiency to be assessed.

Treatment administered for 3 to 4 weeks produced a positive effect. The assessment of treatment efficiency was based on daily urinary estriol excretion and placental enzyme activity, as fetoplacental insufficiency is associated with a twofold drop in estriol excretion, and a twofold rise in heat-stable alkaline phosphatase. In decompensated placental insufficiency, heat-stable alkaline phosphatase drops threefold. If treatment fails to produce an effect within 2 or 3 weeks, these fetoplacental parameters deteriorate dramatically, acting as a predictive sign for preterm delivery.

REFERENCES

1. Nasyrov, A.T. (1984). Placental adaptive mechanisms of carbohydrate metabolism. *Synopsis of Candidate Thesis*, Alma-Ata (Russian)
2. Nasyrov, A.T. (1979). Enzyme methods of the assessment of placental condition and evaluation of preterm newborns. Methodologic recommendations, Alma-Ata (Russian)

Section 4

Gynecological Endocrinology

Part A

Neurotransmitters, neurohormones and neuropeptides in reproduction

58

Neuroendocrine regulation of the prolactin and ACTH response to stress

S.M. McCann, L. Milenkovic, J. Martinovic, G. Pan, G.D. Snyder, C. Franci and V. Rettori

INTRODUCTION

Stresses of various sorts induce a dramatic alteration in the release of anterior pituitary hormones. In man the release of adrenocorticotropin hormone (ACTH), prolactin (PRL) and growth hormone (GH) is increased and the secretion of luteinizing hormone (LH) is decreased. These changes are brought about by altered patterns of release of releasing and inhibiting hormones from the hypothalamus. The responsible factors can vary depending on the type of stress.

DIRECT ACTIONS AT THE PITUITARY TO ALTER PITUITARY HORMONE RELEASE

Early evidence suggested that epinephrine circulating after its release from the adrenal medulla might stimulate ACTH secretion. It is now clear from *in vitro* experiments that such a stimulation can indeed occur[1]. Epinephrine can also evoke ACTH secretion when given intravenously[2]. This action *in vivo* is probably brought about by activation of the hypothalamus since hypothalamic lesions can abolish the response. Alternatively following these lesions which would eliminate the release of other hypophyseotropic factors such as vasopressin and corticotropin-releasing factor (CRF), epinephrine is no longer able to stimulate the corticotropes. There are beta receptors in the gland[3] and consequently it is our current view that epinephrine circulating in the blood to the adenohypophysis from either adrenal medullary and possibly also hypothalamic sources may play a small role in the stress response of ACTH. Short exposure of pituitary cells *in vitro* to epinephrine can also release PRL, so that we have come full circle and the first postulated stimulator has to still be considered as possibly significant in control of the pituitary response to stress.

The next postulated mediator of ACTH release in response to stress was vasopressin since vasopressin is released in response to a variety of stresses and since lesions in the median eminence which impair vasopressin release are usually associated with a blockade of ACTH release. It was also shown that vasopressin could stimulate the release of ACTH both *in vivo* and *in vitro*[4].

There was evidence for another factor in hypothalamic extracts termed CRF; however, its isolation and determination of structure was elusive until 1981 when Vale and co-workers determined the structure of the 41 amino acid CRF[5]. The delay was related to the relatively large size of this peptide on comparison to that of thyrotropin-releasing hormone (TRH), a tripeptide, luteinizing hormone-releasing hormone (LHRH), a decapeptide and somatostatin, a tetradecapeptide. There is now no doubt that CRF plays an important role in control of ACTH release. An interaction between vasopressin and CRF occurs at the pituitary level for vasopressin to augment the response to CRF. This synergism was early shown *in vivo* and has now been confirmed in many additional *in vitro* experiments, so that it is clear that vasopressin and CRF co-operate to stimulate the release of ACTH in stress[4].

Oxytocin had earlier been ruled out as a factor stimulating ACTH release; however, in recent experiments some evidence for a primary releasing action of oxytocin and also for the ability of this peptide to augment the response to CRF has developed[6].

Other peptides have been reported to stimulate ACTH release directly *in vitro*. Angiotensin II is one of these[7]. Conversely, atrial natriuretic peptide can inhibit ACTH release *in vitro*[8].

The release of ACTH from different stresses may depend on different patterns of release of these various putative stimulators into hypophyseal portal blood. For example, it appears that vasopressin is particularly important in the increased ACTH release which occurs following hemorrhage and that it is important in mediating the increased ACTH release which follows adrenalectomy. Both of these conditions are accompanied by increased vasopressin secretion[6,7]. Studies with antisera or antagonists against these various peptides have played an important role in unraveling their physiological significance in control of the ACTH release in stress. New studies of this type support the physiological significance of CRF[5], vasopressin[9] and even oxytocin[10] in mediating the ACTH release from stress; however, no support could be generated for the physiological role of angiotensin II, at least in ether stress, based on studies with the angiotensin antagonist, saralasin and antisera against angiotensin II[10]. It still could play a role in other forms of stress such as hemorrhage which are associated with angiotensin II discharge. On the other hand, oxytocin and vasopressin appear to be important in mediating the ether-induced release of ACTH based on studies in which antibodies directed against each peptide were injected into the third ventricle (3V). Conversely, intraventricular (3V) injection of antibodies against atrial natriuretic peptide resulted in elevated plasma ACTH during stress[10].

The stimulation of PRL release during stress is probably brought about by a number of factors which include possible decrease in dopaminergic inhibitory tone coupled with increased stimulatory effects of oxytocin, vasoactive intestinal peptide (VIP) and possibly peptide histadine isoleucine

(PHI). These conclusions again are based on the demonstration that each of these peptides directly stimulates PRL release and studies with antisera developed against the peptides or with antagonists to their action which partially block stress-induced PRL release. As indicated above epinephrine also has the capability of stimulating PRL release *in vitro* in a perifusion system[11].

Thus, a complex interplay of catecholamines and many peptides mediates the stress-induced changes in anterior pituitary hormone secretion by direct actions on the gland.

HYPOTHALAMIC INTERACTIONS WHICH MEDIATE THE STRESS-INDUCED PATTERN OF ACTH AND PRL RELEASE

The interactions of various transmitters on the hypothalamus are even more complex than those just described for the pituitary gland itself. There is even colocalization of vasopressin and CRF in a number of small neurons with cell bodies in the paraventricular nucleus and axons projecting to the median eminence for release of the peptides into hypophyseal portal capillaries. There is a dramatic cellular response in the adrenalectomized animal with increased euronal accumulation of vasopressin which presumably supports the increased release of vasopressin in this situation to drive ACTH secretion[12].

SHORT-LOOP FEEDBACK OF ACTH TO ALTER ACTH AND PRL RELEASE

Microinjection of ACTH into the third ventricle has little effect on resting ACTH levels; however, it can significantly blunt the stress-induced release of ACTH following ether or restraint stress. At the same time injection of ACTH blunts the PRL release which occurs following these stresses. Thus there is a short-loop negative feedback of ACTH to suppress not only its own release but that of PRL as well. Alpha melanocyte-stimulating hormone (MSH), which is ACTH 1–13, can also suppress PRL release, so it is possible that the PRL suppression induced by ACTH may simply reflect actions of the 1–13 sequence of the molecule. This negative short-loop feedback may operate either by retrograde flow in portal vessels delivering ACTH from the pituitary to the hypothalamus or it may be mediated via release of ACTH from the pro-opiomelanocortin-producing neurons in the arcuate nucleus. It is still not clear whether ACTH itself is actually released from these neurons but certainly either the total pro-opiomelanocortin molecule or fragments thereof are released. The short-loop negative feedback of ACTH has physiological significance since following third ventricular injection of antisera directed against ACTH, there is an augmentation of the ACTH and PRL release from stress. This indicates that in stress ACTH acts within the hypothalamus to blunt its further release[13].

There is also a rapid short-loop feedback of PRL to diminish its own release. This may be mediated via a stimulation of dopamine release. It also is physiologically significant since injection of antisera against PRL into the third ventricle results in augmented stress-induced release of PRL[14].

ULTRASHORT-LOOP FEEDBACK AND THE STRESS RESPONSE

In addition, there appears to be intrahypothalamic action of vasopressin to augment either its own release or that of CRF during stress since intraventricular injection of vasopressin antisera can significantly blunt the ACTH release following ether anesthesia[15]. In contrast to the negative short-loop feedback of ACTH to suppress its own release in stress, there appears to be positive ultra short-loop feedback of CRF to enhance its own release during stress since the intraventricular injection of antisera directed against CRF results in a depression of the ACTH release during stress rather than an augmentation[16]. Furthermore, intraventricular injection of CRF in doses too low to stimulate directly ACTH release enhances ACTH release from stress[17].

ROLE OF OPIOID PEPTIDES IN MEDIATION OF STRESS-INDUCED ACTH AND PRL SECRETION

Resting plasma PRL levels are lowered by the opiate receptor blocker, naloxone, and stress-induced PRL release is also blocked. Similarly, stress-induced PRL release is blocked by intraventricular (3V) injection of antiserum directed against β-endorphin but not α-MSH. Thus, an opioid link is in the chain which leads to PRL release and it is probably mediated by β-endorphin[18]. In contrast, naloxone does not lower, and high doses can even elevate, plasma ACTH and only partially block stress-induced ACTH release which indicates that there are both inhibitory and stimulatory components to the opioid control of ACTH[19].

STRESS OF INFECTION ACTS VIA RELEASE OF MONOKINES FROM IMMUNE CELLS

It has previously been thought that the gland was stimulated only by substances reaching it via the hypophyseal portal vessels; however, many years ago Selye championed the idea of circulating substances, such as histamine, directly stimulating the gland. Recent evidence indicates that in the case of infection, the stress response is mediated at least in part by several monokines released largely from macrophages and monocytes.

It was earlier shown that bacterial endotoxin could induce delayed fever in the dog which was accompanied by ACTH release. At that time evidence was developing for the existence of an endogenous pyrogen coming from monocytes which induced the fever in response to endotoxin by an action on the hypothalamic temperature-regulating centers, resetting hypothalamic temperature to a higher set point. This was the proposed mechanism of action of bacterial endotoxin in the early experiments. We now know that bacterial lipopolysaccharides cause the release of interleukin-1 from monocytes and macrophages. This is a small protein of molecular weight 17 000.

Extensive studies indicate that interleukin-1 can act on the hypothalamus to modulate pituitary hormone release. For example, intravenous injection of interleukin-1 causes ACTH release which is accompanied by an increase in CRF release into portal vessels[20]. Even *in vitro* the protein will cause release of CRF[21]. A direct action of interleukin-1 on the pituitary is controversial. One group reported a release of all pituitary hormones following very low doses of interleukin-1 in a static incubation system[22]; however, others have not found any effect. In our own studies we found that interleukin-1 had a small effect following intraventricular injection to stimulate PRL release; presumably by a hypothalamic action[23].

We have carried out extensive studies with a recently discovered monokine, cachectin (tumor necrosis factor, TNF). Intraventricular injection of TNF induces fever presumably by acting on the temperature regulating centers and can stimulate the release of ACTH, PRL and GH while inhibiting the release of TSH presumably by hypothalamic action[24]. Furthermore, it can directly stimulate the release of ACTH, GH and TSH from pituitary cells incubated *in vitro* at low doses of the order of 10^{-8}–10^{-12} mol/l. TNF did not reproducibly stimulate PRL release except in the presence of somatostatin[25].

We have evaluated the mechanism by which TNF acts on the pituitary and have shown that indomethacin will block the release of the above mentioned pituitary hormones with the exception of ACTH. Cachectin induces a dose-related lowering of cyclic AMP in the pituitary except in the presence of somatostatin. In this instance the lowering is reversed and an elevation occurs with coincubation of somatostatin with cachectin. This is accompanied by PRL release.

Studies currently underway indicate that gamma interferon also has effects on the hypothalamus since following its intraventricular injection we obtained at low but not high doses a stimulation of ACTH and GH release and an inhibition of TSH release with no effect on release of PRL[26]. It is apparent then that a whole series of mediators released by immune cells may have powerful effects to alter the release of pituitary hormones by hypothalamic and pituitary action.

ACKNOWLEDGEMENTS

This work was supported by NIH grant HD09988. We wish to thank Ms Judy Scott for typing the manuscript.

REFERENCES

1. Tilders, F.J.H., Berkenbosch, F., Vermes, I., Linton, E.A. and Smelik, P.G. (1985). Role of epinephrine and vasopressin in the control of the pituitary-adrenal response to stress. *Fed. Proc.*, **44**, 155–60
2. Xu, R.K., Antunes-Rodrigues, J. and McCann, S.M. (1987). Evidence for hypothalamic action of epinephrine to stimulate ACTH secretion in the rat. *Neuroendocr. Lett.*, **9**, 339–44
3. Petrovic, S.L., McDonald, J.K., Snyder, G.D. and McCann, S.M. (1983). Characterization of beta-adrenergic receptors in rat brain and pituitary using a new high-affinity ligand, (^{125}I)iodocyanopindolol. *Brain Res.*, **261**, 249–59
4. McCann, S.M., Lumpkin, M.D. and Samson, W.K. (1982). The role of vasopressin and

oxytocin in control of anterior pituitary hormone secretion. In Baertsche, A.J. and Dreifuss, J.J. (eds). *Neuroendocrinology of Vasopressin, Corticoliberin and Opiomelanocortins*, pp. 319–29. (London: Academic Press)

5. Rivier, J. and Vale, W.W. (1985). Effects of corticotropin-releasing factor, neurohypophyseal peptides and catecholamines on pituitary function. *Fed. Proc.*, **44**, 189–96
6. Gibbs, D.M. (1985). Measurement of hypothalamic corticotropin-releasing factors in hypophyseal portal blood. *Fed. Proc.*, **44**, 203–6
7. Plotsky, P.M. (1985). Hypophyseotropic regulation of adenohypophyseal adrenocorticotropin secretion. *Fed. Proc.*, **44**, 207–13
8. Samson, W.K. and Eskay, R.L. (1986). Endocrine and neuroendocrine actions of cardiac peptides. In Moody, T.W. (ed.) *Neural and Endocrine Peptides and Receptors*, pp. 521–40. (New York: Plenum)
9. Ono, N., Bedran de Castro, J.C., Khorram, O. and McCann, S.M. (1985). Role of arginine vasopressin in control of ACTH and LH release during stress. *Life Sci.*, **36**, 1779–86
10. Franci, C.R., Ono, N. and McCann, S.M. (1989). *Neuroendocrinology*, (submitted)
11. Samson, W.K., Lumpkin, M.D. and McCann, S.M. (1986). Evidence of a physiological role for oxytocin in the control of prolactin secretion. *Endocrinology*, **119**, 554–60
12. Whitnall, M.H., Key, S. and Gainer, H. (1987). Vasopressin-containing and vasopressin-deficient subpopulations of corticotropin releasing factor axons are differentially effected by adrenalectomy. *Endocrinology*, **120**, 2180–2
13. McCann, S.M., Pan, G., Xu, R.J., Martinovic, J. and Rettori, V. (1988). Modulatory hypothalamic action of ACTH on ACTH and prolactin release. In Hoshino, K. (ed.) *Prolactin Gene Family and its Receptors*, pp. 211–18. (Amsterdam: Excerpta Medica)
14. Milenkovic, L., Parlow, A.F. and McCann, S.M. (1989). The physiological significance of the negative short-loop feedback of prolactin. *Neuroendocrinology*, (submitted)
15. Ono, N., Bedran de Castro, J.C., Khorram, O. and McCann, S.M. (1985). Role of arginine vasopressin in control of ACTH and LH release during stress. *Life Sci.*, **36**, 1779–86
16. Ono, N., Samson, W.K., McDonald, J.K., Lumpkin, M.D., Bedran de Castro, J.C. and McCann, S.M. (1985). The effects of intravenous and intraventricular injection of antisera directed against corticotropin releasing factor (CRF) on the secretion of anterior pituitary hormones. *Proc. Natl. Acad. Sci., USA*, **82**, 7787–90
17. Ono, N., Bedran de Castro, J.C. and McCann, S.M. (1985). Ultrashort-loop positive feedback of corticotropin-releasing factor (CRF) to enhance ACTH release in stress. *Proc. Natl. Acad. Sci.. USA*, **82**, 3528–31
18. Bedran de Castro, J.C., Khorram, O., Petrovic, S.L. and McCann, S.M. (1987). Role of opioid peptides in pulsatile release of gonadotropins and prolactin in the rat. *Brain Res. Bull.*, **19**, 539–44
19. Xu, R.J. and McCann, S.M. (1989). Differential effects of naloxone on basal and stress-induced release of ACTH and prolactin in the male rat. *Life Sci.*, (submitted)
20. Sapolsky, R., Rivier, C., Yamamoto, G., Plotsky, P. and Vale, W.W. (1987). Interleukin-1 stimulates the secretion of hypothalamic corticotropin-releasing factor. *Science*, **238**, 522–4
21. Tsagarakis, S., Gillies, G., Rees, L.H., Besser, M. and Grossman, A. (1989). Interleukin-1 directly stimulates the release of corticotrophin releasing factor from rat hypothalamus. *Neuroendocrinology*, **49**, 98–101
22. Bernton, E.W., Beach, J., Holaday, J.W., Smallridge, R.C. and Fein, H.G. (1987). Release of multiple hormones by a direct action of interleukin-1 on pituitary cells. *Science*, **238**, 519–21
23. Rettori, V., Jurcovicova, J. and McCann, S.M. (1987). The central action of interleukin-1 to alter the release of TSH, growth hormone and prolactin in the male rat. *J. Neurosci. Res.*, **18**, 179–83
24. McCann, S.M., Rettori, V., Milenkovic, L., Jurcovicova, J., Snyder, G. and Beutler, B. (1989). Role of interleukin-1 and cachectin in control of anterior pituitary hormone release. In Lakoski, J.M., Perez-Polo, J.R. and Rassin, D.K. (eds) *Neural Control of Reproductive Function*, pp. 333–49. (New York: Liss)
25. Milenkovic, L., Rettori, V., Snyder, G.D., Beutler, B. and McCann, S.M. (1989). Cachectin alters anterior pituitary hormone release by a direct action *in vitro*. *Proc. Natl. Acad. Sci., USA*, (in press)
26. Gonzalez, M.C. (1989). Effects of human recombinant γ interferon on the release of GH, TSH and prolactin in the male rat. Program of the 71st Annual Meeting of the Endocrine Society, p. 63. (Seattle: Endocrine Society)

59

LH pulsatile secretion in normal and in pathological menstrual cycle

A.D. Genazzani, F. Petraglia, F. Facchinetti, F. Baraghini and A.R. Genazzani

INTRODUCTION

Endocrine glands usually secrete hormones in an intermittent or pulsatile pattern and all the hypophyseal hormones obey this rule. The pulsatile secretion as well as the amplitude may transmit information to the target cells, thus inducing the activation or inhibition of their activity.

Many studies have demonstrated that pituitary secretion is controlled by the hypothalamus by the secretion of specific releasing or inhibitory factors, but it is also greatly influenced by the presence of many other substances such as neurotransmitters, neuropeptides and steroid hormones. Luteinizing hormone (LH) secretion is considered to reflect the gonadotropin-releasing hormone (GnRH) secretory pattern[1,2] and since direct sampling for GnRH is not possible in humans, the best way to study the neuroendocrine activity of the hypothalamus on the gonadotropes is to study the gonadotropin secretory pattern. Obviously this approach relies on the assumption that there is a correspondence between GnRH secretion and LH release, as has been demonstrated in monkeys[3]. Although an episodic stimulatory mode is critical for pituitary function, the physiological role of pulsatile gonadotropin stimulation of the gonad has not yet been clarified.

PULSATILE SECRETION STUDY

The secretion of LH in women has been extensively studied using different assay systems and algorithms for pulse detection, both in physiological and pathological circumstances[4–8]. It is obviously important to have a precise and sensitive assay method as well as a sensitive and specific algorithm for pulse detection. In any case two problems have always to be solved for all the studies of hormonal pulsatility: duration of the study and frequency of sampling. Veldhuis *et al.* showed a highly significant dependence of apparent LH pulse frequency on sampling intensity and on duration of the study for both men and women[9]. The reduction of the sampling frequency gives a significant reduction in number of the pulses detected. The wrong choice of sampling interval and/or duration of the study may greatly affect the results of the study.

NORMAL MENSTRUAL CYCLE

Episodic pulsatile secretion of LH changes throughout life. Different LH pulsatile patterns are shown during the menstrual cycle. In a preliminary study the changes of LH secretory pattern during the four phases of the menstrual cycle were studied by sampling every 10 min for 8 h. The time series were analyzed with program DETECT[10]. As other authors reported[6], LH pulsatile frequency remained constant during the early follicular (EFP) and late follicular (LFP) phases (5.7 ± 0.3 and 5.3 ± 1.1 peaks/8 h, respectively; mean $\pm$ SEM) while there was a slight increase of the mean duration from EFP to LFP (58.7 ± 16.3 and 97.8 ± 39 minutes, respectively). During the early luteal phase (ELP) plasma LH showed a lower pulse frequency (3.6 ± 0.3 peaks/8 h) and an increased duration (120 ± 30 minutes). In the late luteal phase (LLP) the LH pulsatile frequency increased again (4.9 ± 0.6 peaks/8 h) while duration showed a slight reduction (75.3 ± 16.4 minutes).

Many of these changes are explained by the contemporary secretion of gonadal steroids and by their feedback action on the hypothalamic–hypophyseal axis. Estrogens are reported to increase the GnRH pulsatile secretion[11] while progesterone induces a slowing of LH pulsatile release[12]. Several other substances may also affect the LH pulsatile release. For example the administration of the opiate receptor antagonist, naloxone, increases LH pulsatile frequency during the luteal phase, demonstrating the influence of endogenous opioids on gonadotropin secretion[13].

The presence of such modifications in LH pulsatile secretion during the normal menstrual cycle suggests the importance that this kind of pattern has in preparing and inducing ovulation as well as in preparing the luteal phase for blastocyst implantation.

HYPOTHALAMIC AMENORRHEA

The term ‘amenorrhea’ indicates the absence of menses and the presence of an abnormal regulation of the menstrual cycle. LH pulsatile frequency is always altered in amenorrheic women and it can be characterized by the complete absence of LH pulses[5] as well as by the reduction of LH pulse amplitude[14]. In primary amenorrhea no evidence of spontaneous LH pulsatile release was found[5,14], even if in some patients a pulsatile pattern was observed during sleep[15]. This last evidence resembles the nocturnal LH pulsatile secretion of the prepubertal period or of delayed puberty. Also anorexia nervosa results in a regression of pulsatile gonadotropin secretion to a prepubertal pattern; resumption of normal weight leads to normalization of pulsatile LH secretion[16].

Amenorrhea has been shown to occur also in long distance runners without weight loss[17] as well as in women after weight loss[18]. Distance runners with secondary amenorrhea had a distinct reduction in spontaneous LH pulse frequency. This slowing in pulse frequency occurred without any significant alterations in plasma concentrations of estradiol. Moreover in these women the capacity of the pituitary gland to release LH was normal in response to exogenous pulses of GnRH[17]. Based upon the available literature several mechanisms may be considered. First, endogenous opioid peptides suppress LH secretion[19] and various types of stress such as physical exercise, increase hypothalamic concentrations of opioids[20]. Secondly, sex steroid hormones, such as progesterone and testosterone, might suppress while estradiol might increase LH pulse frequency[21]. Thirdly, epidemiological studies suggest that nutritional or psychological factors and the effects of energy drain may be implicated as causes of amenorrhea[22].

POLYCYSTIC OVARIAN DISEASE

While several studies have reported a significant increment of LH pulse frequency in patients with polycystic ovarian disease (PCOD)[23,24] other investigators failed to detect a significant difference in LH pulse frequency between women with PCOD and normal women in the follicular phase of the menstrual cycle[8,25]. In a group of seven women, affected by PCOD, sampling for 8 h every 15 min, LH pulse frequency estimated using program DETECT[10] was 5.4 $\pm$ 0.3 peaks/8 h (mean $\pm$ SEM). This frequency is not significantly different from the control group in the EFP; in some of these patients the mean pulse amplitude was higher than that of the control group (Figure 1). The inability to detect an increased LH pulse frequency in PCOD patients fails to support the hypothesis of a hypothalamic pathogenesis of PCOD, although the abnormally high LH pulse amplitudes in PCOD patients may reflect an increased GnRH pulse amplitude[25]. Alternatively, the increased LH amplitude observed in some patients with PCOD could be due to enhanced pituitary sensitivity to GnRH[26].

PREMENSTRUAL SYNDROME

Several endocrinological hypotheses have been proposed to explain premenstrual syndrome (PMS), and the most common finding is the presence of low levels of progsterone[27] which can be present together with a reduction of the nociceptive threshold of the neural system. Often progesterone administration restores the normal condition[27]. Abnormal progesterone plasma levels can be due to an inappropriate receptor synthesis for LH. The low secretion both of follicle stimulating hormone (FSH) and estradiol in the follicular phase or the low LH plasma level in the luteal phase may explain such a change. To characterize better the LH pulsatile release in PMS, a group of five women affected by PMS and five normal women were studied during the luteal phase for 12 h, sampling every 10 min, from 08.00

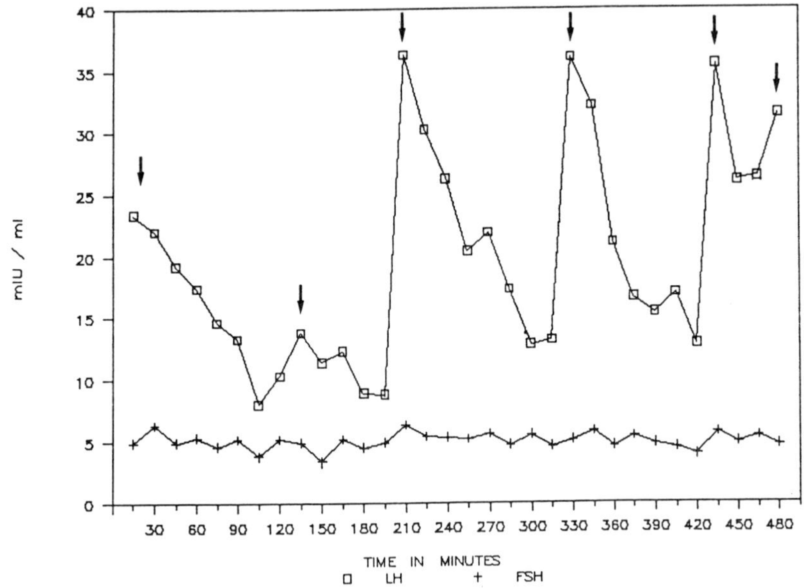

Figure 1 LH (□) and FSH (+) secretory patterns in a subject affected by PCOD. No evidence of pulsatile release was observed on FSH time series

Table 1 LH pulse frequency and duration as estimated on data from controls, PCOD and PMS

	LH pulse frequency	*Duration in minutes*
Controls		
Early follicular phase	5.7 ± 0.3 peaks/8 h	58.7 ± 16.3
Late follicular phase	5.3 ± 1.1 peaks/8 h	97.8 ± 30
Early luteal phase	3.6 ± 0.3 peaks/8 h	120.0 ± 30
Late luteal phase	4.9 ± 0.6 peaks/8 h	75.3 ± 16.4
PCOD	5.4 ± 0.3 peaks/8 h	49.5 ± 5.5
Luteal phase		
Controls	9.7 ± 1.6 peaks/12 h	62.5 ± 11.1
PMS	9.4 ± 1 peaks/12 h	54.6 ± 5.4

to 20.00. Again, time series were analyzed using program DETECT[10]. No significant differences were observed between patients affected by PMS and the control group both for LH pulsatile frequency (9.4 ± 1 and 9.75 ± 1.6 peaks/12 h, respectively; mean ± SEM) and peak duration (62.5 ± 11.1 and 54.6 ± 5.4 minutes, respectively), while, as previously reported[28], pulse amplitude was significantly reduced in patients with PMS (Figure 2).

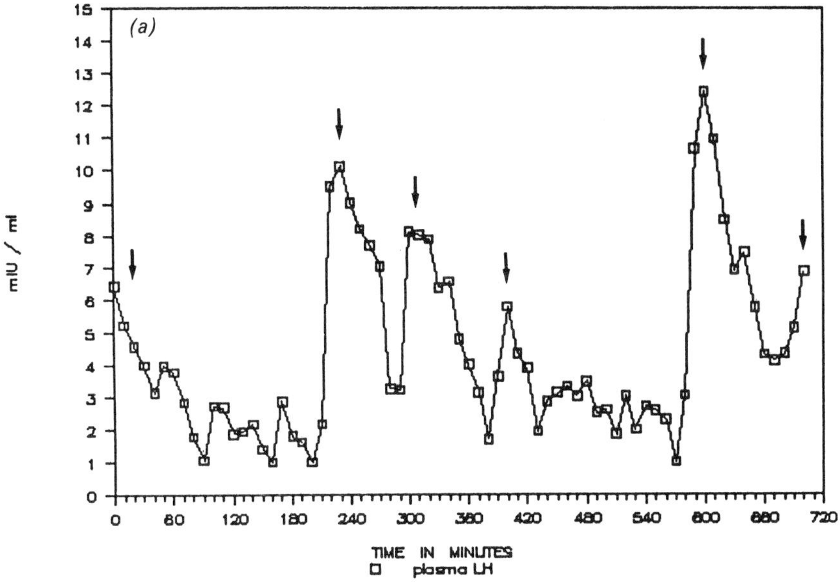

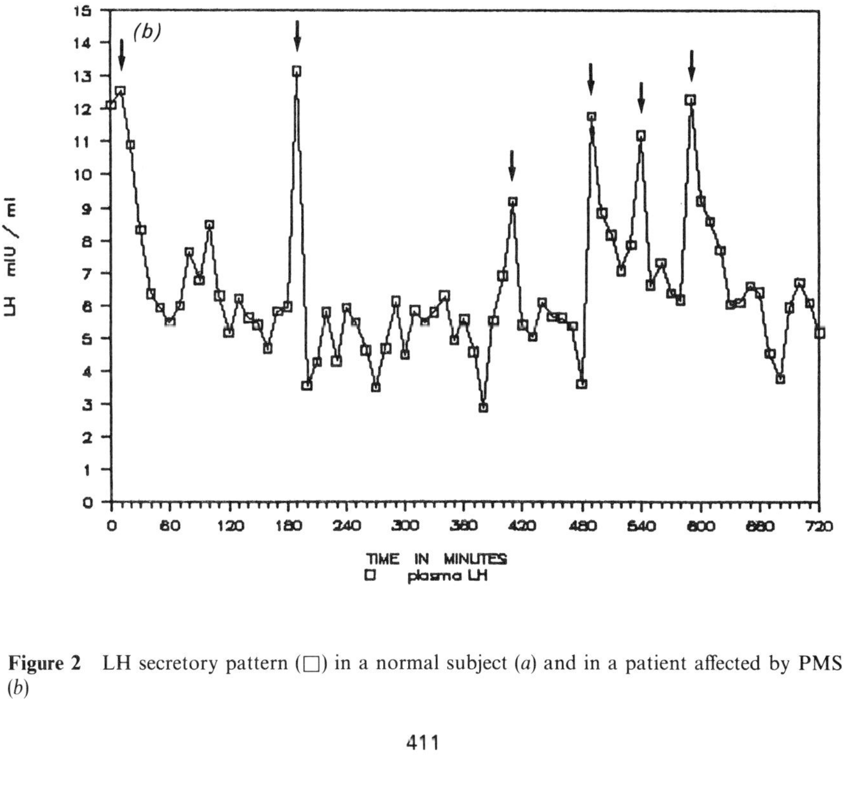

Figure 2 LH secretory pattern (□) in a normal subject (*a*) and in a patient affected by PMS (*b*)

CONCLUSION

The development of a specific, sensitive and statistically based algorithm for pulse detection has greatly improved the interest in chronobiology. The data of this review show how LH pulsatile secretion can be different in some pathological conditions such as in different kinds of amenorrhea where reduced frequency and amplitude or even lack of LH pulses were observed; only a few patients affected by PCOD showed a reduction of LH pulse amplitude, while patients with PMS were all characterized by a significant reduction in LH pulse amplitude but not in pulse frequency. This suggests the importance of the clinical application of the pulsatility studies as the 'tool' for a better definition of the characteristics and intrinsic peculiarity of the pulsatile release of LH both in normal and in abnormal physiopathological conditions.

REFERENCES

1. Levine, J.E. and Ramirez, V.D. (1982). Luteinizing hormone-releasing hormone release during the rat estrous cycle and after ovariectomy, as estimated with push-pull cannulae. *Endocrinology*, **111**, 1439
2. Clarke, I.J. and Cummins, J.T. (1982). The temporal relationship between gonadotropin releasing-hormone (GnRH) and luteinizing hormone (LH) secretion in ovariectomized ewes. *Endocrinology*, **111**, 1737
3. Wilson, R.C., Kesner, J.S., Kaufman, J.M., Uemura, T., Akema, J. and Knobil, E. (1982). Central electrophyiologic correlates of pulsatile luteinizing hormone secretion in the rhesus monkey. *Neuroendocrinology*, **39**, 256
4. Santen, R. and Bordin, C.W. (1973). Episodic luteinizing hormone secretion in man. Pulse analysis, clinical interpretation, physiologic mechanism. *J. Clin. Invest.*, **52**, 2617
5. Crowley, W.F., Filicori, M., Spratt, D. and Santoro, N. (1985). The physiology of gonadotropin-releasing hormone (GnRH) secretion in men and women. *Rec. Progr. Res.*, **41**, 473
6. Filicori, M., Santoro, N., Merriam, G.R. and Crowley, W.F. (1986). Characterization of the physiologic pattern of episodic gonadotropin secretion throughout the human menstrual cycle. *J. Clin. Endocrinol. Metab.*, **62**, 1136
7. Genazzani, A.D., Mercuri, N., Cafarelli, D., Dicecca, M., Fioroni, L. and Genazzani, A.R. (1988). Studio delle secrezioni istantanee (I.S.R.) dell'LH: un nuovo strumento per l'analisi delle secrezioni pulsatili nella sindrome premestruale. Proceedings of *Psicosomatica e Psicoprofilassi in Ostetricia e Ginecologia*, Genazzani, A.R. and Facchinetti, F. (eds.) pp. 333–6. (CIC Publ)
8. Venturoli, S., Porcu, E., Fabbri, R., Magrini, O., Gammi, L., Paradisi, R., Forcacci, M., Bolzani, R. and Flamigni, C. (1988). Episodic pulsatile secretion of FSH, LH, Prolactin, Oestradiol, Oestrone, and LH circadian variations in polycystic ovary syndrome. *Clin. Endocrinol.*, **28**, 93
9. Veldhuis, J.D., Evans, W.S., Johnson, M.L., Wills, M.R. and Rogol, A.D. (1986). Physiological properties of luteinizing hormone pulse signal: impact of intensive and extended venous sampling paradigms on its characterization in healthy men and women. *J. Clin. Endocrinol. Metab.*, **62**, 881
10. Oerter, K., Guardabasso, V. and Rodbard, D. (1986). Detection and characterization of peaks and estimation of Instantaneous Secretory Rate for episodic pulsatile hormone secretion. *Comp. Biomed. Res.*, **19**, 170
11. Karsch, F.J., Foster, D.L., Bittman, E.L. and Goodman, R.L. (1983). A role for estradiol in enhancing luteinizing hormone pulse frequency during the follicular phase of the estrous cycle of the sheep. *Endocrinology*, **113**, 1333
12. Soules, M.R., Steiner, R.A., Clifton, D.K., Cohen, N.L., Aksel, S. and Bremner, W.J. (1984).

Progesterone modulation of pulsatile luteinizing hormone secretion in normal women. *J. Clin. Endocrinol. Metab.*, **58**, 378

13. Van Vugt, D.A., Lam, N.Y. and Ferin, M. (1984). Reduced frequency of pulsatile luteinizing hormone secretion in the luteal phase of the rhesus monkey. Involvement of endogenous opiates. *Endocrinology*, **115**, 378
14. Santoro, N., Wierman, M., Filicori, M. and Crowley, W.F. (1984). The spectrum of abnormal patterns of gonadotropin-releasing hormone (GnRH) secretion in hypothalamic amenorrhea. *Clin. Res.*, **32**, 690A
15. Boyar, R.M., Rosenfeld, R.S., Kapen, S., Finkelstein, J.W., Roffwarg, H.P., Weitzman, E.D. and Hellman, L. (1974). Human puberty: simultaneous segmented secretion of luteinizing hormone and testosterone during sleep. *J. Clin. Invest.*, **54**, 609
16. Boyar, R.M., Kats, J., Finkelstein, J.W., Kapen, S., Weiner, H., Weitzman, E.D. and Hellman, L. (1974). Anorexia nervosa. Immaturity of the 24-hour luteinizing hormone secretory pattern. *N. Engl. J. Med.*, **291**, 861
17. Veldhuis, J.D., Evans, W.S., Demers, L.M., Thorner, M.O., Wakat, D. and Rogol, A.D. (1985). Altered neuroendocrine regulation of gonadotropin secretion in women distance runners. *J. Clin. Endocrinol. Metab.*, **61**, 557
18. Fries, H. and Nillius, S.J. (1973). Dieting, anorexia nervosa and amenorrhea after oral contraceptive treatment. *Acta Psychiatr. Scand.*, **49**, 669
19. Genazzani, A.R., Petraglia, F. and Facchinetti, F. (1988). Opioids and reproduction. In Genazzani, A.R., Petraglia, F., Volpe, A. and Facchinetti, F. (eds). *Advances in Gynecological Endocrinology*, pp. 43–54. (Carnforth: Parthenon Publishing)
20. Genazzani, A.R., Petraglia, F., Monzani, A., Alessandrini, G. and Volpe, A. (1988). Stress and reproduction. In Genazzani, A.R., Petraglia, F., Volpe, A. and Facchinetti, F. (eds). *Advances in Gynecological Endocrinology*, pp. 119–24. (Carnforth: Parthenon Publishing)
21. Goodman, R.L. and Karsch, F.J. (1980). Pulsatile secretion of luteinizing hormone: differential suppression by ovarian steroids. *Endocrinology*, **107**, 1286
22. Knuth, U.A., Hull, M.G.R. and Jacobs, N.S. (1977). Amenorrhea and loss of weight. *Br. J. Obstet. Gynaecol.*, **84**, 801
23. Burger, C.W., Korsen, T., van Kessel, H., van Dop, P.A., Caron, F.J. and Shoemaker, J. (1985). Pulsatile luteinizing hormone patterns in the follicular phase of the menstrual cycle, polycystic ovarian disease (PCOD) and non-PCOD secondary amenorrhea. *J. Clin. Endocrinol. Metab.*, **61**, 1126
24. Filicori, M., Campaniello, E., Michelacci, L., Pareschi, A., Ferrari, P., Bolelli, G.F. and Flamigni, C. (1988). Gonadotropin-releasing hormone (GnRH) analog suppression renders polycystic ovarian disease patients more susceptible to ovulation induction with pulsatile GnRH. *J. Clin. Endocrinol. Metab.*, **66**, 327
25. Kazer, R.R., Kessel, B. and Yen, S.S.C. (1987). Circulating luteinizing hormone pulse frequency in women with polycystic ovary syndrome. *J. Clin. Endocrinol. Metab.*, **65**, 233
26. Rebar, R., Judd, H.L., Yen, S.S.C., Rakoff, J., VandenBerg, G. and Naftolin, F. (1976). Characterization of the inappropriate gonadotropin secretion in polycystic ovary syndrome. *J. Clin. Invest.*, **57**, 1320
27. Zimmerman, A.W., Holden, K.R., Reiter, E.O. and DeKaban, A.S. (1983). Medroxyprogesterone acetate in the treatment of seizures associated with menstruation. *J. Pediatr.*, **83**, 959
28. Facchinetti, F., Sances, G., Romano, G., Fioroni, L., Nappi, G. and Genazzani, A.R. (1988). Alterazioni della pulsatilita' dell'LH in pazienti con sindrome premestruale. In Genazzani, A.R. and Facchinetti, F. (eds). *Psicosomatica e psicoprofilassi in ostetricia e ginecologia*, pp. 33–8. (CIC Publ.)

60

Methionine-enkephalin in human reproduction

F. Petraglia, A. Monzani, G. Fabbri, F. Facchinetti, A. Volpe and A.R. Genazzani

INTRODUCTION

The methionine-enkephalin (ME) sequence is contained in β-endorphin (β-EP), but it is derived from a precursor distinct from that of β-EP: the preproenkephalin A. This precursor is produced by brain, adrenal medulla and other tissues. Preproenkephalin A is the precursor of four copies of ME (five amino acids) and for one copy each of leucine-enkephalin (LE) (five amino acids), ME-arg6-phe7 (seven amino acids) and ME-arg6-gly7-leu8 (eight amino acids). Recently, a new octapeptide has also been described in the carboxy-terminal portion of proenkephalin A, named adenorphin, or metorphamide[1].

The large variety of pharmacological responses to opiates is mediated by interacting with various stereospecific sites in the central nervous system and in peripheral tissues. ME acts on δ-type receptors. Naloxone, the most used opiate antagonist in human studies, at low dose is particularly effective on μ receptors, while at higher doses acts on κ and δ receptors[2].

ME IN BRAIN AND PITUITARY

ME is probably the most widely distributed endogenous opioid peptide in the brain. High concentrations of ME neurons have also been described in the hypothalamus, particularly mediobasal hypothalamus and preoptic area. Furthermore, ME may be involved in modulating sexual behavior since the distribution of ME is similar to that of estrogen and androgen concentrating neurons in the hypothalamus and synthetic ME has been shown to inhibit copulatory behavior[3]. ME concentrations increase in the mediobasal hypothalamus during pregnancy showing the highest hypothalamic concentrations in delivering rats[4]. On the other hand, ME concentrations in the mediobasal hypothalamus of lactating rats decrease, probably for the prolonged hyperprolactinemia[5]. This rise may derive either from the increase in sex steroids and/or from the changes in the turnover of central amines, considering that the hypothalamic concentrations of ME show significant changes after the chronic administration of gonadal steroids[6] or of serotoninergic[7] or dopaminergic drugs[8].

The idea that activation of locomotor activity can be due to ME is mostly supported by the high concentration of this peptide in the basal ganglia, which suggests an involvement in the modulation of the autonomic nervous system. The presence of this peptide in central nuclei regulating autonomic function (nucleus tractus solitarius) supports the contention that ME might also be important in regulating the response to physical and environmental stressful stimuli[9].

Large amounts of ME have been found in the anterior lobe of pituitary, where changes occur during the estrous cycle. The significant rise of anterior lobe ME in the morning of proestrous is probably related to changes of gonadal steroid levels[10]. In humans, pituitary ME content is very high but the pituitary gland does not seem to be responsible for circulating ME, since its plasma concentrations were unaffected by hypophysectomy and glucocorticoids, and did not show any secretory rhythm[9].

The coexistence of ME with classic other neurotransmitters in the same cell bodies, and its low molecular weight, raise the hypothesis that, unlike other opioids, ME could function as a true neurotransmitter. In favor of this concept is the finding of its rapid degradation (less than 1 min) resulting from three different hydrolyzing enzyme systems[10].

ME IN PLASMA

ME circulates in the plasma of normal subjects. Peak values are observed in the morning at 08:00 and 12:00 and the lowest values at 16:00 and 20:00. Dexamethasone treatment suppresses plasma immunoreactive adrenocorticotropic hormone and β-lipotropic pituitary hormone to undetectable levels but does not alter the circulating ME levels significantly[11]. The adrenal glands appear to be the major source of ME. A positive gradient has been demonstrated between adrenal and peripheral venous effluent, and a substantial release of ME is observed upon splanchnic nerve stimulation[9,11]. The processing is limited in yielding a variety of intermediate forms, namely, peptides B, E, F, I, or bovine adrenal medullary peptides, BAM 12P and BAM 22P, have been described in various organs where the precursor is synthesized. It is not known, however, whether these peptides represent end products[1].

Peripherally ME is not only contained in the adrenal medulla but it has also been detected in relatively large amounts in tissue rich in 5-hydroxytryptamine such as the gastrointestinal tract[12] and blood platelets[13]. However, the available experiment evidence does not support the idea that platelet ME is of plasma origin. Bilateral adrenalectomy and hypophysectomy do not affect ME in platelets. One hypothesis is that platelet ME is carried over from the immature stage of the megakaryocyte, or that platelet ME is derived from a presently unknown precursor, either of platelet or of plasma origin.

Spontaneous hypertensive rats have lower platelet concentrations of ME than age-matched normotensive rats[13].

ME concentrations in cerebrospinal fluid are higher than plasma and the variability at different times of the day is more pronounced in the cerebrospinal fluid indicating that the two pools of ME are independently regulated and have different physiological roles. In addition, the rapid variations in concentration suggest that this peptide has a high turnover rate in the cerebrospinal fluid.

ME IN OTHER BIOLOGICAL FLUIDS

The human ovarian follicular fluid and the peritoneal fluid contain significant amounts of ME. The very large difference between its plasma concentrations, which are 10 to 100 lower than those present in follicular and peritoneal fluid, suggest that the ME present in both fluids might derive from local synthesis and secretion[14]. ME concentrations in both follicular and peritoneal fluids do not show significant changes during the menstrual cycle and are very low in postmenopausal women and in patients taking oral contraceptives[15].

ME enhances progesterone production in the presence of follicle-stimulating hormone (FSH) from cultured granulosa cells, considering that ME alone has no effect, it seems evident that the opioid exerts a modulatory role rather than a trophic one[16]. Although, ME follicular levels do not vary throughout the menstrual cycle, their large concentration in the preovulatory follicle could serve as an amplifier system at the moment of the midcycle FSH surge. This may also be related to the preovulatory increase in progesterone biosynthesis in rat ovaries, and to the small preovulatory peak of plasma progesterone levels in the normal menstrual cycle.

ME is also measurable in uterine fluid and concentrations are higher in the secretory than in the proliferative phase of the menstrual cycle, while they are undetectable in postmenopausal women, while increasing during gonadal steroid replacement treatment. The observation that pregnancy- and parturition-related changes are detectable in opiate receptors of rat uterine membranes suggests an influence of opioids on uterine contractility[17].

REFERENCES

1. Facchinetti, F., Petraglia, F. and Genazzani, A.R. (1987). Localization and expression of the three opioid systems. *Sem. Reprod. Endocrinol.*, **2**, 103–13
2. Herz, A. (1984). Multiple opioid receptors. In Delitalia, G., Motta, M. and Serio, M. (eds). *Opioid Modulation of Endocrine Function*, pp. 11–20. (New York: Raven Press)
3. Gessa, G.L. and Paglietti, E. (1979). Induction of copulatory behavior in sexually inactive rats by naloxone. *Science*, **204**, 203–6
4. Petraglia, F., Baraldi, M., Giarrè, G., Facchinetti, F., Santi, M., Volpe, A. and Genazzani, A.R. (1985). Opioid peptides of the pituitary and hypothalamus: changes in pregnant and lactating rats. *J. Endocrinol.*, **105**, 239–45
5. Panerai, A.E., Sawynok, J., La Bella, F.S. and Friesen, H. (1980). Prolonged hyperprolactinemia influences β-endorphin and met-enkephalin in the brain. *Endocrinology*, **106**, 1804–8
6. Hong, J.S., Yoshikawa, K., Hudson, P.M. and Uphouse, L.L. (1982). Regulation of pituitary and brain enkephalin systems by estrogens. *Life Sci.*, **31**, 2181–4

7. Harsing, L.G., Jr, Yang, H.Y.T., Govoni, S. and Costa, E. (1982). Elevation of met^5-enkephalin and β-endorphin hypothalamic content in rats receiving anoretic drugs: differences between d-fenfluramine and d-amphetamine. *Neuropharmacology*, **21**, 141–5
8. Locatelli, V., Petraglia, F., Penalva, A. and Panerai, A.E. (1983). Effect of dopamine drugs on hypothalamic and pituitary immunoreactive β-endorphin concentrations in rat. *Life Sci.*, **33**, 1711–7
9. Clement-Jones, V. and Besser, G.M. (1984). Opioid peptides in humans and their clinical significance. In Udenfriend, S. and Meienhofer, J. (eds). *The Peptides*, pp. 323–72 (New York: Academic Press)
10. Kumar, M.S.A., Chen, C.L. and Muther, T.F. (1979). Changes in the pituitary and hypothalamic content of methionine-enkephalin during the estrous cycle of rats. *Life Sci.*, **25**, 1687–96
11. Clements-Jones, V., Lowry, P.J., Rees, L.H. and Besser, G.M. (1980). Met-enkephalin circulates in human plasma. *Nature*, **283**, 295–7
12. Panerai, A.E., Martini, A. and De Rosa, A. (1982). In Costa, E. and Trabucchi, M. (eds). *Regulatory Peptides: from Molecular Biology to Function*, pp. 139–49. (New York: Raven Press)
13. Di Giulio, A.M., Picotti, G.B., Cesura, A.M., Panerai, A.E. and Mantegazza, P. (1982). Met-enkephalin immunoreactivity in blood platelets. *Life Sci.*, **30**, 1605–14
14. Petraglia, F., Segre, A., Facchinetti, F., Campanini, D., Ruspa, M. and Genazzani, A.R. (1985). β-Endorphin and metenkephalin in peritoneal and ovarian follicular fluids of fertile and postmenopausal. *Fertil. Steril.*, **44**, 615–21
15. Petraglia, F., Di Meo, G., Storchi, R., Segre, A., Facchinetti, F., Szalay, S., Volpe, A. and Genazzani, A.R. (1987). Proopiomelanocortin-related peptides and methionine enkephalin in human follicular fluid: changes during the menstrual cycle. *Am. J. Obstet. Gynecol.*, **157**, 142–6
16. Facchinetti, F., Ruspa, M., Turci, A., Petraglia, F., Segre, A., Forabosco, A. and Genazzani, A.R. (1986). Met-enkephalin enhances follicle-stimulating hormone-dependent progesterone production from cultured granulosa cells. *J. Clin. Endocrinol. Metab.*, **63**, 1222–4
17. Petraglia, F., Facchinetti, F., M'Futa, K., Ruspa, M., Bonavera, J.J., Gandolfi, F. and Genazzani, A.R. (1986). Endogenous opioid peptides in uterine fluid. *Fertil. Steril.*, **46**, 247–51

61

The role of neuropeptide Y in control of gonadotropin release in the rat

S.M. McCann, L. Milenkovic, M. Riedel and V. Rettori

INTRODUCTION

Several reports of the localization of pancreatic polypeptide to neurons within the brain and the hypothalamus prompted us to examine the effects of avian (a) and bovine (b) pancreatic polypeptide (PP) on the secretion of anterior pituitary hormones. In ovariectomized, conscious rats, injection of either aPP or bPP into the third ventricle had a dose-related ability to suppress luteinizing hormone (LH) but not follicle-stimulating hormone (FSH) release. Addition of the peptides to dispersed pituitary cells incubated *in vitro* had no effect[1,2]. Consequently, we assigned a hypothalamic site for the action of PPs to inhibit the release of LH-releasing hormone (LHRH)[2].

Already by this time, Tatemoto and colleagues[3] had isolated and determined structure of a new peptide termed neuropeptide Y (NPY), which was shown to be widely distributed in the central nervous system (CNS), and in particular in the hypothalamus. It had marked sequence homology with PPs and was frequently colocalized with catecholamines both centrally and peripherally. It was soon demonstrated that the immunoreactivity in the brain previously attributed to PP was in all probability due to NPY[4].

Because of the similarity of NPY to PP and the realization that it was indeed found in the hypothalamus, we speculated that it would have similar actions to those of PP on hypothalamic–pituitary function. Indeed, we found that the peptide had exactly similar effects to those previously found with the PPs. In the ovariectomized rat, third ventricular injection of NPY lowered plasma LH in a dose-related fashion with a minimum effective dose (MED) of 5 pmol.

In this case instead of using static incubation of dispersed pituitary cells, we evaluated the effects of NPY in perfused columns of pituitary cells and found to our surprise that it was a potent stimulator of FSH and LH release in a dose-related fashion with a MED of 10^{-9} [5,6]. These actions were opposite to the effects of intraventricular injection of the peptide on LH secretion prompting us to suggest that the peptide had opposite actions at hypothalamic and pituitary sites analogous to the situation with regard to a number of releasing factors previously studied[7].

Subsequent to our initial report on the effects of the PPs, Kalra and Crowley confirmed our finding of suppression of plasma LH in the ovariectomized rat following intraventricular injection of human PP and demonstrated that the response was reversed by priming the animals with ovarian steroids[8]. They went on to evaluate the situation with regard to NPY and reported similar findings to those which they had previously obtained with PP at the same meeting at which we reported our initial findings on NPY[9,10].

Immunocytochemical studies have shown the coexistence of NPY and norepinephrine in brain stem catecholaminergic neurons which may project to the hypothalamus and the existence of NPY in arcuate nuclear neurons which appear to project to the neural lobe and also to the external layer of the median eminence. The finding of NPY terminals in the external layer of the median eminence in close juxtaposition to hypophyseal portal capillaries suggests that it may be released into portal blood[11]. In fact in anesthetized rats higher concentrations of neuropeptide Y have been detected in portal than in systemic blood[11].

Consequently, in the present work we re-evaluated some of the actions of NPY in conscious, male rats and attempted to determine the physiological significance of the peptide in control of gonadotropin secretion by intraventricular injection of highly specific antibodies against NPY in male, ovariectomized and ovariectomized estrogen, progesterone-treated rats.

RESULTS

Effect of third ventricular injection of NPY in conscious male rats

Harfstrand *et al.*[12] had previously studied the effect of intraventricular injection of NPY on anterior pituitary hormone secretion in male rats, whereas our earlier studies had employed ovariectomized females. Consequently, prior to evaluating the effect of passive immunoneutralization of NPY on the secretion of anterior pituitary hormones in male rats, we evaluated a few of the effects of the peptide in conscious, freely moving male rats with third ventricular cannulae. The results demonstrated intraventricular injection of 4 μg of NPY produced a highly significant suppression of prolactin (PRL) release as indicated by a significant decline in plasma PRL, apparent within 15 min of the intraventricular injection of the peptide. The decline became highly significant and persisted for the 120 min duration of the experiment.

The effect of intraventricular injection of NPY antiserum (aNPY) on anterior pituitary hormone release

Since neuropeptide Y itself was capable of lowering LH in ovariectomized animals, it was important to determine if this had physiological significance. Consequently, the antiserum to the peptide was injected at a dilution of 1 to 10 in a volume of 2 μl into the third ventricle and normal rabbit serum

(NRS) at the same dilution served as the control. Neither NRS nor aNPY had a significant effect on plasma levels of LH over a 6 h period in either ovariectomized or ovariectomized, estrogen–progesterone-treated rats. The results were similar in the case of plasma FSH in both the ovariectomized and the ovariectomized, estrogen–progesterone-blocked rats.

In contrast to these results, injection of aNPY in an equivalent dose into male rats had a significant effect to elevate plasma LH beginning at 2 h following its injection and the elevation persisted for the 6 h duration of the experiment. There was no effect of NRS at any time in these animals.

The injection of undiluted aNPY in a volume of 2 μl was followed by no significant change in plasma PRL until 180 min, at which time values were significantly reduced below control. On the other hand in the NRS-injected controls there was no significant change in plasma PRL at any time following the injection.

DISCUSSION

It appears established that NPY has an inhibitory effect on the release of gonadotropins in the ovariectomized female[6] and in the male rat[13]; however, this inhibitory action is converted to a stimulatory effect under the influence of ovarian steroids[12]. There is no doubt that the peptide can stimulate LHRH release *in vitro* in the steroid-primed animal[14,15]. It had no effect on hypothalami of ovariectomized rats; however, these hypothalami were not stimulated with other secretogues[14,15]. That stimulation might be inhibited by the peptide.

We visualize that the brain stem neurons which cosecrete norepinephrine and NPY project to the hypothalamus to inhibit the release of LHRH. These inhibitory actions of NPY on LH release appear to be of significance physiologically in the male in view of the studies with the intraventricular injection of aNPY reported here. Since the antiserum against the peptide failed to affect plasma FSH, it would appear that NPY has no physiological significance under our conditions in the control of FSH in contrast to its role in control of LH release.

The situation in the estrogen-primed animal is reversed in that NPY instead of inhibiting LH release stimulates it. It is already well known that epinephrine and norepinephrine augment the release of LHRH under these conditions[16]. We postulate that brain stem neurons, which contain epinephrine or norepinephrine colocalized with NPY, project to the basal tuberal region to release epinephrine, norepinephrine and NPY which cause an enhanced release of LHRH. Furthermore, NPY, LHRH and epinephrine may be released in enhanced amounts into portal vessels at this time for transport to the pituitary where NPY, LHRH and epinephrine would synergize with each other to produce a dramatic increase in LH release from the gonadotropes. Consequently, the previously held concept that the preovulatory discharge of LHRH is solely responsible for the increased release of LH which occurs on proestrus from the sensitized gonadotropes may need modification. The preovulatory LH discharge may be due to the summation of the actions of NPY and LHRH. Recent studies with intraventricular injection against NPY in ovariectomized, estrogen–progesterone-primed rats have shown that these injections block the proestrous-like surge of LH[17] which supports the physiological role of the stimulatory action of NPY on LH release at this time of the cycle.

Finally, we have confirmed the ability of NPY to suppress PRL release following its intraventricular injection in male rats[12]. We have not studied its possible direct effect on the pituitary to alter prolactin release; however, it has been reported that NPY can stimulate PRL release by monolayer-cultured pituitary cells in static incubation[13]. Again, this is opposite to the action of the peptide itself following intraventricular injection and any direct effect to stimulate must be overpowered by the inhibitory effect. Since NPY has been shown to stimulate dopamine release[12], increased release of dopamine into the portal vessels may mediate the suppression of PRL release. On the other hand, low doses of NPY were reported to stimulate PRL release via decreasing tuberoinfundibular dopamine release[12] and this effect of NPY appears to have physiological significance in the male rat since intraventricular injection of aNPY resulted in a reversal of this action of the peptide itself and a decrease of plasma PRL within 3 h of injection.

It is noteworthy that there was usually a latent period of 2–4 h following injection of antisera before detectable effects on hormone release were seen. We have noted this in the case of other antisera against peptides and we attribute this to time required to be absorbed from the ventricle and to diffuse to the active site within the hypothalamus[18]. The shorter the latency, the closer to the ventricle would be the active site. In the cases where we have observed the effects of antisera, it would appear that they are probably exerted on periventricular structures consistent with the localization of the NPY terminals, particularly in the paraventricular and arcuate nuclear regions.

ACKNOWLEDGEMENTS

This work was supported by NIH grant HD09988. We wish to thank Ms Judy Scott for typing the manuscript.

REFERENCES

1. McDonald, J.K. and Lumpkin, M.D. (1983). Third ventricular injections of pancreatic polypeptides decrease LH and growth secretion in ovariectomized rats. Program of the Meeting of *The Endocrine Society*, Abstract 152, June, San Antonio, Texas
2. McDonald, J.K., Lumpkin, M.D., Samson, W.K. and McCann, S.M. (1985). Pancreatic polypeptides affect luteinizing and growth hormone secretion in rats. *Peptides*, **6**, 79–84
3. Tatemoto, K., Carlquist, M. and Mutt, V. (1982). Neuropeptide Y – a novel brain peptide with structural similarities to peptide YY and pancreatic polypeptide. *Nature*, **296**, 659–60
4. Card, J.P., Brecha, N. and Moore, R.Y. (1983). Immunohistochemical localization of avian pancreatic polypeptide – like immunoreactivity in the rat hypothalamus. *J. Comp. Neurol.*, **217**, 123–36
5. McDonald, J.K., Lumpkin, M.D., Samson, W.K. and McCann, S.M. (1984). Third ventricular injections of neuropeptide Y decrease LH and GH secretion in ovariectomized rats.

Presented at the *Society of Neuroscience*, Abstract 1214, October, Dallas, Texas
6. McDonald, J.K., Lumpkin, M.D., Samson, W.K. and McCann, S.M. (1985). Neuropeptide Y affects secretion of luteinizing hormone and growth hormone in ovariectomized rats. *Proc. Natl. Acad. Sci., USA*, **82**, 561–4
7. McCann, S.M., Samson, W.K., Aguila, C., Bedran de Castro, J., Ono, N., Lumpkin, M.D. and Khorram, O. (1986). The role of brain peptides in the control of anterior pituitary hormone secretion. In Fink, G., Harmer, A.J. and McKerns, K.W. (eds). *Neuroendocrine Molecular Biology*, pp. 101–12 (New York: Plenum Press)
8. Kalra, S.P. and Crowley, W.R. (1984). Differential effects of pancreatic polypeptide on luteinizing hormone release in female rats. *Neuroendocrinology*, **38**, 511–13
9. Kalra, S.P. and Crowley, W.R. (1984). Norepinephrine-like effects of neuropeptide Y (NPY) and human pancreatic polypeptide (hPP) on LH release. Presented at *Society of Neuroscience*, Abstract 1119, October, Dallas, Texas
10. Kalra, S.P. and Crowley, W.R. (1984). Norepinephrine-like effects of neuropeptide Y on LH release in the rat. *Life Sci.*, **35**, 1173–6
11. McDonald, J.K., Koenig, J.E., Gibbs, D.M., Collins, P. and Noe, B.D. (1987). High concentrations of neuropeptide Y in pituitary portal blood of rats. *Neuroendocrinology*, **46**, 538–41
12. Harfstrand, A., Eneroth, P., Agnati, L. and Fuxe, K. (1987). Further studies on the effects of central administration of neuropeptide Y on neuroendocrine function in the male rat: relationship to hypothalamic catecholamines. *Regulatory Pept.*, **17**, 167–79
13. Chabot, J.-G., Enjalbert, A., Pelletier, G. and Dubois, P.M. (1988). Evidence for a direct action of neuropeptide Y in the rat pituitary gland. *Neuroendocrinology*, **47**, 511–17
14. Crowley, W.R., Hassid, A. and Kalra, S.P. (1987). Neuropeptide Y enhances the release of luteinizing hormone (LH) induced by LH-releasing hormone. *Endocrinology*, **120**, 941–5
15. McDonald, J.K., Sabatino, F.D. and Calka, J. (1988). NPY stimulation of LHRH release from rat median eminence: effects of estrogen and calcium. Presented at *Society of Neuroscience*, Abstract, in press, November, Toronto.
16. McCann, S.M. (1982). Physiology and pharmacology of LHRH and somatostatin. *Ann. Rev. Pharmacol. Toxicol.*, **22**, 491–515
17. Wehrenberg, W.B., Corder, R. and Gaillard, R.C. (1988). A physiological role for neuropeptide Y in regulating the estrogen/progesterone induced LH surge in ovariectomized rats. Presented at *The Endocrine Society*, Abstract 1163, June, New Orleans, Louisiana
18. Kentrotri, S., Dees, W.L. and McCann, S.M. (1988). Evidence for a physiological role of hypothalamic gastrin-releasing peptide to suppress growth hormone and prolactin release in the rat. *Proc. Natl. Acad. Sci., USA*, **85**, 953–7

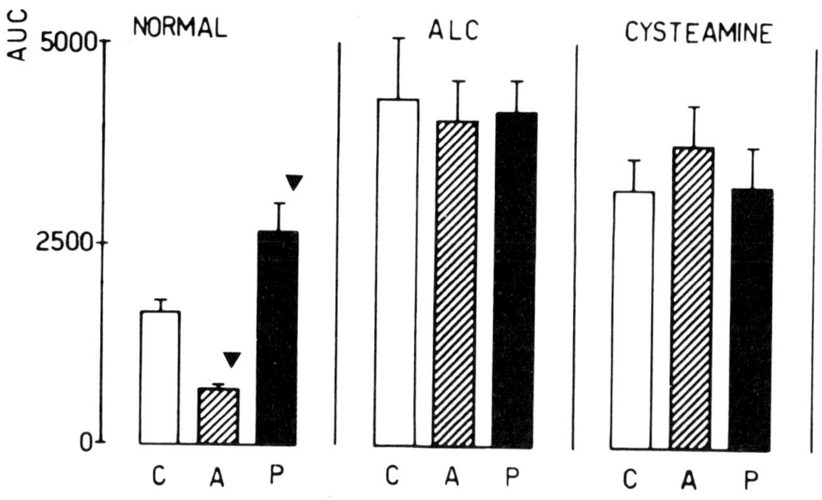

Figure 4 Plasma GH response to GHRH (2 μg/kg i.v.) in normal adult male rats, or rats with hypothalamic GRIH depletion obtained by surgical anterolateral deafferentation of the mediobasal hypothalamus (ALC) or by cysteamine administration. Rats were pretreated with saline or atropine (A, 0.5 mg/kg i.v.) or pilocarpine (P, 2 mg/kg i.v.) $p < 0.05$ vs respective control group (Dunnett's *t* test)

to be of benefit in the inhibition of excessive GH release that occurs in disease states such as diabetes mellitus.

A better understanding of the mechanism of action of different neurotransmitters in GH secretion may rapidly improve the diagnostic use of neuroactive drugs in growth disorders and may disclose novel approaches to therapy.

REFERENCES

1. Frohman, L.A. and Jansson, J.O. (1986). Growth hormone-releasing hormone. *Endocr. Rev.*, **3**, 223–53
2. Müller, E.E. (1987). Neural control of somatotropic function. *Physiol. Rev.*, **67**, 962 1053
3. Wehrenberg, W.B., Brazeau, P., Luben, R., Bohlen, P. and Guillemin, R. (1982). Inhibition of the pulsatile secretion of growth hormone by monoclonal antibodies to the hypothalamic growth hormone-releasing factor (GRF). *Endocrinology*, **111**, 2147–51
4. Tannenbaum, G.S. and Ling, N. (1984). The interrelationship of growth hormone (GH)-releasing factor and somatostatin in generation of the ultradian rhythm of GH secretion. *Endocrinology*, **115**, 1952–7
5. Jansson, J-O., Eden, S. and Isaksson, O. (1985). Sexual dimorphism in the control of growth hormone secretion. *Endocr. Rev.*, **6**, 128–50
6. Terry, L.C. and Martin, J.B. (1981). Evidence for alpha-adrenergic regulation of episodic growth hormone and prolactin secretion in the undisturbed male rat. *Endocrinology*, **108**, 1869–73
7. Cella, S.G., Locatelli, V., De Gennaro, V., Puggioni, R., Pintor, C. and Müller, E.E. (1985). Human pancreatic growth hormone (GH)-releasing hormone stimulates GH synthesis and release in infant rats. An *in vivo* study. *Endocrinology*, **116**, 69–73
8. Szabo, M. and Cuttler, L. (1986). Differential responsiveness of the somatotroph to growth

hormone-releasing factor during early neonatal development in the rat. *Endocrinology*, **118**, 69–73

9. Cozzi, M.G., Zanini, A., Locatelli, V., Cella, S.G. and Müller, E.E. (1986). Growth hormone-releasing hormone and clonidine stimulate biosynthesis of growth hormone in neonatal rats. *Biochem. Biophys. Res. Commun.*, **138**, 1223–30
10. Grossman, A., Savage, M.O., Wess, J.A.H., Lytras, N., Sueiras-Diaz, J., Coy, D.H. and Besser, G.M. (1983). Growth hormone-releasing factor in growth hormone deficiency: demonstration of a hypothalamic defect in growth hormone release. *Lancet*, **ii**, 137–8
11. Pintor, C., Fanni, V., Loche, S., Locatelli, V., Villa, F., Cella, S.G., Minuto, F., Corda, R. and Müller, E.E. (1983). Synthetic hpGRF1-40 stimulates growth hormone and inhibits prolactin secretion in normal children and in children with isolated growth hormone deficiency. *Peptides*, **4**, 929–33
12. Pintor, C., Cella, S.G., Corda, R., Locatelli, V., Puggioni, R., Loche, S. and Müller, E.E. (1985). Clonidine accelerates growth in children with impaired growth hormone secretion. *Lancet*, **i**, 1482–5
13. Massara, F., Ghigo, E., Goffi, S., Molinatti, G.M., Müller, E.E. and Camanni, F. (1984). Blockade of hpGRF-40 induced GH release in normal man by a cholinergic muscarinic antagonist. *J. Clin. Endocrinol. Metab.*, **59**, 1025–6
14. Massara, F., Ghigo, E., Demislis, K., Tangolo, D., Mazza, E., Locatelli, V., Müller, E.E., Molinatti, G.M. and Camanni, F. (1986). Cholinergic involvement in the growth hormone releasing hormone-induced growth hormone release. Studies in normal and acromegalic subjects. *Neuroendocrinology*, **43**, 670–5
15. Locatelli, V., Torsello, A., Redaelli, M., Ghigo, E., Massara, F. and Müller, E.E. (1986). Cholinergic agonist and antagonist drugs modulate in the rat the growth hormone-response to growth hormone releasing hormone. Evidence for mediation by somatostatin. *J. Endocrinol.*, **111**, 271–8

66

Hormonal and auxological assessment in long-term clonidine treatment of short normal children

G. Calzolari, S. Alboni, M. Bonati and P. Riva

INTRODUCTION

The 'short normal' term has been used to indicate two clinical conditions: Genetic Short Stature (GSS) and Constitutional Growth Delay (CGD)[1] whose etiopathology is not related to the endocrine and non-endocrine alterations (Table 1) usually found in typical growth disorders[2–7].

The definition of Neurosecretory Dysfunction (NSD) with various etiologies has recently been introduced[8]; it represents the physiopathological feature

Table 1 Causes of short stature

Intrauterine	*Postnatal* — *Non-endocrine causes*	*Postnatal* — *Endocrine causes*
Malformation syndromes	Chromosomal abnormalities	Hypoparathyroidism–pseudohypoparathyroidism
Genetic skeletal disease	Constitutional skeletal disease	Glucocorticoid excess
Karyotypic disorders syndromes	Chronic disease of organ system	Hypothyroidism
Embryopathy	Malformation and/or dysmorphic syndromes	Hypopituitarism:
Dysmorphic essential dwarfism	Non-dysmorphic, essential dwarfism	panhypopituitarism
Fetal hypotrophy	Psychosocial dwarfism	isolated (GHD)
Intrauterine growth retardation		Congenital
Endocrine neonatal dwarfism		genetic
		disembryogenetic
		idiopathic
		Acquired
		neoplasm
		phlogistic disorders
		following cranial irradiation
		following traumatism
		empty sella
		Biologically inactive GH
		GH resistance
		Decreased IGF_1
		IGF_1 resistance

of many clinical short stature syndromes; it has been described initially in patients previously treated with cranial irradiation or after cranial trauma[9].

The NSD clinical picture is comparable to, and sometimes overlaps with, growth hormone (GH) deficiency and it is now considered a major cause of idiopathic short stature syndromes including the 'short normal' and others of unknown etiology[7].

Most short stature patients referred to endocrinology consultants can be classified as short normal[7]; therefore it is most important for the auxologist to make a differential diagnosis between 'short normal' and GH deficiency especially when the patient has not the pathognomonic expressions of the pituitary dwarfism (Table 2)[1,10–14].

In spite of the validity of parameters considered for the differential diagnosis, our clinical experience suggests that the short stature patients should not be distinctly classified but rather considered varying expression of secretory GH disturbances with clinical overlapping features.

Although these conditions are not considered pathological, a therapeutic approach for 'short normal' has recently been proposed, based on the current knowledge of neuroendocrine regulation of GH secretion and because of the availability of drugs whose rationale has been proved[15–19].

We have studied the therapeutic effect of clonidine, which is a very potent and suitable α_2 agonist[15,17,18,20,21], acting as proximal stimulator[22–24] of GH neuroregulation[25–29].

DATA

Sixteen patients (eight females and eight males) aged 5 to 12 years (mean age 9.5 ± 2.3) have been studied in detail. They were found to have: no systemic disease or endocrinopathy; no pubertal signs (P1 B1); height < the 3rd percentile; growth velocity evaluated during the 6 months before the beginning of the therapy < 5 cm/year; bone age < 11 years.

The auxological data (mean ± SD) of our patients show: pretreatment growth velocity 4.17 ± 0.59 cm/yr; retardation of skeletal age compared with chronologic age 1.9 ± 1.2 years expressed in decimal values; bone

Table 2 Differential characters

	Genetic short stature	*Constitutional growth delay*	*Idiopathic growth hormone deficiency*	*NSD*
Height	≤1.9 S.D. (P_3 correct)	≤1.9 S.D.	<3.5 S.D.	IGHD
Growth velocity	Normal	Normal	<4 cm/year	IGHD
Bone age	<C.A.	Moderate delayed	<C.A.	IGHD
Statural age	S.A. ≤ B.A. = C.A.	S.A. = B.A. < C.A.	S.A. < D.A. < C.A.	IGHD
Family history	Positive	Positive	Negative	IGHD
Clinical feature	Indifferent	Indifferent	Typical	IGHD
Pubertal onset	Normal	Delayed	Delayed	IGHD
Definitive height	= Target height	Normal	< Target height	IGHD
Basal GH	Normal	Normal	Low	Normal
Provocative tests	Normal	Normal	Decreased	Normal
24 h secretion	Normal	Normal	Decreased	Decreased

age/chronologic age ratio < 1 (0.81 ± 0.20).

We submitted all patients to clonidine test and insuline tolerance test (ITT) before treatment; 12 patients were responsive to ITT and clonidine test. Peak value for ITT (mean $\pm$ SD) was GSS $= 10.18 \pm 1.69$ ng/ml, CGD $= 8.11 \pm 1.86$ ng/ml and peak value for clonidine test (mean $\pm$ SD); GSS $= 14.54 \pm 2.91$ ng/ml, CGD $= 10.17 \pm 1.66$ ng/ml.

Two patients were hyporesponsive to ITT (peak value < 8 ng/ml) and other two patients were hyporesponsive to clonidine test (peak value < 10 ng/ml).

The 24 h secretion[14] of GH in two hyporesponsive patients to clonidine was then tested and both subjects showed decreased 24 h secretion: patient A 2.8 ng/ml; patient B 3.2 ng/ml (normal values $\geqslant 3.5$ ng/ml).

Based on our data, seven patients were classified affected by GSS, seven by CGD and two by NSD.

All the 16 patients were treated with clonidine 0.1 mg/m^2/die (one-third of the dose in the afternoon and two-thirds in the evening) *p.o.*[15,17,21] for 12–18 months.

We evaluated auxological, hormonal and laboratory data every 3 months; and X-ray of left hand to evaluate bone age (T.W. 2) every 6 months.

The two initially hyporesponsive patients formerly indicated as patient A and patient B, have been treated for 12 months with clonidine (0.1 mg/m^2/die *p.o.*) because 3 months after the beginning of therapy they showed a significant increase in GH response at clonidine test (peak value after therapy: 8.1 ng/ml patient A; 13.2 ng/ml patient B; peak value before therapy: 1.7 ng/ml patient A; 3.6 ng/ml patient B; $p < 0.01$).

After treatment, clonidine test was repeated in all patients: they showed statistically significant increase in peak values of secretion (seven patients with GSS $= 29.50 \pm 5.25$ ng/ml; $p < 0.01$; seven patients with CGD $= 14.39 \pm 2.10$ ng/ml; $p < 0.01$) (Figure 1).

Even patients initially hyporesponsive, became responsive to clonidine test after therapy.

Auxological data evaluated after treatment showed a significant increase of growth velocity without any important variation of bone age/chronological age ratio, demonstrating a positive growth rate without any interference on potential definitive growth (Table 3).

Patients affected by CGD revealed an improved growth velocity too; although increase in GH response to clonidine test after therapy was lower than in GSS patients.

In these patients we did not find an inverse correlation between growth velocity before and after the treatment as reported by other authors[17,20].

DISCUSSION

The process of growth is subjected to phases of spontaneous changes and it is physiologically influenced by many different variables. Therefore it is difficult to establish the true relationship between the therapy and the improvement of auxological data.

Our longitudinal study, that is neither a follow-up nor a perspective one,

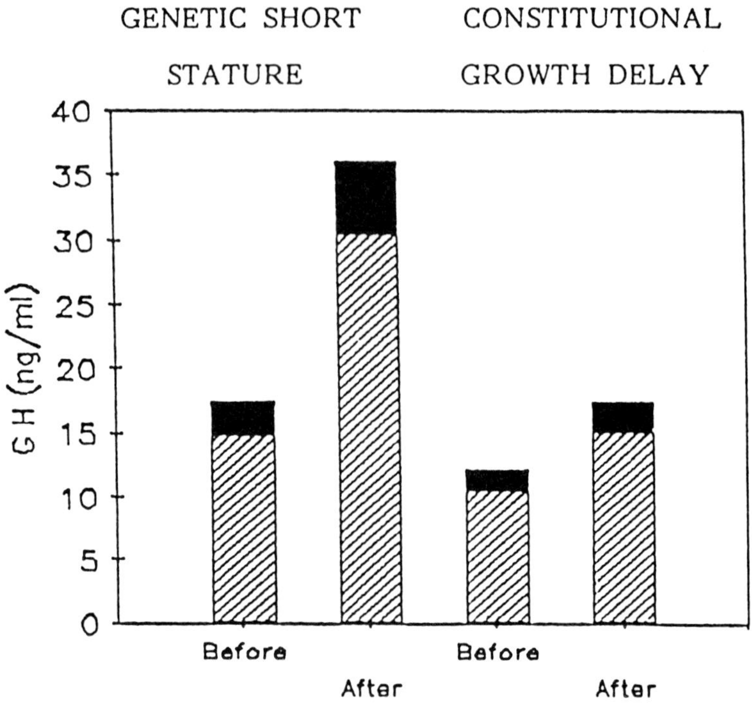

Figure 1

Table 3 Auxological data

	Before clonidine therapy	*After clonidine therapy*
Growth velocity	4.17 ± 0.59	6.62 ± 1.98 $p < 0.001$
BA/CA	0.81 ± 0.20	0.84 ± 0.10 $p = 0.025$

has shown the following results:

(1) The clonidine long-term treatment positively affects the GH secretory and auxological parameters thus supporting its efficacy on nervous system; and

(2) Clonidine may be used in some selected cases of partial GHD and of NSD especially for the non-auxologically urgent patients.

In the latter condition clonidine, which is a physiopathological therapy, aimed to correct altered neurotransmitters pathways and could represent a proximal therapy respectful of the physiological feedback of the GH–growth axis. The drug is suitable for its compliance, absence of significant behavioral, endocrine, biohumoral side-effects and its cost. The positive growth rate during treatment, in the absence of overstimulation on the bone age, would indicate clonidine as a useful drug for long-term therapy of short normal children.

REFERENCES

1. Lanes, R., Bohorques, L., Leal, V., Hernandez, G., Borges, M., Hurtado, E. and Moncada, G. (1986). Growth hormone secretion in patients with constitutional delay of growth and pubertal development. *J. Pediatr.*, **109**, 781–3
2. Job, J.C. (1988). Evolution des rétards de croissance à debut intra-uterin: données cliniques et biologiques. Presented at the *Simposio endocrinologico dell'età evolutiva*, March, Milano.
3. Merimee, T.J., Zapf, J. and Froesch, E.R. (1981). Dwarfism in pygmy. An isolated deficiency of insulin like growth factor I. *N. Engl. J. Med.*, **305**, 965–8
4. Kowarski, A.A. Schneider, J., Ben-Galim, E., Weldom, W. and Daughaday, W.H. (1978). Growth failure with normal serum RIA-GH and low somatomedine activity: somatomedine restoration and growth acceleration after exogenous GH. *J. Clin. Endocrinol. Metab.*, **47**, 461–4
5. Bierich, J.R., Moeller, H. and Ranke, M.B. (1984). Pseudopituitary dwarfism due to resistance to somatomedine: a new syndrome. *Eur. J. Pediatr.*, **142**, 186–8
6. Frazer, T., Gavin, J.R., Daughaday, W.H., Hillman, R.E. and Weldon, V.V. (1982). Growth hormone-dependent growth failure. *J. Pediatr.*, **101**, 12–15
7. Boscherini, B., Spadoni, G.L. and Cianfarani, S. (1987). Le anomalie della crescita. In Muller, E.E. (ed.). *Progressi nella diagnosi e terapia dei disturbi dell'accrescimento*, pp. 175–97. (Roma and Milano: Pythagora Press)
8. Spiliotis, E., August, P., Hung, W., Sonis, W., Mendelson, W. and Bercu, B. (1984). Growth hormone neurosecretory dysfunction. A treatable cause of short stature. *J. Am. Med. Assoc.*, **251**, 2223–30
9. Bercu, B.B., Shulman, D.I. and Root, A.W. (1987). High incidence of prenatal and perinatal complication associated with growth hormone neurosecretory dysfunction (GHND). *Pediatr. Res.*, **224A** (abstract)
10. Tanner, J.M. and Davies, P.S.V. (1985). Clinical longitudinal standards for height and height velocity for North American children. *J. Pediatr.*, **107**, 317–29
11. Zadik, F., Chalew, S.A., Raiti, S. and Kowarski, A.A. (1985). Do short children secrete insufficient quantities of growth hormone? *Pediatrics*, **76**, 355–60
12. Rose, S.R., Ross, J.L., Uriate, M., Barnes, K.M., Cassorla, F.G. and Cutler, G.B. (1988). The advantage of measuring stimulated as compared with spontaneous growth hormone levels in the diagnosis of growth hormone deficiency. *N. Engl. J. Med.*, **319**, 201–7
13. Bercu, B.B., Shulman, D.I., Root, W. and Spiliotis, E. (1986). Growth hormone (GH) provocative testing frequently does not reflect endogenous GH secretion. *J. Clin. Endocrinol. Metab.*, **3**, 709–16
14. Kowarski, A.A., Thompson, R.G. and Migeon, C. (1971). Determination of integrated concentration of true secretion rate of human growth hormone. *J. Clin. Endocrinol. Metab.*, **32**, 356–60
15. Bernasconi, S., Ghizzoni, L., Pellini, C., Volta, C., Petecca, C. and Di Natale, B. (1988). Effect of clonidine administration on linear growth and growth hormone (GH) concentration in children with constitutional delay (CGD). Presented at *International Symposium on Growth Abnormalities*, June, Bologna.
16. Bierich, J.R. (1983). Treatment of constitutional delay of growth and adolescence with human growth hormone. *Klin. Pediatr.*, **195**, 309–16
17. Pintor, C., Cella, S.G., Loche, S., Puggioni, R., Corda, R., Locatelli, V. and Müller, E.E. (1987). Clonidine treatment for short stature. *Lancet*, **i**, 1226–30
18. Rudman, D., Kutner, M.H., Blackstone, R.D., Cushman, R.A., Rain, R.P. and Patterson, J.H. (1981). Children with normal variant short stature: treatment with human growth hormone for six months. *N. Engl. J. Med.*, **305**, 123–31
19. Underwood, L.E. (1984). Growth hormone treatment for short children. *J. Pediatr.*, **104**, 237–9
20. Pescovitz, O.H. and Tan, E. (1988). Lack of benefit of clonidine treatment for short stature in a double-blind, placebo-controlled trial. *Lancet*, **ii**, 874–7

21. Pintor, C., Cella, S.G., Corda, R., Locatelli, V., Puggioni, R., Loche, S. and Müller, E.E. (1985). Clonidine accelerates growth in children with impaired growth hormone secretion. *Lancet*, **i**, 1482–5
22. Massara, F., Mazza, E., Ghigo, E. and Camanni, F. (1987). Il controlle nervoso della secrezione di ormone somatotropo: aspetti clinici. In Müller, E.E. (ed.). *Progressi nella diagnosi e terapia dei disturbi dell'accrescimento*, pp. 71–87. (Roma and Milano: Pythagora Press)
23. The Health Services Human Growth Hormone Committee (1981). Comparison of the intravenous insulin and oral clonidine tolerance tests for growth hormone secretion. *Arch. Dis. Child.*, **56**, 852–4
24. Bernasconi, S., Ragnatela, G., Virdis, R. and Giovannelli, G. (1985). Uso della clonidina per os come test di screening per il deficit di ormone della crescita. *Riv. It. Ped.*, **II**, 430–2
25. Roth, J., Glick, S.M., Yalow, R.S. and Berson, S.A. (1963). Hypoglycemia: a potent stimulus to secretion of growth hormone. *Science*, **140**, 987–8
26. Müller, E.E. (1987). Neural control of somatotropic function. *Physiol. Rev.*, **67**, 962–1053
27. Gertner, J.M., Genel, M., Gianfredi, S.P., Hintz, R.L., Rosenfeld, R.G., Tamborlane, W.W. and Wilson, D.M. (1984). Prospective clinical trial of human growth hormone in short children without growth hormone deficiency. *J. Pediatr.*, **104**, 172–6
28. Ross, J.L., Long, L.M., Loriaux, D.L. and Cutler, G.B., Jr (1985). Growth hormone secretory dynamics in Turner syndrome. *J. Pediatr.*, **10**, 202–6
29. Van Vliet, G., Styne, D.M., Kaplan, S.L. and Grumbach, M.M. (1983). Growth hormone treatment for short stature. *N. Engl. J. Med.*, **309**, 1016–22

67

Ovarian dysgenesis

M. Breckwoldt and P. Wieacker

Ovarian dysgenesis can be interpreted as a consequence of rapid and progressive decline of primordial follicles during fetal development and early childhood resulting in fibrotic transformation of the gonad. Since streak gonads contain no follicular structures to establish negative feedback control of the hypothalamic–pituitary function peripheral follicle-stimulating hormone (FSH) and luteinizing hormone (LH) levels start to rise already in early childhood[1]. Therefore, primary ovarian failure can be classified as hypergonadotropic hypogonadism.

The clinical feature indicative for gonadal dysgenesis is consequently sexual infantilism. Depending on the underlying genetic disorder sexual infantilism can be associated with short stature. Impairment of growth is obviously related to defects or absence of the X chromosome. Turner Syndrome which was originally described by Morgagni more than 200 years ago can be regarded as a classical example. The complete karyotype of 45 XO was almost simultaneously reported in 1959 by Ford *et al.* and by Fraccaro *et al.*[2,3]. The clinical symptomatology is characterized by two obligatory symptoms: sexual infantilism and short stature. Numerous clinical symptoms such as webbed neck, shield chest, pigment naevi and cubitus valgus may or may not be present. During childhood the clinical symptoms are frequently discrete and become more and more prominent as childhood advances. The external and internal genitalia are hypoplastic, the ovaries are transformed into streak structures composed exclusively of connective tissue without any follicular structures. Due to the absence of endogenous sex steroids bone maturation is retarded. Despite normal growth-hormone levels and normal insulin-like growth factor (IGF1) concentrations growth is limited due to the absence of the second X chromosome. The presence of both intact X chromosomes is obviously required for normal growth, normal development of the ovaries and normal ovarian function.

Ovarian dysgenesis is also associated with the mosaic karyotype 45 XO/46 XX. The clinical spectrum of this genetic disorder is variable depending on the ratio of XO to XX cell lines. A high proportion of XO cell lines leads to clinical symptoms indistinguishable from the classical Ullrich–Turner Syndrome. If, however, the proportion of 46 XX cell lines is high, normal pubertal development and normal ovarian function can be observed. In individual cases even pregnancies have been described. However, premature menopause has to be anticipated.

In addition, several groups of mosaic forms have been described as case reports.

Besides abnormalities of the sex chromosomes structural aberrations of the X chromosome have also to be considered. The structural aberrations include the presence of isochromosomes. If the short arm is missing as in the case of 46Xi (Xq) Turner symptoms are well expressed. These patients present with sexual infantilism and impairment of growth. All other symptoms characteristic of this syndrome can also be present[4].

The presence of an isochromosome Xp lacking the long arm has been described in only very few cases. These patients also present sexual infantilism, however, growth is generally unimpaired[5].

Deletion of the terminal segments of the short arm can be associated with normal gonadal function[6]. However, these patients present with growth impairment and clinical symptoms compatible with Turner Syndrome.

Deletions of the lower segments including those of the long arm of the X chromosome are always accompanied with gonadal dysgenesis, impairment of growth in most cases and the expression of Turner Symptoms. Loss of terminal segments may lead to gonadal dysgenesis or premature menopause without affecting growth[7].

From these findings it can be concluded that genetic information for statural determination is localized in the upper regions of the long and the short arm of the X chromosome. Genes coding for normal ovarian development and ovarian function are primarily located in the lower segments of both arms. The genetic regions for statural and ovarian determinations are overlapping as indicated in Figure 1.

Chromosomal translocations from autosomes to the X chromosome can be associated with normal gonadal function but may also lead to primary ovarian failure depending on the translocalized region as presented in Figure 1[8].

In most cases ovarian dysgenesis can be explained by cytogenetic analysis including the banding technique. In certain cases of gonadal dysgenesis, however, cytogenetic analysis provides no helpful information in the diagnostic work up. Pure ovarian dysgenesis is associated with a normal karyotype of 46XX. Swyer Syndrome is characterized by the karyotype of 46XY and a normal female phenotype. Ovarian dysfunction in these syndromes becomes apparent by delayed pubertal development and primary amenorrhea, growth is unimpaired. Endocrinologically these patients can be classified as hypergonadotropic hypogonadism. The internal genitalia, derivatives of the Müllerian ducts, are hypoplastic due to the absence of endogenous sex steroids.

From XX males it is known that the X-chromosomes contain DNA sequences responsible for the induction of testis[7]. This finding explains the male phenotype despite the presence of two X chromosomes. With regard to Swyer Syndrome the karyotype of 46XY and a female phenotype one could expect that the Y chromosome is lacking genetic information coding testicular development. However, so far genetic analysis of the Y chromosome

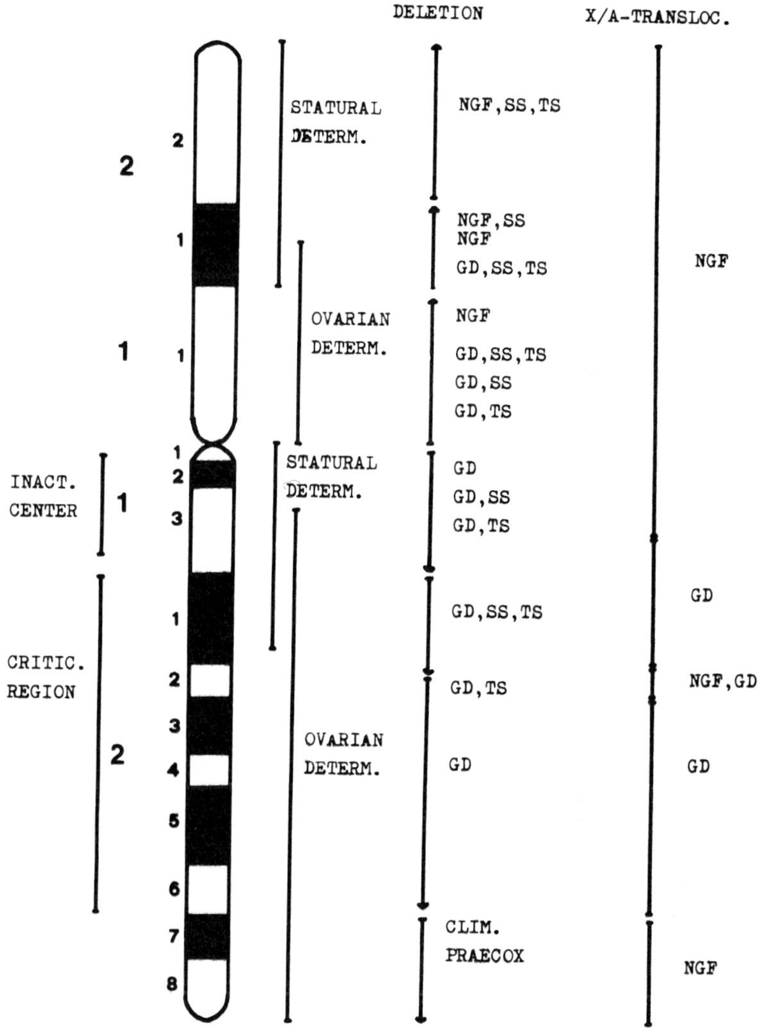

Figure 1 Karyotype/phenotype correlation in X chromosome aberrations

in these individuals failed to provide any evidence to substantiate this assumption. In addition, no genetic defects could be detected in patients presenting with pure gonadal dysgenesis. The etiology of these syndromes has not yet been clarified.

REFERENCES

1. Conte, F.A., Gumbach, M.M. and Kaplan, S.L. (1975). A diphasic pattern of gonadotropin secretion in patients with the syndrome of gonadal dysgenesis. *J. Clin. Endocrinol. Metab.*,

40, 670–4

2. Ford, C.E., Jones, K.W., Polani, P.E., de Almeida, I.C. and Briggs, H.J. (1959). A sex chromosome anomaly in a case of gonadal dysgenesis (Turner's syndrome). *Lancet*, **i**, 711–14
3. Fraccaro, M., Kaijser, K. and Lindsten, J. (1959). Chromosome complement in gonadal dysgenesis (Turner's syndrome). *Lancet*, **i**, 886–9
4. Otto, P.G., Vianne-Morgante, A.M. and Otto, P.A. (1981). The Turner phenotype and the different types of human X isochromosome. *Hum. Genet.*, **57**, 159–64
5. Dewald, G.W. (1983). Isodicentric X chromosomes in humans: origin, segregation behaviour and replication band patterns. In Sandberg, A. A. (ed.) *Cytogenetics of the Mammalian X-Chromosome. Part A Basic Mechanism of X-Chromosome Behaviour*, pp. 405–26 (New York: Academic Press)
6. Wyss, D., De Lozier, C.D., Daniell, J. and Engel, E. (1982). Structural anomalies of the X-chromosome: personal observation and review of non-mosaic cases. *Clin. Genet.*, **21**, 145–9
7. Trunca, C., Thermann, E. and Rosenwaks, Z. (1984). The phenotypic effects of small, distal Xq deletions. *Hum. Genet.*, **68**, 87–9
8. Mattei, M.G., Mattei, J.F., Ayone, S. and Giraud, F. (1982). X-Autosome translocations. Cytogenetic characteristics and their consequences. *Hum. Genet.*, **61**, 295–303
9. Guelleau, G., Casanova, M., Bishop, C., Geldwerth, D., André, G., Fellons, M. and Weissenbach, J. (1984). Human XX males with Y-single-copy DNA fragments. *Nature*, **307**, 172–3

68

Regulation of endocrine cell growth in the hypothalamic–pituitary–pancreatic islet axis

N. Billestrup and J.H. Nielsen

INTRODUCTION

Several endocrine disorders are characterized by hypo- or hyperplasia of the endocrine glands. Although the regulation of the secretion of most hormones is well understood, little is known about the mechanisms involved in the development and growth of the endocrine cells.

When the body mass increases there is an increased demand for insulin. Normally, this is encountered by increase in β-cell mass which is believed mainly to be due to the enhanced glucose load secondary to insulin antagonistic effects of pituitary, adrenal and gonadal hormones[1].

In the following we will review the evidence for existence of hypothalamic–pituitary–pancreatic islet axis in the regulation of the growth of the somatotropes and the β cells.

REGULATION OF PITUITARY SOMATOTROPE GROWTH

A role for hypothalamic regulation of pituitary somatotrope cell proliferation was indicated by studies by Asa *et al.*[2] and by Zafar *et al.*[3]. It was observed that patients with high plasma concentrations of growth hormone (GH) releasing factor (GRF) due to a GRF-secreting tumor exhibited hyperplasia of the pituitary gland. This hyperplasia was caused by an increase in the number of GH-producing cells. In some cases GH-secreting adenomas were observed[4]. These observations led to the hypothesis that GRF can stimulate growth of somatotropic cells in the pituitary and that overproduction of GRF may contribute to cell transformation and subsequent adenoma formation.

A direct stimulatory effect of GRF on somatotrope proliferation has been observed *in vitro*. When pituitary cells from rats are cultured in the presence of GRF a 20-fold increase in somatrope cell proliferation was observed[5]. Interestingly, it was observed that somatostatin was able to inhibit partly the growth-promoting activity of GRF. The ability of GRF to stimulate somatotrope growth *in vitro* strongly suggests that GRF itself is the causative agent in inducing somatotrope hyperplasia under pathological conditions of GRF hypersecretion. The use of long acting somatostatin analogs in the treatment of acromegaly due to GH-secreting adenomas also suggest that somatostatin is able to inhibit growth of GH-producing cells in humans *in vivo*.

The question of whether GRF regulates somatotrope cell growth under normal physiological conditions is still unanswered. However, recent observations in children suffering from isolated GH deficiency suggest that GRF does play a role in normal somatotrope growth and differentiation. The majority of GH deficient children suffer from dysregulation of the pituitary rather than a primary pituitary defect since these children show an increase in GH after GRF administration[6]. This response, however, is often diminished compared to that seen in normal children which may reflect a reduced number of GH-secreting cells. After prolonged treatment with GRF the GH response to GRF gradually increases and in some cases reaches normal levels[7]. These data indicate that in some children suffering from GH deficiency the primary defect is lack of sufficient GRF from the hypothalamus resulting in poor GH secretion and reduced somatotrope growth. Treatment of such children with GRF rather than GH seems to restore somatotrope mass and thus GH secretion to normal levels.

REGULATION OF PANCREATIC β-CELL GROWTH BY GH AND RELATED HORMONES

The association between the pituitary and the endocrine pancreas has long been known. Thus the diabetogenic effect of GH was described by Houssay in the 1920s. This was believed to be due to the insulin antagonistic action of GH on the glucose uptake. Young *et al.* found that the diabetogenic effect depends on age and species[8], and in 1968 Martin *et al.* described a tropic effect of GH on the pancreatic β cell in the rat[9].

We have studied the direct effect of GH and related hormones on the pancreatic islets *in vitro* and found that GH, prolactin (PRL), and placental lactogen (PL) exert a direct mitogenic effect on the β cell (Figure 1)[10].

Since many effects of GH are supposed to be mediated via insulin-like growth factor 1 (IGF-1) produced by the liver or locally in the target tissue[11,12], we looked for the possible role of IGF-1 in the effect of GH on the β cells. IGF-1 did not mimic the GH effect on the β cells and neutralization of IGF-1 with antiserum did not inhibit the stimulatory effect of GH. These results suggest that GH acts as growth factor for the pancreatic β cell. Under conditions where the β cells do not respond to GH, glucose intolerance may occur and diabetes may develop. Such a condition is acromegaly where the incidence of diabetes is markedly increased[13].

Another condition is puberty where the incidence of type 1 diabetes is maximal[14]. Here the rapid increase in somatic growth may not be accompanied by a compensatory increase in the β-cell mass. This may be due to either a pre-existing low β-cell number or the lack of GH responsiveness of the β cells. The latter may be related to the profound changes in hormones

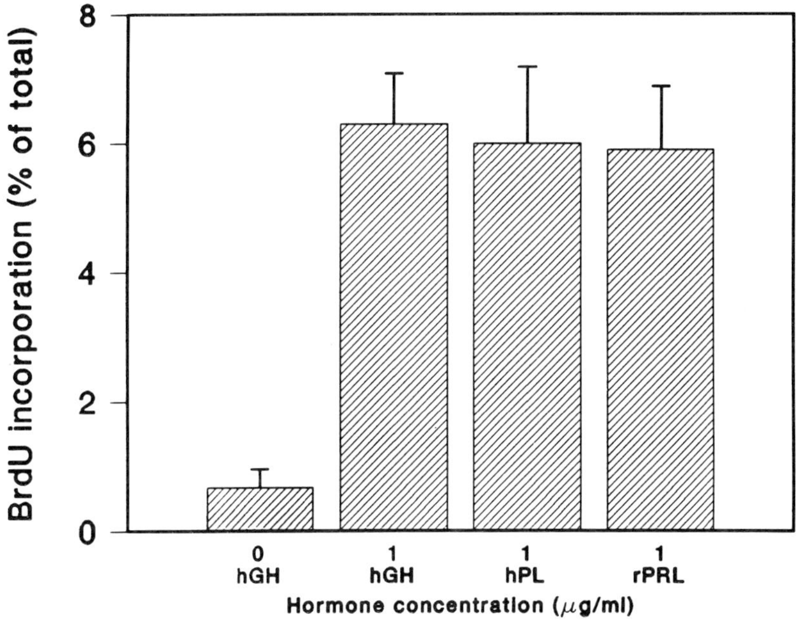

Figure 1 Effect of human growth hormone, human placental lactogen, and rat prolactin on islet β-cell proliferation *in vitro*. Islet cells from newborn rats were cultured in the presence of hormones as indicated. After 14 days cells were labelled with the thymidine analog Bromodeoxyuridine (BrdU). Proliferating β cells were identified by double immunofluorescence staining using insulin and BrdU specific antibodies. The mean $\pm$SD for three experiments is shown

involved in the sexual maturation which also may affect the growth of the β cells.

REGULATION OF β-CELL GROWTH DURING PREGNANCY

Pregnancy is another condition where a rapid increase in the body weight takes place accompanied by an increased demand for insulin. This is normally accomplished by hyperplasia of the islet cells[15], but in 1–3% of all pregnancies glucose intolerance develops, i.e. gestational diabetes. The factors involved in the β-cell growth are not known, but since PL was found to stimulate β-cell replication *in vitro*, it is suggested that this GH-like placental hormone is responsible for the β-cell growth[16]. During the third trimester serum concentrations around 10 μg/ml are found, whereas 0.1 μg/ml gives significant stimulation *in vitro*[10].

PRL which is also increased late in pregnancy may also contribute to the β-cell hyperplasia as it also exerts a mitogenic effect on islet cells *in vitro* (Figure 1)[10].

However, other pregnancy related hormones may influence the growth and function of the β-cells. Thus progesterone increases the glucose sensitivity of the islets but inhibits the proliferation[16]. Estradiol seems not to have

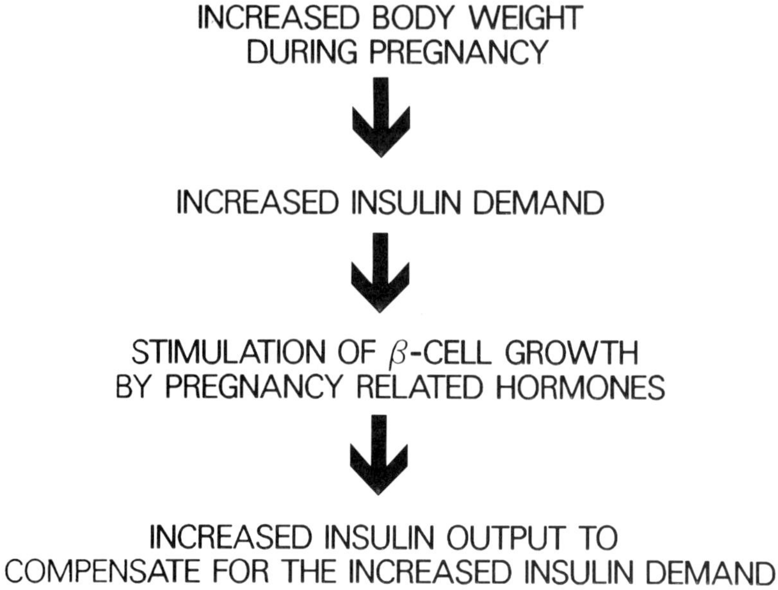

Figure 2 Hypothetical regulation of the β-cell mass during pregnancy

direct effects on the β cells but may increase the responsiveness to the growth promoting hormones by inducing expression of their receptors.

This is in accordance with the observation by Young in the 1940s that although GH is diabetogenic in the adult dog, it is not diabetogenic in puppies and pregnant dogs. Thus these conditions may be characterized by the responsiveness of the β cells to the mitogenic effects of GH and the related hormones PL and PRL.

CONCLUSIONS

The observations reviewed above support the existence of a hypothalamic–pituitary–pancreatic islet axis in the regulation of the growth of the somatotrope in pituitary by GRF and somatostatin, and the mitogenic effect of GH, PRL, and their placental counterpart PL on the growth of the β cells in the endocrine pancreas (Figure 2). Disturbances in these regulatory pathways may give rise to various syndromes, e.g. dwarfism, acromegaly, and diabetes mellitus.

The molecular mechanisms are not known, but as for other growth factors, activation of cellular proto-oncogenes seems to be involved.

REFERENCES

1. Hellerström, C. and Swenne, I. (1985). Growth pattern of pancreatic islets in animals. In Volk, B.W. and Arquilla, E.R. (eds.). *The Diabetic Pancreas*, pp. 53–81. (New York and

London: Plenum Medical Book Company)
2. Asa, S.L., Schlithauer, B.W., Bilbao, J.M., Horvath, E., Ryan, N., Kovacs, K., Randell, R.V., Laws, E.R., Singer, W., Linfoot, J.A., Thorner, M.O. and Vale, W. (1984). A case for hypothalamic acromegaly: a clinicopathological study of six patients with hypothalamic gangliocytomas producing growth hormone-releasing factor. *J. Clin. Endocrinol. Metab.*, **58**, 796–803
3. Zafar, M.S., Mellinger, R.C., Fine, V., Szabò, M. and Frohman, L.A. (1979). Acromegaly associated with a bronchial carcinoid tumor: evidence for ectopic production of growth hormone-releasing activity. *J. Clin. Endocrinol. Metab.*, **48**, 66–71
4. Sano, T., Asa, S.L. and Kovacs, K. (1988). Growth hormone-releasing hormone-producing tumors: clinical, biochemical, and morphological manifestations. *Endocr. Rev.*, **9**, 357–73
5. Billestrup, N., Swanson, L.W. and Vale, W. (1986). Growth hormone-releasing factor stimulates proliferation of somatotrophs *in vitro*. *Proc. Natl. Acad. Sci., USA*, **83**, 6854–7
6. Thorner, M.O., Vance, M.L., Evans, W.S., Blizzard, R.M., Rogol, A.D., Ho, K., Leong, D.A., Burges, J.L.C., Cronin, M.J., MacLeod, R.M., Kovacs, K., Asa, S.L., Horvath, E., Frohman, L., Furlanetto, R., Klingensmith, G.J., Brook, C., Smith, P., Reichlin, S., Rivier, J. and Vale, W. (1986). Physiological and clinical studies of GRF and GH. *Rec. Progr. Horm. Res.*, **42**, 589–640
7. Rochiccioli, P.E., Tauber, M.T., Coude, F.X., Aronone, M., Morre, M., Vboldi, F. and Barbeau, C. (1987). Results of 1-year growth hormone (GH)-releasing hormone-(1-44) treatment on growth, somatomedin C, and 24-hour GH secretion in six children with partial GH deficiency. *J. Clin. Endocrinol. Metab.*, **65**, 268–74
8. Young, F.G. and Korner, A. (1960). Growth hormone. In Williams, R.H. (ed.) *Diabetes*, pp. 216–33. (New York: Paul B. Hoeber)
9. Martin, J.M., Åkerblom, H.K. and Garay, G. (1968). Insulin secretion in rats with elevated hormone due to MtT-W15 tumor. *Diabetes*, **17**, 661–7
10. Nielsen, J.H. (1982). Effects of growth hormone, prolactin and placental lactogen on insulin content and release and deoxyribonucleic acid synthesis in cultured pancreatic islets. *Endocrinology*, **110**, 600–6
11. Green, H., Morikawa, M. and Nixon, T. (1985). A dual effector model of growth hormone action. *Differentiation*, **29**, 195–9
12. Isaksson, O.G.P., Lindahl, A., Nilsson, A. and Isgaard, J. (1987). Mechanism of the stimulatory effect of growth hormone on longitudinal lone growth. *Endocr. Rev.*, **8**, 426–38
13. Luft, R., Cerasi, E. and Hamberger, C.A. (1967). Studies on the pathogenesis of diabetes in acromegaly. *Acta Endocrinol.*, **56**, 593–607
14. Christau, B., Kromann, H., Christy, M., Andersen, O.O. and Nerup, J. (1979). Incidence of insulin-dependent diabetes mellitus (0–29 years at onset) in Denmark. *Acta Med. Scand.*, Suppl., **624**, 54–60
15. Van Assche, F.A., Aerts, L. and Prins, F.D. (1978). A morphological study on the endocrine pancreas in human pregnancy. *Br. J. Obstet. Gynaecol.*, **85**, 818–20
16. Nielsen, J.H., Nielsen, V., Molsted Pedersen, L. and Decekert, T. (1986). Effects of pregnancy hormones on pancreatic islets in organ culture. *Acta Endocrinol.*, **111**, 336–41

69

Insulin-like growth factors and ovarian function

G. Giordano, A. Barreca, A. Volpe and F. Minuto

In the last few years, it has been recognized that, not only the gonadotropins, but also several peptide growth factors (GFs) play a role in the regulation of granulosa cell replication and differentiation. Among these GFs, epidermal growth factor (EGF) and fibroblast growth factor (FGF) have been shown to have a mitogenic effect on bovine, porcine, rabbit and human granulosa cells[1,2]. Both GFs suppress[1,2] follicle-stimulating hormone (FSH)-dependent, luteinizing hormone (LH) receptor induction in serum free culture, and EGF also restrains the follicular development by decreasing the estrogen biosynthesis in a dose related manner[3,4]. The platelet derived growth factor (PDGF), on the contrary, enhances FSH-dependent LH receptor formation *in vitro*, and increases the FSH-stimulated progesterone production[5–7]. Insulin increases glucose transport and cell division in bovine granulosa cells and enhances progestin production as well as FSH-stimulated aromatase activity[8,9]. As most of these effects are obtained with relatively high concentrations of insulin, it is possible that they are achieved by cross-interaction with type I insulin-like growth factor (IGF) receptors. The IGFs or somatomedins are growth promoting peptides belonging to the same family, as they possess insulin-like sulfating and mitogenic activity in a wide range of tissue or cell systems[10]. In particular, insulin-like growth factor I (IGF-I) is a growth hormone-dependent peptide synthesized by many tissues[11,12] and by a variety of normal and tumor-derived cell lines[10,13,14].

It has been recently demonstrated that IGF-I exerts strong stimulatory effects on granulosa cell proliferation[15,16] and differentiation[16–18]. Moreover, the existence of specific type I receptors on porcine[16,19] and murine[20] granulosa cells, and the demonstration of immunoreactive intraovarian IGF-I led to the hypothesis that IGF-I produced by granulosa cells may constitute an intraovarian modulatory signal[21]. It has been shown that IGF-I may also amplify the action of some pituitary hormones on both cell differentiation and replication; in this regard IGF-I potentiates the actions of gonadotropins in rat granulosa ovarian tissue[22–24], and of thyroid-stimulating hormone (TSH) in thyroid cell and human tissue[25–27]. The mechanism by which IGF-I amplifies gonadotropin action is not completely understood, although its ability to synergize with FSH in the production of cAMP[28] and the induction of several cAMP dependent granulosa cell functions has been proved[22-24].

Besides GH, which is the main stimulator of IGF-I secretion by several cell types, EGF has been shown to be a powerful dose dependent stimulator of IGF production by cultured porcine granulosa cells[29]. Gonadal IGF-I secretion can be also stimulated by the main hormones involved in trophic regulation of the ovary. In fact gonadotropins, as well as cAMP, the presumed mediator of their action, and estradiol enhance the secretion of immunoreactive (IR) IGF-I by porcine granulosa cells *in vitro*[30].

Human follicular fluid has been found to contain significant amounts of IGF-II (nearly 2 ng) and of IGF-I[31]; the latter is significantly higher in dominant follicles than in cohort follicles and appears to be related to the follicular volume[32].

As *in vivo* treatment with GH can increase the ovarian response to gonadotropin stimulation in women with ovaries that are relatively resistant to human menopausal gonadotropin hMG therapy[33], and *in vitro* treatment with GH enhances granulosa cell production of IGF-I[34], it seems possible to modify the stimulation of ovarian function by utilizing known endocrine effects in order to affect paracrine control of ovarian function[35].

We have investigated the presence of GH, IGF-I and EGF in the fluids obtained from different ovarian follicles of five patients who could have a superovulation induced only when GH (0.1 U/kg body weight (BW)/day) was added to the gonadotropin therapy. The follicular fluids of three patients who ovulated after treatment with gonadotropin only served as a control.

The results demonstrated the presence in the follicular fluids of GH (M $\pm$ SD: 4.5 $\pm$ 1.8 ng/ml) in significantly higher concentration ($p < 0.001$) than in control follicles (2.1 $\pm$ 0.7), of acid-extractable IGF-I (158.6 $\pm$ 53.5 ng/ml) and of EGF (4.3 $\pm$ 2.3 ng/ml) in concentrations similar to that of control fluids (145.5 $\pm$ 65.8 ng/ml and 4.1 $\pm$ 4.6 ng/ml respectively). A correlation between GH and IGF-I concentration in the follicular fluid was evident only when considering the GH treated subjects ($p = 0.002$). The IGF-I binding protein assay evidenced the presence of considerable amounts of unsaturated binding sites in all fluids (specific binding 12.8 $\pm$ 3.9/0.025 ml).

Gel-filtration of the pooled follicular fluids from GH-treated and control patients revealed the presence of two peaks of IGF-I-like immunoreactivity in both cases. The first peak, which eluted in the void volume, contained specific IGF-I binding activity, the second peak corresponded to the molecular weight of authentic IGF-I. The material eluting in the second peak and synthetic IGF-I showed parallel competition curves in the IGF-I radioimmunoassay. When the material in the first peak was cross-linked by disuccimidylsuberate to radioiodinated IGF-I and analyzed by 10% sodium dodecyl sulfate-polyacrylamide gel electrophoresis, a 35 kDa band was evident. The protein has a monomeric structure, as evidenced by treatment with dithiothreitol and the binding is inhibited by IGF-I excess but it is not influenced by addition of insulin excess.

These results indicate that human follicular fluid contains IGF-I and IGF-I binding protein, and supports the possibility of an IGF-I involvement in the growth and development of human ovarian follicles, in agreement with the finding of its mitogenic effects in cultured rat and porcine granulosa cells.

IGF-I production is known to be stimulated by a number of growth factors, such as fibroblast growth factor (FGF), platelet derived growth factor (PDGF), and epidermal growth factor (EGF) in the presence of PDGF[36]. The finding of a highly significant correlation ($p < 0.001$) between EGF and IGF-I concentration in the follicular fluids, seems to confirm a role for this growth factor in inducing IGF-I production in human ovarian tissue *in vivo*.

As regards the binding activity found in the high molecular weight region, its size and the lack of insulin binding ability exclude the possibility that it is related to cell membrane IGF type I receptors. This binding material formed a 35 kDa complex when reacted with radioiodinated IGF-I. In this regard, it must be recalled that a protein binding the IGFs (mol. wt. 35–40 kDa) has been purified from amniotic fluid[37–39], which behaves similarly to the non-GH-dependent 45 K in different clinical conditions[40,41]. Based on the amino acid sequence homology of the N-terminal segment[42], it appears that this binding protein is the placental protein 12 (PP12).

The higher correlation found between GH and IGF-I in the follicular fluids of GH-treated with respect to those of the non-GH-treated patients, demonstrates the possibility of influencing the IGF-I local synthesis and therefore the growth and maturation of the follicles, by the addition of GH in patients presenting with gonadotropin-resistant anovulation.

The data are consistent with a role of GH and IGF-I in the control of follicular growth and development also in humans, and support the hypothesis of a proliferative and/or permissive effect of IGF-I in ovarian tissue, via an autocrine or paracrine mode of action.

REFERENCES

1. Gospodarowicz, D., Mescher, A.L. and Birdwell, C.R. (1978). Control of cellular proliferation by the fibroblast and epidermal growth factors. *Nat. Cancer. Inst. Monograph.*, **48**, 109
2. Gospodarowicz, D. and Bialecki, H. (1979). Fibroblast and epidermal growth factors are mitogenic agents for culture granulosa cells of rodent, porcine and human origin. *Endocrinology*, **104**, 757
3. Mondschein, J.S. and Schomberg, D.W. (1981). Growth factors modulate gonadotropin receptor induction in granulosa cell cultures. *Science*, **211**, 1179
4. Hsueh, A.J.W., Welsh, T.H. and Jones, P.B.C. (1981). Inhibition of ovarian and testicular steroidogenesis by epidermal growth factor. *Endocrinology*, **108**, 2002
5. Mondschein, J.S. and Schomberg, D.W. (1981). Plateled-derived growth factor enhances granulosa cell luteinizing hormone receptor induction by FSH and serum. *Endocrinology*, **109**, 325
6. Mondschein, J.S. and Schomberg, D.W. (1984). Effects of partially and more highly purified plateled-derived growth factor preparations on luteinizing hormone receptor induction in granulosa cell cultures. *Biol. Reprod.*, **30**, 603
7. Knecht, M. and Catt, K.J. (1983). Modulation of cAMP-mediated differentiation in ovarian granulosa cells by epidermal growth factor and platelet-derived growth factor. *J. Biol. Chem.*, **258**, 2789
8. Garzo, V.G. and Dorrington, J.H. (1984). Aromatase activity in human granulosa cells during follicular development and the modulation by follicle-stimulating hormone and insulin. *Endocr. Rev.*, **148**, 657–62
9. Davoren, J.B. and Hsueh, A.J.W. (1984). Insulin enhances FSH-stimulated steroidogenesis by cultured rat granulosa cells. *Mol. Cell. Endocrinol.*, **35**, 97
10. Van Wyk, J.J. and Underwood, L.E. (1978). The somatomedins and their actions. In

Litwack, G. (ed.), *Biochemical Actions of Hormones*, Vol. V, pp. 101–48 (Academic Press Inc.: New York)

11. Pierson, R.W. and Temin, H.M. (1972). The partial purification from calf serum of a fraction with multiplication stimulating activity for chicken fibroblasts in cell culture and with non-suppressible insulin-like activity. *J. Cell. Physiol.*, **79**, 319–30
12. Dulak, N. and Temin, H.N. (1973). A partially purified polypeptide fraction from rat liver cell conditioned medium with multiplication-stimulating activity for embryo fibroblasts. *J. Cell. Physiol.*, **81**, 153–60
13. Marquardt, H., Todaro, G.J., Henderson, L.E. and Oroszlan, S. (1981). Purification and primary structure of a polypeptide with multiplicating-stimulating activity from rat liver cell cultures. *J. Biol. Chem.*, **256**, 6859–65
14. Nissley, S.P., Adams, S.O., Acquaviva, A.M., Yang, Y.W.H., Bruni, B., Angust, G.P., White, R.M., Foley, T.F. Jr., Moses, A.C., Cohen, K.L. and Rechler, M.M. (1983). Multiplication stimulating activity for cells in culture. In Spencer, E.M. (ed.), *Insulin-like Growth Factors/Somatomedins: Basic Chemistry, Biology, Clinical Importance*. pp. 31–48 (Walter de Gruyter: Berlin/New York)
15. Savion, N. and Lui, G.M. (1981). Factors controlling proliferation and progesterone production by bovine granulosa cells in serum-free medium. *Endocrinology*, **109**, 409
16. Baranao, J.L.S. and Hammond, J.M. (1984). Comparative effects of insulin and insulin-like growth factors on DNA synthesis and differentiation of porcine granulosa cell. *Biochem. Biophys. Res. Commun.*, **124**, 484
17. Adashi, E.Y., Resnick, C.E., Svoboda, M.E. and Van Wyk, J.J. (1984). A novel role for Somatomedin-C in the cytodifferentiation of the ovarian granulosa cell. *Endocrinology*, **115**, 1227–9
18. Adashi, E.Y., Resnick, C.E., Svoboda, M.E., van Wyk, J.J., Hascall, V.C. and Yanagishita, M. (1986). Independent and synergistic action of somatomedin-C in the stimulation of proteoglycan biosynthesis by cultured rat granulosa cells. *Endocrinology*, **118**, 456–8
19. Veldhuis, J.D. and Furlanetto, R.W. (1985). Trophic actions of human somatomedin-C/insulin-like growth factor I on ovarian cells: in vitro studies with swine granulosa cells. *Endocrinology*, **116**, 1235–42
20. Adashi, E.Y., Resnick, C.E., Svoboda, M.E. and van Wyk, J.J. (1986). Follicle-stimulating hormone enhances somatomedin-C binding to cultured rat granulosa cells. Evidence for cAMP dependence. *J. Biol. Chem.*, **261**, 3923–6
21. Adashi, E.Y., Resnick, C.E., D'Ercole, A.J., Svoboda, M.E. and Van Wyk, J.J. (1985). Insulin-like growth factors as intraovarian regulators of granulosa cell growth and function. *Endocr. Rev.*, **6**, 400–20
22. Adashi, E.Y., Resnik, C.E., Svoboda, M.E. and Van Wyk, J.J. (1985). Somatomedin-C synergises with follicle stimulating hormone in the acquisition of progestin biosynthetic capacity by cultured rat granulosa cells. *Endocrinology*, **116**, 2135–42
23. Adashi, E.Y., Resnik, C.E., Brodie, A.M.H., Svoboda, M.E. and Van Wyk, J.J. (1985). Somatomedin-C mediated potentiation of follicle stimulating hormone-induced aromatase activity of cultured rat granulosa cells. *Endocrinology*, **117**, 2313–20
24. Adashi, E.Y., Resnick, C.E., Svoboda, M.E. and Van Wyk, J.J. (1985). Somatomedin-C enhances induction of luteinizing hormone receptors by follicle stimulating hormone in cultured rat granulosa cells. *Endocrinology*, **116**, 2369–75
25. Tramontano, D., Cushing, G.W., Moses, A.C. and Ingbar, S.H. (1986). Insulin-like growth factor-I stimulates the growth of rat thyroid cells in culture and synergizes the stimulation of DNA synthesis induced by TSH and Graves'-IgG. *Endocrinology*, **119**, 940–2
26. Smith, P., Wynford-Thomas, D., Stringer, M.J. and Williams, E.D. (1986). Growth factor control of rat thyroid follicular cell proliferation. *Endocrinology*, **119**, 1439–45
27. Minuto, F., Barreca, A., Del Monte, P., Cariola, G., Torre, G.C. and Giordano, G. (1989). Immunoreactive insulin-like growth factor I (IGF-I) and IGF-I binding protein content in human thyroid tissue. *J. Clin. Endocrinol. Metab.*, **68**, 621–6
28. Adashi, E.Y., Resnick, C.E., Svoboda, M.E. and Van Wyk, J.J. (1986). Somatomedin-C as an amplifier of follicle-stimulating hormone action: enhanced accumulation of adenosine 3′5′-cyclic monophosphate. *Endocrinology*, **118**, 149–55
29. Mondschein, J.S. and Hammond, J.M. (1988). Growth factors regulate immunoreactive insulin-like growth factor-I production by cultured porcine granulosa cells. *Endocrinology*,

123, 463–8
30. Hsu, C.J. and Hammond, J.M. (1987). Gonadotrophins and estradiol stimulate immunoreactive insulin-like growth factor I by porcine granulosa cells *in vitro*. *Endocrinology*, **120**, 198–207
31. Ramasharma, K., Cabrera, C.M. and Li, C.H. (1986). Identification of insulin-like growth factor-II in human seminal and follicular fluids. *Biochem. Biophys. Res. Comm.*, **140**, 536–42
32. Eden, A.J., Jones, J., Carter, G.D. and Alaghband-Zadeh, J. (1988). A comparison of follicular fluid levels of insulin-like growth factor-1 in normal dominant and cohort follicles, polycystic and multicystic ovaries. *Clinical Endocrinol.*, **29**, 327–36
33. Homburg, R., Eshel, A., Abdalla, H.I. and Jacobs, H.S. (1988). Growth Hormone facilitates ovulation induction by gonadotrophins. *Clinical Endocrinology*, **29**, 113–17
34. Davoren, J.B. and Hsueh, A.J.W. (1984). Growth hormone increases ovarian levels of immunoreactive somatomedin-C/insulin-like growth factor I *in vivo*. *Endocrinology*, **118**, 888–90
35. Jia, X.C., Kalmijn, J.K. and Hsueh, A.J. (1986). Growth hormone enhances Follicle-stimulating hormone induced differentiation of cultured rat granulosa cells. *Endocrinology*, **118**, 1401–9
36. Clemmons, D.R. (1984). Multiple hormones stimulate the production of somatomedin by cultured human fibroblasts. *J. Clin. Endocrinol. Metab.*, **58**, 850–6
37. Chochinov, R.H., Mariz, I.K., Hajek, A.S. and Daughday, W.H. (1977). Characterization of a protein in mid-term human amniotic fluid which reacts in the somatomedin-C radioreceptor assay. *J. Clin. Endocrinol. Metab.*, **44**, 902–8
38. Drop, S.L.S., Valiquette, G., Guyda, H.J., Corvol, M.T. and Posner, B.I. (1979). Partial purification and characterization of a binding protein for ILAs in human amniotic fluid: a possible inhibitor of insulin-like activity. *Acta Endocrinol.*, **90**, 505–18
39. Povoa, G., Enberg, G., Jornvall, H. and Hall, K. (1984). Isolation and characterization of somatomedin-binding protein from midterm human amniotic fluid. *Eur. J. Biochem.*, **144**, 199
40. Drop, S.L.S., Kortleve, D.J., Guyda, H.J. and Posner, B.J. (1984). Immunoassay of a somatomedin-binding protein from human amniotic fluid: levels in fetal, neonatal and adult sera. *J. Clin. Endocrinol. Metab.*, **59**, 908–15
41. Povoa, G., Roovete, A. and Hall, K. (1984). Cross-reaction of serum somatomedin-binding protein in a radioimmunoassay developed for somatomedin-binding protein isolated from human amniotic fluid. *Acta Endocrinol.*, **107**, 563–70
42. Koistinen, R., Kalkkinen, N., Huhtala, M.L., Seppala, M., Bohn, H. and Rutanen, E.M. (1986). Placental Protein 12 is a decidual protein that binds somatomedin and has an identical N-terminal amino acid sequence with somatomedin-binding protein from human amniotic fluid. *Endocrinology*, **118**, 1375–8

Section 4 continued

Part C

Dihydroergocriptine and hyperprolactinemia

70

Dihydroergocriptine and prolactin: clinical experience

F. Mailland, P.L. Canonico and A. Zanotti

INTRODUCTION

Dihydroergocriptine (DHEC) is a hydrogenated derivative of a natural ergot alkaloid, with a strong affinity for dopaminergic receptors both in pituitary and in striatal membranes[1,2].

The compound has been shown to suppress either normal or increased prolactin (PRL) secretion in *in vitro* and *in vivo* animal models. In fact, an *in vitro* study[3] reported a concentration-dependent decrease of cAMP formation and PRL release by isolated and dispersed rat pituitary cells, as the result of an activation of dopaminergic receptors on lactotropes, the inhibitory activity of DHEC attaining about 50% at a concentration of 10 nmol/l and being abolished by haloperidol, pimozide and by the cell exposure to pertussis toxin.

On the other hand, the PRL-lowering activity of DHEC was confirmed *in vivo* by investigating the changes of serum PRL profile in intact rats or in animals made hyperprolactinemic by reserpine (2.5 mg/kg i.p.), the increase of serum PRL levels being completely reverted by DHEC 0.2 mg/kg i.p.[4].

CLINICAL EXPERIENCE

In this paper, the PRL lowering activity of DHEC in humans is reported, by reviewing the different conditions being studied, i.e. normal PRL levels, drug-induced PRL rise in serum, puerperium and hyperprolactinemia with or without evidence of pituitary tumors.

Normal PRL levels

DHEC was able to cause a fall of serum PRL levels that was longlasting and dependent on the dose of DHEC administered. In a preliminary study[5], a single 6 mg dose of the drug caused a marked fall in PRL levels in six healthy women. In a second study[4], a single 5 mg dose was significantly more active than 2.5 mg of DHEC in five healthy, young females. The effect on PRL of 5 mg DHEC was similar in extent to that of 2.5 mg bromocriptine in the same subjects and serum PRL levels never returned to baseline even 24 h after the administration of the compound.

Those data have been more precisely confirmed in another experiment (original data) on 12 healthy male volunteers, aged 18 to 45 years (mean $\pm$ SD; 31.1 $\pm$ 7.8), that were given DHEC 5 mg, 3 mg or placebo as single oral doses during the studies on the pharmacokinetics of the compound (Figure 1). Both doses caused a potent and long lasting fall of PRL, that decreased by 31% between 0 and 24 h after 3 mg DHEC in respect to placebo and by 44% after 5 mg DHEC (from area under curve, AUC). After 24 h the serum PRL levels remained lower than baseline, while after 48 h the effect of the drug on PRL was exhausted, the long-lasting activity of DHEC being consistent with the long biological half-life of about 12 h. Data after intravenous administration are also available from the same subjects, with a decrease of PRL AUC in the first 24 h of 52% after 0.25 mg in bolus, and of 60% after 0.5 mg i.v. Thus, a dose–effect relationship was evident for both the parenteral and the oral route and a concentration–effect exponential relationship was also demonstrated between PRL and DHEC AUC.

The PRL lowering effect of DHEC persisted after chronic administration of the drug, while not affecting the circadian rhythm as demonstrated in seven normoprolactinemic, migrainous women (age range: 20–48 yr, mean $\pm$ SEM; 27.6 $\pm$ 3.8) that were given the drug (3 mg b.i.d. for 30 days) or placebo (b.i.d. for 30 days) in a cross-over design as a prophylactic treatment for common migraine headache. As shown in Figure 2, the plasma levels of PRL, measured during the 21st day of the menstrual cycle, were lowest at noon both during chronic DHEC and placebo, the AUCs being decreased by 30% during DHEC in respect to placebo, thus confirming after repeated administration the effect of a single dose above cited in male volunteers.

Finally, a concentration–effect relationship was demonstrated also in patients under repeated treatment with DHEC. In fact, an inverse linear relationship between plasma levels of PRL and DHEC at the steady state ($p < 0.05$) was shown in five patients under chronic treatment with the compound for idiopathic Parkinson disease. The patients were two males and three females aged 61 to 65 years (63 $\pm$ 1.6), treated for 10–12 months with 10 mg twice a day in two cases and three times a day in the other three patients.

Drug-induced PRL rise

The compound was able to suppress dose-dependently the rise of serum PRL levels induced in healthy volunteers by antidopaminergic agents, directly acting, as sulpiride, or indirectly acting, as cimetidine[4].

An injection of sulpiride (10 mg i.m.) caused a 200–1500% increase of serum PRL levels 30 min after administration in eight healthy, young males, who had been given placebo 120 min earlier. The pretreatment with DHEC

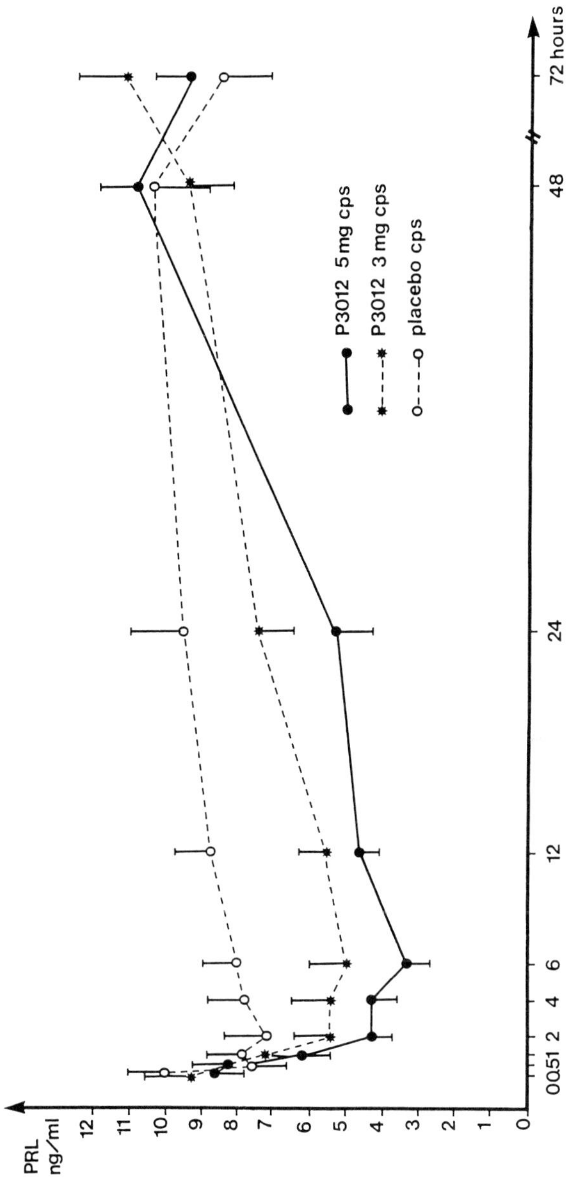

Figure 1 Serum PRL levels in 12 healthy males given DHEC 5 mg, 3 mg or placebo capsules as a single oral dose (mean ± SEM)

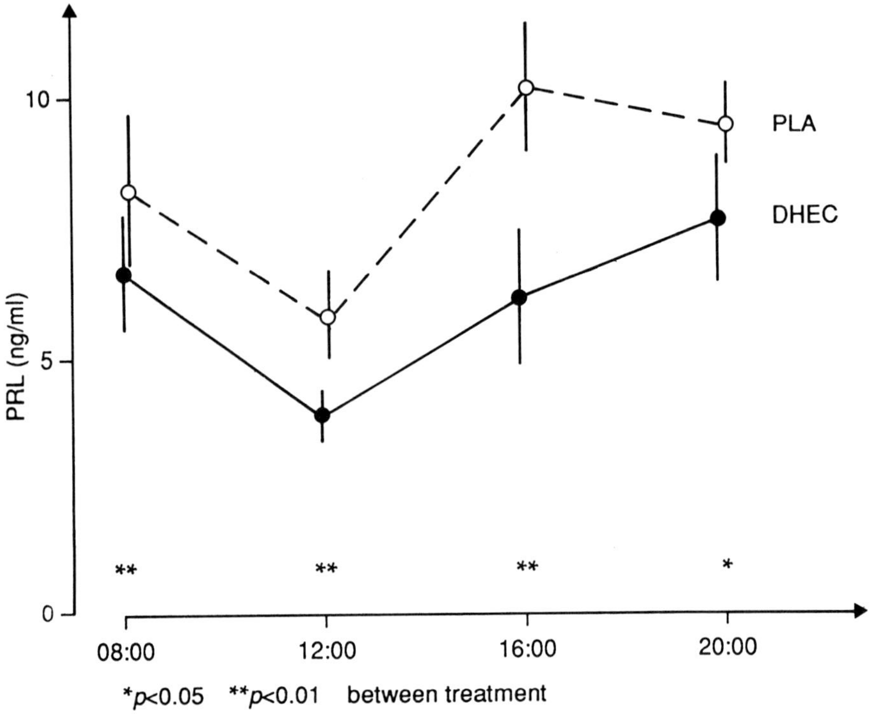

Figure 2 Serum PRL levels in seven normoprolactinemic, migrainous women. Blood samples taken during the 21st day of menstrual cycle, under chronic treatment with DHEC (3 mg b.i.d.) or placebo (mean ± SEM)

(2.5 mg or 5 mg) on two different occasions caused a reduction of sulpiride effect in the same eight subjects with a peak of PRL that reached 50% of that with placebo with the lower dose of DHEC and a complete suppression of sulpiride effect with the higher dose of DHEC (Figure 3).

A similar experiment was reported with cimetidine, that caused a 100–400% increase of serum PRL levels 15 min after i.v. administration (300 mg) in nine healthy males when previously given placebo. The pretreatment with DHEC 90 min before cimetidine injection caused a dose-dependent inhibition of cimetidine effect. The peak of PRL reached 44% or 35% of placebo was respectively completely suppressed after DHEC 2, 3 or 4.5 mg (Figure 3).

Puerperal hyperprolactinemia

From the review of literature, data are available of 85 patients given DHEC to prevent lactation in puerperal women not wishing to breast feed their babies[6–8], (L. Lerro, personal communication).

Serum PRL levels were normalized in 85% of patients after the first 5 mg dose of DHEC, the decrease of PRL amounted to 64% compared to the level 24 h after the delivery. A dose of 10 mg b.i.d. for 7 days was sufficient

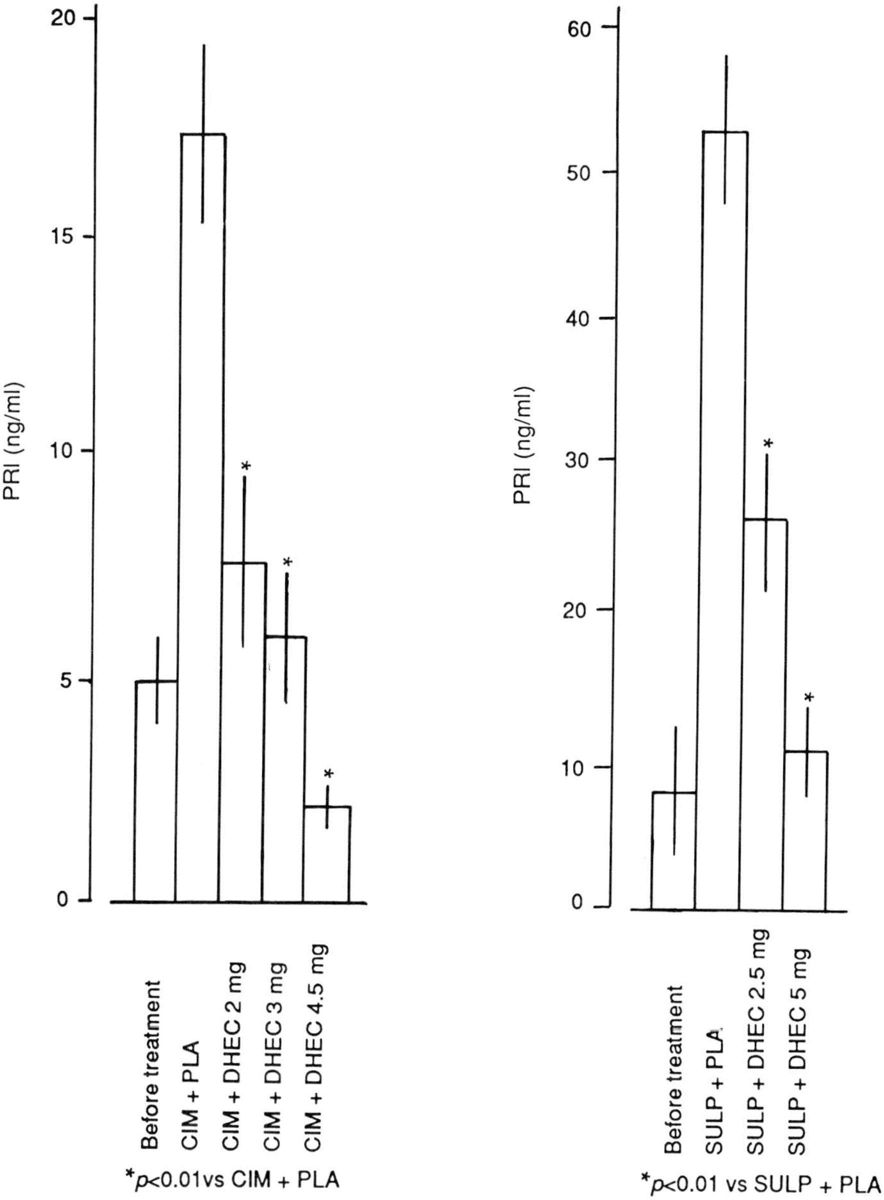

Figure 3 Serum PRL levels in nine healthy males orally given placebo or DHEC 2, 3 and 4.5 mg 90 min before a cimetidine 300 mg i.v. test (on the left). Serum PRL levels in eight healthy males orally given placebo or DHEC 2.5 and 5 mg 120 min before a sulpiride 10 mg i.m. test (on the right)

to prevent milk secretion, breast pain and tenderness in 100% of puerperae. A lower tendency to PRL rebound after stopping DHEC was noted than that seen after bromocriptine in double-blind studies[6,8].

Functional hyperprolactinemia

Many papers reported the effect of DHEC in the management of hyperprolactinemia with amenorrhea–galactorrhea syndrome[6–9], without evidence of pituitary tumors, correctly investigated by standard techniques. Data are available from 51 female patients. After a single DHEC 5 mg dose given to test the responsivity of the patients, serum PRL levels decreased by 60% in respect to basal values. All women who underwent a chronic treatment (43 cases, dose of DHEC 10 mg b.i.d. or t.i.d.) had menstrual cycles within 3 months of therapy, with evidence of ovulation (progesterone levels > 8 ng/ml during the second phase of menstrual cycle) in 39 cases (91%) and serum PRL levels became normal in 100% of cases (from 71.4 ± 6.1 ng/ml at baseline, to 29.4 ± 3.5 ng/ml in acute 5 mg DHEC test and to 8.3 ± 0.7 ng/ml during chronic treatment: Figure 4). Pregnancy was also reported in three patients of this group. Together with the decrease of PRL, galactorrhea disappeared in all women after few days of DHEC therapy.

Pituitary tumors

Data are available from 76 patients, 50 out of them were females with microprolactinoma[6,10] and amenorrhea (45 cases) or anovulation (five cases). Macroprolactinoma was diagnosed in 11 cases, four of them were women with amenorrhea and seven males with impotence and gynecomastia.

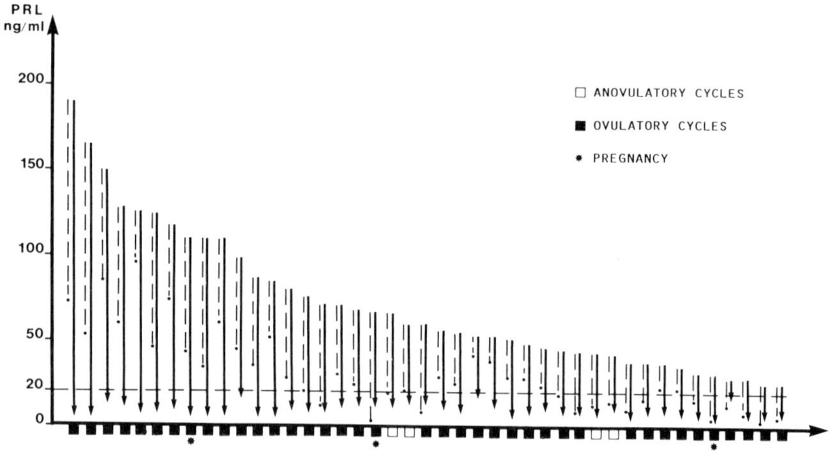

Figure 4 PRL decrease from baseline after 5 mg acute (---) and 20–30 mg/daily chronic treatment (——→) with DHEC and clinical outcome in 43 patients with functional hyperprolactinemia

Headache and ocular symptoms were present in all the macroprolactinoma patients[11]. Acromegaly was diagnosed in 15 cases[5] (G. Faglia, personal communication).

Serum PRL levels at baseline ranged between 15 and 640 ng/ml in microprolactinomas (107.9 ± 17.7) and between 200 and 2350 ng/ml in macroadenomas (727.2 ± 215.9).

On acute DHEC 5 mg testing, serum PRL levels of microadenoma patients decreased by 63%, while during chronic treatment (carried out on 45 women with DHEC 20–40 mg daily), the decrease was 79% of baseline, serum PRL levels being 22.5 ± 5.1 ng/ml and normal levels were reached by 76% of cases (Figure 5). A linear relationship was evident between the serum concentration of drug and per cent decrease of PRL in steady state conditions (Figure 6). Regular menses occurred in all cases, with evidence of ovulation in 78% of patients and two pregnancies. High definition computerized tomography scans (Figure 7) did not show focal hypodense lesions in seven out of 22 patients (32%) followed for 9 months of DHEC treatment[11]; the focal lesions did not reappear in four of them 50 days after drug withdrawal.

In patients with macroadenoma, the acute administration of DHEC 5 mg caused a decrease by 64% of serum PRL levels in 10 cases, while one female was not responsive to therapy.

After long-term treatment normal PRL levels were found in five patients, two females with regular menses (ovulatory in one), and three males. Moreover, three out of seven cases in which the treatment lasted at least 6 months, showed a decrease of the suprasellar or parasellar component of the adenoma[11].

DHEC was also able to suppress PRL secretion in acromegalic patients[5],

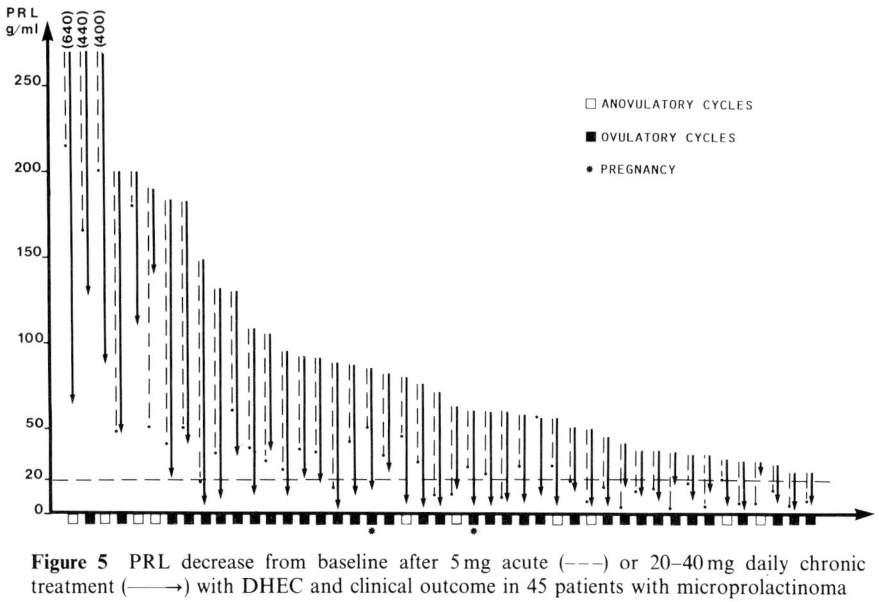

Figure 5 PRL decrease from baseline after 5 mg acute (---) or 20–40 mg daily chronic treatment (——→) with DHEC and clinical outcome in 45 patients with microprolactinoma

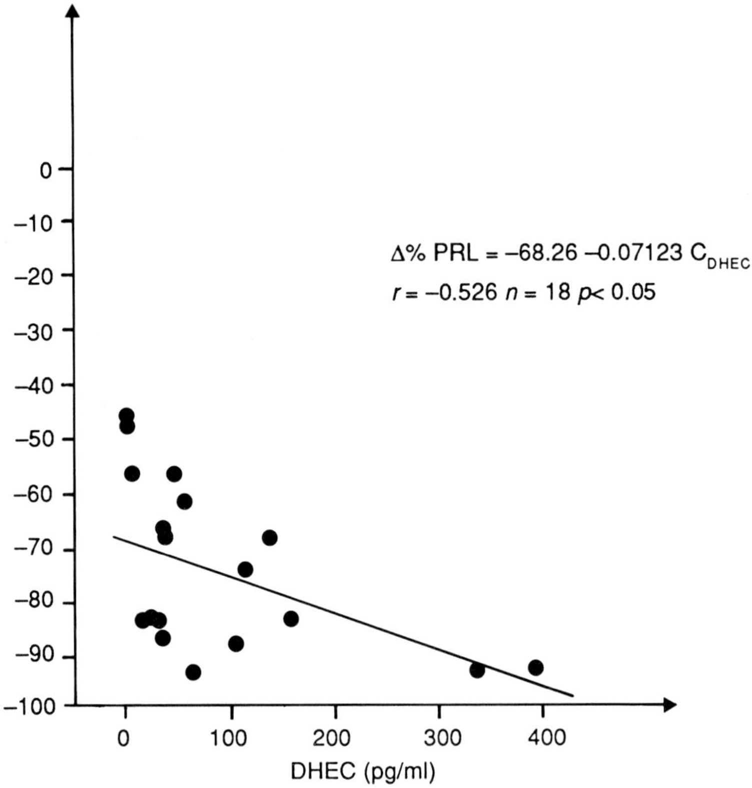

Figure 6 Concentration–effect relationship between DHEC and percentage PRL decrease in patients with microprolactinoma

but it had only minor efficacy on growth hormone secretion and clinical outcome (G. Faglia, personal communication).

Side-effects

DHEC was generally well tolerated by patients both in single dose and chronic studies. Few patients complained of side-effects during DHEC therapy.

The most frequent effects were in the gastrointestinal tract, i.e. mild nausea and gastric pain that never required the discontinuation of treatment. Decrease of blood pressure and dizziness were also reported. Effects on the central nervous system were never reported. The drug was much better tolerated than bromocriptine in comparative studies[4,6,8,10]. In particular, a change to DHEC 30–40 mg daily in six patients who did not tolerate bromocriptine 2.5–7.5 mg daily was not followed by any significant side-effect[10].

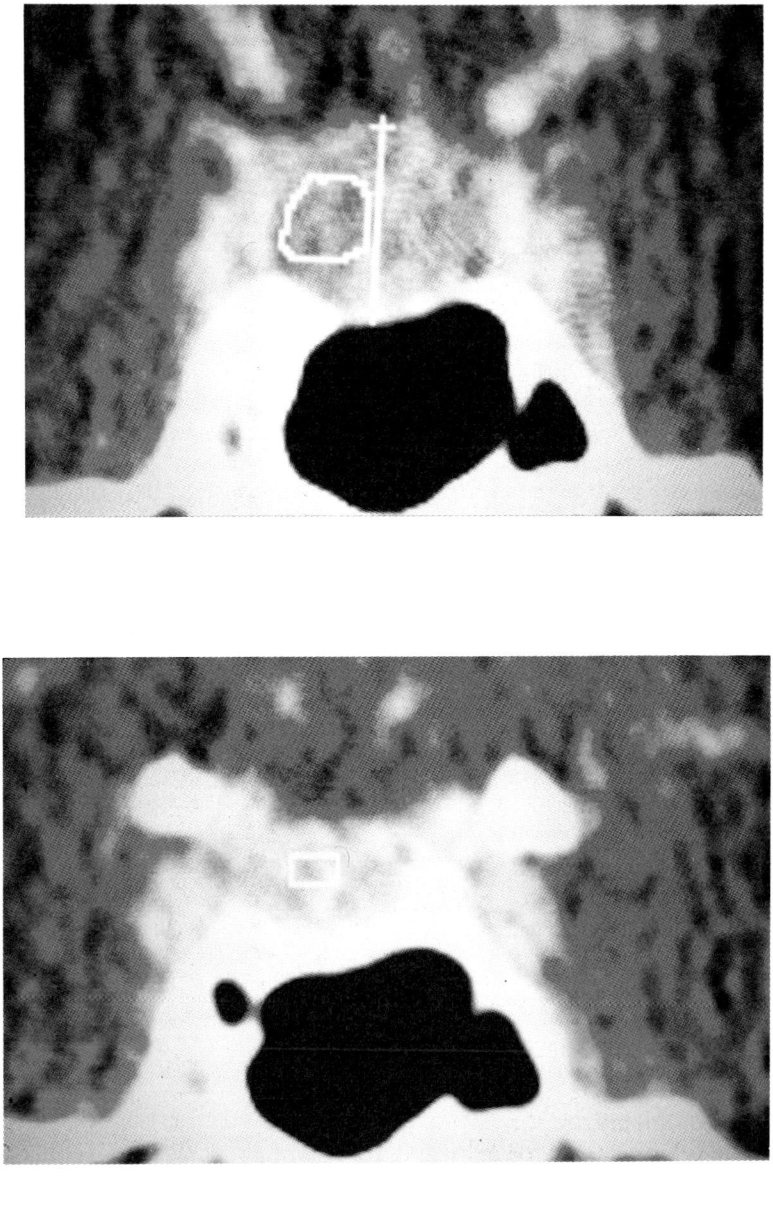

Figure 7 High-definition CT scans of pituitary in a woman with microadenoma and hyperprolactinemia before therapy (top) and disappearance of focal lesion after 9 months of DHEC treatment (bottom)

CONCLUSIONS

DHEC is a hydrogenated ergot alkaloid provided with dopaminergic activity both at pituitary and striatal level. The drug is able to blunt serum PRL levels by an inhibition of dopamine D2-dependent adenylate cyclase on lactotropes. For this reason, it also counteracts the rise of PRL induced by dopamine antagonist agents.

The drug was effective and well tolerated by puerperae and by hyperprolactinemic patients. The drug was able to prevent lactation in 100% of puerperal women when given at a dose of 10 mg b.i.d. for a week without evidence of rebound phenomena after stopping the treatment. In functional hyperprolactinemia, cyclic menses were restored in 100% and fertility in 91% of the women given 20–30 mg daily. In microprolactinoma, cyclic menses were restored in 100% of patients, and fertility in 78% of cases, given 20–40 mg daily of DHEC. The drug was effective and very well tolerated also by patients who did not tolerate more potent dopamine agonists. Therefore, DHEC may be the drug of first choice in the management of hyperprolactinemic states.

The evidence of dose–concentration–effect relationships between DHEC and PRL decrease suggests choosing the final dose of the drug according to PRL levels at baseline. The dose may be maintained for several months or years because tolerance has never been shown even after 3 years of treatment.

ACKNOWLEDGEMENTS

The kind supply of CT scan images by Prof. G. Faglia and V. Bernasconi is gratefully acknowledged.

REFERENCES

1. Libertun, C., Larrea, G.A., Vacas, M.I. and Cardinali, D.P. (1980). [^{3}H]Dihydroergokryptine binding in anterior pituitary and prolactin secretion: further evidence of brain regulation of adenohypophyseal receptors. *Endocrinology*, **107**, 1905–9
2. Groppetti, A., Zambelli, M. and Ferrara, C. (1989). Pharmacology of dihydroergokryptine: neurotransmitters involvement and behavioural aspects. *Gynecol. Endocrinol.*, **3** (Suppl. 1), 3
3. Fiore, L., Scapagnini, U. and Canonico, P.L. (1987). Effect of dihydroergokryptine and dihydroergocristine on cyclic AMP accumulation and prolactin release *in vitro*: evidence for a dopaminomimetic action. *Horm. Res.*, **25**, 171–7
4. Poli, M., Cocchi, D., Mailland, F., Masu, A.M., Landi, G., Craveri, A. and Mueller, E.E. (1986). Prolactin-lowering effect of dihydroergokryptine in rat and in man. *J. Endocrinol. Invest.*, **9**, 31–6
5. Ferrari, C., Rampini, P., Paracchi, A., Boghen, M. and Mailland, F. (1985). Effect of dihydroergokryptine administration on serum prolactin and growth hormone levels in normal, hyperprolactinemic and acromegalic subjects: evidence for potent and long-lasting pituitary dopamine receptor stimulation. *Eur. J. Clin. Pharmacol.*, **27**, 707–11
6. Crosignani, P.G. and Mattei, A.M. (1988). Dihydroergocriptine (DHECP) in physiological and pathological hyperprolactinemia. Abstract of paper presented at the World Congress of Gynecology and Obstetrics, Rio de Janeiro, Brazil, October 23rd–28th, 1988
7. Di Carlo, C., Nappi, C., Colace, G., Affinito, P., Annunziato, L. and Montemagno, U. (1988). Prolactin suppressant effect of dihydroergokryptine in puerperal women. Abstract of paper P-127 presented at the *Vth International Congress on Prolactin*, Kyoto, Japan, July 13–16, 1988

8. Paoletti, A.M., Melis, G.B., Petacchi, F.D., Soldani, R., Mauro, S.A., Maffei, S., Pellegatta, L.C., Zanotti, A. and Fioretti, P. (1990). Dihydroergokryptine (DEK): efficacy and tolerability in the treatment of pathological hyperprolactinemia and inhibition of puerperal lactation. Abstract of paper FC 104 presented at the Second European Winter Conference in Gynecology and Obstetrics, Madonna di Campiglio, March 12th–18th, 1989

9. Venturini, P.L., Fasce, V., Valenzano, M., Ongari, S. and De Cecco, L. (1989). PRL-lowering effect of dihydroergokryptine in hyperprolactinaemic patients: acute and chronic study. Abstract of paper FC 101 presented at the Second European Winter Conference in Gynecology and Obstetrics, Madonna di Campiglio, March 12th–18th, 1989

10. Faglia, G., Conti, A., Muratori, M., Togni, E., Travaglini, P., Zanotti, A. and Mailland, F. (1987). Dihydroergocriptine in Management of Microprolactinomas. *J. Clin. Endocrinol. Metab.*, **65**, 779–84

11. Faglia, G., Muratori, M., Togni, E., Conti, A., Travaglini, P. and Ambrosi, B. (1987). Treatment of prolactinomas with dihydroergokryptine (DHECP). Abstract of paper presented at the Congress "Prolactin 87", Milan, November 6–7, 1987

71

Pharmacokinetics and pharmacodynamics of α-dihydroergocriptine in humans: single dose and steady state

A. Zanotti, G. Coppi and F. Mailland

INTRODUCTION

α-Dihydroergocriptine (DHEC) is the hydrogenated derivative of one of the alkaloids of ergotoxine, with strong dopaminomimetic activity reported by several authors during both *in vitro*[1] and *in vivo*[2] studies. When administered to patients with prolactin-secreting pituitary tumors[3], the drug was able to blunt prolactin (PRL) plasma levels as well as to decrease tremor, rigidity and akinesia in Parkinsonian patients[4].

Our aim was to investigate the blood level profile of DHEC in humans, its oral absorption and bioavailability, and to compare the pharmacokinetics and the pharmacodynamics both in healthy volunteers and patients after single and repeated dosages.

METHODS

Study 1

Five healthy female volunteers aged 22 to 27 years (mean 24.8 ± 1.9 S.D.), weighing 44 to 62 kg (mean 51.8 ± 6.9 S.D.) participated in the preliminary study. The five women received the following randomized treatments, with at least 72 h wash-out: DHEC 2.5 mg (25 drops), DHEC 5 mg (50 drops) and placebo.

The drugs were orally administered in the morning before breakfast. Blood samples were collected at the following times: 09:00, 10:00, 11:00, 12:00, 13:00, 15:00, 17:00, 20:00, 24:00 and 09:00 on the following day. The serum was then obtained by separation for 20 min and centrifugation for 2 min at 2000 r.p.m.

Finally, the supernatant was divided into two samples and frozen at −20°C up to the time of analysis. PRL levels were analyzed by standard radioimmunoassay[5]. DHEC concentrations were also detected by a radioimmunoassay method.

Study 2

Twelve healthy male volunteers aged 18 to 45 years (mean 31.1 $\pm$ 7.8 S.D.) and weighing 67 to 83 kg (mean 72.0 $\pm$ 5.3 S.D.) were included in the second study. The twelve subjects received the following randomized treatments, with 7 days wash-out: DHEC 5 mg (one capsule) DHEC 3 mg (one capsule), DHEC placebo (one capsule), DHEC 0.25 mg ($\frac{1}{2}$ ampoule i.v.) or DHEC 0.5 mg (1 ampoule i.v.).

The treatments were always administered at 09:00 before breakfast. Blood samples were collected at the following times after oral administration: 09:00, 09:30, 10:00, 11:00, 13:00, 15:00, 21:00 and at 09:00 on the three subsequent days. The serum samples were prepared as in study 1.

Study 3

Two groups of patients participated in this study. The first group involved six female patients with amenorrhea and infertility secondary to PRL-releasing pituitary tumor. Informed consent was obtained from all the patients. The patients, aged 19 to 43 years (mean 31.3 $\pm$ 9.9 S.D.) had received DHEC for 2–3 weeks (two capsules of DHEC 5 mg taken together twice a day in four cases or three times daily in two cases). Blood samples were collected at time 0, immediately before drug intake and about 12 or 8 h after the last capsule administration, and then after 1 and 3 h after oral administration of 10 mg of DHEC. Serum samples were stored at -20°C until radioimmunoassay of DHEC and PRL.

The second group included five patients with idiopathic Parkinsonism, all giving their informed consent to the investigation. The patients, two males and three females, aged 61 to 65 years (mean 63.0 $\pm$ 1.6 S.D.), had received DHEC for 10–12 months (two capsules of DHEC 5 mg taken together twice a day in two cases, and three times a day in the other three patients). Furthermore, two patients took DHEC as the only drug while in the other three patients the drug was associated with L-Dopa and decarboxylase inhibitor. Blood samples were collected at time 0, immediately before drug intake and about 12 or 8 h after the last capsule administration, and then 1 h after oral administration of DHEC 10 mg. Serum samples were stored at -20°C until the radioimmunoassay of DHEC and PRL.

ANALYSIS PROCEDURE

Serum levels of DHEC were determined by radioimmunoassay by employing a specific antibody for unmodified drug. Serum samples (500 μl) were mixed with 100 μl tracer solution ^{125}I-labelled derivative of DHEC and allowed to equilibrate for 30 min at 30°C. Then 100 μl of an antiserum dilution (antiserum elicited against conjugates of human serum albumin and the

DHEC component linked via the indole nitrogen of the alkaloid) was added and incubated for 15 min at 30°C and for an additional 15 min at room temperature. After this reaction 500 μl of a charcoal suspension were pipetted into this solution and after 30 min of reaction time in the dark at room temperature a centrifugation of 20 min followed. After this step 1 ml of the supernatant was measured in a γ counter. The sensitivity of the method was 8 pg/ml. All the analyses were made in duplicate. Serum prolactin were determined by a double antibody radioimmunoassay, with the standard technique[5].

RESULTS

Pharmacokinetics

The intravenous and oral administrations of DHEC (Figures 1, 2 and 3) showed plasma levels according to a tricompartmental model. These data are only apparently in contrast with those of Study 1 which, having a mere preliminary value, was interrupted at 24 h and therefore did not allow any thorough analysis of the slow elimination phase. After its i.v. administration DHEC was indeed found to follow a triexponential elimination pattern, while after oral administration it followed an absorption/elimination model of, respectively, the first and the third order. The interpretation of the pharmacokinetics of the drug was correctly performed separately for each subject. The central trend and the variability indices of the pharmacokinetic parameters were reported in Table 1. The interpatient data were found to

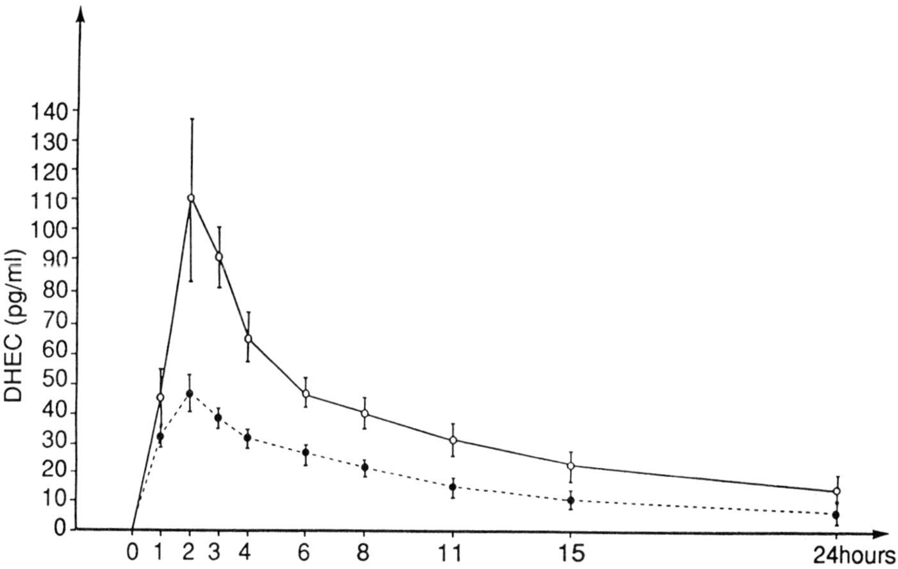

Figure 1 Dihydroergocriptine serum levels in five healthy females after a single oral dose of DHEC drops (mean ± SEM)

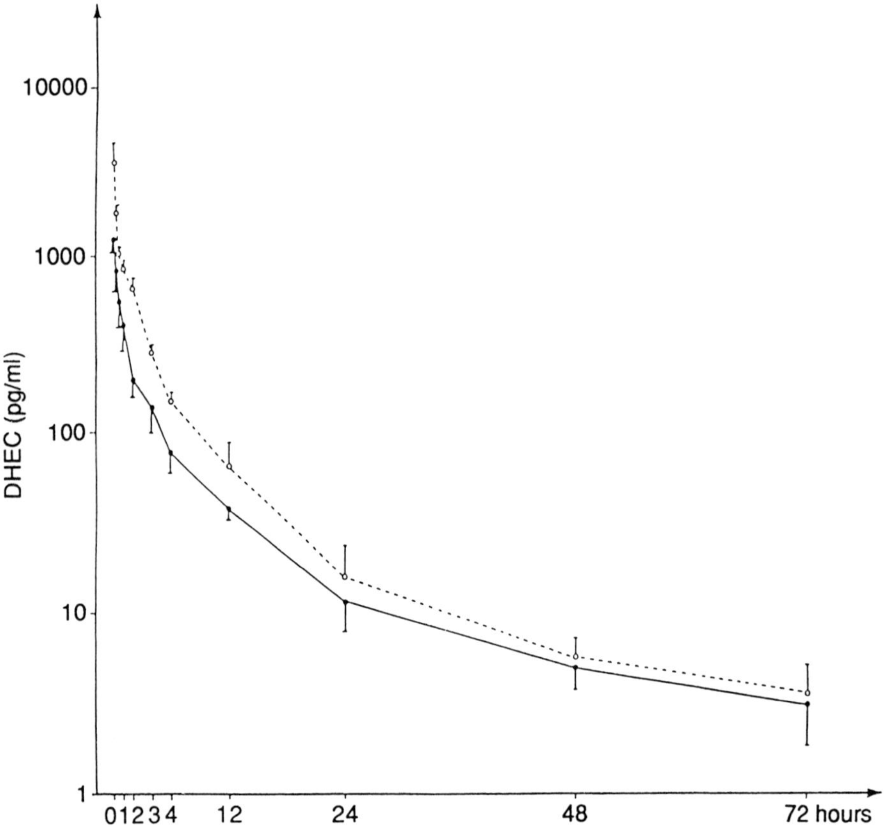

Figure 2 Dihydroergocriptine serum levels in eight healthy males given i.v. DHEC half ampoule (0.25 mg; $n = 6$) or one ampoule (0.5 mg; $n = 2$) (mean ± SEM)

Table 1 α-Dihydroergocriptine pharmacokinetics after single intravenous and oral administration

Pharmacokinetics parameters	*Intravenous administration*		*Oral administration*	
	0.25 mg (n = 6)	*0.5 mg (n = 2)*	*3.0 mg (n = 12)*	*5.0 mg (n = 12)*
Half-life (a) (h)	0.15 ± 0.02		0.13 ± 0.01	0.36 ± 0.02
Half-life (b) (h)	1.79 ± 0.28		0.77 ± 0.09	1.28 ± 0.21
Half-life (c) (h)	12.28 ± 1.34		9.87 ± 0.81	15.02 ± 1.60
$AUC_{0\rightarrow\infty}$ ($pg.h.ml^{-1}$)	2689.22 ± 353.78	5341.89 ± 298.68	846.46 ± 91.05	1223.76 ± 70.41
MRT (h)	9.39 ± 1.75		12.53 ± 1.13	16.50 ± 1.50
Cl_{tot} ($l.h^{-1}.kg^{-1}$)	1.189 ± 0.089		1.078 ± 0.244*	1.114 ± 0.205*
Vd ($l.kg^{-1}$)	21.77 ± 3.70		14.72 ± 2.34*	20.72 ± 1.72*

* corrected for bioavailability

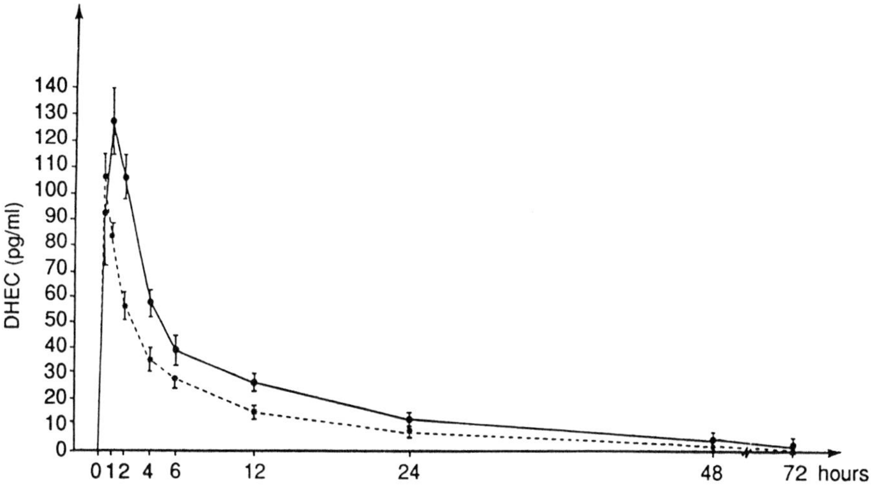

Figure 3 Dihydroergocriptine serum levels in 12 healthy males given a single oral dose of DHEC 5 mg cps or DHEC 3 mg cps (mean ± SEM)

be sufficiently homogeneous. All the plasma curves allowed interpretation according to the same kinetics model. A threefold variation was observed between the minimum and maximum biological half-life values, while a twofold change was found in area under the curve (AUC) (from 0 to ∞) and total clearance values. Finally, the apparent distribution volume, showed a fourfold change, and greatly exceeded the body volume, thus pointing to a mainly extravascular drug distribution (21.8 ± 3.7 l.kg^{-1}, after i.v. administration).

The half-life of the slow phase ranged between 10 and 15 h, being independent of administration route and pharmaceutical formulation. In multiple dose regimen (b.i.d. or t.i.d.) steady state blood levels were reached within 3 days and DHEC serum levels found after 2–3 weeks or 10–12 months were within the expected range (Tables 2 and 3).

Pharmacokinetics and pharmacodynamics relationship

Prolactin levels were reduced by DHEC in a dose-dependent manner. The drug showed a fast absorption with a peak plasma level after 2 h from the absorption while the nadir PRL level was evident between the 3rd and the 6th hour. For this reason, there was no relation between plasma levels of DHEC and PRL after a single dose.

Indeed, there was a significant inverse linear relationship between the $AUC_{0-24\,h}$ of the drug and the $AUC_{0-24\,h}$ of PRL, according to the following equation: $AUC_{PRL} = 292.1 - 0.16478\, AUC_{DHEC}$ ($n = 15$, $c = 0.602$, $p < 0.05$, $F = 7.403$, $p < 0.05$) (Figures 4 and 5).

A concentration/effect linear relationship was evident in steady state condition in patients with Parkinson disease (Figure 6) on a point to point basis, while in patients with microprolactinoma there was a correlation

Table 2 Steady state serum levels of DHEC and PRL in patients with microprolactinoma

						0 h		*1 h*		*3 h*	
Initials	*Age* (yr)	*Sex*	*Dose* (mg/die)	*Total exposure to DHEC* (mg)	*Baseline PRL* (ng/ml)	*PRL* (ng/ml)	*DHEC* (pg/ml)	*PRL* (ng/ml)	*DHEC* (pg/ml)	*PRL* (ng/ml)	*DHEC* (pg/ml)
S.O.	43	♀	10 × 2	252	440	160	10	160	48	115	85
$M.M._2$	41	♀	10 × 2	252	45	7.5	23	7.5	18	7.5	160
B.M.T.	35	♀	10 × 2	252	105	56.5	6	54.5	5	41	68
F.F.	19	♀	10 × 2	252	82	6	65	6	394	6	334
$M.M._1$	28	♀	10 × 3	462	130	44	40	42	56	42	141
T.M.	22	♀	10 × 3	462	108	15	36	17	31	13	105

Table 3 Steady state serum levels of DHEC and PRL in patients with Parkinson disease

			Dose (mg/die)			*0 h*		*1 h*	
Initials	*Age* (yr)	*Sex*	*DHEC*	*1-DOPA*	*Total exposure to DHEC* (mg)	*PRL* (ng/ml)	*DHEC* (pg/ml)	*PRL* (ng/ml)	*DHEC* (pg/ml)
V.A.	63	♂	10 × 3	—	6300	2.1	10	0.5	320
P.R.	65	♀	10 × 3	—	6840	0.9	80	1.4	610
S.S.	61	♀	10 × 3	125	9120	3.4	25	2.1	260
B.C.	64	♀	10 × 2	125	7320	5.6	5	3.0	150
R.L.	62	♂	10 × 2	187.5	6960	3.9	40	3.5	160

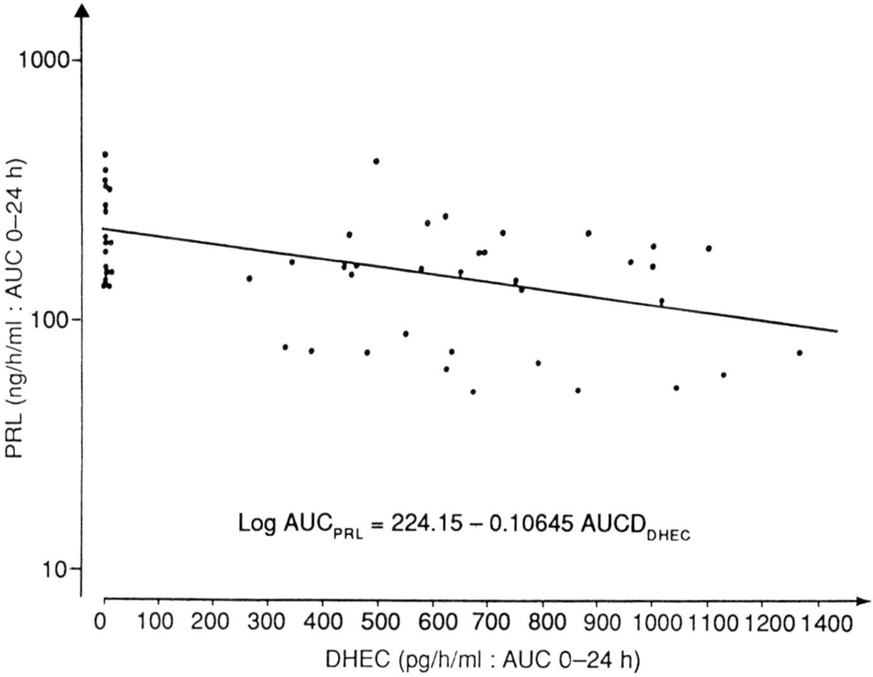

Figure 4 Concentration/effect exponential relationship in 17 healthy volunteers given a single oral dose of DHEC

between DHEC serum levels and per cent PRL decrease. Oral bioavailability (AUC_{DHEC} *per os*/AUC_{DHEC} i.v.) was 2.39 ± 0.50% of the dose for 5 mg capsules and 2.36 ± 0.48% for 3 mg capsules. When however bioavailability was calculated considering the placebo–DHEC differences in prolactinemia (ΔAUC_{PRL} *per os*/ΔAUC_{PRL} i.v.), this was found to be 6.23 ± 0.24% of the dose for 5 mg capsules and 6.65 ± 0.95% of the dose for 3 mg capsules.

The PRL-inhibiting activity of the drug was found to be long-lasting, the maximum effect occurring 3 h after a single oral administration, and thus with a latency of 1–2 h from the appearance of the DHEC peak serum level.

The PRL-lowering effect disappeared within 48 h of the single dose administration. At the steady state, the administration of DHEC twice a day was sufficient to avoid PRL fluctuations.

DISCUSSION AND CONCLUSION

Our data on the pharmacokinetics of DHEC are consistent with a linear dose–plasma concentration/effect relationship by both the oral and the intravenous routes. The drug showed tricompartmental kinetics, with a mean biological half-life of about 12 h, a rapid oral absorption, with a peak plasma level between 30 min and 120 min and an absolute oral bioavailability corresponding to 2.4% of the dose. This amount of drug bioavailable is in

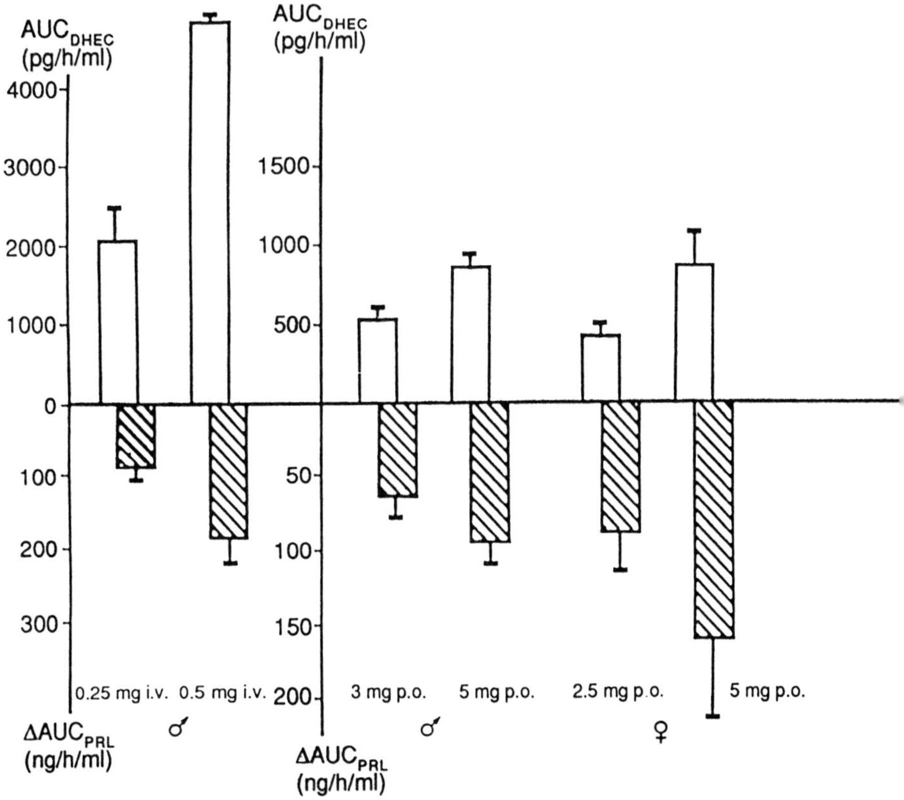

Figure 5 $AUC_{0\to 24h}$ of DHEC and PRL serum levels in healthy volunteers given a single dose of the drug. Data are mean ± SEM. PRL calculated as the difference between placebo and DHEC in the same subject

good agreement with the bioavailability of other hydrogenated ergot alkaloids, such as dihydroergotoxine that has been reported[6] to have an oral bioavailability of about 2% of the administered dose. On the contrary, the total bioavailability of DHEC exceeded 6% of the dose when calculated on the basis of effect on prolactin.

The phenomenon can be accounted for by the evident formation of active metabolites during the first liver transit after oral administration. Such a phenomenon has been widely reported in the literature on ergot alkaloids[7]. Since radioimmunoassay is specific for this kind of drug, bioavailability calculated with the method of drug AUCs is lower than the real value by more than 60%. We can therefore assume that, following oral administration, drug activity is due in the amount of 40% to the molecule unmodified, and in a 60% amount to one or more active metabolites, having an elimination kinetics comparable to that of the unmodified drug.

In multiple dose studies, the steady state serum levels were attained after 3 days and the drug did not accumulate in the central compartment to a

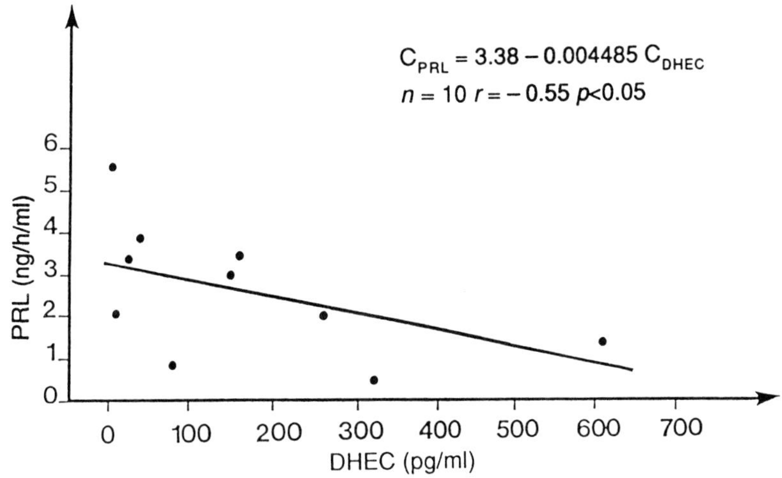

Figure 6 Concentration/effect relationship in Parkinson disease

higher extent than expected. Thus, it seems likely that DHEK does not induce autoinduction phenomena nor accumulation. For this reason, it can also be stated that DHEC does not induce long-term side-effects nor tolerance and therefore that it can be administered for very long periods of time, as is the case of Parkinson disease and hyperprolactinemia.

REFERENCES

1. Fiore, L., Scapagnini, U. and Canonico, P.L. (1987). Effect of dihydroergokryptine and dihydroergocristine on cyclic AMP accumulation and prolactin release *in vitro*: evidence for a dopaminomimetic action. *Horm. Res.*, **25**, 171–7
2. Poli, M., Cocchi, D., Mailland, F., Masu, A.M., Landi, G., Craveri, A. and Müller, E.E. (1986). Prolactin lowering effect of dihydroergokryptine in rat and in man. *J. Endocrinol. Invest.*, **9**, 31
3. Faglia, G., Conti, A., Muratori, M., Togni, E., Travaglini, P., Zanotti, A. and Mailland, F. (1987). Dihydroergokryptine in management of microprolactinomas. *J. Clin. Endocrinol.. Metab.*, **65**, 779
4. Scarzella, L., Cantello, R., Delsedime, M., Gilli, M., Pinessi, L., Riccio, A., Bergamasco, B. and Ruggieri, S. (1985). Clinical trial on the therapeutic activity of dihydroergokryptine in parkinsonism: preliminary results. *Curr. Ther. Res.*, **38**, 432–40
5. Sinha, A.N., Selby, F.W., Lewis, U.J. and Vanerlaan, W.G. (1973). A homologous radioimmunoassay for human prolactin. *J. Clin. Endocrinol. Metab.*, **36**, 500
6. Dominiak, P., Grevel, J., Abisch, E., Grobecker, H., Dennler, H.J. and Welzel, D. (1988). The absolute systemic availability of a new oral formulation of Co-Dergocrine in healthy subjects. *Eur J. Clin. Pharmacol.*, **35**, 53–7
7. Eckert, H., Kiechel, J.R., Rosenthaler, J., Schmidt, R. and Schreier, E. (1978). Ergot alkaloids and related compounds. In: Berde, B. and Schild, H.O. (eds), p. 719. (New York: Springer Verlag)

72

Prolactin-lowering effect of dihydroergocriptine in hyperprolactinemic patients: acute and chronic study

P.L. Venturini, V. Fasce, M. Valenzano, S. Ongari and L. De Cecco

INTRODUCTION

Medical management of patients with hyperprolactinemia using ergot alkaloids with dopaminomimetic or antiserotonergic activity is today a well established and common practice[1-3].

These drugs display a broad spectrum of pharmacological activity having different affinity for adrenergic, dopaminergic and serotonergic receptors[4]. Some of these properties are essential for therapeutic responses while others may contribute to the occurrence of unpleasant side-effects.

Dihydroergocriptine (DHEC) is a dihydrogenated ergot alkaloid known to possess a potent α-adrenergic antagonist action; recently a high affinity binding for dopamine receptors (anterior pituitary and striatum) evidenced by a prolactin-lowering effect has been reported[5-7].

The aim of the study was to evaluate the tolerance of DHEC and the effect of its acute and chronic administration on prolactin (PRL) levels in women with mild functional hyperprolactinemia. Moreover, in order to evaluate DHEC efficacy, expressed as the power of counterbalance to the hyperprolactinemic action of sulpiride, a test with this drug (10 mg i.m.) was performed at the end of the second, third and fourth months of chronic treatment.

PATIENTS AND METHODS

Acute test

Ten women complaining of functional hyperprolactinemia (mean serum PRL level, 54.9 ng/ml), aged 23–42, were selected for the test. All patients were given 5 mg of DHEC in the morning (09:00) following an overnight fast.

After two baseline blood samples had been taken (−15 min and 0 min) further samples for PRL assay were obtained 1, 2, 3, 4, 5 and 6 h after drug administration.

Chronic treatment

Five functional hyperprolactinemic women (mean serum PRL level, 60.3 ng/ml) with previous poor tolerance to other dopamine agonists (minimum washout period 2.5 months) were chosen for a chronic treatment (4 months) with DHEC. All patients complained of amenorrhea (range 2.6–6.3 months). DHEC was administered at a daily dose of 10 mg (5 mg b.i.d.). Two patients needed a higher DHEC daily dose (20 mg) during the second month of treatment in order to lower PRL levels to the normal range (< 20 ng/ml).

Sulpiride test

This test has been performed in the five patients mentioned above (chronic treatment), at the end of the second, third and fourth months of treatment, when PRL levels were similar. Each patient was administered sulpiride, 10 mg i.m., 2 h after DHEC (5 mg p.o.). Blood samples for PRL assay were collected 15, 30, 45, 60, 90 and 120 min after sulpiride administration.

Statistical analysis of data, elaborated as the per cent ratio between the PRL levels at each time period and the baseline, was performed with the Student's *t* test on values obtained 90 min after sulpiride administration (when the hyperprolactinemic action of the drug is higher).

RESULTS

Acute test

Acute administration of DHEC (5 mg) caused a prompt fall of PRL levels (Table 1) showing the following mean per cent decreases of baseline (Figure 1): 27 (at 1 h), 56 (2 h), 66 (3 h), 69 (4 h), 71 (5 h) and 63 (6 h). All patients reached

Table 1 PRL levels (ng/ml) in ten hyperprolactinemic patients after DHEC (5 mg p.o.)

Basal	*1 h*	*2 h*	*3 h*	*4 h*	*5 h*	*6 h*
66.8	55.6	28.5	19.5	20.9	18.3	21.7
58.9	30.2	25.1	13.5	13.1	18.1	28.9
43.1	29.9	17.5	11.1	17.2	22.5	25.9
39.9	33.1	21.0	16.5	17.2	14.3	16.2
55.2	42.9	39.0	33.0	24.2	15.9	15.5
71.1	65.5	40.2	24.2	16.2	11.2	21.9
40.6	31.1	17.2	9.5	8.8	8.3	14.9
55.5	40.1	13.1	13.1	9.5	9.1	13.2
58.0	39.0	20.1	17.5	16.6	12.1	15.5
60.5	33.6	20.3	29.1	28.3	29.2	30.1

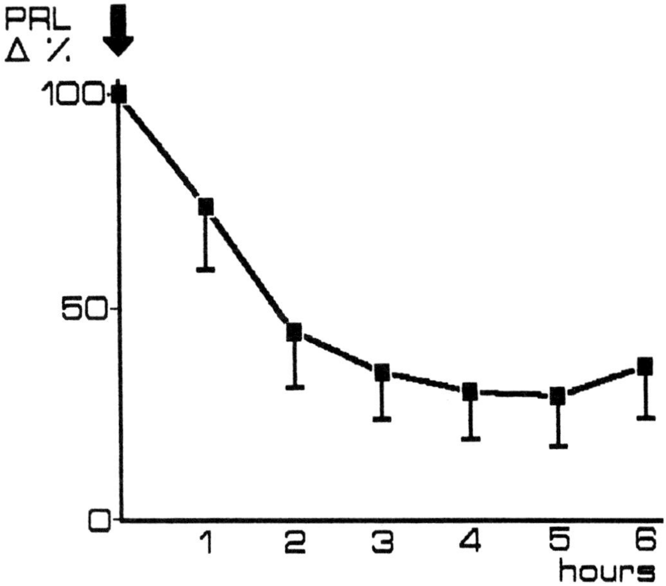

Figure 1 Mean per cent PRL (±SD) in ten hyperprolactinemic patients after DHEC (5 mg p.o.)

normal PRL levels (< 20 ng/ml) 4 h after DHEC administration. No untoward side-effects were observed.

Chronic treatment

PRL levels reached the normal range from the first month of treatment in three of five patients. Two patients needed a higher (20 mg) DHEC daily dose during the second month of treatment. During the third and fourth months of treatment the daily regimen of DHEC was the same for all patients (10 mg). PRL values during treatment are shown in Figure 2. Menstrual cyclicity was restored in all patients in a time ranging from 25 to 48 days after starting treatment. DHEC was very well tolerated.

Sulpiride test

Figure 3 shows the results of the test with sulpiride. We could observe a progressive reduction of the hyperprolactinemic action of sulpiride during the chronic treatment. A statistical evaluation performed on PRL levels 90 min after sulpiride administration indicates a $p < 0.05$ (second against the fourth month) while no significance comparing the second with the third and the third with the fourth month values.

DISCUSSION

The PRL-lowering effect of the acute administration of DHEC is pronounced and long-lasting. Comparing this effect with those obtained with equivalent

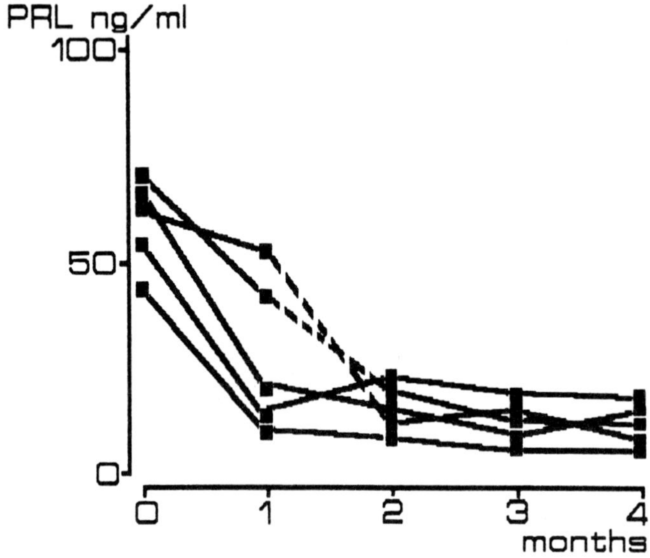

Figure 2 PRL levels (ng/ml) in five patients during treatment with DHEC solid line, 10 mg/die; broken line, 20 mg/die)

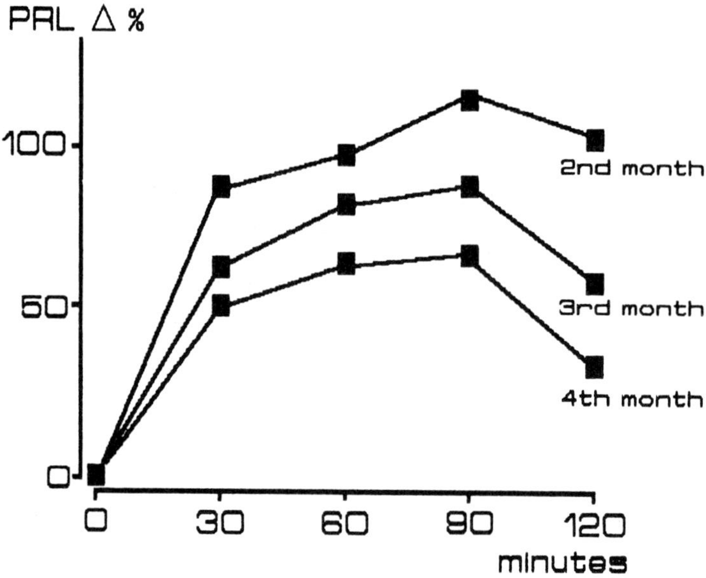

Figure 3 Mean per cent PRL increment after sulpiride (10 mg i.m.) in five hyperprolactinemic patients at the end of the second, third and fourth months of treatment with DHEC (10 mg/die)

doses of other dopamine agonists (i.e. bromocriptine 2.5 mg, lisuride 0.2 mg, transdihydrolisuride 0.2 mg) we can observe a very similar PRL decrease, when expressing values as per cent of baseline[8–10].

The pattern of response to a chronic DHEC administration in mild cases of hyperprolactinemia is very similar to that observed with two other dopaminergic drugs which are very familiar to us (lisuride and trans-dihydrolisuride). In such patients we could often observe a progressive decrease of the dose of drug necessary to maintain PRL suppressed during chronic treatment. Although two of five patients needed a higher DHEC dose during the second month of treatment (20 mg/die), PRL levels remained suppressed for the following 2 months of treatment returning to the starting daily dosage (10 mg). This fact could be ascribed to a progressive increase in sensitivity of the pituitary lactotropes to the drug. In order to confirm this hypothesis we performed the test with sulpiride, reasoning that if such an increased sensitivity to DHEC exists then the hyperprolactinemic action of sulpiride should progressively decrease during the chronic treatment. Our data seem to confirm this hypothesis, though the number of patients is limited and further clinical observations are needed.

In conclusion we can say that DHEC has been shown to be effective in lowering PRL levels both in the acute and in the chronic administration. The drug has been well tolerated and no untoward side-effects were observed. Therefore DHEC seems to possess a high therapeutic index (that is the ratio of the tolerated dose to the effective dose) so that this drug may represent a good choice in patients with mild hyperprolactinemia. Our opinion is that its use in severe forms of this disease should be more extensively investigated and limited to the cases that do not tolerate stronger dopamine agonists.

REFERENCES

1. Vance, M.L., Evans, W.S. and Thorner, M.O. (1984). Diagnosis and treatment, drugs five years later bromocriptine. *Ann. Intern. Med.*, **100**, 78–91
2. Crosignani, P.G., Ferrari, C., Liuzzi, A., Benco, R., Mattei, A., Rampini, P., Dellabonzana, D., Scarduelli, C. and Spelta, B. (1982). Treatment of hyperprolactinaemic states with different drugs: a study with bromocriptine, metergoline and lisuride. *Am. Fertil. Soc.*, **37**, 61
3. Thorner, M.D., Schran, H.F., Evans, W.S., Ragol, A.D., Morris, L. and MacLeod, R. (1980). A broad spectrum of prolactin suppression by bromocriptine in hyperprolactinaemic women: a study of serum prolactin and bromocriptine levels after acute and chronic administration of bromocriptine. *J. Clin. Endocrinol. Metab.*, **50**, 1026–33
4. Fluckiger, E. (1985). Pharmacology of dopaminomimetic drugs. In Del Pozo, E. and Fluckiger, E. (eds), *Dopamine and Neuroendocrine Substances*, pp. 1–10 (London: Academic Press)
5. Fiore, L., Scapagnini, U. and Canonico, P.L. (1987). Effect of dihydroergocryptine on cyclic AMP accumulation and prolactin release *in vitro*: evidence for a dopaminomimetic action. *Horm. Res.*, **25**, 171–7
6. Poli, M., Cocchi, D., Mailland, F., Masu, A.M., Landi, G., Craveri, A. and Muller, E.E. (1986). Prolactin lowering effect of dihydroergokryptine in rat and man. *J. Endocrinol. Invest.*, **9**, 31–6
7. Faglia, G., Conti, A., Muratori, M., Togni, E., Travaglini, P., Zanotti, A. and Mailland, F. (1987). Dihydroergocriptine in management of microprolactinomas. *J. Clin. Endocrinol. Metab.*, **65**, 779–84
8. Venturini, P.L., Horowski, R., Valenzano, M., Costantini, S., Fasce, V., Gorlero, F., Rainer, R. and De Cecco, L. (1986). Effect of terguride on prolactin levels in normal, puerperal and hyperprolactinaemic women. *Eur. J. Clin. Pharmacol.*, **30**, 195–7
9. Horowski, R., Dorow, R., Scholz, A., De Cecco, L. and Schneider, W.H.F. (1984). Lisuride – a new drug for treatment of hyperprolactinaemic disorders. In Rolland, R., Harrison, R.F., Bonnar, J. and Thompson, W. (eds) *Advances in Fertility Control and the Treatment of*

Sterility. Proceedings of a Special Symposium held at the XI World Congress on Fertility and Sterility, pp. 37–49 (Lancaster: MTP Press)

10. De Cecco, L., Venturini, P.L., Ragni, N., Valenzano, M., Costantini, S. and Horowski, R. (1983). Dopaminergic ergots in lactation and cycle disturbances. In Calne, D.B., Horowski, R., McDonald, R.J. and Wuttke, W. (eds) *Lisuride and Other Dopamine Agonists*, pp. 291–9. (New York: Raven Press)

73

Prolactin-lowering effect of dihydroergocriptine in physiological and pathological hyperprolactinemia

A.M. Mattei, A. Zanotti, V. Cavioni, P. Maggioni and P.G. Crosignani

INTRODUCTION

Dopaminergic agents are the standard way to treat hyperprolactinemic disorders[1] and dihydroergocriptine (DHEC) seems to be a very good agent in the management of physiological and pathological hyperprolactinemia[2].

The aims of this study were two: on one side we decided to evaluate the ability of this drug in inhibiting lactation in healthy puerperal women not wishing to breast-feed their babies, on the other side we wanted to verify the efficacy of DHEC in reducing PRL levels into the normal range and in restoring gonadal function in terms of ovulation and menstruation in patients with so called dysfunctional hyperprolactinemia as well as in adenomata subjects.

PATIENTS AND METHODS

Twenty puerperal women with a mean age of 29 years (range between 22 and 40) who did not want or for whom it was contraindicated to breast feed their baby entered this double-blind study.

A single acute administration of 5 mg DHEC was administered to the patients to test responsiveness to the drug.

Furthermore, all the patients were given, randomly, 5 mg DHEC or 2.5 mg bromocriptine every 12 h for 7 days, starting within 48 h after delivery.

Prolactin measurements (by radioimmunoassay) were obtained daily up to the 10th day of treatment. The effect of the drug on puerperal lactation was assessed by the absence of breast-swelling and pain, milk secretion or the evidence of any side-effect linked with the drug intake.

Twenty hyperprolactinemic subjects with a mean age of 30 years (range between 18 and 46) also entered this study. Nine were amenorrheic patients, three were oligomenorrheic while the others showed regular but anovulatory menses.

Fourteen patients showed evidence of a pituitary microadenoma (on the basis of a computerized tomography performed before entering the study), one was carrying a macroadenoma, one already surgically treated showed a relapse of hyperprolactinemia.

All the patients were given 5–40 mg DHEC daily in two administrations; the mean treatment length was 8 months, with a range between 1 and 22.

Plasma PRL levels were verified every 30 days while progesterone levels were measured by radioimmunoassay in the presumptive luteal phase of the cycle.

RESULTS

Among the puerperal patients treated to prevent lactation both the drugs were effective on clinical grounds, without any rebound phenomena. Changes in serum level of PRL during the treatment are shown in Figure 1.

Acute administration of 5 mg DHEC induced a mean PRL level decrease of 64%; all but three patients had a positive response to the test (PRL decrease ≥50% of basal value). Table 1 shows the maximum PRL reduction during chronic treatment in the hyperprolactinemic women. In a group of resistant subjects a further PRL reduction was obtained by increasing the drug doses (Figure 2). The clinical results in terms of restoration of menses, ovulations and pregnancies are summarized in Table 2. No significant side-effect was reported in either of the trials.

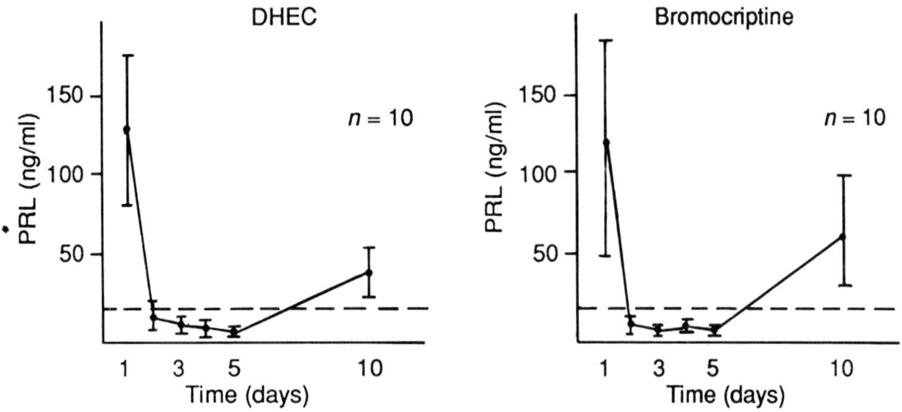

Figure 1 Serum PRL in 20 puerperal women treated with DHEC (left) and bromocriptine (right) to prevent lactation (mean ± SEM)

Table 1 Chronic treatment with DHEC (5–40 mg/day)

		Serum PRL (ng/ml)		
Patients' initials	*Age* (yr)	*Before treatment*	*On treatment*	*Clinical outcome*
Adenoma				
1 P.G.*	41	205	201	no change
2 M.G.	25	200	110	regular menses
3 R.R.	18	41	15	ovulatory menses
4 R.P.	22	25	3	ovulatory menses
5 E.F.	46	91	18	ovulatory menses
6 A.B.**	40	200	48	ovulatory menses
7 V.D.	25	60	4	pregnancy
8 L.G.	23	31	2	ovulatory menses
9 E.B.	44	31	24	regular menses
10 M.S.	22	51	13	ovulatory menses
11 L.L.	39	37	10	ovulatory menses
12 G.I.	39	132	8	ovulatory menses
13 L.L.	35	95	10	ovulatory menses
14 G.G.	21	400	87	regular menses
15 L.M.	23	32	4	regular menses
Idiopathic				
1 A.M.S.	36	42	9	regular menses
2 M.S.	25	67	28	ovulatory menses
3 R.B.	18	35	6	pregnancy
4 M.B.	32	31	3	pregnancy
5 R.O.	29	28	16	ovulatory menses

* Macroadenoma; ** Microadenoma after surgery

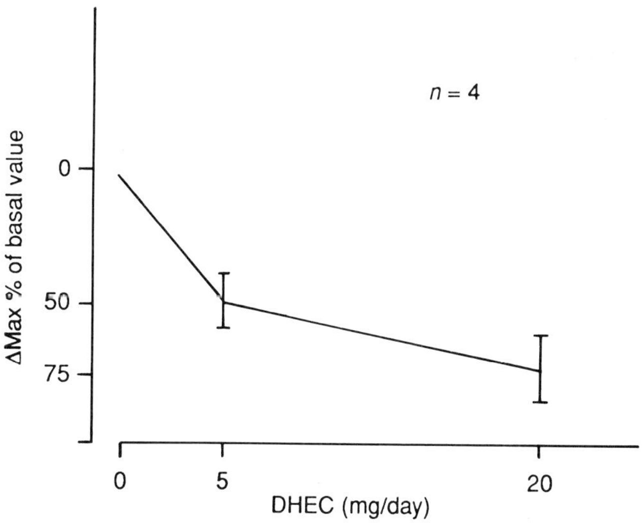

Figure 2 PRL reduction in a group of resistant patients administered with increasing doses of DHEC in mg/day

Table 2 Effect of DHEC on ovarian function in 20 hyperprolactinemic women

Diagnosis	*No. patients treated*	*Ovulation*	*Menstruation*	*No effect*
Adenoma				
Amenorrhea	10	5 (1P)*	4	1
Anovulation	5	5	—	—
Idiopathic				
Amenorrhea	2	1 (1P)	1	—
Anovulation	3	2 (1P)	1	—

* P, pregnancy

DISCUSSION

This new drug proved to be effective in inhibiting puerperal lactation; PRL levels on 10th day of treatment seemed to be lower (mean value 42 ng/ml) in the DHEC group than in the bromocriptine group (mean value 62 ng/ml) although this difference did not reach statistical significance. In non-puerperal women chronic DHEC treatment was able to halve and/or normalize PRL levels in 80% of the patients with a restoration of gonadal function in the great majority of the subjects (90%). In view of the complete lack of any side-effect, with daily doses up to 40 mg, we can conclude that DHEC may be a very effective drug with which to treat hyperprolactinemic disorders.

REFERENCES

1. Crosignani, P.G., Ferrari, C., Galparoli, C., Cavioni, V., Adelasco, P., Zavaglia, C., Spellecchia, D., Scarduelli, C. and Mattei, A. M. (1986). Use of dopaminergic agents in reproduction system disturbances: up to date. In Molinatti, G.M. and Martini, L. (eds). *Endocrinology*, p. 85. (Amsterdam: Elsevier Science Publishers B.V.)
2. Faglia, G., Conti, A., Muratori, M., Togni, E., Travaglini, P., Zanotti, A. and Mailland, F. (1987). Dihydroergokryptine in management of microprolactinomas. *J. Clin. Endocrinol. Metab.*, **65**, 779–84

74

Prolactin-lowering effect of dihydroergocriptine in puerperal women

C. Nappi, F. Votino, G. Colace, C. Di Carlo, G.F. Di Renzo, L. Annunziato, F.G. Tinelli and U. Montemagno

INTRODUCTION

Dihydroergocriptine (DHEC) is a dihydrogenated ergot alkaloid showing a high affinity for α-adrenergic receptors in the central nervous system and pituitary D-2 dopamine receptors[1,2]. Its prolactin (PRL)-lowering effect has been demonstrated both in animals and in humans[3–5]. Therefore, in this study we investigated the effects of DHEC (Poli, Italy) on serum PRL levels and lactation in postpartum women. The results have been compared with those induced by the administration of placebo.

MATERIALS AND METHODS

After giving informed consent, a total of 85 healthy postpartum women aged 19–37 years (mean 27.4 years) who had spontaneously conceived were admitted to the study. No other drug was taken during the present experiment. All the subjects were randomly divided in six groups.

Acute administration

Group 1
Ten puerperal women received a single oral dose of 5 mg of DHEC at 08:00 24–72 h after delivery. Blood samples were taken 0, 30, 60, 90, 120, 180 and 240 min after drug administration.

Group 2
Ten puerperal women received a single oral dose of 10 mg of DHEC at 08:00 24–72 h after delivery. Blood samples were taken 0, 30, 60, 90, 120, 180 and 240 min after drug administration.

Group 3
Ten nursing mothers received a single oral dose of a pharmacologically inactive placebo at 08:00 24–72 h after delivery. Blood samples were taken 0, 30, 60, 90, 120, 180 and 240 min after placebo administration.

Repeated administration

Group 4
Twenty puerperal women asking for suppression of lactation received DHEC (5 mg twice daily *per os* for 7 days) 24–72 h after delivery. Blood samples were taken at 08:00 just before drug administration (day 0 = basal values), and on days 1, 2, 3, 4, 5, 6 and 7 of treatment. An additional morning sample was taken 1 (day 8) and 8 days (day 15) after the end of the treatment.

Group 5
Fifteen puerperal women received, 24–72 h after delivery, DHEC at the dose of 5 mg three times daily *per os* for 7 days. Blood samples were taken at 08:00 just before the drug administration (day 0 = basal values), and on days 1, 2, 3, 4, 5, 6 and 7 of treatment. An additional morning sample was taken 1 (day 8) and 8 days (day 15) after the end of the treatment.

Group 6
Twenty nursing mothers received, 24–72 h after delivery, an oral pharmacologically inactive placebo. Blood samples were collected at 08:00 of days 0 (basal values), 1, 2, 3, 4, 5, 6 and 7 of placebo administration, at least 120 min after suckling had been completed. One (day 8) and 8 days (day 15) after the end of the treatment an additional morning sample was taken.

All blood samples were obtained from an indwelling intravenous catheter placed in the antecubital vein 15 min before the collection of blood samples.

Blood samples were taken after an overnight fast and stored at −20°C. Serum PRL levels were measured by a sensitive double antibody radioimmunoassay kit provided by Biodata (Milan, Italy). Using this PRL kit, normal PRL levels in a large number of controls ranged from 5 to 25 ng/ml. The intra-assay and interassay coefficients of variation were 4.8 and 8.7 respectively. Statistical analysis of results was performed by ANOVA followed by the Newman–Keul's test.

In women of groups 4 and 5 the effectiveness of DHEC treatment was evaluated each day by observing the presence and the extent of breast tenderness, pain, engorgement and milk secretion.

RESULTS

Acute administration

The acute administration of 5 mg of DHEC did not reduce high serum levels of PRL (Figure 1). In contrast, the higher dose of DHEC (10 mg) induced a marked reduction of PRL secretion at all the considered times (Figure 2). No side-effect was observed during this acute treatment.

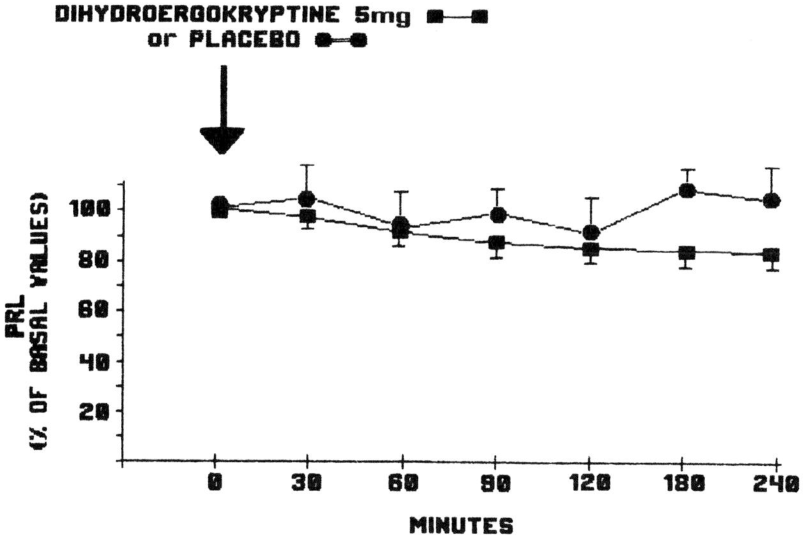

Figure 1 Mean serum PRL levels (± SEM) expressed as percentage of basal values in 10 women receiving a single oral dose of 5 mg of DHEC

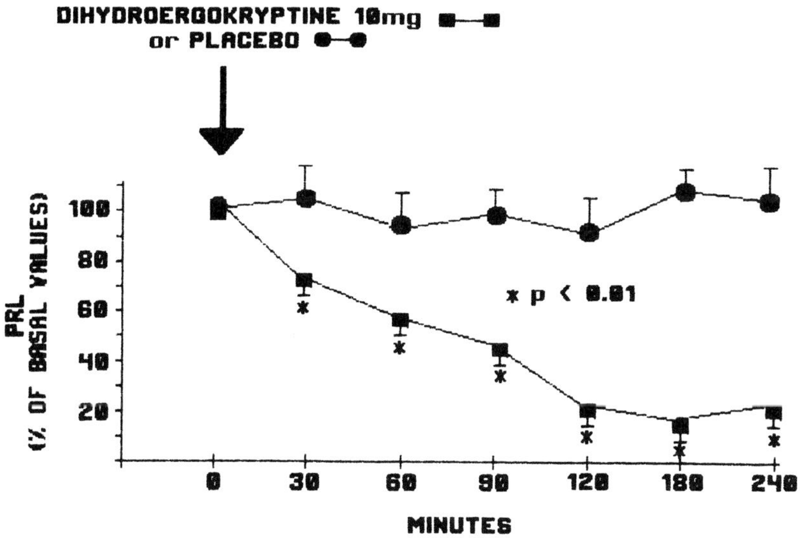

Figure 2 Mean serum PRL levels (± SEM) expressed as percentage of basal values in 10 women receiving a single oral dose of 10 mg of DHEC. *$p < 0.01$ versus basal value at time 0

Repeated administration

The administration of DHEC at the dose of 5 mg twice daily for 7 days, induced a significant decrease of mean PRL levels (Figure 3), which occurred beginning from the 1st day of treatment and lasted for all the time considered

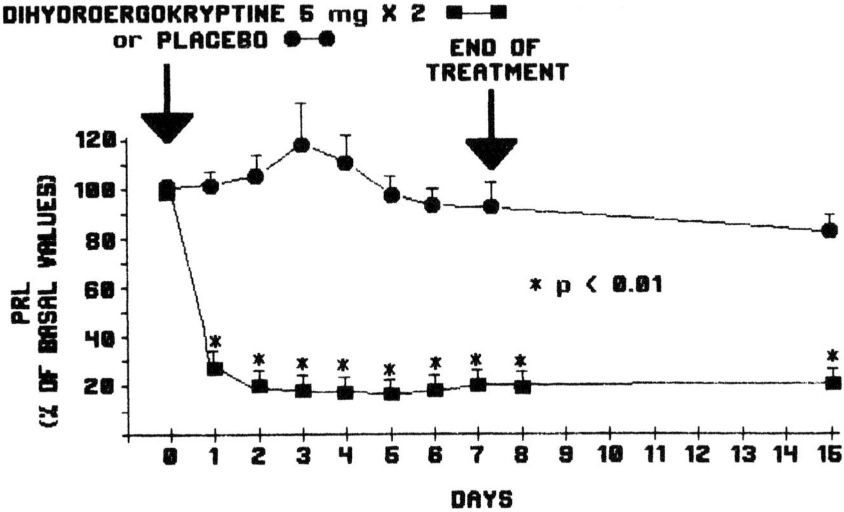

Figure 3 Mean serum PRL levels (± SEM) expressed as percentage of basal values in 20 women receiving DHEC at the daily dose of 10 mg (5 mg × 2) for 7 days. *$p < 0.01$ versus basal value on day 0

in the study.

When DHEC was administered at the dose of 5 mg three times daily, a marked inhibition of PRL secretion was observed (Figure 4). Serum PRL was still inhibited 8 days after the end of the treatment with both doses of

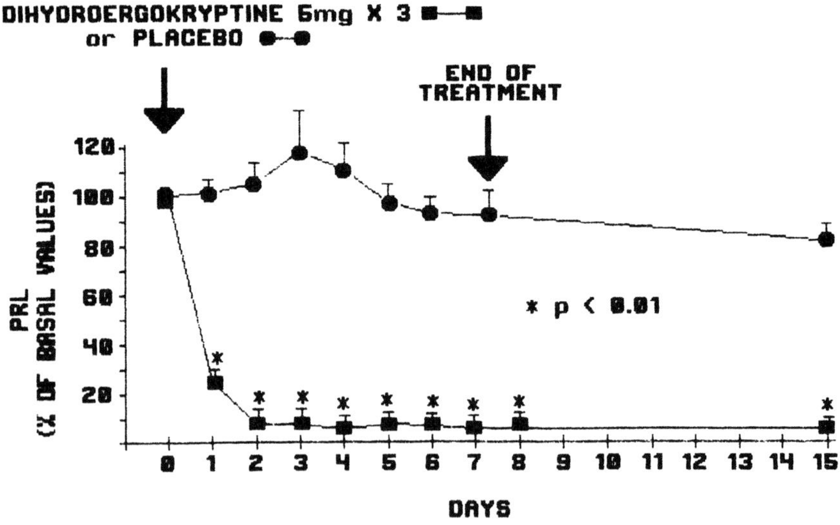

Figure 4 Mean serum PRL levels (± SEM) expressed as percentage of basal values in 15 women receiving DHEC at the daily dose of 15 mg (5 mg × 3) for 7 days. *$p < 0.01$ versus basal value on day 0

the peripheral dopamine agonist.

In puerperal women receiving DHEC (5 mg two or three times daily) the extent of breast tenderness, pain, engorgement and milk secretion progressively decreased from day 1 to 6. The duration of these effects was different in the two groups. In fact these signs and symptoms disappeared on days 4–6 in women treated with 5 mg × 2, whereas they remitted on days 2–4 in subjects receiving 5 mg × 3.

No rebound lactation occurred in any of the puerperal women treated with DHEC. No adverse effect (headache, dizziness, nausea, vomiting, postural hypotension) was observed during the treatment.

DISCUSSION

The results of the present study indicate that DHEC, when administered at the dose of 10 or 15 mg daily significantly lowers PRL levels since the 1st day of treatment. However, the dose of 15 mg produced lower PRL levels and a more precocious suppression of lactation in comparison with the group treated with 10 mg daily of DHEC. The absence of rebound lactation may be attributed to the persistence of low PRL levels until 8 days after the end of treatment.

The acute administration of 5 mg of DHEC did not induce a significant decrease in PRL levels. The lack of effectiveness of this single dose could be due to the fact that it does not produce sufficiently high concentrations of the drug at the level of pituitary dopamine agonist receptors. On the contrary, when 5 mg of DHEC was administered two or three times daily, these critical concentrations could be reached since the half-life of the compound has been reported to be 12 h[7].

Furthermore, it seems interesting to underline that DHEC, at the doses used in the present study, did not induce the side-effects which are characteristic of other ergot alkaloids[8–10].

This lack of side-effects cannot be explained simply in terms of lower dopaminergic activity of DHEC in comparison with other ergot alkaloids. In fact, in other studies, it has been shown that DHEC is also devoid of side-effects when administered at doses able to decrease PRL secretion to the same extent as other ergot alkaloids[5]. It could be hypothesized that DHEC, for its molecular structure, is able to stimulate pituitary dopamine receptors, whereas it is less effective at the level of the cardiovascular and gastrointestinal systems[5].

We conclude that DHEC, at the daily dose of 15 mg, because of its good effectiveness, safety and tolerability, is a good pharmacological approach to the inhibition of puerperal lactation.

REFERENCES

1. Goldstein, M., Lew, J.Y., Hata, F. and Lieberman, A. (1978). Binding interactions of ergot alkaloids with monoaminergic receptors in the brain. *Gerontology*, **24** (Suppl. 1), 76
2. Sibley, D.R. and Creese, I. (1983). Interactions of ergot alkaloids with anterior pituitary D2 dopamine receptors. *Mol. Pharmacol.*, **23**, 585

3. Libertun, C., Larrea, G.A., Vacas, M.I. and Cardinali, D.P. (1980). [^{3}H]Dihydroergokriptine binding in anterior pituitary and prolactin secretion: further evidence of brain regulation of adenohypophyseal receptors. *Endocrinology*, **107**, 1905
4. Poli, M., Landi, G., Masu, A.M., Savi, B., Mailland, F., Del Rosso, R., Barbesti, S. and Craveri, A. (1985). Dihydroergokriptine: effect of a single oral dose on serum prolactin and catecholamines. *J. Endocrinol. Invest.*, **8** (Suppl. 3), 191
5. Poli, M., Cocchi, D., Mailland, F., Masu, A.M., Landi, G., Craveri, A. and Muller, E.E. (1986). Prolactin lowering effect of dihydroergokryptine in rat and in man. *J. Endocrinol. Invest.*, **9**, 31
6. Ferrari, C., Rampini, P., Paracchi, A., Boghen, M. and Mailland, F. (1985). Effect of Dihydroergokriptine administration on serum prolactin and growth hormone levels in normal hyperprolactinaemic and acromegalic subjects: evidence of potent and long-lasting pituitary dopamine receptor stimulation. *Eur. J. Clin. Pharmacol.*, **27**, 707
7. Turba, C. (1990). Farmacocinetica e farmacodinamica nell'uomo della diidroergocriptina. Dosaggio singolo e stato stazionario. (In press)
8. Parlodel. Physicians' Desk Reference, 38th Edition, 1984, p. 1748
9. Franks, S., Horrocks, P.M., Lynch, S.S., Butt, W.R. and London, D.R. (1981). Treatment of hyperprolactinemia with pergolide mesylate: acute effects and preliminary evaluation of long-term treatment. *Lancet*, **ii**, 659
10. Liuzzi, A., Chiodini, P.G., Oppizzi, G., Botalla, L., Verde, G., De Stefano, L., Coluzzi, G., Gräf, K.J. and Horowsky, R. (1978). Lisuride hydrogen maleate: evidence for a long lasting dopaminergic activity in humans. *J. Clin. Endocrinol. Metab.*, **46**, 196

75

Treatment of hyperprolactinemic states with dihydroergocriptine

G.B. Melis, A.M. Paoletti, F.D. Petacchi, G.A. Mauro, R. Soldani, R. Prato, V. Mais, A. Zanotti and P. Fioretti

INTRODUCTION

It is known that elective treatment of hyperprolactinemic states is represented by chronic administration of dopaminergic drugs, such as bromocriptine[1,2] and lisuride[3,4]. These compounds are able to induce a significant inhibition of prolactin (PRL) secretion both in different hyperprolactinemic conditions and in different hyperprolactinemic states[1-7]. In addition, different studies reported the effective antitumoral effects of these drugs with a significant shrinkage of pituitary prolactinoma[8-10]. However, their use is often associated with the appearance of side-effects such as nausea, vomiting and hypotension[11,12]. Thus the research was developed to find other drugs with similar or greater hormonal and clinical efficacy but without the clinical side-effects of dopaminergic drugs.

Dihydroergocriptine (DHEC) is a dihydrogenated ergot alkaloid which has been shown to possess potent dopaminomimetic properties both *in vivo* and *in vitro*[13]. The PRL-inhibiting effect of DHEC is similar to that of bromocriptine and other dopaminergic compounds. However, DHEC is well tolerated by patients, exhibiting a very low incidence of side-effects[13].

The aim of this study therefore was to evaluate clinical efficacy, hypoprolactinemic effect, tolerability and safety of DHEC in different hyperprolactinemic states such as inhibition of puerperal lactation and pathological hyperprolactinemia.

MATERIAL AND METHODS

Inhibition of puerperal lactation

Twenty puerperal women who requested inhibition of lactation, were included in the study. DHEC or bromocriptine was administered randomly using a double-blind experimental protocol at the dose of one capsule every 8 h (three capsules, daily) for 7 days. Each capsule contained 2.5 mg of bromocriptine or

10 mg of DHEC. Plasma PRL levels were measured before treatment, daily during treatment, and 10 days after the end of drug administration. Clinical assessment of mammary symptoms (congestion and milk secretion) was performed every day from the start of treatment until the 10th day after the end of drug administration. The score used to evaluate mammary symptoms was : 0 = absent, 1 = mild, 2 = moderate, 3 = severe. Biochemical analysis was performed before treatment and on the 10th day after the end of drug administration. Blood pressure was measured before treatment, every day during treatment and on the 10th day after the end of drug administration.

Treatment of pathological hyperprolactinemia

Seven hyperprolactinemic women (six with and one without radiological evidence of pituitary adenoma) were included in the study.

Chronic treatment with DHEC was performed for 8 weeks at the initial daily dose of 10 mg (5 mg every 12 h). In four women, this same dose was administered throughout the study. In the remaining three subjects, the dose of DHEC was progressively increased depending on the individual response of PRL secretion. From the beginning of the study plasma PRL concentrations were measured weekly for 10 weeks. Biochemical analysis was performed before and at the end of treatment. Blood pressure was measured before treatment and every week after the initiation of treatment.

RESULTS

Inhibition of puerperal lactation

A significant decrease in PRL secretion was observed in puerperal women treated with bromocriptine. Starting from 50 ± 20 ng/ml, PRL plasma levels decreased to 5 ± 1 ng/ml after only 24 h of drug administration. PRL secretion was significantly inhibited during the treatment and only after 10 days from drug withdrawal, a significant rebound of PRL levels to 20 ± 2 ng/ml was observed (Figure 1). A similar pattern of PRL secretion was observed during DHEC treatment. From basal values of 80 ± 20 ng/ml, PRL concentrations decreased to 7 ± 1 ng/ml after 24 h, remained low during the whole treatment and showed a slight increase to 20 ± 1.2 ng/ml 10 days after drug withdrawal (Figure 1).

As for the clinical results, mammary symptoms (mammary secretion and mammary congestion) were absent during bromocriptine treatment and did not appear at all (Figure 2).

Mammary scores showed a significant reduction during DHEC treatment. Starting from basal values of 0.9 ± 0.05, mammary secretion decreased to 0.4 ± 0.01 after 1 day of treatment, and was 0 from the 3rd day of treatment until the end of observation. Mammary congestion showed a similar decrease. From basal values of 1.8 ± 0.4, the mammary congestion score decreased to 1 ± 0.2 after 1 day of treatment, and was absent (0) from the 3rd day of treatment until the end of observation (Figure 3).

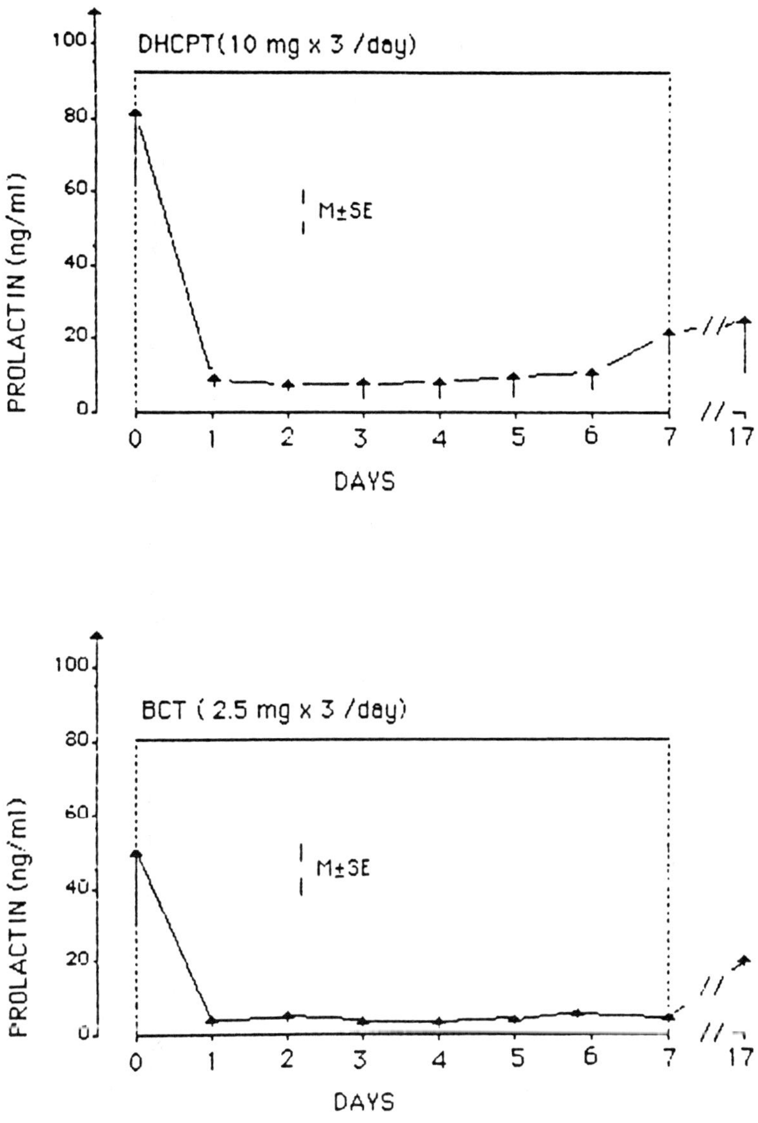

Figure 1 Prolactin-inhibiting effect of chronic DHEC and bromocriptine treatment in puerperal women. Upper panel: A significant decrease in PRL secretion was measured after the first day of DHEC (10 mg × 3/day) treatment. Inhibition of PRL secretion was observed until the end of drug administration. DHEC withdrawal was followed by PRL increase to 20 ng/ml. Lower panel: bromocriptine (2.5 mg × 3/day) induced a significant inhibition of PRL secretion until the end of treatment, whereas a slight increase in PRL levels was observed after 10 days of drug interruption; values are means ± SEM

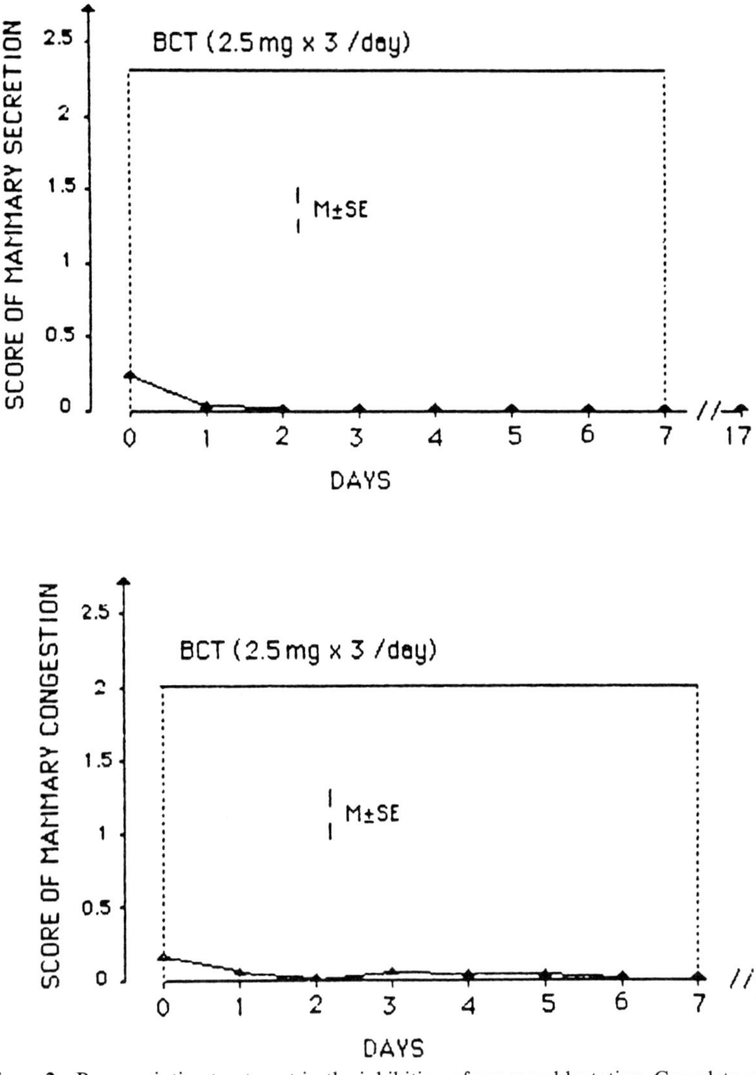

Figure 2 Bromocriptine treatment in the inhibition of puerperal lactation. Complete suppression of mammary secretion and mammary congestion was observed during the treatment and post-treatment periods; values are means ± SEM

Blood pressure levels remained unmodified during both DHEC and bromocriptine treatment. No modifications in biochemical parameters were observed after bromocriptine or DHEC in comparison to those evaluated before the beginning of treatment. No side-effects were reported by the women treated with bromocriptine or DHEC.

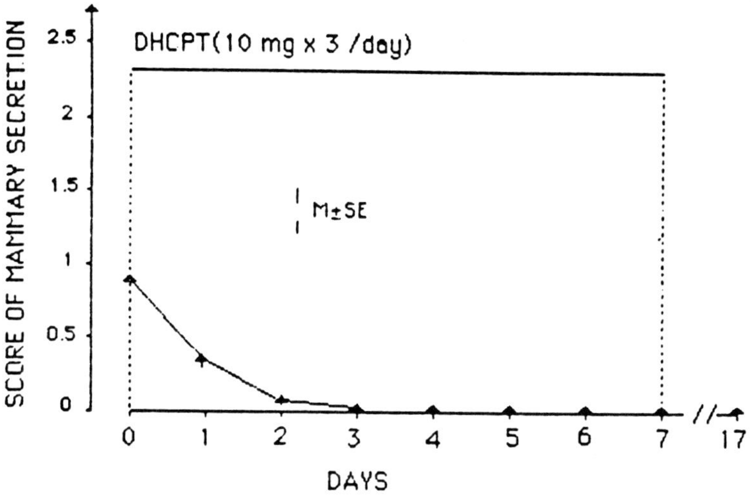

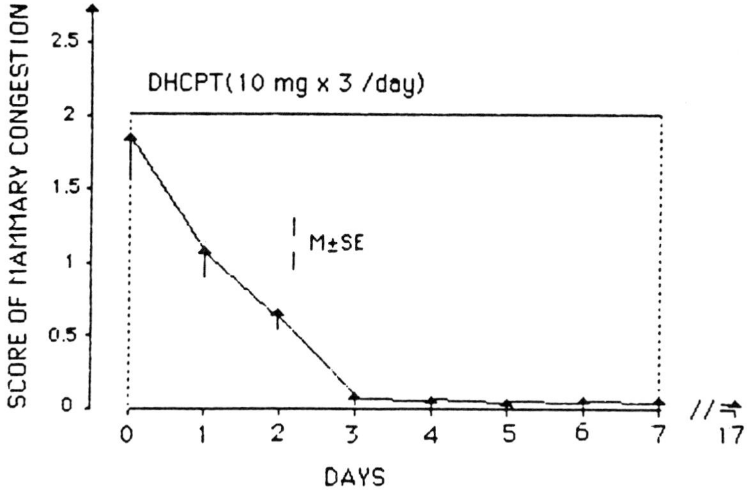

Figure 3 Efficacy of DHEC treatment in the inhibition of puerperal lactation. Complete suppression of mammary secretion and mammary congestion was obtained after 3 days of DHEC treatment and was observed for the entire period of observation; values are means ± SEM

Pathological hyperprolactinemia

Out of the seven hyperprolactinemic subjects, the initial DHEC dose of 5 mg, twice a day was not modified in four subjects since a significant decrease in PRL secretion was observed within the first 3 days of treatment. In these subjects, the initial dose of DHEC was able to induce a rapid inhibition of PRL secretion that from basal values of 42 ± 2 ng/ml decreased to 4 ± 2 ng/ml after 3 days being below the normal range for the entire period of treatment

(Figure 4). At the end of treatment PRL levels increased to 38 ± 4 ng/ml after one week and to 90 ± 25 ng/ml after 2 weeks.

In the remaining 3 subjects daily doses of DHEC higher than 10 mg were used to obtain a significant decrease in PRL secretion (Figures 5–7). In subject PF (40 yr, with secondary amenorrhea and microadenoma), the normalization of PRL secretion was obtained with a daily dose of 20 mg DHEC (Figure 5). After drug withdrawal a rapid PRL rebound was observed within 2 weeks. In patient VA (31 yr, with secondary amenorrhea and microadenoma), starting from the initial daily dose of 10 mg, the DHEC dose was progressively increased to 20, 40 and finally 60 mg/day to obtain a satisfactory decrease in PRL secretion. Values similar to the pretreatment ones were measured within 2 weeks (Figure 6). The highest dosage of DHEC was employed in patient IS (21 yr, secondary amemorrhea and pituitary macroadenoma). In this patient the dose of DHEC was progressively

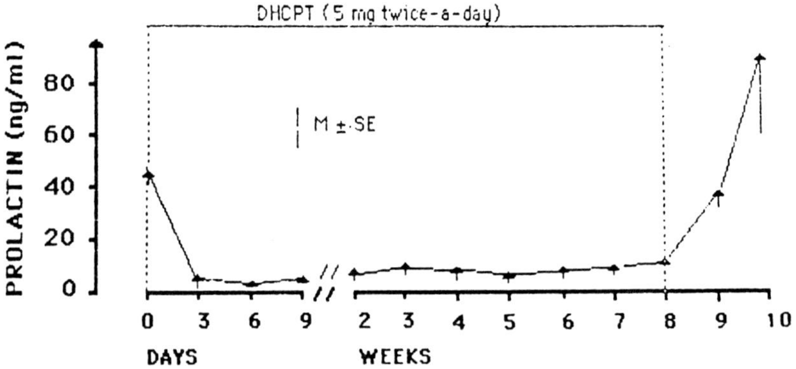

Figure 4 Prolactin-inhibiting effect of DHEC treatment (5 mg, twice a day) in four hyperprolactinemic women. DHEC (5 mg, twice a day) induced a significant decrease in PRL secretion from basal values of 42 ± 2 ng/ml to 4 ± 2 ng/ml, within 3 days of treatment and for the entire period of treatment (8 weeks). A significant increase in PRL secretion was observed after the end of treatment; values are means ± SEM

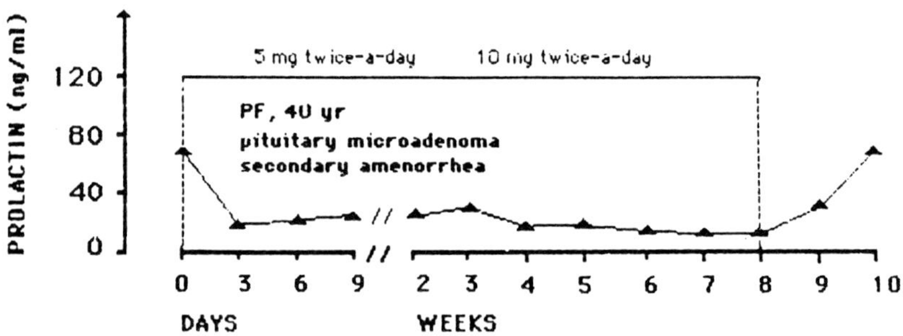

Figure 5 Prolactin-inhibiting effect of DHEC treatment in a hyperprolactinemic woman with secondary amenorrhea and microadenoma. DHEC treatment (5 mg, twice a day) was unable to obtain a sufficient PRL inhibition, whereas the normalization of PRL levels was obtained with a higher regimen of DHEC (10 mg, twice a day)

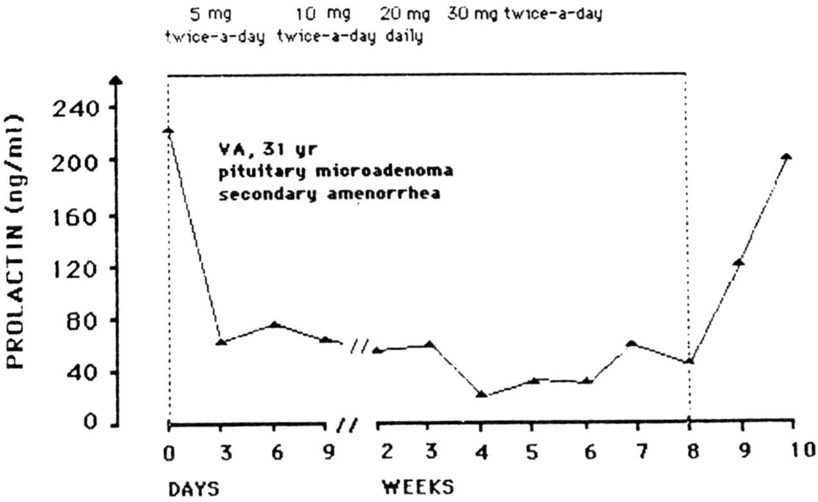

Figure 6 Prolactin-inhibiting effect of DHEC treatment in a hyperprolactinemic woman with secondary amenorrhea and microadenoma. The normalization of PRL levels was obtained with 60 mg of DHEC since the initial dose of 10 mg was unable to induce a significant reduction

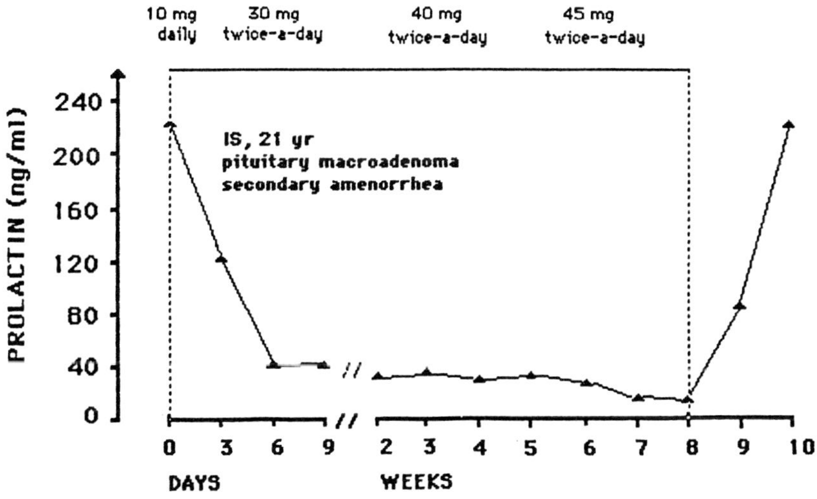

Figure 7 Prolactin-inhibiting effect of DHEC treatment in a hyperprolactinemic woman with secondary amemorrhea and pituitary macroadenoma. A progressive increase of daily dose of DHEC from 10 mg to 90 mg was able to induce the normalization of PRL levels

increased to 60 mg to obtain a decrease of PRL secretion to 40 ng/ml. Only a further increase in the DHEC dosage firstly to 80 mg/day and then to 90 mg/day was able to maintain PRL levels below 40 ng/ml. After drug interruption, an increase in PRL secretion was rapidly observed (Figure 7).

Table 1 Effects of DHEC treatment in hyperprolactinemic women

Subject	*Age*	*Daily dose*	*Menstrual cycle*	*Side-effects*
1	33	10 mg	spontaneous menses	none
2	41	10 mg	spontaneous menses	none
3	38	10 mg	spontaneous menses	none
4	26	10 mg	regular menstrual cycles	none
5	40	10 mg for 3 weeks; 20 mg thereafter	spontaneous menses	none
6	31	10 mg for 1 week; 20 mg for the 2nd week; 40 mg for the 3rd week; 60 mg thereafter	spontaneous menses	none
7	21	10 mg during first 3 days; 60 mg from the 4th day to the 2nd week; 80 mg from the 3rd to the 6th week; 90 mg from the 6th to the 8th week	spontaneous menses	none

In all cases, the decrease in PRL secretion was followed by the normalization of the menstrual cycle (Table 1). In particular, spontaneous menses reappeared in the patients affected by secondary amenorrhea and the normalization to 28 days was reported by the patient with oligomenorrhea.

No modifications in blood pressure or biochemical parameters were observed during the DHEC treatment. No side-effects were reported by the patients (Table 1).

DISCUSSION

DHEC was found to be very effective in preventing lactation and in the inhibition of PRL secretion in puerperal women and in inhibiting PRL secretion in pathological hyperprolactinemia. In puerperal women the effects of DHEC were comparable to those of bromocriptine, that previous studies reported to be very active[7,14]. In addition, our data seem to indicate that a 7-day period of treatment is not only sufficient to induce a significant inhibition of PRL secretion but also to prevent the reappearance of mammary symptoms, whereas other dopaminergic compounds need more than 10 days of treatment to induce complete disappearance of puerperal lactation[14]. Dopaminergic drugs often induce side-effects like nausea, vomiting, dizziness and hypotension[11,12]. These side-efffects are particularly frequent during the first days of treatment and the needed dosages are often reached after many days of progressively increasing doses[14].

Although during puerperium the side-effects are less frequent and intense than in pathological hyperprolactinemia, the short-term treatment does not permit a sufficient period of adaptation. The complete absence of any side-effect makes DHEC particularly suitable to be given at the most efficacous dose. Thus the efficacy associated with a good tolerability and safety of DHEC indicates its usefulness in the suppression of puerperal lactation. The high inhibitory effect of DHEC on prolactin secretion and its tolerability are also observed in patients with pathological hyperprolactinemia. In the majority of subjects, a daily dose of 10 mg was able to normalize PRL secretion within a few days and to keep low the levels of the hormone for the following 2 months. As expected the normalization of PRL levels was also accompanied by the restoration of spontaneous menses in amenorrheic patients and by the normalization of menstrual rhythms in the one having oligomenorrhea. However, since a similar efficacy in inhibiting PRL secretion has also been reported after the administration of other dopaminergic compounds[1-4], the main feature of DHEC treatment seems to be the absolute absence of side-effects also in subjects out of puerperium. Since side-effects may limit the use of dopaminergic compounds, DHEC may represent the drug of choice either for short-term treatments or for the treatment of subjects who present intolerance to bromocriptine. Further studies will demonstrate whether DHEC may be the drug of choice also in the other conditions since its ability to induce ovulations and normal pregnancies has to be applied to a larger population. In fact, in patients with pituitary tumor, doses varying from higher than 10 mg/day to 90 mg/day were necessary to obtain a restoration of normal PRL secretion and spontaneous menstrual cycle. This observation confirms that the efficacy of DHEC, like other similar compounds, is dependent on the dose of the drug and on the endocrine and pathological conditions of the subject[1-7]. Otherwise the need to give high dosages of the drug to obtain a good control of PRL levels, confirms the very interesting tolerability of this drug that did not induce any side-effects also at the higher doses used.

REFERENCES

1. Bergh, T., Nillius, S.J. and Wide, L. (1978). Bromocriptine treatment of 42 hyperprolactinemic women with secondary amenorrhea. *Acta Endocrinol.*, **88**, 435
2. Thorner, M.O., Scharan, H.E., Evans, W.S., Rogol, A.D., Morris, J.L: and MacLeon, R.M. (1980). A broad spectrum of prolactin suppression by bromocriptine in hyperprolactinemic women: a study of serum prolactin and bromocriptine levels after acute and chronic administration of bromocriptine. *J. Clin. Endocrinol. Metab.*, **50**, 1026
3. Bohnet, H. G., Hanker, J.P., Horowski, R., Wickings, E.J. and Schneider, H.P.G. (1979). Suppression of prolactin secretion by lisuride throughout the menstrual cycle and in hyperprolactinemic menstrual disorders. *Acta Endocrinol.*, **92**, 8–19
4. De Cecco, L., Foglia, G., Ragni, N., Rossato, P. and Venturini, P.L. (1978). The effect of lisuride hydrogen maleate in the hyperprolactinemic-amenorrhoea syndrome: clinical and hormonal responses. *Clin. Endocrinol.*, **9**, 491–8
5. Delitala, G., Wass, A.H., Stubbs, W.A., Jones, A., Williams, S. and Besser, G.M. (1979). The effect of lisuride hydrogen maleate, an ergot derivative on anterior pituitary hormone secretion in man. *Clin. Endocrinol.*, **11**, 1–9
6. De Cecco, L., Venturini, P.L., Ragni, N., Rossato, P., Maganza, C., Gaggero, G. and Horowski, R. (1979). Effect of lisuride on inhibition of lactation and serum prolactin. *Br. J. Obstet. Gynaecol.*, **86**, 905–8
7. Solla, E., Murru, S., Onano, A.M. and Melis, G.B. (1978). Inibizione della lattazione con 2-Bromo-Alfa- Ergocriptina (CB 154). *Ann. Ostet. Ginecol. Med. Perin.*, **3**, 199–207
8. Corenblum, B. and Hanley, D.A. (1981). Bromocriptine reduction of prolactinoma size. *Fertil. Steril.*, **36**, 716–19
9. Waas, A.H., Williams, J., Charlesworth, M., Kingsley, D.P.E., Halliday, A.M., Doniach, I., Rees, L.H., McDonald, W.I. and Besser, G.M. (1982). Bromocriptine in management of large pituitary tumours. *Br. Med. J.*, **284**, 1908–11
10. Chiodini, P., Liuzzi, A., Cozzi, R., Verde, G., Oppizzi, G., Dallabonzana, D., Spelta, B., Silvestrini, F., Borghi, G., Luccarelli, G., Rainder, E. and Horowski,, R. (1981). Size reduction

of macroprolactinomas by bromocriptine or lisuride treatment. *J. Clin. Endocrinol. Metab.*, **53**, 737–43
11. Thorner, M.P., Fluckiger, E. and Calne, D.B. (1980). Bromocriptine, *Clinical and Pharmacological Review*
12. Cuellar, F.G. (1980). Bromocriptine mesylate in the management of amenorrhea galactorrhea associated with hyperprolactinemia. *Obstet. Gynecol.*, **55**, 278
13. Poli, M., Cocchi, D., Mailland, F., Masu, A.M., Landi, G., Craveri, A. and Mueller, E.E. (1986). Prolactin lowering effect of dihydroergokryptine in rat and in man. *J. Endocrinol. Invest.*, **9**, 31
14. Duchesne, C. and Leke, R. (1981). Bromocriptine mesylate for prevention of postpartum laction. *Obstet. Gynecol.*, **57**, 464–7

76

Clinical evaluation of dihydroergocriptine in patients with functional hyperprolactinemia and microadenoma

A. Volpe, F. Mercantini, R. Adamo, A. Zanotti, F. Mailland and A.R. Genazzani

INTRODUCTION

Functional hyperprolactinemia is successfully treated with dopamine agonist drugs such as bromocriptine and lysuride, but in some sensitive subjects they cannot be used because of side-effects. This has led to pharmacological research to study new molecules with dopamine agonist activity and reduced side-effects. One of these drugs is dihydroergocriptine (DHEC), a dihydrogenated ergot-alkaloid with dopaminergic agonist and α-adrenergic antagonist properties. This drug is able to suppress prolactin (PRL) secretion[1,2]. A PRL lowering activity of DHEC has also been reported in healthy volunteers and in functional hyperprolactinemia and micro-prolactinomas[3-6]. We studied the efficacy and safety of DHEC in a group of patients with functional hyperprolactinemia and microadenoma.

MATERIALS AND METHODS

Twenty hyperprolactinemic women aged 18–42 years with serum PRL levels ranging between 31 and 218 ng/ml were included in the study, seven presenting hypo-oligomenorrhea, 13 amenorrhea, three cases showed also galactorrhea. In two patients nuclear magnetic resonance showed hypophyseal microadenoma.

They were previously tested with oral acute administration of 5 mg DHEC and blood samples were collected every 15 min during the first 90 min and after 2, 3, 4, 6, 8, 24 and 48 h. During the test blood pressure and side-effects were evaluated.

All patients were treated with oral administration of 5–10 mg daily of DHEC. After 3 months of therapy a second acute test with DHEC was performed. The samples were collected at −15, 0 and after 120, 180, 240 min from oral administration of 5 mg of DHEC.

Every month clinical evaluation, menses and side-effects were recorded. Statistical analysis was performed with ANOVA.

RESULTS

The serum PRL response to acute administration of 5 mg of DHEC is shown in Figure 1. In 18 patients with functional hyperprolactinemia and in one with microprolactinoma we observed a decrease of PRL level from 59.3 ± 9.3 ng/ml to 19.5 ± 4.9 ng/ml after 6 h. The percentage of decrease was 74.5 ± 4.1%. One patient with microprolactinoma was less sensitive (PRL level from 125 to 90 ng/ml). The nadir of PRL decrease was observed 6 h from oral administration of DHEC. During the acute test no modification of blood pressure was observed in 19 of the 20 patients. In the other one the test was stopped after 30 min because of severe hypotension. Mild nausea and cephalalgia were referred by four patients.

Chronic treatment with 5–10 mg daily of DHEC induced a normalization of PRL plasma levels in 17 of 20 patients (18.5 ± 3.5 ng/ml) after 3 months as shown in Figure 2. Three patients did not undergo chronic treatment: one for the mentioned hypotension attack during acute administration, another for weight increase and the last one for reasons not related to the drug (facial hemiparesis). Galactorrhea disappeared in all three patients who

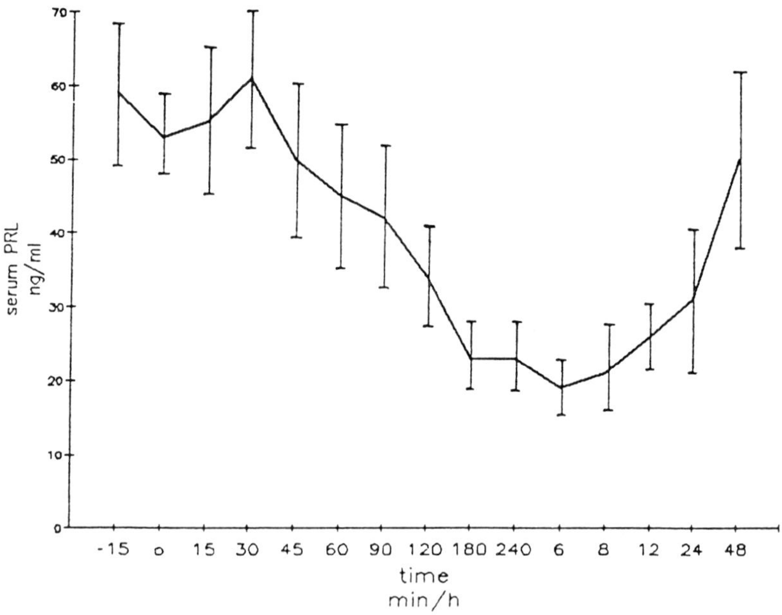

Figure 1 Prolactin plasma level response to acute administration of dihydroergocriptine (5 mg *per os*)

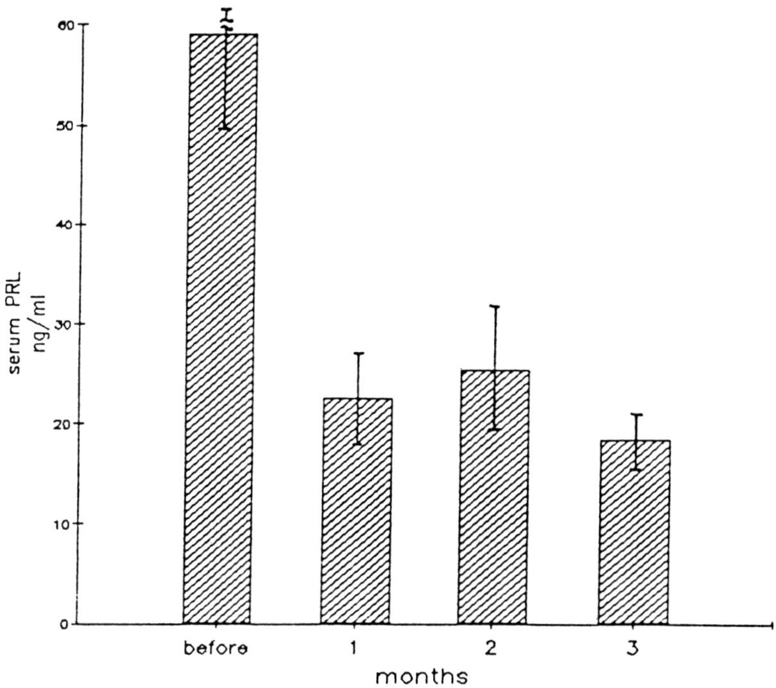

Figure 2 Prolactin plasma level during chronic treatment with dihydroergocriptine (5–10 mg *per os*)

presented this symptom. All women, including the ones with microprolactinoma and supranormal plasma PRL level resumed regular menses and ovulatory cycles.

The acute test performed during chronic treatment showed a decrease of PRL level from 20 ± 4.3 ng/ml to 8.9 ± 3.7 ng/ml (Figure 3).

Chronic treatment did not modify blood pressure values. No side-effects were observed during treatment and mild nausea and cephalalgia initially referred disappeared after a few days (5–10 days) of daily administration of DHEC (Figure 4).

DISCUSSION

Our data, in agreement with some previous reports[6–10] demonstrate that DHEC is a potent and long lasting dopaminergic agent in lowering PRL plasma level. In fact during the acute test the normalization of PRL levels remained for 12–24 h. The effectiveness of DHEC is demonstrated not only by normalization of PRL levels during chronic treatment but also by the excellent clinical effects. All patients resumed regular ovulatory cycles.

The relatively short time of observation does not let us know about the effect of DHEC on size of microprolactinoma: Faglia and co-workers showed a reduction of tumor size with this treatment[6]. In our experience DHEC

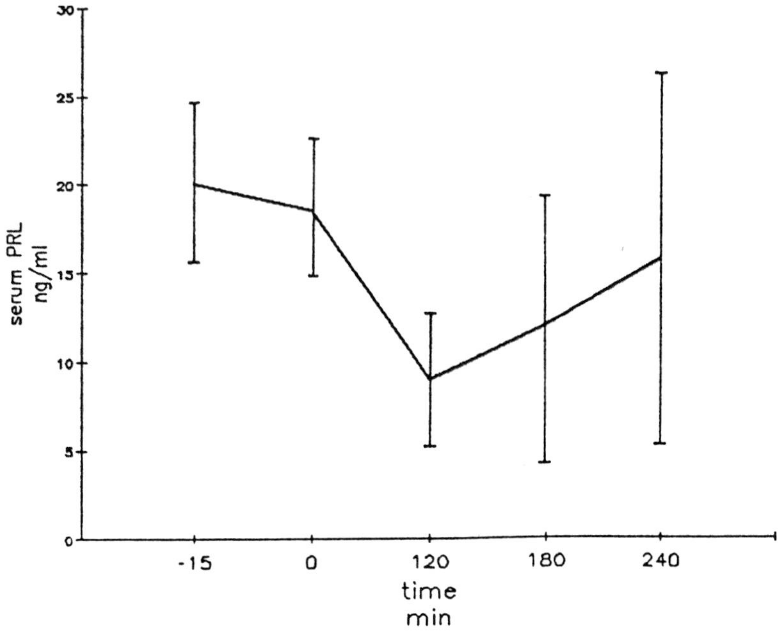

Figure 3 Acute test with dihydroergocriptine during chronic treatment

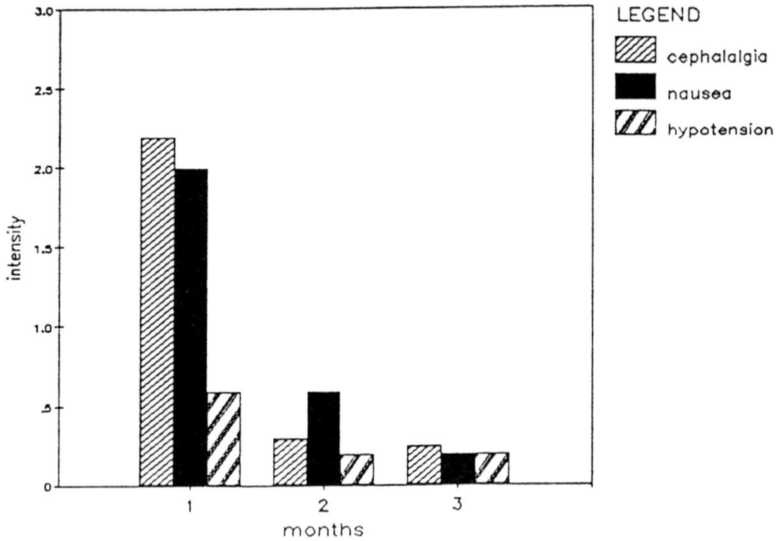

Figure 4 Side-effects during chronic treatment

was very well tolerated without side-effects. Particularly hypotension, nausea, vomiting which are sometimes present during treatment with other dopamine agonists such as bromocriptine, were not observed in our experience. In conclusion DHEC appears to be an effective and well tolerated PRL-lowering drug. It seems effective like other dopamine agonist agents, but without side-effects. Our experience suggests that this is a first choice drug in treating patients with functional hyperprolactinemia and particularly in the patients who tolerate other dopamine agonist drugs badly.

REFERENCES

1. Caron, M.G., Beaulieu, M., Raymond, V., Gagnè, B., Drouin, J., Lefkowitz, R.J. and Labrie, F. (1978). Dopaminergic receptor in the anterior pituitary gland. Correlation of (^{3}H)-dihydroergokryptine binding with the dopaminergic control of prolactin release. *J. Biol. Chem.*, **253**, 2244–53
2. Libertun, C., Larrea, G.A., Vacas, M. I. and Cardinali, D.P. (1980). (^{3}H)-dihydroergokryptine binding in the anterior pituitary and prolactin secretion: further evidence of brain regulation adenohypophyseal receptors. *Endocrinology*, **107**, 1905–9
3. Fluckinger, E. and Del Pozo, E. (1980). Ergot derivatives and pituitary hormones. In Muller, E. E. (ed.) *Neuroactive Drugs in Endocrinology*, pp. 169–90. (Amsterdam: Elsevier North Holland Biomedical Press)
4. Poli, M., Vitali, B., Citella, C., Casati, R., Platti, P.M. and Monti, L.D. (1983). Effect of different hydrogenated ergot-alcaloid on cimetidine-induced prolactin secretion in the normal man. *J. Endocrinol. Invest.*, **6** (suppl 1), 32
5. Poli, M., Cocchi, D., Mailland, F., Masu, A.M., Landi, G., Craveri, E. and Muller, E.E. (1986). Prolactin lowering effect of dihydroergokryptine in rat and in man. *J. Endocrinol. Invest.*, **9**, 31
6. Faglia, G., Conti, A., Muratori, M., Togni, E., Travaglini, P., Zanotti, A. and Mailland, F. (1987). Dihydroergokryptine in management of microprolactinomas. *J. Clin. Endocrinol. Metab.*, **4**, 779–84
7. Ferrari, C., Rampini, P., Paracchi, A., Boghen, M. and Mailland, F. (1985). Effect of dihydroergokryptine administration on serum prolactin and growth hormone levels in normal, hyperprolactinemic and acromegalic subjects: evidence of potent and long-lasting pituitary dopamine receptor stimulation. *Eur. J. Clin. Pharmacol.*, **27**, 707–11
8. Poli, M., Landi, G., Masu, A.M., Savi, B., Mailland, F., Del Rosso, R., Barbesti, S. and Craveri, A. (1985). Dihydroergokryptine: effect of a single oral dose on serum prolactin and catecholamines. *J. Endocrinol. Invest.*, **8**, (Suppl 3)
9. Canonico, P.L. (1987). Diidroergocriptina e meccanismi di trasduzione ipofisari. In Crosignani, P.G. *et al.* (eds). *Prolattina 1987*, (Bologna: Monduzzi)
10. Cavioni, V., Mattei, A.M., Zanotti, A., Spellecchia, D. and Crosignani, P.G. (1987). Terapia degli stati iperprolattinemici e inibizione della lattazione con diidroergocriptina. In Crosignani, P.G. *et al.* (eds). *Prolattina 1987*, (Bologna: Monduzzi)

77

Prolactin-lowering effect of dihydroergocriptine in idiopathic hyperprolactinemia

C. Nappi, G. Colace, P. Affinito, E. T. Goglia, C. Salemme and U. Montemagno

INTRODUCTION

Hyperprolactinemia is a common clinical disorder that has been found in up to 25% of patients with secondary amenorrhea[1,2].

The term of idiopathic hyperprolactinemia indicates the presence of elevated serum prolactin (PRL) levels in the absence of any demonstrable pituitary or central nervous system disease and of any other recognized cause of increased PRL secretion.

Hydrogenated derivatives of natural ergot alkaloids are a well known class of compounds with high affinity for adrenergic, dopaminergic and serotoninergic receptors[3]. In particular, dihydroergocriptine (DHEC) is a C9–C10 hydrogenated alkaloid of the ergot with dopaminergic agonist and α-adrenergic antagonist properties[4]. Indeed, it has recently been demonstrated to suppress PRL release from the pituitary in both *in vitro* and *in vivo* studies[5–7]. Moreover, there is evidence that the PRL-lowering activity of the drug is due to a stimulation of D-2 receptors in hypophyseal mammotropes[3,8].

The aim of the present study was to evaluate the ability of DHEC to normalize serum PRL levels in hyperprolactinemic patients and to lead to the resumption of normal menstrual cycles and ovulation.

MATERIALS AND METHODS

After giving informed consent, six oligoamenorrheic women aged 27–38 years (mean 31.4 years) with serum PRL levels ranging from 53 to 190 ng/ml (mean 111.5 ± 20.9) were admitted to the study. All were in good health with no evidence of cardiovascular, renal, hepatic and other endocrine diseases. High resolution computed tomographic scan (coronal and axial section) of the pituitary fossa did not show evidence of micro- or macroprolactinoma.

In two patients, previous bromocriptine treatment had resulted in severe side-effects leading to discontinuation of the therapy after 2 months.

No other drug was administered during the 6 months before the beginning of this therapy.

The patients were treated with DHEC (Poli, Milan, Italy) for 6 months.

Chronic treatment was preceded by an acute administration test with 5 mg of DHEC in which serum PRL levels were measured 15 min before and 0, 1, 2, 3 and 4 h after drug administration.

The treatment was started with an oral daily dose of 10 mg of DHEC for 2 days. The dose was then gradually increased to 30 mg daily (10 mg × 3/day) during the first week of treatment.

Serum PRL determinations were performed 1 week after the beginning of therapy and then monthly during treatment. Serum progesterone (P) levels were evaluated 21 days after the onset of menses and then in the 21st day of each menstrual cycle. PRL levels were also evaluated 1 month after discontinuation of DHEC.

Blood samples were withdrawn from each patient through an indwelling venous catheter placed in the antecubital vein of the forearm. Serum PRL and P levels were analyzed by a sensitive double antibody radioimmunoassay commercial kit (Biodata, Milan, Italy).

Serum PRL levels were expressed as per cent variations from the baseline values.

Statistical evaluation of data was performed by analysis of variance (ANOVA) followed by Newman–Keul's test.

Pharmacological safety and tolerability of DHEC were evaluated by blood pressure and pulse rate determinations and on the basis of the symptoms referred to by the patients.

RESULTS

The effect of the acute administration of 5 mg of DHEC on serum PRL levels in idiopathic hyperprolactinemic women is shown in Figure 1. A swift inhibition of PRL levels is evident. The decrease was significant ($p < 0.01$)

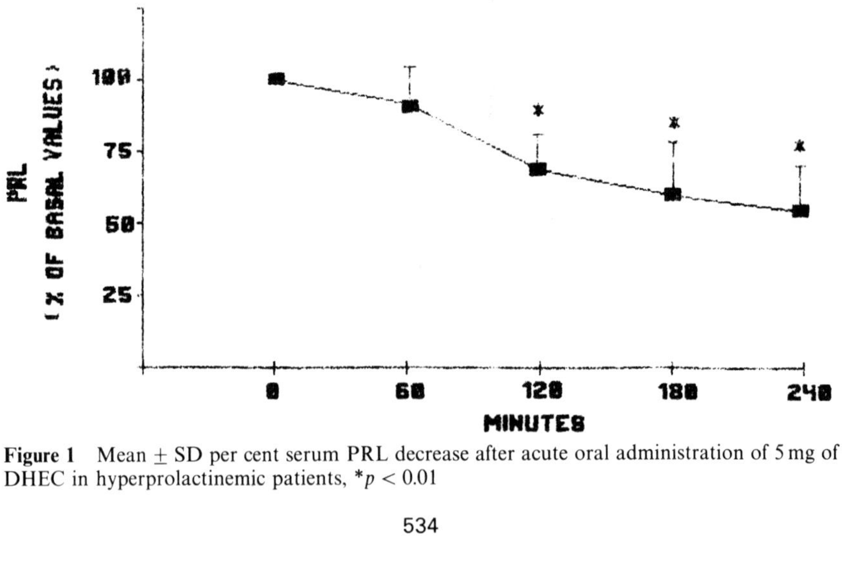

Figure 1 Mean ± SD per cent serum PRL decrease after acute oral administration of 5 mg of DHEC in hyperprolactinemic patients, $*p < 0.01$

120, 180 and 240 min after the administration of the drug. However, in no patient did PRL levels reach the range of normal values.

The results of chronic treatment with DHEC are shown in Figure 2. After the 1st week of treatment, all patients showed normal PRL levels which remained in the normal range for the whole period of therapy. One month after discontinuation of DHEC, in all patients, except one of them who presented a normal PRL value, PRL levels were above normal values but were still significantly ($p < 0.01$) lower than the pretreatment values (47.8% of decrease of PRL).

Resumption of regular menstrual cycles was observed 4–8 weeks after the beginning of treatment.

All the patients presented onset of ovulatory cycles within the 10th week of treatment, as confirmed by the serum P levels.

Disappearance of galactorrhea was observed in all patients after 12–20 days of treatment. One patient became pregnant during the sixth month of therapy. The pregnancy had a normal evolution, with spontaneous delivery at term of a healthy baby.

During treatment patients did not present nausea, vomiting, dizziness, postural hypotension, or pulse frequency changes.

DISCUSSION

The role of dopaminergic drugs in the management of hyperprolactinemic disorders has been well documented[9]. At present, bromocriptine is the most widely used dopaminergic agonist in the treatment of this condition. A low dose of bromocriptine (2.5 mg/day), restores normal PRL levels in 60% of hyperprolactinemic patients. Higher doses are able to normalize PRL levels in 95% of patients[10], but frequently induced adverse side-effects such as

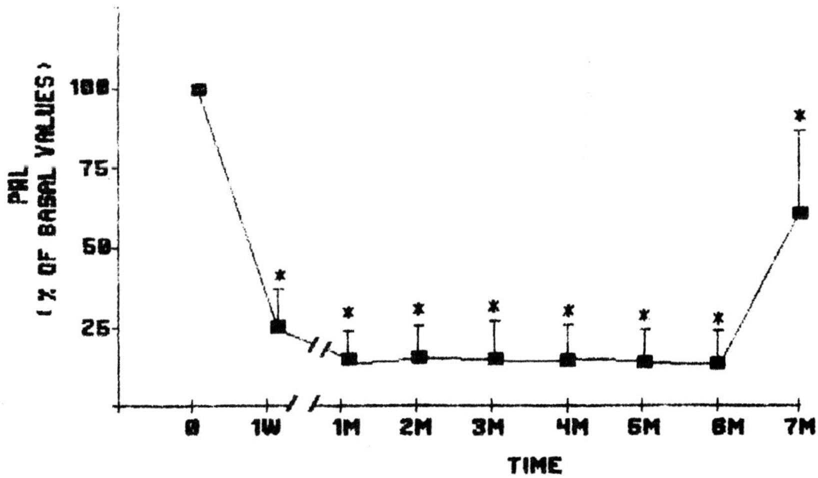

Figure 2 Effects of chronic oral administration DHEC in hyperprolactinemic patients. Data are mean ± SD per cent variations from baseline values, $*p < 0.01$

postural hypotension, dizziness, nausea, vomiting and gallbladder irritability[11]. These adverse reactions may also lead the patients to stop the medication.

Our findings confirm the results of other authors[6,12] showing a marked and prolonged PRL-lowering effect of DHEC in hyperprolactinemic patients.

The swift decrease of PRL levels after the acute administration of 5 mg of DHEC, demonstrates the effectiveness of DHEC in lowering PRL levels also when administered at the dose of 5 mg.

Serum PRL determinations 30 days after DHEC withdrawal showed persistence of its PRL-lowering effect, demonstrating that DHEC has a long duration of action.

It must be pointed out that DHEC administration did not produce any of the side-effects which are characteristic of other dopaminergic compounds. The lack of adverse reactions to DHEC confirms that the effects of this drug on anterior pituitary dopamine receptors may be divorced from those on the cardiovascular and gastrointestinal systems[7].

In summary, DHEC, due to its marked and prolonged PRL inhibitory effect and absence of side-effects, represents an effective and safe drug for long-term treatment of hyperprolactinemic states.

REFERENCES

1. Pepperel, R.J. (1981). Prolactin and reproduction. *Fertil. Steril.*, **35**, 267
2. Tolis, G., Bertrand, G. and Kinch, R. (1983). Hyperprolactinemia: Diagnostic and therapeutic considerations. In Tolis, G. *et al.* (eds). *Prolactin and Prolactinomas*, p. 351. (New York: Raven Press)
3. Fiore, L., Scapagnini, U. and Canonico, P.L. (1987). Effect of Dihydroergokryptine and Dihydroergocristine on cyclic AMP accumulation and prolactin release *in vitro*: evidence for a dopaminomimetic action. *Hormone Res.*, **25**, 171
4. Cronin, M.J., Roberts, J.M. and Weiner, R.I. (1978). Dopamine and dihydroergokryptine binding to the anterior pituitary and other brain areas of the rat and sheep. *Endocrinology*, **103**, 302
5. Caron, M.G., Beaulieum, M., Raymond, V., Gagne, B., Drouin, J., Lefkowitz, R.J. and Labrie, F. (1978). Dopaminergic receptors in the anterior pituitary gland. Correlation of ^{3}[H]dihydroergokryptine binding with the dopaminergic control of prolactin release. *J. Biol. Chem.*, **253**, 2244
6. Fluckiger, E. and Del Pozo, E. (1980). Ergot derivates and pituitary hormones. In Muller, E.E. (ed.). *Neuroactive Drugs in Endocrinology*, p. 169. (Amsterdam: Elsevier/North Holland Biomedical Press)
7. Poli, M., Cocchi, D., Mailland, F., Masu, A.M., Landi, G., Craveri, A. and Muller, E.E. (1986). Prolactin lowering effect of dihydroergokryptine in rat and in man. *J. Endocrinol. Invest.*, **9**, 31
8. Sibley, D.R. and Creese, I. (1983). Interactions of ergot alkaloids with anterior pituitary D2 dopamine receptors. *Mol. Pharmacol.*, **23**, 585
9. Ferrari, C. and Crosignani, P.G. (1986). Review: medical treatment of hyperprolactinaemic disorders. *Hum. Reprod.*, **7**, 507
10. Crosignani, P.G. (1982). Treatment of hyperprolactinemic states with different drugs: a study with bromocriptine, metergoline, and lisuride. *Fertil. Steril.*, **37**, 61
11. Barbieri, R.L. and Ryan, K.S. (1983). Bromocriptine: endocrine pharmacology and therapeutic applications. *Fertil. Steril.*, **39**, 727
12. Ferrari, C., Rampini, P., Paracchi, A., Boghen, M. and Mailland, F. (1985). Effect of dihydroergokryptine administration on serum prolactin and growth hormone levels in normal, hyperprolactinaemic and acromegalic subjects: evidence of potent and long-lasting pituitary dopamine receptors stimulation. *Eur. J. Clin. Pharmacol.*, **27**, 707

Section 4 continued

Part D

Polycystic ovarian syndrome

78

Polycystic ovarian syndrome and adolescence

S. Venturoli, E. Porcu and R. Fabbri

INTRODUCTION

Compared to the first clear cut description, the polycystic ovarian syndrome (PCOS) has become progressively less strictly defined in the past few years. Therefore it is worthwhile to summarize briefly the main elements characterizing the syndrome.

The primary pathophysiological structure consists of the chronic, persistent presence of increased luteinizing hormone (LH) levels with an LH/FSH (follicle-stimulating hormone) ratio greater than three, ovarian hyperandrogenism with relative hyperestrogenism and enlarged polycystic ovaries. The clinical expression of this endocrine structure, such as hirsutism, obesity, hyperinsulinism, acanthosis, are not such crucial elements in defining the syndrome, since they may or may not be present, with wide individual variation, in the number and severity of the symptoms. There is a general agreement on the pubertal onset of PCOS and each author dealing with this syndrome mentions that it originates in adolescence. However, apart from out-of-date overstated hypothesis, acceptable research documenting the first adolescent steps of PCOS is not yet available.

The key questions still arising concern the exact contours of the syndrome in adolescence, the type of pubertal program derangement leading to PCOS, the time of its first appearance and how early a diagnosis can be formulated. In an attempt to answer these questions we planned an experimental design with the aim to identify each of the primary PCOS characteristics in normal adolescents as early as possible.

ANOVULATION

Anovulation is one of the most common features of the developing reproductive system. Thus, it cannot be assumed to have the same meaning as in PCOS. However, we decided to address our investigation precisely in this direction, because of the immaturity of anovulatory adolescents. To our mind, this condition should be the most faithful mirror of the developing reproductive function, including both normal or potentially disordered evolutive patterns.

LH SECRETION

Our first and perhaps most surprising finding was the high percentage (30%) of anovulatory adolescents showing LH levels above the upper normal level[1]. The mean LH levels of these subjects were strikingly similar to that found in our PCOS population (Table 1). Underlying this quantitative similarity in LH secretion we discovered qualitative similarities between adolescent and PCOS LH release. In fact, the pulsatile pattern of anovulatory adolescents with high LH resembles that found in PCOS (Figure 1), both showing

Table 1 Basal plasma steroid, ovarian volume, pulsatile characteristics of LH (values over a period of 8 h) (mean ± SD) and highest levels in 24 h (time of day) in PCOS and in adolescents with high mean plasma levels

	PCOS	*High LH (adolescents)*
Luteinizing hormone (IU/l)	31 ± 9	30 ± 4
Follicle-stimulating hormone(IU/l)	9 ± 3	8 ± 1
Estradiol (pg/ml)	49 ± 26	36 ± 9
Estrone (pg/ml)	48 ± 16	31 ± 6
Androstenedione (ng/dl)	281 ± 112	275 ± 91
Testosterone (ng/dl)	62 ± 32	64 ± 17
Dihydrotestosterone (ng/dl)	23 ± 9	21 ± 6
Dehydroepiandrosterone sulfate (μg/ml)	3.1 ± 1	2.1 ± 0.7
Luteinizing hormone		
Interpulse (min)	62 ± 11	57 ± 8
Amplitude (IU/l)	12 ± 4	12 ± 4
Highest levels (time)	17.20	17.41
Ovarian volume (cm^3)	13.6 ± 5	11.6 ± 5

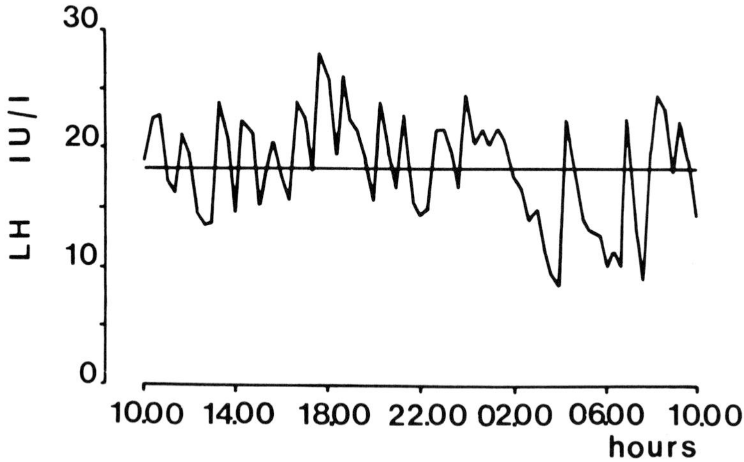

Figure 1 Twenty-four hour profile of luteinizing hormone (LH) secretion in one subject with PCOS. The line indicates the 24 h mean LH value

increased LH pulse amplitude and both being significantly higher than that of normal adolescent and adult controls. No significant differences were seen in pulse frequency between groups though higher values of this parameter are not uncommon in subjects with high LH levels.

A further similarity between PCOS and adolescents was found when evaluating the LH circadian secretion. In a previous paper we described the 24 h LH variations in PCOS[2] and in anovulatory adolescents[3] and the comparison shows that both groups reach the highest circadian production in the afternoon. However, the same is not true for diurnal variations in pulse frequency.

In fact, while PCOS subjects show a nocturnal slowing in pulse frequency very similar to that of adults[2], no circadian variation in the number of pulses can be detected in adolescents. This is probably because of a still persistent neuroendocrine immaturity of these young girls[3].

OVARIAN STEROID SECRETION

Bearing in mind the striking similarity in gonadotropin release between PCOS and a considerable number of anovulatory adolescents, we evaluated the ovarian response to the peculiar gonadotropin condition, discovering a precise relationship linking LH pulse frequency and amplitude and steroid levels in adolescence[4]. In particular, a positive correlation was found between pulse amplitude and levels on the one hand and between pulse frequency and androgen values on the other. Increased androgen levels (testosterone and androstenedione) are present in about 30% of anovulatory adolescents[1] thus demonstrating that a hyperandrogenic condition is quite common at this age. By comparing this endocrine condition with that found in PCOS, we found mean levels of testosterone, dihydrotestosterone and androstenedione almost identical and both significantly higher than those of controls (Figure 2).

A certain degree of relative hyperestrogenism, similar to that of PCOS, is present in adolescents, although to a lesser extent. A reason for this quantitative difference can be found in the higher body mass index of PCOS, whose adipose tissue contributes to estrogenic production.

Dehydroepiandrosterone sulfate (DHEAS) levels appear significantly higher in PCOS and in normal controls than in adolescents (Figure 3). The young chronological age of these girls (16 yr) partly explains this, considering that DHEAS levels progressively increase up to the age of 25. This finding cannot exclude a subsequent DHEAS overproduction in these anovulatory adolescents. Nevertheless it does not confirm the hypothesis of an early adrenal involvement at the root of anovulation and possibly of PCOS.

OVARIAN ASPECTS

Our data on the adolescent ovarian aspects[1,5–9] allow us to affirm that the adolescent, i.e. developmental, ovary is in itself polycystic. This is not a

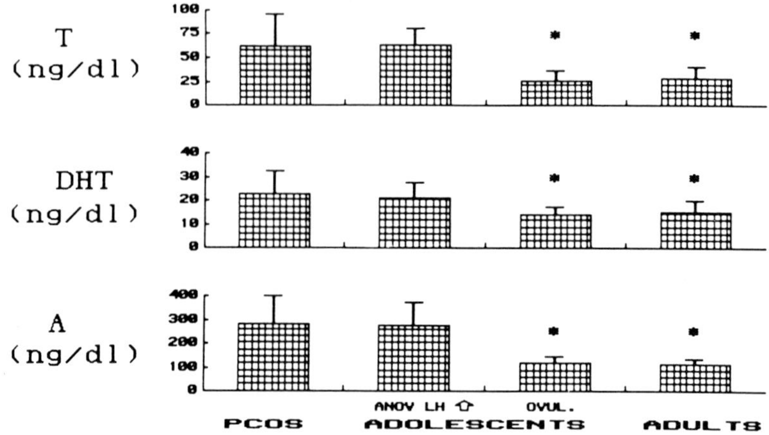

Figure 2 Baseline plasma testosterone (T), 5α-dihydrotestosterone (DHT) and androstenedione (A) values (mean ± SD) of PCOS, anovulatory adolescent with high mean plasma luteinizing hormone (LH) levels, ovulatory adolescent and adult subjects, $*p < 0.05$

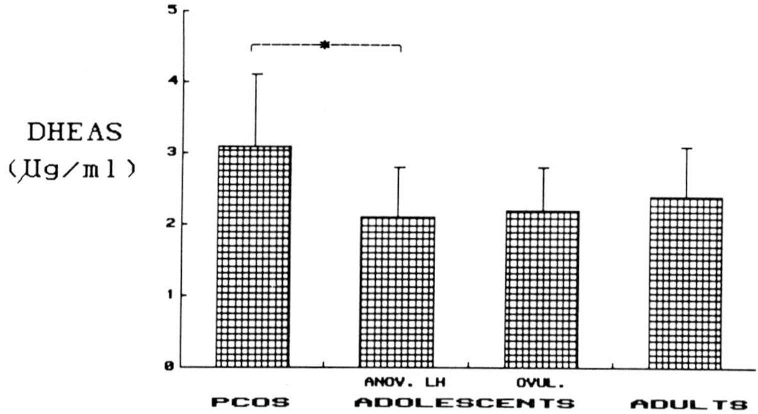

Figure 3 Baseline plasma dehydroepiandrosterone sulfate (DHEAS) values (mean ± SD) of PCOS, anovulatory adolescent with high mean plasma luteinizing hormone (LH) levels, ovulatory adolescent and adult subject, $*p < 0.05$

pathological structure but rather a morphological base waiting for endocrine metabolic events which will decide its final aspect.

The anatomical and histological description of Merril[10] and Peters[11] established that features identical to those found in the PCOS, such as multiple follicles, cystic and atresic follicles, techa hyperplasia and luteinization are common findings in the adolescent ovary. Yet in our investigation we planned to verify this issue in a large number of girls and with a non-invasive technique such as sonographic examinations.

We compared adolescent ovaries with those of adult controls and PCOS. Both PCOS and adolescent ovaries have a greater ovarian volume with respect to adult controls (Figure 4). However, patients with PCOS show

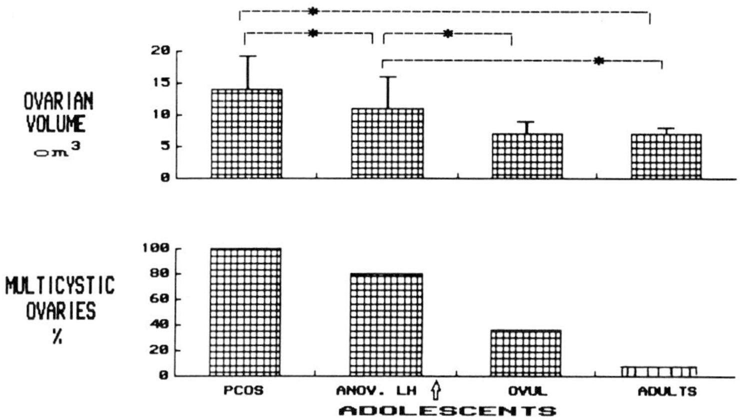

Figure 4 Baseline ovarian characteristics, volume (mean ± SD) and percentage of multicystic ovaries of PCOS, anovulatory adolescent with high mean plasma luteinizing hormone (LH) levels, ovulatory adolescent and adult subjects, $*p < 0.05$

much more enlarged ovaries compared to adolescents with high LH levels, showing that at least a quantitative difference still exists between the two conditions. While all PCOS patients obviously have polycystic ovaries, only 80% of anovulatory adolescents show this structure. Otherwise this percentage is significantly higher than that of controls.

ANALOGIES AND CONTRASTS

The results of our comparison established that crucial pathophysiological aspects such as enhanced LH secretion and hyperandrogenism are shared by both PCOS and anovulatory adolescents. Contrasts are mostly present in secondary aspects, mainly related to the young chronological age, as for example the lower DHEAS levels or the absence of the LH nocturnal slowing in adolescents; or the different body mass index, as for estrone levels; or the longer lasting ovarian effects of the irregular LH secretion, being responsible for the higher ovarian volume and percentage of polycystic structure in PCOS.

ADOLESCENT PCOS: WHAT IS IT?

Despite the impressive coincidence of the most important features in both anovulatory adolescent and PCOS, are we really allowed to classify these girls as PCOS? As much as these girls are adolescents, they cannot be called PCOS in our opinion.

PCOS-like endocrine features in adolescence belong to an endocrine and ovarian functional pathway showing, unlike PCOS, a great plasticity during the developmental period and eventually leading to normal maturity in some subjects. Our longitudinal study is progressively documenting the spontaneous normalization of all the parameters we described, along with the increase of ovulatory frequency. Although conclusive data are not yet available, some individual improvement of both the LH pattern and the ovarian aspect in late adolescence convinced us that PCOS is not PCOS before adult age.

On the other hand the persistence of the PCOS features beyond adolescence probably indicates the irreversible establishment of a disordered endocrine pathway. However, unfortunately, a meaningful biological marker discriminating adolescence from adulthood is still unknown.

REFERENCES

1. Venturoli, S., Porcu, E., Fabbri, R. *et al.* (1986). Menstrual irregularities in adolescents: hormonal pattern and ovarian morphology. *Horm. Res.*, **24**, 269
2. Venturoli, S., Porcu, E., Fabbri, R. *et al.* (1988). Episodic pulsatile secretion of FSH, LH, Prolactin, Oestradiol, Oestrone and LH circadian variations in polycystic ovary syndrome. *Clin. Endocrinol.*, **29**, 93
3. Porcu, E., Venturoli, S., Magrini, O., *et al.* (1987). Circadian variations of luteinizing hormone can have two different profiles in adolescent anovulation. *J. Clin. Endocrinol. Metab.*, **65**, 488
4. Venturoli, S., Porcu, E., Gammi, L. *et al.* (1987). Different gonadotropin pulsatile fashions in anovulatory cycles of young girls indicate different maturational pathways in adolescence. *J. Clin. Endocrinol. Metab.*, **65**, 785
5. Venturoli, S., Porcu, E., Fabbri, R. *et al.* (1983). Ovarian volume and aspects in adolescent menstrual cycles. *Acta Endocrinol. Suppl.*, **256**, 261
6. Venturoli, S., Porcu, E., Fabbri, R. *et al.* (1984). Ovaries and menstrual cycles in Adolescence. *Gynecol. Obstet. Invest.*, **17**, 219
7. Venturoli, S., Porcu, E., Fabbri, R. *et al.* (1986). Ovarian multifollicularity, high LH and androgen plasma levels, and anovulation are frequent and strongly linked in adolescent irregular cycles. *Acta Endocrinol.*, **11**, 368
8. Venturoli, S., Porcu, E., Fabbri, R. *et al.* (1987). Post menarchal evolution of endocrine pattern and ovarian aspects in adolescents with menstrual irregularities. *Fertil. Steril.*, **48**, 1
9. Porcu, E., Venturoli, S. and Flamigni, C. (1987). Multifollicular ovaries in post-puberty. In Massi, G.B. and Bruni, V. (eds) *Pediatric and Adolescent Gynecology*, p. 423 (Rome: CIC Edizioni Internazionali)
10. Merril, J.A. (1961). The morphology of the prepubertal ovary. *South. Med. J.*, **56**, 225
11. Peters, H., Byskov, A.G., Himelstein-Braw, R. *et al.* (1975). Follicular growth: the basic event in the mouse and human ovary. *J. Reprod. Fertil.*, **45**, 559

79

Endocrine and metabolic aspects of polycystic ovarian disease

A. Lanzone, A.M. Fulghesu, C.L. Andreani, R. Muscatello, M. Le Donne, M. Palermo, A. Caruso and S. Mancuso

INTRODUCTION

Hyperinsulinemia and insulin resistance in patients with polycystic ovarian disease (PCOD) has been well documented[1-3].

In these women hyperinsulinemia and hyperandrogenism are positively correlated, but the mechanisms underlying this relationship are still not clarified. Several authors[4-8] speculated that hyperandrogenism could be a primary event leading to hyperinsulinism and insulin resistance; whereas other investigators suggested that insulin resistance may be partially responsible for the excessive androgen production[9,10].

Obesity is frequently a characteristic of patients with PCOD[4] and this condition is often associated with the alteration of insulin secretion[11]. Therefore obese and not obese patients with PCOD were studied in order to investigate the insulin response to oral glucose tolerance test (OGTT) and the effect of hyperinsulinism on ovarian androgen levels.

MATERIALS AND METHODS

Thirty-eight women were studied. They were aged 20–38 years, in good health, not diabetic, euthyroid, and none had taken medications known to affect plasma sex steroid levels or carbohydrate metabolism for at least 3 months before the study. PCO was diagnosed by ultrasound, laparoscopy and endocrine pattern as previously described[12]. Obesity was defined as a weight of 120% or more of the ideal body weight (IBW) according to Lorentz's criteria[13].

Nine non-obese and 12 obese PCOD women were selected for the study. All had experienced the spontaneous onset of puberty and normal sexual development and all had had irregular menses since puberty (oligomenorrhea with intervals of 40–90 days) associated with chronic anovulation. Seven obese and 10 not obese normal women with regular menses of similar age and weight as the two PCOD groups were also studied. Their ovulatory cycles were documented by a biphasic pattern of basal body temperature and by appropriate plasma progesterone (P) levels at midluteal phase of the cycle (at least 8 ng/ml) for three consecutive cycles.

All studies were performed in the mid-follicular phase on cycle days 5–10 after spontaneous or progestin-induced menses.

All women had an OGTT with 75 g glucose load performed at 07:00 after eating a standard diet (300 g carbohydrate) for 3 days and fasting overnight for 10–12 h. Informed consent was obtained from each patient.

Blood was sampled through an indwelling i.v. catheter at −15, 0, 30, 60, 90, 120, 150, 180 and 240 min of the glucose ingestion. At time 0 of an OGTT plasma LH, FSH, prolactin, estradiol (E_2), testosterone (T), androstenedione (A), dehydroepiandrosterone sulfate (DHEAS), insulin (I), cortisol (F) were measured. In all plasma samples of OGTT E_2, T, A, and I, were also measured. Serum glucose levels were determined by the glucose oxidase method. Statistical analysis was performed by paired and unpaired Student's *t* test for the comparison within groups or between two groups, respectively and by analysis of variance for the multiple comparisons.

RESULTS

Table 1 shows the ages, % of IBW, degree of hirsutism and fasting glucose levels for the PCOD women compared to those of the control groups. The ages of the four groups did not differ. The %IBW were similar in both obese groups and in both not obese groups. Hirsutism was similar in the two PCOD groups and was greater than the respective controls. In Table 2 the mean ± SD plasma hormone levels at time of OGTT was indicated.

Polycystic ovarian disease patients showed higher basal values of androgens in respect to control subjects. All patients showed normal fasting glycemic values, and no differences were found between the groups. All patients also showed a normal glycemic response to OGTT (Table 3).

Table 3 shows the mean fasting plasma I levels and values under curve (AUC) in the four groups studied. These two parameters were significantly greater in the obese PCOD women than in the not obese PCOD women,

Table 1 Clinical features of PCOD and controls (mean ± SD)

Patient	*Age*	*% of IBW*	*Hirsutism score*	*Fasting glucose levels* (ng/ml)
PCOD not obese (*n* = 12)	4.3 ± 4.4 (21–36)	101 ± 9	8.7 ± 3.2	85 ± 6
PCOD obese (*n* = 9)	27.1 ± 5.2 (20–34)	142 ± 11	10.2 ± 7.7	86 ± 6
Controls not obese (*n* = 10)	29.8 ± 5.2 (28–38)	98 ± 9	2.5 ± 4.9*††	80 ± 7
Controls obese (*n* = 7)	30.6 ± 5.5 (24–36)	128 ± 9	2.8 ± 1.9*††	80 ± 15

*$p < 0.05$ PCOD obese vs: controls not obese, controls obese
††$p < 0.01$ PCOD not obese vs: controls not obese, controls obese

Table 2 Hormone levels at time of OGTT (mean ± SD)

	Basal			
	PCOD		*Controls*	
	not obese (12)	*obese* (9)	*not obese* (10)	*obese* (7)
LH (mIU/ml)	20.2 ± 8.0	18.9 ± 9.0	14.3 ± 4.8	12.3 ± 5.0†
FSH (mIU/ml)	9.2 ± 3.3	8.0 ± 2.0	10.0 ± 2.7	9.0 ± 1.0
PRL (ng/ml)	11.9 ± 2.3**	15.8 ± 1.7	9.9 ± 3.1**	12.5 ± 4.0*
E_2 (pg/ml)	64.2 ± 15.8	51.0 ± 10.0	68.5 ± 43.2	69.0 ± 43.0
A (ng/ml)	2.4 ± 1.0	1.9 ± 0.8	0.9† ± 0.6*††	0.8 ± 0.3**††
T (ng/ml)	0.5 ± 0.3	0.9 ± 0.5	0.4 ± 0.3*†	0.3 ± 0.0**††
F (ng/ml)	145.3 ± 87	144.1 ± 32	138 ± 37	141.6 ± 7.63
DHEAS (μg/ml)	1.6 ± 1.10	1.41 ± 0.76	1.23 ± 0.9	1.8 ± 0.87

*$p < 0.05$, **$p < 0.01$ PCOD obese vs: PCOD not obese, controls obese, controls not obese
†$p < 0.05$, ††$p < 0.01$ PCOD not obese vs: controls obese, controls not obese

Table 3 Response to OGTT (mean ± SD)

	PCOD		*Controls*	
	not obese (12)	*obese* (9)	*not obese* (10)	*obese* (7)
Glucose peak (mIU/ml)	140.6 ± 28	140.8 ± 31.3	132.5 ± 12.5	145.9 ± 25.3
AUC insulin (mIU/ml)	7267 ± 3128	15 632 ± 6879	4102 ± 883	8529 ± 3824
Insulin (μIU/ml)	11.2 ± 3.3**	15.5 ± 4.7	6.8 ± 1.7**†	9.8 ± 5.9

*$p < 0.05$, **$p < 0.01$ PCOD obese vs: PCOD not obese, controls obese, controls not obese
†$p < 0.05$ PCOD not obese vs: controls obese, controls not obese

the obese and the not obese normal women. Furthermore all PCOD patients showed significantly higher fasting and AUC values of I in respect to all control patients (PCOD patients: I 12.6 ± 5.2 μIU/ml, AUC: 11 226 ± 7442 μIU/ml/240 min control patients; 8.3 ± 4.4 μIU/ml $p < 0.05$, AUC: 6146 ± 3353 μIU/ml/240 min $p < 0.05$).

Hyperinsulinemic responses were eight of nine (89%) in PCOD obese, three of 12 (25%) in PCOD not obese and two of seven (29%) in control obese patients. During OGTT, ovarian steroids remained unchanged in both PCOD and control groups.

Significantly high positive correlation was seen between fasting and AUC I values ($r = 0.58$; $p < 0.01$) and between IBW and plasma fasting I and

AUC I ($r = 0.48$; $p < 0.01$; $r = 0.34$; $p < 0.05$); T and A basal values were also significantly correlated with AUC of I ($r = 0.50$; $p < 0.01$; $r = 0.49$; $p < 0.01$).

DISCUSSION

It is well known that PCOD patients were characterized by hyperandrogenism and insulin resistance. Several investigators[2,9] found that plasma fasting insulin levels correlated with plasma T and A levels. One hypothesis is that hyperandrogenism produces insulin resistance[11]. However the mechanism by which hyperandrogenism could produce insulin resistance remains obscure. In our study it was shown that during OGTT PCOD patients presented a more marked insulin secretion than controls and frequently PCOD obese patients showed both basal and glucose-stimulated increased plasma insulin levels compared to the other groups. The lowest insulin levels were found in the normal not obese women. Similar results have been obtained by Dunaif *et al.*[11].

Other authors found that in PCOD patients who lost weight there was a parallel reduction of the insulin resistant state[1]. Overall, these results suggest that obesity may be considered an important factor associated to insulin resistance: however the presence of such a characteristic in PCOD not obese women indicates that in PCOD factors other than obesity must be involved in promoting insulin resistance.

Results of this study indicate that hyperinsulinism is a heterogeneous feature of PCOD patients; in fact 80% of PCOD obese patients showed an hyperinsulinemic pattern, while this aspect is present in about 30% of control obese and PCOD not obese patients.

Another hypothesis regarding the association between hyperandrogenism and insulin resistance proposes that hyperinsulinemia produces ovarian function disorder, chiefly manifested as hyperandrogenism[14].

In our study no appreciable change of androgen secretion was seen during insulin response to OGTT in both normal and hyperinsulinemic patients. Since obese and not obese PCOD women had similar androgen levels despite a different degree of hyperinsulinemia, these results suggest that insulin does not have a major role in the perpetuation of hyperandrogenic status of PCOD.

In conclusion this study shows that hyperandrogenism, hyperinsulinism and obesity were associated with different modalities in PCOD patients.

REFERENCES

1. Pasquali, R., Venturoli, S., Paradisi, R., Capelli, M., Parenti, M. and Melchionda, N. (1982). Insulin and C-peptide levels in obese patients with polycystic ovarian disease. *Horm. Metab. Res.*, **14**, 284–7
2. Shoupe, D., Kuman, D.D. and Lobo, R.A. (1983). Insulin resistance in polycystic ovary syndrome. *Am. J. Obstet. Gynecol.*, **147**, 588–92
3. Nagamani, H., Van Dinh, T. and Kelver, H.E. (1986). Hyperinsulinemia is hyperthecosis of

the ovaries. *Am. J. Obstet. Gynecol.*, **154**, 384–9

4. Yen, S.S.C. (1980). The polycystic ovary syndrome. *Clin. Endocrinol.*, **12**, 177–207
5. Burghen, C.A., Givens, J.R. and Kitabchi, A.E. (1980). Correlation of hyperandrogenism with hyperinsulinism in polycystic ovarian disease. *J. Clin. Endocrinol. Metab.*, **50**, 113–6
6. Kopelman, P.G., White, N., Pilkington, T.R.E. and Jeffcoate, S.L. (1981). The effect of weight loss on sex steroid secretion and binding in massively obese women. *Clin. Endocrinol.*, **15**, 113–16
7. Chang, R.J., Nakamura, R.M., Judd, H.L. and Kaplan, S.A. (1983). Insulin resistance in non-obese patients with polycystic ovarian disease. *J. Clin. Endocrinol. Metab.*, **57**, 356–9
8. Harlass, F.E., Plymate, S.R., Fariss, B.L. and Belts, R.P. (1984). Weight loss is associated with correction of gonadotropin and sex steroid abnormalities in the obese anovulatory female. *Fertil. Steril.*, **42**, 649–52
9. Barbieri, R.L. and Ryan, K.J. (1983). Hyperandrogenism, insulin resistance, and acanthosis nigricans syndrome: a common endocrinopathy with distinct pathophysiologic features. *Am. J. Obstet. Gynecol.*, **147**, 90–101
10. Barbieri, R.L., Hekris, A. and Ryan, R.J. (1983). Effect of insulin on steroidogenesis in cultured porcine ovarian thecae. *Fertil. Steril.*, **40**, 237–41
11. Dunaif, A., Mandeli, J., Flunk, A. and Dobrjansky, A. (1988). The impact of obesity and chronic hyperinsulinemia on gonadotropin release and gonadal secretion in polycystic ovary syndrome. *J. Clin. Endocrinol. Metab.*, **66**, 131–9
12. Lanzone, A., Fulghesu, A.M., Apa, R., Menini, E., Caruso, A. and Mancuso, S. (1987). Successful induction of ovulation and conception with combined gonadotropin-releasing hormone agonist plus highly purified follicle-stimulating hormone in patients with polycystic ovarian disease. *J. Clin. Endocrinol. Metab.*, **65**, 1253–8
13. Lorentz, F.H. (1929). Ein never constitutios index. *Klin. Wsch.*, **8**, 348–54
14. Taylor, S.I., Dons, R.F., Hernandez, E., Roth, J. and Gorden, P. (1982). Insulin resistance associated with androgen excess in women with autoantibodies to the insulin receptor. *Ann. Intern. Med.*, **97**, 851–5

80

Pulsatile GnRH use in the therapy of ovarian polycystosis

A. Porcelli, N. Surico and G. Ferraris

INTRODUCTION

The existence of a special releasing factor for the hypophyseal gonadotropins was first hypothesized in 1937. Only many years later though, in 1971, was it identified and its biochemical structure defined by Andrew Schally and Roger Guillemin.

The molecular structure of gonadotropin-releasing hormone (GnRH) is that of a decapeptide with pyroglutamic acid in position 1 and glycine in the terminal 10 position.

The particular configurational characteristics and structure are determined by the amino acid sequence 1–6 and 10. The molecule is inactivated by cerebral proteolytic enzymes (peptidases) that lyse the chain in positions 6 and 7. The terminal amino acids give the molecule its biological activity.

GnRH secretion occurs in the arcuate and venteromedial nuclei of the hypothalamus and in the preoptic area.

Substances analogous to GnRH with greater binding potential for specific GnRH receptors, greater resistance to enzymatic degradation, and a longer half-life have been synthesized.

The mechanism for the molecular synthesis of the GnRH analogs is based on the substitution of amino acids on the interior of the original sequence of the GnRH molecule itself. The most important modifications take place at points 2, 3, 6 and 10 of the sequence. Several analogs have nonapeptide structures.

GnRH release into hypothalamic–hypophyseal portal system originates in the median eminence. The hormone is thus transported by the aforementioned route to the adenohypophysis where it stimulates the cells specifically responsible for gonadotropin secretion.

Other areas of GnRH production have been identified and isolated from the cytotrophoblast and from the villous stroma of the human placenta as well as pancreatic cells in the rat.

The half-life of GnRH is 2/8 min and the metabolic clearance is 1028–1640 $\pm$ 59.7 ml/min (values depending upon the radioimmunoassay (RIA) technique used).

GnRH is secreted into the hypothalamic–hypophyseal portal circulation in a pulsatile manner. The frequency and amplitude of the pulsations are of fundamental importance for a correct endocrine equilibrium during the menstrual cycle.

Recent studies found in the literature, cite pulsation ranges between 8 and 14 over 24 h.

Only when there is a pulsatile stimulation of the hypophysis by GnRH is it possible to produce a normal gonadotropic secretion. The optimal stimulation frequency is between 60 and 120 min. A direct correlation between GnRH secretion and hematic levels of luteinizing hormone (LH) has been reported.

Plasmatic levels of GnRH have a direct influence on the hematic concentrations of GnRH receptors (Clayton R.). If the releasing hormone maintains its pulsatility, the continuous infusion induces a down-regulation of the respective receptors, and a corresponding decrease in LH secretion (Figure 1).

Continuous administration of GnRH determines an increase in gonadotropins during the first 4 hours of infusion. After this initial time period one observes a continuous and progressive decline of follicle stimulating hormone (FSH) and LH, for up to 28 h.

Different substances such as the β-endorphins, estradiol (E_2), and progesterone, acting on different sites, can influence the pulsatile characteristics of GnRH (Figure 2).

The most important indications for therapy with GnRH consist of dysfunctional disorders of the hypothalamic–hypophyseal–ovarian axis caused by inadequate production or pulsatility of GnRH.

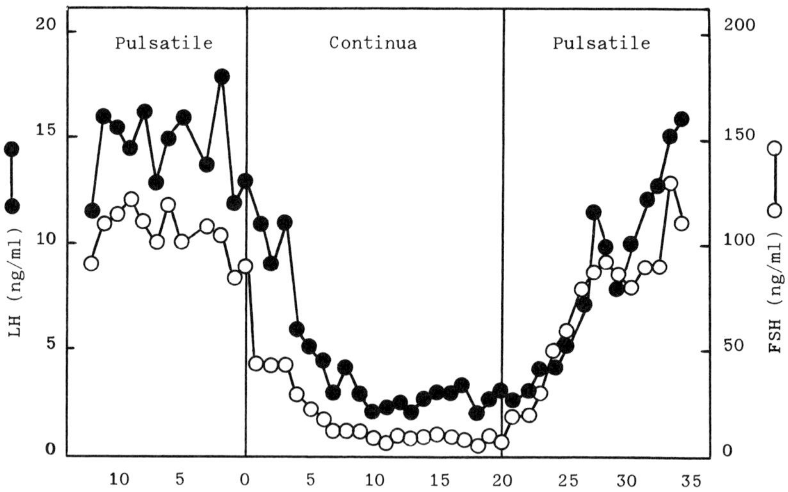

Figure 1 Gonadotropic response to continuous and pulsatile administration of gonadotropin-releasing hormone (taken from Ory, 1983[2])

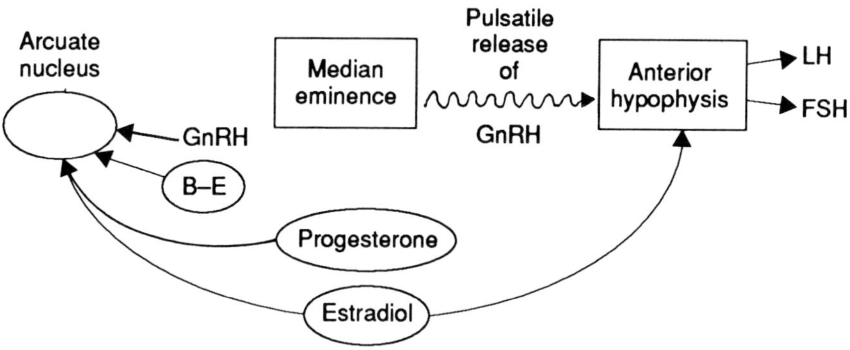

Figure 2 Influence of different substances on the pulsatile characteristics of gonadotropin-releasing hormone

Clinical applications of GnRH and its analogs

GnRH and its analogs are applied in the following areas.

(1) Activation of hypophyseal function:
 Physiological hypogonadotropism of the puerperium,
 Late onset of puberty,
 Cryptorchidism,
 The induction of ovulation in hypogonadotropic amenorrhea, and
 Male hypogonadotropic hypogonadism;

(2) Inhibition of hypophyseal function:
 Precocious puberty,
 Endometriosis,
 Hormone dependent tumors (both breast and prostate), and
 Suppression of ovarian androgen secretion; and

(3) Female contraception:
 Ovulation inhibition,
 Luteolysis induction, and
 Induction of short luteal phase.

In disorders dealing with altered frequency and amplitude of pulsatile GnRH, in the positive sense a disequilibrium of the hypothalamic–hypophyseal axis with a striking increase in LH secretion takes place. The resulting clinical picture is termed ovarian polycystosis.

Ovarian polycystosis is characterized by an altered LH/FSH ratio (> 2), an increased androgen production, and a clinical picture characterized by: anovulation, oligomenorrhea or amenorrhea and various degrees of hirsutism, and obesity.

Polycystic ovarian disease patients have higher LH plasmatic concentrations which in turn stimulate increased quantities of ovarian E_2. This may be interpreted as an increased hypophyseal sensitivity to GnRH which is being released by pulsations having a greater frequency and amplitude.

Under such conditions, therapy with pulsatile GnRH may be influenced by possible LH peaks induced by endogenous stimuli of hypothalamic origin. A consequent therapeutic failure would thus be a possibility.

A pretherapeutic administration of a GnRH analogue causing hypophyseal suppression favors the re-establishment of a normal LH secretory range of frequency and amplitude during the course of therapy with pulsatile GnRH: this phenomenon facilitates the normal follicular recruitment with the consequent selection of the dominant follicle.

MATERIALS AND METHODS

Our study included 37 patients, between the ages of 21 and 35 years with a clinical and or laboratory diagnosis of clomiphene resistant ovarian polycystosis. All cases presented with oligomenorrhea, anovulatory cycles and an altered LH/FSH ratio with LH markedly elevated with respect to FSH. Several patients from the study group underwent pelvic ultrasonography to evaluate ovarian morphology.

In all cases pretherapeutic FSH, LH, E_2 progesterone, prolactin, testosterone, dehydroepiandrosterone sulfate (DEAS-S) and 17-OH progesterone concentrations were measured.

A Zyklomat (Ferring-West Germany) peristaltic pump was used for the pulsatile infusion of GnRH intravenously. A bolus dosage of 5–10 μg/60 min. was administered, and the frequency of administration and the dosage were maintained constant during the cycle. Treatment was continued also during the luteinic phase or until a positive pregnancy test or menstrual flow were obtained.

The therapeutic protocol included daily monitoring of plasma gonadotropin, 17β-estradiol, prolactin and progesterone values. In addition a cervical score and pelvic sonography were performed at 3-day intervals.

All patients also measured basal temperatures daily. Twenty-eight patients underwent two treatment cycles, while in nine patients three cycles of stimulation therapy were performed. The pulsation frequency was maintained at 60 min per bolus.

Patients were subdivided into two groups according to GnRH-A pretreatment. Twenty-one patients were placed in group A (no GnRH-A pretreatment) while 16 patients were placed in group B (pretreatment with GnRH-A).

Buserelin, a GnRH analog was used in the study. The compound is derived from the substitution of glycine in two sites of the amino acid sequence of the natural hormone.

Buserelin was administered to the group B patients at a dosage of 600 μg/day subcutaneously for 8 weeks. Prior to including the patients in the GnRH treatment protocol, GnRH testing was performed, to confirm that hypophyseal suppression had occurred.

RESULTS

The following table depicts the division of the patients into the subgroups A and B based on buserelin pretreatment (Table 1).

Table 2 shows the ovulation and pregnancy percentages obtained in relation to the number of treatment cycles.

In the first group of patients a later FSH elevation, with higher estrogen values in the early follicular phase was observed.

On ultrasonography, multiple ovarian follicles in various stages of maturation were appreciated.

Neither twin pregnancies nor clear indications of hyperstimulation resulted.

In an analogous manner, plasma progesterone levels were observed in the lower average range with respect to the patient group pretreated with GnRH.

Group B, by ultrasonography, more frequently showed the maturation on only one dominant follicle, which correlated with an early rise in the plasma FSH concentration, along with a much slower and progressive LH elevation.

CONCLUSION

From the results obtained in this study it is observed how patients with ovarian polycystosis, treated directly with pulsatile GnRH, frequently underwent anovulatory cycles (68% of the cycles).

In our opinion, this phenomenon is due to a premature increase in plasmatic LH levels resulting in negative effects on follicular growth, and results in absent dominant follicular selection.

This effect is additionally seen at the level of follicular recruitment, where the observed disorganization conditions the cases of absent ovulation.

The causes of the above may be attributable to the pathogenic mechanism of ovarian polycystosis itself, determining a hypothalamic–hypophyseal axis imbalance, expressed as fluctuations of endogenous GnRH secretion. In contrast, the administration of buserelin causes a hypophyseal down-regulation representing a good starting base line for secretory reorganization. Consecutive pulsatile GnRH therapy restores a favorable hypophyseal response with a resulting increase in the plasma FSH and LH concentrations,

Table 1 Characteristics of groups A and B

	Number of patients	*GnRH-A + pulsatile GnRH*	*Total number of treatment cycles with pulsatile GnRH*
Group A	21	no	42
Group B	16	yes	41

Table 2 Post-therapeutic ovulation and pregnancy percentages

	Ovulation	*Pregnancy*
Group A	32% (13 cycles)	5% (2)
Group B	61% (25 cycles)	18% (7)

approaching physiological conditions.

One thus observes a greater percentage of ovulatory cycles (in the cycles evaluated) and a consequent higher probability of conception.

In conclusion, in light of the above, we affirm the validity of this therapeutic protocol in patients with 'clomiphene resistant' ovarian polycystosis, and strongly underline the importance of GnRH analog pretreatment for a more correct and methodical approach to the pathology in question.

BIBLIOGRAPHY

1. Campaniello, E., Filicori, M., Ferrari, P., Meriggiola, M.C., Pareschi, A., Valdiserri, A., Ucci, N., Petrarolo, N. and Flamigni, C. (1988). Induzione dell'ovulazione. In *II Congresso Italiano di Medicina della Riproduzione*, pp. 279–86 (Bologna: Monduzzi Editore)
2. Campaniello, E., Pereschi, A., Meriggiola, M.C., Ferrari, P., Michelacci, L., Valdiserri, A., Cimatti, M., Ucci, N., Petrarolo, N., Flamigni, C. and Filicori, M. (1988). Induzione dell'ovulazione con GnRH pulsatile: prevenzione della complicanze. In *II Congresso Italiano di Medicina della Riproduzione*, pp. 551–4 (Bologna: Monduzzi Editore)
3. Chang, R.J., Laufer, L.R., Meldrum, D.R., DeFazio, J., Lu, J.K.H., Vale, W.W., Rivier, J.E. and Judd, H.L. (1983). Steroid secretion in polycystic ovarian disease after ovarian suppression by a long-acting gonadotropin-releasing hormone agonist. *J. Clin. Endocrinol. Metab.*, **56**, 897–903
4. Charbonnel, B., Krempf, M., Blanchard, P., Dano, F. and Delage, C. (1987). Induction of ovulation in polycystic ovary syndrome with a combination of a luteinizing hormone-releasing hormone analog and exogenous gonadotropins. *Fertil. Steril.*, **47**, 920–4
5. Crowley, W.F., Jr. and McArthur, J.W. (1980). Simulation of the normal menstrual cycle in Kallman's syndrome by pulsatile administration of luteinizing hormone-releasing hormone (LHRH). *J. Clin. Endocrinol. Metab.*, **51**, 173–5
6. D'Ambrogio, G. and Genazzani, A.R. (1984). Induzione dell'ovulazione con LH-RH. *Endocrinologia Ginecologica*, p. 337. (Bologna: Monduzzi Editore)
7. De Leo, V., Bruno, M.G., Mazzarello, E.S., Bilotti, A., Inaudi, P. and D'Antona, N. (1988). Valutazione della secrezione pulsatile dell'LH in pazienti affette da PCO. In *II Congresso Italiano di Medicina della Riproduzione* pp. 387–93. (Bologna: Monduzzi Editore)
3. Filicori, M., Campaniello, E., Michelacci, L., Pareschi, A., Ferrari, P., Bolelli, G. and Flamigni, C. (1988). Gonadotropin-Releasing Hormone (GnRH) Analog suppression renders polycystic ovarian disease patients more susceptible to ovulation induction with pulsatile GnRH. *J. Clin. Endocrinol. Metab.*, **66**, 327–33
9. Grassi, G., Parolini, P., Revelli, A., Mendolicchio, S., Laudadio, A., Alovisi, C., Cenderelli, G. and Massobrio, M. (1988). Induzione dell'ovulazione con GnRH pulsatile. In *II Congresso Italiano di Medicina della Riproduzione*. pp. 451–4. (Bologna: Monduzzi Editore)
10. Hurwitz, A., Rosenn, B., Palti, Z., Ebstein, B., Nar-Nir, R. and Ron, M. (1986). The hormonal response of patients with polycystic ovarian disease to subcutaneous low frequency pulsatile administration of luteinizing hormone-releasing hormone. *Fertil. Steril.*, **46**, 378–83
11. Hammond, C.B., Wiebe, R.H., Haney, A.F. and Yancy, S.G. (1979). Ovulation induction with luteinizing hormone-releasing hormone in amenorrheic, infertile women. *Am. J. Obstet. Gynecol.*, **135**, 924–37
12. Leyendecker, G., Wildt, L. and Hansmann, M. (1980). Pregnancies following chronic intermittent (pulsatile) administration of GnRH by means of a portable pump (Zyklomat). A new approach to the treatment of infertility in hypothalamic amenorrhea. *J. Clin. Endocrinol. Metab.*, **51**, 1214–6
13. Loucopoulos, A., Ferin, M., Vande Wiele, R.L., Dyrenfurth, I., Linkie, D., Yeh, M. and Jewelewicz, R. (1983). Pulsatile administration of gonadotropin-releasing hormone for induction of ovulation. *Am. J. Obstet. Gynecol.*, **148**, 895–900
14. Melega, C., Filicori, M., Pareschi, A., Perigini, A. and Flamigni, C. (1988). Gli analoghi del GnRH per il tratamento della patologia ginecologica. In *II Congresso Italiano di Medicina della Riproduzione*, pp. 83–90. (Bologna: Monduzzi Editore)

15. Ory, S.J. (1983). Clinical uses of luteinizing hormone-releasing hormone. *Fertil. Steril.*, **39**, 577–90
16. Ory, S.J., London, S.N., Tyrey, L. and Hammond, C.B. (1985). Ovulation induction with pulsatile gonadotropin-releasing hormone administration in patients with polycystic ovarian syndrome. *Fertil. Steril.*, **43**, 20–5
17. Reid, R.L., Leopold, G.R. and Yen, S.S.C. (1981). Induction of ovulation and pregnancy with pulsatile luteinizing hormone releasing factor: dosage and mode of delivery. *Fertil. Steril.*, **36**, 553–9
18. Saffan, D. and Seibel, M.M. (1986). Ovulation induction with subcutaneous pulsatile gonadotropin-releasing hormone in various ovulatory disorders. *Fertil. Steril.*, **45**, 475–81
19. Sandow, J. (1982). Clinical applications of LHRH and its analogues. *Clin. Endocrinol.*, **18**, 571–92
20. Santoro, N., Wierman, M.E., Filicori, M., Waldstreicher, J. and Crowley, W.F. (1986). Intravenous administration of pulsatile gonadotropin-releasing hormone in hypothalamic amenorrhea: effects of dosage. *J. Clin. Endocrinol. Metab.*, **62**, 109–16
21. Skarin, G., Nillius, S.J. and Wide, L. (1983). Pulsatile subcutaneous low-dose gonadotropin-releasing hormone treatment of anovulatory infertility. *Fertil. Steril.*, **40**, 454–60
22. Stuckey, B.G.A., Keogh, E.J., Pullan, P.T., Beilby, J.A., Thompson, R.I. and Evans, D.V. (1987). Continuous gonadotropin-releasing hormone for ovulation induction in polycystic ovarian disease. *Fertil. Steril.*, **48**, 1055–7
23. Valdiserri, A., Meriggiola, M.C., Michelacci, L., Cimatti, M., Ucci, N., Perugini, A., Ferrari, P., Campaniello, E., Pareschi, A., Flamigni, C. and Filicori, M. (1988). Sviluppo di cisti ovariche durante l'induzione dell'ovulazione con GnRH pulsatile. In *II Congresso Italiano di Medicina della Riproduzione*, pp. 557–9. (Bologna: Monduzzi Editore)
24. Valdiserri, A., Meriggiola, M.C., Michelacci, L., Ferrari, P., Campaniello, E., Pareschi, A., Cimatti, M., Ucci, N., Flamigni, C. and Filicori, M. (1988). Il GnRH pulsatile per l'induzione dell'ovulazione. In *II Congresso Italiano di Medicina della Riproduzione*, pp. 73–81. (Bologna: Monduzzi Editori)
25. Valdiserri, A., Meriggiola, M.C., Pareschi, A., Campaniello, E., Ucci, N., Cimatti, M., Ferrari, P., Michelacci, L., Flamigni, C. and Filicori, M. (1988). Ruolo della frequenza della pusazioni del GnRH nella dinamica del ciclo mestruale. In *II Congresso Italiano di Medicina della Riproduzione*, pp. 403–6. (Bologna: Monduzzi Editore)
26. Yen, S.S.C. (1983). Clinical applications of gonadotropin-releasing hormone and gonadotropin-releasing hormone analogs. *Fertil. Steril.*, **39**, 257–63

81

Treatment of infertility in polycystic ovarian disease

J. Falck Larsen

INTRODUCTION

It is difficult to present a review on the treatment of infertility in polycystic ovarian disease (PCOD) for several reasons. Firstly, many authors do not mention their *inclusion criteria* for PCOD. Some patient materials are based on clinical findings only, such as anovulation, oligomenorrhea, hirsutism and infertility. The observation period before medication is also important, because many of these patients can have spontaneous ovulations in some periods.

The endocrine criteria may be different. Most authors agree that the patients must have an elevated luteinizing hormone (LH) to follicle-stimulating hormone (FSH) ratio to be included, but the lower limit may be 2, 2.5 or 3. Some authors mention the importance of elevated values of free testosterone and/or androstenedione, but the reference values may be different from hospital to hospital.

An abnormal elevated LH response during a gonadotropin-releasing hormone (GnRH) stimulation test is used for inclusion of the patient by some investigators. Morphological criteria are also difficult to agree upon. Nowadays wedge resections are rare, and biopsies through laparoscope are most often insufficient for a histological diagnosis. The surface of the ovaries can be examined through the laparoscope and be described as enlarged with a smooth capsule.

The ultrasonic diagnosis is attractive but Polson *et al.*[1] found polycystic ovaries in more than 20% of normal women examined by pelvic ultrasound scanning.

Secondly, most of the publications are not based on *controlled clinical trials*. New treatment methods should be compared with established methods in randomized series using a double-blind design. Also it is useful to include a placebo group because of the spontaneous ovulations that may occur in this type of patient.

CLOMIPHENE CITRATE

This is the drug most often used for induction of ovulation in PCOD. It is efficient, safe, and inexpensive compared with most of the newer methods.

With clomiphene the ovulation rates are between 70 and 90% during infertility caused by anovulation. The figures may be lower in patients suffering from PCOD. It has been stated that the pregnancy rate is much lower than the ovulation rate. This observation has been explained by follicular luteinization without rupture (the 'LUF-syndrome'), luteal phase defect or the antiestrogenic effect of clomiphene on the cervical mucus. However, it should be remembered that more than one infertility factor may be present; in patients without other infertility factors than anovulation the pregnancy rate is high.

Nevertheless there is a group of patients with PCOD, who do not ovulate when treated with clomiphene or who do not conceive during this treatment.

A number of different treatments have been introduced during the last few years. It is not possible in a short presentation to discuss all the different schedules, but I have selected some of the methods I find most interesting.

HUMAN MENOPAUSAL GONADOTROPIN (hMG)

If clomiphene treatment fails the next line of treatment in hypothalamic amenorrhea is hMG and this treatment gives good results. The situation is different in PCOD in which the patient has a high baseline serum LH. The stimulation can be difficult and the risk of hyperstimulation and multiple pregnancies is high. Rossmanith *et al.*[2] tried to reduce this risk by giving subcutaneous pulsatile hMG. They needed significantly less hMG with this method compared with the intramuscular route. This method deserves to be tested in a larger trial.

GONADOTROPIN-RELEASING HORMONE

In PCOD the LH secretion is increased as a consequence of increased GnRH pulse frequency and amplitude and enhanced pituitary sensitivity to GnRH promoted by high estrogen levels.

Several studies have shown that it is impossible to override the abnormal pulsatile patterns of GnRH by giving exogenous pulsatile GnRH. A number of investigators have reported that it is possible to induce ovulation with this method but few obtained pregnancies. Wilson *et al.*[3] did not find the method efficient and none of their patients became pregnant. They criticized other investigators for giving insufficient information on their criteria for PCOD.

Somewhat more optimistic results were reported by Eshel *et al.*[4], who treated 48 patients with PCOD with 15 μg subcutaneous GnRH every 90 min. In patients who did not ovulate on subcutaneous GnRH, treatment with clomiphene citrate was added. If this combined treatment was not successful, GnRH was given intravenously. The cumulative conception rate after 6 months was 60%. However, ten of the 23 conceptions ended in miscarriage.

The effect of a temporary suppression of the elevated serum LH has been tested in different ways. Stuckey *et al.*[5] infused synthetic GnRH subcutaneously in six patients. It took 6 to 9 weeks to suppress the gonadotropins. When the GnRH treatment was withdrawn three of the patients ovulated and one conceived on this 'rebound' treatment.

GnRH ANALOGS

The use of GnRH analogs has been promising. After a short period of stimulation the GnRH analog suppresses the LH secretion. The production of a hypogonadotropic–hypogonadal state in these patients results in a predictable LH baseline upon which exogenous gonadotropin therapy can be given[6]. When the serum LH is suppressed the patient can be stimulated with hMG/hCG, FSH/hCG or pulsatile GnRH.

Filicori *et al.*[7] used GnRH analog suppression followed by pulsatile GnRH. They found a more normal response to GnRH after suppression with the GnRH analog and the progesterone values were higher than before the suppression.

BROMOCRIPTINE

There is no agreement on the value of bromocriptine treatment of PCOD. It has been proposed that a dopaminergic component influences LH release in PCOD and that bromocriptine may be useful in the treatment of this disease also in cases with normal prolactin levels.

Two well designed, randomized controlled studies have given different results. El Tabbakh *et al.*[8] carried out a double-blind cross-over study in 20 patients. They were studied for three cycles: a baseline cycle without medication, a placebo cycle, and a bromocriptine cycle. A significant decrease in prolactin, LH/FSH ratio, testosterone and androstenedione occurred during treatment with bromocriptine.

Buvat *et al.*[9] studied 55 patients in another double-blind, randomized study. They gave bromocriptine for 6 months. The only difference they found between the two groups was a lower serum prolactin in the bromocriptine group. They found all the endocrine changes described in other studies, such as suppression of LH- and androgen concentrations restoration of ovulation and regular bleedings. However, they found these changes in the control group, also.

ELECTROCAUTERY OF THE OVARIES

Wedge resection of the ovaries is a well known treatment, which was the standard method of treatment before clomiphene citrate became available. This method is still used in some centers in cases resistant to clomiphene treatment. Wedge resection may result in adhesions, which cause anatomical infertility.

Gjønnaes[10] has introduced a simple method as an alternative to the wedge resection. He suggested the performance of laparoscopic electrocautery of the ovarian capsule. He held the electrode against the ovarian surface for 2–4 seconds and made five to eight holes in the capsule. Ovulation occurred in 92%, and 69% of the infertile patients became pregnant.

Greenblatt and Caspar studied the endocrine changes after electrocauterization and found the same changes as reported after wedge resection[11]. The concentration of testosterone, androstenedione and LH decreased immediately after the electrocautery and the serum LH, followed by a rise in FSH and estradiol.

The method has been modified so the incision in the ovarian capsule is done by a laser beam which may reduce even further the risk of adhesions.

'PURIFIED' FSH (huFSH)

As the PCOD patient has an elevated baseline LH it seems logical to prefer the 'purified' FSH preparation to hMG. This is produced from human urine. Theoretically the LH/FSH should be normalized during treatment with huFSH. The elevated LH concentration in PCOD causes the increased production of androgens, and these may be suppressed if the LH/FSH is corrected by huFSH. It has been claimed that the incidence of hyperstimulation and the potential for multiple births are reduced when huFSH is used for ovarian stimulation.

We carried out a double-blind cross-over study in 12 patients using huFSH- and hMG-stimulation as alternate treatments[12]. We found no significant difference between the endocrine profiles during the two types of stimulation.

CONCLUSION

None of the present methods of treatment seem satisfactory in clomiphene-resistant cases. More randomized controlled clinical trials including placebo are needed to evaluate new methods and compare these with established methods. The use of synthetic GnRH or GnRH analogs is promising. Laparoscopic electrocautery is an interesting method, but the correction of the endocrine dysfunction is probably temporary.

REFERENCES

1. Polson, D.W., Adams, J., Wadsworth, J. and Franks, S. (1988). Polycystic ovaries – a common finding in normal women. *Lancet*, **i**, 870–2
2. Rossmanith, W.G., Sterzik, K. and Wolf, A.S. (1987). Initial experiences with subcutaneous pulsatile human menopausal gonadotropin administration: successful induction of ovulation in patients with polycystic ovarian disease. *Int. J. Fertil.*, **32**, 460–6
3. Wilson, J.M., Traub, A.I., Sheridan, B., Thompson, W. and Atkinson, A.B. (1988). Conventional dose intravenous pulsatile GnRH therapy does not induce ovulation in

polycystic ovarian disease. *Acta Endocrinol.* (Copenh.), **117**, 289–94

4. Eshel, A., Abdulwahid, N.A., Armar, N.A., Adams, J.M. and Jacobs, H.S. (1988). Pulsatile luteinizing hormone-releasing therapy in women with polycystic ovarian syndrome. *Fertil. Steril.*, **49**, 956–60
5. Stuckey, B.G.A., Keogh, E.J., Pullan, P.T., Beilby, J.A., Thompson, R.I. and Evans, D.V. (1987). Continuous gonadotropin-releasing hormone for ovulation induction in polycystic ovarian disease. *Fertil. Steril.*, **48**, 1055–7
6. Fleming, R., Haxton, M.J., Hamilton, M.P.R., McCune, C.S., Black, W.P., McNaughton, M.C. and Coutts, J.R.T. (1985). Successful treatment of infertile women with oligomenorrhea using a combination of an LHRH agonist and exogenous gonadotropins. *Br. J. Obstet. Gynaecol.*, **92**, 369
7. Filicori, M., Campanieello, E., Michelacci, L., Pareschi, A., Ferrari, P., Bolelli, G. and Flamigi, C. (1988). Gonadotropin-releasing hormone (GnRH) analog suppression renders polycystic ovarian disease patients more susceptible to ovulation induction with pulsatile GnRH. *J. Clin. Endocrinol. Metab.*, **66**, 327–33
8. El Tabbakh, G.H., Loutfi, I.A., Azab, I., Rahman, H.A., Southern, L. and Aleem, F.A. (1988). Bromocriptine in polycystic ovarian disease. *Obstet. Gynecol.*, **71**, 301–6
9. Buvat, J., Buvat-Herbaut, M., Marcolin, G., Racadot, A., Fourlinnie, J.C., Beuscart, R. and Fossati, P. (1985). A double blind controlled study of the hormonal and clinical effects of bromocriptine in the polycystic ovary syndrome. *J. Clin. Endocrinol. Metab.*, **63**, 119–24
10. Gjønnæss, H. (1984). Polycystic ovarian syndrome treated by ovarian electrocautery through laparoscope. *Fertil. Steril.*, **41**, 20–5
11. Greenblatt, E. and Casper, R.F. (1987). Endocrine changes after laparoscopic ovarian cautery in polycystic ovarian syndrome. *Am. J. Obstet. Gynecol.*, **156**, 279–85
12. Larsen, T., Falck Larsen, J., Schøler, V., Felding, C. and Bostofte, E. (1990). Comparison of urinary human follicle-stimulation hormone and human menopausal gonadotropin for ovarian stimulation in polycystic ovarian syndrome. *Fertil. Steril.* (in press)

82

In vitro fertilization treatment in polycystic ovarian syndrome

J. Dor, Y. Menashe, A. Shulman, Z. Ben Rafael, D. Levran, E. Rudak and S. Mashiach

INTRODUCTION

Women suffering from polycystic ovarian syndrome (PCOS) which is characterized by anovulation and infertility, can be resistant to treatment by various ovulation-inducing agents. Despite the fact that ovulation can be achieved in more than 76% of the patients treated with clomiphene citrate, pregnancies have been achieved in only 30.3% of those women who ovulated[1]. When human menopausal gonadotropins (hMG) or preparations of urinary follicle-stimulating hormone (FSH) were used, the pregnancy rate reported was 38%, although ovulation was presumed to occur in 91% of the patients[2,3].

Women with PCOS suffer from high basal levels of luteinizing hormone (LH) secretion and in 30% of the cycles where ovulation is induced by exogenous gonadotropins, premature luteinization occurs[4]. In order to prevent an early surge of LH during treatment for ovulation induction, some authors[5,6] have suggested a combined regimen including gonadotropin-releasing hormone (GnRH) analog: gonadotropins were only administered after there was evidence of pituitary LH suppression, and relatively high pregnancy rates of 15–81% have been reported[3,7].

Despite these encouraging figures, a considerable proportion of women with PCOS fail to conceive following ovulation-inducing treatment. It has previously been reported that patients with PCOS can be successfully treated by *in vitro* fertilization (IVF)[8]. Thus, this would appear to be an acceptable alternative of treatment for PCOS patients with intractable infertility.

In this study we present our preliminary results of IVF treatment for PCOS patients. Our objective was to compare the efficiency of treatment of PCOS patients with a second group of women suffering from tubal infertility. We also examined the usefulness of GnRH analog in combination with FSH and hMG as a potential regimen for induction of ovulation in both groups of patients studied.

PATIENTS AND METHODS

Patients

In this study, 16 patients suffering from PCOS underwent 26 treatment cycles in our IVF treatment program. The results we obtained in this group of patients were compared to those of 22 normo-ovulatory women who underwent 29 treatment cycles by IVF within the same time period.

The following criteria were used for diagnosis of women with PCOS: (a) physical characteristics, obesity, hirsutism, (b) menstrual disorders, oligo-menorrhea or amenorrhea, (c) hormonal criteria, high basal LH levels, LH:FSH ratio above 3.0, serum testosterone levels above 0.7 ng/ml. Table 1 shows the basal hormonal study on our two groups of patients.

Induction of ovulation

In the group of PCOS patients, two treatment regimens were used. Group A (12 cycles) was treated with GnRH analog DTRP6 LHRH (Decapeptyl 3.2 mg, Ferring Ltd., Germany) on day 3 of the menstrual cycle to induce pituitary suppression. After suppression was achieved, pure FSH (Metrodin, 75 IU FSH) 150 IU per day was administered for 5 days followed by hMG (Pergonal, 75 IU FSH plus 75 IU LH) 150 IU per day. When the 17β-estradiol (E_2) levels reached above 600 pg/ml and at least two follicles of 16 mm diameter were observed by ultrasonic examination, a dose of 10 000 IU hCG was given intramuscularly. Group B (14 cycles) was treated with FSH (150 IU per day) for 5 days followed by hMG (150 IU FSH plus 150 IU LH) until an adequate response (as described previously) was achieved. The group of patients with tubal infertility was given hMG (150 IU FSH plus 150 IU LH) daily from day 3 of the cycle until an adequate response was achieved.

Our scheme for IVF treatment and laboratory procedures was carried out as has been previously described[9].

RESULTS

The mean serum E_2 levels, progesterone (P) and LH on the day of hCG administration and on the day following hCG administration (day hCG + 1) in the three groups of patients are shown in Table 2. Although the mean E_2 levels were higher in the PCOS patients on day hCG and hCG + 1, the difference was not statistically significant when compared to the control normo-ovulatory women with tubal disease. There was no difference in the

Table 1 Basal hormonal study

	FSH (mIU/ml)	*LH* (mIU/ml)	*LH/FSH*	*T* (ng/ml)
PCOS patients	6.4 ± 3.3	27.7 ± 13.9*	4.3 ± 2.2*	0.92 ± 0.39
Controls	9.2 ± 3.2	7.6 ± 3.3	0.91 ± 0.35	0.53 ± 0.32

*$p < 0.05$ (t test)

Table 2 Mean ± SD hormonal levels during late follicular phase

	Day of hCG			Day of hCG + 1	
	E_2 (pg/ml)	*P* (ng/ml)	*LH* (mIU/ml)	*E_2* (pg/ml)	*P* (ng/ml)
PCOS-A†	1682 ± 588	0.73 ± 0.41	7.32 ± 28	2396 ± 882	3.3 ± 1.6
PCOS-B	1644 ± 702	0.95 ± 0.45	18.2 ± 14.7*	1980 ± 943	4.2 ± 2.0
Control	1198 ± 684	0.76 ± 0.41	10.5 ± 3.02	1326 ± 592	1.6 ± 0.92*

* $p < 0.05$ (analysis of variance)
† PCOS-A = with DTRP6; PCOS-B = without DTRP6

mean E_2 levels of groups A and B of PCOS patients. The mean serum P levels were significantly ($p < 0.05$) lower in the control group when compared to the PCOS patients on day hCG+1, while no difference was observed between the two groups of PCOS patients. The mean serum LH levels were significantly ($p < 0.05$) elevated in the PCOS patients not receiving GnRH treatment (Group B) when compared to Group A PCOS patients receiving the analog and the tubal infertility patients.

The results of the IVF treatment, i.e., oocyte recovery, fertilization, cleavage and pregnancy rates are shown in Table 3. There was a significant difference ($p < 0.05$, analysis of variance) in the mean number of oocytes recovered, being higher in the PCOS patients than in the tubal infertility group. The fertilization and cleavage rates were significantly ($p < 0.05$) lower in the PCOS patient groups. However, there was no significant difference between Group A and Group B cycles. The pregnancy rates were similar in all three patient groups.

DISCUSSION

In this study we have demonstrated that women suffering from PCOS and intractable infertility can be successfully treated by IVF. In our group of PCOS patients the pregnancy rate was similar to that of the group of tubal infertility patients. The use of GnRH agonist to prevent an early LH surge in the PCOS patients followed by ovulation induction with FSH and hMG has proved to be very successful, as reported by Fleming *et al.*[3] This could be explained by the studies of Stanger and Yovich[10] and Howles and

Table 3 Fertilization, cleavage and pregnancy rates

	PCOS-A with analog	*PCOS-B without analog*	*Control*
No. of cycles	12	14	29
No. eggs recovered	152	175	224
Mean no. eggs recovered (±SD)	12.6 ± 7.4	12.5 ± 6.4	7.7 ± 3.4*
No. eggs fertilized (%)	65 (42.7)	77 (44)	149 (66.5)*
No. eggs cleaved (%)	64 (42.1)	72 (41.1)	145 (64.7)*
Pregnancies (%)	6 (50)	5 (35.7)	9 (31)

colleagues[11] who have shown that elevated LH levels, either basal values or in the late follicular phase may exert a deleterious effect on oocyte fertilization, embryonic cleavage and pregnancy rates. In our study, the PCOS patients not treated with GnRH analog showed a significant elevation of serum LH levels on the day of hCG administration. However, this did not selectively affect the oocyte fertilization and cleavage rates between the two groups of PCOS patients and could therefore not be related to treatment with or without GnRH analog. The lower fertilization rates in the PCOS patients when compared to the control group probably could not be directly related to elevation in LH levels during the stimulation period. Our data would appear to be in agreement with those of Salat-Baroux *et al.*[8] who found no difference in pregnancy rates of PCOS patients treated with or without GnRH analog and a control group of patients. We found no difference in pregnancy rate in the two groups of PCOS patients although the higher abortion rate in those women not receiving GnRH analog (40% in Group B and 25% in Group A) could prove to be significant in a larger patient group.

REFERENCES

1. Garcia, J., Jones, G.S. and Wentz, A.C. (1977). The use of clomiphene citrate. *Fertil. Steril.*, **28**, 707–11
2. Calman, P., Seibel, M.M., McArdle, C., Berger, M.J. and Taymor, M.L. (1986). Comparison of intermediate-dose purified urinary follicle-stimulating hormone with and without human chorionic gonadotropin for ovulation induction in polycystic ovarian disease. *Fertil. Steril.*, **46**, 518–21
3. Fleming, R., Jamieson, M.E., Hamilton, M.P.R., Black, W.P., MacNaughton, M.C. and Coutts, J.R.T. (1988). The use of GnRH analogues in combination with exogenous gonadotropins in infertile women. *Acta Endocrinol.*, **288**, 77–84
4. Fleming, R. and Coutts, J.R.T. (1986). Induction of multiple follicular growth in normally menstruating women with endogenous gonadotropin suppression. *Fertil. Steril.*, **45**, 226–30
5. Fleming, R., Haxton, M.J., Hamilton, M.P.R., McCune, G.S., Black, W.P., MacNaughton, M.C. and Coutts, J.R.T. (1985). Successful treatment of infertile women with oligomenorrhea using a combination of LHRH agonist and exogenous gonadotropins. *Br. J. Obstet. Gynaecol.*, **92**, 369–73
6. Haxton, M.J., Fleming, R. and Coutts, R.T.J. (1986). Population study of causes, treatment, and outcome of infertility. *Br. Med. J.*, **292**, 272
7. Charbonnel, B., Krempf, M., Blanchard, P., Dano, F. and Delga, C. (1987). Induction of ovulation in polycystic ovary syndrome with a combination of a luteinizing hormone-releasing hormone analog and exogenous gonadotropins. *Fertil. Steril.*, **47**, 920–4
8. Salat-Baroux, J., Alvarez, S., Antoine, J.M., Cornet, D., Tibi, Ch., Plachot, M. and Mandelbaum, J. (1988). Results of IVF in the treatment of polycystic ovary disease. *Hum. Reprod.*, **3**, 331–5
9. Dor, J., Rudak, E., Mashiach, S., Nebel, L., Serr, D.M. and Goldman, B. (1986). Periovulatory 17 β-Estradiol changes and embryo morphologic features in conception and nonconceptional cycles after human *in vitro* fertilization. *Fertil. Steril.*, **45**, 63–8
10. Stanger, J.D. and Yovich, J.L. (1985). Reduced *in vitro* fertilization of human oocytes from patients with raised basal luteinizing hormone levels during the follicular phase. *Br. J. Obstet. Gynaecol.*, **92**, 385–93
11. Howles, C.M., Macnamee, M.C., Edwards, R.G., Goswamy, R. and Steptoe, P.C. (1986). Effect of high tonic levels of luteinising hormone on outcome of *in vitro* fertilization. *Lancet*, **ii**, 521–2

83

Ovulation induction in polycystic ovarian syndrome

H.G. Burger, H.M. Buckler, D.L. Healy, G.T. Kovacs, J. McDonald, S.E. Phillips and T.-T. Tan

CURRENT PROBLEMS IN THE INDUCTION OF OVULATION

Whilst restoration of ovulation and fertility is usually straightforward in patients with hypothalamic or pituitary disease, the management of anovulatory infertility associated with the polycystic ovarian syndrome (PCOS) is frequently more difficult. The ultrasound findings of multiple peripherally placed cysts, 6–8 mm diameter, with increased stromal echogenicity have been reported in nearly 25% of normal women, in 26% of patients with amenorrhea, 87% with oligomenorrhea and 92% with hirsutism and regular menses[1,2]. Although many chronically anovulatory patients have the characteristics of hirsutism and obesity as classically described in PCOS[3], it is increasingly recognized that many patients presenting for ovulation induction, and found ultrasonically to have polycystic ovaries, are of normal or even reduced weight and have no clinical evidence of androgen excess.

For the purposes of this report, the diagnosis of PCOS is based on the presence of oligomenorrhea or amenorrhea with anovulatory infertility, an inappropriately elevated serum luteinizing hormone (LH) level in the presence of a normal or low follicle-stimulating hormone (FSH) level and follicular phase levels of progesterone[4]. Many, but not all subjects, had recognized PCOS features including hirsutism and increased body mass index. In all patients standard management for chronic anovulation was initiated with clomiphene citrate which is reported to restore ovulation in 70% of PCOS patients, only half of whom conceive[5].

Although a number of factors may contribute to persistent infertility, even after induction of ovulation with clomiphene citrate, there is evidence to suggest that one important contributor may be the elevated levels of serum LH[6]. In attempts to improve the success of ovulation induction regimens in PCOS patients resistant to standard clomiphene, human menopausal and chorionic gonadotropins (hMG and hCG respectively), we have evaluated various regimens in pilot studies which aimed to restore more physiological patterns of LH secretion.

The availability of a specific radioimmunoassay for serum inhibin[7] allowed us to determine the effects of these various approaches on serum inhibin levels and in particular to examine whether highly purified FSH could stimulate ovarian inhibin secretion. We also reviewed the results of ovulation induction in order to evaluate the clinical maxim that obesity affects ovulation and pregnancy rates in PCOS patients treated with gonadotropins.

OVULATION INDUCTION WITH FSH/hCG FOLLOWING PROGESTERONE PRETREATMENT – PURIFIED FSH STIMULATION OF SERUM INHIBIN

Chronic anovulation is associated with absence of the normal luteal phase increase in serum progesterone and inhibin[7]. Because progesterone can inhibit LH secretion[8] and has been reported to induce clomiphene citrate responsiveness in morbidly obese and anovulatory women[9], we initially evaluated the administration of vaginal progesterone prior to ovulation induction with exogenous gonadotropins in 15 women with PCOS[10]. In that study 50 mg of progesterone was administered by vaginal pessary every 12 h and led to serum progesterone concentrations in the lower part of the range seen during the normal luteal phase. Serum LH showed a biphasic response and at the end of 14 days of progesterone treatment had fallen to 79% of control levels. LH pulse frequency was decreased from 7.4 to 4.4 pulses per 6 h. Despite restoration of LH levels towards normal, ovulation occurred in only 56% of cycles and there were no pregnancies. We subsequently treated a further 12 patients using vaginal progesterone, 100 mg twice daily. Because highly purified FSH is theoretically preferable to a mixture of FSH and LH for ovulation induction in patients with an already inappropriately elevated LH level, we used a highly purified preparation of urinary FSH (Metrodin®) free of significant contamination with LH. Mean serum progesterone levels reached 57 mmol/1 after 3–4 days, and remained elevated during the use of the pessaries. Mean serum LH was within the normal range by 13–14 days. Eight patients ovulated at least once with this therapy (total of 24 cycles, 15 of these ovulatory) and there were two pregnancies, one ending in miscarriage.

During FSH administration there were increases in serum FSH, estradiol (E_2) and inhibin but there was no significant change in serum LH. Estradiol and inhibin rose in parallel and were closely correlated. There was a direct correlation between the measured FSH level and inhibin, but there was no correlation between LH and E_2 or FSH. Inhibin and E_2 were correlated with the number of follicles seen on ovarian ultrasound. Estradiol and inhibin levels reached a peak on the day of hCG administration or on the following day, inhibin then fell over the next 2 days in all cycles. In one ovulatory cycle resulting in conception, E_2 and inhibin rose in parallel with progesterone.

It is clear that in this pilot study there was an 80% success in the induction of ovulation on at least one occasion, but a very poor pregnancy rate. The study demonstrated that the previously observed increment in serum inhibin and E_2 during the follicular phase of the cycle in patients treated with hMG is attributable to the FSH component of the hMG[12]. The possibility that unchanging LH levels synergized with FSH cannot be excluded. The data are consistent with previous observations in the immature female rat in which purified FSH was also able to stimulate inhibin specifically[12].

OVULATION INDUCTION WITH LHRH AGONIST AND hMG/hCG

In view of the failure of administered progesterone (50 mg bd) to suppress satisfactorily the inappropriately elevated levels of serum LH in patients with PCOS, we evaluated the effects of the luteinizing hormone-releasing hormone (LHRH) agonist Buserelin® on pituitary and ovarian hormone secretion in a group of 22 patients with PCOS. Buserelin was administered intranasally at a dose of 200 μg six times daily. Ten patients received Buserelin until an estrogen withdrawal bleed occurred while a further 12 received Buserelin for 4 weeks. There was an initial rise in serum LH, FSH, E_2 and inhibin following Buserelin. Serum LH fell to normal by 14 days, but E_2 reached castrate levels only after 28 days of Buserelin administration. Inhibin and both E_2 and FSH were closely correlated throughout Buserelin administration. We compared the results of ovulation induction in these 22 subjects with those in nine undergoing conventional ovulation induction with hMG/hCG. There was no difference in the number of ovulations (52 compared with 66%) or pregnancies (both one) in either group. Similar amounts of hMG were needed in both for ovarian stimulation. In both groups multiple follicular development occurred (more than three follicles, more than 15 mm diameter: 41 v 38%) following hMG administration. Ovarian responsiveness to exogenous gonadotropin was unchanged despite suppression of LH with the LHRH agonist and the sensitivity that occurs in PCOS thus appears to be independent of circulating LH.

We have failed to demonstrate any benefit of pituitary–ovarian suppression with an LHRH agonist on subsequent ovulation induction in subjects with PCOS using hMG/hCG. Ovulation induction using an LHRH agonist and subsequent pulsatile LHRH has also been reported[13]. Prior LHRH agonist administration did not prevent multiple follicular development. Our results contrast with other recent reports suggesting a higher success rate for combinations of LHRH agonist and hMG[14,15]. The reasons for these discrepancies are unclear, though the relatively small numbers of subjects studied may be one important factor. Other approaches to the treatment of PCOS patients have been suggested[16–18].

RESTORATION OF OVULATION FOLLOWING OVARIAN CAUTERY

A classic therapy for ovulation induction in PCOS has been wedge resection of the ovaries, reported to have success rates of 40–70% but with significant risks of postoperative pelvic adhesions[19,20]. Laparoscopic ovarian diathermy has recently been introduced as a new method of therapy[21,22]. Because we had a significant number of patients chronically resistant to all attempts at ovulation induction, we undertook laparoscopic ovarian cautery in 11 patients. Approximately 10 diathermy lesions were made on the surface of each ovary. Multiple hormone measurements were made before and after therapy: the only significant changes were falls in serum testosterone, (from 2.3 to 1.7 nmol/l), and androstenedione (from 4.0 to 3.5 nmol/l). Eight patients ovulated spontaneously within 8 weeks of cautery, four of whom continued to ovulate, with one pregnancy, while the remaining four ceased spontaneous ovulation but became clomiphene-responsive, with one pregnancy. Three patients remained anovulatory but two responded to hMG with one pregnancy. Postoperative adhesion formation in non-pregnant patients was not assessed.

We conclude that laparoscopic ovarian diathermy is a procedure with some benefit for patients chronically resistant to all other forms of ovulation induction. Its place as an earlier or first-line mode of therapy in clomiphene-resistant patients has yet to be evaluated.

OBESITY AND THE RESULTS OF OVULATION INDUCTION IN PCOS

It has been estimated that the incidence of obesity in PCOS is around 41% and may be higher at the time of puberty[4]. Its role in the pathogenesis of PCOS remains controversial. It has been a widespread clinical impression that obesity interferes with attempts at ovulation induction. We therefore examined the records of 43 consecutive patients with clomiphene-resistant PCOS treated with a variety of ovulation induction regimens including human pituitary gonadotropin (hPG), hMG, purified urinary FSH, LHRH, or LHRH agonist plus hMG. Forty-three patients had a total of 199 cycles of which 64% were ovulatory. Seventeen conceived, two of them twice, resulting in 19 pregnancies. The pregnancy percentage rates per cycle and per ovulatory cycle were 9.5 and 15% respectively. There were five spontaneous abortions and one multiple pregnancy. The body mass index (BMI; kg/m^2) ranged from 17.5 to 41.7 with a mean of 26.8. Thirty-five per cent of the patients had a BMI > 30, (i.e. $> 120\%$ of body weight). The BMI tended to be lower in patients who conceived and ovulated than in those who did not, while it tended to be higher in patients who miscarried. However, none of these differences was statistically significant. Comparing patients with BMI < or > 24 (the upper limit of normal) the ovulation rate was higher in the patients with a lower BMI (71%) than in those with BMI > 24 (57%). The percentage conception per ovulatory cycle was similar (14 compared to 15%). The cumulative pregnancy rate in all patients at 6 months was 64.5% with all pregnancies occurring within the first eight cycles of treatment. There was no statistically significant difference in the cumulative pregnancy rate between patients with BMI < 30 and > 30.

We concluded that high BMI clomiphene-resistant PCOS does not decrease clinical outcomes significantly.

OVERALL CONCLUSIONS

We have evaluated various regimens in resistant PCOS in an attempt to improve the results of ovulation induction, but have been unsuccessful despite the achievement of somewhat more physiological conditions than exist spontaneously. Purified FSH specifically stimulates serum inhibin. Obesity does not significantly alter ovulation and conception rates in PCOS. PCOS remains a major challenge to the gynecological endocrinologist both to determine its pathogenesis and to improve methods of therapy.

REFERENCES

1. Polson, D.W., Wadsworth, J., Adams, J. and Franks, S. (1988). Polycystic ovaries – a common finding in normal women. *Lancet*, **ii**, 870–2
2. Adams, J., Polson, D.W. and Franks, S. (1986). Prevalence of polycystic ovaries in women with anovulation and idiopathic hirsutism. *Br. Med. J.*, **293**, 355–9
3. Stein, I.F. and Leventhal, M.L. (1935). Amenorrhoea associated with bilateral polycystic ovaries. *Am. J. Obset. Gynecol.*, **29**, 181–91
4. Yen, S.S.C. (1980). The polycystic ovary syndrome. *Clin. Endocrinol.*, **12**, 177–208
5. Osmond Clarke, F., Murray, M. and Bishop, P.M.F. (1968). The induction of ovulation with clomiphene and its assessment by biological methods. *J. Obstet. Gynecol. Br. Cwlth*, **75**, 531–6
6. Homburg, R., Armar, N.A., Eshel, A., Adams, J. and Jacobs, H.S. (1988). Influence of serum luteinising hormone concentrations on ovulation, conception, and early pregnancy loss in polycystic ovary syndrome. *Br. Med. J.*, **297**, 1024–6
7. McLachlan, R.I., Robertson, D.M., Healy, D.L., Burger, H.G. and de Kretser, D.M. (1987). Circulating immunoreactive inhibin levels during the normal human menstrual cycle. *J. Clin. Endocrinol. Metab.*, **65**, 955–61
8. Soules, M.R., Steiner, R.A., Clifton, D.K., Cohen, N.L., Absel, S. and Bremner, W.J. (1984). Progesterone modulation of pulsatile luteinizing hormone secretion in normal women. *J. Clin. Endocrinol. Metab.*, **58**, 378–83
9. Ayres, A.T. and Ansbacher, R. (1985). Progesterone induction of clomiphene responsiveness in morbidly obese anovulatory women. *Annual Meeting of the American Fertility Society, Abstract 88*. (Birmingham: Am. Fertil. Soc.)
10. Buckler, H.M., Phillips, S.E., Cameron, I.T., Healy, D.L. and Burger, H.G. (1988). Vaginal progesterone administration before ovulation induction with exogenous gonadotrophin in polycystic ovarian syndrome. *J. Clin. Endocrinol. Metab.*, **67**, 300–6
11. McLachlan, R.I., Robertson, D.M., Healy, D.L., de Kretser, D.M. and Burger, H.G. (1986). Plasma inhibin levels during gonadotrophin induced ovarian hyperstimulation for IVF: a new index of follicular function? *Lancet*, **i**, 1233–4
12. Lee, V.W.K., McMaster, J., Quigg, H. and Leversha, L. (1982). Ovarian and circulating inhibin levels in immature female rats treated with gonadotrophin and after castration. *Endocrinology*, **111**, 1849–54
13. Filicori, M., Campaniello, E., Michelacci, L., Pareschi, A., Ferrari, P., Bolelli, G. and Flamigni, C. (1988). Gonadotrophin-releasing hormone (GnRH) analog suppression renders polycystic ovarian disease patients more susceptible to ovulation induction with pulsatile GnRH. *J. Clin. Endocrinol. Metab.*, **66**, 327–33
14. Fleming, R., Haxton, M.J., Hamilton, M.P.R., McCune, G.S., Black, W.P., MacNaughton, M.C. and Coutts, J.R.T. (1985). Successful treatment of infertile women with oligomenorrhea using a combination of an LHRH agonist and exogenous gonadotrophins. *Br. J. Obstet. Gynecol.*, **92**, 369–73
15. Charbonnel, B., Krempf, M., Blanchard, P., Dano, F. and Delage, C. (1987). Induction of ovulation in polycystic ovary syndrome with a combination of a luteinizing hormone-releasing hormone analog and exogenous gonadotropins. *Fertil. Steril.*, **47**, 920–4
16. Yuen, B.H., Pride, S.M. and Sime, M.O. (1984). Successful induction of ovulation and conception with pulsatile intravenous administration of human menopausal gonadotropins

in anovulatory infertile women resistant to clomiphene and pulsatile gonadotropin-releasing hormone therapy. *Am. J. Obstet. Gynecol.*, **148**, 508–12

17. Lanzone, A., Fulghesu, A.M., Conte, M., Apa, R., Caruso, A. and Mancuso, S. (1987). Induction of ovulation by intermittent intravenous purified follicle-stimulating hormone in polycystic ovarian disease. *Fertil. Steril.*, **48**, 1058–61
18. Polson, D.W., Mason, H.D., Saldahna, M.B.Y. and Franks, S. (1987). Ovulation of a single dominant follicle during treatment with low-dose pulsatile follicle stimulating hormone in women with polycystic ovary syndrome. *Clin. Endocrinol.*, **26**, 205–12
19. Kistner, R.W. (1969). Peritubal and peri-ovarian adhesions subsequent to wedge resection. *J. Obstet. Gynecol. Br. Cwlth*, **75**, 1108–12
20. Buttram, V.C. and Vanquero, C. (1975). Post-wedge resection adhesive disease. *Fertil. Steril.*, **26**, 74–6
21. Gjonnaess, H. (1984). Polycystic ovarian syndrome treated by ovarian electrocautery through the laparoscope. *Fertil. Steril.*, **41**, 20–5
22. Greenblatt, E. and Casper, R.F. (1987). Endocrine changes after laparoscopic ovarian cautery in polycystic ovarian syndrome. *Am. J. Obstet. Gynecol.*, **156**, 279–85

84

The diagnostics and therapy of idiopathic hirsutism

M. Szamatowicz and M. Kulikowski

Though a great deal of information has been gathered regarding the physiology of androgens, somatic hyperandrogenization in women still remains a problem open to investigation and presents diagnostic and therapeutic difficulties[1-4].

Hirsutism, one of the symptoms of hyperandrogenization in women, may be due to increased adrenal or ovarian androgen secretion, enhanced peripheral androgen metabolism, a decreased sex hormone-binding globulin (SHBG) concentration, changes in target tissue sensitivity to androgens and the administration of drugs with an androgenic action[1-3,5,6].

In the diagnosis of hirsutism, tests are usually made to reveal androgen overproduction in the adrenal glands or ovaries and higher blood androgen concentrations and a lower plasma SHBG capacity have often been found[4,5,7,8]. These determinations, supplemented by dynamic tests, do not, however, provide an explanation of the cause of hyperandrogenization and in about 35–40% of cases a diagnosis of so-called idiopathic hirsutism is made[2,4,7,9].

Many authors have shown that idiopathic hirsutism is the result of effector hypersensitivity to androgens and are of the opinion that elucidation of its causes requires investigation of the processes taking place within the target organ while, at the same time, taking into account plasma protein steroid binding[3,4,6,10].

Since abnormal hair growth is either stimulated by excess hormone production or is related to follicle sensitivity to androgens the most effective treatment is based upon decreasing blood levels of testosterone and/or minimizing the biological activity of androgens at the target sites[11-14].

In the studies presented here, chosen tests of androgen effector sensitivity were applied in the diagnosis of women with hirsutism in whom it was not possible to establish the ovarian or adrenal source of androgenic hypersensitivity by hormone determinations or dynamic tests. An attempt was also made to evaluate some methods of hirsutism treatment.

MATERIALS AND METHODS

The investigations were carried out in three groups of patients. Group I contained 12 women, 21–37 years of age, with regular menstruation without clinical or biochemical signs of ovulation and with hyperandrogenization symptoms treated with spironolactone in a dose of 50 mg daily from the 5th to 21st day of the cycle and 50 mg of progesterone on the 23rd and 25th days. Group II contained a further 12 women, 23–34 years of age, with irregular menstruation and hirsutism treated with Mestranol in a dosage of 100 μg daily from the 5th to 25th day of the cycle and progesterone administered in phase II in a total dosage of 100 mg. In Groups I and II idiopathic hirsutism was diagnosed by means of estimation of androgen steroids in the blood and using the dynamic tests of adrenal suppression with dexamethasone and ovarian stimulation with hCG[8,9]. A third group contained 11 women, 19–33 years of age, who served as controls.

Blood serum sex hormone binding globulin capacity was determined by the method of Rudd *et al.*[15]. The following were determined in pubic skin samples: dehydroepiandrosterone (DHEA) utilization by the method of Thomas and Oake[16]; DHEA conversion into testosterone (T) and androstenedione (A) by the present authors' method[17]; and cytoplasmic androgen receptor capacity (AR) by the Svensson and Snochowski method[18].

The conversion of T into 5α-dihydrotestosterone (DHT) in the hair follicles from the pubic area was determined by the Schweikert and Wilson method[19].

The results were statistically analyzed by Student's t test.

RESULTS

In Groups I and II and the controls the mean initial values of SHBG capacity were 1.84 ± 0.23, 1.85 ± 0.34 and 2.78 ± 0.25 μg/100 ml, respectively. After treatment, the mean SHBG capacity in Group I was 1.77 ± 0.32 μg/100 ml and in Group II 3.06 ± 0.44 μg/100 ml.

The mean values of DHEA utilization in Groups I and II and the controls were 4.35 ± 1.10, 4.90 ± 1.41 and 2.31 ± 0.63 fmol/mg/h respectively. The differences between Groups I and II and the control group were statistically significant.

The mean values of DHEA conversion into T in Groups I and II and in the controls were 1.77 ± 0.66, 0.72 ± 0.29 and 0.21 ± 0.09 fmol/mg/h respectively and DHEA conversion into A, 1.17 ± 0.54, 1.40 ± 0.65 and 0.44 ± 0.20 fmol/mg/h respectively. The differences between the control and the experimental groups were statistically significant.

The AR capacities in the three groups were 62 ± 35, 76 ± 38 and 18 ± 12 fmol/mg protein respectively.

The conversion of T into DHT in the hair follicles before and after treatment was 0.82 ± 0.55, 0.98 ± 0.61 and 0.12 ± 0.17 fmol/μg DNA/h in the three groups respectively before treatment. After treatment it was reduced to 0.38 ± 0.50 in Group II, and 0.59 ± 0.45 fmol/μg DNA/h in Group I. These differences were statistically significant.

DISCUSSION

These studies show that in women suffering from idiopathic hirsutism with a normal blood testosterone concentration, the SHBG capacity was lower, which may facilitate the entrance of a greater amount of testosterone into the cells of the target tissues[19].

The enhanced DHEA utilization in women with hyperandrogenization symptoms indicates that this androgen of a low biological activity may, in the target tissue, be metabolized into active T[20]. Another possibility is that increased peripheral utilization of preandrogens causes a rise in 5α-reductase activity[4].

The higher activity of enzyme metabolizing precursors of active androgens in the pubic skin of women with hirsutism also suggests an enhanced source of T and A in the target tissues[4,6,16].

In the pubic skin cytosol, the AR capacity is, on average, three to four times greater in women with somatic hyperandrogenization though individual values can vary widely. Similar observations were made by Bonne *et al.*[1] while Mowszowicz *et al.*[21] found the cytoplasmic and nuclear values to be normal.

In diagnosing idiopathic hirsutism, an important step is the determination of enhanced 5α-reductase activity in the skin. For this purpose, however, it is necessary to take quite large sections making repetition of these tests in practice impossible[6,22,23].

In our experiments, increased 5α-reductase activity was demonstrated in hirsute women by evaluating the conversion of T into DHT in pubic hair follicles[24-26]. It was sufficient to take eight to 10 hairs in order to carry out repeated determinations which proved valuable in studying the effectiveness of the treatment applied.

The findings of the studies presented here show that in target sites of women with idiopathic hirsutism, the androgen metabolizing enzyme activity is higher and the AR capacity greater. It would therefore seem that receptor proteins and androgen metabolism enzymes constitute an intracellular system regulating the biological response of the tissue and may determine the so-called hypersensitivity of the tissue effector[4,6,16].

In our opinion the beneficial effect of the estrogen treatment in idiopathic hirsutism is the result of the increased SHBG capacity for T and to a lesser degree of the decreased activity of 5α-reductase of T. Spironolactone acts mainly by diminishing the 5α-reductase activity in hair follicle cells.

CONCLUSIONS

In women with hyperandrogenization, a decrease in the SHBG capacity is observed which increases after treatment with estrogen preparations (e.g. Mestranol). In women with hirsutism, a greater sensitivity of the pubic skin to androgens was noted. This was manifested by: enhanced dehydroepiandrosterone conversion into T and A, increased DHEA utilization, and a greater cytoplasmic AR capacity. In women with hyperandrogenization, intensified conversion of T into DHT occurs in the hair follicles which is reduced after treatment with estrogens and progesterone.

ACKNOWLEDGEMENTS

This research was supported by Ministry of Health and Social Care Research program MZ-VII.

REFERENCES

1. Biffighandi, P., Massucchetti, C. and Molinatti, G.M. (1984). Female hirsutism pathophysiological considerations and therapeutic implications. *Endocr. Rev.*, **5**, 498
2. Givens, J.R. (1976). Hirsutism and hyperandrogenism. *Adv. Intern. Med.*, **21**, 221
3. Kutten, F. and Mauvais-Jarvis, P. (1978). L'hirsutisme. *J. Gynecol. Obstet. Biol. Reprod.* (Paris), **7**, 693
4. Mauvais-Jarvis, P., Kutten, F. and Mowszowicz, I. (1981). Hirsutism. *Monographs in Endocrinology*, no. 19. (Berlin, Heidelberg, New York: Springer Verlag)
5. Kirschner, M.A. and Jacobs, J.B. (1971). Combined ovarian and adrenal vein catheterization to determine the site(s) of androgen overproduction in hirsute women. *J. Clin. Endocrinol. Metab.*, **33**, 199
6. Serafini, P.C. and Lobo, R.A. (1985). Increased 5α-reductase activity in idiopathic hirsutism. *Fertil. Steril.*, **43**, 74
7. Morris, D.V. (1985). Hirsutism. *Clin. Obstet. Gynecol.*, **12**, 649
8. Szamatowicz, M. and Kulikowski, M. (1983). Triiodothyronine in the treatment of hirsute girls. *Exp. Clin. Endocrinol.*, **82**, 15
9. Lopez, J.M., Migeon, C.J. and Jones, G.E.S. (1967). Hirsutism and evaluation of the dexamethasone suppression and chorionic gonadotropin stimulation test. *Am. J. Obstet. Gynecol.*, **98**, 749
10. Serafini, P.C., Catalino, J. and Lobo, R.A. (1985). The effect of spironolactone on genital skin 5α-reductase activity. *J. Ster. Biochem.*, **23**, 191
11. Boisselle, A. and Tremblay, R.R. (1979). New therapeutic approach to the hirsute patient. *Fertil. Steril.*, **32**, 276
12. Givens, J.R. (1985). Treatment of hirsutism with spironolactone. *Fertil. Steril.*, **43**, 841
13. Hammerstein, J., Moltz, L. and Schwartz, U. (1983). Antiandrogens in the treatment of acne and hirsutism. *J. Ster. Biochem.*, **19**, 591
14. Nielsen, P.G. (1982). Treatment of idiopathic hirsutism with spirolactone. *Dermatologica*, **165**, 194
15. Rudd, B.T., Duignan, N.M. and London, D.R. (1974). A rapid method for the measurement of sex hormone binding globulin capacity of sera. *Clin. Chim. Acta*, **55**, 165
16. Thomas, J.P. and Oake, R.J. (1974). Androgen metabolism in the skin of hirsute women. *J. Clin. Endocrinol. Metab.*, **38**, 19
17. Kulikowski, M. (1978). Rola globuliny wiązącej sterydy płciowew przemianie testosteronu i androstendionu w skórze okolicy nadłonowej u kobiet. I. Badania in vitro ze skrawkami skóry. *Endokr. Pol.*, **29**, 191
18. Svensson, J. and Snochowski, M. (1979). Androgen receptor levels in preputial skin from boys with hypospadia. *J. Clin. Endocrinol. Metab.*, **49**, 340
19. Anderson, D.C. (1974). Sex-hormone-binding globulin. *Clin. Endocrinol.*, **3**, 69
20. Faredin, I., Fazekas, A.G., Kokai, K., Toth, I. and Julesz, M. (1967). The *in vitro* metabolism 4-^{14}C dehydroepiandrosterone by human male pubic skin. *Eur. J. Ster.*, **2**, 223
21. Mowszowicz, I., Riahi, M. and Wright, F. (1981). Androgen receptor in human skin cytosol. *J. Clin. Endocrinol.*, **52**, 338
22. Kutten, F., Mowszowicz, I., Schaison, G. and Mauvais-Jarvis, P. (1977). Androgen production and skin metabolism in hirsutism. *J. Endocrinol.*, **75**, 83
23. Serafini, P.C., Ablan, F. and Lobo, R.A. (1985). 5α-reductase activity in the genital skin of hirsute women. *J. Clin. Endocrinol. Metab.*, **60**, 349
24. Glickman, S.P. and Rosenfield, R.L. (1984). Androgen metabolism by isolated hair from women with idiopathic hirsutism is usually normal. *J. Invest. Dermatol.*, **82**, 62
25. Schweikert, H.U. and Wilson, J.D. (1974). Regulation of human hair growth by steroid hormones. I. Testosterone metabolism in isolated hairs. *J. Clin. Endocrinol. Metab.*, **38**, 811
26. Takayasu, S. and Adachi, K. (1972). The conversion of testosterone to 17β-hydroxy-5α-androstan-3-one (dihydrotestosterone) by human hair follicles. *J. Clin. Endocrinol. Metab.*, **34**, 1098

85

Different modalities of gonadotropin administration in the induction of ovulation in polycystic ovarian disease

A. Caruso, A. Lanzone, A.M. Fulghesu, M. Le Donne, C. Guida, C.L. Andreani and S. Mancuso

INTRODUCTION

The clinical approach to the induction of ovulation in patients with polycystic ovarian disease (PCOD) has been widely studied; in fact the therapy usually used, clomiphene citrate or exogenous gonadotropins, needs careful clinical monitoring because of the frequent occurrence of ovarian hyperstimulation syndrome.

On the other hand, factors affecting the response to gonadotropin treatment remain uncertain, but obesity is often associated with abnormal endocrine patterns and anovulation[1,2] and body weight (BW) plays an important role in ovulatory disorders. Many patients with PCOD are obese[3] and this condition may affect a successful therapy. In the present study we have correlated BW and endocrine status with two different gonadotropin treatments.

MATERIALS AND METHODS

Thirty-four PCOD patients were treated for the induction of ovulation with two different modalities of gonadotropin administration. The diagnosis of PCOD was made on the basis of clinical (oligomenorrhea, hyperandrogenism), endocrine [elevated luteinizing hormone (LH) to follicle stimulating hormone (FSH) ratio], echographic and/or laparoscopic findings. None of the patients showed hyperprolactinemia, adrenal pathology or thyroid disorders.

Group A (16 patients, 31 cycles) was treated with pure FSH (Metrodin, 75 i.u. FSH); Group B (18 patients, 19 cycles) were submitted to a pretreatment period (6 weeks) with GnRH agonist (GnRH-A; Buserelin 0.2 mg twice a day s.c.), then a combined GnRH-A plus FSH regimen was given[4]. Two ampoules of FSH/day were administered i.m. to each patient of both groups. In the absence of ovarian response, daily dosage was increased by 1 ampoule every 4 to 5 days of therapy[4,5]. Maximum daily dosage of FSH administered was 300 i.u. in both gonadotropin regimens. Once a follicle was considered to be adequately developed (at least 16 mm diameter), treatment was withheld and after an interval of 24 h 5000 i.u. of hCG (Profasi) were given i.m.

Estradiol (E_2) plasma assay and ultrasound examination of ovaries were performed daily. Retrospectively, plasma androgen levels as well as periovulatory and midluteal progesterone (PG) levels were also assayed. Ovulation time was detected by ultrasound, basal body temperature (BBT) and increase in PG plasma levels. The luteal phase was considered adequate if it lasted more than 12 days with PG levels >6 ng/ml in the mid-luteal phase.

Cycles were also classified as normo- (N) or hyperstimulated (H) according to Rabau *et al.*[6].

Patients were divided in relation to BW, in respect to ideal body weight (IBW) according to Lorentz's criteria[7], into obese (BW $\geq$ 120% IBW) and non-obese (BW $<$ 120% IBW).

RESULTS

In group A, seven patients became pregnant, two twin pregnancies and three abortions occurred. In group B ovulation was achieved in all cycles, five patients became pregnant, two twin pregnancies and one abortion occurred.

In all cycles we found multiple follicular growth. Table 1 shows E_2/ovarian volume and E_2/number of follicles ratios.

Table 2 indicates the dosage and length of FSH treatment required to induce ovulation. Total FSH dosage to induce ovulation successfully was significantly higher in obese patients than in non-obese in both gonadotropin regimens.

Frequency distributions of N and H cycles were: obese patients, N = 66.6%, H = 33.3%; non-obese patients, 85.3% and 14.7%, respectively. The difference was not significant.

When data were displayed for H and N cycles, it was found that in both circumstances obese patients needed a greater amount of FSH to induce ovulation than the others (obese: N 2002 $\pm$ 410 i.u., H 1762 $\pm$ 159 i.u.; non-obese: N 1154 $\pm$ 361 i.u., H 1368 $\pm$ 286 i.u.; $p < 0.01$ and 0.05 respectively),

Table 1 E_2/no. of follicles and E_2/ovarian volume at preovulatory time in FSH (group A) and GnRH-A + FSH (group B) treated women

	E_2/ no. of follicles	*E_2/ ovarian volume*
Group A	514.8 $\pm$ 344.9	20.6 $\pm$ 7.5
Group B	72.7 $\pm$ 91.8	9.0 $\pm$ 7.6
Significance	$p < 0.01$	$p < 0.01$

Table 2 Dosage of FSH therapy and endocrine patterns in patients with PCOD at the start of ovarian stimulation

	Obese		*Non-obese*	
	FSH	*GnRH-A + FSH*	*FSH*	*GnRH-A + FSH*
Dosage (FSH-IU)	2110 ± 431 (a)	1755 ± 234 (b)	1148 ± 327	1400 ± 238
Length (days)	12.6 ± 2.3 (a)	12.4 ± 2.5 (b)	7.8 ± 2.2	9.7 ± 1.9
Testosterone (ng/ml)	0.83 ± 0.42 (x)	0.21 ± 0.11	0.49 ± 0.29 (y)	0.30 ± 0.12
Androstenedione (pg/ml)	2010 ± 870 (y)	690 ± 650	1650 ± 380 (x)	871 ± 315

Significance obese vs non-obese (FSH vs FSH, GnRH-A + FSH vs GnRH-A + FSH) a = $p < 0.01$, b = $p < 0.05$; significance within obese and non-obese (FSH vs GnRH-A + FSH x = $p < 0.01$, y = $p < 0.05$

but no statistical difference within the two classes was seen in relation to the degree of ovarian stimulation.

DISCUSSION

GnRH-A pretreatment permits the achievement of significant reduction of ovarian steroids within a month from the start of therapy.

Normalization of androgens and 17-OH-progesterone (Table 3), in PCOD patients, makes possible a good follicular maturation. In all cycles studied we had a multifollicular growth.

An interesting aspect of this study is that we found a different ratio between plasma E_2 concentrations and ovarian volume or number of follicles, in the patients treated with GnRH-A from those treated with FSH alone: in fact both E_2/ovarian volume and E_2/number of follicles ratios were significantly lower in women who received combined GnRH-A + FSH.

In this study we observed also that the patients with PCOD and excess BW, required a more prolonged stimulation and a higher dosage of FSH than the other patients to achieve ovulation. Furthermore, there was a strong correlation between IBW or BW and the total dosage of FSH used. Similar data have been found by Chong *et al.*[8]. PCOD is a syndrome characterized by excess androgen production and obesity[3], factors which could interfere with ovarian response to gonadotropins. Obese patients generally showed decreased sex hormone binding globulin and elevated levels of androgens.

Table 3 Modifications in plasma levels of androstenedione, 17-OH-progesterone and testosterone under GnRH-A pretreatment

	Basal	*After 6 weeks*
Androstenedione (pg/ml)	1330 ± 620	840 ± 650
17-OH-progesterone (ng/ml)	0.90 ± 0.50	0.49 ± 0.21
Testosterone (ng/ml)	0.44 ± 0.10	0.25 ± 0.10

In this study, in spite of different endocrine milieu obtained with and without GnRH-A pretreatment at the start of FSH therapy (excess or normal androgen levels), the dose-weight relationship is similar in both FSH- and GnRH-A + FSH-treated patients, thus indicating that obesity itself may be considered a factor able to affect ovarian response. In fact after pretreatment with GnRH-A androgen concentrations (testosterone and androstenedione) significantly decreased in respect to those found in basal conditions until normal range values. However, the impact of BW did not appear affected by these long-term endocrine modifications.

However, the superimposable dosage of FSH found in N and H cycles, as well as the incidence of N and H cycles in A and B groups, indicate that, although the effective dosage of FSH to induce ovulation may be estimated in order to avoid further pharmacologically inappropriate stimulus, ovarian response in PCOD patients remains unpredictable because of the hypersensitivity of multifollicular ovaries.

REFERENCES

1. Fishman, J., Boyard, R.M. and Hellman, L. (1975). Influence of body weight on estradiol metabolism in young women. *J. Clin. Endocrinol. Metab.*, **41**, 989–91
2. Louvet, J.P., Harman, S.M., Schreiber, J.R. and Ross, G.T. (1975). Evidence of a role of androgens in follicular maturation. *Endocrinology*, **97**, 366–72
3. Goldzieher, J.W. (1981). Polycystic ovarian disease. *Fertil. Steril.*, **35**, 371–94
4. Lorentz, F.H. (1929). Ein never costitutiosindex. *Klin. Wschr.*, **8**, 348–55
5. Caruso, A., Lanzone, A., Fulghesu, A.M., Apa, R., Guida, C. and Mancuso, S. (1989). Importance of echographic and endocrine monitoring for the assessment of ovulation by follicle stimulating hormone in polycystic ovarian disease. *Int. J. Gynecol. Obstet.*, **28**, 163–9
6. Lanzone, A., Fulghesu, A.M., Spina, M.A., Apa, R., Menini, E., Caruso, A. and Mancuso, S. (1987). Successful induction of ovulation and conception with combined gonadotropin-releasing hormone agonist plus highly purified follicle-stimulating hormone in patients with PCO. *J. Clin. Endocrinol. Metab.*, **65**, 1253–78
7. Rabau, E., Serr, D.M., David, A., Mashiach, S. and Lunenfeld, B. (1975). Human menopausal gonadotropins for anovulation and sterility. *Am. J. Obstet. Gynecol.*, **96**, 92–8
8. Chong, A.P., Rafael, R.P. and Forte, C.C. (1986). Influence of weight in the induction of ovulation with human menopausal gonadotropin and human chorionic gonadotropin. *Fertil. Steril.*, **46**, 599–603

86

The use of buserelin in the treatment of polycystic ovarian disease

C. Di Carlo, M. Mastrocinque, P. Affinito and C. Nappi

INTRODUCTION

The etiology of polycystic ovarian disease (PCOD) is still unclear. However, it is now well known that a pivotal role in its pathogenesis is played by increased luteinizing hormone (LH) pulsatility and by the increased LH to follicle-stimulating hormone (FSH) ratio.

In fact, in 1980 Yen[1] hypothesized the presence of a vicious circle in PCOD. According to his theory the alterations in gonadotropin secretion may be a consequence of the elevated circulating estrone levels deriving from peripheral conversion of the high circulating levels of androstenedione (A) produced by the ovary. In turn, the alterations of gonadotropin secretion may be the cause of the altered ovarian steroidogenesis, leading to hyperandrogenism, altered folliculogenesis and anovulation.

Therapy of PCOD should be aimed towards the reduction of androgen hypersecretion, suppression of unopposed chronic hyperestrogenism, and, if necessary, induction of ovulatory cycles in infertile patients.

SYMPTOMATIC TREATMENT WITH BUSERELIN

In PCOD patients not wishing to conceive, therapy should mainly be aimed towards the reduction of hirsutism, acne and seborrhea (which all cause patient discomfort) and the suppression of endometrial hyperplasia which leads to menstrual irregularities and may evolve into more severe conditions.

The development of gonadotropin-releasing hormone agonists (GnRH-A) provides a new therapeutic approach in PCOD. These peptides, through a desensitization of the pituitary gonadotropes, lead to medical oophorectomy with a decrease in ovarian steroid secretion and may control some of the classical PCOD symptoms[2,3].

Various authors have utilized GnRH-A in the treatment of PCOD symptomatology and all report a decrease of ovarian steroidogenesis in women with PCOD after therapy with GnRH-A[4–11].

We treated eight patients affected by PCOD with the GnRH-A buserelin (Suprefact, Hoechst).

All patients presented the characteristic symptomatology of PCOD (acne, seborrhea, hirsutism, oligoamenorrhea), elevated testosterone (T), A and dehydroepiandrosterone sulfate (DHEA-S) levels, altered LH to FSH ratio and decreased sex hormone-binding globulin (SHBG) levels. Diagnosis of PCOD was confirmed by ultrasonographic examination.

Buserelin was administered at the dose of 200 μg three time daily by intranasal spray for 6 months.

The treatment induced a significant decrease of LH, FSH, estrone (E_1) and estradiol (E_2) (Figure 1), associated with an evident but not significant decrease of A and T (Figure 2). On the other hand DHEA-S and SHBG (Figure 2) were not affected. The lack of effect on DHEA-S, an androgen which is almost exclusively of adrenal origin, demonstrates the selectivity of the GnRH-A-suppressive effect on the pituitary–gonadal axis. Moreover, the inability of buserelin administration to suppress A and T serum levels totally may indicate that in PCOD patients ovarian tissue is excessively sensible to gonadotropin stimulation even at very low concentrations. This suggests the presence of a primary ovarian defect in PCOD[12].

At the end of the treatment these results were reflected by the reduction of hirsutism, acne and skin oiliness. After therapy ultrasonographic examination showed an ovarian size reduction. However, in our reports as well as in others[4–11], the discontinuation of treatment was followed by a relapse of symptoms.

Moreover, a chronic suppression of ovarian function with GnRH-A may involve the risk of alterations of bone mineral content as recently demonstrated[13,14].

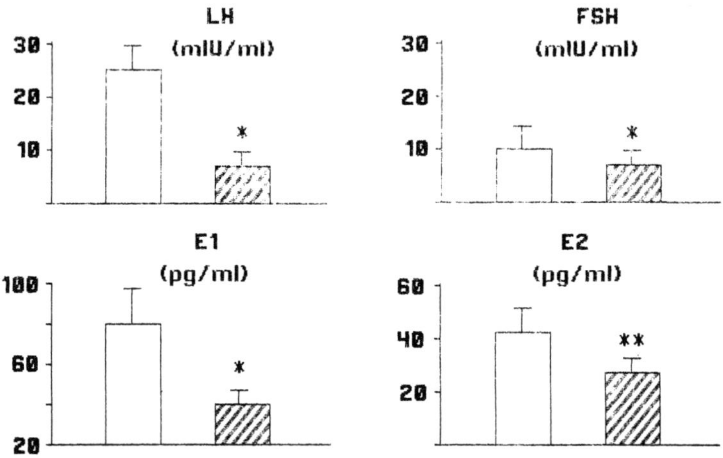

Figure 1 Mean serum concentrations (±SD) of LH, FSH, E_2 and E_1 in eight PCOD patients before (open blocks) and after (hatched blocks) treatment with buserelin nasal spray at the daily dose of 600 μg for 6 months; *$p<0.01$; **$p<0.05$

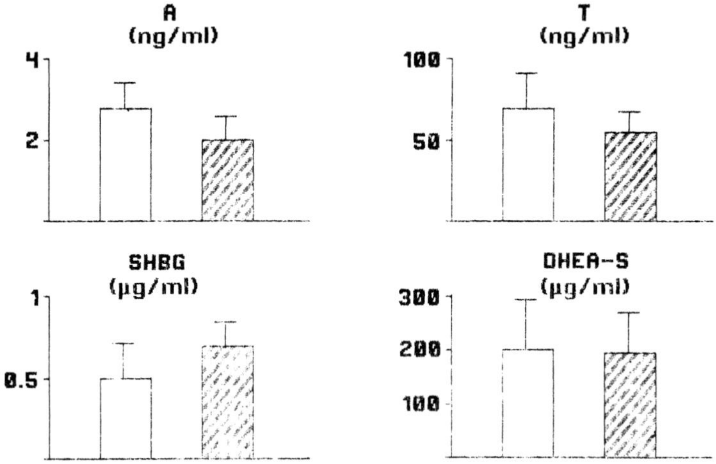

Figure 2 Mean serum concentrations (±SD) of A, T, SHBG and DHEA-S in eight PCOD patients before (open blocks) and after (hatched blocks) treatment with buserelin nasal spray at the daily dose of 600 μg for 6 months

BUSERELIN IN THE INDUCTION OF OVULATION

In PCOD patients wishing to conceive, induction of ovulation presents a high incidence of failure or complications. Clomiphene is reported to have a successful ovulation induction rate ranging from 55% to 99% and a pregnancy rate of 52–76%[15,16].

Infertile PCOD patients unresponsive to clomiphene are generally treated with exogenous gonadotropins. However, since women with PCOD show an increased LH pulsatility, which can interfere with exogenous gonadotropin, this treatment is associated with a high incidence of ovarian hyperstimulation, multiple births, premature follicular luteinization and early miscarriages[17–19].

Moreover, in these patients pulsatile GnRH therapy is often ineffective due to the occurrence of spontaneous LH surges which may induce premature follicular luteinization with reduced pregnancy rate and increased rate of early miscarriage[20,21].

Furthermore, the risk of ovarian hyperstimulation and multiple pregnancy may also be a rather rare complication of pulsatile GnRH therapy in PCOD[22].

The use of GnRH agonists, in association with exogenous gonadotropins, in the induction of ovulation in PCOD patients, is effective in suppressing endogenous gonadotropin secretion, blocking spontaneous LH surges, without interfering with the action of exogenous gonadotropins on the ovary[23]. In other words the use of GnRH agonists gives the opportunity to transform a PCOD patient into a hypogonadotropic subject thus avoiding the complications due to the presence of a functional pituitary gland. Various authors have employed this approach reporting an improvement in the response to exogenous gonadotropins[23–31].

More recently Filicori *et al.*[32,33] and our group[34–36] have reported the use of pulsatile GnRH in the induction of ovulation in PCOD after pituitary suppression with GnRH agonists. Here we present a comparison of the results we have achieved in the induction of ovulation in PCOD patients with either exogenous gonadotropins or pulsatile GnRH after ovarian suppression with buserelin.

In our study we treated 16 infertile patients affected by PCOD selected on the basis of the absence of any other cause of couple infertility. Diagnosis of PCOD was confirmed by hormonal data and ovarian ultrasonography.

All patients had previously failed to respond to clomiphene and had presented premature follicular luteinization, ovarian hyperstimulation, or ovarian stimulation failures to gonadotropin or pulsatile GnRH treatment.

Nine patients (Table 1) were treated for a total of 18 cycles with the GnRH agonist buserelin administered intranasally at the dose of 200 μg twice daily in four cycles or 200 μg three times daily in 14 cycles, until suppression of endogenous gonadotropin was achieved and then with buserelin plus human menopausal gonadotropin (hMG) in six cycles or buserelin plus human FSH (hu-FSH) in 12 cycles. The doses of gonadotropins varied according to the ovarian response assessed by daily plasma E_2 measurement and ovarian ultrasound scannings.

Treatment was stopped when at least one follicle reached 18 mm in diameter and plasma E_2 levels exceeded 400 pg/ml. Ovulation was then induced within 48 hours by a single intramuscular injection of human

Table 1 Protocol of treatment and results achieved in nine PCOD patients treated for a total of 18 cycles with buserelin and exogenous gonadotropins

Patient	*Daily dose of buserelin*	*Gonadotropin utilized*	*Pregnancy*	*Abortion*	*OHS*	*PL*
1	400 μg i.n.	hMG	–	–	+	–
	400 μg i.n.	hMG	+	–	–	–
2	400 μg i.n.	hMG	–	–	–	–
	400 μg i.n.	hMG	–	–	–	–
3	600 μg i.n.	FSH	–	–	+	–
	600 μg i.n.	FSH	+	–	–	–
4	600 μg i.n.	FSH	–	–	–	–
	600 μg i.n.	FSH	–	–	–	–
	600 μg i.n.	FSH	+	+	–	–
5	600 μg i.n.	FSH	–	–	+	–
	600 μg i.n.	FSH	+	–	–	–
6	600 μg i.n.	hMG	–	–	+	–
	600 μg i.n.	FSH	–	–	–	–
7	600 μg i.n.	FSH	–	–	+	–
	600 μg i.n.	FSH	+*	–	–	–
8	600 μg i.n.	hMG	–	–	–	–
	600 μg i.n.	FSH	–	–	+	–
9	600 μg i.n.	FSH	+	+	–	–

OHS, ovarian hyperstimulation; PL, premature follicular luteinization; hMG, human menopausal gonadotropin

*Multiple pregnancy

chorionic gonadotropin (PROFAS; HP 2000, Serono). Luteal phase was supported by exogenous gonadotropins.

The initial increase of FSH, LH and E_2 levels, with corresponding increase of ovarian size, was followed by a decrease of all these parameters. Suppression of the pituitary–ovarian axis was achieved in about 20 days.

Induction of ovulation with exogenous gonadotropins induced follicular maturation and high values of E_2 in all cycles.

Neither spontaneous LH surges nor premature follicular luteinization was observed. Six patients conceived and one multiple pregnancy occurred. However, multiple follicular developments were observed in 10 cycles and a moderate ovarian hyperstimulation was observed in six cases.

The other seven patients (Table 2) were treated, for a total of 11 cycles, with buserelin followed by pulsatile GnRH administration.

Three patients received buserelin intranasally with a daily dose of 600 μg until suppression was achieved.

In the other four patients we administered buserelin subcutaneously at a

Table 2 Protocol of treatment and results achieved in seven PCOD patients treated for a total of 12 cycles with buserelin followed by pulsatile GnRH

Patient	*Daily dose of buserelin*	*Dose GnRH* (90 min)	*Pregnancy*	*Abortion*	*OHS*	*PL*
1	600 μg i.n.	10 μg	+	–	–	–
2	600 μg i.n.	10 μg	–	–	–	–
3	600 μg i.n.	10 μg	–	–	–	–
	600 μg i.n.	10 μg	–	–	–	–
4	1500 μg s.c. + 600 μg i.n.	10 μg	–	–	–	–
	1500 μg s.c. + 600 μg i.n.	10 μg	+	–	–	–
5	1500 μg s.c. + 600 μg i.n.	10 μg	–	–	–	–
	1500 μg s.c. + 600 μg i.n.	10 μg	–	–	–	+
	1500 μg s.c. + 600 μg i.n.	10 μg	–	–	–	–
6	1500 μg s.c. + 600 μg i.n.	10 μg	–	–	–	–
	1500 μg s.c. + 600 μg i.n.	10 μg	+	+	–	–
7	1500 μg s.c. + 600 μg i.n.	10 μg	+	–	–	–

OHS, ovarian hyperstimulation; PL, premature follicular luteinization

Table 3 Comparison of the results achieved with the two different treatment protocols

	Buserelin + *exogenous gonadotropins*	*Buserelin* + *pulsatile GnRH*
Patients	9	7
Cycles	18	11
Pregnancies	6	4
Abortions	2	1
Ovarian hyperstimulation	6	0
Multiple follicular development	10	2
Twin pregnancy	1	0
Premature follicular luteinization	0	1

daily dose of 1500 μg for 10 days and then intranasally at the daily dose of 600 μg until a state of hypogonadotropic hypogonadism was achieved.

The day after buserelin had been stopped, pulsatile GnRH administration was started in both groups with a portable computerized intravenous infusion pump (Zyklomat, Ferring), at the dose of 10 μg every 90 minutes, until ovulation was achieved. In all patients the luteal phase was supported with exogenous human chorionic gonadotropin (Profasi HP 2000 i.m., Serono).

Patients treated with 600 μg of buserelin daily showed a significant suppression of LH and FSH after about 28–42 days of treatment. Pulsatile GnRH administration was followed by ovulation and a sufficient luteal phase in all patients and by a pregnancy in one of them.

In the other group, a significant suppression was achieved after 20–28 days of treatment. Successive pulsatile GnRH administration was followed by ovulation in each case. Three pregnancies were achieved. During pulsatile GnRH administration one premature luteinization was observed. Neither ovarian hyperstimulation nor multiple pregnancies was observed. A summary of the results is reported in Table 3.

Similar pregnancy rates were achieved with the two protocols. However, the use of pulsatile GnRH leads to a reduced incidence of ovarian hyperstimulation and multiple follicular developments.

In conclusion, we confirm that the induction of a state of hypogonadotropic hypogonadism in patients with PCOD allows the achievement of higher pregnancy rates after ovulation induction with either exogenous gonadotropins or pulsatile GnRH administration. However, the use of pulsatile GnRH seems to be free of hyperstimulation and multiple ovulation risks.

REFERENCES

1. Yen, S.S.C. (1980). The polycystic ovary syndrome. *Clin. Endocrinol.*, **12**, 177
2. Filicori, M. and Flamigni, C. (1988). GnRH agonists and antagonists. Current clinical status. *Drugs*, **35**, 63
3. Andreyko, J.L., Marshall, L.A., Dumesic, D.A. and Jaffe, R.B. (1987). Therapeutic uses of gonadotropin-releasing hormone analogs. *Obstet. Gynecol. Surv.*, **42**, 1
4. Chang, R.J., Laufer, L.R., Meldrum, D.R., De Fazio, J., Lu, J.K.H., Vale, W.W., Rivier, J.E. and Judd, H.L. (1983). Steroid secretion in polycystic ovarian disease after ovarian suppression by a long acting gonadotropin-releasing hormone agonist. *J. Clin. Endocrinol.*

Metab., **56**, 897

5. Fleming, R., Black, W.P. and Coutts, J.R.T. (1985). Effects of LH suppression in polycystic ovary syndrome. *Clin. Endocrinol.*, **23**, 683
6. Mongioi, A., Maugeri, G., Macchi, M., Calogera, A., Vicari, E., Coniglione, F., Aliffi, A., Sipione, C. and D'Agata, R. (1986). Effect of gonadotropin releasing hormone analog (GnRH-A) administration on serum gonadotropin and steroid level in patients with polycystic ovarian disease. *Acta Endocrinol.*, **111**, 228
7. Calogero, A., Macchi, M., Montanini, B., Mongioi, A., Maugeri, G., Vicari, E., Coniglione, F., Sipione, C. and D'Agata, R. (1987). Dynamics of plasma gonadotropin and sex steroid release in polycystic ovarian disease after pituitary-ovarian inhibition with an analog of gonadotropin releasing hormone. *J. Clin. Endocrinol. Metab.*, **64**, 980
8. Steingold, K., De Ziegler, D., Cedars, M., Meldrum, D.R., Lu, J.K.H., Judd, H.L. and Chang, R.J. (1987). Clinical and hormonal effects of chronic gonadotropin releasing hormone agonist treatment in polycystic ovarian disease. *J. Clin. Endocrinol. Metab.*, **65**, 773
9. Couzinet, B., Le Strat, N., Brailly, S. and Schaison, G. (1986). Comparative effect of ciproterone acetate or a long-acting gonadotropin releasing hormone agonist in polycystic ovarian disease. *J. Clin. Endocrinol. Metab.*, **63**, 1031
10. Faure, N. and Lemay, A. (1988). Acute pituitary–ovarian response during chronic luteinizing hormone releasing hormone agonist administration in polycystic ovarian syndrome. *Clin. Endocrinol.*, **29**, 403
11. Rittmaster, R.S. (1988). Differential suppression of testosterone and estradiol in hirsute women with the superactive gonadotropin releasing hormone agonist Leuprolide. *J. Clin. Endocrinol. Metab.*, **67**, 651
12. Montemagno, U. and Nappi, C. (1988). Polycystic ovarian disease: a pathogenic problem. In Genazzani, A.R., Montemagno, U.C., Nappi, C. and Petraglia, F. (eds). *The Brain and Female Reproductive Function*, pp. 395–410 (Carnforth: Parthenon Publishing)
13. Matta, W.H., Shaw, R.W., Hesp, R. and Evans, R. (1988). Reversible trabecular bone density loss following induced hypo-oestrogenism with the GnRH analogue buserelin in premenopausal women. *Clin. Endocrinol.*, **29**, 45
14. Johansen, J.S., Riis, B.J., Hassager, C., Moen, M., Jacobson, J. and Christiansen, C. (1988). The effect of a gonadotropin-releasing hormone agonist analog (nafarelin) on bone metabolism. *J. Clin. Endocrinol. Metab.*, **67**, 701
15. Lobo, R.A., Gysler, M., March, C.M., Goebelsmann, U. and Mishell, D.R. (1982). Clinical and laboratory predictors and clomiphene response. *Fertil. Steril.*, **37**, 168
16. Gysler, M., March, C.M., Mishell, D.R. and Bailey, E.J. (1982). A decade's experience with an individualized clomiphene treatment regimen including its effect on the postcoital test. *Fertil. Steril.*, **37**, 161
17. Wang, G.F. and Gemzell, C. (1980). The use of human gonadotropins for the induction of ovulation in women with polycystic ovarian disease. *Fertil. Steril.*, **33**, 479
18. Seibel, M.M., McArdle, C., Smith, D. and Taymor, M.L. (1985). Ovulation induction in polycystic ovary syndrome with urinary follicle stimulating hormone or human menopausal gonadotropin. *Fertil. Steril.*, **43**, 703
19. Nappi, C. (1987). Urinary follicle stimulating hormone in clomiphene-resistant anovulatory women with polycystic ovarian disease. In Genazzani, A. R., Volpe, A. and Facchinetti, F. (eds). *Gynecological Endocrinology*. p. 335. (Carnforth: Parthenon Publishing)
20. Eshel, A., Abdulwahid, N.A., Arman, A.A., Adams, J. and Jacobs, H.S. (1988). Pulsatile luteinizing hormone-releasing hormone therapy in women with polycystic ovary syndrome. *Fertil. Steril.*, **49**, 956
21. Ory, S.J. (1988). Pulsatile luteinizing hormone-releasing hormone therapy in women with polycystic ovary syndrome. *Fertil. Steril.*, **49**, 941
22. Filicori, M., Michelacci, L., Ferrari, P., Campaniello, E., Pareschi, A. and Flamigni, C. (1986). Triplet pregnancy after low-dose pulsatile gonadotropin releasing hormone in polycystic ovarian disease. *Am. J. Obstet. Gynecol.*, **155**, 768
23. Fleming, R., Haxton, M.J., Hamilton, M.P.R., McCune, G.S., Black, W.P., Macnaughton, M.C. and Coutts, J.R.T. (1985). Successful treatment of infertile women with oligomenorrhea using a combination of an LHRH agonist and exogenous gonadotropins. *Br. J. Obstet. Gynaecol.*, **92**, 369
24. Tan, S.L., Armar, N.A., Adams, J., Abdulwahid, N.A., Honour, J.W. and Jacobs, H.S. (1986).

The use of superactive LHRH analogue with FSH – a new method for induction of ovulation in patients with polycystic ovarian syndrome. *Singapore J. Obstet. Gynecol.*, **17**, 93

25. Dodson, W.C., Hughes, C.L., Whitesides, D.B. and Haney, A.F. (1987). The effect of leuprolide acetate on ovulation induction with human menopausal gonadotropins in polycystic ovary syndrome. *J. Clin. Endocrinol. Metab.*, **65**, 95
26. Fleming, R., Yates, R.W.S., Haxton, M.J., Coutts, J.R.T., Hamilton, M.P.R. and Conaghan, C. (1987). Ovulation induction using the combination of buserelin and exogenous gonadotropins in women with functional pituitaries. *Br. J. Clin. Pract.*, **41**, 34
27. Charbonnel, B., Krempf, M., Blanchard, P., Dano, F. and Delage, C. (1987). Induction of ovulation in polycystic ovarian syndrome with combination of a luteinizing hormone-releasing hormone analog and exogenous gonadotropins. *Fertil. Steril.*, **47**, 920
28. Lanzone, A., Fulghesu, A.M., Spina, M.A., Apa, R., Menini, E., Caruso, A. and Mancuso, S. (1987). Successful induction of ovulation and conception with combined gonadotropin-releasing hormone agonist plus highly purified follicle-stimulating hormone in patients with polycystic ovarian disease. *J. Clin. Endocrinol. Metab.*, **65**, 1253
29. Weise, H.C., Fiedler, K. and Kato, K. (1988). Buserelin suppression of endogenous gonadotropin secretion in infertile women with ovarian feed-back disorders given human menopausal/human chorionic gonadotropin treatment. *Fertil. Steril.*, **49**, 399
30. Nakamura, Y., Yoshimura, Y., Tamaoka, Y., Ubukata, Y., Yoshida, K., Yamada, H., Iizuka, R. and Suzuki, M. (1988). Treatment of polycystic ovarian disease by inducing ovulation with pulsatile subcutaneous administration of human menopausal gonadotropin associated with luteinizing hormone-releasing hormone analogue. *Clin. Endocrinol.*, **29**, 395
31. Ayalon, D., Ben-David, M., Wohl, R., Jaffe, R., Vagman, I., Eckstein, N., Limor, R., Comaru-Schally, A.M. and Schally, A.V. (1988). Induction of ovulation with D-Trp 6-LHRH combined with purified FSH in patients with polycystic ovarian disease. *Gynecol. Endocrinol.*, **2**, 319
32. Filicori, M., Ferrari, P., Michelacci, L., Pareschi, A., Campaniello, E., Vizziello, G., Valdiserri, A., Meriggiola, C., Ucci, N., Sorgi, F., Bovicelli, L. and Flamigni, C. (1988). Combined gonadotropin-releasing hormone (GnRH) analog and low dose pulsatile GnRH for induction of ovulation in polycystic ovarian disease. In Genazzani, A.R., Montemagno, U., Nappi, C. and Petraglia, F. (eds). *The Brain and Female Reproductive Function*, pp. 525–31 (Carnforth: Parthenon Publishing)
33. Filicori, M., Campaniello, E., Michelacci, L., Pareschi, A., Ferrari, P., Bolelli, G. and Flamigni, C. (1988). Gonadotropin-releasing hormone (GnRH) analog suppression renders polycystic ovarian disease patients more susceptible to ovulation induction with pulsatile GnRH. *J. Clin. Endocrinol. Metab.*, **66**, 327
34. Mastrocinque, M., Minutolo, M., Colace, G., Cudemo, V. and Nappi, C. (1988). A new treatment protocol for the induction of ovulation in polycystic ovarian disease. In Genazzani, A.R., Montemagno, U., Nappi, C. and Petraglia, F. (eds). *New Trends in Brain and Female Reproductive Function* p. 251. (Rome: CIC Edizioni Internazionali)
35. Mastrocinque, M., Di Carlo, C., Colace, G., Affinito, P., Nappi, C. and Montemagno, U. (1988). Induction of ovulation in PCOD with pulsatile GnRH therapy after suppression of gonadotropins by a GnRH agonist. In Genazzani, A.R., Petraglia, F. and Volpe, A. (eds). *Recent Research on Gynecological Endocrinology*, p. 555. (Carnforth: Parthenon Publishing)
36. Nappi, C., Petraglia, F., Mastrocinque, M., Di Carlo, C., De Chiara, B.M., Genazzani, A.R. and Montemagno, U. (1988). Treatment of PCOD by a GnRH agonist and pulsatile intravenous administration of GnRH. Abstracts of the *XII World Congress of Gynecology and Obstetrics*, Rio de Janiero, 23–8 October

Section 4 continued

Part E

New aspects on the use of monoclonal antibody in the pituitary gonadotropin assays

87

Clinical approach to LH and FSH results obtained with monoclonal antibodies assay

P.L. Venturini, V. Remorgida, V. Aguggia, and L. De Cecco

INTRODUCTION

It is fundamental in reproductive physiology and related disorders to detect plasma levels of circulating gonadotropin accurately. Our actual knowledge in the field of gynecological endocrinology, either in terms of accurate diagnosis or appropriate therapies, is mostly dependent on this information.

For many biological substances a physiological variation of structure and potency is known to exist. Luteinizing hormone (LH) belongs to this group and many isoelectrofocusing studies have shown the charge heterogeneity of human LH in the pituitary, in blood and also in the international standards used for antisera preparation[1]. The oligosaccharide content and structure, mainly sialic acid, appear to be responsible for the charge microheterogeneity of the LH molecule. An association between isoelectrofocusing characteristics and biological potencies has been suggested[2] and variations in the biological activity of the immunoassayed circulating LH have been shown during the menstrual cycle[3] and under specific hormonal environments[4].

Recently, technology employed in the production of monoclonal antibodies has been applied to the development of radioimmunometric assays to be used in laboratory routine.

The aim of this study was to evaluate how the monoclonal approach might influence everyday analysis of gonadotropins, mainly LH, and to compare these results with those provided by our previous assay. We have tested its efficacy in a physiological setting and in some endocrinological situations, where changes in LH concentration or molecules are known to occur.

MATERIAL AND METHODS

Origin of the samples

Our blood samples came from two categories of women. Normally menstruating women ($n=51$) volunteered to give at least five samples during a menstrual cycle. Confirmation of ovulation was performed by means of ultrasound scan of the ovaries (dominant follicle) around midcycle. Based on menstrual history, values have been analyzed and plotted on a hypothetical 28-day cycle. From this pool of data we selected those originating from early follicular (days 2–4, $n=21$) middle follicular (days 7–10, $n=21$) and late luteal phase (days 20–24, $n=21$) to be used for comparison purposes.

In 12 normal subjects a gonadotropin hormone-releasing hormone (GnRH) test (100 μg i.v. as a bolus) was performed within the first 7 days of the cycle. Blood samples were taken before and 20, 40 and 60 min after the injection.

Patients referred to our Endocrine and Infertility Unit for hormonal evaluation constituted the basis from which we selected our group of functional hypothalamic amenorrheic women ($n=19$) and our polycystic ovarian patients ($n=27$). Patients suffering from endometriosis or uterine fibroids ($n=13$) and treated with a minimum daily dosage of 600 μg s.c. of a gonadotropin hormone-releasing hormone analog (LHRH-A) constituted the sources of blood samples from a medically induced hypogonadotropism.

Hormonal assay

The assay tested in this work is the Maiaclone produced by Ares Serono (Milano, Italy). The standards of the assay are calibrated against WHO, 1st International Reference Preparation (IRP) for human LH (68/40). This assay combines three features: radioimmunometry, monoclonal technology and magnetic solid phase. A detailed description of the monoclonal antibody used in this preparation has been published[5].

The other assay used for comparison is a polyclonal system (Ter, Ares Serono) based on the principle of the double antibody separation technique. This assay has been used in our Department for several years and its characteristics have already been published[6]. Its standards are calibrated against the 2nd International References Preparation for human LH (69/104).

The follicle-stimulating hormone (FSH) determination was based solely on the Maiaclone assay, which is identical in principle with that described for LH. The monoclonal antibody was raised against 2nd International Reference Preparation (IRP) for human FSH) (78/549).

Statistical analysis and graphical representation

Statistical evaluation used a software package (Statgrafic 1.2, STSC, Inc) run on an IBM personal computer. Tests performed were: *t* test for paired and unpaired data and linear regression with coefficient of correlation.

RESULTS

The mean LH and FSH values found with the monoclonal assay during normal menstrual cycles in our normal women, the presence of an LH and FSH peak around midcycle, the former larger than the latter, is consistent with our knowledge of gonadotropin dynamics. The LH/FSH ratio with the monoclonal assay was <1 until the periovulatory phase and close to 1 during the luteal phase.

In order to facilitate comparison, although not formally correct because of the known differences existing between the two international standards[7], all data originating from the 2nd international standard (the polyclonal assay) were multiplied by 0.50. This number has been calculated as the conversion factor between 2nd and 1st standard for that assay. This figure was generated on the basis of the National Quality Control Program performed by the CNR (National Research Council)[8,9].

Overal results of the groups considered in this study are shown in Figures 1 and 2 where a box display of the data gives a simple descriptive statistical analysis. It is visible from the figures how the average values resulting from the two methods, both for total and each of the group analyzed, is lower when the monoclonal assay is used.

Student t test performed on the whole data showed that there was a significant difference ($p<0.001$) between the results provided by the two assays even though a large overlap existed. When the same test was performed on each of the groups considered, we noticed that in data collected throughout the menstrual cycle this difference was lost (p=n.s.). GnRH test results are in accordance with those observed in the normal cycle (p=n.s.). On the other hand the amenorrheic patients were differently discriminated by the two assays ($p<.001$).

This difference was striking in the LHRH-A treated patients. In this group the dispersion of data was dramatically reduced with the monoclonal assay.

Data collected in patients with polycystic ovaries at basal condition revealed, unlike the other categories discussed, the presence of a lower value for the polyclonal assay with $p<0.001$ statistical difference.

CONCLUSION

It has been stated that 'Immunometric assays, using monoclonal antibodies, will supersede radioimmunoassay for FSH and LH during the next few years'.[10]. For this reason, when this type of assay became commercially available we thought it would be valuable to test its effectiveness in clinical practice.

We decided to compare the answers provided by the two assays in physiological conditions such as the normal menstrual cycle and in specific endocrine situations like functional hypothalamic amenorrhea, polycystic ovarian disease and treatment with LHRH-A.

The profile of the normal cycle was comparable to that described in previous work[11].

It is important to remember that the two assays used in this study were raised against international standards which are known to be very different[7]. In order to facilitate comparison we introduced the 'conversion factor' for the old assay. Notwithstanding this limitation, it is clear that values obtained with the immunoradiometric assay were lower than those obtained with the previous system.

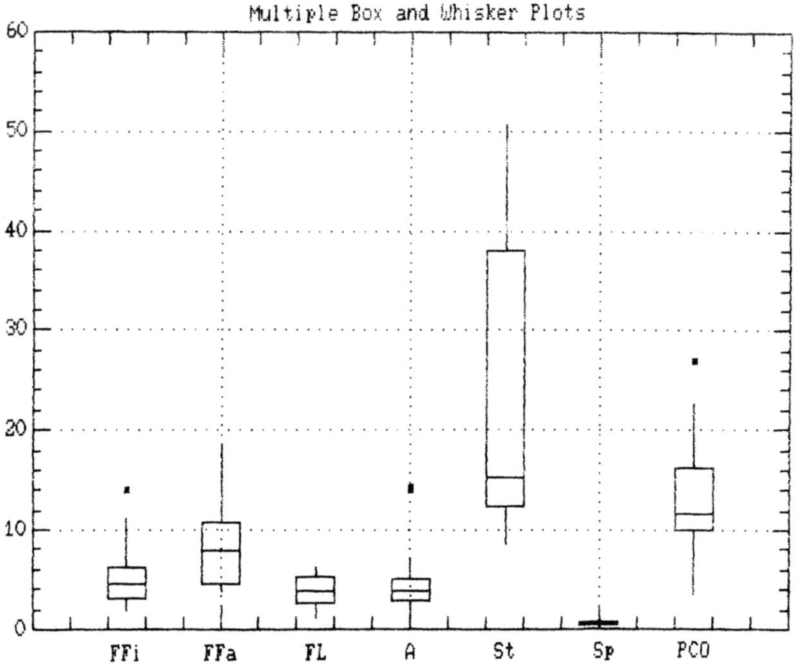

Figure 1 Display of LH values obtained with monoclonal assay. On the y axis is the LH concentration (mIU/ml). On the x axis the groups considered in the study (FFi = early follicular phase; FFa = midfollicular phase; FL = luteal phase; A = functional hypothalamic amehorrhea; St = GnRH challenge test; Sp = LHRH-A treatment; PCO = polycystic ovarian disease). The box plots allow a summary display of the distribution of the data. The upper and lower quartile are portrayed by the top and bottom of the rectangle, the median by an horizontal line segment within the rectangle. Solid lines (whiskers) extend from the ends of the box to the adjacent values which are defined to be the longest observation that is less than or equal to the interquartile range (IQR) × 1.5. If any data falls outside the range of the two adjacent values it is considered an outsider value and it is plotted as an individual point

The comparison of the results obtained during the physiological menstrual cycle has shown that a good correlation between the two methods is present. This equivalence is lost when the sample is instead originating from ovulatory disorders such as amenorrhea. This might be taken as an evidence that assorted LH molecules are circulating in the blood and are differently detected by the two assays, as the monoclonal system is specific only to the intact molecule. For instance cross-reaction from the α chain of the LH molecules was not discriminated with the polyclonal assay.

When we analyzed data collected in patients with a medical hypogonadotropinism[12] under LHRH-A therapy we noticed how the monoclonal assay correctly displayed the achievement of this condition while the polyclonal assay was still falsely detecting circulating LH molecules. As it has been clearly shown that the pituitary GnRH receptor down-regulation operated by this kind of drug results in discharge of α-LH chains[13], it is highly suggestive of a discriminating ability of the monoclonal antibodies between the intact molecule and its chains.

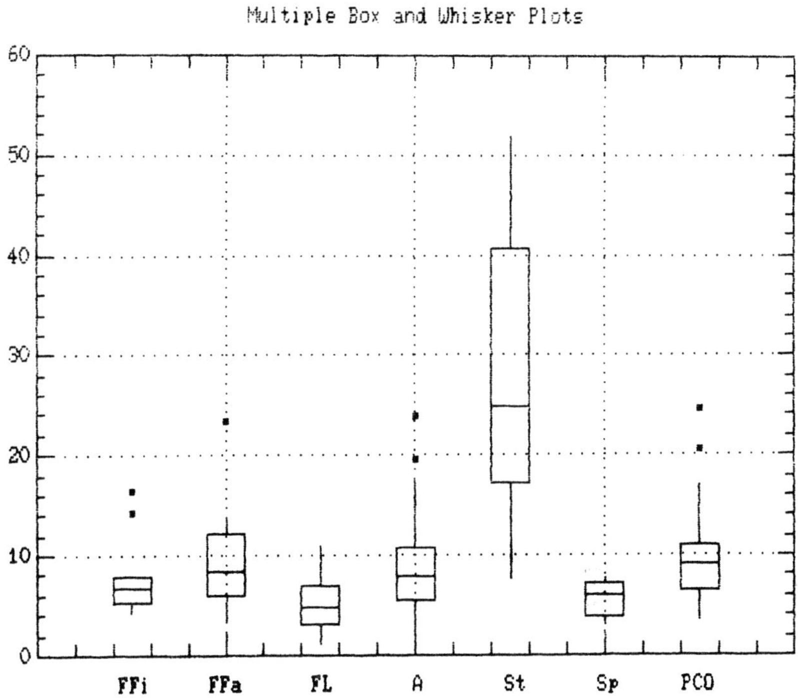

Figure 2 Display of LH values obtained with polyclonal assay. On the y axis is the LH concentration (mIU/ml). On the x axis the groups considered in the study (FFi = early follicular phase; FFa = midfollicular phase; FL = luteal phase; A = functional hypothalamic amenorrhea; St = GnRH challenge test; Sp = LHRH-A treatment; PCO = polycystic ovarian disease). The box plots allow a summary display of the distribution of the data. The upper and lower quartile are portrayed by the top and bottom of the rectangle, the median by an horizontal line segment within the rectangle. Solid line (whiskers) extend from the ends of the box to the adjacent values which are defined to be the longest observation that is less than or equal to the interquartile range (IQR) × 1.5. If any data falls outside the range of the two adjacent values it is considered an outsider value and it is plotted as an individual point

In polycystic ovarian disease patients we observed a good overlapping between the two populations with a tendency to higher LH values with the monoclonal assay after the standard transformation. This is in agreement with previous work showing that LH from these patients is fully biologically active[14].

In conclusion, the monoclonal assay has been shown to possess a good specificity toward the molecule enabling better discrimination in clinical conditions characterized by a qualitative variation of the LH molecule.

Polyclonal assay must still be considered effective for heavy everyday routine work. However, for the clinician who is more and more frequently involved with drugs interacting with the reproductive endocrine environment, the information provided by monoclonal assay represents a useful support either for pretreatment evaluation or for monitoring the response to therapy.

REFERENCES

1. van Ginkel, L.A. and Loeber, J.G. (1987). Heterogeneity of human luteinizing hormone. *Acta Endocrinol. (Copenh)*, **114**, 572–6
2. Dufau, M.L., Catt, K.J. and Tsuruhara, T. (1971). Retention of *in vitro* biological activities by desialylated human luteinizing hormone and chorionic gonadotropin. *Biochem. Biophys. Res. Comm.*, **44**, 1022–9
3. Veldhuis, J.D., Beitins, I.Z., Johnson, M.L., Serabian, M.A. and Dufau, M.L. (1984). Biologically active luteinizing hormone is secreted in episodic pulsations that vary in relation to stage of the menstrual cycle. *J. Clin. Endocrinol. Metab.*, **58**, 1050–8
4. Evans, R.M., Doelle, G.C., Lindner, J., Bradley, V. and Rubin, D. (1984). A luteinizing hormone-releasing hormone agonist decreases biological activity and modified chromatographic behavior of luteinizing hormone in men. *J. Clin. Invest.*, **73**, 262–6
5. Siddle, K., Gard, T.G., Soos, M.A., Gray, I.P. and Hales, C.N. (1986). Immunoradiometric assay of polypeptide hormones using monoclonal antibodies. In Forti, G., Serio, M. and Lipsett, M.B. (eds). *Monoclonal Antibodies: Basic Principles, Experimental and Clinical Applications in Endocrinology*, pp. 49–57. (New York: Serono Symposia Raven Press)
6. Remorgida, V., Venturini, P.L., Anserini, P., Lanera, P. and De Cecco, L. (1989). Administration of pure follicle-stimulating hormone during gonadotropin-releasing hormone agonist therapy in patients with clomiphene resistant polycystic ovarian disease: hormonal evaluation and clinical perspectives. *Am. J. Obstet. Gynecol.*, **160**, 108–13
7. Khan, S.A., Qazi, M.H. and Diczfalusy, E. (1984). The significance of *in vitro* bioassays for the estimation and characterization of human luteinizing hormone (LH). *J. Endocrinol. Invest.*, **7**, (suppl.3), 1–22
8. Albertini, A., Iacobello, C., Pizzocolo, G., Signorini, C. and Tosoni, S. (1984). Suppliers of kits for lutropin, follitropin, and prolactin should all use the same calibrators. *Clin. Chem.*, **30**, 1723–4
9. Albertini, A., Iacobello, C., Pilo, A., Pizzocolo, G., Signorini, C. and Zucchelli, G.C. (1982). CNR external quality control program for LH, FSH and CG: first semester experience. *J. Nucl. Med. All. Sci.*, **26**, 285–90
10. Beastall, G.H., Ferguson, K.M., O'Reilly, D.S.T.J., Seth, J. and Sheridan, B. (1987). Assay for follicle stimulating hormone and luteinising hormone: guidelines for the provision of a clinical biochemistry service. *Ann. Clin. Biochem.*, **24**, 246–62
11. Landgren, B.M., Unden, A.L. and Diczfalusy, E. (1980). Hormonal profiles in the cycles in 68 normally menstruating women. *Acta Endocrinol. (Copenh)*, **94**, 89–98
12. McLachlan, R.I., Healy, D.L. and Burger, H.G. (1986). Clinical aspects of LHRH analogues in gynaecology: a review. *Br. J. Obstet. Gynaecol.*, **93**, 431–54
13. Meldrum, D.R., Tsao, Z., Monroe, S.E., Braunstein, G.D., Sladek, J., Lu, J.K.H., Vale, W., Rivier, J., Judd, H.L. and Chang, R.J. (1984). Stimulation of LH fragments with reduced bioactivity following GnRH agonist administration in women. *J. Clin. Endocrinol. Metab.*, **58**, 755–9
14. Lobo, R.A., Kletzky, O.A., Compeau, J.D. and Di Zerega, C.S. (1983). Elevated bioactive luteinizing hormone in women with the polycystic ovary syndrome. *Fertil. Steril.*, **39**, 674–7

88

The use of gonadotropin assays in the diagnosis of polycystic ovary syndrome

S. S. Lynch, M. Obhrai, W. Robinson and W. R. Butt

INTRODUCTION

The polycystic ovary syndrome (PCOS) is a common cause of infertility in women presenting with amenorrhea and oligomenorrhea[1]. In the past the definitive diagnosis depended upon laparoscopy or laparotomy with ovarian biopsy to detect histologically multiple follicular cysts and increased stroma. Advances in high resolution ultrasonography have now enabled diagnosis of the syndrome to be made without the need for invasive techniques. In conjunction with ultrasonography, hormonal analysis to detect any hormonal abnormalities is useful as this may give guidance on the subsequent treatment which is most appropriate.

The hormones most commonly found to be abnormal are the androgens and luteinizing hormone (LH). Elevated LH was found in 49 of 76 patients (64.5%) presenting with typical PCOS in a recent study[2]. Follicle stimulating hormone (FSH) however, tends to be within the normal range or on the low side so that the LH:FSH ratio is raised and 52 of the above 76 patients (68.4%) had elevated ratios. Gonadotropins are measured in different laboratories with widely differing reagents using antibodies which may be polyclonal or monoclonal and with tracers which may be radioactive or non-radioactive. Not surprisingly results on the same samples may differ widely and badly affect results such as the LH:FSH ratio[3]. The objective of the present study was to determine serum LH, FSH and LH:FSH ratio by five different assay methods in women with PCOS diagnosed ultrasonically to gain information on the likely variation in results.

PATIENTS AND METHODS

The patients with PCOS diagnosed by ultrasound were divided into four groups (P1–P4) according to their menstrual histories[2]. Group P1 consisted of 10 patients who presented with fairly regular but anovular cycles, P2 were 49 patients with oligomenorrhea with periods not less than 42 days apart, P3 were eight patients with primary or secondary amenorrhea and P4 were nine found to have raised progesterone at the time of the hormonal assays.

The analyses were performed on samples of blood taken in the first 7 days of the menstrual cycle where possible or when patients attended the clinic in those with amenorrhea. The methods used were the routine laboratory radioimmunoassays and four commercially available kits based on immunoradiometric methods:

(1) Routine (R) LH and FSH radioimmunoassays[4] using polyclonal antibodies, separation by magnetizable particles and ^{125}I tracer.

(2) Serono MAIAClone (M) LH and FSH immunoradiometric assays using monoclonal antibodies, separation by magnetizable particles and ^{125}I tracer.

(3) Serono Serozyme (S) LH and FSH immunoenzymatic assays using monoclonal antibodies and separation by magnetizable particles with spectrophotometric end-point.

(4) Amersham Amerlite (A) LH and FSH immunochemiluminescent assays using monoclonal (LH first antibody, FSH second antibody) and polyclonal (LH second antibody, FSH first antibody) antibodies, separation by well-adhesion and chemiluminescent end-point.

(5) LKB Delfia (D) LH and FSH immunofluorometric assays using monoclonal antibodies, separation by well adhesion and fluorometric end-point.

Results were analyzed by standard statistical techniques using Student *t* tests and regression analysis.

RESULTS

The average age of the patients was 26.4 years with a range of 17–37 years. There were no significant differences between the mean ages of the four groups of patients and their age ranges were similar.

There was an excellent correlation between LH assays by method R and each of the other methods ($r = 0.83$–0.95; $p < 0.001$): an example is shown in Figure 1. The correlation between FSH assays by method R and each of the other methods was also significant ($r = 0.64$–0.88; $p < 0.001$) although there was more scatter than for LH: an example is shown in Figure 2.

The mean LH values assayed by the R method were greater than the mean values for any of the other methods for each group of patients (Table 1). There were no significant differences between these kit methods themselves. FSH results were closer to one another and the R estimates did not differ significantly from the kit methods (Table 2). The LH : FSH ratio was therefore higher estimated from the R results than by the other methods except for groups P2 and P4 where the A method results were not significantly different (Table 3).

The control ranges for LH and FSH assays by the R method and the quoted control ranges by the other methods are given in Table 4. In the

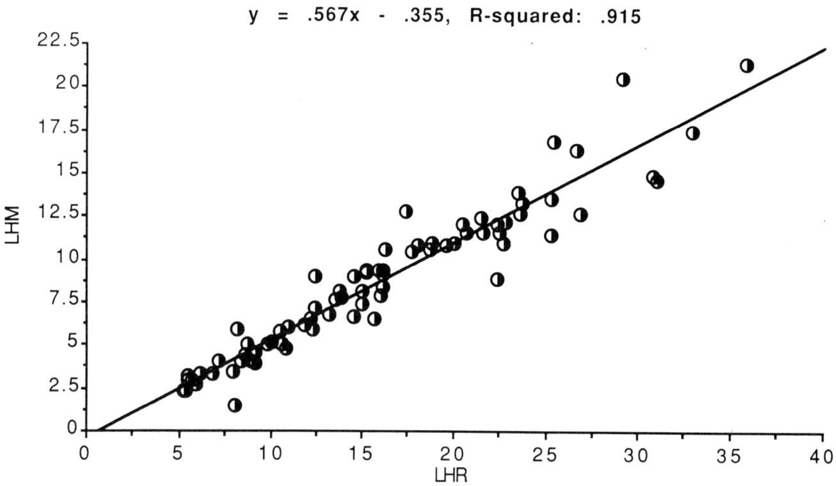

Figure 1 Correlation between the results of LH assays by Method R and Method M

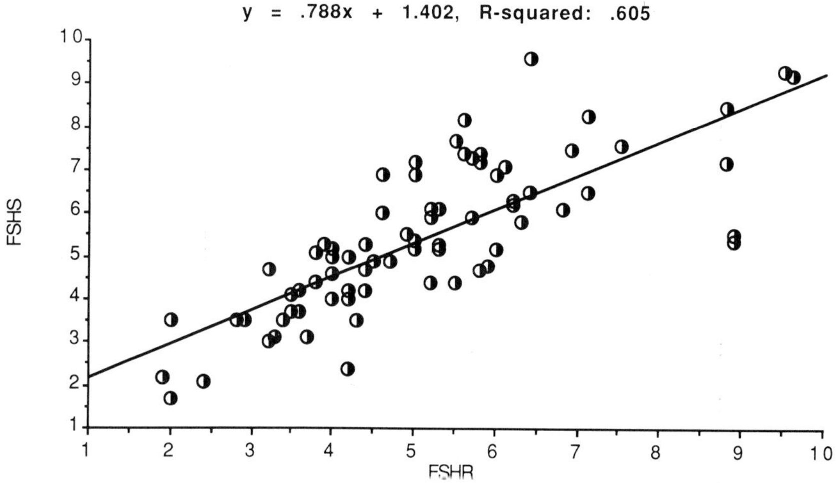

Figure 2 Correlation between the results of FSH assays by method R and method S

Table 1 Mean values for LH (u/l) in the PCOS patients by five methods of assay

Method of assay	*Patient group*			
	P1	*P2*	*P3*	*P4*
R	11.8	17.0	16.7	11.4
M	6.7	9.3	9.5	6.5
S	6.9	9.3	9.7	6.9
A	9.3	13.5	14.8	8.3
D	6.3	9.6	9.1	7.4

The mean values for each group of patients assayed by method R were significantly greater than the mean values by the other methods ($p < 0.001$)

Table 2 Mean values for FSH (u/l) in the PCOS patients by the five methods of assay

Method of assay	*Patient group*			
	P1	*P2*	*P3*	*P4*
R	5.3	5.4	4.9	3.0
M	6.4	5.6	4.8	3.2
S	6.3	5.6	4.8	3.6
A	5.4	4.9	5.5	2.7
D	5.4	4.8	4.7	3.2

Table 3 Mean values for the LH:FSH ratio in the PCOS patients by the five methods of assay

Method of assay	*Patient group*			
	P1	*P2*	*P3*	*P4*
R	2.14	3.22	3.46	3.65
M	1.02	1.74	2.08	2.11
S	1.05	1.73	2.10	1.87
A	1.69	3.02	2.82	3.15
D	1.11	2.22	2.02	2.34

The mean values for each group of patients assayed by method R were significantly ($p < 0.001$) greater than the mean values by the other methods except for the method A results in Groups P2 and P4

Table 4 Quoted control ranges for the five methods of assay

Method	*LH (IRP 68/40)*		*FSH (2nd IRP 78/549)*	
	Follicular	*Luteal*	*Follicular*	*Luteal*
R	1–12	1–12	1–9	1–9
M	1.8–13.4	0.7–19.4	3–12	2–12
S	1.2–12.5	0.4–19	3.2–10	1.3–11
A	0.5–12	0.5–12	0.5–10	0.5–10
D	2–12	5–15	2–12	2–12

follicular phase of the cycle these ranges are similar for the various methods. The results in the 76 patients were examined alongside these control ranges and the number of patients with results above the range for LH were R = 59, M = 17, S = 27, A = 50 and D = 19. No FSH value was outside the control range.

In the absence of a control group of normal patients the patients who were menstruating regularly but were not ovulating, group P1, were considered to be the nearest to normal. They were used as a control group against which to compare the other groups. Their mean LH:FSH ratios (Table 3) were significantly lower than the mean ratios in the other groups by each method of assay. The number of patients with ratios greater than the mean for P1 for each method were R = 53, M = 52, S = 55, A = 53 and D = 56 with 92% correspondence.

DISCUSSION

This study has demonstrated that LH determined in samples from PCOS patients by different immunological techniques varies considerably. This is unexpected considering the similar control ranges quoted for each method. The results between methods however, showed significant correlations. FSH did not vary as much so that the LH : FSH ratio, often used in the diagnosis of PCOS, differed in level between the methods of assay. Similar variation was found by others[3].

These results are not unexpected when the variety of antisera used in the assays is considered. The epitopes recognized by polyclonal antibodies as used in method R for instance, may not recognize the epitopes to monoclonal antibodies in the other methods. It is important therefore, that the reference ranges for each hormone be assessed for each method and that an upper normal limit for the LH : FSH ratio should not be quoted without stating the method.

A problem which arises in studies of this kind is to be sure of the stage of the cycle in patients who have only occasional periods. The LH : FSH ratio may change if follicular development and the occasional ovulation occurs. It is recommended therefore that samples be taken within 7 days of a menstrual period in those with fairly regular cycles and by 7 days after a progestogen-induced bleed in the others.

ACKNOWLEDGEMENTS

This work was supported financially by Serono Diagnostics UK and by the Central Birmingham Health Authority Trust Funds. We thank Mr G Holder for the statistical analyses and Mrs Rachel Round for technical assistance.

REFERENCES

1. Hull, M.G.R. (1987). Epidemiology of infertility and polycystic ovarian disease: endocrinological and demographic studies. *Gynecol. Endocrinol.*, **1**, 235–45
2. Obhrai, M., Lynch, S.S., Holder, G., Jackson, R., Tang, L. and Butt, W.R. (1990). Hormonal studies on women with the polycystic ovary syndrome diagnosed by ultrasound. *Clin. Endocrinol.* (in press)
3. Robinson, S., Rodin, D.A., Deacon, A. and Clayton, R.D. (1988). Is the LH/FSH ratio of value in diagnosis of polycystic ovary syndrome? *J. Endocrinol.*, **117**, (Supplement Abstract) 139
4. Lynch, S.S., Reay, P. and Bluck, M. (1988). The extraction and purification of human pituitary follicle-stimulating hormone and luteinizing hormone. *Acta endocrinol.* (*Copenh.*), **119**, (Supplement 228,) 12–19

89

Significance of specific LH patterns for success in an IVF/ET program

H. Zech, P. Weiss, H. Fritzsche and H. Schönholzer

INTRODUCTION

Due to organizational reasons most oocyte collections for either IVF or gamete intrafallopian transfer are timed by the injection of an ovulatory dose of human chorionic gonadotropin (hCG). Irrespective of the stimulation protocol for ovarian augmentation, monitoring of follicular growth is based on one or more of the following criteria[1,2]: the predicted day of ovulation, number of follicles, follicle growth rate, follicular size, level and rate of rise of serum estradiol (E_2), progesterone (P) or 17-hydroxyprogesterone (17-OH-P) determinations in plasma prior to hCG application, luteinizing hormone (LH) concentrations in plasma or urine around the day of hCG application.

There is some controversy with regard to the continuation of therapy in case of a premature LH rise. While some investigators suggest cancelling cycles in which there are LH rises because of a poor prognosis for pregnancy[3], others successfully use an endogenous LH surge for ovulation induction timing with an improvement of both oocyte maturation and endometrial transformation[4].

Our experience of the importance of a specific endogenous LH surge around the day of hCG application for the establishment of a pregnancy after stimulation for IVF/ET has been demonstrated earlier[5] and was supported by reports of other investigators[6]. The preovulatory LH surge, which induces final follicular maturation with the resumption of the second meiotic division of the oocyte is the result of well balanced positive and negative feedback mechanisms of ovarian steroids as well as of non-steroidal ovarian factors on the release of gonadotropins[7,8]. In order to elucidate further the significance of this gonadotropin for the establishment of pregnancy we retrospectively examined these LH patterns and correlated them to the outcome of therapy.

MATERIAL AND METHODS

One hundred and five consecutive patients with proven tubal infertility, ovulatory spontaneous cycles and with a normal sperm count of their husbands (concentration > 20 Mio/ml, motility > 40%, > 40% normal forms) have been stimulated for IVF/ET with a combination of Clomiphene Citrate (Cl) (Clomiphen®, Arcana), pure follicle–stimulating hormone (FSH) (Fertinorm®, Serono) and hCG (Pregnyl®, Organon) as described earlier[5].

Depending on the length of the unstimulated cycle, therapy was either started on cycle day 5 (> 28 days), 4 (25–27 days) or 3 (spontaneous cycle length < 24 days) with 100 mg/d of Cl for 5 days, when the stimulation with FSH (150 IU/d) was continued until the leading follicle reached 18 mm. At 08.00 the following day the collection of representative urine samples every 4 h was started and continued until 24.00 when an ovulatory dose of 10 000 IU of hCG was given. After this hCG application urine collection was continued every 6 h until 06.00 on the day of follicle puncture (Figure 1).

Follicular growth was monitored with an intravaginal ultrasound transducer (Model IVT 5.0 MHz, SMS).

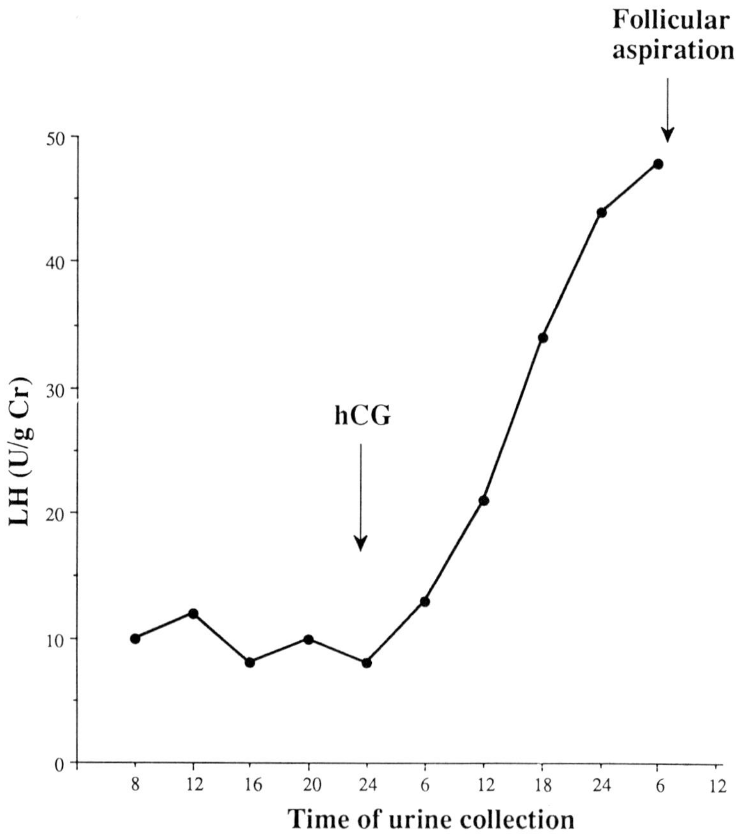

Figure 1 Urinary LH concentrations in relation to hCG application and follicular aspiration

The recent development of a rapid serum/urine LH radioimmunoassay (MAIAclone, Serono Diagnostics) which uses monoclonal antibodies and does not therefore cross-react with hCG, allows the monitoring of LH to continue after the injection of hCG.

In order to facilitate the organization and to exclude sources of errors with volume and time interval documentations the LH concentrations were correlated to the urinary creatinine concentrations and expressed as LH units per gram creatinine (LH u/g Cr)[9].

Follicles were aspirated transvaginally under a mild neuroleptanalgesia on an outpatient basis. For embryo culture a modified Earle's medium supplemented with 10% (v/v) heat inactivated serum was used. Conceptus transfer was performed in a total volume of 15–20 μl 20–44 h after insemination. The corpus luteum phase was supported with 20 mg dydrogesteron (Duphaston®, Duphar), 14 and, where there was a positive result, again 16 days after ovulation induction β-hCG levels for the detection of implantation were determined.

All data were stored in a computer (PS 80, PC Math. Lab., IBM). For each LH concentration (10 per cycle) of all patients variables were calculated and analyzed by the linear discriminant analysis[10].

RESULTS

Of 105 stimulations in patients with classical tubal infertility 31 cycles (30%) had to be cancelled mainly due to pathological LH patterns as evaluated in an earlier investigation[5]: nine patients had very low (< 5 LH u/g Cr) and 12 patients markedly increased (> 20 LH u/g Cr) LH concentrations with no characteristic surge (mean basal concentration + 2 SD) after hCG. The LH profiles of 10 patients revealed significant fluctuations both prior to and after hCG; two of these patients additionally suffered from acute influenza with mild temperature rises.

A mean number of 2.4 oocytes per patient was aspirated. The fertilization rate was 86%, the cleavage rate 76%, irrespective of the LH profile. Of the 74 patients with follicular aspirations 29 showed rising β-hCG levels on days 14 and 16 after ovulation induction respectively.

The application of the discriminant analysis for the LH patterns of each patient enabled the determination of the value 'd' of the discriminant function. 'd' is a real number characterized by the attribute that as a rule pregnant [P] patients have negative, the not pregnant [NP] patients positive values. In order to be able to arrange patients into two groups, 'g' was calculated. Thus, the line through the separation point could be determined. The variance analysis of the LH profiles enabled the discrimination of these two groups: Group 1 – pregnant [P] with a smaller value 'd' of the discriminant function than 'g' and Group 2 – not pregnant [NP] with a larger value 'd' (Figure 2).

The retrospective analysis of these data demonstrated that of the total of 74 patients 69 (93%) could be assigned to the correct group. Twenty-seven (93%) of the 29 patients in Group 1 were assigned to the correct group, two

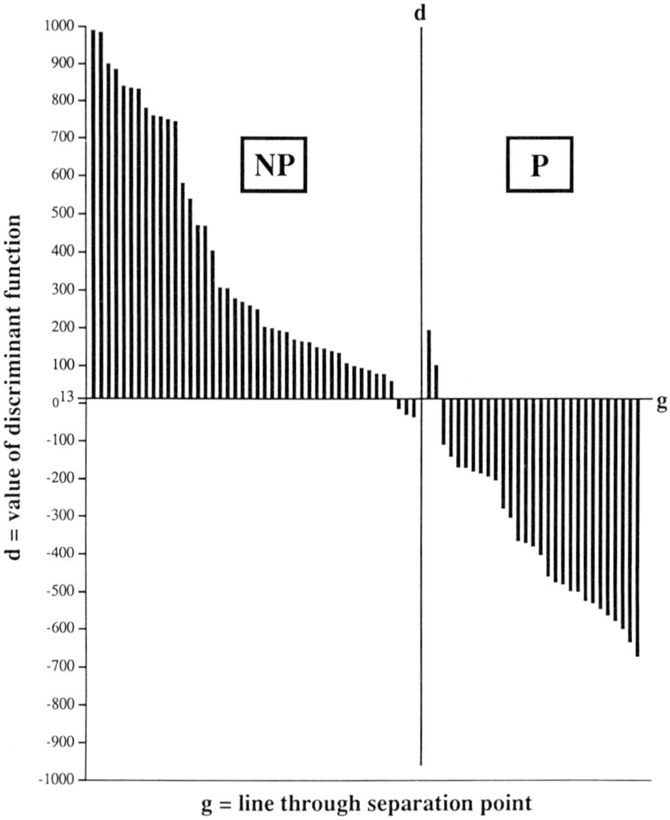

Figure 2 Linear discriminant analysis for binary data collected from two groups. Group 1 = urinary LH values from pregnant (P) patients. Group 2 = urinary LH values from not pregnant (NP) patients

(7%) patients to the wrong group. The same percentage of correct and wrong grouping respectively could be calculated in Group 2: in 42 (93%) of these 45 cycles allocation to the correct group was possible, in three (7%) cycles grouping with this method was wrong.

DISCUSSION

These data, obtained through the use of frequent LH determinations before and after ovulation induction with hCG permitted detailed investigations of the influence of LH on the establishment of a pregnancy after stimulation for IVF/ET.

The preovulatory high levels of E_2 finally led to a sharp increase in the pituitary output of LH. Within the mature follicle, the LH surge triggers a complex set of events that finally result in ovulation and luteinization.

Due to organizational reasons, ovulation induction in stimulated cycles is carried out by the application of hCG. All patients in this study received the same dose of 10 000 u hCG to induce final maturation of the follicular structures.

The retrospective analysis of the LH profiles of all patients showed very clearly that for the establishment of a pregnancy specific endogenous LH influences on the follicular structures are necessary. There was no difference in the fertilization and cleavage rate between pregnant and not pregnant patients. Therefore, it is likely, that a certain endogenous LH surge-pattern is mandatory for the establishment of an intact corpus luteum. Although hCG can also be used to stimulate corpus luteum function, other mechanisms seem to exist which are LH-dependent. They may be important for the early and late corpus luteum formation. Whether there also exists an influence on the oocyte, not only to cleave but to implant, is not yet clear.

The concomitant rise of E_2 and P reflects the acquisition of LH receptors in the granulosa cells and, therefore, the ability to initiate the biosynthesis of 17-OH-P and P. The elevation of circulating P which begins approximately 12 h before the onset of the LH rise may augment the timing, amplitude and duration of the LH surge[11–17].

Preovulatory oocytes irrespective of the LH profiles could be found in aspirates of all patients. This may indicate that apart from other reasons for the failure to establish a pregnancy, in cycles with implantation particular LH responses are imperative. The detection of these surge patterns retrospectively may confirm the quality of the follicular phase.

These LH profiles have been studied by the discriminant analysis. It was possible to separate LH patterns which are mandatory for the establishment of a pregnancy from LH profiles which fail to induce these effects on the granulosa cells and to respond to rising E_2 and the augmentation of P.

In summary, the data presented provide relatively precise information on the importance of particular LH patterns for the establishment of a pregnancy in stimulated cycles. Further, the present observations suggest that for the monitoring of these patients statistical analysis of LH concentrations which retrospectively confirm the quality of the follicular phase may help to select the right patient at the right time for the IVF/ET procedure and to increase the pregnancy rate with this therapy.

REFERENCES

1. Miron, P., Hay, D.L., Johnston, W.I.H., McKenna, M. and McBain, J. C. (1988). Midcycle changes of 17-OH-progesterone levels in women superovulated with clomiphene citrate and human menopausal gonadotropin for *in vitro* fertilization. *Fertil. Steril.*, **49**, 843–7
2. Trounson, A.O. and Calabrese, R. (1984), Changes in plasma progesterone concentrations around the time of the luteinizing hormone surge in women superovulated for *in vitro* fertilization. *J. Clin. Endocrinol. Metab.*, **59**, 1075–80
3. Maroulis, G.B., Emery, M., Verkauf, B. and Cohen, A. (1987). Significance of serum LH before and after hCG in low dose pergonal follicular stimulation for IVF. In *5th World Congress on In Vitro Fertilization and Embryo Transfer*. pp. 24. (Norfolk: Am. Fertil. Soc.)
4. Janecek, P., Pexieder, T. and Boillat, E. (1987). Use of endogenous LH surge for ovulation induction timing and monitoring in gonadotropin stimulated IVF/ET cycles. In *5th World Congress on In Vitro Fertilization and Embryo Transfer*. pp. 23. (Norfolk: Am. Fertil. Soc.)

5. Zech, H., Weiss, P., Zerlauth, M. and Fritzsche, H. (1988). Bedeutung spezifischer LH-Muster vor und nach Ovulationsinduktion mit hCG im Rahmen der *In vitro* Fertilisierung und deren vereinfachte Diagnostik. *Geburtsh. Frauenheilk.*, **48**, 404–8
6. Osborn, J.C., Sharman, D., Burslem, R.W., Liebermann, B.A. and Lowe, B. (1987). Does continued monitoring of LH after hCG injection allow a retrospective assessment of hCG timing? In *3rd Meeting of the European Society of Human Reproduction and Embryology*. pp. 47. (Cambridge: European Society of Human Reproduction and Embryology)
7. Hoff, J.D., Quigley, M.E. and Yen, S.S.C. (1983). Hormonal dynamics at midcycle: A reevaluation. *J. Clin. Endocrinol. Metab.*, **57**, 792–6
8. Littman, B.A. and Hodgen, G.D. (1984). Human menopausal gonadotropin stimulation in monkeys: blockade of the luteinizing hormone surge by a highly transient ovarian factor. *Fertil. Steril.*, **41**, 440–7
9. Vought, R.L., London, W.T., Lutwak, L. and Dublin, T.D. (1963), Reliability of estimates of serum inorganic iodine and daily fecal and urinary iodine excretion from single causal specimens. *J. Clin. Endocrinol. Metab.*, **23**, 1218
10. Flury, B. and Riedwyl, H. (1983). *Angewandte multivariable Statistik*. (Stuttgart: Fischer)
11. Leyendecker, G., Wildt, L., Gips, H., Nocke, W. and Plotz, E.J. (1976). Experimental studies on the positive feedback effect of progesterone. 17α-dihydroprogesterone on the pituitary release of LH and FSH in human female. *Arch. Gynaekol.*, **221**, 29
12. March, C.M., Goebelsmann, U., Nakamura, R.M. and Mishell J. (1979). Roles of estradiol and progesterone in eliciting the midcyle luteinizing hormone and follicle stimulating hormone surges. *J. Clin. Endocrinol. Metab.*, **49**, 507
13. Odell, W.D. and Swerdloff, R.S. (1968). Progesterone induced luteinizing and follicle stimulating hormone surge in postmenopausal women: a simulated ovulatory peak. *Proc. Natl. Acad. Sci., USA*, **61**, 629
14. Rakoff, J.S. and Yen S.S.C. (1968). Progesterone induced acute release of prolactin in estrogen primed ovariectomized women. *J. Clin. Endocrinol. Metab.*, **47**, 918
15. Aono, T., Miyake, A., Kinugasa, T. and Kurachi, K. (1976). Progesterone advancement of estrogen induced luteinizing hormone release during the midfollicular phase in normal cyclic women. *J. Endocrinol.*, **71**, 451
16. McNatty, K.P., Smith, D.M., Makris, A., Osathanondh, R. and Ryan, K.J. (1979). The microenvironment of the human antral follicle: interrelationship among the steroid levels in antral fluid, the population of granulosa cells, and the status of the oocyte *in vivo* and *in vitro*. *J. Clin. Endocrinol. Metab.*, **49**, 851
17. McNatty, K.P., Makris, A., Grazia, C., Osathanondh, R. and Ryan, K.J. (1979). The production of progesterone, androgens and estrogens by human granulosa cells, thecal tissue and stromal tissue from human ovaries *in vitro*. *J. Clin. Endocrinol. Metab.*, **49**, 851

90

Pituitary gonadotropins in peri- and postmenopause: monoclonal antibody technique

V. De Leo, D. Lanzetta, P. Inaudi, A. Voltolini, S. Danero, M.G. Ricci and N. D'Antona

INTRODUCTION

Several years before the end of menstrual cyclicity, there is a significant reduction in estrogen and progesterone plasma levels and first an increase in follicle stimulating hormone (FSH) and later also in luteinizing hormone (LH)[1,2]. These changes often occur when the menstrual cycle is still ovulatory: the FSH increase in most cases, is not accompanied at once by that of LH[3,4]. In this period, the ovary must be less responsive to gonadotropin stimulation. FSH increase marks the beginning of a period of variable duration, which leads to menopause.

The factors which cause an FSH increase unaccompanied by a rise in LH are not yet well understood. A reduction in the number and activity of ovarian follicles causes a drop in estrogen levels, and particularly estradiol (E_2) which no longer exerts its negative feedback effect on gonadotropin release and particularly that of FSH, in the hypothalamus–pituitary axis[5]. To this is added a reduced production of inhibin which selectively inhibits the release of FSH during the female reproductive period. After menopause FSH and LH levels remain high: FSH levels are very stable and those of LH are more variable. Polyclonal antibody assay methods show an FSH/LH ratio > 1 in postmenopause.

The study of LH and FSH pulsatility in postmenopausal women by assaying blood samples taken every 10 min for a number of hours, has shown that there is higher FSH pulsatility in these subjects than in fertile women[6,7]. The different behavior of the two gonadotropins in peri- and postmenopause is a sign that LH and FSH are regulated by different mechanisms. This difference is particularly evident in postmenopause when LH and FSH levels are higher, however it probably also exists in the other phases of reproductive life in women but is masked by negative feedback mechanisms and low plasma concentrations. The new assay techniques using monoclonal antibodies have revealed that the differences between peri- and postmenopausal levels of these two hormones are even greater than previously appeared.

The aim of this study was to investigate the pattern of the two gonadotropins by monoclonal antibody techniques, in perimenopause, and after surgical and physiological menopause. Steroid hormones were also assayed.

MATERIALS AND METHODS

Subjects

The total number of women examined was 255, composed as follows: 190 in physiological postmenopause (age 52–59 years) and 65 in premenopause (42–49 years). Twenty of the latter underwent hysterectomy with bilateral ovariectomy. In all subjects a basal blood sample was taken for the determination of plasma FSH, LH, E_2, progesterone (P), androstenedione (A), testosterone (T) and dehydroepiandrosterone sulfate (DHEA-S). In the patients undergoing ovariectomy, the blood sample was repeated after an interval of a week. In eight of the 20 fertile patients in premenopause, spontaneous LH and FSH pulsatility was evaluated by means of blood samples taken every 10 min for 4 h, before (in follicular phase) and 1 week after ovariectomy.

Radioimmunoassay

Plasma LH and FSH concentrations were measured by double antibody RIA in all samples. Serono (Rome, Italy) kits were used. Each sample was assayed in duplicate, at two different dilutions. All samples from a given subject were assayed together. Quality control pools at low, normal and high LH and FSH levels were used in each assay. The assay sensitivities were 2.5 miu/ml for LH and FSH. Inter- and intra-assay coefficients of variation were 6.5% and 5.0%.

LH and FSH pulsatility was analyzed by a modified version of the method of Santen and Bardin[8]. An FSH or LH peak was defined as an increase in plasma levels which exceeded the previous nadir by at least 20% and followed a progressive increase in at least two preceding values.

Statistical analysis

The data is presented as mean $\pm$ SEM and was analyzed using Student's t test for the comparison of different groups.

RESULTS

In the women in natural postmenopause, FSH levels were much higher than those of LH. The FSH/LH ratio was greater than 2 (Figure 1*a*). In the fertile

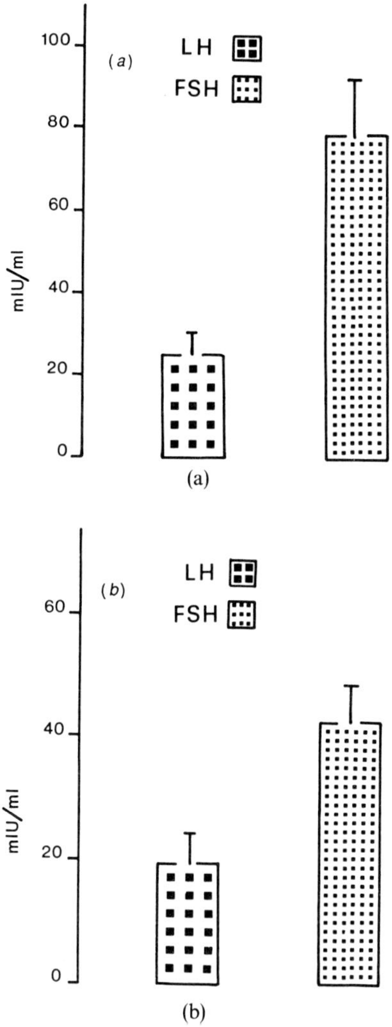

Figure 1 (*a*) FSH and LH basal levels (mean ± SEM) in women in natural postmenopause. The FSH/LH ratio was greater than 2; (*b*) FSH and LH basal levels (mean ± SEM) in fertile premenopausal women

premenopausal women, FSH levels were significantly higher than in young women but LH levels were normal (Figure 1*b*). Basal FSH levels in fertile premenopausal subjects were significantly higher 1 week after ovariectomy; LH concentrations were practically unchanged and E_2 levels were very low (< 10 mg/ml) (Figure 2).

FSH pulsatility, both as number of peaks and peak amplitude, was significantly higher 1 week after ovariectomy than before the operation ($p < 0.01$). The pulsatility of LH was found to be only slightly increased,

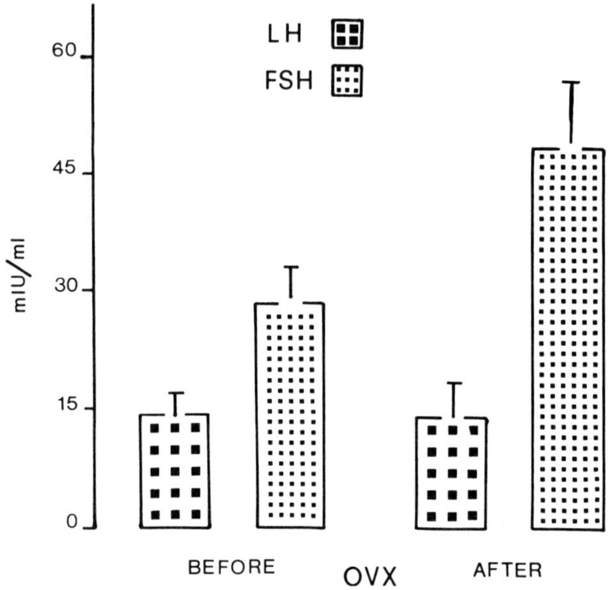

Figure 2 FSH and LH basal levels (mean ± SEM) in fertile premenopausal subjects before and after ovariectomy. FSH levels were significantly higher 1 week after ovariectomy

confirming the behavior of basal levels which did not follow the increase observed for FSH (Figure 3).

DISCUSSION

The most important finding in the menopausal subjects was the increase in FSH levels accompanied by a drop in estradiol concentrations. The use of monoclonal antibodies revealed that the difference between the two pituitary gonadotropins is already detectable in premenopause. The observation of FSH levels double those of LH in postmenopause, suggests that the two hormones are regulated by different mechanisms: the cessation of ovarian function and low E_2 levels remove the negative feedback control mechanism of FSH but LH continues to be controlled by the still functional hypothalamus.

In previous studies[9] we found another difference in the behavior of the two gonadotropins: both LH and FSH diminished during infusion of dopamine but only LH increased after metoclopramide stimulation. In premenopause, the significant increase in FSH but not LH in follicular phase, in the presence of normal concentrations of E_2, suggests that reduced ovarian secretion of inhibin, known to inhibit only FSH, is responsible for this increase[10,11].

The pulsatility of FSH, both as peak number and height, had already risen only 1 week after ovariectomy, whereas LH pulsatility did not significantly change. This is further evidence that the two gonadotropins are under different control mechanisms, because ovariectomy eliminates the inhibitory

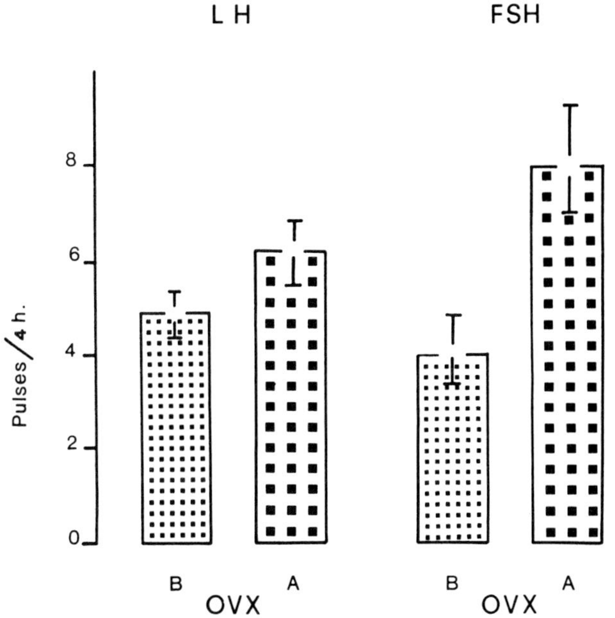

Figure 3 FSH pulsatility, as number of peaks (mean ± SEM) was significantly higher 1 week after ovariectomy. The pulsatility of LH was only slightly increased

control of E_2 and inhibin on FSH. The later increase in LH seems due to modifications at hypothalamic neuromodulator level caused by the drop in estrogen levels[12,13].

Our patients did not complain of hot flushes 1 week after the operation. This symptom is correlated with LH peaks when the pulsatile frequency of this gonadotropin undergoes modification[14,15] and was not reported by our patients until later.

In conclusion, the use of monoclonal antibodies in the evaluation of gonadotropin patterns in premenopause and physiological and surgical postmenopause, provides evidence of the different regulation mechanisms of LH and FSH, particularly evident when their levels rise in menopause.

REFERENCES

1. Sherman, B.W., West, J.H. and Korenman, S.G. (1976). The menopause transition: Analysis of LH, FSH, estradiol, and progesterone concentrations during menstrual cycles of older women. *J. Clin. Endocrinol. Metab.*, **42**, 629
2. Metcalf, M.G., Donald, R.A., and Livesey, J.H. (1981). Pituitary ovarian function in normal women during the menopausal transition. *Clin. Endocrinol.*, **14**, 245
3. Van Look, P.F.A., Lothian, H., Hunter, W.M., Michie, E.S. and Baird, D. (1977). Hypothalamic-pituitary-ovarian function in perimenopausal women. *J. Clin. Endocrinol. Metab.*, **7**, 13
4. Medina, M., Scaglia, A.E., Vazques, G., Alatorre, S. and Pèrez-Palacios, G. (1976). Rapid oscillation of circulating gonadotropins in post-menopausal women. *J. Clin. Endocrinol.*

Metab., **43**, 1015

5. Monroe, S.E., Jaffe, R.B. and Midgley, A.R. (1972). Regulation of human gonadotropins. XIII. Changes in serum gonadotropins in menstruating women in response to oophorectomy. *J. Clin. Endocrinol. Metab.*, **34**, 420
6. Yen, S.S.C., Tsai, C.C., Naftolin, F., Vandenberg, G. and Ajabar, L. (1972). Pulsatile patterns of gonadotropin release in subjects with and without ovarian function. *J. Clin. Endocrinol. Metab.*, **34**, 671
7. Jasonni, V.M., Filicori, M., Naldi, S., Capelli, M., Baraghini, G.F. and Flamigni, C. (1988). Secrezione pulsatile delle gonadotropine in postmenopausa. In Filicori, M., Flamigni, C. and Crowley, W.F. (eds.) *Bioritmi endocrino, fisiologia, diagnostica ed applicazioni terapeutiche.*
8. Santen, R.J. and Bardin, C.W. (1973). Episodic luteinizing hormone secretion in man: Pulse analysis, clinical interpretation, physiological mechanisms. *J. Clin. Invest.*, **52**, 2617
9. De Leo, V., Petraglia, F., Bruno, M.G., Lanzetta, D., Inaudi, P. and D'Antona, N. (1989). Different dopaminergic control of plasma luteinizing hormone, follicle-stimulating hormone and prolactin in ovulatory and postmenopause women: effect of ovariectomy. *Gynecol. Obstet. Invest.*, **27**, 94
10. Ling, N., Ying, S.Y., Ueno, N., Shimasaki, S., Esch, F., Hotta, M. and Guillemin, R. (1986). Pituitary FSH is released by a heterodimer of the β-subunits from the two forms of inhibin. *Nature*, **321**, 780
11. Marder, M.L., Channing, C.P. and Schwartz, N.B. (1977). Suppression of serum follicle stimulating hormone in intact and acutely ovariectomized rats by porcine follicular fluid. *Endocrinology*, **101**, 1639
12. Judd, S.J., Rigg, L.A. and Yen, S.S.C. (1979). The effects of ovariectomy and estrogen treatment on the dopamine inhibition of gonadotropin and prolactin release. *J. Clin. Endicrinol. Metab.*, **49**, 182
13. Knobil, E. (1980). The neuroendocrine control of the menstrual cycle. *Recent. Prog. Horm. Res.*, **36**, 53
14. Treloar, A.E. (1981). Menstrual cyclicity and the premenopause. *Maturitas*, **3**, 249
15. Casper, R.F., Yen, S.S.C. and Wilkes, M.M. (1979). Menopausal flushes a neuroendocrine link with pulsatile LH secretion. *Science*, **205**, 823

Section 4 continued

Part F

Infertility and sterility

91

Software for data storage and retrieval for GIFT centers

P. Anserini, V. Azzarini, V. Remorgida, G. L. Capitanio and L. De Cecco

INTRODUCTION

Gamete intrafallopian transfer (GIFT), *in vitro* fertilization and embryo replacement (IVF–ER) and intrauterine insemination (IUI) are some of the several techniques developed to assist infertile couples. Every treatment cycle performed with one of these techniques, produces a large quantity of data arising from different disciplines (echotomography, endocrinology, embryology, andrology, surgery). An extensive registration of this information is necessary both for everyday routine and research purposes. With the widespread diffusion of personal computers this time-consuming work has become easier and faster to perform.

Unfortunately the few programs already developed were designed either as a comprehensive data base, very useful in clinical practice but unaccessible for statistics, or for the storage and retrieval of a limited set of basic data with the only aim of research[1–3]. We therefore felt the need to develop our own program trying to match clinical and research requirements. This program, now in its third version, has been used for the last 2 years in our department.

TECHNICAL CHARACTERISTIC

For the creation of the program we originally employed the DBase III, a software written by Wayne & Ratliff for Ashton-Tate and running on IBM personal computers (PC, XT, AT) or compatible brands with the hard disk configuration. For the latest version we have adopted the update release of DBase III, DBase III plus. This program uses data base files (.dbf) for storage of data according to a predetermined structure, and program files (.prg) containing a sequence of DBase III commands. Program files are responsible for the creation of menus and screen displays for input and output. The choice for this programming language was based on its possibility to store a large quantity of data in different data base files and to link them to each other. This results in a simple interaction between the computer and the user.

System design

The program is menu-driven and primarily divided in two sections, easily accessible from the main menu: one is devoted to data collection and storage (Database Section) and the other to data processing. Utilities and services programs can also be called from the main menu (Figure 1).

Data base

The data base was designed to be as comprehensive as possible so that it could be adopted by any other GIFT or IVF-ER group. To fulfil this requirement, we faced the difficulty of saving more than a 1000 pieces of information for one couples' cycle of therapy. We were therefore forced to split this enormous amount of information into 38 different data files, all relinked together. In order to allow an easier input and retrieval of the information a modular structure was selected: in other words, data concerning each couple are divided into the following options accessible from the data base menu:

(1) Patient's Registration Information
(2) Follicular recruitment and monitoring
(3) Oocyte recovery
(4) GIFT
(5) Embryo Laboratory Observations
(6) Embryo replacement
(7) Semen analysis
(8) Freezing
(9) Luteal phase.

```
DEPARTMENT OF OBSTETRIC AND GYNAECOLOGY
UNIVERSITY OF GENOA

* G . I . F . T .   C E N T E R *

M A I N   M E N U

P = Patient data entry
S = Patient search
H = Husband search
I = Patient index
M = Media quality control
D = Data processing
U = Utilities
E = Exit

Enter selection :
```

Figure 1 Screen display of the main menu. Points defined as P, S, H, I constitute the data base

Each section is made of one or more pages: the pages can be scrolled up and down and on each page data entry, correction or just visualization can be performed. This modular structure presents several advantages. Data entry can be done day by day as each of the pages can be addressed separately and each member of the team can manage the section of his competence independently from the other members. Moreover, as techniques constantly evolve, it is highly likely that new parameters will need to be recorded in the future. The modular structure allows the addition of a new module whenever the necessity to process new information is felt. The newly inserted module will interact with the already existing ones and enable new data processing, connections between modules being very easy. As the number of possible users is large, we have introduced a severe control of the inputs. We used numeric and data fields when necessary and coded fields whenever possible, limiting character field to a minimum as they are not subsequently available for statistics. All codifications are displayed at user's need on help windows; it is only necessary to digit the number and the corresponding information will be automatically recorded thus avoiding possible mistyping. Whenever a yes/no answer is contemplated, choosing the no answer is linked to an automatic skip of all the inputs related to the affirmative possibility.

Data processing section

This section, like the previous one, is menu-driven and relatively simple though a little practice is needed for its extensive use. The first option of the data processing menu allows display or printing of all variables available for data retrieval and statistical computation. The base of this section is an accessory data file (.dbf) developed in order to manage the whole amount of information recorded in the data base without limitations. Program files (.prg) of this section refer totally to this working file. The structure of this working file is made of eight fields. The first one contains the detailed description of one variable, i.e. 'number of transferred oocytes'. The second field contains the name of the variable as recorded in the original .dbf file, i.e. 'ovotrasf'. The third field defines whether this variable is recorded as character (1), number (2) or date (3) field; in our example this is 2. The fourth field defines the maximal length of that variable (i.e. 1 digit). The fifth and sixth fields record respectively the data (.dbf) and index (.ndx) files where the variable is originally stored (i.e. Modul3A.dbf, Rifer3A.ndx). The last two fields define position and numbers of codes in the file where definitions of codifications are recorded.

From the data processing menu different options can be called. Any stored variable can be sorted out separately or along with others. Selections of subsets of patients can be performed on the basis of any parameters, as long as it was saved in the data base. Fields, apparently unrelated to each other, can be examined extensively. Moreover data can be analyzed with statistical packages external to the system. Our present choice is Abstat, Anderson-Bell Co., 1984, a commercially available statistical package, which reads DBase files.

CONCLUSIONS

The greatest difficulty encountered in the creation of this program has been the establishment of a structure able to store the extraordinarily large mass of data generated in every cycle of assisted reproduction. To obviate this limitation the data base has been subdivided in several archives. This solution unfortunately has the disadvantage to make the retrieval of data much more complex.

On the other hand, being not still aware of the real influence played by each factor on the final result, we thought it unreasonable to perform a preselection of the information to be stored. Moreover, we aimed to create a tool that could be used by other Infertility Centers that are not necessarily adopting our procedures. This has resulted in a further increase of possible recordable data. The ultimate version of the program will perform the patient's report, to be given at the dismissal.

Though there is no possibility of totally substituting the paper records, our 2-year experience has resulted in a positive appreciation of this tool. We are now able to retrieve and analyze in a short period of time thousands of data, an event that is difficult to repeat with a paper archive. Finally, besides giving real time evaluation of the ongoing stimulatory cycles, constitutes a severe control system of our activities.

REFERENCES

1. Quigley, M.M. (1984). Data management in an *in vitro* Fertilization and Embryo Transfer program. In Wolf, P. and Quigley, M.M. (eds). *Human in Vitro Fertilization and Embryo Transfer*, pp. 383–41. (New York: Plenum Press)
2. Wilkes, C. (1986). Data storage and retrieval. In Jones, H.W., Jones, G.S., Hodgen, G.D. and Rosenwaks, Z. (eds). *In Vitro Fertilization-Norfolk*. (Baltimore: Williams and Wilkins)
3. Riss, P.A. and Reinthaller, A. (1986). A simple database system for an *in Vitro* Fertilization programme using commercial software. *Br. J. Obstet. Gynaecol.*, **93**, 999–1001

92

STER-Expert: microcomputer-based decisional support for the management of female endocrine infertility

P.L. Venturini, V. Fasce, F. Gorlero and L. De Cecco

INTRODUCTION

Computer-based medical decisional supports have been developed in the area of artificial intelligence and possess some features of expert systems. They simulate the human decision process and are designed to support the physicians complementing their natural ability to make judgements with the computer's memory, reliability and processing capabilities.

STER-Expert is a microcomputer-based decisional support designed to aid the clinician in the assessment and treatment of female endocrine infertility. This program offers one or more working diagnoses together with a therapeutic suggestion and also allows the gathering of all clinical information (including diagnostic studies, laboratory findings and treatments) about patients presenting with this disease.

The program is built as a framework of questions and answers which follow the traditional diagnostic process. The recording of the answers to different questions (medical history and physical examination) leads the program to a preliminary assessment and a suggestion of the investigations which are needed to reach a firm diagnosis. These studies include: evaluation of hormonal status, dynamic hormonal tests, imaging techniques (ultrasound, laparoscopy, hysteroscopy, etc.) and karyotype. Thereafter, entering the results of the appropriate studies leads the program to an intermediate and final level of diagnosis together with the therapeutic option. The proper therapeutic regimen is related to the patient's wish for pregnancy and considers the hormonal status.

A special part of the program is designed for the follow-up of therapies, particularly for those which require a close monitoring of follicular growth and estrogen levels (gonadotropins).

The program provides a final score for the different causes of female endocrine infertility (final diagnoses) which are divided into three groups:

(1) For patients complaining of primary amenorrhea the final diagnoses are: functional hypothalamic, isolated gonadotropin deficiency, hypo-

pituitarism, hyperprolactinemia, polycystic ovary syndrome (PCOS), Turner syndrome, other X deletions (mosaicism), chromosomally competent ovarian failure, uterovaginal agenesis, other Müllerian defects, Morris syndrome and pseudohermaphroditism.

(2) For patients complaining of secondary amenorrhea the final diagnoses are: functional hypothalamic, hyperprolactinemia, PCOS, precocious menopause, idiopathic, anorexia nervosa, anatomical defects (uterine) and secondary to endocrinological diseases.

(3) For patients who keep menstrual function the final diagnoses are anovulation or luteal insufficiency due to: hypothalamic dysfunction, hyperprolactinemia, PCOS, endocrinological diseases and resistant ovary.

All the answers to the different questions (including numerical data) represent the variables of the program. Each variable has been related to the above mentioned different causes of female endocrine infertility through the attribution of numerical weights which reflects the degree of negative or positive correlation between the findings and the disease. The zero value indicates no correlation. These values have been obtained through a heuristic procedure based on the current literature and the authors' experience, taking into account both frequency and the evocatory strength of findings for each disease. The final score is also provided through a series of production rules (such IF → THEN or inclusion/exclusion criteria). The structure of the program is shown in Figure 1.

TECHNICAL DETAILS

STER-Expert has been developed in C, under MS/DOS; it is implementable on IBM-compatible PC, in the hard disk configuration, with a minimum of 512 kbytes of RAM.

Figure 1 Structure of the program

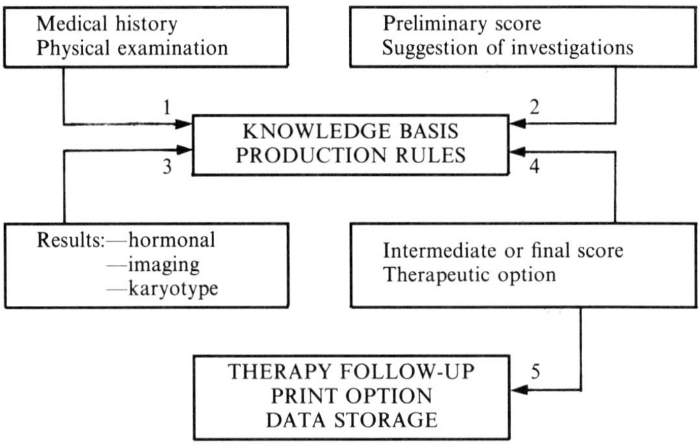

The program includes 2230 variables and 198 production rules. Thirty-one months/man of work have been necessary to complete the program.

VALIDATION

A group of 232 patients selected among those who referred to the Endocrinology Unit of the Institute of Obstetrics and Gynecology of the University of Genoa, classified with diagnosis of secondary amenorrhea, primary amenorrhea and anovulation or luteal insufficiency, were retrospectively evaluated for the present study.

The patient's clinical data were entered into the program by a resident doctor who reported the resulting diagnosis after history, physical examination and laboratory findings (first and second levels) and the final diagnosis (resulting from the integration of all the investigation data).

The program's diagnostic hypotheses were then compared with the previous evaluation of an expert physician. A statistical evaluation of results has been performed and both specificity and sensibility of the program as decisional support were calculated. The specificity is the ratio of true negatives to true negative + false positive cases. The sensibility is the ratio of true positive to true positive + false negative cases.

RESULTS

The results of the validation study are shown in Tables 1, 2 and 3.

Of 134 patients with secondary amenorrhea, 104 (77%) and 116 (85%) were correctly predicted by the program respectively at the first and final diagnostic level. Both sensibility and specificity were highly satisfactory with values ranging from 0.71 to 0.91 and 0.84 to 0.94 respectively at the first and final diagnostic level (Table 1).

Table 1 Secondary amenorrhea

Type of amenorrhea	*Clinical diagnosis*	*1st diagnosis*	*Final diagnosis*
Functional hypothalamic	59	47 (79%)	50 (84%)
PCOS	42	31 (73%)	36 (85%)
Hyperprolactinemic	21	15 (71%)	19 (90%)
Uterine	1	1	1
Precocious menopause	4	3	4
Anorexia nervosa	2	2	2
Secondary to endocrine disease	4	4	4
Idiopathic	0	1	0
Total	134	104 (77%)	116 (85%)
Functional hypothalamic	sensibility	0.79	0.84
	specificity	0.84	0.90
PCOS	sensibility	0.73	0.85
	specificity	0.90	0.94
Hyperprolactinemic	sensibility	0.71	0.90
	specificity	0.91	0.89

Of the 31 cases with primary amenorrhea, 27 (77%) and 29 (93%) were correctly predicted by program respectively at the first and final diagnostic level. Neither sensibility nor specificity were evaluated because of the small numbers of cases (Table 2).

Finally 67 cases presenting with anovulation or luteal insufficiency, 49 (73%) and 58 (86%) were correctly predicted by the program. Both sensibility and specificity were highly satisfactory with values ranging from 0.71 to 0.92 and 0.82 to 0.95 respectively at the first and final diagnostic level (Table 3).

DISCUSSION

The diagnosis of female endocrine infertility is often the result of an integrated approach by the physician, when we consider that he or she has to deal not only with specific problems of woman's reproduction but also with other pathological conditions, some of which are fairly unfamiliar.

Moreover the knowledge concerning the physiopathology of these diseases

Table 2 Primary amenorrhea

Type of amenorrhea	*Clinical diagnosis*	*1st diagnosis*	*Final diagnosis*
Functional hypothalamic	8	7 (87%)	8 (100%)
Isolated gonadal deficiency	1	0	1
Hypopituitarism	1	1	1
Hyperprolactinemic	7	5 (71%)	6 (85%)
PCOS	4	3 (75%)	3 (75%)
Turner syndrome	3	2	3
Other X deletions	0	1	0
Chromosome competent ovarian failure	0	0	0
Uterovaginal agenesis	3	2	3
Other Müllerian defects	2	2	2
Morris syndrome	2	1	2
Pseudohermaphroditism	0	0	0
Total	31	24 (77%)	28 (93%)

Table 3 Anovulation/luteal insufficiency

Type of Diagnosis	*Clinical diagnosis*	*1st diagnosis*	*Final diagnosis*
Hypothalamic dysfunction	24	17 (70%)	20 (83%)
Hyperprolactinemia	21	15 (71%)	18 (85%)
PCOS	18	15 (83%)	17 (94%)
Endocrine diseases	3	3	3
Resistant ovary	1	0	0
Total	67	49 (73%)	58 (86%)
Hypothalamic dysfunction	sensibility	0.77	0.85
	specificity	0.82	0.89
Hyperprolactinemia	sensibility	0.77	0.87
	specificity	0.87	0.91
PCOS	sensibility	0.85	0.94
	specificity	0.91	0.95

has greatly developed together with the availability of new diagnostic procedures and therapies.

For these reasons our computerized program can also be considered useful to bring the physician up-to-date.

The results of the validation study indicate that the program is highly reliable. This reliability of the program and its logical diagnostic iteration can thus be considered characteristic of an educational tool.

BIBLIOGRAPHY

Batson, E. (1984). Computer as a consultant. Application of artificial intelligence in diagnosis. *Postgrad. Med.*, **75**, 211–14

De Vries, P.H. and De Vries, P.F. (1984). An overview of medical expert system. *Meth. Inf. Med.*, **24**, 57–64

Gorry, G.A. (1973). Computer-assisted clinical decision-making. *Meth. Inf. Med.*, **12**, 45–59

Kulinowski, A. (1985). Artificial Intelligence methods for expert medical consultant systems. *Mt Sinai J. Med. (NY)*, **52**, 87–93

Shortliffe, E.H. (1983). Hypothesis generation in medical consultation systems: artificial intelligence approaches. *MEDINFO 83.*, pp. 480–3. (Amsterdam: North Holland Press)

Kunz, J.C., Shortliffe, E.H., Buchanan, G.B. and Feigenbaum, E.A. (1984). Computer-assisted decision making in medicine. *J. Med. Philos.*, **9**, 135–60

Kleinmunts, B. (1984). Diagnostic problem solving by computer: a historical review and the current state of the science. *Comput. Biol. Med.*, **14**, 255–70

Sandel, H.S. and Bourne, J.R. (1985). Expert systems in medicine: a biomedical engineering perspective. *Crit. Rev. Biomed. Eng.*, **12**, 95–129

Shortliffe, E.H. (1984). Reasoning methods in medical consultation systems: artificial intelligence approaches. *Comput. Prog. Biomed.*, **18**, 5–13

Gross, R. (1985). Can computers replace a physician's abilities? (Editorial). *Wien Med. Wochenschrift.*, **135**, 315–17

Tuhrim, S. and Reggia, J.A. (1985). An introduction to computer-assisted medical decision making. *Computing*, **2**, 28–36

Venturini, P.L., Fasce, V., Gorlero, F., Arnulfo, G. and Mortola, G.P. (1987). Results on the application to a retrospective series of patients of computerized system for diagnosis and management of amenorrhea. *7th International Congress of the European Federation for Medical Informatics.* Supplement to the Proceedings, pp. 21–25

93

Pulsatile gonadotropin-releasing hormone by intradermal–subcutaneous route for ovulation induction in cases of hypothalamic amenorrhea or of clomiphene-unresponsive polycystic ovary syndrome

C. Campagnoli, L. Belforte, D. Botta, M.M. Di Sario, M.G. Lanza, R. Olivero, E. Pedrini, P. Tuninetti and C. Peris

INTRODUCTION

The use of subcutaneous or intravenous pulsatile gonadotropin-releasing hormone (GnRH) infusion is the most valid therapeutic approach for the treatment of hypothalamic amenorrhea in patients desiring children. More recently it has been proposed for the treatment of anovulation in women with polycystic ovarian disease.

Even though this type of treatment is more effective than traditional therapy with exogenous gonadotropins in determining high ovulation and pregnancy rates with minimal ovarian hyperstimulation and multiple pregnancy risks, it is not yet clear which route of administration is more practical.

A recent review of published data confronting therapy with adequate doses of GnRH administered intravenously (i.v.) or subcutaneously (s.c.) did not show significant differences in ovulation and pregnancy rates between the two routes of administration[1]. The subcutaneous route is simpler, free of complications and well tolerated by the patient because it permits continuing normal work activity even in cases of heavy manual labor. The need of higher dosages is undoubtedly one of the disadvantages of the subcutaneous route. It is still controversial as to whether the ovulatory response is less predictable and less efficient. Data dealing with the efficacy of s.c. administration differ greatly.

Leyendecker and Wildt[2] reported a 60% ovulation rate with s.c. treatment compared to a 100% with i.v. therapy; in 1986 the same authors[3] reported an 85% ovulation rate with s.c. administration compared to 95% with the i.v. route. Blunt and Butt[4] reported no difference between the two routes of administration.

It should be noted that in Leyendecker's first experiences an infusion catheter was introduced in the subcutaneous adipose tissue of the abdominal area; his more recent and more favorable studies were carried out by positioning a butterfly needle more superficially.

Blunt's data refer to the positioning of the needle in the hypodermis of the deltoid area which is much thinner than that of the abdominal area. The site of infusion, characterized by an adequate vascularization, influences the entity and velocity of drug absorption and therefore the biological validity of the 'pulse'. We chose to insert the butterfly needle, generally, in the peri-umbilical area, so that the tip of the needle remained in the dermis or in the immediately underlying hypodermis. Such a position takes advantage of the rich vascularization that characterizes the deepest layer of the dermis and the immediately underlying hypodermis.

MATERIALS AND METHODS

We administered pulsatile GnRH subcutaneously to 15 patients presenting primary hypothalamic amenorrhea (PHA) in 34 cycles; to five presenting secondary hypothalamic amenorrhea (SHA) in 10 cycles; and to six with polycystic ovarian syndrome (PCOS), not responsive to adequate doses of clomiphene, in 10 cycles: a total of 54 treatment cycles in 26 patients.

The average age of the 15 patients with PHA was 29 (range 23–40); of the patients with SHA, 27 (range 24–29); of the patients with PCOS, 30 (range 29–33).

In the hypothalamic amenorrhea group the severity of hypothalamic failure was determined on the basis of the gonadotropic response to an acute test with GnRH (100 μg i.v.). All patients with PHA were placed in group 3 of Leyendecker's classification (nine in group 3a and six in 3b). The degree of hypothalamic failure in patients with SHA was variable in time, as often seen in such cases, being related to underlying etiopathogenetic factors (stress, variations in weight, etc.): upon initiation of pulsatile GnRH therapy all SHA patients had negative results to the progestin test. Thyroid and adrenal function and plasma prolactin were normal in all hypothalamic amenorrhea patients. No patient was overweight. Radiological examinations of the sella turcica were within normal limits in all cases. The partners of nine patients presented semen abnormalities.

All PCOS patients presented euthyroidism. Two presented slight hyperprolactinemia. One presented a slight late-onset adrenal 21-hydroxylase defect, treated with dexamethasone 0.5 mg/day; however, anovulation persisted. The partners of three patients presented semen abnormalities.

In 25 cycles we used the Zyklomat (Ferring, Kiel, West Germany) pump which administers a 50 μl/pulse in 1 min. In 29 cycles we used the Microjet CD4 Hormon (Canè Elettronica Medicale, Collegno, Italy) pump which administers a 125 μl/pulse in 1–2 seconds.

In the majority of cases, the 25 gauge Butterfly needle was inserted 1–2 mm in the peri-umbilical area so that the drug was released in the deeper layers of the dermis or in the immediately underlying hypodermis. In some cases the needle was positioned in the deltoid area.

Patients with hypothalamic amenorrhea were treated with GnRH pulses at the dosage of 5–20 μg, with a frequency of 1 pulse every 90 min; the frequency was not changed after ovulation. Pulsatile GnRH therapy was continued for 2–8 days (average: 4.6) after ovulation.

In five of the six patients with PCOS, pulsatile GnRH treatment was preceded by administration of an estrogen–progestin contraceptive 'pill' for 2 to 3 months; during the last cycle of this treatment a GnRH analog, Buserelin, was added and continued for another 2 weeks. Buserelin was administered intranasally at 07:00, 11:00, 15:00, 19:00 and 23:00 in two patients for a total dosage of 1000 mg. In the remaining three patients 200 mg of Buserelin was given at 07:00, 15:00 and 23:00, for a total of 600 mg/day. Once gonadotropin secretion was suppressed, as shown by ultrasound examination (linear endometrium and resting ovaries) and by serum estradiol levels (< 30 pg/ml), intradermal subcutaneous pulsatile GnRH administration was initiated and Buserelin administration suspended. The dosage of pulsatile GnRH varied between 10 and 25 μg/pulse at a frequency of 1 pulse every 120 min, later changed to 1 pulse every 90 min during the late follicular phase. In three cases the frequency was and remained 1 pulse every 90 min. Pulsatile GnRH therapy continued for 5–13 days (average 8.1 $\pm$ 1.7) after ovulation. Hypophyseal desensitization with Buserelin was not used in one case; in this case the pump was applied after a progestogen-induced withdrawal bleeding. In three cycles the pump was applied immediately after the start of uterine bleeding following the preceding treatment.

As support during the luteal phase in patients with hypothalamic amenorrhea 2000 IU of human chorionic gonadotropin (hCG) (1 ampoule) were administered intramuscularly every 2 days, starting on day two of the temperature rise, for a total of 4 ampoules. In patients with PCOS, 2000 IU (1 ampoule) of hCG were administered intramuscularly every 3 days for a total of three ampoules.

RESULTS

The results obtained in the group of patients with hypothalamic amenorrhea were as follows. Ovulation occurred in 14 of the 20 women (70%); in nine of the 15 with PHA (60%) and in all five of those with SHA (100%); in 35 of the 44 treatment cycles (79.5%). In the patients with PHA ovulations occurred in 27 of the 34 treatment cycles and two follicles developed in four of these (14.8% of the ovulations); two cycles presented luteinized unruptured follicles (LUF). In the patients with SHA ovulation occurred in eight of ten cycles; two follicles matured in two cases (25% of the ovulations). Six women with PHA did not respond to treatment continued for an average of 26 days (range 19–37). Two patients with SHA had an anovulatory cycle, even though some follicular maturation occurred.

Pregnancy was obtained in 12 of the 20 women (60%), for a total of 14 pregnancies: in nine patients with PHA (two pregnancies occurring in the same woman) and in five SHA (two pregnancies in the same woman). The pregnancy rate for treatment cycle was 26.5% in the PHA group and 50% in the SHA group. It is interesting to note that the majority of the pregnancies were achieved in the first three treatment cycles, even in the presence of a male factor: two pregnancies resulted in the first cycle and two in the second cycle; in the remaining cases with concomitant male factors, pregnancy occurred in the 5th, 6th and 8th cycle, respectively. Four pregnancies resulted in miscarriage (two with 'blighted egg'); one pregnancy is currently ongoing in the second trimester; nine achieved term, of which one was a twin pregnancy: of the ten babies born five were male and five were female.

Figure 1 shows the main characteristics of the ovulatory cycles occurring in patients with PHA and SHA, distinguishing the cycles in which two follicles developed. The duration of preovulatory treatment was longer in the PHA group but the difference was not statistically significant. There was no difference in the estradiol peak, in progesterone levels and in the duration of the luteal phase. There was no significant difference between the cycles in which pregnancies were obtained, considering only those which evolved regularly to term, and the ovulatory cycles not resulting in pregnancy (Figure 2).

The response was generally constant in the cases requiring more than one treatment cycle, as in one case of PHA which resulted in pregnancy (presently ongoing) during the 8th cycle; ovulation occurred in all previous cycles (with one pregnancy resulting in miscarriage). There was one exception; a patient with PHA (probably not idiopathic, but rather an outcome of meningitis during infancy) who presented one anovulatory cycle, two with inadequate luteal phase, one of which presented marked inadequate luteal phase and LUF, and two ovulatory cycles, and who finally obtained a pregnancy during the 6th treatment cycle.

Table 1 summarizes the results obtained in the group of patients with PCOS. Ovulation was induced in eight of ten cycles (80%) and precisely in the cycle without pretreatment with Buserelin (luteal phase defect), in five of six cycles with pretreatment (one with luteal phase defect) and in two of three cycles immediately following a first (after pretreatment) ovulatory cycle. It is interesting to note the course of these last three cycles (Figure 3). In one patient adequate ovulation with two follicles was achieved in the first cycle, and with one follicle in the second cycle. In another patient both cycles were ovulatory, but with a luteal phase defect in the second. In a third patient, an adequate ovulatory response was followed by an anovulatory cycle.

No significant differences were observed between the follicular phase duration, preovulatory estradiol levels and midluteal progesterone levels of the ovulatory cycles in the patients with PHA, SHA and PCOS. Only the two patients with PCOS presenting ovulation of two follicles had a longer follicular phase and a significantly higher preovulatory estradiol level compared with the patients with HA presenting double ovulation (Figure 4).

DISCUSSION

The results obtained in patients with hypothalamic amenorrhea and PCOS document the efficacy of pulsatile GnRH therapy administered by intra-

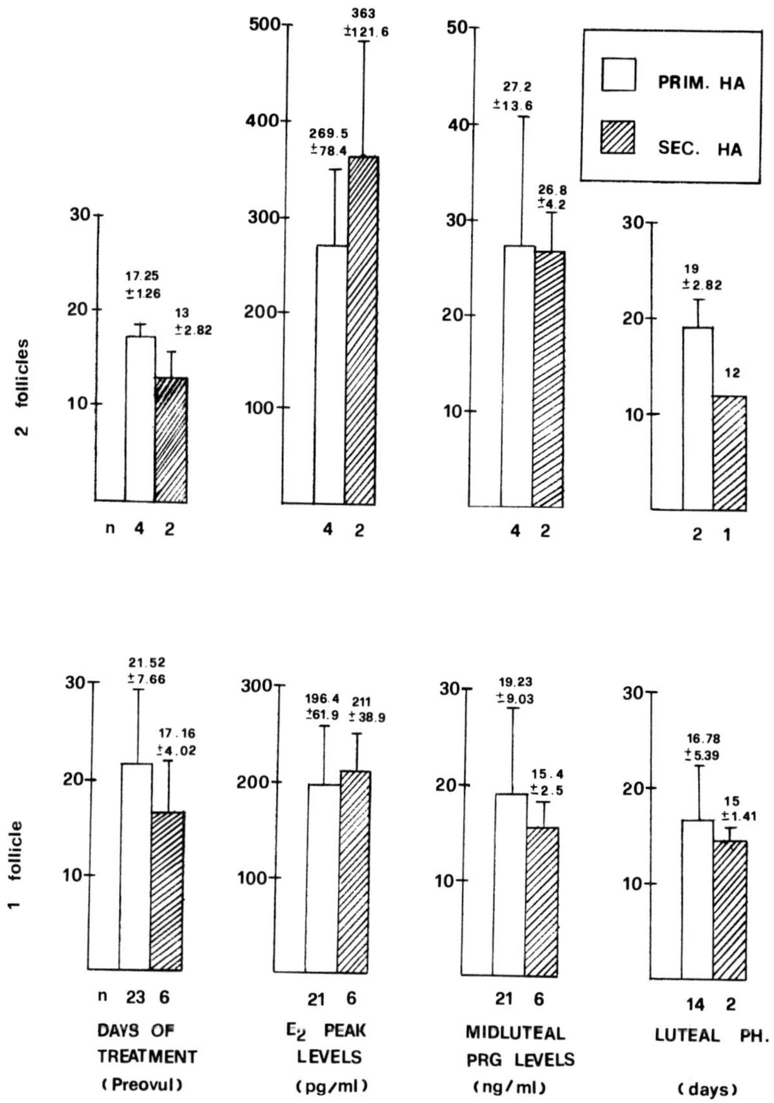

Figure 1 Main characteristics of ovulatory cycles obtained by GnRH pulsatile treatment in patients with primary (open blocks) or secondary (hatched blocks) hypothalamic amenorrhea

dermal–subcutaneous route. The ovarian response to equal doses differs according to the degree of hypothalamic failure. A dose which is too low may be insufficient to induce hypophyseal stimulation, and a dose which is too high may provoke hyperstimulation with multiple follicular maturation. Published data concerning hypothalamic amenorrhea report a high percentage of ovulatory cycles obtained with doses between 5 and 20 μg every 90 to 120 min i.v. and 15–20 μg/90 min s.c., using lower doses for grades 2 and

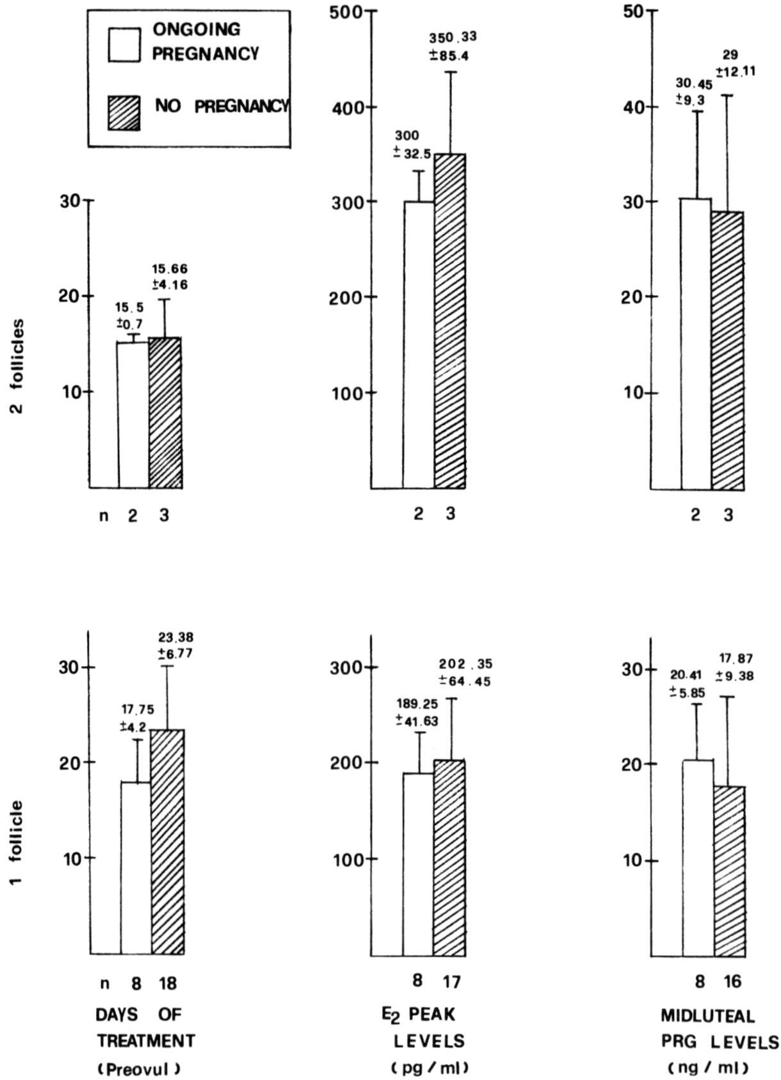

Figure 2 Comparison of the main characteristics of ovulatory cycles followed (open blocks) or not followed (hatched blocks) by pregnancy in patients with hypothalamic amenorrhea treated with pulsatile GnRH

3a and higher doses for 3b and 3c of Leyendecker's classification[5]. At the beginning of our experience, we used low doses (5–10 μg/pulse) in some cycles in patients with PHA; these dosages were insufficient to induce follicular maturation which was obtained by increasing the dosage progressively to 20 μg/pulse. Subsequently, on the basis of the clinical responses observed, we considered 20 μg/90 min as the optimal starting dose for patients with primary amenorrhea and 10 μg/90 min for those with secondary amenorrhea.

Table 1 Pulsatile GnRH by the intradermal–subcutaneous route in clomiphene-unresponsive PCOS patients

	Ovulation	
Results	*No*	*Yes*
1 p. 1 cycle without pretreatment		1 (LPD)*
1 p. 2 cycles with pretreatment		2
1 p. 1 cycle with pretreatment	1	
3 pp. 1 cycle with pretreatment		3
and 1 further immediate non-pretreated cycle	1	2 (1 LPD)*
TOTAL	2	8 (80%)

* Luteal Phase Defect

In the latter group we found it best to initiate therapy with relatively low doses which were subsequently increased if necessary. This criterion was followed because the degree of hypothalamic failure in SHA is often variable in time and is less severe than in PHA[6].

If ovulation fails to occur, it can be induced by increasing dosages per pulse, as reported by Caruso *et al.*[7] using the i.v. route: by increasing the dose from 2.5 μg/pulse to 12.5 μg/pulse they obtained 100% ovulation cycles while obtaining 80% ovulation cycles with low doses. Recently, Blunt and colleagues[8] underlined that the same was also true for s.c. administration.

In five out of six patients with PCOS, pulsatile GnRH therapy was preceded by a GnRH analogue which lowers endogenous luteinizing hormone (LH) levels. In PCOS cases, persistent high levels of LH have been considered to be the cause not only of the discrepancies occurring between ovulations and the number of pregnancies obtained with the various medical treatments, but also the cause of the high percentage of miscarriage (up to 40% of the pregnancies). In fact, it has been suggested that the penetration of high quantities of LH in the follicle induces the premature completion of the first meiotic division of the oocyte which normally occur 36–48 h before ovulation; the exact timing of this event is a prerequisite of fertilization and regular development of the embryo[9]. In cases of ovulation induction with pulsatile GnRH therapy, LH levels during the follicular phase were higher in patients with PCOS than in patients with hypothalamic hypoestrogenic amenorrhea[10]; this could explain the fewer successes in terms of ovulation, pregnancies and term pregnancies seen in almost all studies[9,11-16]. Using a GnRH analogue as pretreatment to pulsatile GnRH therapy, Filicori *et al.*[17,18] found success rates in patients with PCOS similar to those obtained in cases of hypothalamic amenorrhea. Even in our limited experience, the administration of pulsatile GnRH after pretreatment with a GnRH analogue as therapy for cases of PCOS non-responsive to clomiphene appears to give satisfying results. No pregnancy was achieved; however, it should be noted that five ovulation cycles were obtained in the three patients whose partners presented semen defects. The response obtained in the three patients treated for two consecutive cycles (Figure 3) is probably significant in that the positive biological effects reached with the GnRH analog pretreatment are quickly lost with time. In fact, pulsatile GnRH therapy can induce ovulation; however it is not able to correct the intrinsic defect of PCOS[19].

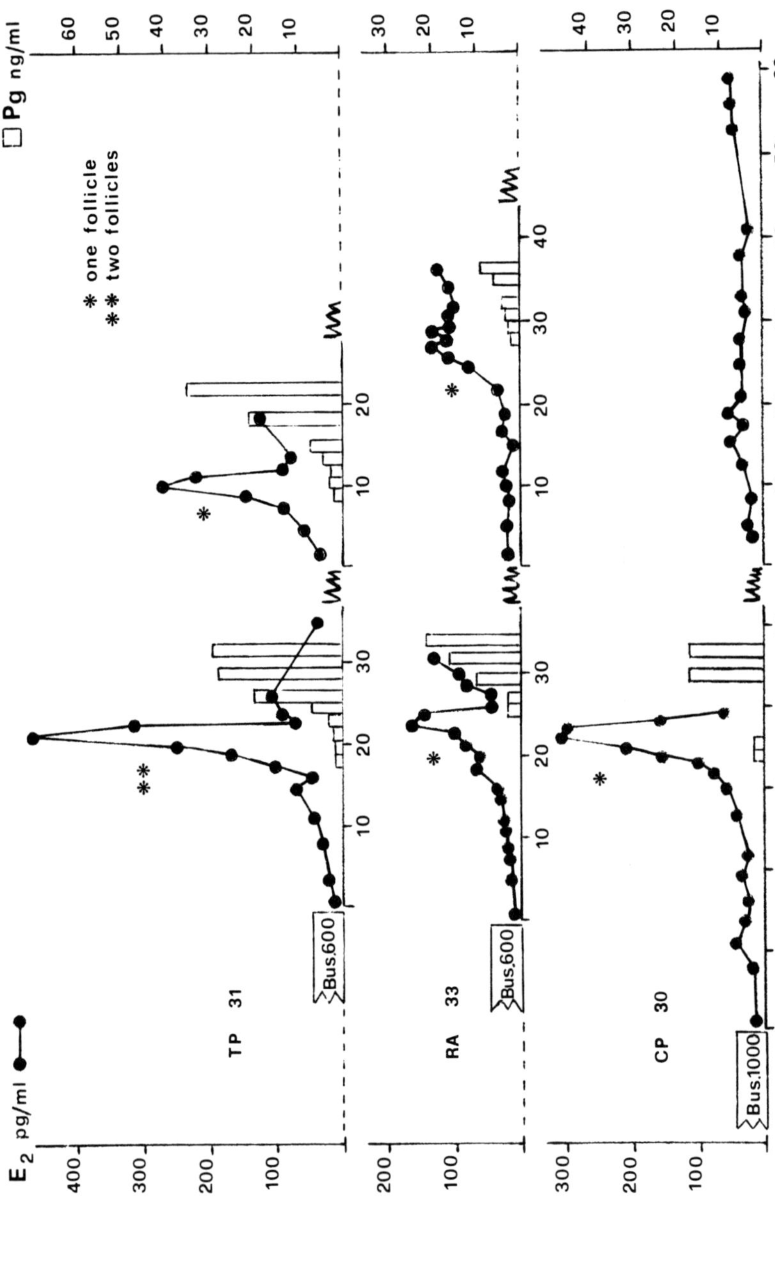

Figure 3 Treatment with pulsatile GnRH in three PCOS patients: comparison between the first cycle after pretreatment with Buserelin and the immediately following cycle

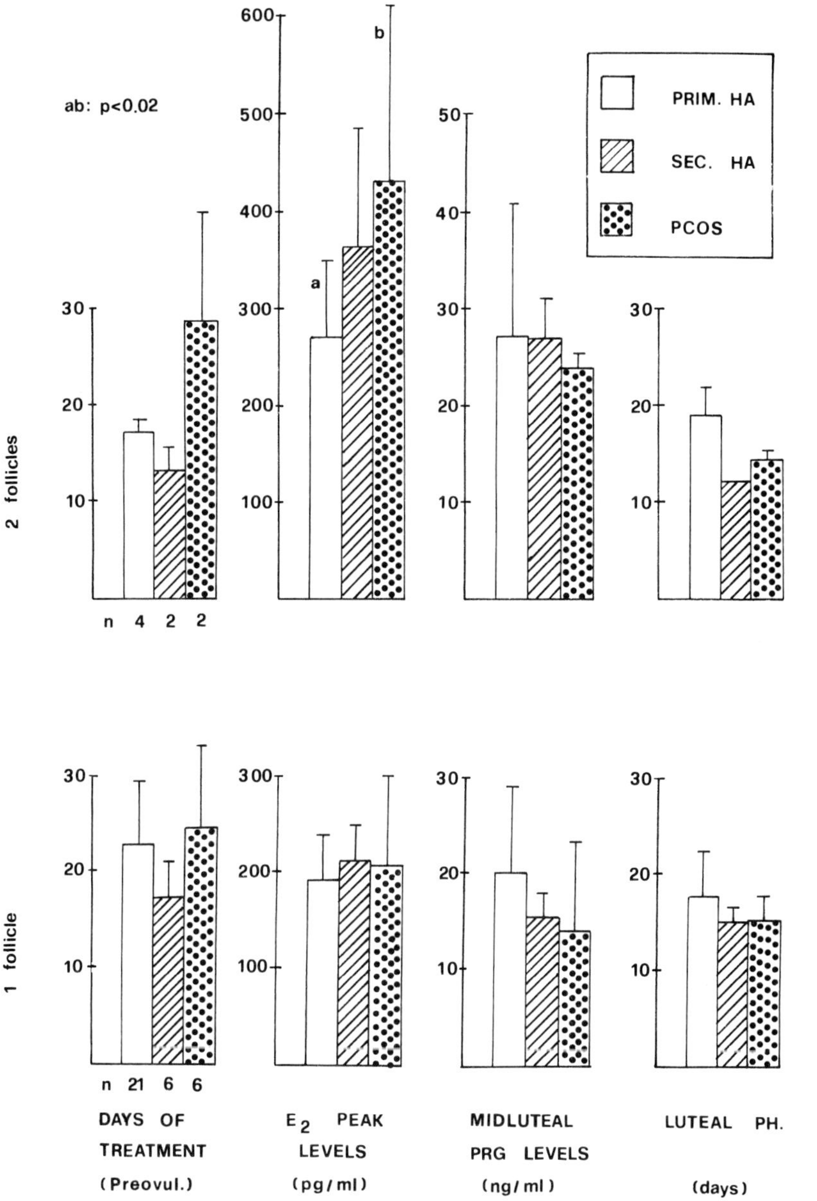

Figure 4 Comparison of the main characteristics of ovulatory cycles obtained by GnRH pulsatile treatment in patients with primary hypothalamic amenorrhea (open blocks), secondary hypothalamic amenorrhea (hatched blocks) and PCOS (stippled blocks)

Conflicting results have been reported regarding route of administration efficacy. Soules *et al.*[20] reported an ovulation rate varying from 85% to 100% in some studies and between 0% and 30% in others, with the s.c. route. However, Phansey *et al.*[1] did not report significant differences between the s.c. and i.v. routes. Blunt *et al.*[4,8] documented that the positioning of the infusion needle in a well-vascularized area is very important for an adequate response; they reserve the i.v. route for patients who do not respond to s.c. administration, in that the latter is safer and more readily accepted by the patient.

REFERENCES

1. Phansey, S.A., Toffle, R., Curtin, J., Nagel, T.C., Tagatz, G.E., Barnes, M.A. and Nair, R. (1985). Alternative indications for pulsatile gonadotropin-releasing hormone therapy in infertile women. *Fertil. Steril.*, **44**, 589–94
2. Leyendecker, G. and Wildt, L. (1984). Pulsatile administration of GnRH in hypothalamic amenorrhea. *Uppsala J. Med. Sci.*, **89**, 19–32
3. Leyendecker, G. and Wildt, L. (1986). Induction of ovulation and pregnancy by pulsatile administration of GnRH. In *Atti della Società Italiana di Fertilità e Sterilità*, pp. 3–21. XIII Congresso Nazionale–Salsomaggiore Terme, 22–24 maggio
4. Blunt, S.M. and Butt, W.R. (1988). Pulsatile GnRH therapy for the induction of ovulation in hypogonadotropic hypogonadism. *Acta Endocrinol.*, **288**, 58–65
5. Leyendecker, G. and Wildt, L. (1983). Induction of ovulation with chronic intermittent (pulsatile) administration of GnRH in women with hypothalamic amenorrhea. *J. Reprod. Fertil.*, **69**, 397–409
6. Mais, V., Melis, G.B., Antinori, D., Paoletti, A.M., Strigini, F., De Ruggiero, A. and Fioretti, P. (1988). Terapia dei disordini dell'ovulazione con GnRH a dosaggi personalizzati. In *Riassunti II° Congresso Nazionale di Scienze Ginecologiche ed Ostetriche*, p. 68. Isola d'Elba, 12–19 giugno
7. Caruso, A., Lanzone, A., Fulghesu, A.M. and Mancuso, S. (1987). The impact of dosage on ovulation induction by pulsatile gonadotropin-releasing hormone (GnRH) in hypothalamic amenorrhea. *J. Endocrinol. Invest.*, **10**, 513–16
8. Blunt, S.M., Clayton, R.N. and Butt, W.R. (1986). Effect of injection site on the pharmacokinetics and pharmacodynamics of subcutaneously administered luteinizing hormone releasing hormone. *Clin. Endocrinol.*, **25**, 589–96
9. Jacobs, H.S. (1987). Polycystic ovaries and polycystic ovary syndrome. *Gynecol. Endocrinol.*, **1**, 113–31
10. Abdulwahid, N.A., Adams, J., Van Den Spouy, Z.M. and Jacobs, H.S. (1985). Gonadotropin control of follicular development. *Clin. Endocrinol.*, **23**, 613–26
11. Hurley, D.M., Brian, R., Outch, K., Stockdale, J., Fry, A., Hackman, C., Clarke, I. and Burger, H.G. (1984). Induction of ovulation and fertility in amenorrheic women by pulsatile low-dose gonadotropin-releasing hormone. *N. Engl. J. Med.*, **310**, 1069–74
12. Mason, P., Adams, J., Morris, D.V., Tucker, M., Price, J., Voulgaris, Z., Van Der Spuy, Z. M., Sutherland, I., Chambers, G.R., White, S., Wheeler, M.J. and Jacobs, H.S. (1984). Induction of ovulation with pulsatile luteinizing hormone releasing hormone. *Br. Med. J.*, **288**, 181–5
13. Burger, C.W., Korsen, T.J.M., Hompes, P.G.A., Van Kessel, H. and Schoemaker, J. (1986). Ovulation induction with pulsatile luteinizing releasing hormone in women with clomiphene citrate-resistant polycystic ovary-like disease: clinical results. *Fertil. Steril.*, **46**, 1045–54
14. Saffan, D. and Seibel, M.M. (1986). Ovulation induction with subcutaneous pulsatile gonadotropin-releasing hormone in various ovulatory disorders. *Fertil. Steril.*, **45**, 475–82
15. Hurwitz, A., Rosenn, B., Palti, Z., Ebstein, B., Har-Nir, R. and Ron, M. (1986). The hormonal response of patients with polycystic ovarian disease to subcutaneous low frequency pulsatile administration of luteinizing hormone-releasing hormone. *Fertil. Steril.*, **46**, 378–89

16. Homburg, R., Armar, N.A., Eshel, A., Adams, J. and Jacobs, H.S. (1988). Influence of serum luteinizing hormone concentrations on ovulation, conception and early pregnancy loss in polycystic ovary syndrome. *Br. Med. J.*, **297**, 1024–6
17. Filicori, M. and Flamigni, C. (1987). The use of pulsatile GnRH and GnRH analogs for induction of ovulation in polycystic ovarian disease *Gynecol. Endocrinol.*, **1**, 355–60
18. Filicori, M., Ferrari, P., Pareschi, A., Michelacci, L., Campaniello, E., Valdiserri, A., Meriggiola, C., Ucci, N., Cimatti, M. and Flamigni, C. (1988). L'uso del GnRH pulsatile e degli analoghi del GnRH nella terapia dei disordini ovulatori. In *Abstracts — Secondo Congresso Nazionale di Scienze Ginecologiche ed Ostetriche*, p. 67. Isola d'Elba, 12–19 giugno
19. Burger, C.W., Hompes, P.G.A., Korsen, T.J.M. and Schoemaker, J. (1989). Ovulation induction with pulsatile luteinizing hormone-releasing hormone in women with clomiphene citrate-resistant polycystic ovary-like disease: endocrine results. *Fertil. Steril.*, **51**, 20–9
20. Soules, M.R., Southworth, M.B., Norton, M.E. and Bremner, W.J. (1986). Ovulation induction with pulsatile gonadotropin-releasing hormone: a study of the subcutaneous route of administration. *Fertil. Steril.*, **46**, 578–85

94

Ovulation induction with clomiphene citrate: a reassessment

Z. Shoham, C. Pariente and B. Lunenfeld

Clomiphene citrate (CC) is a non-steroidal, triphenylethylene compound with both estrogenic and antiestrogenic properties. The commercial preparations of CC currently available are composed of a mixture of two isomers: Enclomiphene (En) 62% (with antiestrogenic properties) and Zuclomiphene (Zu) 38% (with mild estrogenic activity). A comparison of the pharmacokinetic disposition of the two isomers revealed that each has its own characteristic profile. The En isomer is absorbed faster and eliminated more completely than the Zu isomer. In a study of 23 healthy, female volunteers, it was found that the plasma concentrations of Zu isomer were much higher than those of the En isomer after administration of one 50 mg tablet of CC[1].

It is claimed that the main effect of clomiphene is due to competition with estrogen for binding sites on the acceptor molecules which complex the receptor to deoxyribonucleic acid (DNA). The stereoscopic configuration of CC is sufficiently similar to that of estradiol (E_2) to compete with it for available estrogen receptor sites in all estrogen-dependent target cells in the hypothalamus, pituitary, ovary, uterus and cervical epithelium. The hypothalamus–pituitary axis will respond to CC by increasing gonadotropin output[2,3]. Due to these properties it has been extensively used over the last 20 years to induce ovulation. The overall mean ovulation rate following CC treatment as reported by various authors, was 70% or higher[4]. However, the mean pregnancy rate reported in the same compilation of 8843 patients was only 33.1%[4]. The striking difference between ovulation and pregnancy rate has been attributed to the antiestrogenic effect of CC on the cervical mucus and endometrium. It has been found that approximately half the responsive patients will undergo enhanced follicular development with excessive E_2 production that will counteract the antiestrogenic effect on the cervix and endometrium and will facilitate conception.

The antiestrogenic effect on the cervical mucus, when present, is expressed by a low cervical score which occurs despite the relatively high levels of estrogen in the circulation. In about half the patients given clomiphene, the cervical mucus production is not suppressed, since the antiestrogen effect on the hypothalamus results in elevated follicle-stimulating hormone (FSH) and luteinizing hormone (LH) levels. The elevated gonadotropin levels induce multifollicular development, which, in turn, enhances estrogen production. The elevated estrogen, two to three times higher than in normal cycles, may mask the antiestrogen effect on the cervix and endometrium. The exaggerated levels are probably the result of multifollicular development and a direct effect on the ovary. We have recently shown that similar to diethylstilbestrol (DES), CC, Zu and En isomers increased FSH-stimulated production of E_2 in rat granulosa cells *in vitro* in a dose-related manner (Figure 1).

The maximal stimulatory effect on aromatase activity as expressed by E_2 production, was obtained with 100 nm CC, Zu and En clomiphene (1411 ± 113, 1198 ± 127 and 1710 ± 68 E_2 pg/ml). At this dose the stimulatory effect of CC and its isomers was significantly greater ($p < 0.05$) than that of DES at the same concentration (607 ± 108 E_2 pg/ml). The effects of Zu or CC were similar, however, significantly lower than that of En ($p < 0.05$) (Figure 1).

Since all these factors cannot fully explain the discrepancy between the ovulation and pregnancy rate we attempted to look for additional factors by assessing and comparing the hormonal profile following administration of CC in women who conceived and those who did not.

The study sample comprised 41 oligomenorrheic patients who were normoprolactinemic and non-hirsute and exhibited no other endocrine disorders or any mechanical factors. Their husbands were normospermic. Of 41 patients, treated during a single cycle with 100 mg/day of CC for 5 days, ovulation was assumed to have occurred in 28 patients. In all the 28 patients

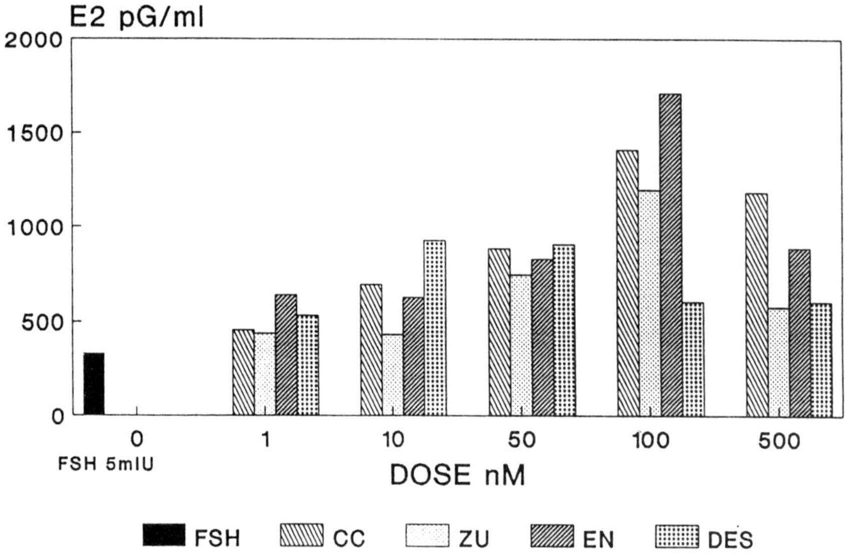

Figure 1 Rat granulosa cells were incubated with 5 mIU follicle-stimulating hormone (FSH) in the absence or presence of different doses (1 nM–500 nM) of diethylstilbestrol (DES), clomiphene citrate (CC), Zu and En isomers. After 48 hours of incubation estradiol (E_2) content in the spent media was measured by radioimmunoassay (RIA)

prior to administration of CC (day 5), follicular development, as determined by ultrasonography, was similar and the LH/FSH ratio was less than 1.5. Following the last day of CC administration (day 9), two distinct patterns of LH/FSH secretion emerged. In one group (17 patients), designated as the 'normal responsive group' (NR) five clinical pregnancies occurred (29.4%). In this group of patients the secretory patterns of LH, FSH, E_2 and progesterone were similar in those who conceived and those who did not conceive. The LH/FSH ratio was not significantly different from that on day 5 and its mean never exceeded 2 and remained constant until the occurrence of the ovulatory LH peak. The LH peaks were of similar duration and height and occurred within 24 h of the E_2 peak. At the same time as the LH peak progesterone levels never exceeded 0.6 ng/ml. This secretory pattern constituted the normal response (NR) to CC administration.

The second group of 11 patients showed a distinctly different hormonal pattern and in this group no clinical pregnancy occurred. In this group, mean LH and E_2 levels during the follicular phase (until day 12 of the cycle) were significantly higher than in the NR group (Figure 2). The LH/FSH ratios from day 9 were above 2.5 and continued to increase until the LH peak occurred (Figure 3). The mean LH peak in this group was significantly lower ($p<0.02$) and the mean E_2 level significantly higher ($p<0.001$) than in the NR group (Figure 2). At the time of the LH peak more follicles were observed in the AR group than in the NR group (3.6 ± 1.2 and 2.7 ± 1.4 respectively), but the difference was not significant.

In five of these abnormally responding patients serum LH and FSH between day 10 to 13 were measured in another cycle of CC therapy. The

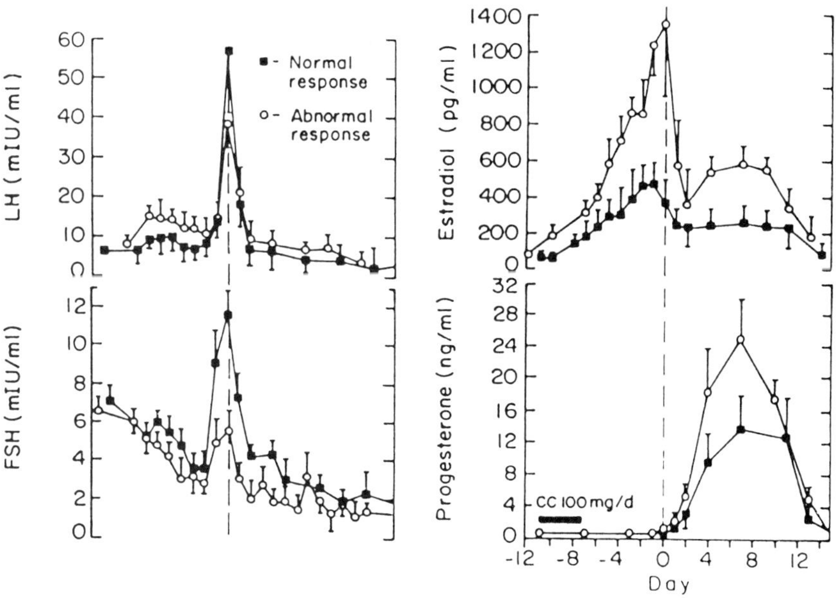

Figure 2 Patterns of hormonal secretion in patients exhibiting normal response and abnormal response to clomiphene citrate (CC)

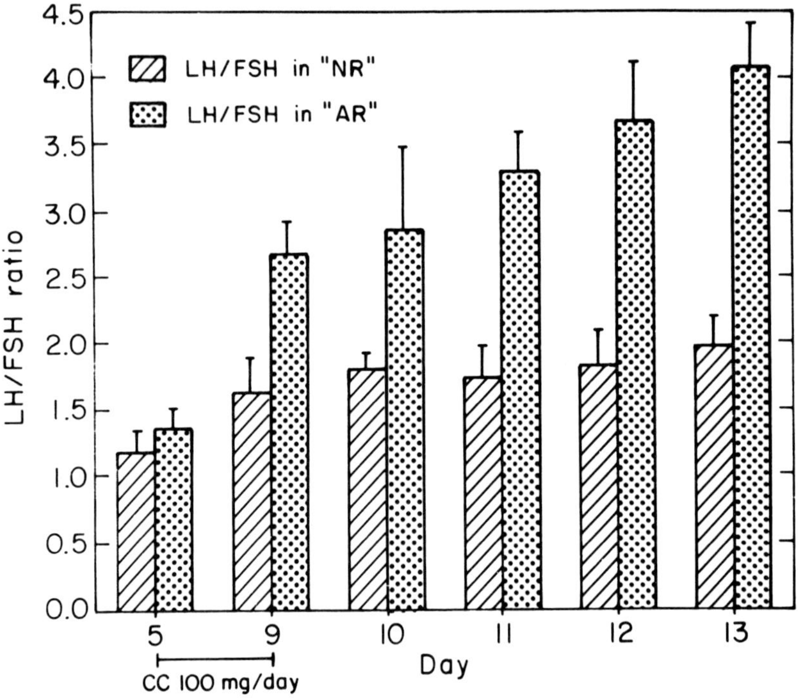

Figure 3 Luteinizing hormone (LH)/follicle stimulating hormone (FSH) ratio in patients exhibiting normal response (NR) and abnormal response (AR) to clomiphene citrate (CC). The LH/FSH ratios on day 5 were similar. From day 9 to 12 the LH/FSH ratio was significantly higher in the AR group (day 9–10, $p<0.05$; day 11–12, $p<0.001$)

elevated serum LH and LH/FSH ratio were similar to those of the previous cycle (mean 13.8 ± 1.8 versus 14.4 ± 2.3 and 2.8 ± 0.8 versus 3.1 ± 0.4 respectively, with no significant difference).

These results are compatible with the emerging hypothesis that overexposure to LH during the follicular phase, may be detrimental to fertilization and contribute to early pregnancy loss. It may be speculated that the elevated LH during the follicular phase may be responsible for:

(1) Excessive androgen and estrogen production.
(2) Premature luteinization of the follicle(s) as demonstrated by elevation of progesterone prior to the LH peak.
(3) Decrease of the pituitary reserve of LH resulting in a diminished LH peak compatible with corpus luteum insufficiency.
(4) Excessive LH milieu may inhibit the meiosis inhibiting factor resulting in aging of the oocytes prior to ovulation.

This hypothesis is strengthened by other authors[5-7]. Howles *et al.*[5] claimed that patients stimulated for *in vitro* fertilization, who did not conceive had significantly higher urinary LH output prior to human chorionic gonadotropin (hCG) administration than those who conceived. Stanger and Yovich[6] demonstrated that patients with exaggerated basal serum LH levels undergoing *in vitro* fertilization had a significantly reduced fertilization rate of mature oocytes. They suggested that a high level of LH may represent a potential cause of infertility, despite adequate follicular growth and E_2 production. Homberg *et al.*[7] indicated that raised basal serum luteinizing hormone concentration during the time of follicular growth significantly interferes with conception, thus they claim that concentration of LH during the follicular phase in women with polycystic ovarian disease (PCOD) have a deleterious effect on rate of conception. They suggest that in patients with exaggerated LH levels during the follicular phase premature maturation may occur[7]. The above authors based their hypothesis on the fact that LH is a potent inhibitor of the meiosis inhibiting factor as previously suggested by Tsafriri and Pomerantz[8] and Dekel[9]. High concentration of LH may penetrate the follicle and allow the oocyte to mature prematurely. This will result in ovulation of physiologically aged oocytes. These oocytes are less likely to be fertilized or tend to produce embryos that implant poorly[10–12].

As far as we are aware, this study demonstrates for the first time that CC administration may be followed by at least two patterns of gonadotropic response. In our limited study of 28 women who were assumed to ovulate in response to CC treatment, nearly a third exhibited, during the follicular phase, excessive LH and E_2 secretion and a decreased amplitude of the LH peak. Within this group not a single clinical pregnancy occurred. If patients belonging to this group were to be identified following their first treatment cycle and offered alternative therapy, the overall pregnancy rate in this population might be increased.

REFERENCES

1. Mikkelson, T.J., Kroboth, P.D., Cameron, W.J., Dittert, L.W., Chungi, V. and Manberg, P.J. (1986). Single-dose pharmacokinetics of clomiphene citrate in normal volunteers. *Fertil. Steril.*, **46**, 392–6
2. Kerin, J.F., Liu, J.H., Pillipou, G. and Yen, S.S.C. (1985). Evidence for a hypothalamic site of action of clomiphene citrate in women. *J. Clin. Endocrinol. Metab.*, **61**, 265–8
3. Vandenberg, G. and Yen, S.S.C. (1973). Effect of anti-estrogen action of clomiphene during the menstrual cycle: Evidence for a change in the feedback sensitivity. *J. Clin. Endocrinol. Metab.*, **37**, 356–65
4. Blankstein, J., Mashiach, S. and Lunenfeld, B. (1986). *Ovulation Induction and In Vitro Fertilization.* pp. 122. (Year Book Medical Publishers: Chicago)
5. Howles, C.M., Macnamee, M.C., Edwards, R.G., Goswamy, R. and Steptoe, P.C. (1986). Effect of high tonic levels of luteinizing hormone on outcome of in-vitro fertilization. *Lancet*, **ii**, 521–3
6. Stanger, J.D. and Yovich, J.L. (1985). Reduced in-vitro fertilization of human oocytes from patient with raised basal luteinising hormone levels during the follicular phase. *Br. J. Obstet. Gynaecol.*, **92**, 385–93
7. Homberg, R., Armar, N.A., Eshel, A., Adams, J. and Jacobs, H.S. (1988). Influence of serum luteinizing hormone concentrations on ovulation, conception and early pregnancy loss in polycystic ovary syndrome. *Br. Med. J.*, **297**, 1024–6
8. Tsafriri, A. and Pomerantz, S.H. (1986). Oocyte maturation inhibitor. *Clin. Endocrinol. Metab.*, **15**, 157–70
9. Dekel, N. (1986). Hormone control of ovulation. In Litwack, G. (ed.) *Biochemical Actions of Hormones.* Vol. 13, pp. 57–90. (Academic Press: Orlando, Florida)
10. Hunter, R.H., Cook, B. and Baker, T.G. (1976). Dissociation of response to injected

gonadotropin between the Graafian follicle and oocyte in pigs. *Nature*, **260**, 156–8
11. Austin, C.R. (1981). The egg. In Austin, C.R., Short, R.E. (eds). *Reproduction in Mammals. Part I. Germ cells and fertilization.* 2nd edn, p. 58. (Cambridge University Press: Cambridge)
12. Guerrero, R.J. and Rojas, O.I. (1975). Spontaneous abortion and ageing of human ova and spermatozoa. *N. Engl. J. Med.*, **293**, 573–5

95

Induction of ovulation in hypothalamic amenorrhea by GnRH therapy

J. Schoemaker and D.D.M. Braat

INTRODUCTION

It is well established that the pulsatile secretion of luteinizing hormone (LH), and to a certain extent of follicle-stimulating hormone (FSH), from the pituitary, is stimulated by gonadotropin-releasing hormone (GnRH), secreted in a pulsatile fashion from the hypothalamus[1,2]. Secretion patterns have been extensively studied in regularly cycling women[3], as well as in women with hypothalamic amenorrhea and polycystic ovarian disease (PCOD)[4]. The latter study showed that in PCOD the pulse frequency and the pulse amplitude were higher than during the follicular phase, while in hypothalamic amenorrhea the pulse frequency was the same as in PCOD but the pulse amplitude was lower than in the follicular phase. Hypothalamic amenorrhea can thus be depicted as a syndrome which is caused by a deficient secretion of GnRH, while in PCOD the syndrome is rather depicted as associated with a dysregulation of GnRH secretion. It therefore stands to reason that the indication for substitutional therapy with GnRH is hypothalamic amenorrhea, rather than PCOD.

Continuous infusion of GnRH leads to desensitization of the pituitary and therefore to a discontinuation of the release of LH and FSH[5]. Only pulsatile infusion with pulse intervals of at least 30 min will ensure sustained release. Leyendecker[6] was the first to introduce pulsatile GnRH administration as a therapy for clomiphene-resistant hypothalamic amenorrhea. The pulsatile infusion is accomplished by portable infusion pumps, most of which can be programmed to different pulse volumes and pulse intervals. By varying the concentration of GnRH in the syringe the pulse dose can be modified. Both subcutaneous and intravenous application is practiced. Highly sophisticated pumps have been developed over the past 10 years and are now readily available.

THE PULSE DOSE

Several authors have studied the effect of the pulse dose on the outcome of ovulation induction. In our own studies[7] we showed that if the administration of GnRH was interrupted during the night, no difference in estrogen excretion between cycles induced with 20 or 100 μg per pulse could be shown. Neither was there a difference of these two groups with the estrogen excretion of spontaneously cycling women. FSH levels, however, were lower in the 100 μg group, both during the follicular and the luteal phase (Figure 1) suggesting that a greater number of follicles may have been recruited initially.

Leyendecker and Wildt[8] developed their classification of hypothalamic amenorrhea on the basis of the patients' response to functional tests such as the clomiphene test, the progesterone challenge test and the luteinizing hormone-releasing hormone (LHRH) test. They concluded that the correct dose for patients with hypothalamic amenorrhea with a negative clomiphene test is 2.5–5 μg per pulse unless the LHRH test shows no response at all. In the latter case a dose of 15–20 μg per pulse should be used.

Santoro *et al.*[9] concluded that a dose of 25 ng/kg per pulse was marginal in inducing follicular growth in women with hypothalamic amenorrhea. On the other hand a dose of 100 ng/kg per pulse, which equals approximately 5–6 μg per pulse, showed already multifollicular development in her group of patients.

Finally Braat and co-workers[10], in a large multicenter study on the outcome of pregnancies in GnRH-induced cycles, showed that the incidence of multiple pregnancies is significantly higher in cycles induced with 11–20 μg GnRH per pulse than in cycles induced with 6–10 μg per pulse or even less than 5 μg per pulse. Therefore the selection of the correct dose may help to avoid multiple pregnancies.

A reasonable approach seems to be that, in general, ovulation induction should be started at a dose of 5–10 μg per pulse while, if no follicular growth has been noted to occur on ultrasound monitoring after 2 weeks, the dose should be increased to 15–20 μg per pulse.

PULSE INTERVAL

Few studies have addressed the influence of the pulse interval in GnRH-induced cycles.

Braat *et al.*[10] found no significant difference in the incidence of multiple pregnancies comparing cycles induced with a pulse interval of 60–90 min versus those induced with 120 min intervals. Bringer *et al.*[11] neither found any difference in the endocrinology or outcome of cycles induced with a pulse interval of 64, 90 or 120 min, neither in anorexia nervosa patients, nor in women with unexplained anovulation or PCOD.

Our own study[7] showed the FSH levels to be marginally lower, although significantly lower between days −3 and +7 in patients treated with a pulse interval of 90 min instead of those treated with a pulse interval of 120 min. However, neither of the other endocrine parameters did show a difference. Moreover, in this study it was shown that lowering the pulse frequency to one pulse every 240 min during the luteal phase does not adversely affect

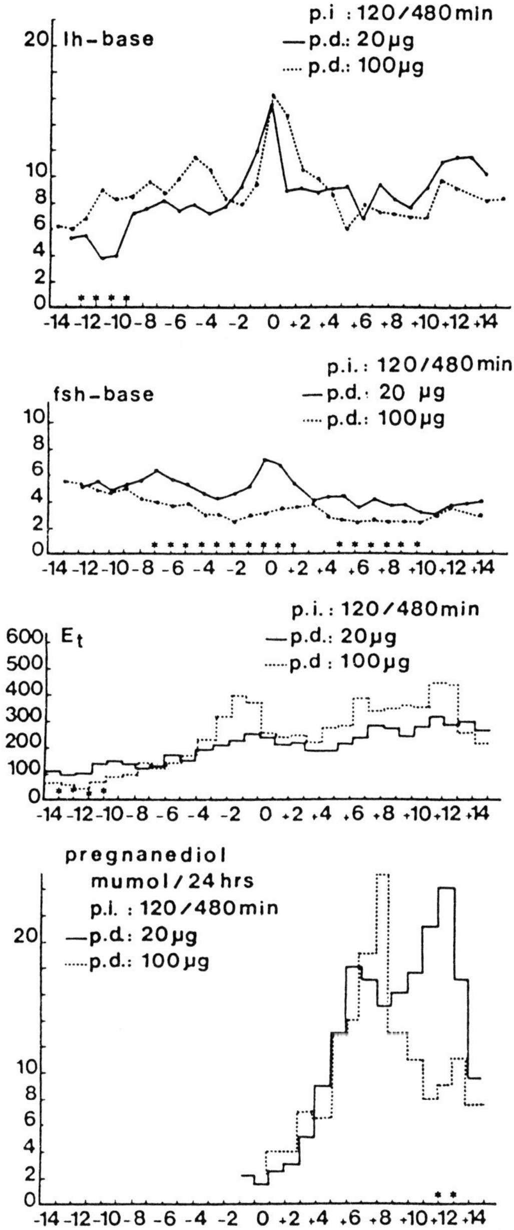

Figure 1 Comparison of the endocrinology of cycles induced with a pulse dose of 20 (solid line) or 100 (dotted line) μg. Pulse interval 120 min. Interruption during the night from 23:00 till 07:00. Lines connect median values per day in each group. Asterisks on the abscissa indicate day where differences are statistically significant (Wilcoxon Rank sum test, $p < 0.05$), luteinizing hormone (LH) and follicle-stimulating hormone (FSH) in IU/l. Total urinary estrogen excretion (E_t) in nmol/24 h, normalized to a daily excretion of 10 μmol creatinine. Pregnanediol in μmol/24 h. (from reference 7 with permission from the author)

steroid production of the corpus luteum. Comparison of cycles which were induced with a pulse frequency of one pulse every 120 min during the entire day and night with cycles induced with the same pulse frequency but with a daily interruption of treatment from 23:00 to 07:00 showed that this interruption impaired the steroidogenic potential of the growing follicle and therefore probably the development of the follicle itself.

As the pulse interval seems to have little bearing on the outcome of induced cycles, it seems wise to use a pulse interval of 120 min during the follicular phase and 240 min during the luteal phase, as those probably give the best benefit/cost ratio.

ROUTE OF ADMINISTRATION

The choice is between the subcutaneous (s.c.) and the intravenous (i.v.) routes. Intravenous stimulation is more effective and more reliable because McIntosh and McIntosh[12] demonstrated that the response of the pituitary to GnRH stimulation is dependent on the steepness of the increase of GnRH concentration in plasma.

Handelsman *et al.*[13] indeed demonstrated that the slope, with which the plasma GnRH concentration increases, is steeper after an i.v. bolus injection than after an s.c. bolus. The dose, necessary to induce ovulation, therefore is an estimated 4–5 times higher using the s.c. route compared to the i.v. route. Another drawback of the s.c. route is the possibility of developing antibodies to GnRH. This phenomenon has not yet been described using the i.v. route. Obviously the i.v. route carries the risk of bacteremia and sepsis. Therefore, if it is used, one should be alert that a sepsis might occur. In case of fever, the needle should always be removed as soon as possible even if it seems obvious that the fever is caused by something else. The choice of the route therefore is dependent on the monitoring possibilities available at the treatment center.

RESULTS

All authors report highly favorable results of this treatment in patients with hypogonadotropic amenorrhea. Few reports have so far reported on the fecundity rate per cycle of induction. Figure 2 shows the cumulative pregnancy rate, calculated according to the life table method, based on 272 cycles induced in 49 patients with hypogonadotropic and normogonadotropic amenorrhea. After 12 months a cumulative pregnancy rate in this group of patients has been reached of 92%. The figure also shows that the curve of the cumulative pregnancy rate of the population that has not conceived after 6 months remains the same for the next 6 months. As the monthly fecundity does not really change over the first 12 months, it is thus well worth continuing treatment for 12 months before changing to a different therapy. Significant differences in fecundity could be demonstrated between the population without additional infertility factors and with other factors, as well as between patients with primary and those with secondary amenorrhea,

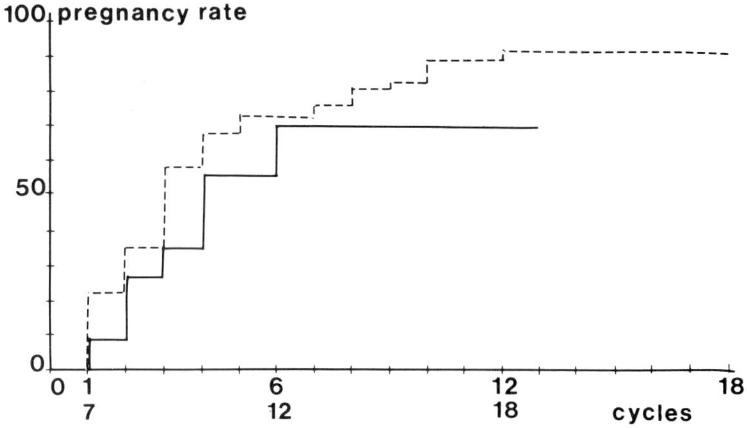

Figure 2 Cumulative pregnancy rates of all patients (broken line) and of patients who had not become pregnant yet after 6 months of treatment (solid line). No significant difference in fecundity rate during the first and second 6 months

the latter showing a better prognosis than the former.

There was no difference between patients with normoestrogenic and hypoestrogenic amenorrhea. Body weight did not seem to influence the results, although patients who had been anorexic in the past seemed to have a better fecundity than those who had not been underweight. In 49 patients with hypogonadotropic or normogonadotropic amenorrhea 55 pregnancies were achieved in 272 cycles. Of these 55 pregnancies five were multiple (four twins, one triplet). This high multiple pregnancy rate (9.1%), observed by several investigators, was the reason to initiate a multicenter survey, to examine the pregnancy outcome of GnRH induced cycles[10].

The most important results from this study are that of 174 pregnancies in patients with hypogonadotropic amenorrhea 26 (14.9%) were multiple. Of 12 pregnancies in patients with normogonadotropic amenorrhea one (8.3%) was multiple and in 24 pregnancies in patients with PCOD, none were multiple. Of 27 multiple pregnancies two aborted early (twins). Of the remaining 25, one quadruplet, two triplets and 14 twins were born prematurely, six twins were born at term and two were still ongoing at the time of closurc of thc study.

As mentioned above the multiple pregnancy rate appeared to be dose-dependent, the higher rates with the higher doses. There was a significantly higher multiple pregnancy rate in first induced cycles compared to later cycles. In 206 children born, four major congenital abnormalities were observed and one minor.

CONCLUSION

Induction of ovulation in patients with clomiphene resistant hypothalamic amenorrhea has proven to be a very effective safe and easy to perform therapy. The initial dose should be 5–10 μg per pulse unless the LHRH test shows no response, in which case the dose should be 15–20 μg per pulse. A pulse interval of 120 min before and 240 min after ovulation gives the best cost/benefit ratio, without affecting the effectiveness of the therapy. The route of administration should be chosen on the basis of the monitoring possibilities of the center. The results are excellent and the side-effects are minimal with exception of the risk of multiple pregnancies, which is approximately 15%. This high rate is dose-dependent. The incidence of multiple pregnancies is higher in the first cycle of treatment compared to subsequent cycles. The outcome of pregnancies shows a high rate of prematurity due to the high rate of multiple pregnancies. The abortion rate is normal, as is the incidence of congenital anomalies.

REFERENCES

1. Levine, J.E., Pau, K.-Y.F., Ramirez, V.D. and Jackson, G.L. (1982). Simultaneous measurement of luteinizing hormone-releasing hormone release in unanesthetized sheep. *Endocrinology*, **111**, 1449
2. Clarke, I.J. and Cummins, J.F. (1982). The temporal relationship between gonadotropin releasing hormone (GnRH) and luteinizing hormone (LH) secretion in ovariectomized ewes. *Endocrinology*, **111**, 1737
3. Filicori, M., Santoro, N., Merriam, G.R. and Crowley, W.F. Jr. (1986). Characterization of the physiological pattern of episodic gonadotropin secretion throughout the human menstrual cycle. *J. Clin. Endocrinol. Metab.*, **61**, 1136–43
4. Burger, C.W., Korsen, T., van Kessel, H., van Dop, P.A., Caron, F.J.M. and Schoemaker, J. (1985). Pulsatile Luteinizing Hormone patterns in the follicular phase of the menstrual cycle, polycystic ovarian disease (PCOD) and non-PCOD secondary amenorrhea. *J. Clin. Endocrinol. Metab.*, **61**, 1126–32
5. Knobil, E. (1980). The neuroendocrine control of the menstrual cycle. *Rec. Progr. Horm. Res.*, **36**, 53–88
6. Leyendecker, G. and Wildt, L. (1978). The pathophysiology of hypothalamic ovarian failure. Diagnostic and therapeutic considerations. *Eur. J. Obstet. Gynecol. Reprod. Biol.*, **9**, 175–86
7. Schoemaker, J., Korsen, T.J.M. and van Kessel, H. (1986). Reflections on pulse dose and pulse interval. In Coelingh Bennink, H.J.T., Dogterom, A.A., Lappöhn, R.E., Rolland, R. and Schoemaker, J. (eds). *Pulsatile GnRH 1985*, pp. 131–7 (Ferring Publication: Haarlem, Netherlands)
8. Leyendecker, G. and Wildt, L. (1983). Induction of ovulation with chronic intermittent (pulsatile) administration of GnRH in women with hypothalamic amenorrhea. *J. Reprod. Fert.*, **69**, 379–409
9. Santoro, N., Wierman, M.E., Filicori, M. Waldstreicher, J. and Crowley, W.F. Jr. (1986). Intravenous administration of pulsatile gonadotropin releasing hormone in hypothalamic amenorrhea: effects of dosage. *J. Clin. Endocrinol. Metab.*, **62**, 109–16
10. Braat, D.D.M., Ayalon, D., Blunt, S.M., Bogchelman, D., Coelingh Bennink, H.J.T., Handelsman, D.J., Heineman, M.J., Lappohn, R.E., Lorijn, R.H.W., Rolland, R., Willemsen, W.N.P. and Schoemaker, J. (1989). Pregnancy outcome in luteinizing hormone releasing hormone induced cycles: a multicenter study. *Gynecol. Endocrinol.*, **3**, 35–44
11. Bringer, J., Hedon, B., Jaffiol, C., Nicolou, S., Gibert, F., Cristol, P., Orsetti, A., Viola, J.L. and Mirouze, J. (1985). Influence of the frequency of gonadotropin-releasing hormone (GnRH) administration on ovulatory responses in women with anovulation. *Fertil. Steril.*, **44**, 42
12. McIntosh, R.P. and McIntosh, J.E.A. (1983). Influence of the characteristics of pulses of gonadotropin releasing hormone on the dynamics of luteinizing hormone release from perfused sheep pituitary cells. *J. Endocrinol.*, **98**, 411
13. Handelsman, D.J., Jansen, R.P.S., Boylan, L.M., Spaliviero, J.A. and Turtle, R.J. (1984). Pharmacokinetics of gonadotropin-releasing hormone: comparison of subcutaneous and intravenous routes. *J. Clin. Endocrinol. Metab.*, **59**, 739

96

Hormonal and endometrial parameters in periovulatory gonadotropin stimulated cycles in women included in an *in vitro* fertilization–embryo transfer program

H. Meden-Vrtovec

The effectiveness of *in vitro* fertilization and embryo transfer (IVF–ET) procedure depends on numerous factors only a few of which are known and determined: the method of ovulation induction[1–4], the type of estradiol (E_2) rise[5,6] and gonadotropin increase and, above all, premature luteinizing hormone (LH) increase[7,8]. The quality and number of oocyte and spermatozoa define embryo quality and its implantation ability[9]. The endometrial quality, maturity and receptiveness[10–12] are also important factors contributing to the success rate of the IVF procedure.

As in the IVF–ET procedure embryo transfer is performed at least 2 days before the embryo reaches the uterus in natural cycles[13], it is possible that the endometrium is not adequately prepared for implantation. Therefore, the objective of our study was to define the relation between periovulatory $E_2$and progesterone (P) concentrations, and endometrial quality 2 days after ovulation, i.e. in the period of ET.

MATERIALS AND METHODS

Patients

Twenty-five patients, admitted to the IVF–ET procedure at the University Department of Obstetrics and Gynecology Ljubljana in 1986/87 included in the study. In those patients embryo transfer was not carried out for various reasons, therefore endometrial morphological analysis in the period when ET should normally be performed was possible.

The patients were divided into three groups according to E_2 concentrations in the period of chorionic gonadotropin administration.

In the first group there were patients in whom E_2 concentration did not exceed 3.0 nmol/l, in the second those with E_2 value from 3–6 nmol/l, in the third patients in whom at the administration of human chorionic gonadotropin (hCG) E_2 value exceeded 6 nmol/l.

In the first group there were seven patients, aged 26–38 years (average 34.0 ± 5.29 years), in the second seven patients, aged 29–38 years (average 34.8 ± 3.54 years), and in the third group 11 patients, aged 30–39 years (average 33.27 ± 2.83 years).

In all the patients human menopausal gonadotropin (hMG) Pergonal (Serono) was used for the stimulation of ovulation; the daily dose was adjusted to a patient's individual reactiveness. In the first group 10 to 32 ampoules ($\bar{x} = 23.42 \pm 8.12$) were used, in the second 14 to 32 ampoules ($\bar{x} = 21.0 \pm 8.67$), and in the third group 16 to 39 ampoules ($\bar{x} = 24.0 \pm 7.34$). Ovarian follicle growth and maturation were monitored by daily E_2 determination and ultrasound folliculometry. Besides E_2 concentration, serum P concentration was defined as well.

Methods of work

Serum E_2 and P values were determined by the radioimmunoassay (RIA) method with the Biodata reagents kit.

Normal E_2 values for follicular phase of the cycle are 0.11–0.33 nmol/l, for luteal phase 0.29–0.85 nmol/l, in preovulatory peak 0.58–1.28 nmol/l.

Normal P values for follicular phase are 0.64–10.0 nmol/l for luteal phase 16.0–64.01 nmol/l.

Student's *t* test was used in the statistical analysis of the data.

Endometrial biopsy (BE) was performed 2 days after the ovulation (after laparoscopic aspiration of oocytes) with Novak's curette without dilatation and without anesthesia. Endometrial samples were evaluated by a pathologist, who was not informed about the data concerning E_2 and P concentrations.

Reference group

To compare hormonal analyses and conditions of the endometrium in patients in stimulated cycles to the ones in untreated cycles, a reference group of 23 patients was formed. BE and P determination were adjusted for the second day after the elevation of basal body temperature (BBT) of 0.5 to 0.8°C (i.e. day 16 or 17 of the cycle).

RESULTS

Average E_2 value in the first group of patients (E_2 to 3 nmol/l) was at the time of hCG administration 2.33 ± 0.72 nmol/l ($\bar{x} \pm SD$) and 2 days after ovulation it was 1.057 ± 0.418 nmol/l. The average P concentration after ovulation in this group of patients was 41.5 ± 29.72 nmol/l.

The average number of oocytes obtained was 1.57 ± 1.98. Bioptical endometrial sample analysis showed in four patients (57.1%) initial, and in three (42.9%) early secretory endometrial transformation.

In seven patients with moderate E_2 elevation (from 3 to 6 nmol/l) the value of E_2 at the time of hCG administration was 4.53 ± 1 .08 nmol/l, and 2 days after ovulation 1.94 ± 0.98 nmol/1. Average P concentration after ovulation was 82.3 ± 30.66 nmol/l, and average aspirated oocyte number was 5.14 ± 4.4.

In two patients morphological pattern of endometrium showed early, (28.6%) and in five patients initial secretory endometrium (71.4%).

In 11 patients from the third group (E_2 above 6 nmol/l) average E_2 value at the hCG administration was 9.75 ± 4.22 nmol/l, and after ovulation 2.609 ± 1.057 nmol/l.

The average P concentration 2 days after ovulation was 146.8 ± 57.6 nmol/l. With laparoscopic aspiration an average of 5.7 ± 3.39 oocytes was obtained. Bioptic endometrial sample analysis showed a uniform pattern (100%) of early secretory endometrium. Average number of aspirated oocytes, P concentration and morphological characteristics of endometrium in the three groups of patients are shown in Figures 1, 2 and 3.

Bioptic endometrial sample analysis in 23 patients of the reference group showed proliferative endometrium in nine patients (39.1%), initial secretory endometrium in five patients (21.7%), early secretory endometrium in six patients (26.1%), and late secretory endometrium in three patients (13.1%).

In patients with proliferative endometrium the average concentrations

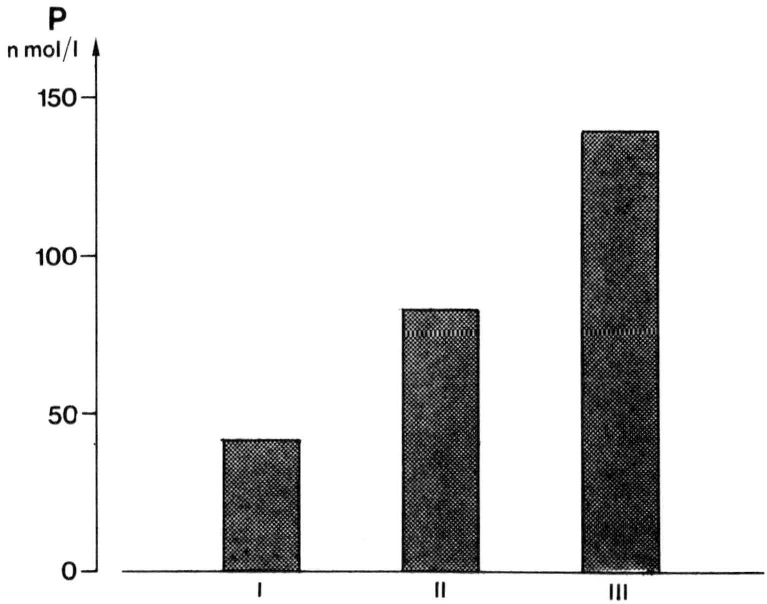

Figure 1 Mean progesterone concentrations 2 days after ovulation in three groups of patients: I, patients with E_2 rise to 3 nmol/l; II, patients with E_2 rise from 3 to 6 nmol/l; and III, patients with E_2 rise > 6 nmol/l

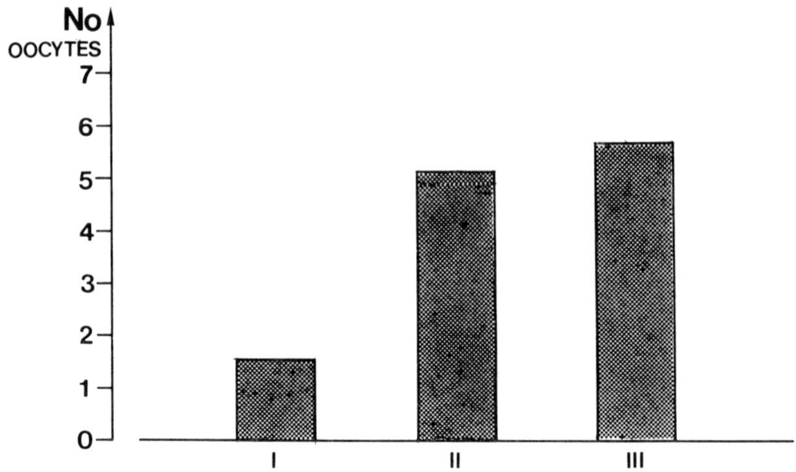

Figure 2 Mean number of oocytes recovered in three groups of patients: groups as in Figure 1

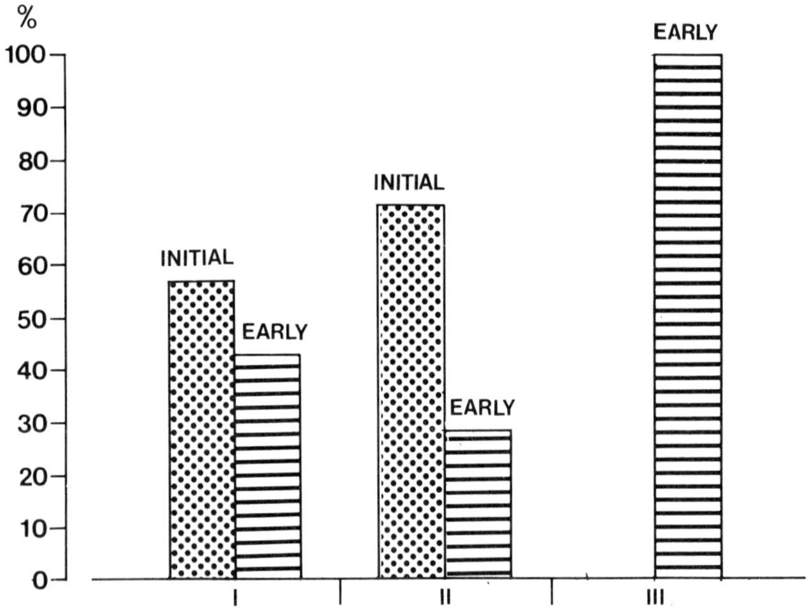

Figure 3 Morphological analysis of endometrium in three groups of patients: groups as in Figure 1

were E_2: 0.55 ± 0.44 nmol/l, and P: 0.87 ± 1.61 nmol/l at the time of bioptic sample taking.

The average E_2 value in patients with initial secretory endometrium was 0.78 ± 0.70 nmol/l, P value was 18.65 ± 8.03 nmol/l. Patients with early secretory endometrium had an average E_2 value 0.38 ± 0.12 nmol/l, P value was 27.1 ± 13.1 nmol/l. In three patients with late secretory endometrium average E_2 value was 0.68 ± 0.50 nmol/l, P value was 26.8 ± 5.7 nmol/l.

Morphologically ideal early secretory phase was related to the E_2 concentration 0.39 nmol/l and P 38.8 nmol/l. The results are shown in Figure 4.

Absolute comparison between P and E_2 concentrations is not possible as in stimulated cycles more follicles grow and mature and after the aspiration they develop into an arbitrary number of corpora lutea leading to higher hormone concentrations. When comparing stimulated and natural cycles only relations between E_2 and P concentrations can be established. The relation between E_2 and P is in the reference group 1:24 in initial secretory transformation, 1:71 in the early one, and 1:39 in the late secretory transformation of endometrium. The ideal early endometrium transformation is carried out in the ratio: E_2:P = 1:99.

In patients of the study group endometrial phases with low and moderate E_2 concentrations were overlapping, so E_2:P ratio could have been determined only in the group with high E_2 responsiveness in which a uniform pattern of endometrium, early secretory endometrium, was found. In those patients the ratio was E_2:P = 1:56.

DISCUSSION

Corpus rubrum is present already 1 h after ovulation[14] and initial steroid activity is present 48 h after ovulation. Then the initial secretory endometrium

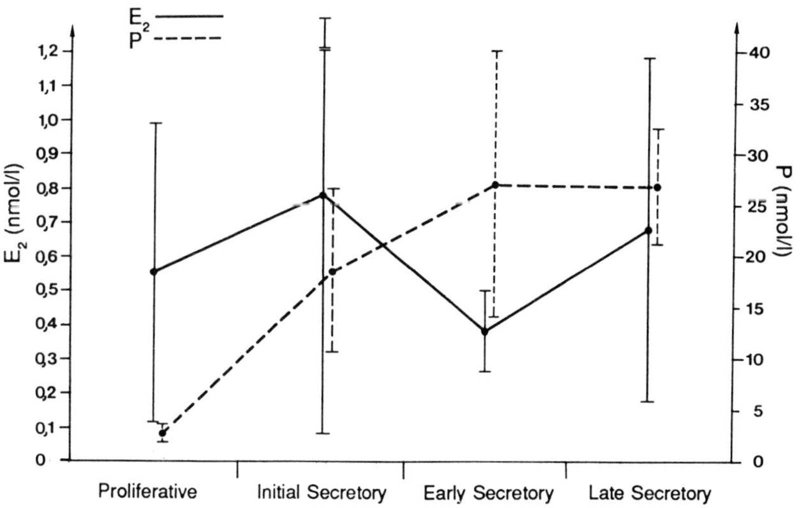

Figure 4 Concentrations of E_2 and P in different stages of endometrial development in patients of the reference group

transformation is expected.

Endometrial samples in patients with low E_2 responsiveness did not esssentially differ from the one in patients with moderate E_2 responsiveness, in the latter P concentration being significantly higher than in patients with low ovarian responsiveness.

Patients with high E_2 responsiveness (3rd group) exhibited a uniform endometrial pattern of an early secretory transformation of endometrium which is anticipated in the phase of the cycle that corresponds also to higher P values, found normally in the midluteal phase. High E_2 concentration is indirectly related to the aspiration of a greater number of oocytes, but at the same time it represents a possibility for a premature luteinization of granulosa cells leading to the aspiration of oocytes of poor quality.

These findings accord with the results, stated by Dirnfeld[15] which ascertain pregnancy rate in 28% of patients with moderate E_2 responsiveness. Premature and therefore out of phase development of the endometrium can theoretically represent a favorable surrounding for the embryo arriving into uterus from 24 to 48 h earlier than in natural conception. Garcia[13] states that P concentrations in a group of patients with advanced endometrium are on the same level as in patients who have conceived. On the other hand some authors establish that the anticipation of endometrium, carried out at high P and E_2 concentrations, represents an unsuitable surrounding for implantation[10,16–19].

Relations of endometrial samples and hormonal concentrations can be clarified taking the patterns of the natural cycle to be physiological.

Comparing the relationship between E_2 and P concentrations in patients with natural cycles with early secretory endometrium to the E_2 and P relationship in patients with early secretory endometrium in stimulated cycles it can be observed that in natural cycles the relationship between E_2 and P is 1:71 and in stimulated cycles 1:56. Such proportions point to the inadequate ratio E_2:P – on account of a higher E_2 concentration – considering the fact that the identical picture of the early secretory phase of endometrium was established in all patients with E_2 concentration exceeding 6 nmol/l.

Early secretory phase in natural cycles, 2 days after ovulation, is anticipated according to the cycle phase, but is nevertheless understandable according to the manner of timing BE (BBT, day of the cycle). In the study group ovulation (i.e. aspiration of follicles) is exactly programmed and temporally determined and E_2, P, BE correspond to the 2nd day after ovulation. This is not exactly valid for the reference group.

Endometrial anticipation in stimulated cycles with high E_2 responsiveness represents aberration from the criteria that are valid for natural cycles because of the modified E_2 and P relationship. Although the endometrium does not morphologically differ from the one in natural cycles, its altered quality and receptiveness are the factors which can prevent implantation because of the modified steroid ratio.

ACKNOWLEDGEMENT

I wish to thank Professor Dr Srečko Rainer for his kind help in performing all analyses of endometrial bioptic samples.

REFERENCES

1. Lunenfeld, B., Serr, D.M., Maskach, S., Delsner, G., Blaukstein, J., Dor, J., Frenkel, Y., Ben-Raphael, Z., Tikotzy, D. and Suyder, M. (1980). Therapy with gonadotropins: where are we today. Analysis of 2890 mezotropin treatment cycles in 915 patients. In Insler, V. and Bettendorf, G. (eds). *Advances in Diagnosis and Treatment of Infertility*, pp. 27–31. (Amsterdam: Elsevier, North Holland)
2. Bettendorf, G., Braendie, W. Sprotte, C.M., Weise, C.M. and Zimmerman, R. (1980). Overall results of gonadotropin therapy. In Insler, V. and Bettendorf, G. (eds). *Advances in Diagnosis and Treatment of Infertility*, pp. 20–6. (Amsterdam: Elsevier, North Holland)
3. Stanger, J.D. and Yovich, J.L. (1985). Reduced in vitro fertilization of human oocytes from patients with raised basal luteinizing hormone levels during follicular phase. *Br. J. Obstet. Gynaecol.*, **92**, 385–93
4. Wu, C.H. (1984). A rational and practical approach to clomiphene therapy. *Clin. Obstet. Gynecol.*, **27**, 953–6
5. Pittaway, D.E. and Wentz, A.C. (1983). Evaluation of the exponential rise of serum estradiol concentrations in human menopausal gonadotropin induced cycles. *Fertil. Steril.*, **40**, 763–67
6. Diamond, M.P. and Wentz, A.C. (1986). Ovulation induction with human menopausal gonadotropins. *Obstet. Gynecol. Survey*, **41**, 480–4
7. Zeleznik, A.J. and Hiller, S.G. (1984). The role of gonadotropins in the selection of the preovulatory follicle. *Clin. Obstet. Gynecol.*, **27**, 927–40
8. Wood, C., Master, Mc. R., Rennie, G., Trousson, A. and Leeton, J. (1985). Factors influencing pregnancy rates following in vitro fertilization and embryo transfer. *Fertil. Steril.*, **43**, 245–50
9. Ferraretti, A.P., Garcia, J.E., Acosta, A.A. and Jones, G.S. (1983). Serum luteinizing hormone during ovulation induction with human menopausal gonadotropin for in vitro fertilization in normally menstruating women. *Fertil. Steril.*, **40**, 742–6
10. Glissant, A., Mouzon, de J., and Frydman, R. (1985). Etude de l'endometre par ultrasons au cours des cycles de fecondation in vitro. *Gynecologie*, **36**, 107–11
11. Dallenbach-Hellweg, G. (1984). The endometrium of infertility. *Pathol. Res. Pract.*, **178**, 527–37
12. Cornillie, F.J., Lauweryns, J.M. and Brosens, I.A. (1985). Normal human endometrium, an ultrastructural survey. *Gynecol. Obstet. Invet.*, **20**, 113–29
13. Garcia, J.E., Acosta, A.A., Hsiu, J.G. and Jones, H.W. (1984). Advanced endometrial maturation after ovulation induction with human menopausal gonadotropin/human chorionic gonadotropin for in vitro fertilisation. *Fertil. Steril.*, **41**, 31–5
14. Cherney, de, A.H. and Laufer, N. (1984). The monitoring of ovulation induction using ultrasound and estrogen. *Clin. Obstet. Gynecol.*, **27**, 993–1003
15. Dirnfeld, M., Lejeune, B., Campus, M., Vekemans, M. and Leroy, F.(1985). Growth rate of follicular estrogen secretion in relation to the outcome of in vitro fertilization and embryo transfer. *Fertil. Steril.*, **43**, 379–84
16. Shepard, M.K. and Senturia, Y.D. (1977). Comparison of serum progesterone and endometrial biopsy for confirmation of ovulation and evaluation of luteal function. *Fertil. Steril.*, **28**, 541–8
17. Vargyas, J., Kletzky, O. and Marrs, R.P. (1986). The effect of laparoscopic follicular aspiration on ovarian steroidogenesis during the early preimplantation period. *Fertil. Steril.*, **45**, 221–5
18. Johannisson, E., Parker, R.A., Landgren, B.M. and Diczfalusy, E. (1982). Morphometric analysis of the human endometrium in relation to peripheral hormone levels. *Fertil. Steril.*, **38**, 546–71
19. Frydman, R., Testart, J., Giacomini, P., Imbert, M.C., Martin, E. and Nahoul, K. (1982). Hormonal and histological study of the luteal phase in women following aspiration of the preovulatory follicle. *Fertil. Steril.*, **3**, 312–17

97

Prevention and management of ovarian hyperstimulation syndrome

J.G. Schenker

The most common complication of induction of ovulation in cases of anovulation and in cases of stimulation of ovaries for *in vitro* fertilization and other assisted reproductive techniques are ovarian hyperstimulation syndrome (OHSS), high multiple gestation, and high rate of spontaneous abortions[1].

RISK FACTORS FOR OHSS

The incidence of OHSS varies with the different clinical conditions in which ovulation is induced, the types of preparation administered and the dose and protocol of therapy.

The pharmacological preparations currently used for induction of ovulation and their combinations are shown in Table 1. The incidence of OHSS with clomiphene therapy is less than following induction of ovulation with human menopausal gonadotropin (hMG), follicle-stimulating hormone (FSH) or FSH/hMG.

In our experience[2] combined therapy of hMG/dexamethasone and hMG/bromocriptine were more frequently associated with OHSS. The

Table 1 Preparations used for induction of ovulation

Clomiphene citrate
hMG
FSH
GnRH analogs
1. Usually with hCG
2. Combination of different preparations
Clomiphene citrate–hMG–hCG
hMG–dexamethasone–hCG
hMG–bromocriptine–hCG
FSH–hMG–hCG
GnRH–hMG–hCG

combination of hMG/dexamethasone was administered in cases of polycystic ovarian disease (PCOD) with a relatively hyperandrogenic state, whereas the combination of hMG/bromocriptine was administered to patients with hyperprolactinemia who did not respond to bromocriptine therapy alone. Ovarian hyperstimulation syndrome seems to occur more frequently when luteinizing hormone-releasing hormone (LHRH) agonists with hMG or FSH are administered for follicular stimulation in *in vitro* fertilization (IVF) cases.

Our group has shown that anovulatory patients, who develop OHSS, are younger, with low mean weight. Parameters like height, duration of infertility and type of infertility – primary or secondary did not contribute to the development of OHSS. The syndrome was more frequently observed in patients from group 2 compared to group 1 according to the classification of the World Health Organization (WHO). Patients who are prone to developing OHSS have a special hormonal profile before induction of ovulation as assessed in the early follicular stage. Patients who develop OHSS have higher luteinizing hormone (LH), prolactin, estradiol, androstenedione and testosterone levels (Figures 1,2,3).

CLINICAL SIGNS AND SYMPTOMS

Symptoms and signs of OHSS vary according to the clinical grading of the syndrome.

Chemical hyperstimulation is a very common accompaniment of ovulation induction. It is of little clinical concern, and usually resolves with the onset

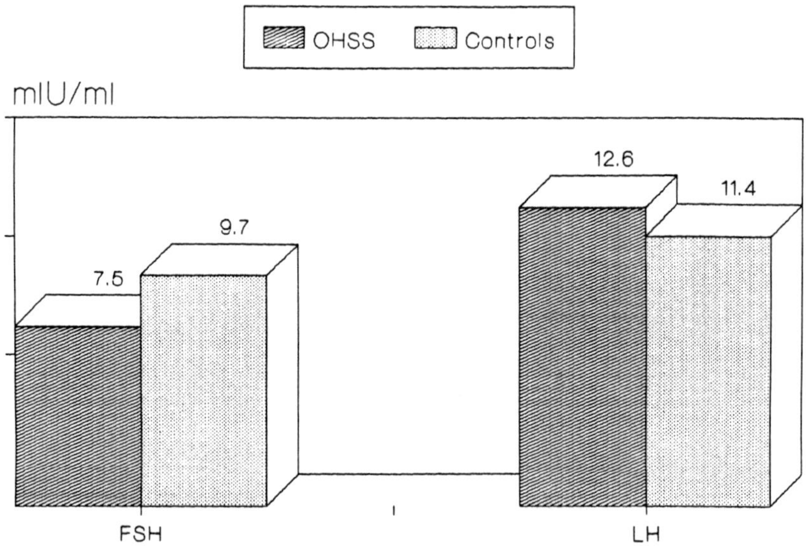

Figure 1 Serum of luteinizing hormone (LH) and follicle-stimulating hormone (FSH) in early follicular phase of patients who developed ovarian hyperstimulation syndrome (OHSS) compared with controls

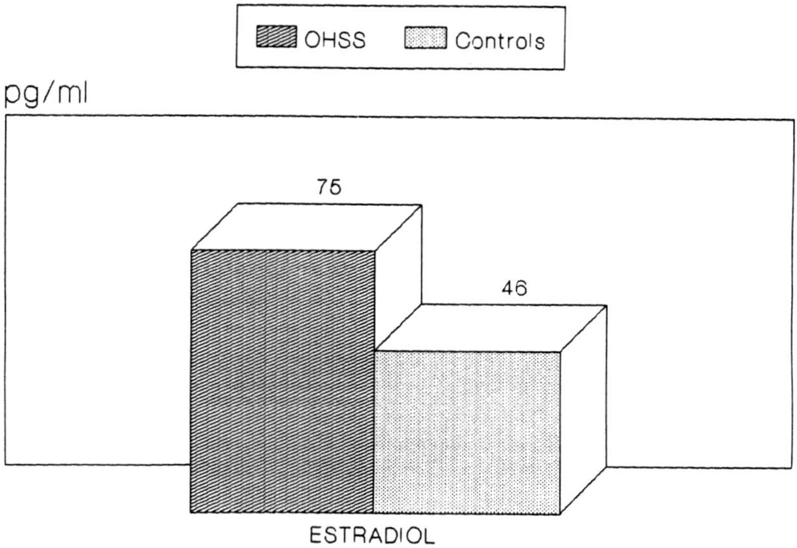

Figure 2 Serum estradiol (E_2) in early follicular phase in patients with ovarian hyperstimulation syndrome (OHSS) compared to controls

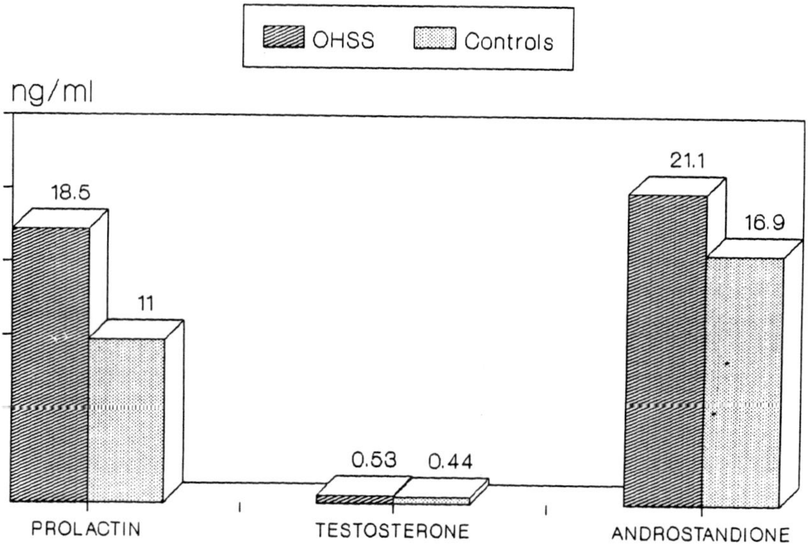

Figure 3 Serum prolactin, testosterone and androstenedione in patients with ovarian hyperstimulation syndrome (OHSS)

of menses. Chemical hyperstimulation may usually follow human chorionic gonadotropin (hCG) administration or even occur with hMG, FSH or gonadotropin-releasing hormone (GnRH) alone.

The mild form of this syndrome presents as a feeling of abdominal heaviness, tension, swelling and pain. The physical findings are bilateral ovarian enlargement by multiple follicular and corpus luteum cysts, measuring up to 5 × 5 cm. The symptoms and physical findings or enlarged ovaries usually begin 3 to 6 days after hCG administration. If pregnancy does not occur, the ovarian enlargement gradually declines until menses, after which there is an accelerated decline. If conception occurs, further ovarian enlargement generally follows late in the cycle because of additional endogenous hCG administration, and this may persist during the first trimester of pregnancy.

In cases of moderate hyperstimulation, the abdominal discomfort is more pronounced. Gastrointestinal symptoms such as nausea, vomiting and, less frequently, diarrhea are present. There is some gain in weight, and the ovaries are enlarged (up to 12 × 12 cm). Symptoms of moderate severity usually subside spontaneously with bed rest for 2 to 3 weeks.

Severe OHSS is a serious complication of therapy given to a previously healthy woman. The clinical manifestations include ascites, pleural effusion, electrolyte imbalance, hypovolemia, oliguria and even hypovolemic shock. The ovaries are greatly enlarged.

Recently a case of death occurred in Israel of a 42-year-old woman who was treated with hMG/hCG and developed OHSS, characterized by clinical signs of thrombosis of internal carotid artery.

PATHOPHYSIOLOGICAL CHANGES IN OHSS

The main pathological findings in severe hyperstimulation syndrome are multiple ovarian cysts, more than 10 cm in diameter, follicular cysts, corpora lutea and severe edema of the stroma. Massive enlargement of the ovaries is accompanied by different degrees of acute body fluid shift, with ascites formation, hydrothorax and sometimes anasacra. The sudden body fluid shift seems to be due to increased capillary permeability, especially of the ovarian vessels, as was demonstrated in our experimental studies[3]. The evidence that increased capillary permeability is the pathogenic mechanism of severe OHSS is supported by the fact that the values for electrolytes in blood and ascitic fluid are similar. This demonstrates that ascitic fluid has transudated. The cause of increased permeability in OHSS is still not clearly understood. It was demonstrated that indomethacin, a blocker of prostaglandin synthesis, can prevent the fluid shift associated with the ascites, pleural effusion and hypovolemia seen in this syndrome[4].

RENIN ANGIOTENSIN SYNTHESIS IN THE OVARY

There are sufficient data in the literature to indicate that renin–angiotensin system is locally active in the human ovary[5,6]. A tenfold rise of prorenin occurs early in pregnancy. It reaches maximal levels 4 weeks following conception. Prorenin measurement during menstrual cycles shows the following timing: during the follicular phase there is no rise in the level of prerenin; it increases about two-fold at the time of LH surge and a second peak is observed during the mid-luteal phase. Studies on primates demonstrated that prorenin is secreted from the ovary. Ovarian secretion of prorenin is stimulated following administration of hCG. In cases of induction of ovulation, the levels of plasma protein are directly related to the number of developing follicles in the ovaries. The concentration of prorenin in the follicular fluid is about 10–40 times higher than its concentration in the plasma. Low prorenin values were detected in the fluid of premature follicles. Higher levels of active renin, angiotensin I and angiotensin II were found in follicular fluid compared to plasma levels.

We recently determined the presence of angiotensin converting enzyme activity (ACE) in the human preovulatory follicular fluid which converts angiotensin I into angiotensin II. The ACE activity in the follicular fluid was similar to its activity in the plasma. Correlations were sought between follicular fluid ACE and both serum and follicular fluid estradiol (E_2) and progesterone (P). A highly significant correlation was found between ACE activity in the follicular fluid and follicular P. No linear correlation could be demonstrated between serum and follicular fluid ACE activity and between ACE activity and serum E_2 and P or follicular E_2.

PREVENTION OF OVARIAN HYPERSTIMULATION

Theoretically OHSS may be eliminated, provided careful monitoring is experienced, and hCG is withheld whenever the physiological range of ovarian response is exceeded. There are, however, numerous reasons why even with the most careful and painstaking preventive measures, OHSS could not be eliminated. First of all, if the physiological range is considered an adequate ovarian response, the efficiency of gonadotropin treatment is markedly reduced. The probable explanation for the difference between physiological estrogen levels in spontaneous cycles verus the higher minimal effective level in stimulated cycles is due to the multiple follicles which reach a more advanced stage of maturation under both clomiphene and gonadotropin induction of ovulation. A direct proof for that statement is evident from studies in *in vitro* fertilization. The number of fertilizable ova under clomiphene treatment which are retrieved during follicular aspiration is usually two to three, while under hMG stimulation it may reach six or eight. The overlap which exists between the minimal effective dose in terms of conception, and the dose which causes ovarian hyperstimulation is another reason for the inability of eliminating OHSS. However, the incidence of OHSS may be significantly reduced by clinical, biochemical and bioelectronic methods used in monitoring induction of ovulation.

Since direct observation of follicular maturation is impossible, we follow measurable parameters which reflect, as accurately as possible, follicular maturation. Some of the parameters, which reflect indirectly total estrogen activity are of academic interest, i.e. the karyopyknotic index in vaginal cytology.

We have used the indirect method of assessment of estrogen activity by examination of the cervical score. This evaluation includes the quantity of cervical mucus, mucus crystalization (fern test), spinnbarkeit, and the changes in the appearance of the external cervical os. We found, as others have done, that the gradual development of copious mucus with maximal ferning and changes in the external os are good indicators of follicular ripeness. During treatment, the cervical parameters must be estimated frequently enough to determine the expected day of follicular maturation. It usually takes from 1 to 5 days from the initial cervical reaction until the follicles can respond to hCG by ovulation. A positive effect is already found at estrogen values of 10 to 20 μg/24 h, whereas about 50 μg/24 h there may not be additional changes in cervical score.

Individual responses of the endocervical glands may vary considerably. Some patients will respond with high cervical scores when the estrogen levels are still very low, while others will fail to respond at high estrogen levels.

Clomiphene citrate, because of its anti-estrogenic activity, may block altogether the response of the cervical glands to high levels of circulating estrogens.

The sensitivity of an individual patient's endocervical glands may be determined by the administration of an estrogen preparation prior to gonadotropin therapy. In view of the above disadvantages of cervical scoring, this method alone is considered unsatisfactory; furthermore, the predictive value of impending ovarian hyperstimulation is poor, if it exists at all.

Total urinary estrogens and later serum estrogen values established their effectiveness in monitoring induction of ovulation. Total estrogens were above 150 μg/24 h.

The advantage of measuring serum levels, which provide a measure of endogenous E_2 production on the same day as hMG administration, over determining urinary estrogens, which represent the previous day's levels, is seen as sufficiently important to justify incidence of OHSS than when hCG overlapped.

It is well established today that by monitoring the estrogen levels daily during administration of hMG or FSH, and by withholding hCG when the estrogen levels are too high, severe OHSS can be prevented.

In our series, mean serum estradiol levels were 1041 $\pm$ 381 on day of hMG administration in cases of OHSS compared to a control group (Fig. 4).

Serial ultrasonographic measurements of follicular size reflect maturation as well as the number of follicles. At present no conclusive data were reported of repeated ultrasonographic measurement of follicles which can predict the development of OHSS. There is a strong positive correlation between the total number of follicles and the occurrence of OHSS. Mean number of immature follicles below 12 mm in diameter, small follicles 12–14 mm and large follicles >18 mm were observed on day of hCG administration in patients who developed OHSS.

TREATMENT OF OHSS

Mild and moderate hyperstimulation does not require any active therapy other than observation, whereas patients with severe OHSS require hospitaliz-

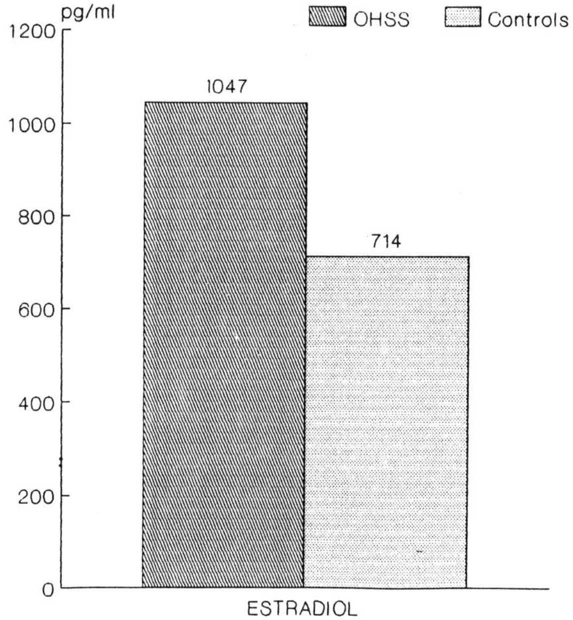

Figure 4 Mean serum levels at day 0 (day of human chorionic gonadotropin hCG administration) in patients with severe ovarian hyperstimulation syndrome (OHSS)

ation and prompt treatment. On the premise that the basic disturbance of this syndrome is an acute shift in fluids from the intravascular compartment to the peritoneal and pleural cavities, management should be conservative, consisting essentially of monitoring plasma volumes and their correction.

On admission, fluid intake and output are carefully assessed. Basal blood studies, including blood count and clotting parameters, are performed. Blood and urine osmolarity are measured. In some severe cases blood volume estimations are carried out and central venous pressure is monitored.

In order to prevent hypovolemia – which may lead to hemoconcentration, decreased renal perfusion, and even shock – we infuse our patients with low molecular weight dextran (Macrodex), 400 ml to 1000 ml/24 h, and appropriate electrolytic solutions. In most cases, the low infusion of low molecular weight dextran is continued for 4 to 7 d, with good results.

Diuretics are ineffective in evacuating fluid accumulated in the peritoneal and pleural cavities, and moreover are contraindicated, as a steeper decrease in the volume of the already contracted intravascular compartment may even induce hypovolemic shock.

Anticoagulant therapy is indicated in cases in which there is clinical evidence of thromboembolic phenomena, or laboratory findings of hypercoagulability.

On the basis of our concept of prostaglandin mediation in OHSS, supported by our experimental animal model, indomethacin, a blocker of prostaglandin biosynthesis, was given. Indomethacin may be contraindicated because of possible teratogenicity. Nevertheless, we believe that indomethacin therapy is justified in severe OHSS, even if the patient has conceived.

Our studies, which show that the renin–angiotensin system is also involved in OHSS, may offer new possibilities for therapy by administration of Captopril, a specific competitive inhibitor of angiotensin converting enzyme.

Some authors propose abdominal paracentesis for drainage of ascites, a practice not favored by us. Pleural effusions should be drained for respiratory distress, and sometimes repeated punctures are required. Surgical intervention should be avoided. The indications for surgery being either signs of intraperitoneal bleeding due to rupture of an ovarian cyst, or torsion of an ovarian cyst. Surgery, if necessary, should be as conservative as possible, a tedious task in view of the hyperemic edematous and friable ovarian tissue encountered during laparotomy.

HIGH MULTIPLE PREGNANCIES AND OHSS

There are conflicting data on the association between OHSS and multiple pregnancy, despite the obvious common denominator to both entities, namely production of multiple follicles and multiple corpora lutea.

The management of OHSS associated with multiple pregnancy is based on the concept of the pathogenetic mechanism of OHSS as detailed in the previous section. Increased fetal wastage in multiple pregnancy is mainly attributed to either an increased abortion rate or the consequences of prematurity. With modern treatment, a fetal loss of 100% is expected in sextuplets, 44% in quintuplets, 40% in quadruplets and 30% in triplets.

High multiple pregnancies may be prevented by ultrasonically guided aspiration of oocytes before administration of hCG.

REFERENCES

1. Schenker, J.G. and Weinstein, D. (1978). *Fertil. Steril.*, **30**, 255
2. Navot, D. *et al.* (1988). *Am. J. Obstet. Gynecol.*, **159**, 210
3. Schenker, J.G. and Polishuk, W.Z. (1979). *Eur. J. Obstet. Gynecol.*, **53**, 580
4. Schenker, J.G. (1989). In Iizuka, R. and Semm, K. (eds). *Human Reproduction*, pp. 355, (Amsterdam: Elsevier *Excerpta Medica*)
5. Navot, D. *et al.* (1987). *Fertil. Steril.*, **48**, 57
6. Fernandez, L.A. *et al.* (1985). *Fertil. Steril.*, **44**, 219

98

Combined gonadotropin plus growth hormone treatment for induction of superovulation in the *in vitro* fertilization program

A. Volpe, P.G. Artini, M. Silferi, G. Coukos, F. Minuto, A. Barreca and A.R. Genazzani

INTRODUCTION

Induction of superovulation during an *in vitro* fertilization–embryo transfer (IVF–ET) program is at the present time performed by means of gonadotropins, clomiphene citrate plus human menopausal gonadotropin (hMG) or luteinizing hormone-releasing hormone (LHRH) analog and gonadotropins. According to our experience and to that of others, there has been no observed difference, in terms of follicular recruitment and growth[1], as well as of oocyte recovery and fertilization rate[2] and incidence of pregnancy[3], between different schedules of treatment. It is a common experience that a more pronounced ovarian response follows a higher dosage treatment in most patients. Some women however, are very resistant to gonadotropin treatment for induction of superovulation[4]. In these patients, cycles are cancelled because of poor or abnormally delayed ovarian response despite strong stimulation. These observations suggest that ovarian activity other than that depending on gonadotropins might also be influenced by other factors.

Recent *in vitro* studies show that some growth factors may have an important role in modulating the ovarian reponse to gonadotropins. Among them, insulin-like growth factor-I (IGF-I) seems to be an important stimulatory factor of granulosa cell differentiation. In fact, the response of cultured rat and porcine granulosa cells to stimulation by follicle-stimulating hormone (FSH) can be increased by co-incubation with IGF-I[5–9]. *In vivo* studies demonstrate that exogenous administration of growth hormone (GH) is followed by an increase of plasma IGF-I of probable hepatic origin[10]. Moreover, *in vivo* studies show that GH administration in hypophysectomized estrogen-treated female rats increases ovarian tissue IGF-I levels[11]. Growth hormone is also capable of potentiating the FSH-induced differentiation of rat granulosa cells *in vitro*[12].

On the basis of this evidence and the preliminary report of Hombourg *et al.*[13], we studied the efficacy of combined gonadotropins and GH treatment for induction of superovulation in some low responding patients.

MATERIALS AND METHODS

We have treated 11 patients, aged 26–41 years, who had proved resistant to gonadotropin therapy in a previous cycle. Six patients were 26–35 years old, three of them were obese. Five patients, aged 39–41 years, were also treated; one of them was obese.

All patients had been treated in a previous cycle with purified menofollitropin (Metrodin, Serono, 150 IU FSH), 6–17 ampoules/cycle, and hMG (Pergonal, Serono, 75 IU FSH + 75 IU LH), 34–80 ampoules/cycle. All previous cycles were cancelled within 9–12 days because of low estrogen plasma levels and/or poor follicular recruitment or follicular growth.

In all patients pituitary GH response to exogenous growth hormone-releasing factor (GRF) was tested before starting the second treatment cycle. From the group of younger patients, three of them, two obese and one of normal body weight, did not respond to the GRF-stimulatory test. From the other group, one patient out of four obese, did not respond to the GRF-test.

During the second cycle all patients were administered approximately the same dosage of gonadotropins as the previous cycle plus a standard dosage of GH 0.1 U/kg of body weight/day, subcutaneously (Grormone, Kabi, Stockholm, Sweden). When at least one follicle reached 16 mm of average diameter and plasma estradiol was approximately 200 pg/ml/follicle human chorionic gonadotropin (hCG) (Profasi 10 000, Serono, hCG) was administered; follicular aspiration was performed 36 h after hCG administration.

The response to treatment was monitored through daily plasma estradiol measurement radioimmunoassay (RIA) and ultrasound transvaginal follicular evaluation, starting from day 5 of the stimulatory cycle. Follicular growth is expressed as the total follicular volume day by day, i.e. the daily sum of the volume values of all single follicles of both ovaries. The follicular volumes were obtained by the mathematical computation of a sphere or ellipssoid volume, i.e. $V = 1/6\, d^2$ or $V = 1/6\, a\, b\, c$, respectively (where d = the diameter of the sphere and a,b,c = the main diameters of the ellipssoid).

RESULTS

In the first stimulatory cycle we did not obtain a satisfactory ovarian response in any of the 11 patients. All cycles were cancelled between day 9 and 12 of stimulatory cycle.

The second cycle with combined GH and gonadotropins was also cancelled in five patients because of unsatisfactory ovarian response. All of them were above 39 years of age.

In the six remaining patients, all between 26 and 35 years, the association of GH to gonadotropin stimulation induced a satisfactory ovarian response with a better follicular recruitment (average nine, range seven to 16 follicle/patient) and oocyte recovery (average 6.6 oocyte/patient). The fertilization rate in these six patients was three oocyte/patient. No pregnancy was obtained (Figure 1).

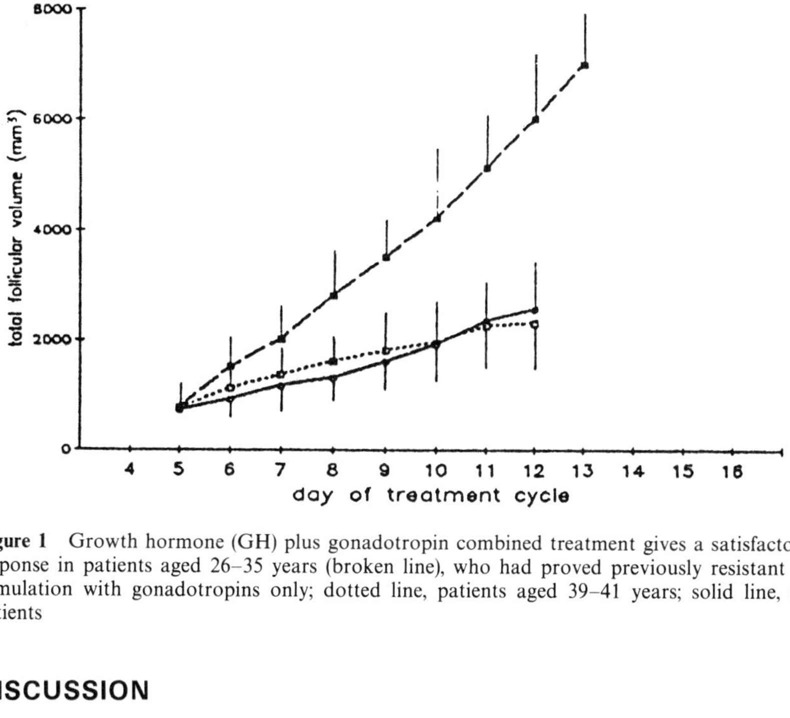

Figure 1 Growth hormone (GH) plus gonadotropin combined treatment gives a satisfactory response in patients aged 26–35 years (broken line), who had proved previously resistant to stimulation with gonadotropins only; dotted line, patients aged 39–41 years; solid line, all patients

DISCUSSION

Our results show that GH administration can increase the ovarian response to gonadotropins in women under 35 years who are relatively resistant to gonadotropins superovulation induction. Our data confirm the previous report of Hombourg *et al.*[13], showing that the addition of GH significantly enhanced the ovarian response in seven patients previously resistant to gonadotropins treatment.

Our data may be supported by the *in vitro* and *in vivo* evidence concerning the growth factors involvement in the ovarian function. In fact, GH deficiency in female rats reduces the ovarian steroidogenic response to hCG and delays the onset of puberty. Replacement of GH in these animals restores the ovarian progesterone production in response to gonadotropins and re-advances the onset of puberty[14]. *In vitro* studies show that GH potentiates the differentiative response to FSH of rat granulosa cells[15]. GH administration in rats increases the ovarian tissue content of IGF-I[11]. Besides, IGF-I has been

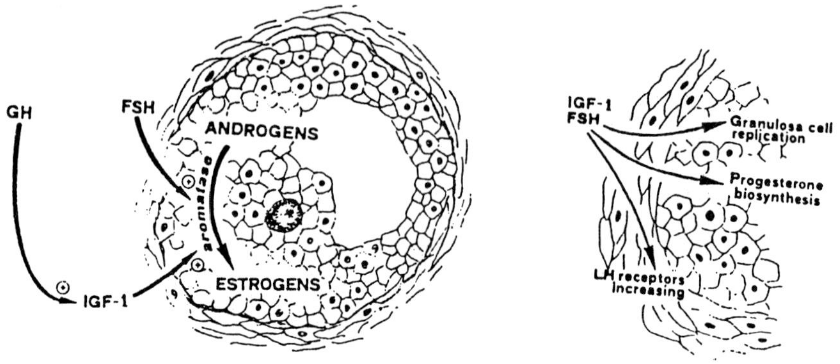

Figure 2 Growth hormone and insulin-like growth factor-1 (IGF-I) potentiate the effects of follicle-stimulating hormone (FSH) on granulosa cells

shown to enhance the aromatase-inducing effect of FSH in rat granulosa cells *in vitro*[8] as well as the FSH-induced differentiation of cultured rat and porcine granulosa cells[5–7,9] (Figure 2).

It has been shown that GH administration induces an increase of plasma IGF-I levels in humans[10]. In some of our patients GH administration significantly improved the ovarian response to gonadotropins. This effect can be possibly attributed to a plasma or ovarian IGF-I increase.

We cannot explain the different response to GH administration between the two different age subgroups of our patients. It is known, however, that after 35 years of age a decrease in fertility potentiality is observed and a decrease in IVF treatment success has been reported in patient above 37–38 years of age[16].

REFERENCES

1. Mahadevan, M.M., Fleetham, J., Taylor, P.J., Leader, A. and Pattinson, A.H. (1987). The effect of the day of initiation of ovarian stimulation in the day of luteinizing hormone surge and outcome of in vitro fertilization. *Fertil. Steril.*, **47**, 976
2. Trounson, A.J. and Wood, C. (1984). In vitro fertilization results 1979–1982, at Monash University, Queen Victoria, and Epworth Medical Centers. *J. Vitro. Fert. Embryo Transfer*, **1**, 42
3. Fishel, S.B., Edwards, R.G., Purdy, J.M., Steptoe, P.C. *et al.* (1985). Implantation, abortion, and birth after in vitro fertilization using the natural menstrual cycle or follicular stimulation with Clomiphene Citrate and Human Menopausal Gonadotropin. *J. Vitro Fert. Embryo Transfer*, **2**, 123
4. Pellicer, A., Lightman, A., Diamond, M.P., Russel, J.B. and De Cherney, A.H. (1987). Outcome of in vitro fertilization in women with low response to ovarian stimulation. *Fertil. Steril.*, **47**, 812
5. Davoren, J.B., Hsueh, A.J.W. and Li, C.H. (1985). Somatomedin C augments FSH-induced differentiation of cultured rat granulosa cells. *Am. J. Physiol.*, **249**, E26
6. Adashi, E.Y., Resnick, C.E., Svoboda, M.E. and Van Wyk, J.J. (1984). A novel role for somatomedin-C in the cytodifferentiation of the ovarian granulosa cell. *Endocrinology*, **115**, 1227
7. Adashi, E.Y., Resnick, C.E., Svoboda, M.E., Van Wyk, J.J., Hashal, V.C. and Yanagishita, M. (1986). Independent and synergistic actions of somatomedin-C in the stimulation of

proteoglycan biosynthesis by cultured rat granulosa cells. *Endocrinology*, **118**, 456

8. Adashi, E.Y., Resnick, C.E., Brodie, A.M.H., Svoboda, M.E. and Van Wyk, J.J. (1985). Somatomedin-C mediated potentiation of follicle-stimulating hormone-induced aromatase activity of cultured rat granulosa cells. *Endocrinology*, **117**, 2313
9. Maruo, T., Hayashi, M., Matsuo, H., Ueda, Y., Morikawa, H. and Mochizuki, M. (1988). Comparison of the facilitative roles of insulin and insulin-like growth factor 1 in the functional differentiation of granulosa cells: in vitro studies with the porcine model. *Acta Endocrinol.* (*Copenh.*), **117**, 230
10. Zapf, J., Rinderknecht, E., Humbel, R.E. and Froesch, E.R. (1978). Nonsuppressible insulin-like activity (NSILA) from human serum: reaccomplishments and their physiological implications. *Metabolism*, **27**, 1803
11. Davoren, J.B. and Hsueh, A.J.W. (1986). Growth hormone increases ovarian levels of immunoreactive somatomedin C/insulin-like growth factor *in vivo*. *Endocrinology*, **118**, 888
12. Jia, X.C., Kalman, J. and Hsueh, A.J.W. (1986). Growth hormone enhances follicle-stimulating hormone-induced differentiation of cultured rate granulosa cells. *Endocrinology*, **118**, 1401
13. Homburg, R., Eshel, A., Abdalla, H.I. and Jacobs, H.S. (1988). Growth hormone facilitates ovulation induction by gonadotrophins. *Clin. Endocrinol.*, **29**, 113
14. Advis, J.P., White, S.S. and Ojeda, S.R. (1981). Activation of growth hormone short loop negative feedback delays puberty in the female rat. *Endocrinology*, **108**, 1343
15. Sheikholislam, B.M. and Stempfel, Jr, R.S. (1972). Hereditary isolated somatotropin deficiency: effects of human growth hormone administration. *Pediatrics*, **49**, 362
16. Edwards, R.G. and Steptoe, P.C. (1983). Current status of in vitro fertilization and implantation of human embryos. *Lancet*, **2**, 1265

99

GnRH and central control of reproductive function: mechanism of secretory responses to GnRH

S. S. Stojilković, S.-I. Izumi and K. J. Catt

INTRODUCTION

The control of reproductive function is exerted through the actions of hypothalamic peptides which regulate the secretory activity of gonadotropin-secreting cells of the anterior pituitary gland[1]. While gonadotropin-releasing hormone (GnRH) is the major hypothalamic factor in the control of gonadotrope differentiation and pulsatile gonadotropin secretion release, other peptides including substance P, neuropeptide Y and neurohypophyseal hormones have been found to modulate gonadotropin secretion[2]. GnRH regulates pituitary function and gonadotropin secretion by binding to specific, high-affinity receptors in the gonadotrope plasma membrane[3]. The mechanism of receptor-mediated activation in gonadotropes involves the integrated actions of several intracellular messenger systems, including phosphoinositide breakdown and mobilization of intracellular calcium, as well as influx of extracellular calcium[4–7]. This paper describes the role of different second messenger systems in the genesis of the biphasic gonadotropin response to GnRH, and the participation of these systems in the initiation of refractoriness to prolonged or frequent stimulation by GnRH.

BIPHASIC ACTIVATION OF CYTOSOLIC FREE CALCIUM AND GONADOTROPIN RESPONSES BY GnRH

In primary cultures of rat pituitary cells, GnRH stimulates rapid peak increases in $[Ca^{2+}]_i$ and luteinizing hormone [LH] release, followed by lower but sustained elevations of both $[Ca^{2+}]_i$ and hormone secretion[7] (Figure 1). The total duration of the acute phase of both responses was 2.5 min; the maximum $[Ca^{2+}]_i$ occurred within 20 s, and the peak in gonadotropin release in 35 s. Omission of extracellular Ca^{2+} decreased the peak of $[Ca^{2+}]_i$ by 20% and prevented the prolonged increases in $[Ca^{2+}]_i$. However, the amount of LH released during the peak phase was reduced by

40% and the second phase was stongly attenuated but not abolished under extracellular Ca^{2+}-deficient conditions (Figure 1). Three biochemical events are important for the understanding of the peak and sustained phases of $[Ca^{2+}]_i$:

(1) GnRH causes a rapid and progressive rise in the formation of inositol 1,4,5-trisphosphate ($InsP_3$) and of higher polyphosphoinositols corresponding to inositol tetrakisphosphate and pentakisphosphate[4].

(2) Specific $InsP_3$ receptors sites with high affinity and rapid binding kinetics are present in pituitary membrane preparations, in which $InsP_3$-induced Ca^{2+} release is also demonstrable[5]. The $InsP_3$ binding sites appear to represent the specific intracellular receptors through which the calcium mobilization response to phosphoinositide hydrolysis is expressed in response to GnRH.

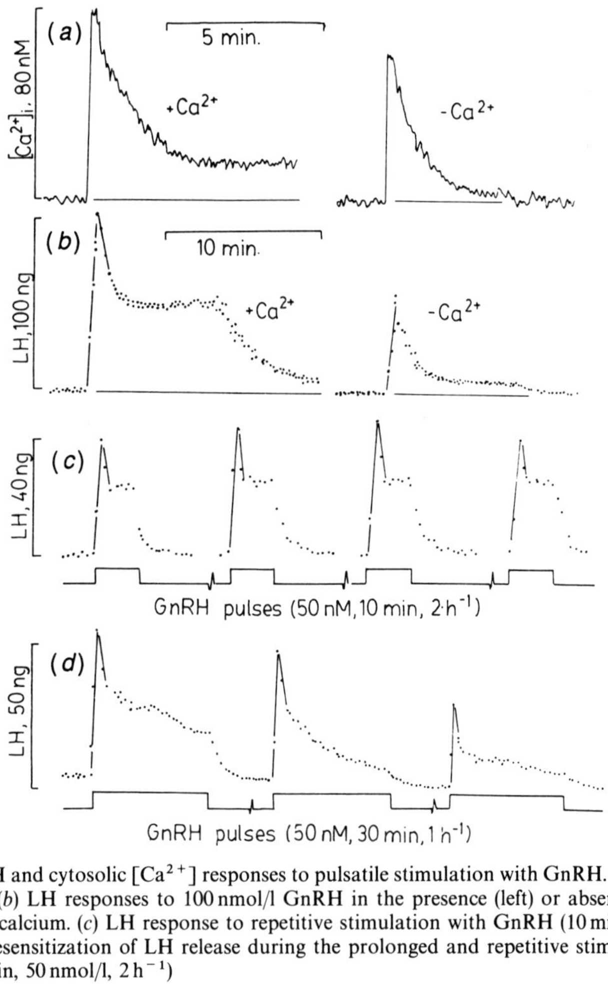

Figure 1 LH and cytosolic $[Ca^{2+}]$ responses to pulsatile stimulation with GnRH. (*a*) Cytosolic $[Ca^{2+}]$ and (*b*) LH responses to 100 nmol/l GnRH in the presence (left) or absence (right) of extracellular calcium. (*c*) LH response to repetitive stimulation with GnRH (10 min, 50 nmol/l, $2\,h^{-1}$). (*d*) Desensitization of LH release during the prolonged and repetitive stimulation with GnRH (30 min, 50 nmol/l, $2\,h^{-1}$)

(3) The extracellular Ca^{2+}-dependent pathway participates in both the peak and sustained phases, and influx of calcium occurs through voltage-sensitive calcium channels (VSCC). The ability of the non-specific depolarizing action of high K^+ to evoke a cytosolic $[Ca^{2+}]$ rise and LH release (Figure 2) supports the presence of this type of channel in the plasma membrane of gonadotropes. Further, specific Ca^{2+} channel agonist (BK 8644) and antagonist (nifedipine and nicardipine) analogs respectively enhance or reduce the $[Ca^{2+}]_i$ and LH responses to both GnRH and K^+, indicating the presence and the role of dihydropyridine-sensitive Ca^{2+} channels during GnRH action (Figure 2*c* and *d*, Figure 3*b*). However, nifedipine does not completely inhibit the entry of Ca^{2+} (Figure 3*a*), indicating that another kind of channel, in addition to that mediating dihydropyridine-sensitive Ca^{2+} influx, participates in GnRH action.

CO-ORDINATE ACTIONS OF PROTEIN KINASE C AND ARACHIDONIC ACID

Comparison of the $[Ca^{2+}]_i$ and the amount of LH released in the presence or absence of extracellular Ca^{2+} supports the idea that Ca^{2+}, as a second messenger, correlates with gonadotropin release in response to GnRH. However, this does not occur in a simple linear manner, and the Ca^{2+} signal is amplified during both phases of GnRH action[8]. Such amplification

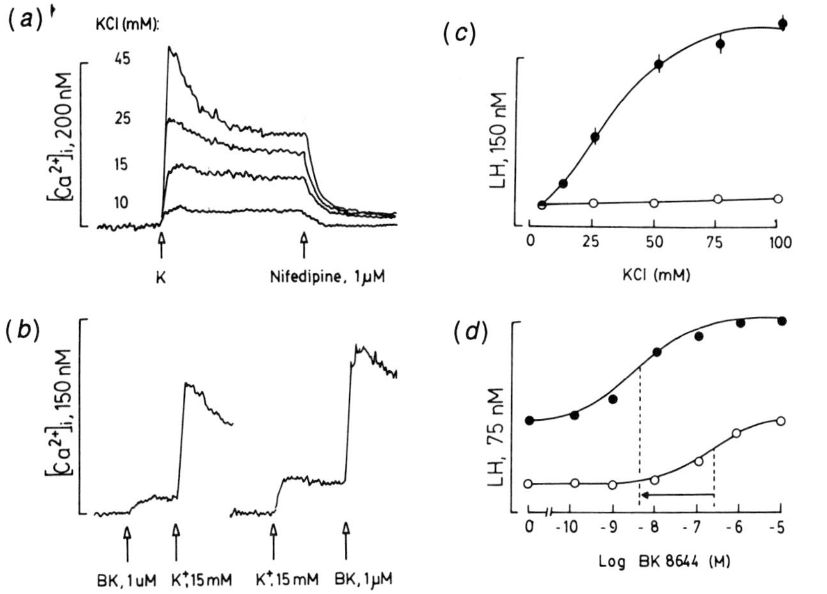

Figure 2 The effects of high K^+ and calcium channel agonist, BK 8644, on cytosolic $[Ca^{2+}]$ and LH release. (*a*) Dose-dependent effect of K^+ on $[Ca^{2+}]_i$ and (*b*) LH release. Additive effects of BK 8644 on high K^+ induced $[Ca^{2+}]_i$ (*c*) and LH release (*d*)

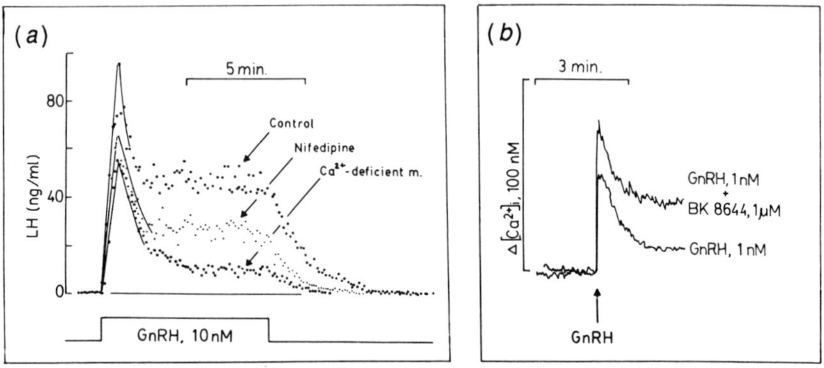

Figure 3 Modulatory effects of dihydropyridines on GnRH action. (*a*) Inhibitory action of the calcium channel blocker, nifedipine, on LH release. (*b*) Potentiation of GnRH action on $[Ca^{2+}]_i$ in the presence of BK 8644

may occur through the action of diacylglycerol, another product of phosphoinositide metabolism in activated gonadotropes[9]. In the presence of extracellular Ca^{2+}, diacylglycerol as well as phorbol esters activate protein kinase C, and this action induces an increase in LH release. Phorbol esters promote Ca^{2+} entry, but they also mediate secretory responses without changes in calcium influx and $[Ca^{2+}]_i$[10]. Further, in our hands protein kinase C-depleted gonadotropes showed significant reduction in the actions of GnRH and phorbol ester (TPA) on LH release and synthesis[11].

In addition to activating protein kinase C, the diacylglycerol released from phosphatidylinositol bisphosphate may also be cleaved by diacylglycerol lipase to yield a 2-arachidonyl acid monoacylglycerol, which can be metabolized to glycerol with the release of arachidonic acid[9], another proposed mediator of GnRH action. Arachidonic acid itself, and its lipoxygenase metabolites including 5-hydroxyeisatetraenoic acid (5-HETE) and leukotriene C_4, have been reported to stimulate LH secretion[12]. In contrast, other free fatty acids including palmitate and stearate and non-metabolizable analogs of arachidonic acid were ineffective in evoking LH release[13].

ELECTROPHYSIOLOGICAL CHARACTERIZATION OF TWO TYPES OF CALCIUM CHANNELS IN THE PITUITARY GONADOTROPES

The properties of calcium channels in cultured rat pituitary gonadotropes have been analyzed by the patch clamp technique. The inward Ca^{2+} current, recorded in the presence of 5.2 mmol/l Ca^{2+} or Ba^{2+}, included a fast, transient component with activation–inactivation kinetics, and a delayed component with slower activation[14]. The rate of inactivation of the first component was strongly voltage dependent. On the other hand, the size of the delayed component of the Ca^{2+} current remained constant during long-lasting (100–200 ms) low-frequency depolarizing voltage clamp pulses[15]. The rapidly inactivating current appears to be attributable to a transient (T-type) channel and the slow-inactivating current to the L (dihydropyridine-sensitive), type channel described in excitable tissues. The calcium current is also sensitive to Co^{2+}. However, comparison between the effects of Co^{2+} on LH release and calcium current indicated that this ion not only caused blockade of the voltage-sensitive calcium currents, but also inhibited LH secretion at an intracellular locus[8].

CORRELATION BETWEEN ACTIVATION–INACTIVATION KINETICS OF DIHYDROPYRIDINE-SENSITIVE CALCIUM CHANNELS AND GONADOTROPIN RELEASE

In general, T channels are activated by small depolarizing steps and show fast voltage-dependent inactivation (less than 100 ms). In contrast, L channels have a higher threshold of activation, a slower activating and very slow inactivating phase[16] (in minutes). The difference in the activation–inactivation kinetics of these channels suggests that high K^+-induced Ca^{2+} entry and LH release predominantly correspond to the activation of L channels[6,17]. In perifused rat pituitary cells, a transient K^+ pulse evokes a typical *on–off* response in dose-dependent manner. Early rapid LH and $[Ca^{2+}]_i$ peaks occur during the first 35 s of stimulation (*on* response) followed by an exponential attenuation of the secretion of the *steady state* level during the next 3 min (Figure 4*a* and *b*). Removal of stimulation induces a further rapid (*off*) response followed by an exponential decrease to the basal level of LH secretion. The secretory profile of LH follows the status of L channels; the ascending part of the *on* phase correlates with increase in the number of VSCC in open state, followed by decreasing phase which represent inactivation of these channels. The *steady state* level represents the equilibrium between the open and inactivated state. Inactivation of dihydropyridine-sensitive Ca^{2+} channels depends on $[Ca^{2+}]_i$, under extracellular calcium-deficient conditions the effects of high K^+ are abolished and the subsequent elevation of $[Ca^{2+}]_e$ during the K^+ pulse is followed by restoration of the typical *on* response (Figure 4*c*, Stojilković, Virmani, Rojas, and Catt, unpublished observations).

PITUITARY DESENSITIZATION BY GnRH IS INITIATED BY INACTIVATION OF VOLTAGE-SENSITIVE CALCIUM CHANNELS

The frequency, and the ratio between frequency, amplitude and duration, of GnRH pulses are critical factors in the generation of the two phases of the LH responses, as well as for the development of tolerance to GnRH. As shown in Figure 1c, repetitive applications of GnRH pulses (50 nM) of short duration (10 min) and low frequency ($2\,h^{-1}$) evoked similar LH secretory profiles. However, increasing the duration of the GnRH pulse from 10 min to 30 min and maintaining the recovery period between pulses constant at 30 min, markedly impaired LH release (Figure 1*d*). The analysis of the LH

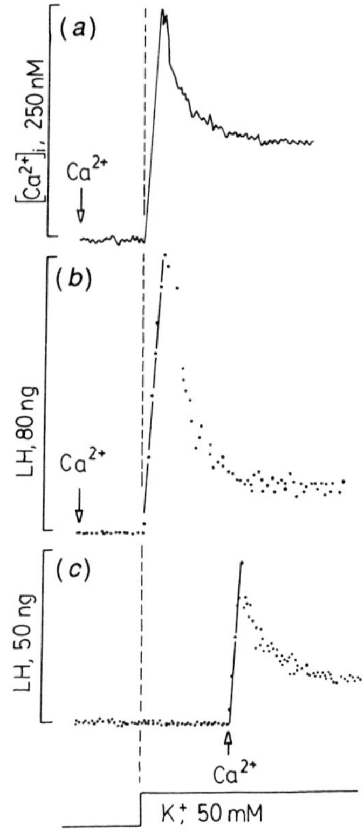

Figure 4 Stimulation of cytosolic [Ca^{2+}] and LH release from perifused rat pituitary cells by high K^+. (*a*) effects of 50 mmol/l K^+ on cytosolic [Ca^{2+}] and (*b*) LH release.

secretory profile and $[Ca^{2+}]_i$ in the presence and absence of calcium are consistent with the conclusion that increased cytosolic Ca^{2+} is required for such agonist-induced desensitization[18]. Measurement of membrane calcium current revealed significant impairment of VSCC activity in gonadotropes during desensitization by GnRH. In cells with high K^+-induced prolonged inactivation of L channels, the secretory responses to GnRH are reduced and vice versa[18]. These data suggest that inactivation of VSCC is a calcium-dependent process. Further, inactivation of L type calcium channels during GnRH action appears to be a primary factor in the onset of desensitization in pituitary gonadotropes.

REFERENCES

1. Catt, K.J. and Pierce, J.G. (1986). Gonadotropic hormones of the adenohypophysis (FSH, LH, and prolactin). In Yen, S.S.C. and Jaffe, R.B. (eds). *Reproductive Endocrinology.* (Philadelphia: W.B. Saunders)
2. Moore, R.Y. (1986). The central nervous system and the neuroendocrine regulation of reproduction. In Yen, S.S.C. and Jaffe, R.B. (eds). *Reproductive Endocrinology.* (Philadelphia:

W.B. Saunders)
3. Loumaye, E., Naor, Z. and Catt, K.J. (1982). Binding affinity and biological acitivity of gonadotropin releasing hormone agonist in isolated pituitary cells. *Endocrinology*, **111**, 730–6
4. Morgan, R.O., Chang, J.P. and Catt, K.J. (1986). Novel aspects of gonadotropin-releasing hormone action on inositol polyphosphate metabolism in cultured pituitary gonadotrophs. *J. Biol. Chem.*, **262**, 1166–71
5. Guillemette, G., Balla, T., Baukal, A.J. and Catt, K.J. (1987). Inositol 1,4,5-trisphosphate binds to a specific receptor and releases microsomal calcium in the anterior pituitary gland. *Proc. Natl. Acad. Sci., USA*, **84**, 8195–9
6. Chang, J.P., Stojilković, S.S., Graeter, J.S. and Catt, K.J. (1988). Gonadotropin-releasing hormone stimulates luteinizing hormone secretion by extracellular calcium-dependent and -independent mechanisms. *Endocrinology*, **122**, 87–97
7. Tasaka, K., Stojilković, S.S., Izumi, S.-I. and Catt, K.J. (1988). Biphasic activation of cytosolic free calcium and LH responses by gonadotropin-releasing hormone. *Biochem. Biophys. Res. Comm.*, **154**, 398–403
8. Stojilković, S.S., Torsello, A., Dufour, S., Stutzin, A., Rojas, E. and Catt, K.J. (1989). Biochemical, pharmacological and electrophysiological characterization of biphasic $[Ca^{2+}]_i$ and gonadotropin response to GnRH. *Biology of Cellular Transduction Signals* '89, *Washington, D.C.*
9. Chang, J.P., Morgan, R.O. and Catt, K.J. (1988). Dependence of secretory responses to gonadotropin-releasing hormone on diacylglycerol metabolism. *J. Biol. Chem.*, **263**, 18614–20
10. Stojilković, S.S., Chang, J.P., Izumi, S.-I., Tasaka, K. and Catt, K.J. (1988). Mechanism of secretory responses to gonadotropin-releasing hormone and phorbol esters in cultured pituitary cells. *J. Biol. Chem.*, **262**, 17301–6
11. Stojilković, S.S., Chang, J.P., Ngo, D. and Catt, K.J. (1988). Evidence for the role of protein kinase C in luteinizing hormone synthesis and secretion. *J. Biol. Chem.*, **263**, 17307–11
12. Catt, K.J., Loumaye, E., Wynn, P.C., Iwashita, M., Hirota, K., Morgan, R. and Chang, J.P. (1985). GnRH receptors and actions in the control of reproductive function. *J. Steroid Biochem.*, **23**, 677–89
13. Naor, Z. and Catt, K.J. (1981). Mechanism of action of gonadotropin-releasing hormone. *J. Biol. Chem.*, **256**, 2226–9
14. Stojilković, S.S., Stutzin, A., Catt, K.J. and Rojas, E. (1989). *Biophys. Soc. Mtg.* (Abstracts)
15. Stutzin, A., Stojilković, S.S., Catt, K.J. and Rojas, E. (1989). Characteristics of two types of calcium channels in the plasma membrane of rat pituitary gonadotropes. *Am. J. Physiol.* (submitted)
16. Miller, R.J. (1987). Multiple calcium channels and neuronal function. *Science*, **235**, 46–52
17. Stojilković, S.S., Izumi, S.-I. and Catt, K.J. (1988). Participation of voltage-sensitive calcium channels in pituitary hormone release. *J. Biol. Chem.*, **263**, 13054–61
18. Stojilković, S.S., Rojas, E., Stutzin, A., Izumi, S.-I. and Catt, K.J. (1989). Desensitization of pituitary gonadotropin secretion by agonist-induced inactivation of voltage-sensitive calcium channels. *J. Biol. Chem.* (in press)

Section 4 continued

Part G

Premenstrual syndrome: neuroendocrine correlations and therapeutic strategies

100

Clinical and epidemiological aspects of premenstrual symptoms

L. Fioroni, S. Montorsi, G. Sances and F. Facchinetti

INTRODUCTION

The premenstrual syndrome (PMS), first described by Frank in 1931[1], is still vaguely defined today. This haziness is due to difficulty in the recording of symptoms and several self-administered questionnaires have been proposed, both retrospective and prospective.

Among the retrospective questionnaires many authors used the 'Menstrual symptom questionnaire'[2] and the 'Premenstrual assessment form'[3]. However, in retrospective compilations there is an overevaluation, about 15% of symptoms are decreased in comparison with prospective studies, both in severity and quantity. For the prospective way Moos proposed the Menstrual Distress Questionnaire (MDQ)[4] and today several authors agree on its application. The MDQ's efficiency was proven by test–retest[5] and by comparison with other tests such as the Minnesota Multiphasic Personality Inventory (MMPI)[6], the Hamilton Rate Scales for Anxiety and Depression[7] and Zung Scales[8].

As far as the epidemiology of PMS is concerned data from several general population studies have been collected. The first large population study was reported in 1963 by Coppen and Kessel in England[9]. This was followed by Lehert and Van Keep in France[10], and Andersch and colleagues in Sweden[11]; these studies were carried out in different countries, using different instruments to assess symptoms, but they all suggested that while women suffered from premenstrual symptoms, fewer than 10% experience symptoms which were severe in nature.

Social and cultural aspects in the development of the pain compliance should also be taken into account.

In fact Most *et al.* in a study on Israeli women found that only 30% reported premenstrual symptoms[12], while in European and American studies the range was 25–92%[9,10,15].

In the present study the PMS symptomatology was recorded in a prospective way, by using the MDQ. Our population was composed of suffering women who had good grounds for going to the physician.

MATERIALS AND METHODS

Subjects

We selected 53 patients, 22–49 years old (mean 35 years), affected by PMS for 2–19 years (mean 6.5). Dysmenorrhea was present in the personal history of 42 cases and 19 cases had irregular menstrual cycle. In the obstetric history they generally had one or two pregnancies (12 and 18 cases respectively). All the patients were out of therapy, including oral contraceptives, and they were free from endocrine, metabolic or psychiatric (DSM III criteria) disorders.

Methods

The MDQ was administered in a prospective way. In 20 cases the MDQ was administered at two different times, 2–6 months apart. All the symptoms were self-reported every 2 days during the cycle, the intensity of the symptomatology was evaluated from 0 to 3: 0 = none, 1 = slight, 2 = mild, 3 = severe.

Statistical analysis of data was made with the Student's t test on premenstrual (PM: -7 to -1 days) versus intermenstrual (IM: $+10$ to $+17$ days) scores using the SPSS-PC package. Coefficients of correlation were calculated according to Pearson's Rank correlation.

RESULTS

The item negative affect represented the most prevalent symptom (34%) followed by water retention and concentration (32%) (Figure 1). By means of frequencies analysis, using mean $\pm$ 1 SD of the premenstrual score reported in the item control with the maximum level for the exclusion criteria (0.4). The severity of symptomatology was thus classed into four categories: 0–0.4, none; 0.41–1.2, slight; 1.21–2, mild; and >2, severe.

Considering the peripheral symptoms we found severe PMS in the 13.2% of patients claiming for pain, while 25.9% had a mild PMS for water retention (Figure 2). When central symptoms were considered it appeared that 13.2% of patients suffered from negative affect in a severe way, and 18.2% had a mild PMS for concentration.

According to the gynecological history, patients previously suffering dysmenorrhea showed higher scores at behavioral changes, concentration, negative affect and arousal ($p < 0.01$) (Figure 3). A good correlation between the two evaluations was obtained when comparing PM scoring at first and second MDQ retesting; statistical analysis with paired t test gave negative results, and this equality was confirmed by correlation according to Pearson's Rank test that showed $p < 0.001$ for all the items (Figure 4).

DISCUSSION

The present population is composed of women who are really suffering in premenstrual phase and who have applied to our center because of their

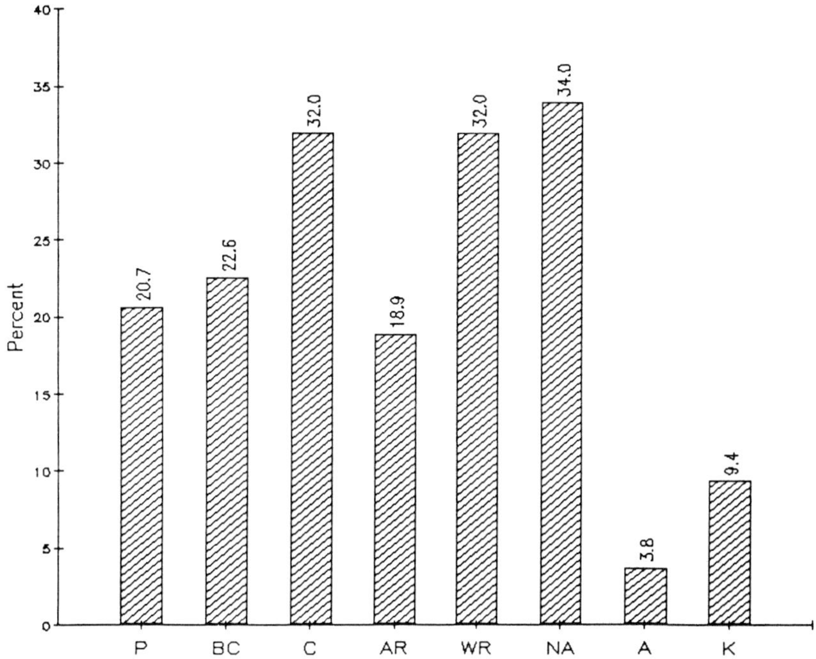

Figure 1 Prevalence of symptoms. P = pain, BC = behavioral changes, C = concentration, AR = autonomic reactions, WR = water retention, NA = negative affect, A = arousal, K = control; Student *t* test of PM against IM

symptoms. The statistical analysis we proposed, i.e. the Student's *t* test for all the items between PM and IM phases, has never been used in the literature for population studies. Moreover all the epidemiological and clinical studies so far reported have a backlog, i.e. the retrospective symptomatology recording, which allow overestimation. The data presented here thus differ from any other study since they were obtained in patients with PMS, they were prospectively collected and submitted to a statistical analysis inside each case. Following these criteria, we found that the prevalent symptoms were negative affect and water retention in agreement with other studies[4,10]. However, the symptoms worsening familial and social interactions were limited to pain and negative affect. Indeed, out of the 53 patients about 13% could not tolerate premenstrual pain and swinging mood. A similar figure (3–15%) was reported by another study[13].

Considering the influence of biological variables in the development of PMS we analyzed age, pregnancy and previous dysmenorrhea. PMS was more represented in the third decade but, in agreement with other authors, without statistical correlation[10,11,14,15].

Similarly, the number of pregnancies does not influence the symptomatology; but in 80% of those patients suffering PMS, previous dysmenorrhea was present. This finding was actually in discussion because of the contradictory results reported in the literature[16,17]. It should be noted that the

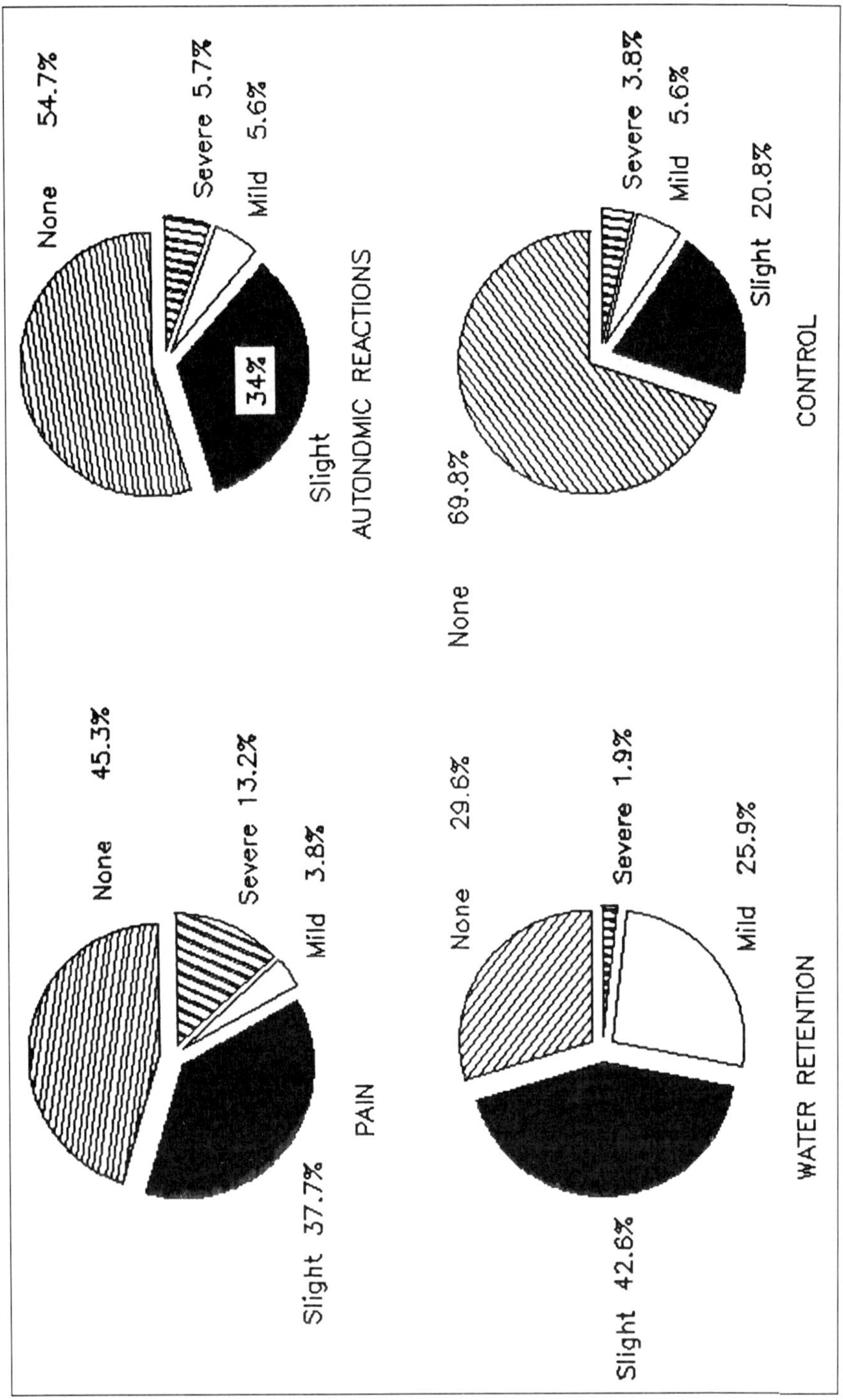

Figure 2 Segmental analysis of the peripheral symptoms

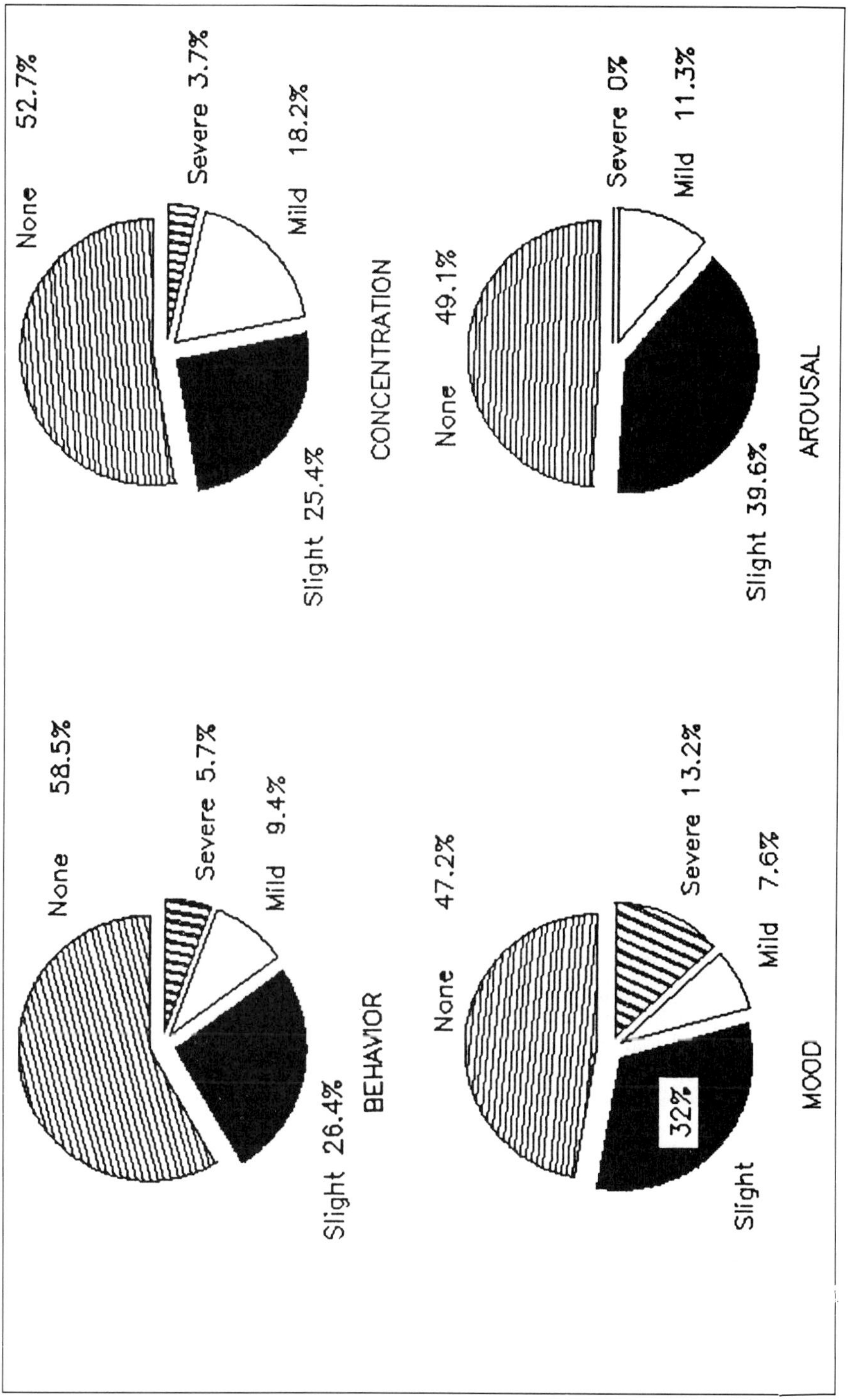

Figure 3 Segmental analysis of the central symptoms

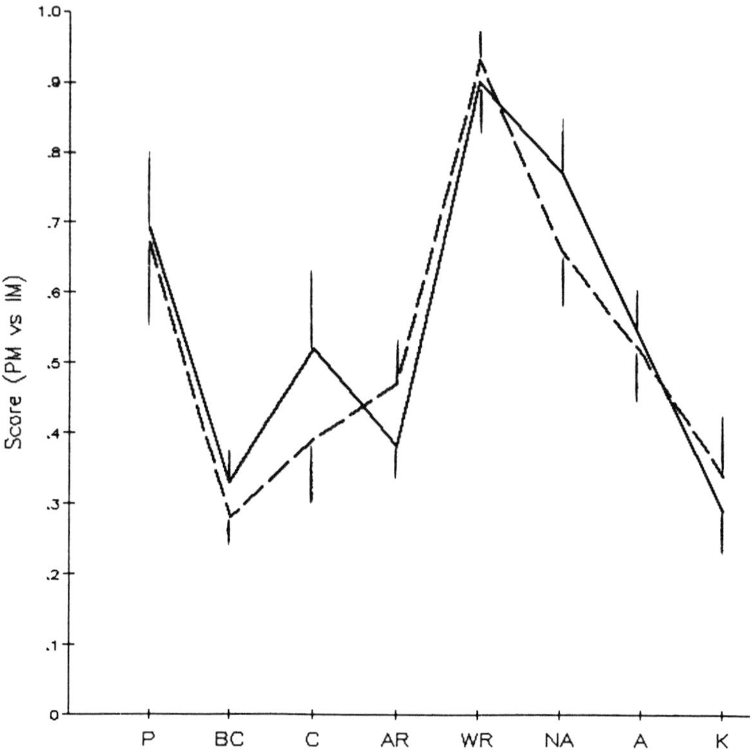

Figure 4 Reliability. P = pain, BC = behavioral changes, C = concentration, AR = autonomic reactions, WR = water retention, NA = negative affect, A = arousal, K = control; solid line, basal line 1; broken line, basal line 2

presence of menstrual pain represents a negative factor affecting only symptoms originating in the central nervous system. Probably the connection has to be looked for in the patient's attitude in facing distressing events connected with reproductive life.

Among several hypotheses raised to explain the etiopathogenesis of PMS many authors proposed it as a simple reaction in women with a hypocondriac trait[18]. This idea was apparently sustained by the elevated variability in symptom recording, both in quality and in quantity[19]. However, the good reliability in the self-readministration of MDQ showed by our patients indicates that their claiming of a symptom or a group of symptoms is apparently true and really interferes with the patient's life.

REFERENCES

1. Frank, R.T. (1931). The hormonal causes of premenstrual tension. *Arch. Neurol. Psychiatr.*, **26**, 1052
2. Hargrove, J.T. and Abraham, G.E. (1982). The incidence of premenstrual tension in a gynaecologic clinic. *J. Reprod. Med.*, **27**, 721

3. Halbreich, U. and Endicott, J. (1986). Premenstrual changes: pattern and correlates of daily ratings. *J. Affect. Disord.*, **10**, 127
4. Moos, R.H. (1968). The development of a menstrual distress questionnaire. *Psychosom. Med.*, **30**, 853
5. Markum, R.A. (1976). Assessment of the reliability and the effect of neutral instruction on the symptoms ratings on the MDQ. *Psychosom. Med.*, **38**, 163
6. Gruba, G.J. and Rohrbaug, M. (1975). MMPI correlates of menstrual distress. *Psychosom. Med.*, **37**, 265
7. Chuong, C.J., Colligan, R.E., Coulam, C.B. and Bergstralh, E.J. (1988). The MMPI as an aid in evaluating patients with premenstrual syndrome. *Psychosom. Med.*, **29**, 197
8. Sances, G., Martignoni, E., Facchinetti, F., D'Avola, G., Rosettino, G., Costa, A. and Nappi, G. (1986). MDQ e le scale di Zung nella valutazione dei cambiamenti affettivo-comportamentali. In Genazzani, A.R. *et al.* (eds). *Endocrinologia Ginecologica*, pp. 9–13. (Bologna: Monduzzi Edizione)
9. Coppen, A. and Kessel, H. (1963). Menstruation and personality. *Br. J. Psychiatr.*, **109**, 711
10. Lehert, P. and Van Keep, P.A. (1981). The premenstrual syndrome: an epidemiological and statistical exercise. In Van Keep, P. and Utian, W. (eds). *The Premenstrual Syndrome*, p. 31. (Lancaster: MTP Press)
11. Andersch, B., Wenderstan, C. and Hahn, L. (1986). Premenstrual complaints: prevalence of premenstrual symptoms in a swedish urban population. *J. Psychosom. Obstet. Gynaecol.*, **5**, 39
12. Most, A.F., Woods, N.F., Dery, G.K. *et al.* (1981). Distress associated with menstruation among Israeli women. *Int. J. Nurs. Stud.*, **18**, 61
13. Palma, E., Maruotti, G. and Aragona, C. (1988). Premenstrual syndromes. In Genazzani, A.R., Nappi, G., Facchinetti, F. and Martignoni, E. (eds) *Pain and Reproduction*, pp. 89–98. (Carnforth: Parthenon Publishing)
14. Reid, R.L. and Yen, S.S.C. (1981). Premenstrual syndrome. *Am. J. Obstet. Gynecol.*, **139**, 84
15. Johnson, S.R., McChesney, C. and Bean, A.J. (1988). Epidemiology of premenstrual symptoms in a non-clinical sample. *J. Reprod. Med.*, **33**, 340
16. Steege, J.F., Stout, A.L. and Rupp, S.L. (1985). Relationships among premenstrual symptoms and menstrual cycle characteristics. *Obstet. Gynecol.*, **65**, 398
17. Metcalf, M.G., Livesey, J.H., Hudson, S.H. and Wells, E.J. (1988). The premenstrual syndrome; moods, headaches and physical symptoms in 133 cycles. *J. Psychosom. Obstet. Gynaecol.*, **8**, 31
18. Rees, W.L. (1976). Stress, distress and disease. *Br. J. Psychiatr.*, **128**, 3
19. Ruble, D.N. (1977). Premenstrual symptoms: a reinterpretation. *Science*, **197**, 291

101

Effects of dihydroergocriptine on dopaminergic neurons. A rationale for its use in premenstrual syndrome?

A. Groppetti, G. Ceresoli, C. Ferrara, M. Zambelli and M. Parenti

Premenstrual syndrome (PMS) is characterized by several symptoms ranging from breast tenderness, weight gain and abdominal bloating to headache, anxiety, craving for sweet or salty foods, fatigue, irritability, depression and emotional lability[1]. Estrogen–progesterone imbalance, prolactin, aldosterone, prostaglandins, β-endorphins and pyridoxine are among the causes which have been postulated to be related to PMS[1–5]; but the precise physiological mechanisms underlying the syndrome remain unclear.

The lack of a basic understanding of the etiology of PMS has, as a consequence, encouraged the use of a wide range of drugs including diuretics, progestogens, tranquilizers, analgesic anti-inflammatories and dopamine agonists[5,7–9].

The rationale for using this last family of drugs in PMS originates from the knowledge that activation of central and/or peripheral dopaminergic circuits affects emotional behavior, increases diuresis and sodium excretion while food intake and fatigue are decreased[10]. Also the secretions of prolactin, gonadotropin-releasing hormone, β-endorphin, aldosterone[11] and, as recently demonstrated in cultured pituitary cells, arachidonic acid[12], the prostaglandin precursor, are depressed.

Unfortunately, in spite of these positive characteristics, the benefits deriving from dopamine agonist therapy in PMS have been modest, as for most of the other families of drugs so far tried.

However, the possibility that the cause for the disappointing therapeutic efficacy could be an unsuitable biodisposition or affinity for the population of dopamine receptors involved in the control of the clinical signs, has encouraged the search for new molecules.

In the present study we have investigated the putative dopaminergic properties of dihydroergocriptine (DHEC), an ergot derivative which has been demonstrated to ameliorate the symptoms of Parkinson disease and to lower serum prolactin levels[13,14].

MATERIALS AND METHODS

Experiments were carried out on male Sprague-Dawley albino rats (Charles River) weighing 150–180 g. Intranigral injections were performed stereotaxically using co-ordinates based on the König and Klippel Atlas[15]. For the intranigral 6-hydroxydopamine (6-OHDA) injections (8 μg) the animals were kept under pentobarbital anesthesia and the coordinates were as follows: A–P = 3.2; L = 1.4; V = 7.6.

The following compounds were used: 6-OHDA–HBr and apomorphine–HCl (Sigma), L-sulpiride (a gift from Ravizza), SCH-23390 and [^{3}H]SCH-23390 (a gift from Schering), bromocriptine (a gift from Sandoz), dihydroergocriptine (DHEC) (a gift from Poli), SKF-38393 (a gift from Smith, Kline & French), haloperidol (Janssen), [^{3}H]spiperone (New England Nuclear).

Bromocriptine and DHEC were administered twice a day for 2 weeks. The single doses were 0.25 mg/kg for bromocriptine and 0.5 mg/kg for DHEC. The animals were killed 3 days after the last treatment.

Adenylate cyclase activity and the binding of [^{3}H]SCH-23390 or [^{3}H] spiperone were assayed in washed striatal particulate fractions according to the procedure described by Groppetti *et al.*[16]. Protein concentration was measured by the method of Bradford[17].

RESULTS

In vitro studies

The interactions with dopamine receptors have been evaluated on partially purified striatal membranes. Similarly to dopamine and SKF-38393, DHEC displaced [^{3}H]SCH-23390, a marker for D-1 receptors, from its binding sites (Figure 1a). The efficacy of DHEC was of the same order of dopamine, but about tenfold less than the D-1 agonist SKF-38393.

The findings that the displacement of [^{3}H]SCH-23390 by DHEC was not GTP-dependent (data not shown) and that the dose–response curve of dopamine-stimulated adenylate cyclase was shifted toward the right in the presence of DHEC 10 μM (Figure 1b), strongly suggest that the ergot derivative acts on D-1 receptors as an antagonist. Similar results have been found for bromocriptine. The data in Figure 2a show that DHEC also displaced [^{3}H]spiperone, a marker for D-2 receptors, from its binding sites. In this respect, the efficacy of DHEC was markedly weaker than bromocriptine. The finding that DHEC inhibited the basal activity of adenylate cyclase (Figure 2b), indicates the agonist nature of the interaction of this drug with D-2 receptors.

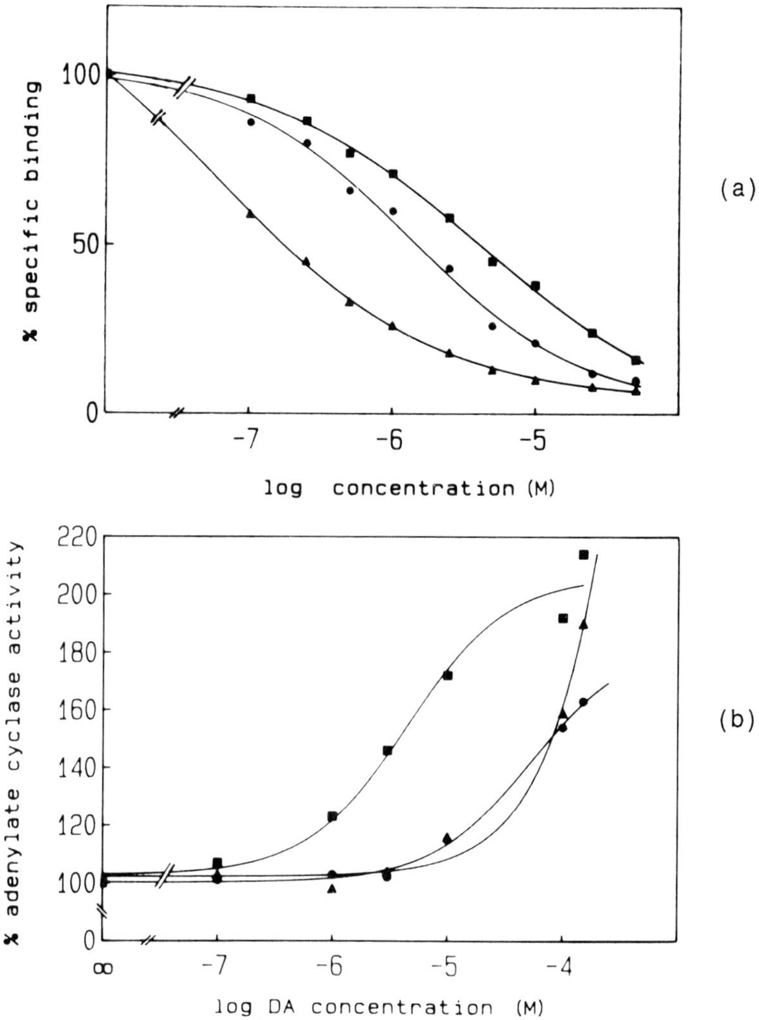

Figure 1 (a) Inhibition of [^{3}H]SCH-23390-specific binding by increasing concentrations of dopamine (■), SKF-38393 (▲) and DHEC (●). (b) Effect of different concentrations of dopamine on adenylate cyclase activity in the presence of vehicle alone (■), DHEC (10 μM) plus L-sulpiride (10 μM) (▲) or bromocriptine (10 μM) plus L-sulpiride (10 μM) (●). Assays were performed on partially purified striatal membranes

In vivo studies

The findings from *in vivo* studies further support the agonist and the antagonist properties, on D-2 receptors and D-1 receptors respectively, of DHEC.

In fact, DHEC (0.5 mg/kg) inhibited the rotations induced by the D-1 agonist SKF-38393, in rats lesioned by a monolateral injection of 6-OHDA

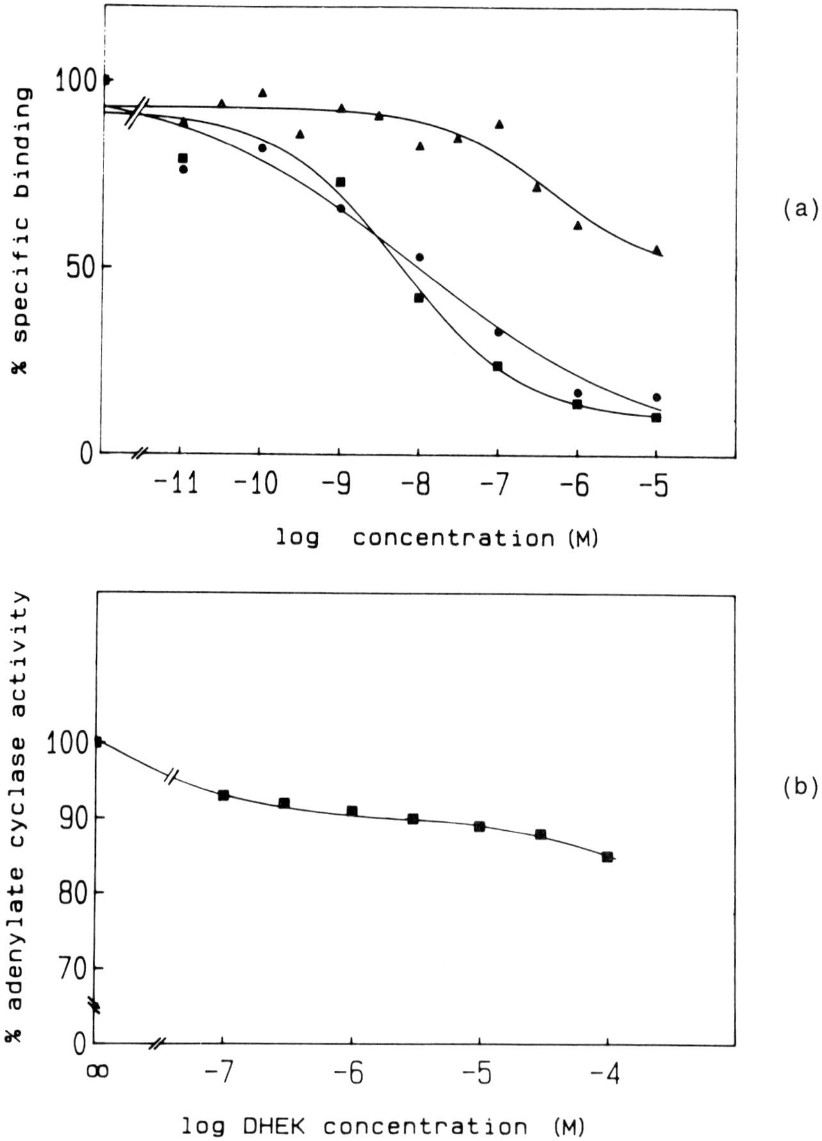

Figure 2 (a) Inhibition of [^{3}H]spiperone-specific binding by increasing concentrations of haloperidol (■), bromocriptine (●) or DHEC (▲). (b) Effect of different concentrations of DHEC on adenylate cyclase activity in presence of SCH-23390 (0.1 μM). Assays were performed on partially purified striatal membranes

into the substantia nigra (Figure 3). Similar effect was observed after bromocriptine (0.25 mg/kg) pretreatment.

On the other hand the data in Figure 4a indicate that in striata of rats treated daily for 14 days with DHEC, the binding of [^{3}H]spiperone was

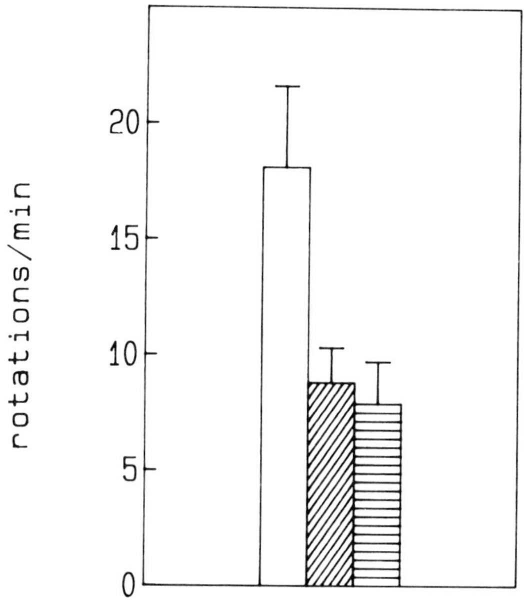

Figure 3 Effect of DHEC or bromocriptine pretreatments on SKF-38393-induced contralateral rotations in rats monolaterally lesioned with intranigral 6-OHDA injections (8 μg). DHEC (0.5 mg/kg; hatched block) or bromocriptine (0.25 mg/kg; horizontally hatched block) were given 15 min before SKF-38393 (10 mg/kg) treatment. Results from rats given saline alone are shown by the open block

markedly decreased. Bromocriptine, given at a dose of 0.25 mg/kg, produced a similar effect (Figure 4b). The binding studies were performed 3 days after the last treatment with the two drugs.

DISCUSSION

Evidence indicates that ergot derivatives act on central and peripheral dopaminergic neurons[10,11].

Disorders such as Parkinson disease, hyperprolactinemia, acromegaly, characterized by a deficit of dopaminergic tone, are currently treated with these drugs.

The data reported here show that the dihydrogenated ergopeptine derivative DHEC interacts with both families of dopamine receptors being an agonist for the D-2 subpopulation and mostly an antagonist or partial agonist for the D-1 subpopulation. Both, *in vitro* and *in vivo* studies seem to support this evidence. On the other hand these findings are in line with previous reports showing that DHEC improves Parkinson disease symptoms, decreases hyperprolactinemia and binds to dopamine receptors[13,14,18].

In this respect the data indicate that the pharmacological profile is similar for DHEC and bromocriptine, another ergopeptine derivative that has also been demonstrated to act as an agonist and antagonist on dopamine

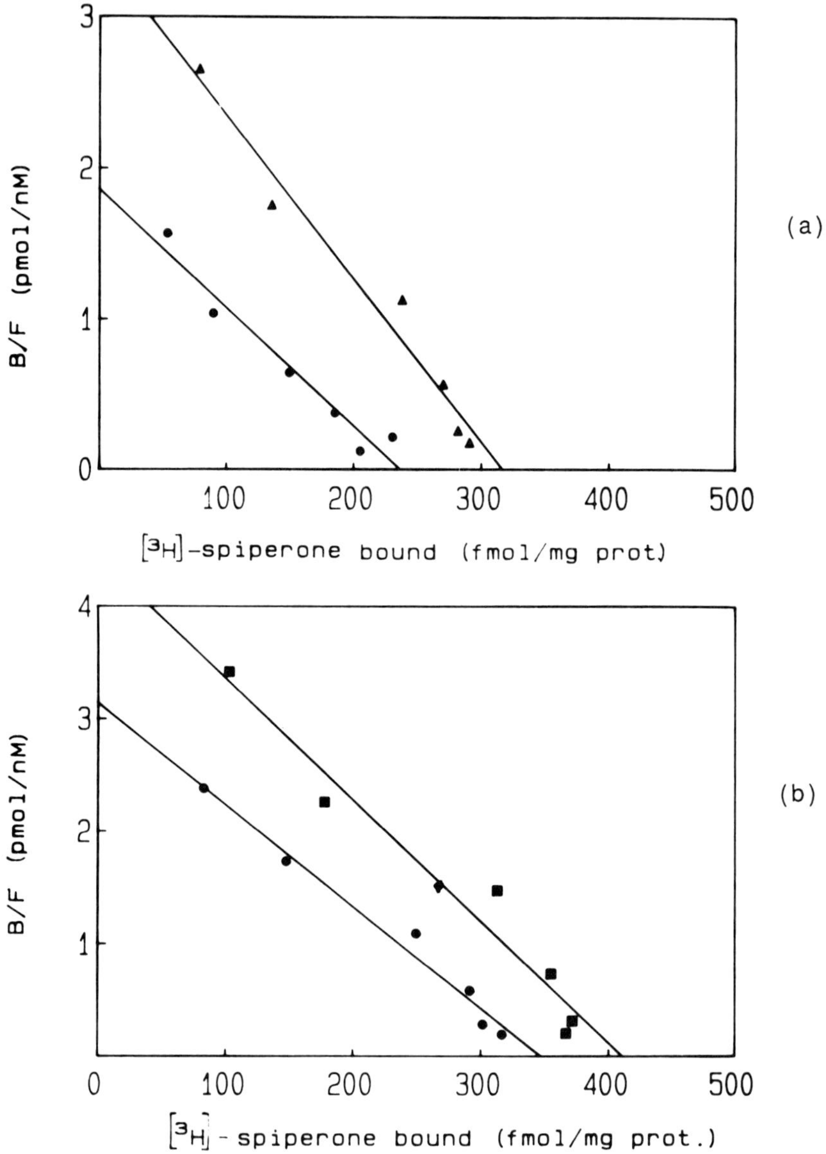

Figure 4 $[^3H]$Spiperone binding in striatal membrane preparations from rats chronically treated with DHEC (●) or control (▲) (a) or bromocriptine (●) or control (■) (b). The single doses were 0.5 mg/kg and 0.25 mg/kg for DHEC and bromocriptine respectively. The two drugs were given twice a day for 2 weeks. Animals were killed 3 days after the last treatment

receptors[19]. Differences between the two ergots could be found only when the degree of their interaction with each of the two receptor populations is considered. In the present work where the effects on the dopaminergic nigrostriatal system have been studied, DHEC was less potent than bromocriptine as a D-2 agonist, while the efficacy for inhibiting D-1 receptors was of the same order of magnitude for the two drugs.

The finding that DHEC has a minor impact with striatal D-2 receptors than bromocriptine is in agreement with reports showing that in rats lesioned with a monolateral injection of 6-OHDA into substantia nigra DHEC induces rotations only at doses tenfold higher than bromocriptine[20].

An opposite condition seems to be present in the anterior pituitary gland where the relative potency for inhibiting prolactin release or for binding to membrane preparations indicates that DHEC is at least fivefold more active than bromocriptine[21]. On the other hand, also in striatum the different potency between the two compounds on D-2 receptors seems greatly attenuated after chronic treatments. In fact, DHEC and bromocriptine given to rats in a ratio of 2 to 1 for 2 weeks show the same efficacy in reducing the number of D-2 binding sites in striatum.

Therefore the differences between DHEC and bromocriptine in affecting dopamine D-1 and D-2 receptor activity, seem to be related to the tissue, acute or chronic treatment and probably animal species. The preference for the clinical use of one or the other compound is therefore difficult to establish on the basis of experimental findings alone. In fact, therapeutic benefits and side-effects of these ergot derivatives depend primarily upon their complex interactions with dopamine receptors although their pharmacokinetics and the ability to interfere with other neurotransmitters, such as noradrenaline and serotonin, should also be considered.

REFERENCES

1. Gonzalez, E.R. (1981). Premenstrual syndrome: an ancient woe deserving of modern scrutiny. *J. Am. Med. Assoc.*, **245**, 1393–6
2. Greene, R. and Dalton, K. (1953). The premenstrual syndrome. *Br. Med. J.*, **1**, 1007–13
3. Munday, M.R., Brush, M.G. and Taylor, R.W. (1981). Correlations between progesterone, oestradiol and aldosterone levels in the premenstrual syndrome. *Clin. Endocrinol.*, **14**, 1
4. O'Brien, P.M.S. and Symonds, E.M. (1982). Prolactin levels in the premenstrual syndrome. *Br. J. Obstet. Gynaecol.*, **89**, 303
5. Budoff, P.W. (1987). Use of prostaglandin inhibitors in the treatment of PMS. *Clin. Obstet. Gynecol.*, **30**, 443–64
6. Reid, R.L. and Yen, S.S.C. (1981). Premenstrual syndrome. *Am. J. Obstet. Gynecol.*, **139**, 85–104
7. O'Brien, P.M.S. (1982). The premenstrual syndrome: a review of the present status of therapy. *Drugs*, **24**, 140
8. Shapiro, S.S. (1988). Treatment of dysmenorrhoea and premenstrual syndrome with non-steroidal anti-inflammatory drugs. *Drugs*, **36**, 475–90
9. Ho, K.Y. and Thorner, M.O. (1988). Therapeutic applications of bromocriptine in endocrine and neurological diseases. *Drugs*, **36**, 67–82
10. Fuxe, K., Agnati, L.F., Kalia, M., Goldstein, M., Andersson, K. and Harfstrand, A. (1985). Dopaminergic systems in the brain and pituitary. In Fluckinger, E., Muller, E.E. and Thorner, M. (eds.). *The Dopaminergic System*, pp. 11–25 (Berlin: Springer-Verlag).
11. Clark, B.J. (1985). The role of dopamine in the periphery. In Fluckinger, E., Muller, E.E. and Thorner, M. (eds). *The Dopaminergic System*, pp. 27–39. (Berlin: Springer-Verlag)
12. Canonico, P.L. (1988). Dopamine and the inhibition of prolactin secretion: involvement of multiple intracellular signals. In Spano, P.F., Biggio, G., Toffano, G. and Gessa, G.L. (eds). *Central and Peripheral Dopamine Receptors: Biochemistry and Pharmacology*, pp. 237–45 (Berlin: Springer-Verlag)

13. Scarzella, L., Cantello, R., Delsedime, M., Gilli, M., Pinessi, L., Riccio, A., Bergamasco, B. and Ruggeri, S. (1985). Clinical trial on the therapeutic activity of dihydroergokryptine in parkinsonism: preliminary results. *Curr. Ther. Res.*, **38**, 432–40
14. Poli, M., Cocchi, D., Mailland, F., Masu, A.M., Landi, G., Craveri, A. and Muller, E.E. (1986). Prolactin lowering effect of dihydroergocriptine in rat and in man. *J. Endocrinol. Invest.*, **9**, 31–6
15. Konig, J.F.R. and Klippel, R.A. (1963). *The Rat Brain: a Stereotaxic Atlas of the Forebrain and Lower Parts of Brain Stem.* (Baltimore: Williams & Wilkins)
16. Groppetti, A., Flauto, C., Parati, E., Vescovi, A. and Parenti, M. (1986). Dopamine receptors changes in response to prolonged treatment with L-DOPA. *J. Neural Transm.*, **225**, 33–45
17. Bradford, M.M. (1976). A rapid and sensitive method for the quantification of microgram quantities of protein using the principle of protein-dye binding. *Anal. Biochem.*, **72**, 248–54
18. Davis, J.N., Strittmatter, W.J., Hoyler, E. and Lefkowitz, R.J. (1977). [^{3}H]dihydroergokryptine binding in rat brain. *Brain Res.*, **132**, 327–36
19. Trabucchi, M., Spano, P.F., Tonon, G. and Frattola, L. (1976). Effect of bromocriptine on central dopaminergic receptors. *Life Sci.*, **19**, 225–32
20. Loew, D.M., van Deusen, E.B. and Meier-Ruge, W. (1978). Effects on the central nervous system. In Berde, B. and Schild, H.O. (eds). *Ergot Alkaloids and Related Compounds*, pp. 421–531. (Berlin: Springer-Verlag)
21. Caron, M.G., Beaulieu, M., Raymond, V., Gagne, B., Drouin, J., Lefkowitz, R.J. and Labrie, F. (1978). Dopaminergic receptors in the anterior pituitary gland. *J. Biol. Chem.*, **253**, 2244–53

102

Abnormal luteinizing hormone pulsatile pattern in patients suffering from premenstrual syndrome

F. Facchinetti, G. Romano, A.D. Genazzani, S. Stanzani and A.R. Genazzani

INTRODUCTION

Premenstrual syndrome (PMS) still represents a clinical problem that must be totally defined both in its pathogenetic and therapeutic aspects. The interest raised by PMS for its social costs in USA has induced several authors to write review papers in order to summarize the main features of PMS. Nevertheless many aspects remain obscure. In fact we do not have accurate diagnostic instruments and we do not know the real prevalence of PMS nor its etiology[1-4].

Besides the lack of good methodology in most studies about therapy, the few double-blind controlled studies performed have shown a remarkable therapeutic efficacy of placebo. So we need further knowledge about causes, development and treatment of this syndrome.

Up to now hormonal changes have been considered among the main causal factors of PMS. However, since ovarian hormones cannot explain central effects like behavioral, mood and nociceptive sensitivity changes, many authors began taking into account neurotransmitter systems (especially neuropeptidergic ones) which represent a target for gonadal secretion.

The study of opioid system activity and of its fluctuations during the menstrual cycle demonstrates a lower opioid tone in the follicular phase, a rise at ovulation and a peak at midluteal phase[5]. During the premenstrual phase PMS patients show a sharp decrease of both peripheral and central opioids while in controls they remain steady[6,7]. This phenomenon is related with progesterone/estradiol ratio decrease which occurs from midluteal phase up to the menses[8].

Hypothalamic opioids inhibit luteinizing hormone-releasing hormone (LHRH) and consequently pituitary luteinizing hormone (LH) release and this action is controlled by gonadal steroids[5]. In fact naloxone fails to be effective in modifying plasma LH levels in postmenopause, prepuberty and hypogonadotropic hypogonadism. On the contrary a response to naloxone is present in both castrate males and females upon replacement hormonal therapy[9,10] demonstrating how the steroid milieu affects opioid activity.

Opioids are considered one of the main regulating factors of hypothalamic LH pulsatility and they even seem to be its cause[11].

It is well known that LH secretion is under both a tonic and phasic control. The phasic secretion parameters (amplitude and frequency) change during the menstrual cycle. The follicular phase is characterized by lower amplitude spikes with a frequency of one spike/hour; in the periovulatory period the frequency remains stable while amplitude rises significantly; finally during the luteal phase a lower frequency (one spike every 3–4 hours), with very high amplitude (even tenfold the basal value) can be observed.

So we decided to evaluate LH pulsatile secretion in PMS patients in order to verify if the neuroendocrine disorders described in these patients could affect this biological phenomenon, so fundamental to reproduction.

MATERIALS AND METHODS

Subjects

Seven patients suffering from PMS for at least 3 years (aged from 27 to 33 years) have been studied. They presented regular cycles lasting 24–31 days. None of them were under hormonal or psychopharmacological therapy. No patient had a personal or familial history positive for psychiatric diseases. Moos' Menstrual Distress Questionnaire (MDQ) was used for the diagnosis[12].

Six healthy volunteers (aged from 24 to 32 years) with regular menstrual cycles (26–30 days) were taken as controls. In these subjects premenstrual complaints were completely absent.

Protocol

Both patients and controls recorded basal temperature and were asked to reach the endocrine ward 8 days after temperature rise. A catheter was inserted into the brachial vein at 07:30 and then kept pervious with saline. Blood samples (3 ml) were taken every 10 min for 12 h (73 samples in total). During the trial the subjects could walk and eat at their usual times. The plasma, obtained by centrifugation, was stored at $-20°C$ until the assay.

LH and prolactin (PRL) radioimmunoassays (double antibody) were performed using commercial kits (Radim, Rome). Every pulsatility was measured in the same assay in order to reduce the intra-assay coefficient of variation (C.V.) which varied by 6.5–7.2% depending on technicians. The radioimmunoassays were performed in duplicate.

Prolactin was measured in the first six samples of every pulsatility.

Statistical analysis

The results were analyzed using two different algorithms: 'Towers' by Capelli, Valastro and Filicori, which is a modified version by Santen and Bardin[13] and 'Detect' recently proposed by Dr Rodbard[14]. For both softwares the following parameters were evaluated: spike number, frequency per 12 hours, amplitude (subtracted from basal value) and per cent increase at peak.

'Towers' identifies a peak when the LH value at one point is more than three times the C.V. of the LH in the previous one.

RESULTS AND DISCUSSION

The summary of data of the plasma LH pulsatile pattern is reported in Table 1. In controls, both softwares used, reveal a similar number of peaks/12 hours; i.e. about nine. It is well known that the LH pulsatile pattern changes during the menstrual cycle, endogenous opioids, steroids and dopamine being the main regulators of frequency[5,11,15]. However, the premenstrual period has been poorly studied.

In the midluteal phase, the frequency of LH peaks is at its lowest level due to the maximal presence of both opioid and progesterone (P) inhibition. The corpus luteum regression and the consequent decrease of P levels allow the LH pulses to increase. This is why the subjects studied here, in the presence of P levels below 3 ng/ml, showed a frequency almost double that observed in the midluteal phase. Interestingly, the amplitude of the LH peaks remained similar to that described in midluteal phase[16] suggesting the existence of different factors that regulate the pituitary synthesis and secretion of LH.

Neither 'Detect', nor 'Towers' indicate any difference in LH frequency between controls and PMS patients. A deeper investigation of LH pulses through the instant secretion rate calculation reaches the same conclusion (Table 1).

On the contrary, the study of LH pulse amplitude offers to consider important differences between patients and controls. The mean amplitude of LH secretion in PMS patients is reduced twofold with respect to controls. 'Towers' software is unable to find such a difference and this may be due to the lower threshold used for peak detection. Indeed 'Towers' reveals more peaks than 'Detect', perhaps including also peaks of very small amplitude that are not included in the calculation by 'Detect'. In this way, the mean amplitude of controls becomes artifactually reduced. The difference of peak

Table 1 Number and amplitude of spontaneous plasma LH peaks (means ± SD) in controls and patients with premenstrual syndrome. These parameters were calculated using two softwares: 'Towers' and 'Detect'. The instant secretion rates (ISR) were calculated from the deconvolution of 'Detect' analysis[14]

	Number of peaks			*Peak amplitude* (mIU/ml)		
	Towers	*Detect*	*ISR*	*Towers*	*Detect*	*ISR*
Controls ($n = 7$)	10.2 ± 4.1	9.0 ± 3.1	8.5 ± 4.3	4.1 ± 3.7	4.0 ± 1.0	3.3 ± 1.7
PMS ($n = 9$)	10.0 ± 3.4	9.9 ± 2.1	9.3 ± 4.3	3.4 ± 2.9	7.2 ± 4.4	6.7 ± 5.5
p	NS	NS	NS	NS	0.05	0.10

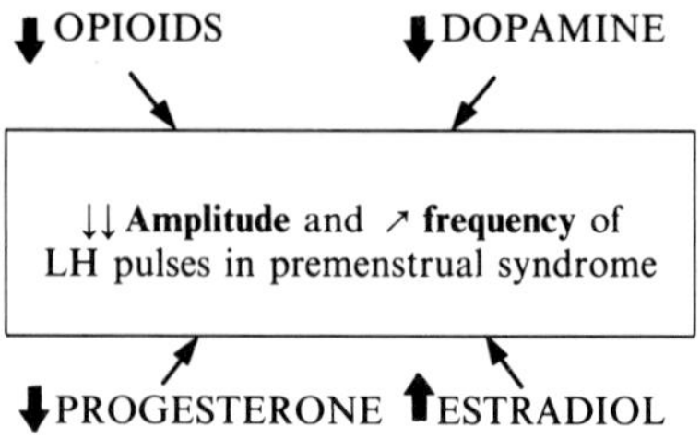

Figure 1 The reduced amplitude and the trend toward increased frequency of LH pulsatility in PMS patients could be a consequence of several neuroendocrine disorders affecting circulating steroids and both opioid and dopaminergic systems

analysis of the two softwares is emphasized also by the observation that no correlation exists between individual spikes of LH as measured by 'Towers' and 'Detect' ($r = 0.325$).

The reduced amplitude of LH peaks in PMS patients could be linked to several neuroendocrine findings characterizing these subjects. Progesterone levels should first be taken into consideration. In the present series of patients, confirming previously reported data, the P levels are reduced in comparison with controls[7,17]. Moreover PMS shows a transient reduction of central opioid tone in the premenstrual period[6–8]. This finding could therefore condition the activity of hypothalamic LHRH discharge[18]. Finally, prolactin levels have been reported to be abnormally elevated in the luteal phase of PMS patients[1–4,19] suggesting a reduction of dopaminergic activity. This finding is confirmed also by the actual data. Indeed, patients show a mean value (18.9 ± 11.2 ng/ml, mean $\pm$ SD) which is significantly higher than in controls (11.7 ± 5.9, $p < 0.05$ at Mann-Whitney) (Figure 1). Such a finding could also be related to the abnormal pulsatile LH pattern of PMS in view of the dopaminergic inhibition of LH secretion during the menstrual cycle[15].

In conclusion, these data indicate an abnormal LH pulsatility during the late luteal phase in patients suffering from premenstrual syndrome, i.e. in the symptomatic period. This neuroendocrine finding remains to be elucidated, and several defined hormonal systems could be responsible for these changes. Nevertheless, these data allow the definition of PMS as a psychoneuroendocrine disorder.

REFERENCES

1. Reid, R.L. and Yen, S.S.C. (1981). Premenstrual syndrome. *Am. J. Obstet. Gynecol.*, **139**, 85–101
2. Rubinow, D.R. and Byrne, P.R. (1984). Premenstrual syndrome: overview from a methodologic perspective. *Am. J. Psychiatr.*, **141**, 163–84
3. Vaitukaitis, J.L. (1984). Premenstrual syndrome. *N. Engl. J. Med.*, **21**, 1371–3
4. O'Brien, P.M.S. (1985). The premenstrual syndrome: a review. *J. Reprod. Med.*, **30**, 113–126
5. Ferin, M. (1984). Endogenous opioid peptides and the menstrual cycle. *Trends Neurosci.*, **3**, 194–8
6. Facchinetti, F., Martignoni, E., Petraglia, F., Sances, M.G., Nappi, G. and Genazzani, A.R.

(1987). Premenstrual fall of plasma β-endorphin in patients with premenstrual syndrome. *Fertil. Steril.*, **47**, 570–3

7. Facchinetti, F., Martignoni, E., Sola, D., Petraglia, F., Nappi, G. and Genazzani, A.R. (1988). Transient failure of central opioid tonus and premenstrual symptoms. *J. Reprod. Med.*, **33**, 633–8
8. Facchinetti, F., Nappi, G., Petraglia, F., Volpe, A. and Genazzani, A.R. (1983). Estradiol/progesterone imbalance and the premenstrual syndrome. *Lancet*, **ii**, 1302
9. Petraglia, F., Comitini, G., D'Ambrogio, G., Volpe, A., Facchinetti, F., Alessandrini, G. and Genazzani, A.R. (1985). Short-term effects of ovariectomy: the opioid control of LH secretion in fertile, climacteric and postmenopausal women. *J. Endocrinol. Invest.*, **8**, 325–30
10. De Feo, M.L., Maggi, M., Guardabasso, V., Rodbard, D., Delitala, G., Fazzi, V., Genazzani, A.R., Facchinetti, F. and Forti, G. (1986). Naloxone administration does not affect gonadotropin secretion in agonadal men either basally or during treatment. *J. Clin. Endocrinol. Metab.*, **63**, 257–61
11. Veldhuis, J.D., Guardabasso, V., Rogol, A.D., Evans, W.S., Oerter, K.E., Johnson, M.L. and Rodbard, D. (1987). Appraising the nature of luteinizing hormone secretory events in men. *Am. J. Physiol.*, **252**, E599–605
12. Moos, R.H. (1968). The development of a menstrual distress questionnaire. *Psychosom. Med.*, **30**, 853–64
13. Santen, R.J. and Bardin, C.W. (1973). Pulse analysis, clinical interpretation physiological mechanism. *J. Clin. Invest.*, **52**, 2617–28
14. Oerter, K.E., Guardabasso, V. and Rodbard, D. (1986). Detection characterization of peaks and estimation of instantaneous secretory rate for episodic hormone secretion. *Comp. Biomed. Res.*, **19**, 170–91
15. Yen, S.S.C. and Jaffe, R.B. (1986). *Reproductive Endocrinology*. (Philadelphia: W.B. Saunders Company)
16. Filicori, M., Butler, J.P. and Crowley, W.F. (1984). Regulation of the hypothalamic-pituitary-ovarian axis during the luteal phase of the human menstrual cycle. *J. Clin. Invest.*, **73**, 1638–46
17. Munday, M.R., Brush, M.G. and Taylor, W. (1981). Correlations between progesterone, oestradiol and aldosterone levels in the premenstrual syndrome. *Clin. Endocrinol.*, **14**, 1–10
18. Crowley, W.F., Jr, Filicori, M., Spratt, D. and Santoro, N. (1985). The physiology of gonadotropin releasing hormone (GnRH) secretion in men and women. *Rec. Prog. Horm. Res.*, **41**, 473–96
19. Varma, T.R. (1984). Hormones and electrolytes levels in the premenstrual syndrome. *Int. J. Gynecol. Obstet.*, **22**, 51–7

103

Dihydroergocriptine treatment: behavior changes in premenstrual syndrome

A. Levi Minzi, G. Zavattini and D. De Maio

INTRODUCTION

Many aspects of the premenstrual syndrome (PMS) still give rise to much controversy[1]. There is confusion about its definition, diagnosis and etiology. The lack of a basic understanding of the pathophysiology of the syndrome has slowed progress in its treatment. In fact no standard therapy exists at present for PMS. Treatments recommended include dietary manipulation, vitamin therapy, hormone supplements particularly progesterone[2–5], diuretics[6], psychotropic drugs, non-steroidal anti-inflammatory drugs[7–11] and, in particular, a dopamine agonist, bromocriptine[12–17].

Therapeutic trials with bromocriptine were undertaken in the belief that abnormal dopamine synthesis and resulting hyperprolactinemia were important etiological factors[18–21]. The results of these trials suggest that bromocriptine is active only on some symptoms, i.e. mastodynia[16,17], irritability[12] and depression[13] but this may be due to the difficulty of reliable analysis. The activity of bromocriptine cannot be increased by giving higher dosages because of the onset of side-effects[22].

The possibility of using dihydroergocriptine (DHEC), a new dopamine receptor stimulating agent, at higher dosages without side-effects[23] and new sources of information such as the 'Diagnostic and Statistical Manual of Mental Disorders' (DSM-III-R) of the American Psychiatric Association[24] which define the pathology and aid in more precise diagnosis, encouraged us to undertake a clinical trial. The aim was to assess the effects of DHEC on mood, behavior and physical symptoms associated with the luteal phase of the menstrual cycle, in a group of women selected for PMS according to the DSM-III-R criteria.

PATIENTS AND METHODS

The design of this prospective study was randomized, double-blind and placebo-controlled. Subjects were accepted for the study if they fulfilled the following criteria:

(1) Age between 18 and 45 years with regular periods and a cycle length of 24–32 days;
(2) Personal history of severe PMS for at least 2 years;
(3) No other medical or psychiatric disorders;
(4) Use of adequate non-hormonal methods of contraception;
(5) Total score on Menstrual Distress Questionnaire (MDQ) ⩾ 22;
(6) Diagnosis of PMS according to DSM-III-R.

Recently, PMS has been termed Late Luteal Phase Dysphoric Disorder (LLPDD) on the basis of the development of operational criteria adopted for its definition[24].

Given the controversy whether LLPDD is a gynecological or a psychiatric disorder, the decision was taken to include this syndrome in the Appendix to the revision of the third edition of the DSM-III-R until further research resolves the question. We used the definition and diagnostic criteria of inclusion for LLPDD for our patients.

The 26 women admitted to the study were asked to start with placebo or medication, a tablet of DHEC 10 mg/day on the evening of the predicted day 18 of their cycle, that is 10 days before the expected data of menses, and continue until the onset of menstruation (Figure 1). Cycles with 65% tablet-compliance or higher were accepted for analysis. The compliance was ascertained by counting the number of tablets returned by the subjects at the end of each cycle and comparing this number with the number that should have been taken. The trial included four menstrual cycles for each patient: first, a control cycle without medication, including vitamins, then three treatment cycles, in which each patient received at random DHEC or placebo.

PMS patients were interviewed according to a modified Moos Menstrual Distress Questionnaire (MDQ)[25], consisting of 30 adverse symptoms scored on the 15th day of every cycle, on a scale from 0 to 4 (no symptoms to invalidating symptom). Because of the wide range of symptomatology, the symptoms are grouped into four 'clusters'.

The interviews were taken on day 15 ± 2 before the start of menstruation, in the afternoon, at the same place, by the same investigator.

Fully informed consent was obtained from each patient after a detailed explanation of the study protocol.

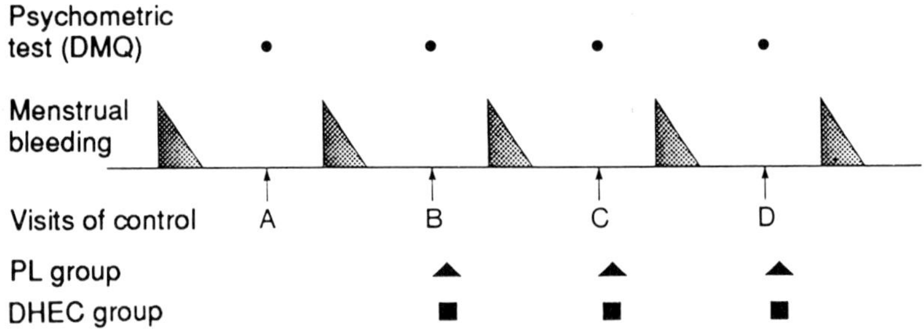

Figure 1 Experimental design

At the end of the study the trialist gave a global assessment of the efficacy of the treatment.

STATISTICAL ANALYSIS

Ordinal scale data and transformation variables were analyzed with χ^2, Mann–Whitney, Friedman and Wilcoxon tests to estimate between treatments and among observation's times within treatment difference.

Chemistry parameters were analyzed within treatment group using a paired samples t test.

RESULTS

Twenty-six patients completed the study; there were no drop-outs. Demographic data on the study subjects are given in Table 1. The mean age of the patients was 32.9 (range 20–41) years. In the DHEC group, the mean duration of PMS before treatment was 5.4 ± 2.2 years and five women reported previous unsuccessful treatment for PMS. In the placebo group, six cases reported a previous treatment for PMS.

The characteristics of the two groups, including baseline scores from MDQ, were similar.

Using a graphical representation of the MDQ symptom profile, the two groups were seen to be comparable for the quality and quantity of correlates of the PMS (Figure 2).

The overall efficacy on symptoms (decrease in total score for each item) was high in DHEC patients but not all symptoms were completely relieved in some placebo patients and a few obtained no relief (Figure 3).

A study of the effect of medication or placebo on overall mean severity of symptoms, reported by each patient showed there was significant clinical improvement after DHEC. A decrease was also observed during placebo treatment but to a lesser degree. Only four out of 13 patients (30.7%) gave final scores below 22, which was the minimum for a patient to be eligible for admission (Figure 4).

Analysis of the prospective symptom ratings showed a significantly better activity of DHEC over placebo after three cycles, also for the four symptom

Table 1 Characteristics of patients before treatment

	DHEC	*Placebo*
No. of patients	13	13
Age (years)	32.8 ± 6.3	33.1 ± 7.4
Married	6	7
Employed	10	7
Duration of PMS (years)	5.4 ± 2.2	5.8 ± 2.5
Duration of flow (days)	4.9 ± 0.5	4.9 ± 0.3
Duration of symptom/cycle (days)	8.0 ± 1.7	8.1 ± 1.9
Previously treated for PMS	5	6
MDQ* (mean score)	28.6 ± 4.6	28.9 ± 4.4

* Menstrual Distress Questionnaire

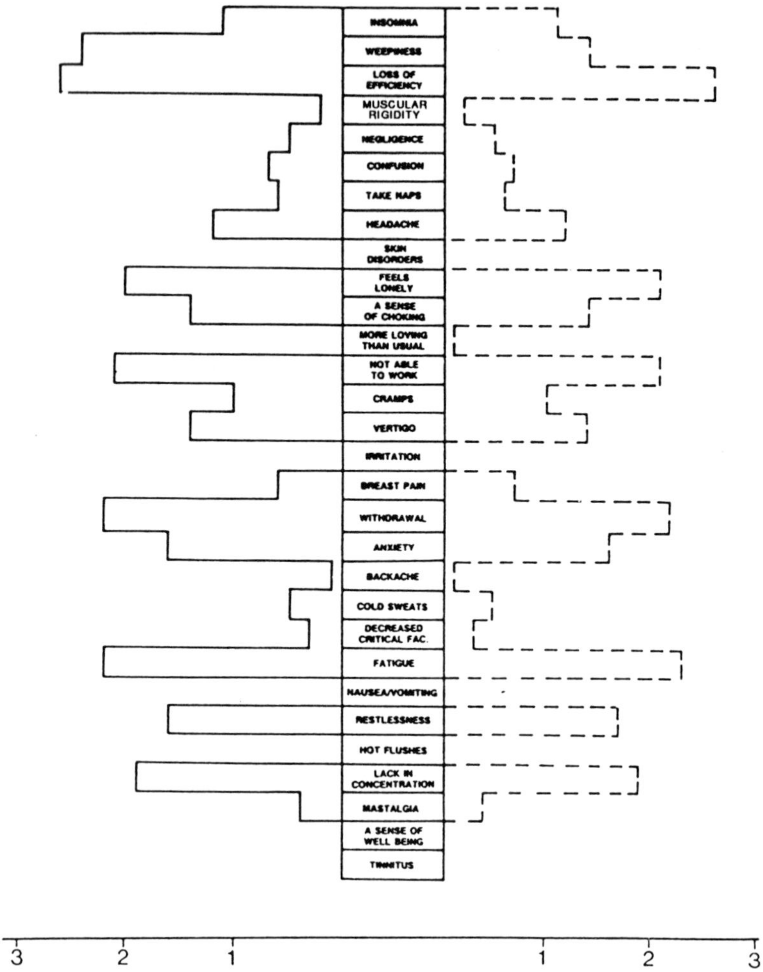

Figure 2 Profile of baseline MDQ symptoms in patients treated with dihydroergocriptine (left) and placebo (right) (mean values)

clusters in the MDQ: social relationships/behavior, physical symptoms, increase of anxiety and mood/depression (Figure 5).

DHEC was particularly effective on the physical symptoms of PMS, with significant relief of headache. Table 2 is a statistical summary of the data in Figure 5. Statistical significance was always in favor of DHEC treatment over the symptom clusters although an active response to placebo was also seen. Many of these patients admitted to problems with personal, family and sexual relationships and it is this aspect of their distress that we believe responds to placebo.

According to the investigator, treatment with DHEC or placebo had a beneficial effect (very good plus adequate) in respectively 77% and 23% of

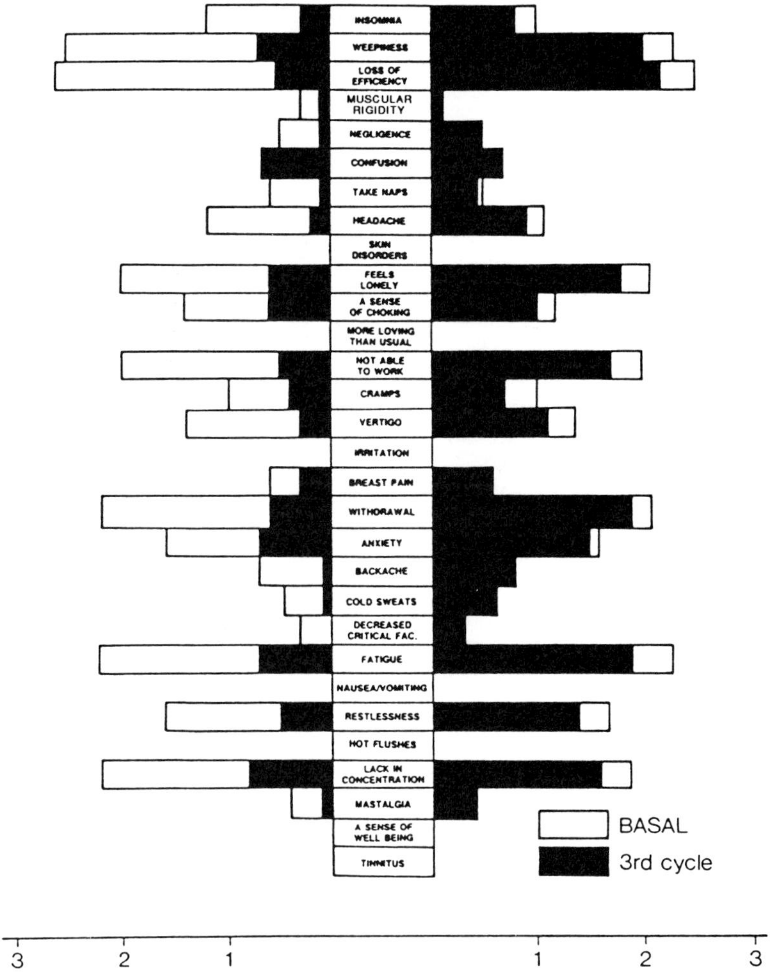

Figure 3 Profile of MDQ symptoms in patients treated with DHEC (left) or placebo (right) (mean values) at baseline and after the third cycle

the patients at the end of the trial. These frequencies are significantly different for the two groups ($\chi^2 = 10.77$; $p < 0.01$) (Figure 6).

DISCUSSION

The design of this study overcomes many of the problems found in earlier reported trials of PMS drug treatment. First of all we used the DSM-III-R to define the pathology and make diagnosis more precise; second, the women were carefully 'screened' to exclude psychiatric and physical illness; third, the study was prospective (i.e. it did not depend on retrospective recall of symptoms) and subjects were studied for one cycle during which they took

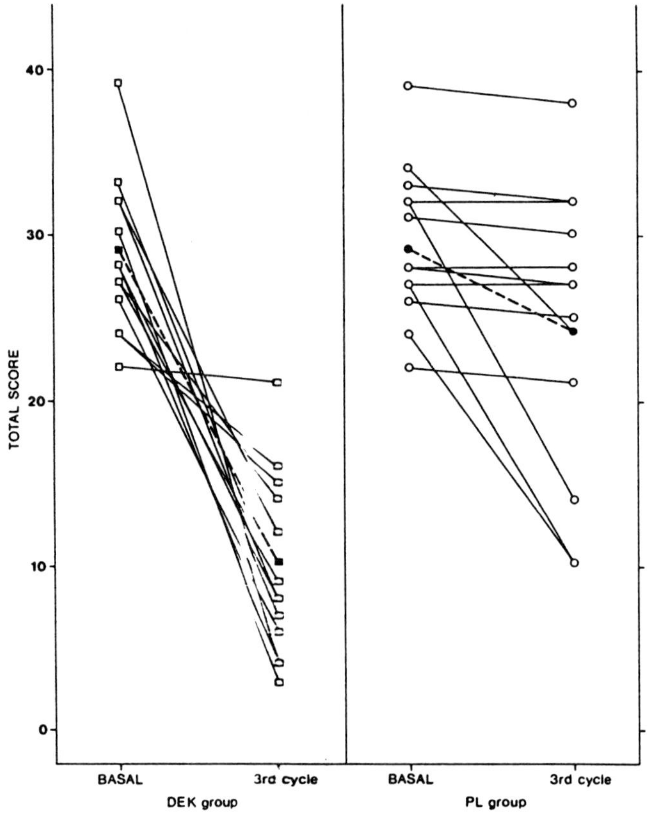

Figure 4 Responses to treatment: (□) individual patients' mean values (DHEC); (○) individual patients' mean values (placebo); (■) group mean (DHEC); (●) group mean (placebo)

no medication. Finally, the active treatment (DHEC) was compared with placebo.

The results suggest that treatment with DHEC was well tolerated and appeared effective for severe cases of PMS. From the clinical point of view, the impression is that positive results were obtained only with regard to physical symptoms (see headache) and the beneficial effects on the other symptom clusters may appear only as a consequence.

Through its natriuretic action, demonstrated in animals, DHEC might possibly reduce the fluid retention that causes edema of various organs, with the resulting symptoms: mastodynia, headache, abdominal tension and others. In the rat oral DHEC markedly raised urinary sodium output[26].

We are planning further trials with larger number of patients and longer treatment, so as to see whether any initial improvement is sustained and to confirm our hypothesis.

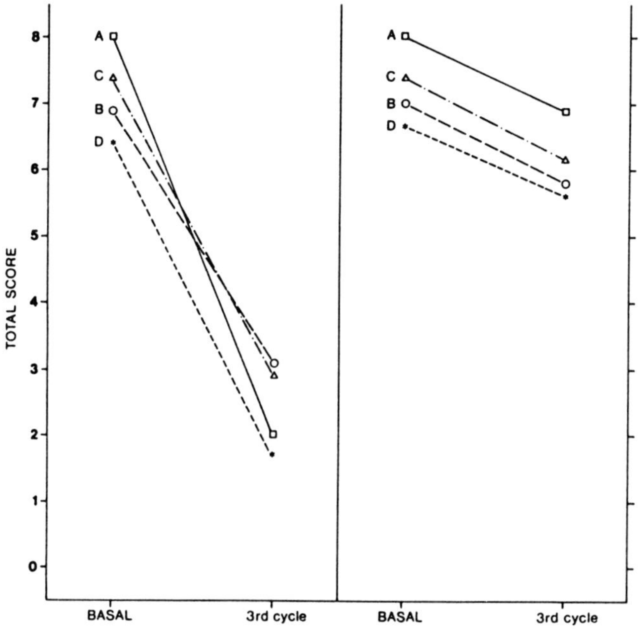

Figure 5

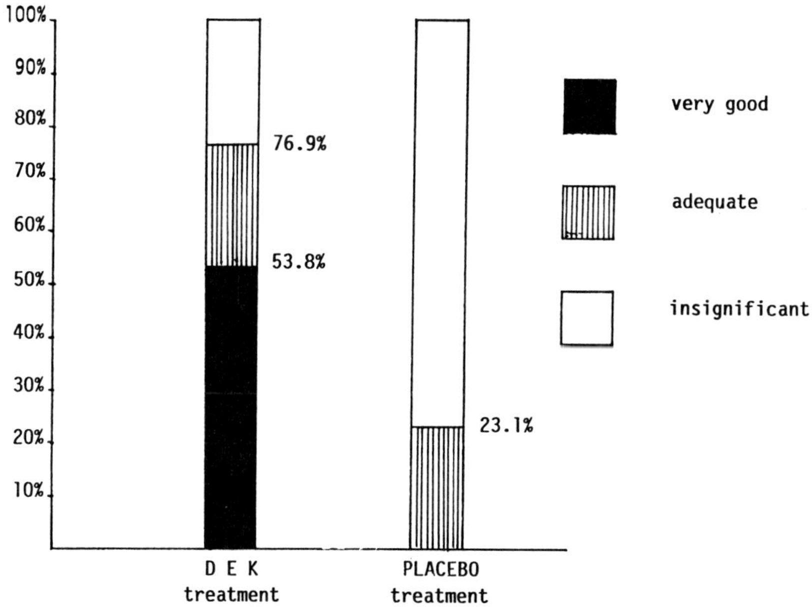

Figure 6 Physician's overall assessment of therapeutic response during DHEC (left) and placebo (right) treatment; open areas, insignificant response; hatched areas, adequate response and solid area, very good response

Table 2 Statistical analysis between times and groups of MDQ clusters; A = social relationships/behavior; B = physical symptoms; C = increase of anxiety; D = mood/depression

Clusters	*DHEC* $T_0 \rightarrow T_t$	*Placebo* $T_0 \rightarrow T_t$	*DHEC* → *placebo*
A	$p < 0.01$	$p < 0.05$	$p = 0.01$
B	$p < 0.01$	$p < 0.05$	$p < 0.05$
C	$p < 0.01$	NS	$p = 0.02$
D	$p < 0.01$	$p < 0.05$	$p < 0.05$

ACKNOWLEDGEMENT

The authors are grateful to Miss Tacchelli for her secretarial assistance.

REFERENCES

1. Gath, D. and Iles, S. (1988). Treating of premenstrual syndrome. *Br. Med. J.*, **297**, 237–8
2. Maddocks, S., Hahn, P., Moller, F. and Reid, R.L. (1986). A double-blind placebo-controlled trial of progesterone vaginal suppositories in the treatment of premenstrual syndrome. *Am. J. Obstet. Gynecol.*, **154**, 573–81
3. Dennerstein, L., Morse, C., Brown, J., Smith, M., Oats, J. and Burrows, G. (1985). Hormonal treatment for premenstrual complaints. *Gynecol. Endocrinol.*, 205–9
4. Sampson, G.A. (1979). Premenstrual syndrome: a double-blind controlled trial of progesterone and placebo. *Br. J. Psychiatr.*, **135**, 209–15
5. Van Der Meer, Y.G., Benedek-Jaszmann, L.J. and Van Loenen, A.C. (1983). Effect of a high-dose progesterone on the premenstrual syndrome: a double-blind cross-over trial. *J. Psychosom. Obstet. Gynaecol.*, **2**, 220
6. Baden, W.F. and Lizcano, H.R. (1964). Evaluation of a new diuretic drug (Quinethazone) in the premenstrual tension syndrome. *J. New Drugs*, **3**, 167–71
7. Budoff, P.W. (1987). Use of prostaglandin inhibitors in the treatment of PMS. *Clin. Obstet. Gynecol.*, **30**, 443–64
8. Puolakka, J., Makarainen, L., Viinikka, L. and Ylikorkala, O. (1985). Biochemical and clinical effects of treating the PMS syndrome with prostaglandin synthesis precursors. *J. Reprod. Med.*, **30**, 149–53
9. Wood, C. and Jakubowicz, D.L. (1980). The treatment of premenstrual symptoms with mefenamic acid. *Br. J. Obstet. Gynaecol.*, **87**, 627–30
10. Jakubowicz, D.L., Godard, E. and Dewhurst, J. (1984). The treatment of premenstrual tension with mefenamic acid: analysis of prostaglandin concentrations. *Br. J. Obstet. Gynaecol.*, **91**, 78–84
11. Mira, M., McNeil, D., Fraser, I.S., Vizzard, J. and Abraham, S. (1986). Mefenamic acid in the treatment of premenstrual syndrome. *Obstet. Gynecol.*, **68**, 395–8
12. Andersch, B. (1983). Bromocriptine and premenstrual symptoms: a survey of double-blind trials. *Obstet. Gynecol. Surv.*, **38**, 643–6
13. Elsner, C., Buster, J., Ruth, A., Schindler, L.V.N., Nessim, S.A. and Abraham, G.E. (1980). Bromocriptine in the treatment of premenstrual tension syndrome. *Obstet. Gynecol.*, **56**, 723–5
14. Ghose, K. and Coppen, A. (1977). Bromocriptine and premenstrual syndrome: controlled study. *Br. Med. J.*, **1**, 147–8
15. Benedek-Jaszmann, L.J. and Hearn-Stuztevant, M.D. (1976). Premenstrual tension and functional infertility. *Lancet*, 1095–8
16. Andersen, A.N., Larsen, J.F., Steenstrup, O.R., Svendstrup, B. and Nielsen, J. (1977). Effect of bromocriptine on the premenstrual syndrome. A double-blind clinical trial. *Br. J. Obstet. Gynaecol.*, **84**, 370
17. Massil, H.Y. and O'Brien, S. (1987). Approach to the management of premenstrual syndrome. *Clin. Obstet. Gynecol.*, **30**, 443–52

18. Rubinow, D.R. and Roy-Byrne, P. (1984). Premenstrual syndrome: overview from a methodologic perspective. *Am. J. Psychiatr.*, **141**, 163–72
19. Sharma, V. (1982). Premenstrual syndrome. *Practitioner* **226**, 1091–8
20. Reid, R.L. and Yen, S.S.C. (1981). Premenstrual syndrome. *Am. J. Obstet. Gynecol.*, **139**, 85–104
21. Ferrari, C., Rampini, C., Paracchi, A., Boghen, M. and Mailland, F. (1985). Effect of dihydroergokryptine administration on serum prolactin and growth hormone levels in normal, hyperprolactinaemic and acromegalic subjects: evidence of potent and long-lasting pituitary dopamine receptor stimulation. *Eur. J. Clin. Pharmacol.*, **27**, 707–11
22. Ho, K.Y. and Thorner, M.O. (1988). Therapeutic applications of bromocriptine in endocrine and neurological diseases. *Drugs*, **36**, 67–82
23. Faglia, G., Conti, A., Muratori, M., Togni, E., Travaglini, P., Zanotti, A. and Mailland, F. (1987). Dihydroergokryptine in management of microprolactinomas. *J. Clin. Endocrinol. Metab.*, **65**, 779–84
24. The American Psychiatric Association (1987). *Diagnostic and Statistical Manual of Mental Disorders*, Third Edition, Revised. (Washington D.C.: The American Psychiatric Association)
25. Moos, R.H. (1968). The development of a Menstrual Distress Questionnaire. *Psychosom. Med.*, **30**, 853–66
26. Coppi, G., Barchielli, M., Faini, D., Falcone, A. and Turba, C. (1988). Antihypertensive activity of alpha-dihydroergokryptine by stimulation of peripheral dopamine receptors. *Pharmacol. Res. Commun.*, **20** (Suppl. II), 112

104

Dihydroergocriptine in the treatment of premenstrual syndrome

G.B. Melis, A.M. Paoletti, R. Soldani, G.A. Mauro, F.D. Petacchi, F. Strigini, A. Zanotti and P. Fioretti*

INTRODUCTION

Several physical and psychological symptoms which begin in the luteal phase characterize a particular gynecological syndrome known as the premenstrual syndrome (PMS)[1].

A high percentage of women report that their symptoms are severe enough to be an impediment to daily business and social activities. While edema, mammary tension, nervousness and irritability are the more frequent premenstrual symptoms, other discomforts, such as headache, abdominal pain, skin alterations, etc. are also reported by women affected by PMS[1].

The observation that the blockage of ovarian function using non-steroidal compounds such as gonadotropin-releasing hormone (GnRH) agonist analogs is followed by a significant regression in the PMS syndrome implies that the etiopathogenesis of the syndrome is related to ovarian function[2]. Indeed, many observations suggest that the appearance of PMS symptoms is related to the phases of the menstrual cycle[3] and is characterized by an imbalanced estradiol/progesterone secretion[4,5]. The prevalence of estradiol activity may explain the appearance of the major premenstrual symptoms like edema, mammary tension and headache[6]. However, other data seem to suggest that normal ovarian function may be present in subjects with PMS[7–9]. In addition, some behavioral symptoms, such as nervousness, irritability and depression may probably depend on the impairment of different neuroendocrine systems at a central level more than on peripheral hormonal alterations[5,6]. Although the peripheral and central alterations may be interdependent, the function of opioidergic system may be decreased in women affected by PMS in comparison to normal controls, independently from other endocrine alterations[10,11]. In addition to the well known anatomical and functional correlations between opioidergic and other neurotransmitter systems, other studies seem to suggest that the imbalance of the dopaminergic system may also be involved in PMS pathogenesis, mainly because enhanced prolactin levels were measured in PMS patients[12–16]. Based on these data, different therapeutic strategies of PMS have been proposed like progesterone supplementation and/or progestin treatments, anti-inflammatory drugs and antidepressant agents. Interestingly dopamine agonist drugs, such as bromocriptine, are also effective in the therapy of PMS. The majority of the studies report a significant remission of PMS symptoms with bromocriptine in comparison with placebo[15–18]. However, the high incidence of side-effects with bromocriptine motivates a search for new dopaminergic compounds which are effective in the treatment of premenstrual syndrome and which have fewer side-effects. Dihydroergocriptine (DHEC) is a dihydrogenated ergot alkaloid which has been shown to possess potent dopaminomimetic properties both *in vivo* and *in vitro*[19]. The prolactin-inhibiting effect of DHEC is similar to that of bromocriptine whereas DHEC seems to induce a lower incidence of side-effects and consequently it is better tolerated by patients[20].

The aim of this study was therefore to compare the efficacy of DHEC in the management of premenstrual syndrome using a randomized placebo-controlled double-blind study design.

MATERIALS AND METHODS

Clinical and endocrine assessment

Twenty women with premenstrual syndrome, aged 19–37 years, were included in the study.

Each woman was instructed to indicate the intensity with which she experienced the most common premenstrual symptoms like edema, breast pain and tension, nervousness, irritability, depression, etc. on a special diary chart. The scoring system used to evaluate these PMS symptoms was: 0 when the symptoms were absent, 1 in the presence of mild symptoms (therapy not required), 2 when the symptoms were moderate (therapy not mandatory) and 3 when the symptoms were severe (therapy required). Objective evaluation of premenstrual symptoms was performed by the mean score of physical and psychological symptoms calculated for each woman during the last 10 days of her cycle.

Basal levels of prolactin (PRL), estradiol (E_2) and progesterone (P) were evaluated in serial blood samples collected during the luteal phase in the group of PMS women and in a group of 20 healthy women. The ratio between the values of progesterone and estrogens (P/E_2) measured during the luteal phase was also calculated using the formula: $PEL = [P(pg/ml)/E_2(pg/ml)] \times 0.01$.

The PEL index was obtained according to Mauvais-Jarvis *et al.*[21] and was used as an index of corpus luteum activity. Placebo or 10 mg of DHEC (1 tablet twice-a-day) in capsule form was randomly administered to the group of 20 women suffering from PMS in a double-blind experimental design. Capsules were administered from day 15 of the cycle until day 1 of the following cycle. The treatment was repeated for three cycles. In each patient, the same clinical and endocrine assessments performed before treatment were repeated during the treatment and during the first cycle after stopping treatment with placebo or DHEC.

Statistical analysis of results was performed by two factor Anova, χ^2, or Student's t test, as appropriate.

RESULTS

Prior to treatment, the mean luteal value of P was 6.1 ± 0.71 ng/ml in the group of PMS women. This value was significantly lower ($p < 0.05$; t test) than that measured in the control group (10.2 ± 0.61 ng/ml) (Figure 1). No significant difference was observed between the values of E_2 in PMS women (118 ± 9.7 pg/ml) and in control women (144.1 ± 11.65 pg/ml) (Figure 1). In PMS women, the pretreatment PEL index (0.6 ± 0.08) was significantly lower ($p < 0.05$; t test) than that calculated for the control group (0.79 ± 0.05) (Figure 1). In women suffering from PMS, the mean luteal PRL value before treatment was 17 ± 1.6 ng/ml. This value did not differ significantly from that of the control group (14.6 ± 1.1 ng/ml) (Figure 2).

Placebo treatment was unable to modify PRL secretion, which was similar before beginning treatment (22.5 ± 3.5 ng/ml), during all treatment cycles (the range was 11.5 ± 2.9–19.2 ± 2.1 ng/ml) and after the end of therapy

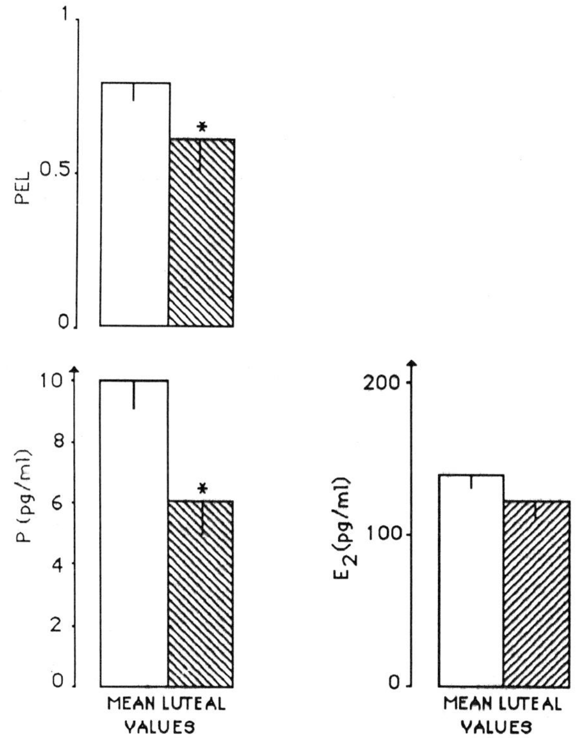

Figure 1 17-β-estradiol (E_2) and progesterone (P) blood levels and progesterone/estradiol ratio (PEL index) during the luteal phase in control women (open blocks) and in women suffering from PMS (hatched blocks); means ± SEM; $p < 0.05$

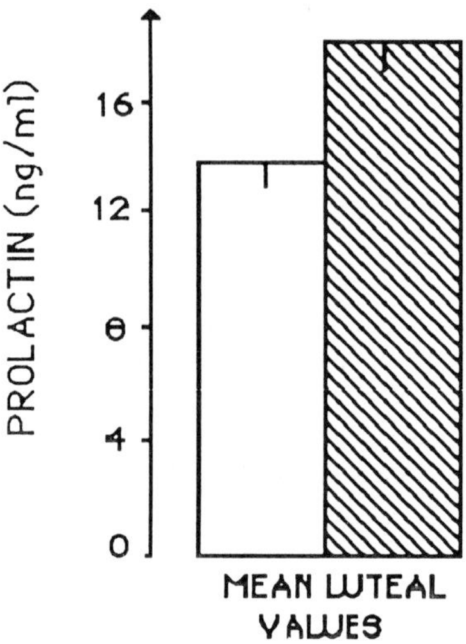

Figure 2 Prolactin secretion measured during the luteal phase in control women (open block) and in women suffering from PMS (hatched block); means ± SEM

(16.5 ± 3.2 ng/ml) (Figure 3). In the group of subjects who underwent DHEC therapy, PRL concentrations were normal before treatment, with mean values of 15.3 ± 2.7 ng/ml, similar to those of control group. As expected, the drug induced a significant decrease of PRL levels, which ranged from 3.3 ± 0.4 ng/ml to 4.3 ± 1 ng/ml during the therapy, and was followed by the restoration of PRL pretreatment values on the first month after stopping the therapy, with mean PRL values of 21.6 ± 7.7 ng/ml. No significant difference was found between the values of luteal P measured in the groups of PMS women who underwent placebo treatment (7.5 ± 1.1 ng/ml) or DHEC treatment (6 ± 0.8 ng/ml) (Figure 4). No modifications of P plasma levels were detected during and after placebo treatment (6.8 ± 0.6–7.2 ± 1.0 ng/ml) (Figure 4). During DHEC treatment, a significant increase ($p < 0.01$) in mean progesterone levels was found in all treatment cycles (8 ± 1.3–9.4 ± 1.5 ng/ml) and after the withdrawal of DHEC (9.9 ± 0.9 ng/ml) (Figure 4).

The values of E_2 levels did not vary significantly in the two groups of PMS patients taking DHEC or placebo before, during and after stopping treatment (109.6 ± 2.6 pg/ml–121.7 ± 20.6 pg/ml) (Figure 5). As for the PEL index, no significant difference was found in the values measured in women treated with placebo (0.6 ± 0.1) and those treated with DHEC (0.5 ± 0.1). In comparison to pretreatment values, no variations were observed during the 3 months of placebo administration nor after withdrawal (values ranging from 0.6 ± 0.1 to 0.4 ± 0.08 (Figure 5).

In the women treated with DHEC, the mean PEL index showed a significant increase ($p < 0.01$) during the 3 months of treatment, ranging from 0.7 ± 0.1 to 0.9 ± 0.1) (Figure 6). A persistence in the elevated PEL

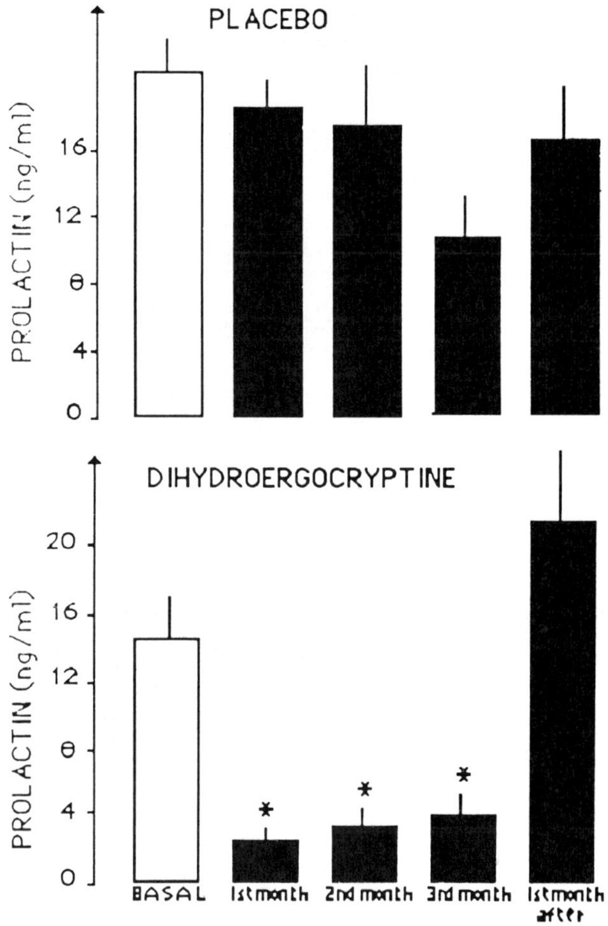

Figure 3 The effect of placebo and dihydroergocriptine on prolactin secretion in women suffering from PMS; means $\pm$ SEM, $*p < 0.01$

index was also observed after the interruption of DHEC administration (Figure 6).

Clinical results

Before the administration of placebo or DHEC, no significant difference in the mean score for premenstrual tension, premenstrual edema and psychological symptoms was observed between the two treatment groups (Figures 7 to 9). Placebo treatment was unable to modify the premenstrual edema (Figure 7), premenstrual tension (Figure 8) and psychological symptom scores (Figure 9) both during the 3 months of treatment and after the interruption of treatment.

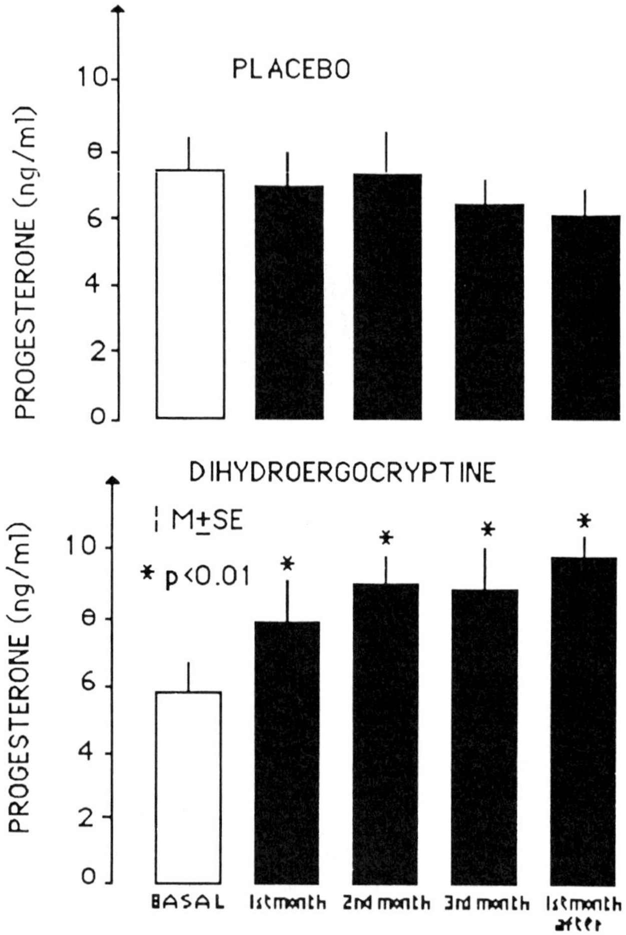

Figure 4 The effect of placebo and dihydroergocriptine treatment on luteal progesterone secretion in women suffering from PMS; means ± SEM, $*p < 0.01$

However, a significant reduction in the score of premenstrual edema was observed during each month of DHEC treatment. From pretreatment values of 2.5 ± 0.2, premenstrual edema showed a significant decrease ($p < 0.05$) to 0.9 ± 0.2 during the first month of treatment, to 0.5 ± 0.2 during the second month of treatment, and to 0.2 ± 0.2 during the third month of treatment (Figure 7). Premenstrual edema values were also significantly lower ($p < 0.05$) after the interruption of DHEC administration (0.6 ± 0.2) (Figure 7). The premenstrual tension score was unmodified during placebo administration whereas a significant reduction ($p < 0.05$) in premenstrual tension was observed during DHEC administration (Figure 8). An initial significant decrease was observed during the first month of treatment (from 2.7 ± 0.2 to 1.1 ± 0.3). In the last months of treatment, premenstrual tension values

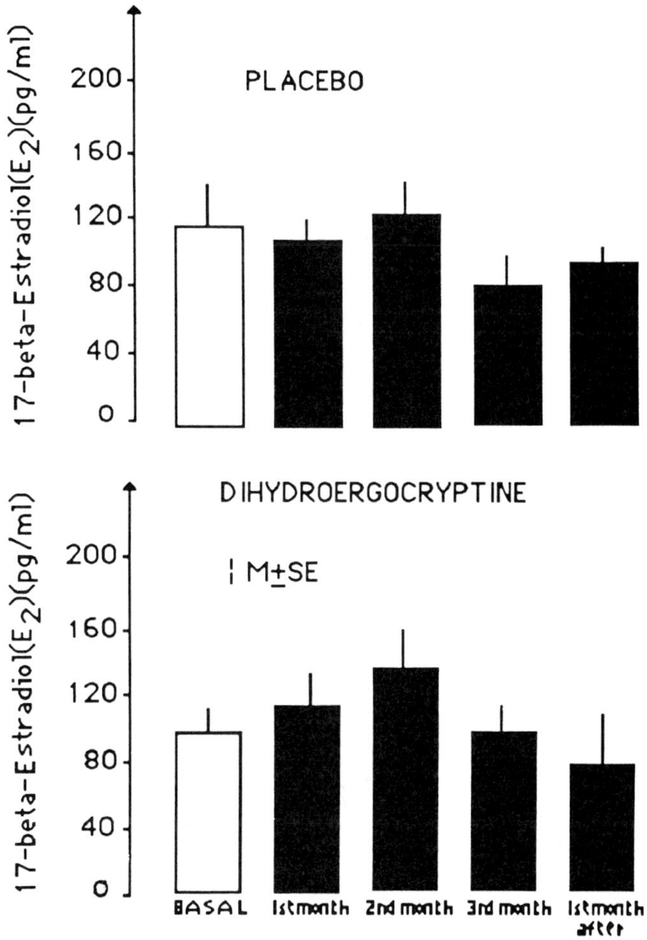

Figure 5 Effect of placebo and dihydroergocriptine on luteal 17β-estradiol secretion in women affected by PMS; means $\pm$ SEM

were often decreased with values of 1.1 ± 0.2 during the second month and 1.1 ± 0.35 during the third month of treatment (Figure 8). The premenstrual tension score was still reduced after the interruption of DHEC treatment (0.9 ± 0.3). In addition, a significant reduction ($p < 0.05$) in the psychological symptom scores was observed during DHEC treatment.

From basal values of 2.2 ± 0.2, the mean scores of the psychological symptoms decreased to 1.2 ± 0.2 during the first month. A significant reduction in psychological symptoms in comparison to basal values was also observed during the second and third months. A reduction in the intensity and/or the frequency of psychological symptoms was also observed after the interruption of treatment (Figure 9).

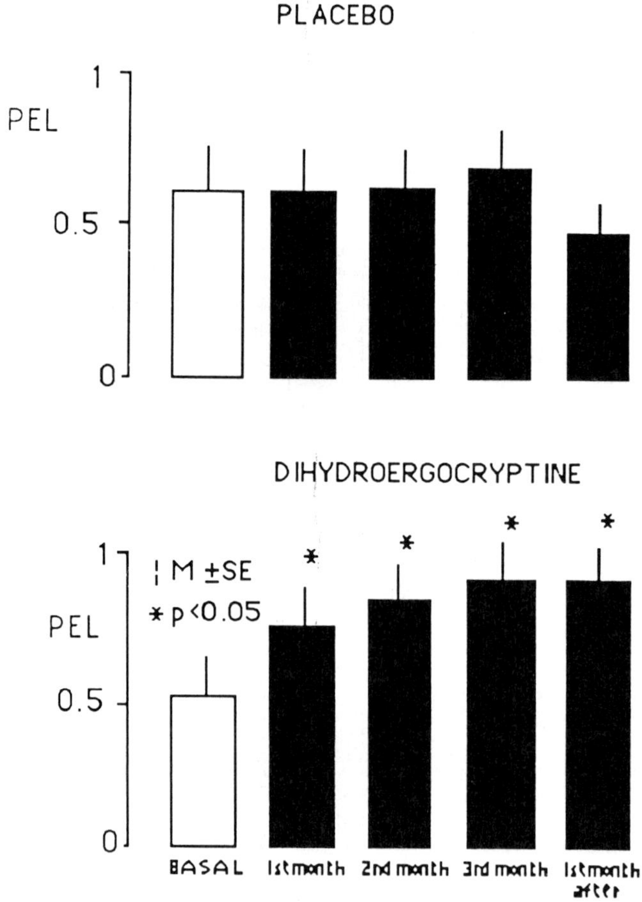

Figure 6 Progesterone/estradiol ratio (PEL index) in women affected by PMS during treatment with placebo or dihydroergocriptine; means ± SEM, $*p < 0.05$

DISCUSSION

The present data seem to confirm previous studies demonstrating that inadequate luteal phase is often present in women with PMS[4,5]. The results of this imbalance of luteal function, which is also confirmed by the impairment of PEL index, is represented by the increase of estrogenic activity due to the relative decrease of P secretion[6]. Consequently, many symptoms like cyclical edema, premenstrual tension, breast tension, cyclical pain and others may be justified by relative hyperestrogenism. It may be suggested that peripheral hormones can also induce modifications on central neuroendocrine systems, although the possibility that an imbalance in the neuroendocrine system is primary and not secondary cannot be excluded. In fact the regression in premenstrual symptoms in women treated with DHEC suggests that a reduced central dopaminergic activity is present in women with PMS, but

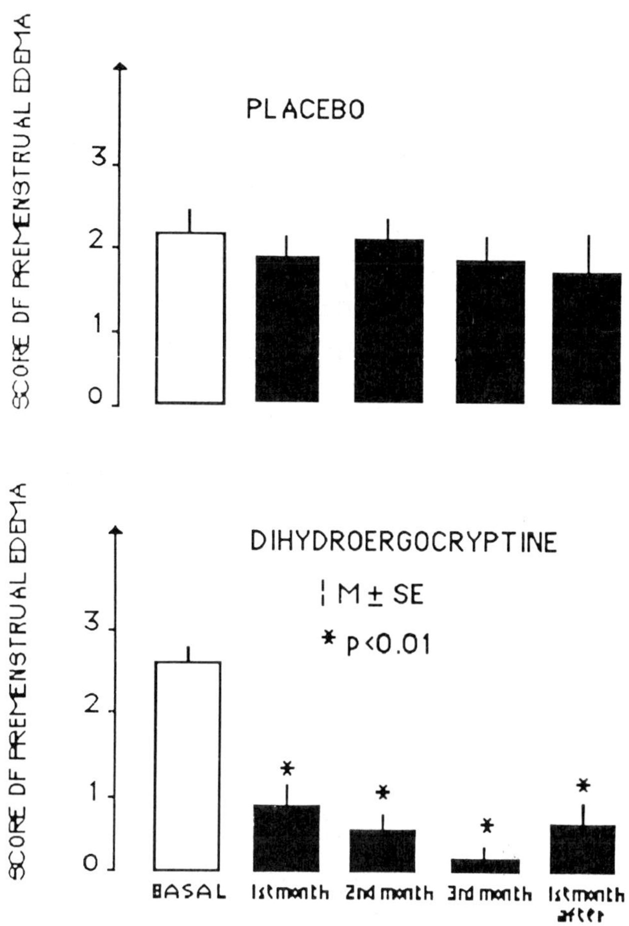

Figure 7 Effects of placebo and dihydroergocriptine on the premenstrual edema in women affected by PMS; means ± SEM, $*p < 0.01$

the origin of dopaminergic impairment is not completely understood. According to previous results obtained in patients with PMS treated with bromocriptine[15-18], DHEC also induced a significant modification in PRL and P secretion. In particular, DHEC treatment is associated not only with the expected significant reduction of PRL secretion, but also with a significant increase in P secretion which was not observed in placebo-treated women. It may then be hypothesized that normalization of the E_2/P ratio imbalance, namely the pathological reduction of the PEL index, may represent the major mechanism in the remission of PMS symptoms. However, we cannot exclude the possibility that the remission of PMS symptoms was due to the direct effects of the drug on impaired dopaminergic activity. This last hypothesis is suggested by a previous study from our laboratory demonstrating that chronic intermittent treatment with a luteinizing releasing factor

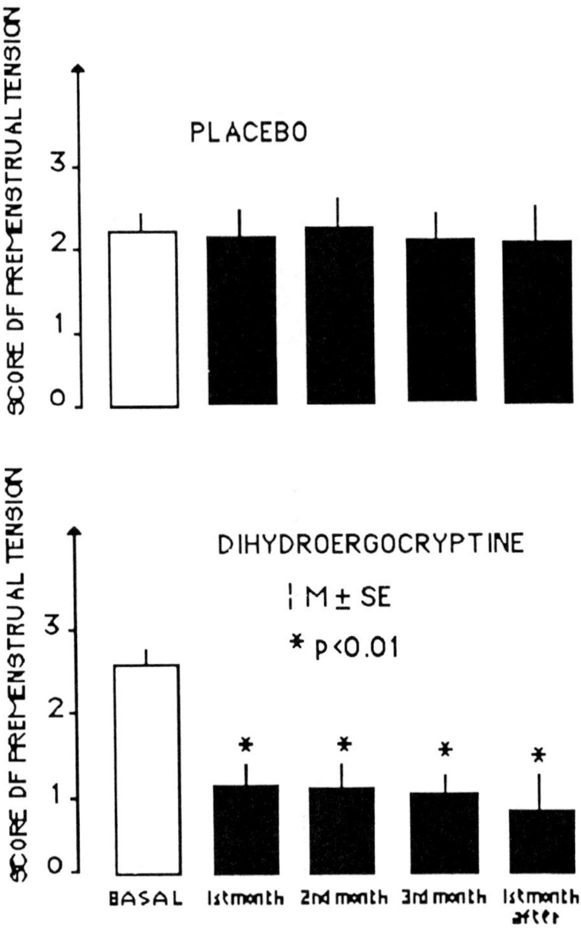

Figure 8 Effects of placebo and dihydroergocriptine on premenstrual tension in women affected by PMS; means ± SEM, $*p < 0.01$

(LRF) agonist drug induced a significant remission of PMS symptoms in conjunction with a significant reduction of progesterone secretion[22]. This paradoxical beneficial effect of the luteolytic activity of this compound seems to suggest a central action of LRF analog on behavior and neuroendocrine homeostasis. Although other data seem to be necessary to clarify the exact DHEC mechanism involved in PMS, it is evident that its administration is followed by a remission of premenstrual symptoms, as is observed with the use of bromocriptine. Since the efficacy of DHEC treatment in PMS syndrome is not associated with the appearance of side-effects, which are present in a high percentage of women treated with bromocriptine, the treatment with DHEC offers a better alternative to bromocriptine in the treatment of PMS syndrome.

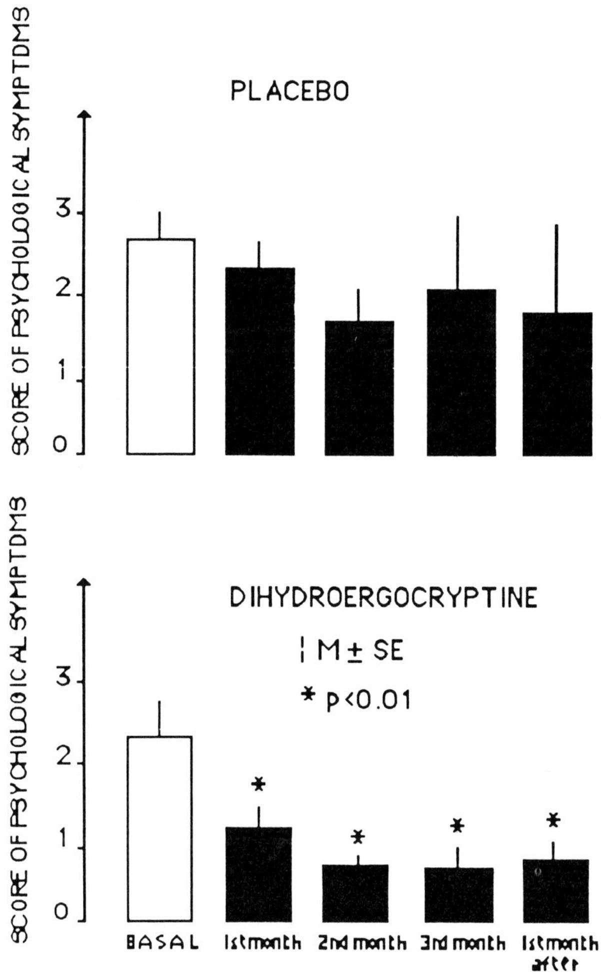

Figure 9 Effects of placebo and dihydroergocriptine on the premenstrual psychological alterations in women affected by PMS; means ± SEM, $**p < 0.01$

REFERENCES

1. Reid, R.L. and Yen, S.S.C. (1981). Premenstrual syndrome. *Am. J. Obstet. Gynecol.*, **139**, 85
2. Muse, K.N., Cetel, N.S., Futerman, L.A. and Yen, S.S.C. (1984). The premenstrual syndrome. Effects of medical ovariectomy. *N. Engl J. Med.*, **311**, 1345
3. Reid, R.L. (1983). Endogenous opioid activity and the premenstrual syndrome. *Lancet*, **ii**, 786
4. Bäckström, T. and Mattsson, B. (1975). Correlation of symptoms in premenstrual tension to oestrogen and progesterone concentrations in blood plasma. *Neuropsychobiology*, **1**, 80
5. Munday, M., Brush, M.G. and Taylor, R.W. (1977). Progesterone and aldosterone levels in premenstrual tension syndrome. *J. Endocrinol.*, **73**, 21 P
6. Morton, O., Frisk, M., Tenhunen, T. and Hartling, H. (1967). Gynecological findings in adolescence: A study of 514 patients. *Acta Obstet. Gynecol. Scand.* (suppl. 10) **46**, 10
7. Faratian, B., Gasper, A., O'Brien, P.M.S. *et al.* (1984). Premenstrual syndrome: weight,

abdominal swelling and perceived body image. *Am. J. Obstet. Gynecol.*, **150**, 200

8. Ying, Y., Soto-Albors, C.E., Randolph, J.E., Walters, C.A. and Riddick, D.H. (1987). Luteal phase defect and premenstrual syndrome in an infertile population. *Obstet. Gynecol.*, **69**, 96
9. Rubinow, D.R., Hoban, M.C., Grover, G.N., Galloway, D.S., Roy-Byrne, P., Andersen, R. and Merriam, G.R. (1988). Changes in plasma hormones across the menstrual cycle in patients with menstrually related mood disorder and in control subjects. *Am. J. Obstet. Gynecol.*, **158**, 5
10. Choung, C.J., Coulam, C.B., Kao, P.C., Bergstralh, E.J. and Go, V.L. (1985). Neuropeptide levels in premenstrual syndrome. *Fertil. Steril.*, **44**, 760
11. Facchinetti, F., Martignoni, E., Petraglia, F., Sanchez, M.G., Nappi, G. and Genazzani, A.R. (1987). Premenstrual fall of plasma beta-endorphin in patients with premenstrual syndrome. *Fertil. Steril.*, **47**, 570
12. Melis, G.B., Cagnmacci, A., Gambacciani, M., Paoletti, A.M., Caffi, T. and Fioretti, P. (1988). Chronic bromocriptine administration restores luteinizing hormone response to Naloxone in postmenopausal women. *Neuroendocrinology*, **47**, 159
13. Rasmussen, D.D., Liu, J.H., Wolf, P.F. and Yen, S.S.C. (1983). Gonadotropin releasing hormone neurosecretion in the human hypothalamus: in vitro regulation by dopamine. *J. Clin. Endocrinol. Metab.*, **57**, 1107
14. Halbreich, U., Assael, M., Ben-David, M. *et al.* (1976). Serum prolactin in women with premenstrual syndrome. *Lancet*, **i**, 654
15. Andersch, B., Hahn, L., Wendstam, C. *et al.* (1978). Treatment of premenstrual tension syndrome with bromocriptine. *Acta Endocrinol.* (suppl. 216), **88**, 165
16. Eslner, C.W., Buster, J.E., Schindler, R.A., Nessim, S.A. and Abraham, G.E. (1980). Bromocriptine in the treatment of premenstrual tension syndrome. *Obstet. Gynecol.*, **56**, 723
17. Durning, P. and Sellwood, R.A. (1982). Bromocriptine in severe cyclical breast pain. *Br. J. Surg.*, **69**, 248
18. Mansel, R.E., Preece, P.E. and Hughes, L.E. (1978). A double blind trial of the prolactin inhibitor bromocriptine in painful benign breast disease. *Br. J. Surg.*, **65**, 724
19. Fluckiger, E. and Del Pozo, E. (1980). Ergot derivatives and pituitary hormones. In Muller, E. E. (ed.). *Neuroactive Drugs in Endocrinology*, p. 169. (Amsterdam: Elsevier/North-Holland Biomedical Press)
20. Poli, M., Cocchi, D., Mailland, F., Masu, A.M., Landi, G., Craveri, A. and Mueller, E.E. (1986). Prolactin lowering effect of dihydroergokryptine in rat and in man. *J. Endocrinol. Invest.*, **9**, 31
21. Sitruk-Ware, R., Sterkers, N. and Mauvais-Jarvis, P. (1979). Benign Breast Disease I: Hormonal investigation. *Obstet. Gynecol.*, **53**, 457
22. Gambnacciani, M., Paoletti, A.M., Melis, G.B., Nepi, G., Mais, V. and Fioretti, P. (1983). Effetti paradossi degli analoghi agonisti dell 'LHRH nella donna. In Fioretti, P., Melis, G.B. and Paoletti, A. M. (eds). *Problematiche Diagnostiche e Terapeutiche in Fisiopatologia della Riproduzione*, p. 343. (Pisa: Pacini Editore)

105

The role of magnesium in the premenstrual syndrome

R. A. Sherwood and B. F. Rocks

INTRODUCTION

Women with the premenstrual syndrome (PMS) present with a wide variety of symptoms, both psychological and physical. These symptoms have been grouped into four categories by Abraham[1] as shown in Table 1. Many patients have symptoms from more than one group. It is interesting to note that some signs of magnesium deficiency, for example cardiac dysrhythmias, tremor, cramps and depression, are featured among the list of symptoms of PMS.

Magnesium was first implicated in PMS in the early 1960s by Durlach and co-workers in France[2]. They used magnesium nitrate to treat sufferers of PMS and essential dysmenorrhea, with some success. Although this work was published in the French scientific literature the use of magnesium for the treatment of PMS was largely ignored until Abraham and Lubran in 1981[3] showed that 26 patients with PMS had lower erythrocyte magnesium concentrations than did nine normal premenopausal women. There was, however, no significant difference in the plasma magnesium concentrations between the two groups of subjects. As magnesium is primarily an intracellular cation, the erythrocyte concentration should be a more sensitive indicator of body stores of magnesium than plasma magnesium measurements. The numbers of patients and controls involved in the Abraham and Lubran study were small and a larger study of blood magnesium concentrations in PMS was needed to confirm their findings.

Table 1 Abraham's classification of PMS[12]

PMS-A	*PMS-H*	*PMS-C*	*PMS-D*
Nervous tension	Weight gain	Headaches	Depression
Mood swings	Swelling of extremities	Craving for sweets	Crying
Irritability	Breast tenderness	Increased appetite	Forgetfulness
Anxiety	Abdominal bloating	Heart pounding	Confusion
		Fatigue	Insomnia
		Dizziness/fainting	

THE BRIGHTON STUDY

One hundred and five women whose PMS was assessed using a modified Moos questionaire[4] were included in the study from two sources (57 from a 'Clinic of Natural Medicine' and 48 from a Well Woman Clinic). Plasma and erythrocyte magnesium were assayed using atomic absorption spectroscopy[5]. For the erythrocyte measurement the hematocrit of the whole blood specimen was determined and then an aliquot (10 μl) of whole blood was added to 2 ml of 1% ethylenediamine tetra-acetic acid (EDTA) and the cells were lysed using a commercially available solution (Zapoglobin). The magnesium concentrations in the resulting supernatant and in a sample of plasma (20 μl in 2 ml of EDTA) were determined. After multiplying the whole blood result by two to correct for the smaller sample volume the erythrocyte magnesium concentration could be calculated using the following formula: $E = \{[(W - P) \times 100]/H\} + P$ where E = erythrocyte magnesium (mmol/l); W = whole blood magnesium (mmol/l); P = plasma magnesium (mmol/l); H = hematocrit (%).

Plasma and erythrocyte magnesium were also measured in a control group of 50 premenopausal women without symptoms of PMS. Normal ranges had previously been established for plasma and erythrocyte magnesium by this laboratory[6] – plasma magnesium 0.7–1.0 mmol/l and erythrocyte magnesium 2.0–3.0 mmol/l.

RESULTS

The results for the plasma and erythrocyte magnesium concentrations in the PMS patients and the control group are shown in Table 2. The mean erythrocyte magnesium concentration found in the PMS patients was significantly different ($p < 0.01$, Student's t test), from that of the control group. There was no significant difference in the plasma magnesium concentration between the two groups. There was a considerable overlap in the erythrocyte magnesium concentrations between the groups (controls, 1.87–3.07, PMS, 1.56–2.56) but 45% of the PMS patients had levels below the lower limit of our laboratory's normal range (<2.0 mmol/l). There was no significant difference between the patients from the two sources, one of which – the 'Clinic of Natural Medicine' might have been expected to have a higher proportion of women taking 'over the counter' vitamin or mineral preparations.

Table 2 Blood magnesium concentrations in women with PMS

	Control subjects	*Women with PMS*
No of subjects	50	105
Mean age (yr)	36 ± 9.5	38 ± 8
Plasma magnesium (mmol/l)	0.82 ± 0.05	0.79 ± 0.06
Erythrocyte magnesium (mmol/l)	2.47 ± 0.3	2.06 ± 0.25

OTHER STUDIES

Two other studies have reported concentrations of plasma and erythrocyte magnesium in patients with PMS[3,7]. The results from these studies are shown in Table 3.

The differences in the ranges of plasma and erythrocyte magnesium concentrations found in the control groups may be due to methodological differences in the assays. Both studies however show significantly lower erythrocyte magnesium concentrations in PMS patients compared to the control group. The study by Stewart and Howard shows a lower mean plasma magnesium concentration in the PMS group but the spread of results in the control group means the difference is not statistically significant[7].

TREATMENT

The Brighton study did not attempt to assess the benefits of magnesium administration to PMS patients but a number of the women reported significant improvements in their symptomatology after taking magnesium supplements (200–300 mg of elemental magnesium per day in the form of magnesium nitrate or magnesium amino acid chelate). Repeat analysis of these patients erythrocyte magnesium concentrations after 3–6 months showed that most had increased to around the lower limit of the normal range. In many patients the length of time they needed magnesium supplementation before their erythrocyte magnesium was normalized was greater than 3 months.

In 1973 Nicholas[8] reported that a high proportion of PMS patients with various symptoms showed an improvement after taking magnesium nitrate. The percentage who improved depended on the symptoms being considered as shown in Table 4. The greatest benefits were experienced by PMS-A and PMS-H patients.

Table 3 Other studies that have investigated erythrocyte magnesium status in PMS

	Abraham and Lubran[3]		*Stewart and Howard*[7]	
	Controls	*PMS*	*Controls*	*PMS*
No of subjects	9	26	—	17
Plasma magnesium (mmol/l)	0.70 ± 0.02	0.74 ± 0.02	0.9 ± 0.15	0.75 ± 0.05
Erythrocyte magnesium (mmol/l)	1.85 ± 0.1	1.28 ± 0.1	2.2 ± 0.2	1.67 ± 0.08

Table 4 Effect of magnesium nitrate on PMS in 192 patients[8]

	Patients with symptoms		*Favorable response*	
Symptoms	*Number*	*% of total*	*Number*	*% of total*
Nervous tension	179	93	159	89
Mastalgia	162	84	155	96
Weight gain	62	32	59	95
Headache	37	19	16	43

A double-blind, cross-over study by Chakmakjian *et al.*[9] showed a beneficial effect on PMS symptoms and the correction of hormonal abnormalities sometimes associated with PMS[10] by the administration of Optovite (a multivitamin/multimineral preparation giving 300 mg of Vitamin B_6 and 250 mg of elemental magnesium daily).

PATHOPHYSIOLOGY

The reason for an apparent magnesium deficit in the erythrocytes of women with PMS is not yet understood. There are four possible mechanisms which could lead to this relative cellular deficiency:

(1) Decreased intake,
(2) Reduced absorption from the gastrointestinal tract,
(3) Increased urinary excretion, and
(4) Impaired cellular transport mechanisms.

It may well be that it is a combination of two or more of these factors that leads to the reduced erythrocyte magnesium concentration. The normal plasma magnesium concentration in PMS sufferers might indicate an impaired magnesium transport mechanism or might just be due to the preservation of plasma levels at the expense of cell concentrations.

There is some evidence for an interaction between vitamins and magnesium. Vitamin B_6 at a dosage of 200 mg daily increased subnormal erythrocyte magnesium levels in a group of premenopausal women[11]. The mechanism by which this occurred was not clear.

Abraham has proposed several hypotheses to account for the symptoms of the different categories of PMS described in Table 1[12]. The role of magnesium deficiency in the production of the symptoms is discussed below.

PMS-A

It has been proposed that B vitamin deficiency could cause the hyperestrogenemia seen in patients in this category due to reduced hepatic clearance of estrogens[13]. The luteolytic effect of these estrogens results in hypoprogestrogenemia. Estrogens influence monoamine oxidase (MAO) activity selectively by inhibition of type A MAO (which deactivates noradrenaline, adrenaline, dopamine and serotonin) whilst increasing type B MAO (which deactivates only dopamine and phenylethylamine)[14]. Therefore hyperestrogenemia could cause a relative imbalance of the biogenic amines, with excess serotonin, noradrenaline and adrenaline and a relative deficiency of dopamine. Adrenaline triggers anxiety, noradrenaline promotes hostility and irritability whilst serotonin at high levels causes nervous tension, water retention and impairs an individual's ability to concentrate. Dopamine is believed to balance out the effects of these three amines by inducing relaxation and increasing mental awareness[15]. Thus an imbalance in the biogenic amines could trigger PMS-A symptoms. The role of magnesium in PMS-A may be by the depletion of brain dopamine without affecting brain serotonin or noradrenaline caused by magnesium deficiency[16]. This would exacerbate the imbalance caused by B vitamin deficiency.

PMS-H

The symptoms of PMS-H are similar to those produced by increased extracellular fluid (ECF) volume secondary to sodium chloride and water retention. The control of ECF volume is primarily mediated by aldosterone, the secretion of which is under the influence of ACTH and angiotensin. Magnesium deficiency increases aldosterone secretion and hence sodium and water retention. As aldosterone itself increases the urinary excretion of magnesium a vicious circle exists perpetuating magnesium deficiency which can only be broken by increasing magnesium intake.

PMS-C

Abraham proposes that the symptoms of PMS-C can be caused by an increase in carbohydrate tolerance in the luteal phase resulting in increased intake, increased insulin secretion and attacks of hypoglycemia[12]. The way in which magnesium may influence this is by its involvement in prostaglandin synthesis. Magnesium is a cofactor in the enzymic conversion of *cis*-linoleic acid to γ-linoleic acid which is the rate limiting step in prostaglandin (PG)E_1 synthesis. PGE_1 inhibits glucose-induced insulin secretion thus preventing hypoglycemia. Stebbing *et al.*[18] reported low erythrocyte magnesium in 14 women with reactive hypoglycemia but did not state at which point in the menstrual cycle the samples were taken.

PMS-D

Abraham has suggested that magnesium deficiency may cause the depression seen in women with PMS in the PMS-D category by promoting chronic lead intoxication by increasing intestinal lead absorption and by reducing renal excretion[11]. There is little evidence of increased lead levels in patients with PMS and this mechanism must be doubtful.

CONCLUSION

The premenstrual syndrome has such a wide spectrum of symptoms that its cause is likely to be multifactorial. A relative deficiency of magnesium in the erythrocytes of patients with PMS has now been shown by several groups. This study contained a large number of women with PMS over 40% of whom had an erythrocyte magnesium concentration below the laboratory's normal range.

Further investigations are needed to ascertain how a cellular magnesium deficit could occur in these patients. It is by no means certain that a cellular magnesium deficiency is not a result of PMS rather than being a causal factor. Assessment of urinary magnesium excretion after a magnesium load and the examination of the transport mechanisms for cations across the erythrocyte membrane to determine whether any differences exist between normal women and those with PMS might help to understand further the role of magnesium in the syndrome.

REFERENCES

1. Abraham, G.E. (1980). Premenstrual tension. *Curr. Problems Obstet. Gynecol.*, **3**, 5
2. Durlach, J. and Lemierre, L. (1962). Dysmenorrhea essentielle et deficit magnesium menstrual. *Gynecol. Obstet.*, **61**, 408
3. Abraham, G.E. and Lubran, M.M. (1981). Serum and red cell magnesium levels in patients with premenstrual tension. *Am. J. Clin. Nutr.*, **34**, 2364
4. Moos, R.H. (1969). Typology of menstrual cycle symptoms. *Am. J. Obstet. Gynecol.*, **103**, 390
5. Sherwood, R.A., Rocks, B.F., Stewart, A. and Saxton, R.S. (1986). Magnesium and the premenstrual syndrome. *Ann. Clin. Biochem.*, **23**, 667
6. Sherwood, R.A., Ariyanayagam, R.P., Rocks, B.F. and Mankikar, G.D.M. (1986). Hypomagnesaemia in the elderly. *Gerontology*, **32**, 105
7. Stewart, A. and Howard, J. (1986). Magnesium and potassium deficiencies in women with premenstrual syndrome. Presented at the *2nd European Congress on Magnesium*, Stockholm
8. Nicholas, A. (1973). Traitement du syndrome pre-menstruel et de la dysmenorrhee par l'ion magnesium. In Durlach, J. (ed.) *1st International Symposium on Magnesium Deficiency in Human Pathology*, p. 261. (Paris: Springer-Verlag)
9. Chakmakjian, Z.H., Higgins, C.E. and Abraham, G.E. (1985). The effect of a nutritional supplement Optovite for women, on premenopausal tension syndromes. *J. Appl. Nutr.*, **37**, 12
10. Fuchs, N., Hakim, M. and Abraham, G.E. (1985). The effect of a nutritional supplement Optovite for women, on premenstrual tension syndromes. *J. Appl. Nutr.*, **37**, 1
11. Abraham, G.E., Schwartz, U.D. and Lubran, M.M. (1981). The effect of vitamin B_6 on plasma and red blood cell magnesium in premenopausal women. *Ann. Clin. Lab. Sci.*, **11**, 333
12. Abraham, G.E. (1983). Nutritional factors in the etiology of the premenstrual tension syndrome. *J. Reprod. Med.*, **28**, 446
13. Biskind, M.S. and Biskind, G.R. (1945). Effect of vitamin B complex deficiency on inactivation of estrone in the liver. *Endocrinology*, **32**, 97
14. Briggs, M. (1972). Relationship between monoamine oxidase activity and sex hormone concentration in human blood plasma. *J. Reprod. Fertil.*, **29**, 447
15. Boshes, B. and Arbit, J. (1970). A controlled study of the effect of L-dopa upon selected cognition and behavioural functions. *Trans. Am. Neurol. Assoc.*, **55**, 59
16. Barbeau, A., Rojo-Ortega, J.M., Brecht, H.M. *et al.* (1973). Deficience en magnesium et dopamine cerebrale. In Durlach, J. (ed.) *1st International Symposium on Magnesium Deficiency in Human Pathology*, (Paris: Springer-Verlag)
17. Horton, J. and Biglieri, E.G. (1962). Effect of aldosterone on the metabolism of magnesium. *J. Clin. Endocrinol.*, **22**, 1187
18. Stebbing, J.B., Turner, M.O. and Franz, K.B. (1982). Reactive hypoglycaemia and magnesium. *Magnesium Bull.*, **4**, 131

Section 4 continued

Part H

Contraception

106

Effect of a new low-dose estrogen oral contraceptive combination on endocrine parameters

L. Falsetti and M.R. Schivardi

INTRODUCTION

The first oral contraceptives used contained high levels of estrogens and progestogens. These doses were then gradually reduced. Beside the reduction of the total dose, the molecular characteristics of each single component were also modified. These changes were aimed at reducing the side-effects observed during the first 10 years of oral contraceptive use[1].

The most serious side-effect linked with the use of oral contraceptives is represented by cardiovascular disease[2–4]. Though the exact mechanisms of this undesirable effect have not yet been thoroughly clarified, it is reasonable to suppose that metabolic modifications, especially of the lipid pattern, may be involved[5,6]. Numerous data suggest that estrogens and progestogens have, in many aspects, antagonistic effects[7]. However, it has been shown that the metabolic effects depend upon the doses of the steroids used. This is especially true for estrogens, while the effects of the progestogens depend principally on their intrinsic characteristics[8].

The estrogenic component of the last generation pill is entirely made up of ethinylestradiol used in average doses of 30–35 μg. The progestogens on the other hand are different. Among these, desogestrel is a progestin which has low androgenic activity. This progestin does not abolish the estrogen-induced increase of high-density lipoprotein cholesterol (HDL-C) when used in combination with ethinylestradiol[9].

The aim of this study was to evaluate the contraceptive effectiveness and the overall tolerance of a new oral contraceptive containing a very low dose of ethinylestradiol (20 μg) together with desogestrel (150 μg).

MATERIALS AND METHODS

Thirty-nine women aged between 18 and 38 years were admitted to the study. The subjects were volunteer, normal, healthy, menstruating women without contraindications to oral contraceptive use. They took a new fixed-dose combination containing only 20 μg of ethinylestradiol (EE) with 150 μg of desogestrel (DOG). Treatment was planned to run for 12 consecutive cycles. During the week before the anticipated start of their next menstrual period, hormonal profiles and biochemical data were measured. Oral contraceptive intake started on the 1st day of the menstrual period. During the third, the sixth and the 12th treatment cycle, laboratory data were measured again. Besides these, a few clinical parameters were periodically checked such as weight (pretreatment weight: 56.4 ± 7.7 kg), blood pressure and possible side-effects. Venous samples of blood were taken at approximately 09.00 from the cubital vein after an overnight fast for the assay and the measurement of the following parameters: gonadotropins (luteinizing hormone, LH; follicle-stimulating hormone, FSH), prolactin (PRL), estradiol (E_2), total testosterone (T-Te), free testosterone (F-Te), androstenedione (A), dehydroepiandrosterone sulfate (DHEAS), sex hormone-binding globulin (SHBG), corticosteroid-binding globulin (CBG). Hormonal parameters were measured by radioimmunoassay using commercial kits (Serono–Biodata, Italy). The method employed for F-Te determination in serum was a solid-phase ^{125}I radioimmunoassay (DPC, Coat-A-count, LA-CA-USA). Serum concentrations of SHBG were determined using a non-competitive 'liquid phase' immunoradiometric assay (Farmos–Diagnostica, Finland). Radioimmunoassay using a double monoclonal antibody was used to measure CBG.

The statistical significance was analyzed by Student's *t*-test.

RESULTS

Table 1 shows the variations of hormonal parameters. It is clear that the oral combination utilized induced a significant reduction of gonadotropins, estrogens and androgens.

LH and FSH underwent a significant decrease ($p<0.01$) between initial levels and those at the third cycle. LH showed a further reduction between the latter and those at 12th cycle ($p<0.01$). PRL presented a low incidence at the 12th cycle rising from 12.1 ± 5.1 ng/ml to 14.1 ± 6 ng/ml. E_2 decreased significantly ($p<0.01$) from initial levels (69.5 ± 28.6 ng/ml) to those at the third cycle (28 ± 12.5 ng/ml). T-Te and A underwent a significant decrease after three cycles of pill intake ($p<0.01$). A showed a further reduction

Table 1 Variations of hormonal parameters during pill intake

		Pretreatment	*Third cycle*	*Sixth cycle*	*12th cycle*
LH	mUI/ml	11.8 ± 3.9	7.5 ± 4.8**	7.0 ± 2.6	5.8 ± 2.1**
FSH	mUI/ml	8.3 ± 3.7	5.7 ± 3.0**	5.4 ± 2.6	4.0 ± 2.1
PRL	ng/ml	12.1 ± 5.1	13.8 ± 8.2	13.3 ± 6.5	14.1 ± 6.0
E_2	ng/ml	69.5 ± 28.6	28.0 ± 12.5**	22.2 ± 12.2	21.1 ± 9.8
T-Te	pg/ml	0.6 ± 0.2	0.4 ± 0.3**	0.3 ± 0.1	0.3 ± 0.1
A	ng/ml	1.4 ± 0.6	1.0 ± 0.4**	0.9 ± 0.5	0.8 ± 0.4*
F-Te	pg/ml	2.1 ± 1.1	1.4 ± 0.7**	0.8 ± 0.4	0.8 ± 0.3**
DHEAS	μg/ml	1.9 ± 0.8	1.3 ± 0.5**	1.2 ± 0.5	1.1 ± 0.4

* $p<0.05$; ** $p<0.01$

at the 12th cycle ($p<0.01$). DHEAS, adrenal androgen, decreased from 1.9 ± 0.8 μg/ml to 1.3 ± 0.5 μg/ml at third cycle ($p<0.01$). F-Te underwent a significant decrease after three cycles ($p<0.01$) and a further reduction at the 12th cycle ($p<0.01$).

In Table 2 the levels of the SHBG and CBG are reported. SHBG showed a significant increase ($p<0.01$) between initial levels and those at the third cycle and between the latter and those as the 12th cycle ($p<0.01$). Their increase at 12th cycle was 144%. CBG underwent a significant increase ($p<0.01$) during the first three cycles. Their increase at 12th cycle was 49%.

In the course of the observation period no pregnancies occurred. None of the 39 women of the study discontinued usage of this new low-dose combination pill. No variations were observed in weight (12th cycle $= 57.1 \pm 7.1$ kg) and arterial pressure values, nor were other important side-effects noted.

Some women reported breast tenderness during the first three cycles of pill intake (10%). Spotting occurred in seven women during the first cycle of intake (17.9%), in three during the second cycle (7.6%) and only one woman during the third (2.5%).

DISCUSSION

The study of hormonal parameters and of SHBG and CBG during oral contraceptive intake is important because it allows an evaluation of the degree of inhibition of the pituitary–ovarian axis, the hormonal environment of the oral combination and the biological activity of the progestin component.

As the pill studied induces a marked reduction of both the gonadotropin concentrations, especially LH, and the ovarian steroids, it is efficient in suppressing the pituitary–ovarian activity and therefore results in an effective contraceptive effect. The significant reduction of DHEAS reflects the inhibitory capacity of the oral contraceptives in general on the adrenal androgen secretion[10]. SHBG and CBG levels reflect the estrogenicity of the oral combination, an expression of estrogen–progestin balance of the specific preparations. The estrogenic effect on SHBG is contrasted by the progestin component in relation to degree of androgenicity[11]. Desogestrel is characterized by having a weak androgenic activity, incapable of cancelling the effect of the estrogens. CBG reflects the general estrogenicity of the oral combination which also depends by antiestrogenic effect on the progestin component. The significant increase of SHBG and CBG and the corresponding reduction of F-Te observed during this study, reflect the estrogenic environment of the pill utilized and the low androgenicity of desogestrel, in spite of the reduced dose of ethinylestradiol employed (20 μg/ml)[12].

Table 2 Variations of SHBG and CBG during pill intake

		Pretreatment	*Third cycle*	*Sixth cycle*	*12th cycle*
SHBG	(nmol/l)	57.3 ± 18.6	128.6 ± 70.0**	146.1 ± 39.5	140.2 ± 20.0**
CBG	(μg/ml)	53.6 ± 8.9	87.8 ± 20.4**	96.5 ± 19.4	80.0 ± 17.5

** $p<0.01$

We have confirmed these considerations about the estrogenicity of the studied pill with the results obtained from a study on lipoproteins during which plasma levels of total cholesterol, triglycerides, LDL-C and HDL2-C were not statistically significantly altered[13]. It is also documented that this pill has no effect on coagulation factors[14] and on glucidic metabolism[15].

In conclusion, this monophasic combination low-dose pill, (dose/cycle 0.420 versus 0.630 of other oral contraceptives), resulted in an optimal subjective tolerability with a negligible incidence of side-effects.

REFERENCES

1. Royal College of General Practitioners. (1977). Oral contraception study: mortality among oral contraceptive users. *Lancet*, **ii**, 727
2. Fraser, I.S. and Health, A. (1986). Perspective of hormonal contraceptives. *Acta Obstet. Gynecol. Scånd. Suppl*, **134**, 33
3. Plunkett, E.R. (1982). Contraceptive steroid, age and the cardiovascular system. *Am. J. Obstet. Gynecol.*, **142**, 747
4. Vessey, M.P., McPherson, K. and Johnson, B. (1977). Mortality among women participating in Oxford Family Planning Association contraceptive study. *Lancet*, **ii**, 731
5. Fotherby, K. (1985). Oral contraceptives, lipids and cardiovascular disease. *Contraception*, **31**, 367
6. Wynn, V. and Nithyanathan, R. (1982). The effect of progestins in combined oral contraceptives on serum lipids with special reference to high-density lipoproteins. *Am. J. Obstet. Gynecol.*, **142**, 766
7. Bradley, D.D., Wingerd, J., Petitti, D.B., Krauss, R.H. and Rancharan, S. (1978). Serum high-density lipoprotein cholesterol in women using oral contraceptives, estrogens and progestins. *N. Engl. J. Med.*, **299**, 17
8. Powell, M.G., Hedlin, A.M., Cerskus, I., Kakis, G., Prudham, D. and Rosenrot, P. (1984). Effects of oral contraceptives of lipoprotein lipids: a prospective study. *Obstet. Gynecol.*, **63**, 764
9. Bergink, E.W., Holma, P. and Pyorala, T. (1983). Effects of oral contraceptive combination containing levonorgestrel or desogestrel on serum proteins and binding. *Scand. J. Clin. Lab. Invest.*, **41**, 663
10. Wiebe, R.H. and Morris, C.V. (1984). Effect of an oral contraceptive on adrenal and ovarian androgenic steroids. *Obstet. Gynecol.*, **63**, 12
11. El Makhazangy, M.N. and Lawrence, D.M. (1979). Sex hormone binding globulin capacity as an index of estrogenicity in women on oral contraceptive steroids. *Clin. Endrocrinol.*, **10**, 39
12. Falsetti, L., Schivardi, M.R., Galbignani, E. and Rubessa, S. (1988). Sex hormone binding globulin and corticosteroid binding globulin during treatment with various oral contraceptives. *Gynecol. Endocrinol.*, **2**, (suppl. 2) 140
13. Falsetti, L., Schivardi, M.R. and Prandini, B.D. (1987). A new low-dose estrogen oral contraceptive combination: effect on endocrine parameters and lipid status. *Contraception*, **36**, 489
14. Miccoli, R., Orlandi, M.C., Fruzzetti, F., Melis, G.B. and Fioretti, P. (1987). Effetti metabolici di tre contraccettivi orali contenenti desogestrel, gestodene o ciproterone acetato: glicemia e insulinemia dopo OGTT a sei mesi di follow-up. In Fioretti, P. and Melis, G.B. (eds). *Aggiornamenti in Scienze Ginecologiche e Ostetriche* p. 505. (CIC ED. Int.)
15. Fioretti, P., Melis, G.B., Fruzzetti, F. and Ricci, C. (1988). Effect of a monophasic pill containing 20 μg ethinylestradiol (EE) plus 150 μg desogestrel (DOG) on coagulation factors. *Gynecol. Endocrinol.*, **2**, (suppl 2) 52

107

Effects of ethinylestradiol reduction in oral contraceptives on thrombin generation

S. Pinto, C. Rostagno, M. Costanzo, G. Costanzo, V. Bruni, D. Rosati and R. Abbate

INTRODUCTION

The contribution of estrogens to the increased risk of cardiovascular disease in women on oral contraceptives has been suggested by both laboratory investigations and epidemiological studies. Meade *et al.*[1] referred to hemostatic changes of lower degree in women treated with formulations containing 30 μg estrogen in comparison to those receiving 50 μg estrogen. The administration of a low-dose estrogen contraceptive pill was associated with significantly lower incidence of ischemic heart disease[2] and a reduced risk of venous thromboembolism[3].

The purpose of this study was to investigate the behavior of the hemostatic system during the administration of a new oral contraceptive with greatly reduced estrogen content (20 μg ethinylestradiol (EE) – 150 μg desogestrel) in order to evaluate the occurrence of blood clotting activation and changes in the functional activity of physiological inhibitors of coagulation.

MATERIALS AND METHODS

Subjects

The study was performed on 13 healthy women aged between 20 and 45 yr (mean age 37 ± 8 yr). The subjects were selected on the basis of no history of thrombotic disorders or varicose veins, normal dietary and life habits, no excess weight, no pregnancy or contraceptive treatment for at least 9 months. Four of the 13 were mild smokers (5–10 cigarettes/day).

All subjects were treated with the combination of 20 μg EE and 150 μg desogestrel. Blood samples were withdrawn before starting and after one, three and six cycles of treatment between the 25th and 28th day of the menstrual cycle from overnight fasting subjects. No subjects had taken any other drug during the 2 weeks preceding blood sampling.

Materials

Fibrinopeptide A (FPA) concentration was measured in platelet poor plasma by ELISA (Boehringer Mannheim, FRG) according to Soria *et al.*[4]. Antithrombin III (ATIII) activity was measured by amidolytic assay[5] using automated equipment (Allied Instrumentation Laboratory, Milan, Italy). Protein C activity was determined by coagulant assay (Behringwerke Marburg, FRG)[6]. Platelet count and megathrombocyte count were performed in whole blood by Platelet Analyzer 810 (Baker Instruments, Allentown PA, USA). Platelet aggregate ratio (PAR) was performed according to Wu and Hoak[7]. Routine blood clotting tests were assayed using automated equipment (Allied Instrumentation Laboratory, Milan, Italy).

Statistical analysis

The statistical analysis of the results was carried out by the Student's t test for paired data. Results are reported as mean ± standard deviation.

RESULTS

After the 1st month of pill administration FPA plasma concentrations were found to be increased (from 1.2 ± 0.4 to 2.2 ± 1.2 ng/ml, $p < 0.005$, Figure 1) in all women but two and 10 of 13 FPA values were outside the confidence limits (99%). At the end of three cycles of treatment FPA levels were intermediate (1.7 ± 1.2 ng/ml) between basal and first cycle values. Six of 13 values were outside the confidence limits (99%). After 6 months FPA plasma concentrations were slightly higher (1.6 ± 0.7 ng/ml) than before treatment and significantly lower than after one cycle ($p < 0.02$). Four of 13 were out of the confidence limits (99%).

No significant differences in ATIII activity were observed throughout the study (baseline values $97.9 \pm 6.5\%$, first cycle $98.4 \pm 6.9\%$, third cycle $99.8 \pm 8.4\%$, sixth cycle $98.7 \pm 7\%$, Figure 2).

The activity of protein C was found unchanged at all observations (baseline values $100.5 \pm 11.5\%$, first cycle $102.4 \pm 12.4\%$, third cycle $99.4 \pm 10.6\%$, sixth cycle $103.3 \pm 11.2\%$, Figure 3).

No significant differences in circulating platelet aggregate were observed during the 6 months of treatment (baseline values 0.94 ± 0.05, first cycle 0.93 ± 0.07, third cycle 0.95 ± 0.07, sixth cycle 0.94 ± 0.08).

Platelet and megathrombocyte count and routine blood clotting tests were found unmodified during the treatment.

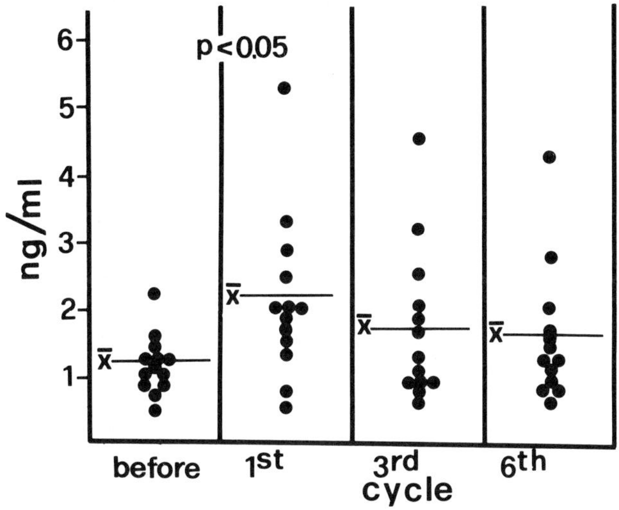

Figure 1 Fibrinopeptide A plasma levels before and after one, three and six cycles of 20 μg EE – 150 μg desogestrel treatment

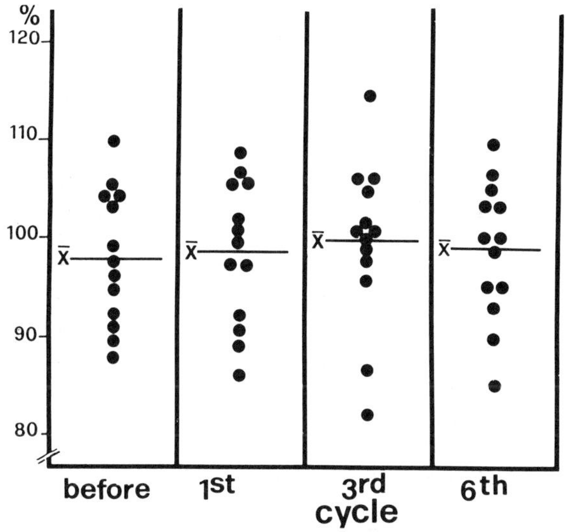

Figure 2 Antithrombin III activity before and after one, three and six cycles of 20 μg EE – 150 μg desogestrel treatment

DISCUSSION

The changes in the hemostatic system observed during treatment with oral contraceptives have been principally attributed to the estrogen content. The

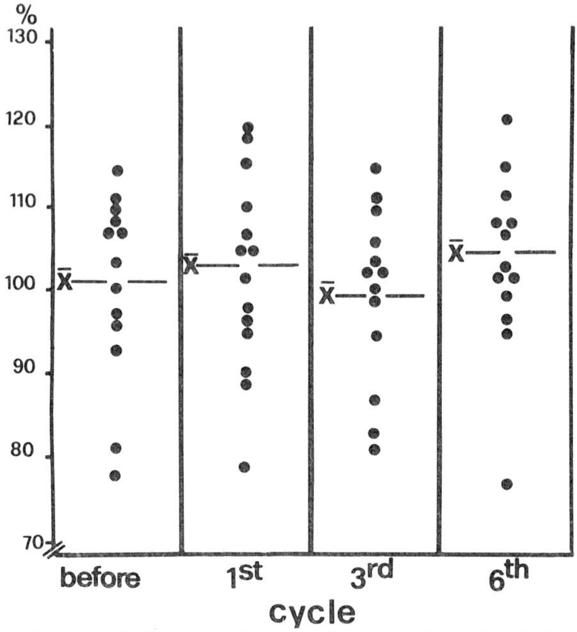

Figure 3 Protein C activity before and after one, three and six cycles of 20 μg EE – 150 μg desogestrel treatment

introduction of low-dose estrogen preparations has notably reduced both the hemostatic alterations[1,8,9] and the risk of thrombotic disease[10].

In this study the occurrence of a hypercoagulable state has been evaluated by investigating FPA, the first fragment split from fibrinogen by trace amounts of thrombin[11]. We also planned the study of the two most important physiological blood clotting inhibitors, ATIII and protein C, by methods based on functional activity and not on immunological techniques. Sex hormones in fact may stimulate the hepatic synthesis of these proteins and immunological assays may detect higher levels due to circulating non-functional protein[12].

Our findings show that during the administration of a pill with further reduced estrogen content (20 μg EE–150 μg desogestrel) an early, but transitory, increase of FPA plasma levels occurs. In fact FPA was found to be significantly increased after the first month of treatment but subsequently FPA values showed a tendency to decrease and after 3 and 6 months they did not significantly differ from basal levels, even if they were found to be slightly higher. Other authors[13] reported a significant increase of FPA values after 6 months. However from this study it is not possible to infer the time-course of FPA enhancement.

The FPA increase observed in our study at the first month of treatment was of limited degree and notably lower in comparison to that reported during the administration of 30 or 50 μg EE–desogestrel preparations.

Inauen *et al.*[14] found a fourfold increase of FPA when women were on 50 μg estrogen pill and a twofold enhancement was referred to by Melis *et al.*[15] and our group[16] during the administration of the association with 30 μg EE.

The small degree of thrombin generation increase accounts for the absence of modifications of physiological inhibitors, ATIII and protein C, so suggesting that no consumption of these proteins occurs. Similarly the absence of platelet changes is in keeping with a thrombin concentration lower than 0.01 iu/ml, which represents the amount able to trigger platelet activation[12].

In conclusion these findings seem to indicate that the further reducton of EE content in oral contraceptives can contribute to limit the changes of the hemostatic system, affecting thrombin generation minimally.

REFERENCES

1. Meade, T.W., Haines, A.P., North, W.R.S., Chakrabarti, R., Howarth, D.J. and Stirling, Y. (1977). Haemostatic, lipid and blood pressure profiles of women on oral contraceptives containing 50 μg or 30 μg of oestrogen. *Lancet*, **ii**, 948–51
2. Meade, T.W., Greenberg, G. and Thompson, S.G. (1980). Progestogens and cardiovascular reactions associated with oral contraceptives and a comparison of the safety of 50 and 30 oestrogen preparations. *Br. Med. J.*, **280**, 1157–61
3. Vessey, M., Mant, D., Smith, A. and Yeates, D. (1986). Oral contraceptives and venous thromboembolism: findings in a large prospective study. *Br. Med. J.*, **292**, 526
4. Soria, J., Soria, C. and Ryckewaert, J.J. (1980). A solid phase immunoenzymological assay for the measurement of human Fibrinopeptide A. *Thromb. Res.*, **20**, 425–9
5. Philo, R.D. and Gaffney, P.J. (1982). Comparison of antithrombin III assays using biological and chromogenic substrates. *Br. J. Haematol.*, **50**, 147–56
6. Bertina, R.M., Broekmans, A.W., Krommenhoek-Van Es, C. and Wijngarden, A. (1984). The use of a functional and immunologic assay for Protein C in the study of heterogeneity of congenital Protein C deficiency. *Thromb. Haemost.*, **51**, 1–5
7. Wu, K.K. and Hoak, J.K. (1974). A new method for the quantitative detection of platelet aggregates in patients with arterial insufficiency. *Lancet*, 923–4
8. Bruni, V., Rosati, D., Abbate, R., Pinto, S., Bucciantini, S., Verni, A., Costanzo, G. and Costanzo, M. (1986). Platelet and coagulation functions during triphasic oestrogen-progestogen treatment. *Contraception*, **33**, 39–46
9. Bruni, V., Bucciantini, S., Rosati, D., Abbate, R. and Pinto, S. (1987). Long term study of the effects of a combination of cyproterone acetate and ethinylestradiol on the hemostatic system. *Fortschr. Med.*, **3**, 51–6
10. Meade, T.W. (1988). Risks and mechanisms of cardiovascular events in users of oral contraceptives. *Am. J. Obstet. Gynecol.*, **158**, 1646–52
11. Nossel, H.L., Buther, V.P., Canfield, R.D., Yudelman, I., Ti, M., Spanondis, K. and Soland, T. (1975). Potential use of fibrinopeptide A measurements in the diagnosis and management of thrombosis. *Thromb. Diath. Haemorrh.* (*Stuttgart*), **33**, 426–34
12. Cohen, H., Mackie, I.J., Walshe, K., Gillmer, M.D.G. and Machin, S.J. (1988). A comparison of the effects of two triphasic oral contraceptives on haemostasis. *Br. J. Haematol.*, **69**, 259–63
13. Fioretti, P., Fruzzetti, F., Navalesi, R., Ricci, C., Miccoli, R., Cerri, M., Orlandi, M.C. and Melis, G.B. (1987). Clinical and metabolic study of a new pill containing 20 μg ethinylestradiol plus 0.150 mg desogestrel. *Contraception*, **35**, 229–43
14. Inauen, W., Baumgartner, H.R., Haeberli, A. and Straub, P.W. (1987). Excessive deposition of fibrin, platelets and platelet thrombi on vascular subendothelium during contraceptive drug treatment. *Thromb. Haemostas.*, **57**, 306–9
15. Melis, G.B., Fruzzetti, F., Paoletti, A., Carmassi, F. and Fioretti, P. (1984). Fibrinopeptide A plasma levels during low-estrogen oral contraceptive treatment. *Contraception*, **30**, 575–83
16. Bruni, V., Rosati, D., Bucciantini, S., Verni, A., Abbate, R., Costanzo, M., Pinto, S. and

Costanzo, G. (1987). Desogestrel in monophasic E/D combination: monitoring of endocrine parameters and evaluation of hemostatic function. *Acta Eur. Fertil.*, **18**, 277–80
17. Kaplan, K.L., Nossel, H.L., Drillings, M. and Lesznik, G. (1978). Radioimmunoassay of platelet factor 4 and thromboglobulin: development and application to studies of platelet release in relation to Fibrinopeptide A generation. *Br. J. Haematol.*, **39**, 129–46

108

Multicenter clinical trial on the new oral contraceptive containing 20 μg ethinylestradiol

P. Bilotta and M. Casanica

INTRODUCTION

A long-standing attempt has been made to render oral contraception not only safe and effective but also a method willingly accepted by the woman. So far, however, the pill has been associated with side-effects although these have been greatly reduced through the use of low hormonal dosages and non-androgenic progestogens[1].

The emphasis is no longer on an increased thromboembolic risk nor, for the last 10 years, on a higher incidence of cardiovascular diseases[1-6]. Nevertheless, pill and tolerability are still buzzwords, i.e. although safe and without serious sequelae, oral contraception is sometimes associated with minor complaints which make it tolerable but not fully accepted.

The pill is a very peculiar pharmaceutical product, because its use for contraceptive purposes does not make it a therapeutic instrument. If it makes sense to tolerate the side-effects of a drug that has been prescribed to fight a disease, it is less reasonable to accept the unpleasant effects of a product which is not a cure. Weight increase, cellulitis, nausea, vomiting, headaches, mastodynia and other subjective ailments, are still frequent complaints among the users of oral contraceptives, and they are mainly ascribed to the estrogen component of the pill[7,8].

Furthermore, while non-androgenic progestogens have favorable effects on the lipidic and the glucidic metabolism, low estrogen dosages still have an influence on the hemostatic equilibrium. In fact, there is biochemical evidence that the 30 μg of ethinylestradiol (EE) contained in the latest generation pills affect the fibrinopeptide A plasma level, one of the most sensitive hemocoagulation indices[9]: hence the attempt to obtain an optimal estrogen dosage without any effect on coagulation.

Experience shows that it is not desirable to eliminate estrogen in the oral contraceptives. In fact, pills with progestogen alone have proved less effective and provide insufficient control of the cycle[10,11]. Hence the search for an estroprogestin combination to reach the most favorable estrogen level and greater compliance with physiological metabolism.

An estroprogestin combination, containing 20 μg of EE and 150 μg of desogestrel (Mercilon; Organon), has been formulated. According to metabolic studies on hemostatic parameters[12], this oral contraceptive has no effect on coagulation; in fact, a slight increase of fibrinopeptide A was reported during the first intake cycle only, with a subsequent return to pretreatment levels. An extended clinical trial was conducted in order to evaluate the clinical characteristics of the new formulation.

MATERIAL AND METHODS

One thousand and sixty-eight women entered the study aged between 18 and 45 (Table 1); 740 of them had not used oral contraceptives in the 3 months preceding the start of the survey (new users), 328 switched directly from another estroprogestin to the new formulation (switchers). Before the treatment each woman underwent an accurate historical investigation, gynecological examination, weight, height and blood pressure measurements, and a blood sample to determine the following hematological parameters: total cholesterol, high density (HDL) and low-density (LDL) lipoprotein cholesterol, total triglycerides, transaminases (SGOT and SGPT), total bilirubin, γ-GT, glycemia, total proteins. Further information was collected about contraceptive methods previously used.

The women were instructed to take the pill for 21 consecutive days, starting from the 1st day of their menstrual period.

Each was provided with a diary in which she had to report whether she had not taken one or more pills, the characteristics of any bleeding occurring during the intake days; in this connection, the woman had to specify the day of the cycle on which the bleeding occurred, its duration in days and the number of sanitary towels used per day.

The follow-ups were scheduled at the end of the first, third and sixth cycles; 170 women were followed for 12 cycles. At the follow-up visits, the woman had to submit the diary duly completed, and the results of hematochemical tests made between the 18th and 21st days of the treatment cycle. Body weight, blood pressure and any disorder spontaneously reported were carefully evaluated. In drop-out cases, the reason for leaving was indicated.

In line with the international nomenclature for cycle control, the following definitions were used:

Table 1 Age distribution of women included in the study

Age	*Women*	%
<20	107	10.0
20–25	373	34.9
26–29	223	20.9
30–34	190	17.8
35–39	125	11.7
>39	50	4.7

(1) *Spotting* Slight bleeding occurring during intake days, that does not require any special hygienic measure, or, at most, a sanitary towel/day.

(2) *Breakthrough bleeding (BTB)* Irregular bleeding occurring during intake days which calls for more than one sanitary towel/day.

(3) *Withdrawal bleeding* Bleeding similar to a menstruation which begins in the non-intake period.

Statistical evaluations were performed according to the Anova 1 way test.

RESULTS

Of the 1068 women entering the study; 170 were followed up to the 12th cycle, 1004 women completed six treatment cycles. Of the 170 women followed for 12 cycles, 156 completed the study. Altogether, 7127 cycles were studied.

Data were collected on the total number of women examined and separately, on the new users and switchers.

The contraceptive methods used before the study are listed in Table 2.

Hematochemical parameters

Fasting glycemia, protidemia, and liver function indices (bilirubin, γ-GT, SGOT, and SGPT) did not change significantly.

Lipid profile

During treatment the LDL levels significantly decreased ($p<0.005$), while HDL levels significantly increased ($p<0.005$) (Figure 1).

Contraceptive effectiveness

During the 7127 cycles studied, no pregnancy occurred, with a Pearl Index equal to 0.00, even though in 234 cycles (3.3%) at least one pill had been forgotten. The number of pills forgotten in each cycle versus the total number of women, is illustrated in Table 3.

Table 2 Contraceptive methods used before the treatment

	Number	%
None	326	30.5
Oral	328	30.7
IUD	110	10.3
Others	304	28.5

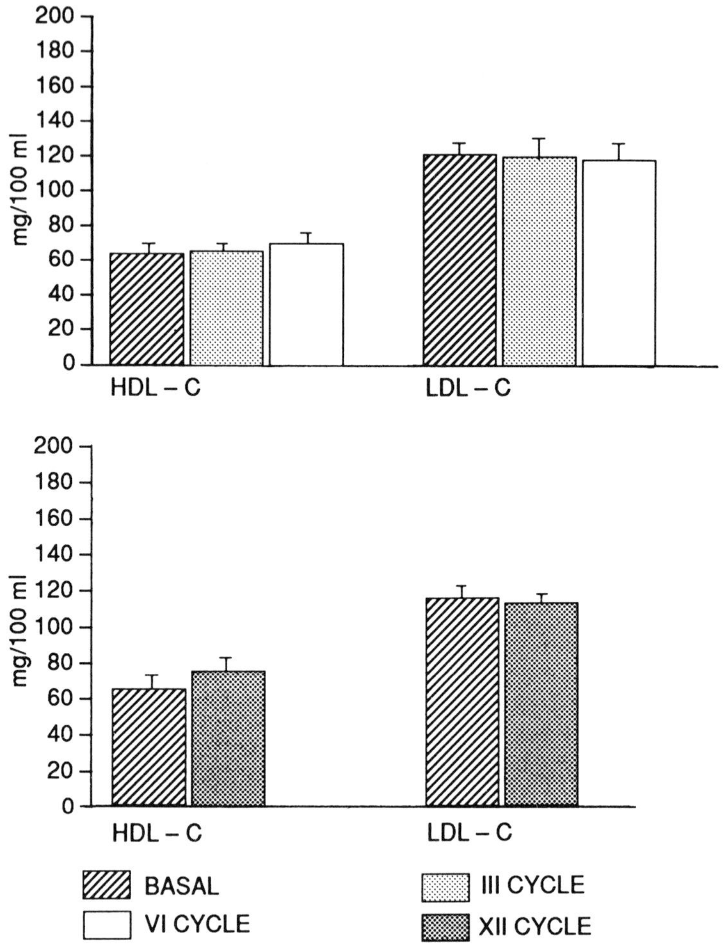

Figure 1 Lipid profiles of HDL and LDL cholesterol (a) a comparison between basal levels and the third and sixth cycles and (b) a comparison between basal levels and the 12th cycle; * $p<0.005$

Table 3 Pills forgotten

Pills forgotton per cycle	*Cycles*						
	I	*II*	*III*	*IV*	*V*	*VI*	*XII*
1	48	36	20	24	36	20	2
2	12	8	4	12	—	4	—
3	3	—	—	4	—	—	—
>3	1	—	1	—	—	—	—

Cycle control

Cycle control proved effective from the first treatment cycle and was comparable to that of higher dosage formulations[13–19] (Tables 4 and 5).

Among switchers, the incidence of irregular bleeding was lower than among new users. The incidence of spotting and BTB, starting from the first cycle, was lower than the pretreatment values. In many studies, the incidence of irregular bleeding is calculated according to the total number of cycles studied. According to this criterion, the incidence of spotting and BTB during treatment with the new estroprogestin, is comparable to that of other oral contraceptives of the new generation[13–19].

In fact, spotting and BTB occurred in 5.8% and in 1.7% respectively of the first six cycles of treatment, with an overall incidence of irregular bleeding equal to 7.4%. Withdrawal bleeding appeared in 99.6% of the women studied, with a prevalence of moderate flows, and a duration of 4–6 days (Table 6).

Side-effects

The women studied did not suffer from any serious side-effects. Subjective symptoms such as nausea, vomiting, headache, breast tension, etc. were

Table 4 Cycle control in total number of women, switchers and new users and the average duration of irregular bleeding

		Cycle						
	Basal	*I*	*II*	*III*	*IV*	*V*	*VI*	*XII*
Total no. of women								
Spotting (%)	5.4	16.5	8.8	4.3	2.0	1.5	1.2	0.8
BTB (%)	1.3	4.1	2.9	1.2	0.8	0.5	0.4	—
Switchers								
Spotting (%)	6.4	13.8	6.1	2.8	0.9	0.9	0.9	—
BTB (%)	1.8	3.4	2.2	1.2	—	0.6	—	—
New users								
Spotting (%)	5.0	17.8	9.7	4.9	2.4	1.8	1.3	1.3
BTB (%)	1.1	4.4	3.2	1.1	1.1	0.4	0.6	—
Average duration (days)								
Spotting	—	3.19	2.93	2.91	2.69	2.68	2.61	2.00
BTB	—	3.61	3.17	3.14	3.07	3.02	2.97	—

Table 5 Percentage of irregular bleeding-free days

Cycles	%
I	97.46
II	98.72
III	99.41
IV	99.72
V	99.80
VI	99.85
XII	99.95

Table 6 Duration and amount of withdrawal bleeding in cycles III, VI and XII compared with basal values

	Basal	*III*	*VI*	*XII*
Amount of bleeding (%)				
Slight	12.2	16.7	22.3	33.3
Moderate	62.1	71.5	74.7	66.7
Abundant	27.6	11.8	3.0	—
Duration of bleeding (%)				
<4 days	14.1	17.3	20.9	30.1
4–6 days	79.7	79.0	77.6	69.9
>6 days	6.3	3.8	1.5	—

largely reported before the treatment and they were greatly reduced during the study. Occurrence of these complaints for the first time during treatment was very rare and they disappeared from the sixth cycle onwards (Table 7). Headache, nausea and vomiting decreased during the treatment and there was marked improvement in cases of acne and hirsutism.

Blood pressure

The percentage distribution of systolic and diastolic pressure did not change nor did the range of the values (Table 8).

Body weight

The women were sub-divided into four groups: (underweight, normal weight, overweight and obese), according to their body weight and height. The results show that the new combination does not affect body weight (Table 9).

Reasons for drop-out

During the first six cycles of treatment, 64 women gave up the treatment. Of the 170 subjects studied up to the 12th cycle, 14 did not complete the protocol.

Table 7 Minor side-effects (%) in total (T), pre-existing (P) and new (N) cases

		Cycle I			*Cycle III*			*Cycle VI*			*Cycle XII*		
	Basal	*T*	*P*	*N*	*T*	*P*	*N*	*T*	*P*	*N*	*T*	*P*	*N*
Nausea	2.3	3.2	2.2	1.0	0.6	0.4	0.2	0.3	0.3	—	—	—	—
Vomiting	1.5	0.5	0.3	0.2	0.3	0.2	0.1	—	—	—	—	—	—
Breast tension	7.8	7.4	6.3	1.1	3.6	3.3	0.3	1.9	1.9	—	13	1.3	—
Nervousneess	12.0	3.7	3.3	0.4	1.1	0.9	0.2	0.2	0.2	—	—	—	—
Headache	7.0	4.8	3.5	1.3	0.9	0.8	0.1	0.1	0.1	—	—	—	—
Acne	5.1	4.8	4.1	0.7	4.1	3.9	0.2	3.4	3.4	—	1.9	1.9	—
Hirsutism	2	1.8	1.4	0.4	1.5	1.3	0.2	1.3	1.3	—	1.3	1.3	—

Table 8 Percentage distribution of systolic and diastolic pressure

	Basal	*III*	*VI*	*Basal*	*XII*
Systolic pressure					
<120	3.9	3.7	3.5	5.8	3.2
120–130	72.5	72.8	73.0	73.7	72.4
131–140	23.3	23.2	23.2	19.5	23.1
141–150	0.2	0.2	0.2	—	0.6
151–160	0.1	0.1	0.1	0.6	0.6
>160	—	—	—	—	—
$\bar{x}$	127.01	127.02	127.04	126.60	127.28
SD	4.98	4.95	4.90	5.37	5.26
Range	100–155	100–155	100–150	100–155	100–150
Diastolic pressure					
<85	96.6	96.5	96.3	96.8	95.9
86–90	3.0	3.2	3.4	1.9	3.9
91–95	0.2	0.1	0.1	—	0.6
96–100	0.1	0.1	0.1	1.3	0.6
>100	0.1	0.1	0.1	—	—
$\bar{x}$	77.31	77.31	77.32	77.38	77.31
SD	1.80	1.79	1.75	2.29	2.33
Range	65–105	65–105	65–100	65–95	65–95

Table 9 Body weight (percentage distribution) during treatment compared with basal values

	Underweight	*Normal*	*Overweight*	*Obese*
Basal	21.8	54.2	22.3	1.7
III	21.8	55.2	21.5	1.5
VI	20.7	56.6	21.5	1.2
Basal	21.2	54.7	22.9	1.2
XII	19.2	60.9	19.2	1.3

The low incidence of drop-outs and the reasons related show that the new formulation is largely acceptable (Table 10).

DISCUSSION

The results show that 20 μg EE and 150 μg desogestrel are a highly effective, well tolerated and fully balanced combination with good cycle control, negligible incidence of minor complaints and no effect on metabolic parameters.

No woman in the study became pregnant, not even those who forgot to take three or more pills during the same treatment cycle.

Spotting and BTB were at the same level as in other oral contraceptives and tended to decrease considerably as early as the second treatment cycle[13–19]. If the incidence of irregular bleeding is calculated over the number of cycles studied in the first 6 months of therapy, spotting accounts for about 5.8% and BTB for around 1.7%, with an overall incidence of irregular bleeding (spotting + BTB) equal to 7.4%. Amenorrea occurred in only 4 women (0.6%). In the remaining 99.4% there was regular withdrawal bleeding

Table 10 Reasons for drop-out

Cycles	*I*	*III*	*VI*	*XII*
Headache	1	1	2	—
Nausea/vomiting	2	1	1	1
Nervousness	—	2	2	—
Depression	—	1	—	—
Weight gain	—	2	—	1
Desire to become pregnant	—	2	7	2
Amenorrea	1	3	—	—
Spotting	5	3	2	2
Personal reason	—	3	10	3
Lost to follow-up	1	4	8	5
Total	10	22	32	14

which improved over time. In fact, the amount and duration of flow steadily decreased during therapy with regularization of overabundant and overextended flows.

The incidence of subjective complaints was negligible, while the pretreatment ailments were significantly reduced.

Similarly, desogestrel does not hamper estrogen-dependent synthesis of HDL in the liver and does not increase that of LDL, thus providing a favorable lipid profile even in women over 35 years of age who are traditionally more exposed to lipid metabolic disorders. This clinical evidence is supported by the results of studies on sex hormone-binding globulin (SHBG) plasma levels during treatment with 20 μg of EE and 150 μg of desogestrel[23-25]. In fact, this formulation was shown to increase SHBG considerably.

The simultaneous decrease in the percentages of the underweight, overweight and obese women, show the neutral effect of the new combination on the body weight.

As shown by the unchanged distribution and range of the values, the new combination does not effect blood pressure.

The liver function parameters studied (bilirubin, γ-GT, SGOT and SGPT) did not show significant variations and glycemia was always at normal levels.

The new preparation is well accepted, thanks to the good cycle control and the very low incidence of minor side-effects; in addition it has complete metabolic safety, thanks to the unmodified hemostatic equilibrium and the favorable lipid profile[12].

Therefore, because of its peculiar characteristics, the new combination is expected to improve oral contraception, allowing a wide number of women to adopt a highly effective, safe and comfortable contraceptive method.

REFERENCES

1. Rekers, H. and Kloosterboer, H.J. (1988). The new generation of monophasic oral contraceptives. In Keller, P.J. and Sirtori, C. (eds). *Contraception into the Next Decade*, pp. 13–23. (Carnforth: Parthenon Publishing)
2. Stadel, B.V. (1981). Oral contraceptives and cardiovascular disease. *N. Engl. J. Med.*, **305**, 612–18

3. Vessey, M.P. *et al.* (1986). Oral contraceptives and venous thromboembolism: findings in a large prospective study. *Br. Med. J.*, **292**, 526
4. Vessey, M.P. (1984). Oral contraception and stroke: findings in a large prospective study. *Br. Med. J.*, **289**, 530–1
5. Graeff, H. *et al.* (1977). Evaluation of hypercoagulability in users of oral contraceptives. *Klin. Wochenschr.*, **55**, 175–9
6. Böttiger, L.E. *et al.* (1980). Oral contraceptives and thromboembolic disease: effects of lowering the oestrogen content. *Lancet*, **i**, 1097–101
7. Guillebaud, J. (1985). *Contraception – Your questions answered.* (London: Pitman Publishing)
8. Mishell, D.R. (1976). Current status of oral contraceptive steroids. *Clin. Obstet. Gynecol.*, **19**, (4) 749–50
9. Melis, G.B. *et al.* (1984). Fibrinopeptide A (FPA) levels during oral contraceptive treatment. *Contraception*, **30**, 575–83
10. Ross, A. and Zanconato, G. (1983). *La contraccezione – Fondamenti scientifici* – p. 181. (Verona: Edizioni Libreria Cortina)
11. Maneschi and Martorana (1986). *Ginecologia Endocrinologica – Clinica e Terapia*, 2nd Edn, p. 268. (CIC)
12. Abbate, R. *et al.* (1989). Effects of low dose (20mcg) ethinyl-estradiol oral contraceptive on hemostasis. *Gynecol. Endocrinol.*, **3**, (Suppl. 1) 83
13. Dieben, T. (1984). A comparative study of the clinical efficacy of Marvelon and a triphasic combination. *Organorama*, **21**, 1–4
14. Rekers, H. (1988). Multicenter trial of a monophasic oral contraceptive containing ethinylestradiol and desogestrel. *Acta Obstet. Gynecol. Scand.*, **67**, 171–4
15. Upton, V. (1983). Clinical experience with triphasic oral contraceptive. In Elstein, M. (ed.) *Update on Triphasic Oral Contraception*, pp. 54–74. (Amsterdam: Excerpta Medica)
16. Allen, H. *et al.* (1983). A Canadian multicenter trial of a triphasic oral contraceptive. In Elstein, M. (ed.) *Update on Triphasic Oral Contraception*, pp. 82–99. (Amsterdam: Excerpta Medica)
17. De Cecco, L. *et al* (1981). The efficacy of triphasic oral contraceptives. In *New Considerations in Oral Contraception.* (New York: Biomedical Informations)
18. Lachnit-Fixson, U. (1980). Clinical comparison between a monophasic preparation and a triphasic preparation. In Rolland, R. (ed.) *Advances in Fertility Control and Treatment of Sterility*, pp. 71–79. (Lancaster: MTP Press)
19. Rabe, T. *et al.* (1987). Clinical and metabolic effects of two low dose combined pills for oral contraception containing gestodene (SHD 356C) or levorgestrel (Microgynon) In Genazzani, A.R., Volpe, A. and Facchinetti, F. (eds). *Gynecological Endocrinology*, pp. 503–16. (Carnforth: Parthenon Publishing)
20. Bounds, W. *et al.* (1979). A randomized double-blind trial of two low-dose combined oral contraceptives. *Br. J. Obstet. Gynaecol.*, **86**, 325–9
21. Preston, S.N. (1972). A report of a collaborative dose-response clinical study using decreasing doses of combination oral contraceptives. *Contraception*, **6**, 17–35
22. Preston, S.N. (1974). A report of the correlation between the pregnancy rates of low estrogen formulations and pilltaking habits of females. *J. Reprod. Med.*, **13**, 75–7
23. Tuimala, R. *et al.* (1987). Effects of the oral contraceptive combination 0.150 mg desogestrel plus 0.020 mg ethinylestradiol on serum lipids, SHBG, glycosylated proteins and plasma antithrombin III activity in healthy women. *Acta Obstet. Gynecol. Scand.* suppl., **114**, 37–9
24. Kloosterboer, H.J. *et al.* (1987). Effects of three low-dose oral contraceptives on sex hormone binding globulin, corticosteroid binding globulin and antithrombin III activity on healthy women. *Acta Obstet. Gynecol. Scand.* suppl. **144**, 41–4
25. Falsetti, L. *et al.* (1987). A new low-dose estrogen oral contraceptive combination: effects on endocrine parameters and lipid status. *Contraception*, **36**, 489–97
26. Hassold, T. and Chui, D. (1985). Maternal age-specific rates of numerical chromosome abnormalities with special reference to trisomy. *Hum. Genet.*, **70**, 11–17
27. Vessey, M.P. *et al.* (1977). Mortality among women participating in the Oxford/Family Planning Association contraception study. *Lancet*, **ii**, 731

APPENDIX – RESEARCHERS INVOLVED IN THE STUDY

Prof. Giorgio Cagnazzo 1st Obstetric and Gynecological Department, University of Bari
Prof. Luigi De Cecco and Prof. Gianluigi Capitanio 2nd Obstetric and Gynecological

Department, University of Genoa
Prof. Leopoldo Falsetti Obstetric and Gynecological Department, University of Brescia
Prof. Piero Fioretti and Prof. Gianbenedetto Melis Obstetric and Gynecological Department, University of Pisa
Prof. Carlo Flamigni and Dr Liviana Gammi Obstetric and Gynecological Department, University of Bologna
Prof. Andrea R. Genazzani and Prof. Annibale Volpe Obstetric and Gynecological Department, University of Modena
Prof. Antonio Martorana Endocrinological Gynecology Department, University of Palermo
Prof. Luigi Marzetti and Dr Gianfranco Marcellini 3rd Obstetric and Gynecological Department, University of Rome, "La Sapienza"
Prof. Giovanbattista Massi and Prof. Vincenzina Bruni Obstetric and Gynecological Department, University of Florence
Prof. Giovacchino Mollica and Dr Francesco Pansini Obstetric and Gynecological Department, University of Ferrara
Prof. Ugo Montemagno and Prof. Carmine Nappi 1st Obstetric and Gynecological Department, University of Naples
Prof. Giuseppe Palumbo and Dr Antonio Cianci Endocrinological Gynecology Department, University of Catania
Prof. Nino Pasetto and Prof. Emilio Piccione Obstetric and Gynecological Department, University of Rome "Tor Vergata"
Prof. Clemente Pulle and Prof. Domenico Granese Obstetric and Gynecological Department, University of Messina
Prof. Carlo Romanini and Dr Herbert Valensise Obstetric and Gynecological Department, University of Ancona
Prof. Bruno Salvadori and Prof. Alberto Bacchi-Modena Obstetric and Gynecological Department, University of Parma
Prof. Tullio Wierdis and Dr Antonio Rizzitiello Obstetric and Gynecological Department, University of Torino
Prof. Lucio Zichella and Dr Giuseppina Perrone 1st Obstetric and Gynecological Department, University of Rome

109

Effects of two monophasic oral contraceptives containing 150 μg desogestrel in combination with 20 or 30 μg ethinylestradiol in adolescents with oligomenorrhea and ovarian hyperandrogenism

C. Nappi, F. Leone, A. Nicotra, M.J. Farace, C. Di Carlo and U. Montemagno

INTRODUCTION

The early postmenarchal years of adolescent girls are characterized by a high incidence of irregular menstrual cycles and anovulation, associated frequently with clinical signs of hyperandrogenism including hirsutism and acne[1-4]. Both the ovarian morphology and the endocrine pattern of these adolescents are often difficult to distinguish from those of the polycystic ovarian disease (PCOD) in adults. In fact, increased ovarian volume and multifollicularity[3,5] are associated with increased luteinizing hormone (LH), androstenedione (A), testosterone (T) and decreased sex hormone-binding globulin (SHBG) plasma concentrations[1-6].

This condition of ovarian hyperandrogenism is secondary to a state of immaturity of the entire hypothalamic–pituitary–ovarian axis[7], and is usually reversible with the onset of regular ovulation[8]. On the contrary, adolescents with persistent ovarian hyperandrogenism are predisposed to the onset of PCOD in adulthood[4,9].

Treatment of symptomatic ovarian hyperandrogenism of adolescents with combined oral contraceptives, reducing the high LH and androgen levels, may have therapeutic and/or preventive value in order to stop the evolution of the morphofunctional ovarian process inducing PCOD[6,10,11]. Moreover, combined oral contraceptives are sufficient to improve the cosmetic manifestations of hyperandrogenism (hirsutism, acne and seborrhea) and provide contraceptive protection.

It has been shown that low-dose oral contraception preparations have a favorable short-term effect on the hyperandrogenic picture of oligomenorrheic girls[12]. Besides, we have recently demonstrated that the association of 30 μg ethinylestradiol (EE) and 150 μg desogestrel is able to decrease the elevated LH and androgen levels and reduce the hyperandrogenic signs in adolescents with ovarian hyperandrogenism[3].

In this study we compared the clinical and hormonal effectiveness of two monophasic low-dose oral contraceptive combinations containing different amounts of EE (20 μg or 30 μg) and the same amount of desogestrel (150 μg) in adolescents with ovarian hyperandrogenism.

MATERIALS AND METHODS

Fourteen adolescents with clinical and hormonal signs of ovarian hyperandrogenism between 14 and 19 years of age were studied. Informed consent was obtained. None had been treated with any hormonal preparation for 12 months before the study, and no contraindications for the use of oral contraceptives were present. Breast development and pubic hair were at 4–5 pubertal stage.

The subjects were affected by oligomenorrhea (intermenstrual intervals ranging from 45 to 180 days) associated with hormonal and clinical signs of ovarian hyperandrogenism. In fact, they showed elevated plasma LH, A, and free and total T, low follicle-stimulating hormone (FSH) and SHBG concentrations, associated with mild hirsutism and/or acne and seborrhea. Hirsutism was graded using the Ferriman and Gallway scale[13] (index ranging from 8 to 14). Obesity, defined as weight to height greater than the 90th percentile of fatness, was present in six patients.

Androgen-secreting tumors, congenital adrenal hyperplasia and hyperprolactinemia were ruled out. All hyperandrogenic adolescents had enlarged and microcystic ovaries as diagnosed by ultrasound. Diagnosis of polycystic ovaries was confirmed by laparoscopy and/or ovarian biopsy in seven subjects.

The girls were divided in two groups of seven subjects. One (Group A) was treated with the association of 20 μg EE and 150 μg desogestrel (Organon, The Netherlands) and one (Group B) with 30 μg EE and 150 μg desogestrel (Organon, The Netherlands), both in double-blind study. The treatment lasted 21 days starting on the 1st day of menstrual bleeding, and was continued for 6 consecutive months. The subsequent courses of pill administration were to begin after a 7-day treatment-free interval. No other hormonal medication was used during the study. All patients were asked to eat a 1000–1200 kcal/day diet.

The two groups were similar according to age, height/weight, age at menarche, gynecological age, length of cycle (Table 1), and endocrine and ovarian features (Table 2). All these basal parameters were compared to those of a control group (Group C) consisting of ten healthy and eumenorrheic (intermenstrual interval ranging between 26 and 32 days in the last 12 months) adolescents with ovulatory cycles without clinical and hormonal signs of hyperandrogenism.

Table 1 Mean age, height/weight ratio, age at menarche, gynecological age and length of the cycle (±SD) in adolescents with ovarian hyperandrogenism treated with oral contraceptives containing 20 μg EE + 150 μg desogestrel (Group A) or 30 μg EE + 150 μg desogestrel (Group B) and in control adolescents (Group C)

	Group A	*Group B*	*Group C*
Age (yr)	17.4 ± 1.2	17.1 ± 1.3	16.5 ± 1.2
Height/weight ratio	3.1 ± 0.4	3.0 ± 0.3	3.2 ± 0.4
Age of menarche	13.2 ± 1.4	12.9 ± 1.3	12.8 ± 1.4
Gynecological age (yr)	4.5 ± 1.3	4.6 ± 1.4	4.2 ± 1.5
Length of cycle	55 ± 15	57 ± 20	28.7 ± 1.7

Table 2 Mean basal hormonal concentrations and ultrasonographic findings (±SD) in adolescents with ovarian hyperandrogenism treated with oral contraceptives containing 20 μg EE + 150 μg desogestrel (Group A) or 30 μg EE + 150 μg desogestrel (Group B) and in control adolescents (Group C)

	Group A	*Group B*	*Group C*
FSH (mIU/ml)	7 ± 2.2	6.3 ± 1.7	8.5 ± 2.3
LH (mIU/ml)	14 ± 2.5**	16 ± 2.6**	7.5 ± 1.5
A (ng/ml)	2.5 ± 0.7**	2.8 ± 1**	1.6 ± 0.6
Total T (ng/ml)	1 ± 0.2*	1.1 ± 0.3*	0.7 ± 0.1
Free T (pg/ml)	2.4 ± 0.5**	2.2 ± 0.6**	1.3 ± 0.8
DHEA-S (μg/dl)	260 ± 48	280 ± 55	240 ± 58
SHBG (μg/dl)	0.6 ± 0.1**	0.8 ± 0.1**	1.3 ± 0.2
PRL (ng/ml)	10 ± 3.1	12 ± 2.9	11 ± 3.3
Ovarian volume (cm^3)	12 ± 2**	13 ± 3**	7 ± 1.5
Number of cysts	4.8 ± 0.6**	4.9 ± 0.8**	1.6 ± 0.3

In comparison with Group C: *$p < 0.05$; **$p < 0.01$

In normal and hyperandrogenic subjects basal blood samples were drawn between 08.00 and 09.00 on the 5th to 7th day of the menstrual cycle.

In hyperandrogenic subjects additional blood samples were obtained during oral contraceptive administration (between days 18 and 21 of the third and sixth cycles of treatment). The blood samples were collected in heparinized tubes and centrifuged. Plasma was separated and stored at −20 °C until analysis. Plasma determinations were carried out for FSH, LH, free and total T, A, dehydroepiandrosterone sulfate (DHEA-S), SHBG and prolactin (PRL). Ultrasonographic evaluations of ovarian volume and morphology were performed before and during therapy on the same days of the hormonal determinations, using a CGR scanner in B-mode and real time with a 3.5 MHz transducer. The ovarian volume (V) was calculated according to the formula of Gohari *et al.*[14].

Before and during therapy, the patients were monitored monthly by hirsutism scoring.

FSH, LH, T and PRL concentrations were assayed using radioimmunoassay (RIA) kits from Biodata (Italy). The Diagnostic Products Corporation (Los Angeles, California) kits were used for free T detection. Determinations of A were performed after petroleum ether extraction, using RIA kits purchased from Bio-Merieux (France). The DHEA-S assay was directly performed using Bio-Merieux kits. SHBG concentrations were measured according to procedures of Nisula *et al.*[15]. All results obtained were statistically analyzed by the Student's *t* test for paired and unpaired data.

RESULTS

Before treatment, the oligomenorrheic adolescents (Groups A and B) showed high basal LH, A, total and free T, and DHEA-S concentrations compared with control subjects (Group C). In Groups A and B SHBG levels were significantly lower than in control group. FSH and PRL values were similar in both hyperandrogenic groups (Table 2). Moreover, all oligomenorrheic girls showed greater mean ovarian values and multifollicularity with at least four echo-free cystic structures.

The administration of the two monophasic oral contraceptives containing different amounts of EE (20 μg or 30 μg) and the same amount of desogestrel (150 μg) induced a significant decrease in LH, FSH (Figure 1), free T and A, associated with a significant increase in SHBG (Figure 2). The reduction in total T (Figure 2) and DHEA-S (Figure 3) was not significant in both groups. No change in PRL values occurred.

At the sixth cycle of treatment in both groups of adolescents treated, a significant decrease of the total ovarian volume was observed, with a reduced number or disappearance of echo-free cystic follicles in both ovaries (Figure 4).

Moreover, a significant decrease in the Ferriman–Gallway index, compared to initial values, was noticed in the two treatment groups after 6 months of treatment (Figure 5). No significant difference between the two groups was evident. In particular, in all subjects a decrease of hirsutism and frequency of depilation within 3 months, and a progressive improvement of the entire hyperandrogenic picture up to 6 months of treatment were observed. An evident improvement of seborrhea and acne occurred in adolescents who showed these symptoms before treatment.

Irregular bleeding occurred in two adolescents of Group A and in one of

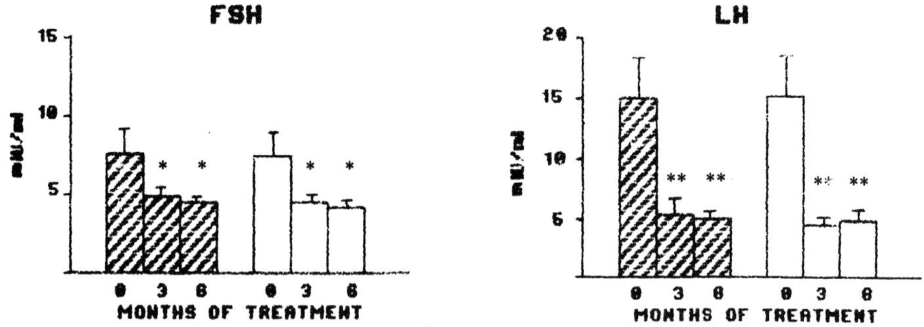

Figure 1 Mean plasma FSH and LH (±SD) concentrations before and during (third and sixth cycles) treatment with the two oral contraceptives containing 20 μg EE/150 μg desogestrel (hatched blocks) or 30 μg EE/150 μg desogestrel (open blocks) in adolescents with ovarian hyperandrogenism; in comparison with basal values: $*p < 0.05$; $**p < 0.01$

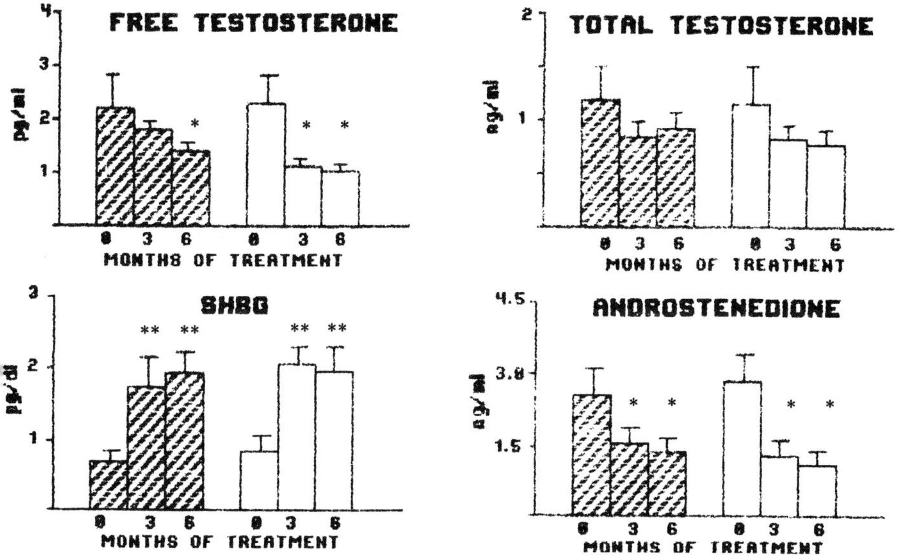

Figure 2 Mean plasma free and total T, SHBG and A (±SD) concentrations before and during (third and sixth cycles) treatment with the two oral contraceptives containing 20 μg EE/150 μg desogestrel (hatched blocks) or 30 μg EE/150 μg desogestrel (open blocks) in adolescents with ovarian hyperandrogenism; in comparison with basal values: $^*p < 0.05$; $^{**}p < 0.01$

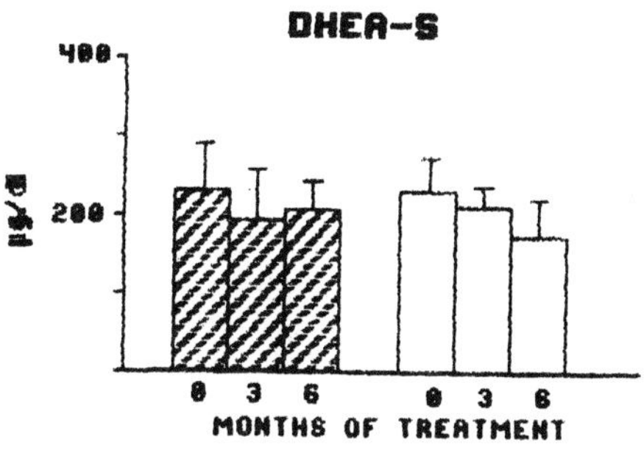

Figure 3 Mean plasma DHEA–S (±SD) concentrations before and during (third and sixth cycles) treatment with the two oral contraceptives containing 20 μg EE/150 μg desogestrel (hatched blocks) or 30 μg EE/150 μg desogestrel (open blocks) in adolescents with ovarian hyperandrogenism

Group B, in the initial months of use, but after 6 months only one in Group A reported irregular bleeding. Withdrawal bleeding occurred in all adolescents. No evidence of body weight gain was present in both treatment groups.

With both preparations the frequency of minor side-effects such as nausea, headaches, nervousness and breast tenderness was low. In general, these subjective complaints occurred exclusively in the initial treatment cycles.

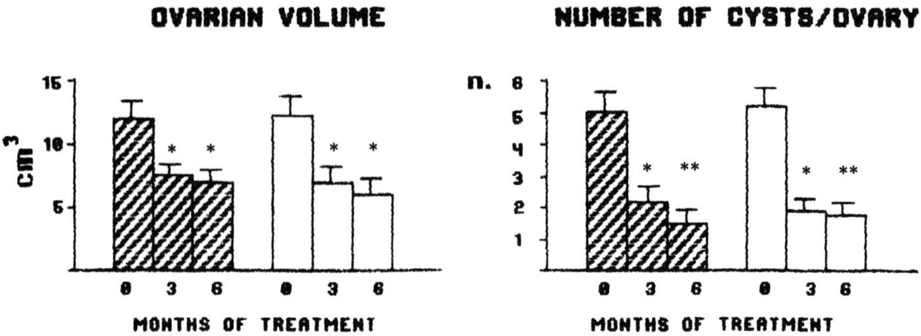

Figure 4 Mean ovarian volume and number of cysts/ovary (±SD) before and during (third and sixth cycles) treatment with the two oral contraceptives containing 20 μg EE/150 μg desogestrel (hatched blocks) or 30 μg EE/150 μg desogestrel (open blocks) in adolescents with ovarian hyperandrogenism; in comparison with basal values: $*p < 0.05$; $**p < 0.01$

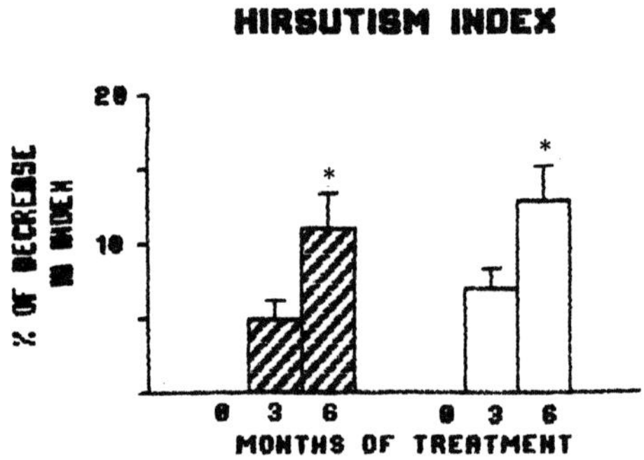

Figure 5 Mean per cent decrease in hirsutism index (±SD) during (third and sixth cycles) treatment with the two oral contraceptives containing 20 μg EE/150 μg desogestrel (hatched blocks) or 30 μg EE/150 μg desogestrel (open blocks) in adolescents with ovarian hyperandrogenism; in comparison with basal values: $*p < 0.05$

DISCUSSION

Our results confirm several reports[1–6] indicating that the background of irregular cycles in the first years after menarche is an LH-dependent ovarian hyperandrogenism. It is characterized by high LH, A and T, and low SHBG plasma concentrations associated with enlarged and polyfollicular ovaries. This condition of ovarian hyperandrogenism is due to the immaturity of the hypothalamic–pituitary–ovarian axis of adolescents[7], including a peripubertal 'desynchronization of the LH clock'[16] which results in repetitive positive feedback stimulating the ovarian theca to produce androgen excess.

There is considerable evidence suggesting that adolescents with persistent irregular menses after menarche, along with high LH and androgen levels, and enlarged polyfollicular ovaries, may maintain this condition of ovarian hyperandrogenism and are predisposed to the onset and persistence of PCOD[4,9]. The long-term androgen induces thickening of the tunica albuginea and basal membrane which then produces follicular alterations[17].

It is probable that reduction of high LH and androgen endogenous levels may be appropriate as an early medical approach able to prevent and/or stop the evolution of the morphofunctional process, which is characteristic of PCOD[6]. In fact, ovarian suppression may possibly avoid any further evolution of the pathological ovarian picture, although there is no confirmation of this from controlled longitudinal studies.

Complete suppression of excessive androgen production from the ovary depends upon suppression of LH levels into the normal range induced by the inhibitory action of the progestin component in the pill. The estrogen component gives further benefit in hyperandrogenism increasing SHBG levels, which leads to a decrease in free T. Low-dose oral contraceptives are as effective as high-dose preparations in increasing SHBG and decreasing total and free T[11].

In our study the administration of the two monophasic oral contraceptives containing 150 μg desogestrel and different doses of EE (20 μg or 30 μg) induced a decrease in LH, FSH, free and total T, A and DHEA-S associated with a significant SHBG increase. No significant difference was evident between the two treated groups with respect to all these hormonal variations. Moreover, both combinations showed favorable short-term effect on the hyperandrogenic clinical picture, a good cycle control and an excellent patient compliance.

It is probable that the low estrogen content of the oral contraceptives which we used may induce fewer antiandrogenic effects than the higher estrogen content of other oral contraceptives. But desogestrel is a progestin with a high gestagen activity and a lower intrinsic androgenicity[18] than other derivates of 19-nortestosterone and therefore does not inhibit but instead emphasizes the positive antiandrogenic effects of the estrogen component. In fact, some recent reports indicate the administration of oral contraceptives containing desogestrel as being effective in patients with hirsutism[19] or PCOD[20] and also in normal women who are prone to hirsutism and acne[21].

In particular, because of its lower estrogen and desogestrel content, the 20 μg EE/150 μg desogestrel combined preparation may be the most rational and effective therapeutic and contraceptive approach in oligomenorrheic adolescents with clinical and hormonal signs of ovarian hyperandrogenism. In fact, an oral contraceptive which contains low doses of components is always preferable in young girls, inducing a low rate of 'post pill amenorrhea'[22] and having no effect on the postpubertal growth and development of the adolescents[23].

In conclusion, our study indicates that, because of its lower estrogen content, the 20 μg EE/150 μg desogestrel combination may be both a therapeutic and contraceptive approach for oligomenorrheic adolescents with clinical and hormonal signs of ovarian hyperandrogenism. We suggest that its administration may also be appropriate and widespread in sexually-active non-hyperandrogenic girls who still have an incomplete maturation of the reproductive axis and are prone to androgenic side-effects of the pill.

REFERENCES

1. Apter, D. (1980). Serum steroids and pituitary hormones in female puberty: a partly longitudinal study. *Clin. Endocrinol.*, **12**, 107–20

2. Siegberg, R., Nilsson, C.G., Stenman, U.K. and Widmola, Q. (1986). Endocrinologic features of oligomenorrheic adolescent girls. *Fertil. Steril.*, **46**, 852–6
3. Nappi, C., Farace, M.J., Leone, F., Minutolo, M., Tommaselli, A.P. and Montemagno, U. (1987). Effect of a combination of ethinylestradiol and desogestrel in adolescents with oligomenorrhoea and ovarian hyperandrogenism. *Eur. J. Obstet. Gynecol. Reprod. Biol.*, **25**, 209–19
4. Venturoli, S., Porcu, E., Fabbri, R., Magrini, O., Paradisi, R., Pallotti, G., Gammi, L. and Flamigni, C. (1987). Postmenarchal evolution of endocrine pattern and ovarian aspects in adolescents with menstrual irregularities. *Fertil. Steril.*, **48**, 78–85
5. Venturoli, S., Porcu, E., Fabbri, R., Paradisi, R., Orsini, L.F. and Flamigni, C. (1984). Ovaries and menstrual cycles in adolescents. *Gynecol. Obstet. Invest.*, **17**, 219–22
6. Emans, S.J., Grace, E. and Golstein, D.P. (1980). Oligomenorrhea in adolescent girls. *J. Pediatr.*, **97**, 815–19
7. Baird, D.T. (1976). Pituitary-ovarian relationships in disorders of menstruations. In James, V.H.T., Serio, M. and Guisti, G. (eds.) *The Endocrine Function of the Human Ovary*, p. 349. (New York: Academic Press)
8. Moll, G.W. and Rosenfield, R.L. (1983). Plasma free testosterone in the diagnosis of adolescent polycystic ovary syndrome. *J. Pediatr.*, **102**, 461–4
9. Venturoli, R., Porcu, E., Fabbri, R., Paradisi, R., Flamigni, C. (1981). Hyperandrogenism in postmenarchal oligomenorrhea: a stage of polycystic ovary? *Acta Endocrinol. (Copenh.)*, **97**, (Suppl. 243), 72
10. Jung-Hoffmann, C. and Kuhl, H. (1987). Divergent effects of two low-dose oral contraceptives on sex hormone binding-globulin and free testosterone. *Am. J. Obstet. Gynecol.*, **156**, 199–203
11. Raj, S.G., Raj, M.H.G., Talbert, L.M., Sloan, C.S. and Hicks, B. (1982). Normalization of testosterone levels using a low estrogen-containing oral contraceptive in women with polycystic ovarian disease. *Obstet. Gynecol.*, **60**, 15–19
12. Siegberg, R., Nilsson, C.G., Stenman, U.H. and Whidholm, O. (1984). Sex hormone profile in oligomenorrheic adolescent girls and the effect of oral contraceptive. *Fertil. Steril.*, **41**, 888–93
13. Ferriman, D. and Gallwey, J.D. (1961). Clinical assessment of body hair in women. *J. Clin. Endocrinol. Metab.*, **21**, 1440–7
14. Gohari, P., Berkowits, R.L. and Hobbins, J.C. (1987). Predictions of intrauterine growth retardation by determination total intrauterine volume. *Am. J. Obstet. Gynecol.*, **127** (3), 255–60
15. Nisula, B.C., Loriaux, D.L. and Wilson, Y.A. (1978). Solid phase method for measurements of binding capacity of testosterone-estradiol binding globulin in human serum. *Steroids*, **31**, (5), 681–90
16. Zumoff, B., Freeman, R., Coupey, S., Saengdsc, P., Markowitz, M. and Kream, J. (1983). A chronobiologic abnormality in LH secretion in teenage girls with polycystic ovary syndrome. *N. Engl. J. Med.*, **309**, 1206–9
17. Amirikia, H., Savoy-Moore, R.T., Sundareson, A.S. and Moghissi, K.S. (1986). The effects of long-term androgen treatment. *Fertil. Steril.*, **45**, 202–8
18. Bergink, E.W., Hamburger, A.D., De Jager, E. and Van der Vies, J. (1981). Binding of contraceptive progestogen ORG 2969 and its metabolites to receptor proteins and human SHBG. *J. Steroid Biochem.*, **14**, 175–83
19. Dewis, P., Petsos, P., Newman, M. and Anderson, D.C. (1985). The treatment of hirsutism with a combination of desogestrel and ethinylestradiol. *Clin. Endocrinol. (Oxf).*, **22**, 29–36
20. Cullberg, G. (1985). Low-dose desogestrel-ethinylestradiol combination on hirsutism, androgen and sex hormone binding globulin in women with polycystic ovary syndrome. *Acta Obstet. Gynecol. Scand.*, **64**, 195–202
21. Hammond, G.L., Langley, M.S., Robinson, P.A., Nummi, S. and Lund, L. (1984). Serum steroid binding protein concentration, distribution of progestogens, and bioavailability of testosterone during treatment with contraceptives containing desogestrel or levonorgestrel. *Fertil. Steril.*, **42**, 44–51
22. Rey-Stocker, I., Zufferey, M-M., Lemarchand, M-T. and Rais, M. (1980). Sensibilitat der hypophyse der gonaden und der schiddruse beim jungen madchen vor und nach kombinierten oralen kontrazeption. *Gynaekol. Rundsch.*, **20**, 135–61
23. Prader, A. and Zachmann, M. (1979). Treatment of excessively tall girls and boys with sex hormones. *Pediatrics*, **62**, 1202–10

110

Advantages of a 20 μg ethinylestradiol oral contraceptive administration in older women

A. Volpe, F. Petraglia, A. Maietta Latessa, V. Santoro, M. Silferi and P. Pozzo

INTRODUCTION

Safety is an important factor in the choice of an oral contraceptive in older women. In the past, oral contraception was advised against in women over 35. The risks were due to the two components, estrogenic and progestinic, of the combination pill[1–5]. Progestins present in the oral contraceptive preparation can negatively influence lipid metabolism; some progestins, those with androgenic activity, increase low density lipoprotein (LDL) and apolipoprotein (Apo) B plasma levels which are directly related to an elevated risk of cardiovascular disease, while high-density lipoprotein (HDL) and Apo A levels, which normally protect against atheromatic disease, decrease[6–9]. Synthetic estrogens in the oral contraceptive increase clotting factors such as fibrinogens VII, VIII, IX, X, and decrease antithrombin III[10,11]; therefore during the administration of oral contraceptives an unfavorable condition develops: the coagulative system increases and the fibrinolytic system decreases. Age is synergic with these two unfavorable effects; on the one hand the relative reduction of estrogenic levels in preclimacteric women could induce a decrease in the HDL plasma levels; on the other, the greater age of the women could be synergic with synthetic estrogens in increasing the activity of clotting factors.

The effects of both estrogens on lipid metabolism and progestins on the clotting system are dose-dependent. Therefore in recent years pharmacological and clinical research has been directed towards the reduction of the dosage of ethinylestradiol and progestin present in the oral contraceptive and towards the synthesis of new progestins without any androgenic activity and without any metabolic side-effect.

At present there is general agreement about the possibility of using the recently developed oral contraceptives until the age of 45 where there are no risk factors such as smoking, obesity or hypertension. It is worth noting that smoking is the most significant cause of any alteration in clotting factors in the presence of oral contraceptives, in fact the oral contraceptives used by women over 40 do not modify coagulative parameters[12]. Recently a new combination has been proposed; 150 μg desogestrel, a progestin with a very weak androgenic activity, consequently without effects on the lipid metabolism and only 20 μg ethinylestradiol. The use of a low dosage of estrogen in this combination could provide better control over clotting factors especially in women over 40.

MATERIALS AND METHODS

We studied the association of a low androgenic activity progestin, desogestrel (150 μg/die) and of a low dosage estrogen, ethinylestradiol (20 μg/die) in 47 patients, aged 35–45 years.

Treatment lasted for 12 months in all patients, while 11 patients continued for 24 cycles, three patients for 36 cycles and two patients for 42 cycles for a total number of 900 cycles.

We included women with proved fertility, regular menses, enjoying good health with no contraindication to oral contraception. Eleven of the women included were smokers, with an average of 10 cigarettes per day.

Baseline control was made before therapy and after three, six, 12, 24, 36, 42 cycles. Lipid metabolism, clotting factors, side-effects, blood pressure were evaluated. In addition each month breakthrough bleeding characteristics were registered.

RESULTS

The average duration of menstrual cycle was standardized after the second cycle of treatment at 26 ± 1 days and duration of menses was 4 ± 1 days (Figure 1*a* and *b*). Spotting occurred in 18% of the women during the 1st month of treatment, progressively decreasing thereafter; was present in 12% of patients at 3 months of treatment, absent at the 6th month. It was present in 5% of patients at 12 months.

Withdrawal bleeding did not occur in 1–3% of patients during the period of observation.

We did not observe any significant variation in HDL and LDL nor in Apo A and B plasma levels. Mastodynia occurred in 12% of patients in the first cycle, in 8% in the 3rd month, 7% in the 6th month and then disappeared in the following months.

Nausea was present in 2% of patients in the first cycle and 1% in the 3rd month. Headache was observed in 5% of patients (Figure 1*c*).

All these side-effects were slight and in no case was it necessary to interrupt treatment. No women gained weight.

Therapy did not modify the coagulation markers such as prothrombin time, partial thromboplastin time, fibrinogen, antithrombin III and fibrinopeptide A.

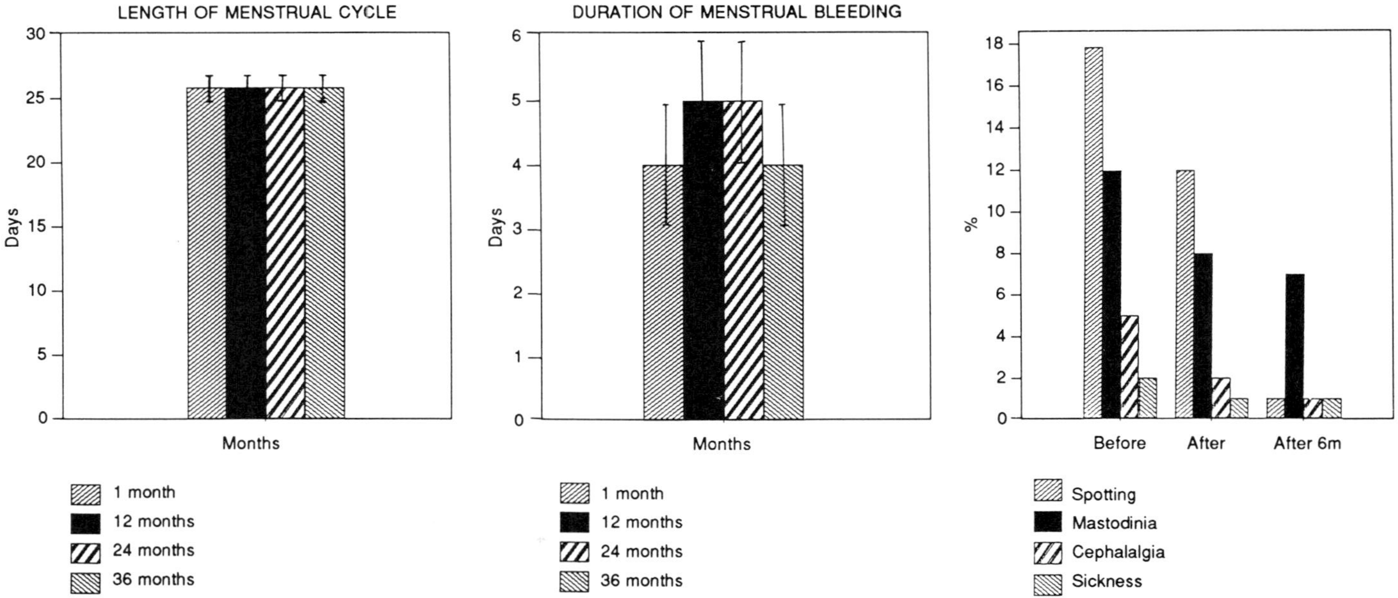

Figure 1 (*a*) Length of menstrual cycle after 1, 12, 24 and 36 months of treatment; (*b*) duration of menstrual bleeding and 1, 12, 24 and 36 months of treatment; and (*c*) side-effects before and after 3 to 6 months of treatment

No significant modification of high density and low density lipoprotein nor of apolipoproteins A and B occurred.

DISCUSSION

The use of oral contraceptives in the preclimacteric and climacteric period is favorable for women because it favors satisfactory sexual activity, controls menstrual cycle related symptoms (such as dysmenorrhea, ovulatory pains etc.) and reduces the incidence of gynecological pathological diseases which are frequent in this period of life.

In older women, in fact, most cycles are anovulatory and only sometimes are ovulatory or with luteal deficiency and this reflects on target organs with a long estrogenic stimulation unbalanced by progesterone. Combined oral contraceptives, especially the preparation we used, are effective on treating and preventing this abnormality, but they are not usually prescribed.

Cardiovascular complications are the most important reason for advising against the use of oral contraceptives in women aged between 40 and 50.

It is well known that this risk is linked to the androgenic activity of the progestin[13]. Paradoxically progestins or danazol are more frequently used, drugs which are known to have unfavorable effects on lipid metabolism and therefore to increase the cardiovascular risk.

Moreover some estro–progestin associations for climacteric symptom treatment contain higher daily dosages of progestin than the new combined oral contraceptives[14]. Thus the risk is linked not only to the progestin but also to the synthetic estrogen which alters the clotting factors.

The combination 150 μg desogestrel + 20 μg ethinylestradiol with a low dosage estrogen and a low atherosclerotic risk progestin, could be used until the age of 45, on the condition that other risk factors, especially smoking (over 10 cigarettes/day), are absent. In our experience this association showed absolute contraceptive efficiency, good tolerance and lack of side-effects.

In this association the presence of desogestrel, which also blocks gonadotropins, allowed the use of 20 μg of ethinylestradiol for the first time. This fact makes this association the pill of first choice, which is also suitable for use by preclimacteric and estrogen-sensitive women.

REFERENCES

1. Cartwright, A. (1976). *How many children*? p. 90. (London: Routledge and Kegan Paul)
2. Gray, R.H. (1979). Biological and social interactions in the determination of late fertility. *J. Biosoc. Sci.*, **97**, 115
3. Jansen, R.P. (1984). Fertility in older women. *IPPF Med. Bull.*, **18**, 4
4. Beard, R.J. (1979). Risks and problems for the older parent. In Roberts, D.F. and Chester, R. (eds). *Changing Patterns of Conception and Fertility*. (London: Academic Press)
5. Kay, C.R. (1983). Do changes in HDL-cholesterol have any clinical relevance? *Novum*, **23**, 3
6. Wingrave, S.J. (1982). Progestogen effects and their relationship of lipoprotein changes. *Acta Obstet. Gynecol. Scand.*, **105**, 33
7. Bradley, D.D., Wingerd, J., Petitti, D., Krauss, R.M. and Ramcharan, S. (1978). Serum high-

density-lipoprotein cholesterol in women using oral contraceptives, estrogens and progestins. *N. Engl. J. Med.*, **17**, 299
8. Wahl, P., Walden, C., Knopp, R., Hoover, J., Wallance, R., Heiss, C. and Rifkind, B. (1981). Effect of oestrogen-progestin potency on lipid-lipoprotein cholesterol. *N. Engl. J. Med.*, **308**, 862
9. Hirvonen, E., MalRonen, M. and Manninen, V. (1981). Effects of different progestogens on lipoproteins during post-menopausal replacement therapy. *N. Engl. J. Med.*, **304**, 560
10. Meade, T.W. (1982). Oral contraceptives, clotting factors and thrombosis. *Obstet. Gynecol.*, **42**, 758
11. Conarad, J., Cazenave, B., Samama, M., Hollerou, M.H., Zorn, J.R. and Neau, C. (1980). AT III content and antithrombin activity in oestrogen-progestogen and progestogen-only treated women. *Thromb. Res.*, **18**, 675
12. Notelowitz, M. *et al.* (1985). The effects of low-dose oral contraceptives on coagulation and fibrinolysis in two high-risk populations: young female smokers and older premenopausal women. *Am. J. Obstet. Gynecol.*, **15**, 995
13. Stadel, B.V. (1981). Oral contraceptives and cardiovascular disease. *N. Engl. J. Med.*, **305**, 612 and 672
14. Guillebaud, J. (1985). Contraception for the older women. *J. Obstet. Gynecol.*, **5**, (Suppl) 70

Section 4 continued

Part I

Endometriosis

111

The biological and clinical significance of endometrial proteins in reproductive endocrinology

T. Chard and R. J. S. Howell

The human endometrium produces a number of specific proteins, some of which may be of considerable functional significance in the process of reproduction[1]. Two of these proteins were originally isolated from extracts of whole placentae and hence were given the designation 'placental protein 12' and 'placental protein 14' (PP12 and PP14)[2]. However, it is now apparent that they arise from the maternal endometrium rather than the fetal trophoblast. Furthermore, both PP12 and PP14 have proven to be identical with a number of proteins isolated from other sites by different groups of workers. This has led to some confusion in the nomenclature (Tables 1 and 2). Because much of the work on the reproductive aspects of these proteins has been carried out using materials supplied by Bohn, his original nomenclature will be used here.

SOURCES OF PP12 AND PP14

The proteins orginally described by Bohn and Kraus[2] were obtained from extracts of whole placenta. Obviously this included tissues of both fetal origin (trophoblast etc.) and maternal origin (decidua). It is now universally agreed that the materials known as PP12 and PP14 arise from the endometrium in

Table 1 Proteins extracted from various sources which are either identical or very similar to PP12

Reference	*Protein*
Bohn and Kraus[2]	Placental protein 12
Bohn *et al.*[20]	
Bell *et al.*[48]	α-1 pregnancy-associated endometrial protein
	Endometrial protein 14
Koistinen *et al.*[17]	34 kDa IGF-binding protein

Table 2 Proteins extracted from the placenta or uterus which are either identical or very similar to PP14. The full range of materials secreted by the human endometrium in pregnancy and the menstrual cycle has been reviewed by Bell (1988)[1]

Reference	*Protein*
Petrunin *et al.*[55,56]	Chorionic α2 microglobulin
Bohn and Kraus[2] Bohn *et al.*[20]	Placental protein 14
Sutcliffe *et al.*[57]	α-uterine protein
Joshi *et al.*[58]	
Sutcliffe *et al.*[59] Julkunen *et al.*[4]	Progestogen-dependent endometrial protein
Bell *et al.*[3,48]	Pregnancy-associated endometrial α2 globulin
	Endometrial protein 15
Huhtala *et al.*[23]	β-lactoglobulin

both the pregnant and the non-pregnant state. In particular, cultured explants of endometrium can incorporate labelled amino acids (methionine) into materials with the properties of PP12 and PP14[3–6].

Immunohistochemical studies indicate that PP12 arises from the decidualized decidua compacta region of the endometrium[7,8]. In the non-pregnant state the main source of circulating PP12 is probably tissues other than the genital tract (e.g. the liver). It is also secreted in small amounts by granulosa cells[9].

Both biochemical and immunohistochemical observations[10] have shown that PP14 is the most abundant protein product of the late secretory endometrium. The secretory cells appear to be the glandular epithelium of the functional zone[11], and PP14 is actively secreted into the uterine lumen[12]. The circulating levels increase 20-fold from the late secretory phase to early first trimester whereas tissue levels rise only twofold; this suggests that much of the rise is due to the increase in the mass of the decidua[1]. PP14 has also been demonstrated in seminal plasma[13–15], and in ovarian follicular fluid[16].

THE CHEMISTRY OF PP12 AND PP14

The material described by Bohn and Kraus[2] as PP12 had a molecular weight of 25 kDa or 51 kDa, a carbohydrate content of 4.3% and the electrophoretic mobility of an α-1-globulin. Later estimates of molecular weight place this closer to 34 kDa. The N-terminal amino acid sequence of PP12 is identical to that of the small insulin-like growth factor (IGF)-binding protein[17].

Placental protein 12 binds IGF-I with high affinity. Two groups[18,19] have isolated a cDNA clone and an mRNA corresponding to PP12. These studies show that PP12 consists of 259 amino acids with a 25-amino acid signal peptide. The mature protein has a predicted molecular mass of 25 293 Da.

The material described by Bohn and Kraus[2] as PP14 had a molecular weight of 42 000 and a carbohydrate content of 17.5%[20]. The electrophoretic mobility is that of an α-2-globulin and the isoelectric point is 4.8[21]. A number of workers have shown that PP14 is similar to the β-lactoglobulins (βLG)[22–24]. Huhtala and colleagues showed a 59.1% sequence identity between the

N-terminal sequence of PP14 and horse βLG and similar homologies with the βLG of other species[23]. The intramolecular disulfide bridges characteristic of the βLG are all conserved in PP14[25]. There is also a 22.7% sequence identity between PP14 and retinol-binding protein, and homologies with carrier proteins in amphibia and insects[26]. Julkunen and colleagues[25] have identified a cDNA clone and an mRNA corresponding to PP14. These studies show that PP14 contains 180 amino acids, 18 of which correspond to a signal peptide. The predicted molecular mass is 20 555 for prePP14 and 18 787 for the mature protein.

BIOLOGICAL FUNCTIONS OF PP12 AND PP14

It is now clear that PP12 is chemically and biologically identical to the small (34kDa) IGF-binding protein. The functions must therefore include transport of IGF in the blood. In addition, the IGF-binding proteins play an integral role in the binding of the IGFs to their cell receptors. The effect may be either to enhance or inhibit the action of the IGFs and it has been proposed that the endometrial synthesis of an IGF-binding protein provides a defence mechanism whereby maternal tissues in the uterus are protected against invasion by the trophoblast[27]. In support of this suggestion, it has been demonstrated that maternal PP12 levels are elevated in pregnancies associated with fetal growth retardation[28].

The chemical similarity of PP14 to βLG and retinol-binding protein suggests that PP14 might have functions in the transport of small hydrophobic molecules within or across tissues. This could be of obvious importance to the developing embryo and fetus. However, no such binding of retinol by PP14 has been demonstrated. Extracts of first trimester endometrium have been shown to inhibit the mixed lymphocyte reaction and mitogen-induced lymphocyte proliferation; immunochemical evidence suggested that the material responsible for this was PP14[29,30]. However, this has not been confirmed with other preparations of this material[1]. The fact that maternal PP14 levels remain unchanged during abortion induced by administration of the progesterone antagonist, RU486, indicates that PP14 is not a pre-eminent factor in the maintenance of early pregnancy[31].

THE CONTROL MECHANISMS OF PP12 AND PP14

The PP12 of endometrial origin appears to be primarily under the control of progesterone[6]. Levels of PP12 are rapidly reduced following administration of the progesterone receptor antagonist RU486[32]. However, it is now obvious that many other tissues secrete an identical material (IGF-binding protein). The levels of 'non-endometrial' IGF-binding protein relate closely to nutritional status, and to growth hormone and insulin[33–35]. The levels increase after prolonged exercise[36].

PP14 levels are elevated in the luteal phase of the cycle, suggesting that the synthesis and secretion of this protein might be under the control of progesterone. This is supported by the fact that oral administration of progesterone increases the serum PP14 concentration in normal women[37,38]. However, a low level of PP14 is found in the blood of postmenopausal women, even after hysterectomy. Thus PP14 cannot be absolutely specific for either endometrium or progesterone.

Administration of estrogen–progesterone to postmenopausal women produces a 45% rise in PP14 levels in women with an intact uterus, but only an 8% rise in women who have had a hysterectomy[26]. Prolonged treatment with danazol, a progesterone antagonist, produces a fall in PP14 levels[39]. But a number of factors suggest that progesterone may only have an indirect effect on PP14 secretion. First the substantial gap between the rise in progesterone and the rise in PP14 is untypical of most tissue responses to steroids which tend to occur in hours rather than days. Second, there is no fall of PP14 levels following administration of the progesterone receptor antagonist RU486[31]. Finally, the relationship to progesterone does not explain the very rapid fall in PP14 levels after 9 to 10 weeks of pregnancy, a time when progesterone levels are continuing to rise. The latter phenomenon is better explained by the appearance and regression of a particular group of secretory cells[1].

LEVELS OF PP12 AND PP14 IN NON-PREGNANT SUBJECTS

The most notable feature of circulating PP12 levels in the non-pregnant state is the extraordinarily striking diurnal variation with a nadir at 10:00–11:00[34]. Surprisingly, there is no apparent variation during the menstrual cycle[40]. Following hysterectomy there is a small decline, returning to normal within 3 to 4 weeks, confirming that the endometrium is not a major source in the non-pregnant state. However, ovarian hyperstimulation can lead to an increase in PP12[26].

In ovulatory cycles the values of PP14 rise in the last week of the luteal phase; high levels are maintained for the first days of the next period and eventually fall in the mid to late proliferative phase[38,41–44]. There is no rise in anovulatory women.

LEVELS OF PP12 AND PP14 IN PREGNANT SUBJECTS

Levels of PP12 start to rise at 8 weeks gestation. There is a major peak at 18–24 weeks and a smaller rise at 36–40 weeks[45,46]. In cord serum the concentrations are similar to those in the mother, whereas amniotic fluid levels are 100-fold higher or more.

Circulating levels of PP14 start to rise 1 week after ovulation. In a fertile cycle the levels continue to rise steeply until weeks 8–10 of pregnancy and decline thereafter, a pattern similar to human chorionic gonadotropin[21,41,47,48]. A similar pattern is observed in the endometrium[48]. At term PP14 levels in the fetus correlate with but are 10-fold less than, those in the mother[48]. The PP14 concentration in amniotic fluid is 100 to 1000-fold higher than in maternal or cord blood[49]. The highest levels in amniotic fluid are found at weeks 8–10 of pregnancy[21].

CLINICAL APPLICATION OF MEASUREMENT OF PP12 AND PP14 LEVELS

In non-pregnant women, measurement of PP12 may be of value in the monitoring of ovarian hyperstimulation[26]. Elevated PP12 levels have been reported in advanced ovarian cancer[26] and in patients with primary liver cancer[50], and reduced levels in women with polycystic ovarian disease[51]. However, the specificity is low and it is unlikely that these will become useful clinical tests.

In late pregnancy, elevated levels of PP12 are found in association with pre-eclampsia[45,52]. There is also an *inverse* relationship to the weight of the fetus in both normal and pre-eclamptic pregnancies[28]. The practical clinical significance of these findings needs to be re-evaluated with *timed* samples, in the light of the very major diurnal rhythm of this protein.

Because there is virtually no overlap in late luteal PP14 levels between ovulatory and anovulatory cycles, it has been suggested that PP14 measurement might be a useful retrospective test for ovulation[43]. In subjects considered to have an inadequate luteal phase on the basis of endometrial histology the serum concentration of progestogen-dependent endometrial protein (identical to PP14) shows a smaller rise than in normal ovulatory cycles[42]. However, there are cases in which there is no rise in PP14 despite an apparently normal pattern of progesterone secretion[38]. Studies in IVF–ET pregnancies show that a rise in PP14 is associated with implantation[38]. However, the difference between successful and unsuccessful attempts is only apparent 21 days after the LH surge[52].

Small amounts of PP14 can be found in peritoneal fluid. As would be expected, the amount is greatly increased in association with endometriosis during the secretory phase[38]. Administration of progesterone can stimulate PP14 secretion in some but not all cases of endometrial carcinoma[38]; whether this is a guide to the potential usefulness of progestogen therapy in an individual patient requires further investigation. Circulating PP14 is increased in association with trophoblastic tumors, the levels being much higher in benign (hydatidiform mole) than in malignant disease (choriocarcinoma)[54].

In late pregnancy there is no relationship between maternal PP14 levels and the sex or birthweight of the child, and age or parity of the mother[53]. In hypertensive pregnancies PP14 levels have variously been described as elevated[60], or reduced.

REFERENCES

1. Bell, S.C. (1988). Secretory/endometrial decidual proteins and their function in early pregnancy. *J. Reprod. Fertil.*, Suppl. **36**, 109–25
2. Bohn, H. and Kraus, W. (1980). Isolierung und charakterisierung eines neue plazentaspezi-

fischen proteins. *Arch. Gynekol.*, **229**, 279–91

3. Bell, S.C., Patel, S., Hales, M.W., Kirwan, P.H. and Drife, J.O. (1985). Immunochemical detection and characterisation of pregnancy associated endometrial alpha-globulin, and alpha-globulins secreted by the human endometrium. *J. Reprod. Fertil.*, **74**, 261–70
4. Julkunen, M., Raikar, R.S., Joshi, S.G., Bohn, H. and Seppala, M. (1986). Placental protein 14 and progestagen-dependent endometrial protein are immunologically indistinguishable. *Hum. Reprod.*, **1**, 7–8
5. Rutanen, E.M., Koistinen, R., Wahlstrom, T., Bohn, H., Ranta, T. and Seppala, M. (1985). Synthesis of placental protein 12 by decidua. *Endocrinology*, **116**, 1304–9
6. Rutanen, E.M., Koistinen, R., Sjoberg, J., Julkunen, M., Wahlstrom, T., Bohn, H. and Seppala, M. (1986). Synthesis of placental protein 12 by human endometrium. *Endocrinology*, **118**, 1067–71
7. Wahlstrom, T. and Seppala, M. (1984). Placental protein 12 (PP12) is induced in the endometrium by progesterone. *Fertil. Steril.*, **41**, 781–4
8. Waites, G.T., James, R.F.L. and Bell, S.C. (1989). Human 'pregnancy-associated endometrial alpha-1-globulin', an insulin-like growth factor-binding protein: immunohistological localization in the decidua and placenta during pregnancy employing monoclonal antibodies. *J. Endocrinol.*, **120**, 351–7
9. Suikkari, A.M., Jalkanen, J., Koistinen, R., Butzow, R., Ritvos, O., Ranta, T. and Seppala, M. (1989). Human granulosa cells synthesise low molecular weight insulin-like growth factor-binding protein. *Endocrinology*, **124**, 1088–90
10. Wahlstrom, T., Koskimies, A.I., Tenhunen, A., Rutanen, E.M., Yki-Karvinen, H., Julkunen, M. and Seppala, M. (1985). Pregnancy proteins in the endometrium after follicle aspiration for in vitro fertilization. *Ann. N.Y. Acad. Sci.*, **442**, 402–7
11. Waites, G.T., Wood, P.L., Walker, R.A. and Bell, S.C. (1988). Immunohistological localization of human endometrial secretory protein, 'pregnancy-associated endometrial alpha-2-globulin' (α2-PEG) during the menstrual cycle. *J. Reprod. Fertil.*, **82**, 665–72
12. Bell, S.C. and Dore-Green, F. (1987). Detection and characterization of human secretory 'pregnancy-associated and endometrial alpha-2-globulin' (α-2-PEG) in uterine luminal fluid. *J. Reprod. Fertil.*, **11**, 13–29
13. Julkunen, M., Wahlstrom, T., Seppala, M., Koistinen, R., Koskimies, A., Stenman, U.H. and Bohn, H. (1984). Detection and localization of placental protein 14-like proteins in human seminal plasma and in the male genital tract. *Arch. Androl.*, **12** (Suppl.), 59–67
14. Bolton, A.E., Pinto-Furtado, L.G., Andrew, C.E. and Chapman, M.G. (1986). Measurement of the pregnancy-associated proteins, placental protein 14 and pregnancy-associated plasma protein A in human seminal plasma. *Clin. Reprod. Fertil.*, **4**, 233–40
15. Bell, S.C. and Patel, S.R. (1987). Immunochemical detection, physicochemical characterization and levels of human secretory pregnancy-associated endometrial alpha-2-globulin (α-2-PEG) on seminal plasma in men. *J. Reprod. Fertil.*, **80**, 31–42
16. Seppala, M., Koskimies, A.E. and Tenhunen, A. (1985). Pregnancy proteins in seminal plasma, seminal vesicles, preovulatory follicular fluid and ovary. *Ann. N.Y. Acad. Sci.*, **442**, 212–26
17. Koistinen, R., Kalkkinen, N., Huhtala, M.L., Seppala, M., Bohn, H. and Rutanen, E.M. (1986). Placental protein 12 is a decidual protein that binds somatomedin and has an identical N-terminal amino acid sequence with somatomedin-binding protein from human amniotic fluid. *Endocrinology*, **118**, 1375–8
18. Julkunen, M., Koistinen, R., Aalto-Setala, K., Seppala, M., Janne, O.A. and Kontula, K. (1988). Primary structure of human insulin-like growth factor binding protein/placental protein 12 and tissue-specific expression of its mRNA. *FEBS Letters*, **236**, 295–302
19. Grundman, U., Nerlich, C., Bohn, H. and Rein, T. (1989). Cloning of cDNA encoding human placental protein 12 (PP12): binding protein for IGF I and somatomedin. *Nucl. Acids Res.*, **16**, 8711
20. Bohn, H., Kraus, W. and Winckler, W. (1982). New soluble placental tissue proteins: their isolation, characterization, localization and quantification. In Klopper, A. (ed.), *Immunology of Human Placental Proteins*, pp. 67–81. (Eastbourne: Praeger)
21. Julkunen, M., Rutanen, E.M., Koskimies, A., Ranta, T., Bohn, H. and Seppala, M. (1985). Distribution of placental protein 14 in tissues and body fluids during pregnancy. *Br. J. Obstet. Gynaecol.*, **92**, 1145–51

22. Bell, S.C., Keyte, J.W. and Waites, G.T. (1987). Pregnancy-associated endometrial alpha-2-globulin (α-2-PEG), the major secretory protein of the luteal phase and first trimester pregnancy endometrium, is not glycosylated prolactin but related to beta-lactoglobulins. *J. Clin. Endocrinol. Metab.*, **65**, 1067–71
23. Huhtala, M.L., Seppala, M., Narvanen, A., Palomaki, P., Julkunen, M. and Bohn, H. (1987). Amino acid sequence homology between human placental protein 14 and beta-lactoglobulins from various species. *Endocrinology*, **120**, 2620–2
24. Westwood, O.M.R., Chapman, M.G., Totty, N., Philp, R., Bolton, A.E. and Lazarus, N.R. (1988). N-terminal sequence analysis of human placental protein 14 purified in high yield from decidual cytosol. *J. Reprod. Fertil.*, **82**, 493–500
25. Julkunen, M., Seppala, M. and Janne, O.A. (1988). Complete amino acid sequence of human placental protein 14: a progesterone-regulated uterine protein homologous to beta-lactoglobulins. *Proc. Natl. Acad. Sci., USA*, **85**, 8845–9
26. Seppala, M., Riitinen, L., Julkunen, M., Koistinen, R., Wahlstrom, T., Iino, K., Alfthan, H., Stenman, U.H. and Huhtala, M.L. (1988). Structural studies, localization in tissue and clinical aspects of human endometrial proteins. *J. Reprod. Fertil.*, Suppl. **36**, 127–41
27. Rutanen, E.M., Pekonen, F. and Makinen, T. (1988). Soluble 34K binding protein inhibits the binding of insulin-like growth factor I to its cell receptors in human secretory phase endometrium: evidence for autocrine/paracrine regulation of growth factor action. *J. Clin. Endocrinol. Metab.*, **66**, 173–80
28. Howell, R.J.S., Perry, L.A., Choglay, N.S., Bohn, H. and Chard, T. (1985). Placental protein 12 (PP12): a new test for the prediction of the small-for-gestational-age infant. *Br. J. Obstet. Gynaecol.*, **92**, 1141–4
29. Bolton, A.E., Pockley, A.G., Clough, K.J., Mowles, E.A., Soker, R.J., Westwood, O.M.R. and Chapman, M.G. (1987). Identification of placental protein 14 as an immunosuppressive factor in human reproduction. *Lancet*, **i**, 593–5
30. Bolton, A.E., Pockley, A.G., Stoker, R.J., Westwood, O.M.R. and Chapman, M.G. (1988). Biological activity of placental protein 14. In Chapman, M., Grudzinskas, M. and Chard, T. (eds). pp. 135–144. (London: Springer-Verlag)
31. Howell, R.J.S., Olajide, F., Teisner, B., Grudzinskas, J.G. and Chard, T. (1989). Circulating levels of placental protein 14 and progesterone following RU38486 and Gemeprost for termination of first trimester pregnancy. *Fertil. Steril.*, **52**, 66–8
32. Olajide, F., Howell, R.J.S., Wass, J.A.H., Holly, J.M.P., Bohn, H., Grudzinskas, J.G., Chapman, M.G. and Chard, T. (1989). Circulating levels of placental protein 12 and chorionic gonadotropin following RU38486 and Gemeprost for termination of first trimester pregnancy. *Hum. Reprod.*, **4**, 337–40
33. Suikkari, A.M., Koivisto, V.A., Rutanen, E.M., Yki-Jarvinen, H., Karonen, S.L. and Seppala, M. (1987). Insulin regulates the serum levels of low molecular weight insulin-like growth factor-binding protein. *J. Clin. Endocrinol. Metab.*, **66**, 266–72
34. Holly, J.M.P., Biddlecombe, R.A., Dunger, D.B., Edge, J.A., Amiel, S.A., Howell, R., Chard, T., Rees, L.H. and Wass, J.A.H. (1988). Circadian variation of GH-dependent IGF-binding protein in diabetes mellitus and its relationship to insulin. A new role for insulin. *Clin. Endocrinol.*, **29**, 667–75
35. Suikkari, A.M., Koivisto, V.A., Koistinen, R., Seppala, M. and Yki-Karvinen, H. (1989). Dose-response characteristics for suppression of low molecular weight plasma insulin-like growth factor-binding protein by insulin. *J. Clin. Endocrinol. Metab.*, **68**, 135–40
36. Suikkari, A.M., Sane, T., Seppala, M., Yki-Jarvinen, H., Karonen, S.L. and Viovisto, V.A. (1989). Prolonged exercise increases serum insulin-like growth factor binding protein concentrations. *J. Clin. Endocrinol. Metab.*, **68**, 141–4
37. Seppala, M., Ronnberg, L., Karonen, S.L. and Kauppila, A. (1987). Micronized oral progesterone increases the circulating level of endometrial secretory PP14/beta lactoglobulin homologue. *Hum. Reprod.*, **2**, 453–5
38. Joshi, S.G. (1987). Progestin-dependent human endometrial protein: a marker for monitoring human endometrial function. *Adv. Exp. Med. Biol.*, **230**, 167–96
39. Than, G., Seppala, M., Julkunen, M., Szabo, D., Bodis, J., Szilagyi, A. and Csaba, I. (1987). The effect of danazol on the circulating levels of 34K insulin-like growth factor binding protein and endometrial beta-lactoglobulin in cultured decidual and chorionic villus cells. *Hum. Reprod.*, **2**, 431–4

40. Suikkari, A.M., Rutanen, E.M. and Seppala, M. (1987). Circulating levels of immunoreactive insulin-like growth factor-binding protein in non-pregnant women. *Hum. Reprod.*, **6**, 297–300
41. Joshi, S.G., Bank, J.F., Henriques, E.S., Makarachi, A. and Matties, G. (1982). Serum levels of progestagen-associated endometrial protein during the menstrual cycle and pregnancy. *J. Clin. Endocrinol. Metab.*, **55**, 642–8
42. Joshi, S.G., Rao, R., Henriques, E.E., Raikar, R.S. and Gordon, M. (1986). Luteal phase concentration of a progestagen-associated endometrial protein (PEP) in the serum of cycling women with adequate or inadequate endometrium. *J. Clin. Endocrinol. Metab.*, **63**, 1247–9
43. Julkunen, M., Apter, D., Seppala, M., Stenman, U.H. and Bohn, H. (1986). Serum levels of placental protein 14 reflect ovulation in non-conceptual menstrual cycles. *Fertil. Steril.*, **45**, 47–50
44. Rutanen, E.M., Bohn, H. and Seppala, M. (1982). Radioimmunoassay of placental protein 12: levels in amniotic fluid, cord blood and serum of healthy adults, pregnant women and patients with trophoblastic disease. *Am. J. Obstet. Gynecol.*, **144**, 460–3
45. Than, G.N., Csaba, I.F., Szabo, D.G., Arany, A.A., Bognar, Z.J. and Bohn, H. (1984). Serum levels of placenta-specific tissue protein 12 (PP12) in pregnancies complicated by pre-eclampsia, diabetes or twins. *Arch. Gynecol.*, **236**, 41–5
46. Bell, S.C., Jackson, J., Dore-Green, F., Kirwan, P.H. and Drife, J.O. (1987). Development and validation of a radioimmunoassay for human secretory 'pregnancy associated endometrial alpha-2-globulin' (α-2-PEG) and detection in serum during pregnancy. *Hum. Reprod.*, **2**, 387–9
47. Than, G.N., Tatra, G., Bohn, H., Szabo, D.G., Csaba, I.F. and Arnold, I. (1987). Placental protein 14 serum levels following conception. *Med. Sci. Res.*, **15**, 1243–4
48. Bell, S.C., Hales, M.W., Patel, S.R., Kirwan, P.H. and Drife, J.O. (1985). Protein synthesis and secretion by the human endometrium and decidua during early pregnancy. *Br. J. Obstet. Gynecol.*, **92**, 793–803
49. Bolton, A.E., Dawkins, K.P., Stoker, R.J., Rubenstein, E., Obiekwe, B.C. and Chard, T. (1985). The relationship of placental protein 14 (PP14) in the mother and fetus to specific products of the human placenta. *Placenta*, **6**, 1–4
50. Rutanen, E.M., Wahlstrom, T., Koistinen, R., Sipponen, P., Jalanko, H.R. and Seppala, M. (1984). Placental protein 12 in primary liver cancer and cirrhosis. *Tumour Biol.*, **5**, 95–102
51. Suikkari, A.M., Ruutiainen, K., Erkkola, R. and Seppala, M. (1989). Low levels of low molecular weight insulin-like growth factor-binding protein in patients with polycystic ovarian disease. *Hum. Reprod.*, **2**, 136–9
52. Iino, K., Sjoberg, J. and Seppala, M. (1986). Elevated circulating levels of decidual protein, placental protein 12 in pre-eclampsia. *Obstet. Gynecol.*, **68**, 58–60
53. Howell, R.J.S., Bolton, A.E. and Chard, T. (1986). Placental protein 14 (PP14) in late pregnancy. *Arch. Gynecol.*, **239**, 27–9
54. Than, G.N., Tatra, G., Szabo, D.G., Csaba, I.F. and Bohn, H. (1988). Beta lactoglobulin homologue placental protein 14 (PP14) in serum of patients with trophoblastic disease and non-trophoblastic gynecologic malignancy. *Arch. Gynecol. Obstet.*, **243**, 131–7
55. Petrunin, D.D., Gryaznova, I.M., Petrunina, Y.A. and Tatarinov, Y.S. (1976). Immunological identification of organ specific placental alpha-1-globulin and its content in amniotic fluid. *Bull. Exp. Biol. Med. USSR*, **82**, 994–6
56. Petrunin, D.D., Gryaznova, I.M., Petrunina, Y.A. and Tatarinov. Y.S. (1976). Comparative immunochemical characteristics of human chorionic alpha-1 and alpha-2 microglobulins. *Bull. Exp. Biol. Med. USSR*, **85**, 658–661
57. Sutcliffe, R.G., Bolton, A.E., Sharp, F., Nicholson, L.V.B. and Mackinnon, R. (1980). Purification of human alpha uterine protein. *J. Reprod. Fertil.*, **58**, 435–42
58. Joshi, S.G., Ebert, K.M. and Swartz, D.P. (1980). Detection and synthesis of a progestagen-dependent protein in human endometrium. *J. Reprod. Fertil.*, **59**, 273–85
59. Sutcliffe, R.G., Joshi, S.C., Patterson, W.F. and Bank, J.F. (1982). Serological identity between human alpha uterine protein and human progestagen-dependent endometrial protein. *J. Reprod. Fertil.*, **65**, 207–9
60. Iino, K., Julkunen, M., Sjoberg, J. and Seppala, M. (1986). Is decidua affected in gestational hypertension? Indication by elevated PP14 levels. *Acta Obstet. Gynecol. Scand.*, **65**, 367–70

112

New therapeutic approaches to endometriosis

C. O'Herlihy

INTRODUCTION

The frequency with which pelvic endometriosis is diagnosed in gynecological patients appears to be increasing, particularly in those women presenting for investigation of infertility[1]. Certainly more widespread use of laparoscopy and heightened public awareness of subfertility assessment are influencing this trend, together with later age of childbearing in some societies. Most women experiencing a delay in conception in association with endometriosis have mild disease with no significant pelvic adhesions and American Fertility Society (AFS) scores in single figures. Retrograde menstruation is a universal phenomenon in normal women but also represents the pathogenic mechanism of endometriosis[2], although the pelvic promoting factors in susceptible subjects have not been elucidated.

MILD ENDOMETRIOSIS AND INFERTILITY

While extensive endometriosis undoubtedly reduces fecundity, the causal relationship with mild endometriosis is much less certain, despite proven disturbance of peritoneal and ovarian function[3] (Table 1). The increased local prostaglandin levels[4] have been blamed for premature luteolysis and failure of oocyte release following the LH surge. Increased peritoneal fluid volume, macrophage overactivity[5] and both cellular and humoral immune disturbances have all been documented, as have circulating antiendometrial autoantibodies[6] and deficient local T-lymphocyte function.

Table 1 Postulated mechanisms of infertility with mild endometriosis

Luteal phase insufficiency
Intraperitoneal macrophage overactivity
Peritoneal fluid embryo toxicity
Luteinized unruptured follicle syndrome
Autoantibody activity

Experimental endometriosis models in animals[7] and 'soft' epidemiological evidence suggest that mild disease causes reduced fertility in a proportion of cases and most clinicians provide anecdotal support for this hypothesis. However, it must be conceded that a significant proportion of patients with non-adhesive disease will conceive if observed untreated for 1–2 years from the time of diagnosis[8,9]. The data to support a causal role for endometriosis is generally uncontrolled. Visible pelvic deposits may constitute only a small proportion of the total microscopically affected pelvic tissues, making firm diagnosis and assessment of therapy treacherous[10]. Nevertheless, this key question as to whether scattered deposits represent the cause or merely the result of delayed conception will only be satisfactorily answered by a large (probably multicentered) randomized trial of early suppressive therapy compared with a control cohort untreated for 12 months or more after diagnosis.

Our own observational experience in 62 patients with mild disease (AFS scores 1–6) and other infertility factors excluded, illustrate this need for randomized data (Table 2). These patients were treated with either danazol or gonadotropin-releasing hormone analogs for 6 months, except for four patients who conceived before starting planned therapy. The satisfactory pregnancy rates in both immediate and delayed treatment groups fail to shed light on the causal significance of their endometriosis, although the negative significance of ovarian deposits has also been noted by others.

NON-INVASIVE DISEASE MARKER

Because of its almost exclusive pelvic localization, endometriosis can generally be conclusively diagnosed only by direct surgical inspection. More importantly in clinical practice, the disease response to therapy is similarly difficult to monitor non-invasively. Individual susceptibility to drug treatment appears to vary considerably but, in the absence of 'second-look' laparoscopy, persistence or recurrence of disease and duration of treatment for the most part must depend on guesswork. The potential advantages of a reliable circulating index of endometriotic activity would therefore be considerable.

CA-125 is an antigen associated with a high molecular weight glycoprotein, which is expressed in human celomic epithelium[11]. Using the monoclonal

Table 2 The outcome in terms of fertility in 62 patients presenting with mild endometriosis and infertility

Pretreatment interval (< 6 months)	22
(i) conceived before treatment	4 (18%)
(ii) conceived within 18 months*	14 (64%)
No pretreatment interval	40
(i) conceived within 12 months*	25 (63%)
(ii) conceived within 18 months*	30 (75%)
Conceived following ovarian deposits*	13/28 (46%)

*All these patients completed 6 months of therapy

antibody OC-125, elevated circulating levels have been documented in association with ovarian carcinoma, pregnancy (with very high concentrations in amniotic fluid) and pelvic inflammation.

In normal subjects, CA-125 values below 16 μg/ml are usual, although a physiological increase occurs during menses[12]. Basal levels in women with advanced endometriosis generally exceed 35 μg/ml and are also raised at menstruation[13]. In cases of mild endometriosis CA-125 seems less discriminant, with considerable overlap with values in normal women, and analysis of peritoneal fluid samples does not enhance its sensitivity[14].

Serum concentrations fall during various forms of medical therapy towards normal values (below 20 μg/ml)[15]; early evidence suggests that levels which remain low for 8 weeks after completing treatment are associated with a better prognosis and lower relapse rate than if an early 'rebound' occurs[16]. Another interesting application for this marker involves radiolabelled OC-125 immunoscintigraphy of pelvic endometriotic deposits when serum CA-125 levels are normal; this technique may provide information on disease activity, in addition to its localization[17]. The relatively low sensitivity on the assay suggests that CA-125 is not ideal as a screening technique, although its values rise progressively with the extent of endometriosis; it probably offers more as an index of response to treatment.

THE ROLE OF GONADOTROPIN-RELEASING HORMONE ANALOGS

Danazol is currently the most widely used medical therapy for endometriosis, acting through a combination of antigonadotropic and antiestrogenic/mildly androgenic activity[18]. Danazol may also have a direct immune-mediated effect on deposits[19]. It has been shown that induction of amenorrhea on treatment correlates with regression of pelvic deposits and to achieve this, daily dosages of 600 mg or more are needed in women of average body mass[20]. In such a dosage, unwanted effects may provoke cessation of therapy in a small proportion of cases.

This disadvantage has lead to a reappraisal of danazol with the advent of analog agonists of the hypothalamic decapeptide, gonadotropin-releasing hormone (GnRH-a). These agents cause a down regulation of anterior pituitary and thus ovarian function and induce a state of reversible hypoestrogenism which permits regression of endometriotic deposits[21]. Because of rapid digestive degradation, agonist treatment must be parenteral and was initially given either by subcutaneous injection or intranasal spray. These routes necessitate frequent administration and will suppress circulating estradiol to early follicular phase levels.

More recently a biodegradable copolymer agonist preparation (Zoladex) can be given as a single monthly depot injection. This induces a more profound ovarian suppression, together with observable improvement in endometriosis. The menopause-like vasomotor symptoms, common to all patients on GnRH-a treatment, vary widely in individuals but may be longer lasting and more incapacitating with profound estradiol suppression to levels below 25 pg/ml. Reduced libido and vaginal dryness are less commonly problematic than flushes during a 6-month course of therapy. Reductions in bone mineral density invariably occur with hypoestrogenic states of this duration but appear to be reversible on completion of treatment[22].

Data comparing the efficacy of 6 months of therapy with GnRH-a and danazol in clearing endometriosis are inconclusive to date, although large studies are in progress. In terms of cost, both agents are expensive and both induce troublesome symptoms in a proportion of patients. Danazol causes some bone accretion in contrast with the osteoporotic effects of the analogs but the longer term relevance of this side-effect is uncertain in women who resume regular menstruation. The appeal of once-monthly dosage to those with endometriosis may come to outweigh the menopausal effects if abolition of pelvic pain and pregnancy rates are shown to be comparable with danazol.

REFERENCES

1. Olive, D. and Haney, A.F. (1986). Endometriosis – associated infertility: a critical review of therapeutic approaches. *Obstet. Gynecol. Surv.*, **41**, 538–55
2. Geist, S.H. (1979). The viability of fragments of menstrual endometrium. *Am. J. Obstet. Gynecol.*, **125**, 751–4
3. Muse, K.N. and Wilson, E.A. (1982). How does mild endometriosis cause infertility? *Fertil. Steril.*, **38**, 145–52
4. Dawood, M.Y., Kahn-Dawood, F.S. and Wilson, L. (1984). Peritoneal fluid prostaglandins and prostanoids in women with endometriosis, chronic pelvic inflammatory disease and pelvic pain. *Am. J. Obstet. Gynecol.*, **148**, 391–5
5. Haney, A.F., Muscato, J.J. and Weinberg, J.B. (1981). Peritoneal fluid cell populations in infertility patients. *Fertil. Steril.*, **35**, 696–9
6. Halme, J. and Mathur, S. (1987). Local autoimmunity in mild endometriosis. *Int. J. Fertil.*, **32**, 309–11
7. Dizerega, G.S., Barber, D.L. and Hodgen, G.D. (1980). Endometriosis: role of ovarian steroids in initiation, maintenance and suppression. *Fertil. Steril.*, **33**, 649–53
8. Garcia, C.R. and David, S.S. (1977). Pelvic endometriosis: infertility and pelvic pain. *Am. J. Obstet. Gynecol.*, **129**, 740–4
9. Collins, J.A., Writom, W., Janes, L.B. and Wilson, E.H. (1983). Treatment-independent pregnancy among infertile couples. *N. Engl. J. Med.*, **309**, 1201–3
10. Murphy, A.A., Green, W.R., Bobbie, D., De La Cruz, Z. and Rock, J.A. (1986). Unsuspected endometriosis documented by scanning electron microscopy in visually normal peritoneum. *Fertil. Steril.*, **46**, 522–6
11. Niloff, J.N., Knapp, R.C., Schaetzl, E., Reynolds, C. and Bast, R.C. (1984). CA-125 antigen levels in obstetric and gynaecological patients. *Obstet. Gynecol.*, **64**, 703–7
12. Pittaway, D.E. and Fayez, J.A. (1987). Serum CA125 antigen levels increase during menses. *Am. J. Obstet. Gynecol.*, **156**, 75–6
13. Patton, P.E., Field, C.S., Harms, R.W. and Coulam, C.S. (1986). CA-125 levels in endometriosis. *Fertil. Steril.*, **45**, 770–3
14. Moretuzzo, R.W., Di Lauro, S., Jenison, E., Chen, S.L., Reindollar, R.H. and McDonough, P.G. (1988). Serum and peritoneal lavage fluid CA-125 levels in endometriosis. *Fertil. Steril.*, **50**, 430–3
15. Irvine, L.M., Burford, G., Acien, P. and Shaw, R.W. (1988). The assessment of the role of CVA-125 in the diagnosis, prognosis and efficiency of treatment in endometriosis. *Br. J. Obstet. Gynaecol.*, **95**, 726
16. Takahashi, K., Yoshino, K., Nagata, H., Kusakari, M. and Kitao, M. (1988). CA-125 is an effective marker for patients with external endometriosis and on danazol: case reports. *Fertil. Steril.*, **50**, 173–5

17. Kennedy, S.H., Soper, N., Mojiminiyi, O.A., Shepstone, B.J. and Barlow, D.H. (1988). Immunoscintigraphy of ovarian endometriosis. A preliminary study. *Br. J. Obstet. Gynaecol.*, **95**, 693–7
18. Barbieri, R.L. and Ryan, K.L. (1981). Danazol: endocrine pharmacology and therapeutic applications. *Am. J. Obstet. Gynecol.*, **141**, 453–8
19. El-Roeiy, A., Dmowski, W.P., Gleicher, N., Radwanska, E., Harlow, L., Binor, Z., Tummon, I. and Rawlins, R.G. (1988). Danazol but not gonadotropin-releasing hormone agonists suppresses autoantibodies in endometriosis. *Fertil. Steril.*, **50**, 864–6
20. Biberoglu, K.O. and Behrman, S.J. (1981). Dosage aspects of danazol therapy in endometriosis: short term and long term effectiveness. *Am. J. Obstet. Gynecol.*, **139**, 645–9
21. McLachlan, R.I., Healy, D.L. and Burger, H.G. (1986). Clinical aspects of LHRH analogues in gynaecology: a review. *Br. J. Obstet. Gynaecol.*, **93**, 431–54
22. Tummon, I.S., Ali, A., Pepping, M.E., Radwanska, E., Binor, Z. and Dmowski, W.P. (1988). Bone mineral density in women with endometriosis before and during ovarian suppression with gonadotropin releasing hormone agonists or danazol. *Fertil. Steril.*, **49**, 792–6

113

Does medical treatment influence the reproductive potential of patients with minimal or mild endometriosis?

G.B. Candiani, L. Fedele, P. Vercellini, S. Bianchi, L. Arcaini and F. Parazzini

Endometriosis is one of the commonest gynecological disorders in women of reproductive age. Its association with infertility is generally accepted, and a conservative therapeutic approach is required. This explains the continuing attempts to identify an effective medical treatment for the forms without adhesions or anatomically altered pelvic structures. The recent observation of microscopic and subperitoneal disease[1,2] makes the requirement for medical treatment even more important. Endometriosis is a sex steroid-dependent disorder, as shown by its manifestations according to different phases of a woman's reproductive life and by animal studies[3]. Progestogens alone or combined with estrogens have therefore been used to treat endometriosis with the aim of inducing pseudodecidualization and atrophy of the implants. Other treatments administered include danazol, a compound able to induce a hypoestrogenic and hyperandrogenic environment, gestrinone, a steroid with progestogenic action and marked androgenic activity, and lastly gonadotropin releasing hormone (GnRH) analogs, which induce a state of more or less marked hypogonadotropic hypogonadism similar to prepuberty.

In this study we evaluated the impact of danazol, gestrinone and a GnRH agonist, buserelin, on infertility associated with minimal and mild endometriosis, comparing the pregnancy rates obtained with the various treatments with that of a control group of untreated patients.

MATERIAL AND METHODS

We studied 115 infertile women with laparoscopic diagnosis of R-AFS[4] stage I or II endometriosis made at the 1st Department of Obstetrics and Gynecology of Milan University. Before laparoscopy a complete infertility work-up was performed including semen analysis of the partner, postcoital test, evaluation of ovulation of basal body temperature and serum progesterone, prolactin determination, hysterosalpingography, and an endometrial biopsy in the luteal phase. Patients with bilateral tubal occlusion or whose partner had severe dyspermia were excluded from the study as were women who had been treated with sex hormones in the previous 6 months and those with severe systemic or endocrine diseases. During the diagnostic laparoscopy no attempt was made to remove or cauterize the endometriotic lesions.

The patients were allocated to one of the following four treatment groups:

(1) Expectant treatment ($n = 29$);
(2) Danazol 600–800 mg daily for 6 months ($n = 41$);
(3) Gestrinone 2.5 mg two or three times weekly for 6 months ($n = 13$);
(4) Intranasal buserelin 1200 μg daily for 6 months ($n = 32$).

At the end of the treatment the women were followed for at least 6 months.

In the patients who received expectant treatment, and during follow-up in all the other women, adequate therapeutic measures were performed to correct any other infertility factors present.

Restoration of fertility was analyzed with the life-table method. χ^2 analysis was used to compare the groups.

RESULTS

At the diagnostic laparoscopy 62 patients had stage I endometriosis and 53 had stage II. The mean age, parity, duration of infertility and extent of the disease did not differ significantly in the four treatment groups (Table 1). The mean follow-up was 16 months (range 8–40). The crude, corrected and cumulative pregnancy rates at 18 months are shown in Table 2. The differences among the groups were not significant although the patients given

Table 1 Clinical data of 115 patients with minimal or mild endometriosis

Treatment groups	*No. of patients*	*Age* (mean ± SD)	*Parity*	*Months of infertility* (mean ± SD)	*Stage I*	*Stage II*
Danazol	41	30.8 ± 4.1	3	47.9 ± 23.4	21	20
Gestrinone	13	28.6 ± 3.9	—	52.3 ± 14.7	6	7
Buserelin	32	30.1 ± 3.7	2	40.4 ± 27.6	17	15
Expectant management	29	31.3 ± 4.8	4	54.1 ± 35.7	18	11

Table 2 Recovery of fertility in 115 women with minimal or mild endometriosis

Treatment groups	*No. of patients*	*Pregnancies*			
		No.	*Crude rate**	*Corrected rate**	*Cumulative rate†*
Danazol	41	16	39%	47%	44%
Gestrinone	13	4	31%	40%	34%
Buserelin	32	14	44%	54%	48%
Expectant management	29	15	52%	60%	54%

*Not significant by χ^2 analysis
†Cumulative pregnancy rates at 18 months follow-up; not significant by life-table analysis

expectant treatment showed the best results in terms of restored fertility.

The cumulative pregnancy rate in the patients with stage I endometriosis did not differ from that in the women with stage II disease.

DISCUSSION

The choice of the most appropriate therapeutic modality for infertile women with minimal or mild endometriosis is still a difficult problem for the gynecologist. The surgical approach is very controversial, but it is an invasive procedure that has not been found superior to medical treatment in increasing the possibility of conception[5]. In the last years pharmacological research has made various compounds available to the gynecologist, all able to induce a remission of the pain symptoms and regression of the disease at repeat laparoscopy. However, a precise evaluation of their efficacy in the treatment of infertility associated with endometriosis still cannot be made despite the numerous studies published[6]. This is due primarily to the methodological flaws of the clinical trials performed until now, such as the lack of a control group, of randomization procedures, and of adequate statistical analysis of the results.

In patients with endometriosis, especially at the initial stages, spontaneous recovery of fertility is relatively frequent. Therefore, a treatment for endometriosis should, if effective, result in a better pregnancy rate than that observed with the so-called expectant management. Various reports have been published on the results of expectant treatment after a laparoscopic diagnosis of mild endometriosis[7–14]. The pregnancy rates obtained are relatively high, varying from 22.2 to 72.2%, although the monthly pregnancy rate is notably lower than that of the general population. In the largest study published so far a pregnancy rate of 41% was reported in 244 patients with minimal or mild endometriosis according to the R-AFS classification, who have received expectant treatment for a year after laparoscopy[13].

The present study demonstrated that treatment with danazol, gestrinone or buserelin in infertile women with minimal or mild endometriosis did not offer any advantage over expectant treatment when the outcome was considered in terms of restored fertility. Our findings agree with those of the only two randomized controlled trials reported until now, one of danazol[10] and the other of gestrinone[15] as well as with the results of the recent large comparative studies of Hull[12] and Badawy *et al.*[16]. Given the relatively small number of patients included in the randomized studies, a partial impact of danazol and gestrinone on the reproductive prognosis of women with minimal or mild endometriosis cannot be definitively excluded, but it appears improbable that these drugs confer a real advantage. As regards the GnRH agonists, no sufficiently large controlled study has yet been published with which to compare our results, but they seem not to contradict the preliminary data reported[17].

The reasons for the scanty efficacy of medical treatment of infertility associated with endometriosis warrant careful consideration. On the one hand, the administered drugs' real effect on endometriotic lesions, i.e. their capacity to cure the disease, is still unclear, and on the other the relation between endometriosis and infertility is also uncertain. The efficacy of treatment has usually been evaluated by laparoscopy. However, it is now evident that this procedure is inadequate to detect the real extent of the disease, especially if performed at the end of a period of hypogonadism[18,19]. More important information is instead obtained from morphological studies. Ultrastructural investigations have demonstrated that danazol[20] and gestrinone[21] can induce inactivity and cellular degeneration of endometriotic implants. However, this effect seems to occur only in 25% of the lesions, and does not appear to be increased by prolonging the treatment[18]. A recent study has shown that gestrinone, buserelin and lynestrenol do not induce disappearance of the glandular epithelium of ovarian implants nor impede mitosis[22]. On the other hand, ectopic endometrium does not present the same cyclic modifications as eutopic endometrium[23], and the frequency and distribution of the sex steroid receptors of endometriotic implants differ markedly from those of endometrial receptors[24,25]. These data clearly indicate that hormonal control of endometriotic tissue is different from that of endometrium[26], which may explain why the disease is relatively resistant to endocrine treatment. Such treatment is probably able to induce a remission of endometriosis but not a cure, as suggested also by the high frequency of recurrence of pain symptoms and the constant persistence of the disease in patients undergoing a second laparoscopy a year after suspension of danazol treatment[27].

There is no scientific evidence to support the hypothesis that minimal and mild endometriosis causes infertility[9,28]. Various factors have been implicated including prostaglandin and peritoneal macrophage abnormalities, immune phenomena and endocrine dysfunctions, but no one theory satisfactorily explains the relation between the disease and difficulty in conception. Thomas and Cooke have reported that in their patients with complete elimination of the disease after treatment with gestrinone the recovery of fertility was no better than in the women with persistent disease at follow-up laparoscopy, as it should have been if the endometriosis were the direct cause of their problem[29]. In a recent study of 21 infertile women with minimal endometriosis who underwent donor insemination for a severe male problem, the monthly probability of conception was similar to that of the general population[14]. These observations seem to suggest that infertility is independent of the presence of endometriosis and that therefore patients with initial stages of the disease should be considered in the same way as women with unexplained infertility.

In conclusion, according to the analyzable data available, medical treatment does not seem able to improve the reproductive prognosis of infertile women with minimal endometriosis, but large randomized trials are required to confirm this impression. In addition, studies are needed to ascertain the relation between endometriosis and infertility, and hormonal regulation of the growth and maintenance of endometriotic implants should also be investigated with the aim of providing specific treatment.

Correction of any associated infertility factors and careful monitoring of ovulatory function could constitute the first approach for an infertile woman with minimal or mild endometriosis, with medical treatment reserved for persistent infertility after 1 year and for patients with pain symptoms.

REFERENCES

1. Murphy, A.A., Green, W.R., Bobbie, D., Cruz, Z.C. and Rock, JA. (1986). Unsuspected endometriosis documented by scanning electron microscopy in visually normal peritoneum. *Fertil. Steril.*, **46**, 522–5
2. Vasquez, G., Cornillie, F. and Brosens, I. (1984). Peritoneal endometriosis: scanning electron microscopy and histology of minimal pelvic endometriotic lesions. *Fertil. Steril.*, **42**, 696–703
3. Dizerega, G.S., Barber, D.L. and Hodgen, G.D. (1980). Endometriosis: Role of ovarian steroids in initiation, maintenance and suppression. *Fertil. Steril.*, **33**, 649–53
4. American Fertility Society (1985). Revised American Fertility society classification of endometriosis: 1985. *Fertil. Steril.*, **43**, 351–2
5. Guzick, D.S. and Rock, J.A. (1983). A comparison of danazol and conservative surgery for the treatment of infertility due to mild or moderate endometriosis. *Fertil. Steril.*, **40**, 580–4
6. Olive, D.L. and Haney, A.F. (1986). Endometriosis-associated infertility: A critical review of therapeutical approaches. *Obstet. Gynecol. Surv.*, **41**, 538–55
7. Acosta, A.A., Buttram, V.C. Jr., Bresh, P.K., Malinak, L.R., Franklin, R.R. and Vanderheyden, J.D. (1973). A proposed classification of pelvic endometriosis. *Obstet. Gynecol.*, **42**, 19–25
8. Garcia, C.R. and David, S.S. (1977). Pelvic endometriosis: infertility and pelvic pain. *Am. J. Obstet. Gynecol.*, **129**, 740–7
9. Schenken, R.S. and Malinak, L.R. (1982). Conservative surgery versus expectant management for the infertile patient with mild endometriosis. *Fertil. Steril.*, **37**, 183–7
10. Seibel, M.M., Berber, M.J., Weinstein, F.G. and Taymor, M.L. (1982). The effectiveness of danazol on subsequent fertility in minimal endometriosis. *Fertil. Steril.*, **38**, 534–7
11. Portuondo, J.A., Echanojauregui, A.D., Herran, C. and Alijarte, I. (1983). Early conception in patients with untreated mild endometriosis. *Fertil. Steril.*, **39**, 22–5
12. Hull, M.E., Moghissi, K.S., Magyar, D.F. and Hayes, M.F. (1987). Comparison of different treatment modalities of endometriosis in infertile women. *Fertil. Steril.*, **47**, 40–4
13. Inoue, M., Kobayashi, Y., Honda, I., Hara, I., Uchimura, M. and Fujii, A. (1988). Expectant therapy for infertile patients with endometriosis: analysis of 26 cases. In Ichinoue, K., Segal, S.J. and Mastroianni, L. (eds). *Preservation of Tubo-Ovarian Function in Gynecologic Benign and Malignant Diseases*, pp. 503–13. (New York: Raven Press)
14. Rodriguez-Escudero, F.J., Neyro, J.L., Corcostegui, B. and Benito, J.A. (1988). Does minimal endometriosis reduce fecundity? *Fertil. Steril.*, **50**, 522–4
15. Thomas, E.J. and Cooke, I.D. (1987). Successful treatment of asymptomatic endometriosis: Does it benefit infertile women? *Br. Med. J.*, **294**, 1117–9
16. Badawy, S.Z.A., El Bakry, M.M., Samuel, F. and Dizer, M. (1988). Cumulative pregnancy rates in infertile women with endometriosis. *J. Reprod. Med.*, **33**, 757–60
17. Fedele, L., Bianchi, S., Arcaini, L., Vercellini, P. and Candiani, G.B. (1988). GnRH agonists in the treatment of endometriosis. *Acta Eur. Fertil.*, **19**, 5–12
18. Brosens, I.A., Verleyen, A. and Cornillie, F. (1987). The morphologic effect of short-term medical therapy of endometriosis. *Am. J. Obstet. Gynecol.*, **157**, 1215–21
19. Evers, J.L.H. (1987). The second look laparoscopy for evaluation of the result of medical treatment of endometriosis should not be performed during ovarian suppression. *Fertil. Steril.*, **47**, 502–4
20. Schweppe, K.W., Dmowski, W.P. and Wynn, R.M. (1981). Ultrastructural changes in endometriotic tissue during danazol treatment. *Fertil. Steril.*, **36**, 20–3
21. Cornillie, F.J., Vasquez, G. and Brosens, I.A. (1985). The response of human endometriotic implants to the antiprogesterone steroid R 2323: a histologic and ultrastructural study. *Pathol. Res. Pract.*, **180**, 647–50
22. Nisolle-Pochet, M., Casanas-Roux, F. and Donnez, J. (1988). Histologic study of ovarian endometriosis after hormonal therapy. *Fertil. Steril.*, **49**, 423–6
23. Schweppe, K.W. and Wynn, R.M. (1981). Ultrastructural changes in endometriotic implants

during the menstrual cycle. *Obstet. Gynecol.*, **58**, 465–9

24. Janne, O., Kauppila, A., Kokko, E., Lantto, T., Ronnberg, L. and Vihko, R. (1981). Estrogen and progestin receptor in endometriosis lesions: comparison with endometrial tissue. *Am. J. Obstet. Gynecol.*, **141**, 562–6
25. Vierikko, P., Kauppila, A., Ronnberg, L. and Vihko, L. (1985). Steroidal regulation of endometriosis tissue; lack of induction of 17α-hydroxysteroid dehydrogenase activity by progesterone, medroxyprogesterone acetate, or danazol. *Fertil. Steril.*, **43**, 218–21
26. Kauppila, A, Isomaa, V., Ronnberg, L., Vierikko, P. and Vihko, L. (1985). Effect of gestrinone in endometriosis tissue and endometrium. *Fertil. Steril.*, **44**, 466–70
27. Fayez, J.A., Collazo, L.M. and Vernon, C. (1988). Comparison of different modalities of treatment for minimal and mild endometriosis. *Am. J. Obstet. Gynecol.*, **159**, 927–32
28. Muse, K.N. and Wilson, E.A (1982). How does mild endometriosis cause infertility? *Fertil. Steril.*, **38**, 145–9
29. Thomas, E.J. and Cooke, I.D. (1987). Impact of gestrinone on the course of asymptomatic endometriosis. *Br. Med. J.*, **294**, 272–4

114

Treatment of endometriosis with a GnRH analog (Buserelin)

M. Massobrio, D. Guidetti, A. Laudadio, A. De Filippi, G. Grassi, G. Breccia, G. Cenderelli and G.F. Trossarelli

INTRODUCTION

Endometriosis is a pathological condition characterized by the proliferation of endometrial tissue external to the uterine cavity, situated mainly in the pelvis, but also outside this area. Endometriosis of uterine muscle is defined as adenomyosis.

The therapeutic effect of ovariectomy and the almost constant regression of this disease during the menopause[1] suggests that the role of ovarian steroids is important in the maintenance of endometriosis. This is further corroborated by the fact that during pregnancy and menopause the ectopic endometrium undergoes the same modifications as the normal endometrium.

On the basis of these physiopathological statements, the treatment of endometriosis may be performed by inducing a pharmacological pseudopregnancy through continuous administration of estroprogestins or through the induction of a pseudomenopause. The latter may be achieved either using steroids like danazol or gestrinone, which unfortunately cause androgenic side-effects, or using long-acting gonadotropin-releasing hormone (GnRH) agonists.

In view of their prolonged pharmacological effect, the hyperactive GnRH agonists are as effective as continuous GnRH infusion in causing the long-lasting and steady occupation of receptors and the progessive desensitization of gonadotropic cells. Initially the GnRH have a stimulating effect on the gonadotropic function, but the repetitive and prolonged administration of high doses causes the down regulation of the pituitary receptors in their neurohormone and, as a consequence, an inhibiting effect on the pituitary gonadotropic function and ultimately on gonadal function.

The first reports about the treatment of endometriosis with GnRH agonists were published in 1980. Many methods of administration have been proposed:

continuous infusion by osmotic micropumps, subcutaneous injection and intranasal spray. The aim of the current studies is to identify therapeutic practices able to provide an effective suppression of the hypothalamus–pituitary–ovarian axis which are practical and available for wide clinical use.

We report here the results of a trial which employs the intranasal administration of buserelin for the treatment of endometriosis.

MATERIALS AND METHODS

Sixty-four patients (mean age 31 ± 6.4 years, range 21–43) with pelvic endometriosis were given buserelin, a GnRH agonist analog, for 6 months. Grouping of disease stages was made according to the classification of the American Fertility Society (RAFS), revised in 1985, by means of celioscopy performed before and after the course of treatment.

Nine patients were at the first stage, 35 at the second and 17 at the third. Cysts larger than 3 cm in diameter were removed by surgery in 14 patients. However, endometrial implants with scores above 5 (RAFS) persisted at the end of the operation. These cases were treated with buserelin and the results were evaluated by celioscopy at the end of 6 months.

Two patients with rectum–vaginal septum endometriosis and one with sigmoid endometriosis were also included. Clinical diagnosis was confirmed by histology. Thirty-five patients started therapy during the early follicular phase and 29 during the late luteal phase. Over the first 5 days, the patients were given 200 μg of buserelin subcutaneously every 12 h; and then 400 μg every 8 h intranasally for the remaining 24 weeks. Before starting the treatment, follicle stimulating hormone (FSH), luteinizing hormone (LH), prolactin, estradiol, progesterone, plasma testosterone, salivary testosterone, and sex hormone-binding globulin (SHBG) levels were measured weekly for the first month and monthly for the following 5 months. Gonadotropic assay was performed both by polyclonal radioimmunoassay (BIODATA-TER) and by monoclonal immunoradiometric assay (DELFIA). The former, as it also measures free α-subunits and fragments of hormonal subunits, is not so specific as the latter which solely measures the molecule as a whole. Thyroid (tri-iodothyronine, thyroxine, thyrotropin) and adrenal (08.00 cortisol) functions were examined every 2 months. Blood glucose, urea, creatinine, uric acid, aspartate aminotransferase, alanine aminotransferase, glutamyl transferase, alkaline phosphatase, calcium, phosphorus, total cholesterol, high-density and low-density lipoprotein cholesterol, triglycerides were checked every 2 months. Stimulation with GnRH (100 μg i.v., BIODATA) and polyclonal assay of LH and FSH (−15 min; 0 min; +20 min; +30 min; +60 min; +90 min; +120 min) was performed before the start of treatment and during the 3rd month of therapy. Before the beginning and after 6 months of treatment Nordin test (Ca_u/Cr_u;OHp_u/Cr_u), plasma osteocalcin and lumbar (L2–L4) double photonic ray osteodensitometry were carried out. Statistical analysis was achieved by Student t testing for paired data.

RESULTS

In the patients who received buserelin in the early follicular phase the average LH concentrations evaluated by polyclonal radioimmunoassay (Figure 1*b*) showed a significant rise ($p<0.001$) after the 1st week of treatment. After the 2nd week LH levels still remained significantly higher than the basal ones

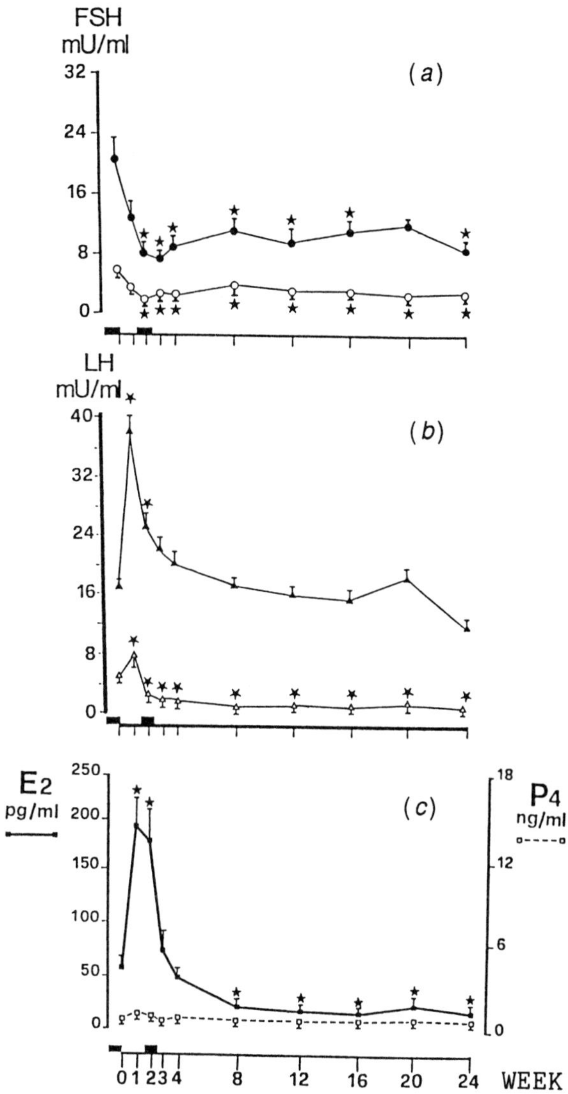

Figure 1 FSH, LH, estradiol (E_2) and progesterone (P_4) patterns of patients who began therapy in the early follicular phase; open symbols, monoclonal assay; filled symbols, polyclonal assay (in *a* and *b*); * indicates results significantly different from each other and blocks on x axis indicate periods of spotting

($p<0.005$), but remarkably lower than those measured during the 1st week. During the following 6 weeks, LH levels progressively decreased becoming lower, but not significantly, than the baseline level. From the 3rd month of treatment LH levels remained in the range of the early follicular phase. Mean baseline or in-treatment LH levels measured with monoclonal immunoradiometric assay were remarkably lower than those detected by polyclonal radioimmunoassay. During the 1st week of buserelin a significant rise in LH ($p<0.05$) was encountered once again using this method; afterwards LH levels significantly decreased, being invariably under the baseline values during the remaining period of therapy. A fall in the hormonal levels had been noted through both polyclonal and monoclonal FSH (Figure 1*a*) since the 1st week of treatment. This reduction became significant after the 2nd week. Only the polyclonal FSH levels of the 5th month were not significantly lower than the basal ones. The lack of gonadotropic reaction to GnRH stimulation during the 3rd month of treatment (ΔFSH = 1.5 mUI/ml, ΔLH = 2.7 mUI/ml) confirmed the suppression of the pituitary response capacity to the neurohormone.

Estradiol levels (Figure 1*c*) rose significantly after the 1st and 2nd weeks of treatment ($p<0.001$), then showed a marked decrease during the 2nd month ($p<0.001$) and thereafter. In 12 patients, occasional rises of estradiol levels beyond the menopausal range were observed together with vaginal bleeding. In three cases the intranasal administration was withdrawn due to severe blood loss and a subcutaneous method was adopted whereupon the bleeding stopped.

Progesterone monitoring (Figure 1*c*) showed the absence of ovulation in all the patients during the entire period of treatment. Patients who began treatment during the late luteal phase displayed a different pattern of average LH and FSH levels. During and after the 1st week of therapy, LH levels measured using the monoclonal method progressively decreased becoming significantly lower than the baseline values during the remaining 23 weeks of therapy (Figure 2*a*).

FSH levels tested by the monoclonal method fell after the 1st week of treatment but a statistical difference in relation to the baseline values was never found (Figure 2*a*).

After the 1st week there was a reduction of estradiol levels which became statistically significant during the remaining 23 weeks of therapy (Figure 2*b*). A significant drop in progesterone levels was observed during the 1st week of treatment when breakthrough bleeding occurred; these levels were maintained for the following 6 months (Figure 2*b*).

The assay of plasma and salivary testosterone, sex hormone binding globulin and the other hormonal parameters did not show significant variations. Neither did hematochemical tests performed during the treatment, show significant alterations; total cholesterol and low density lipoprotein cholesterol levels rose very slightly while triglycerides showed an insignificant decrease.

Nordin test, osteocalcin assay and bone mineral content assessed by osteodensitometry did not change during treatment (Table 1). Modifications of symptoms during the treatment are reported in Table 2. At the second

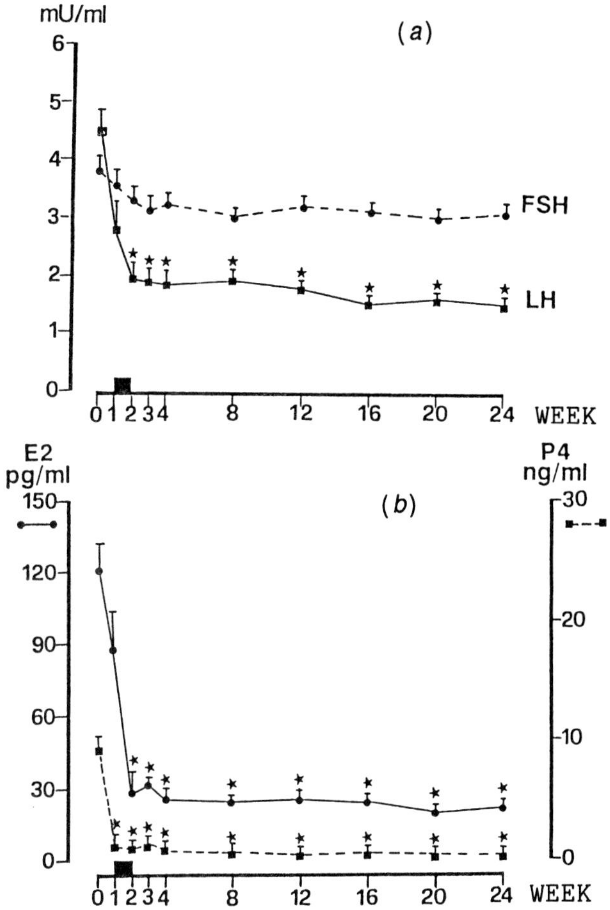

Figure 2 FSH, LH, estradiol (E_2) and progesterone (P_4) patterns of patients who began therapy in the late luteal phase; * indicates significant differences, filled blocks on x axis indicate periods of spotting

laparoscopy, performed at the termination of the therapy, endometriosis implants were not detected in 23 patients (36%), 19 cases (30%) showed a partial regression of endometriosis, whereas no variation was observed in 22 (34%). Total mean score of endometriosis decreased from 18.6 to 8.8 but the score reduction is more significant if adhesions are not considered (from 15 to 5.7). The grouping of the patients according to the stage of disease and the results of the therapy are reported in Table 3. Follow-up on 34 patients took place during the 6 months after the end of therapy in order to compare the symptoms before and after the treatment. A significant improvement of dysmenorrhea (−69%), pelvic pain (−69%) and dyspareunia (−12%) was found. Seventy-three per cent of these patients had ovulatory cycles with a pregnancy rate of 27% (three pregnancies out of 11 patients wishing to be pregnant).

Table 1 Hormonal hematochemical and bone metabolism tests before and during treatment with buserelin

	Basal		*2nd month*		*4th month*		*6th month*	
	x	*SD*	*x*	*SD*	*x*	*SD*	*x*	*SD*
Tri-iodothyronine (ng/dl)	107	27	120	18	125	21	116	21
Thyroxine (μg/dl)	7.9	1.4	8.4	1.3	8.5	1.7	8.4	0.3
Thyrotropin (mUI/ml)	1.4	0.8	1.4	0.7	1.3	0.7	1.7	0.9
Prolactin (ng/dl)	10	5.7	8.5	5.5	7.9	4.7	7.0	4.0
Plasma testosterone (ng/ml)	0.4	0.1	0.3	0.1	0.3	0.1	0.3	0.2
Salivary testosterone (ng/dl)	2.1	0.8	1.9	0.8	1.7	0.4	1.8	1.1
Sex hormone-binding globulin (nmol/l)	49	21	45	23	45	28	43	21
Cortisol (μg/dl)	14	5.5	15	5.8	14	3.1	14	5.6
Total cholesterol (mg/dl)	205	35	210	34	219	40	235	40
High-density lipoprotein C (mg/dl)	71	18	72	16	69	19	71	11
Low-density lipoprotein C (mg/dl)	116	10	124	10	135	13	148	3.0
Triglycerides (mg/dl)	91	38	71	35	74	37	82	56
Blood glucose (mg/dl)	82	5.1	87	6.3	85	5.6	86	6.3
Urea (mg/dl)	27	4.2	41	5.3	27	7.4	26	6.1
Creatinine (mg/dl)	0.6	0.2	0.6	0.08	0.7	0.05	0.6	0.03
Uric acid (mg/dl)	3.2	0.7	3.2	0.9	3.0	0.9	3.2	0.8
Aspartate aminotransferase (U/l)	8.0	1.7	9.8	2.7	8.5	2.7	8.9	2.5
Alanine transferase (U/l)	7.8	2.5	10.6	2.7	8.8	2.1	8.6	3.4
Glutamyl transferase (U/l)	6.5	2.6	6.6	1.7	6.3	1.0	6.4	1.8
Alkaline phosphatase (U/l)	102	32.2	98	12.5	95	22.9	94	28.0
Calcium (mg/dl)	9.5	0.2	9.5	0.5	9.8	0.24	9.7	0.4
Phosphorus (mg/dl)	3.6	0.5	3.8	0.4	4.0	0.6	3.8	0.9
Bone mineral content (gHA/cm)*	4.26	0.7	—		—		4.23	0.4
Plasma osteocalcin (ng/ml)	3.4	0.12	—		—		3.7	0.17
Nordin test								
Ca_u/Cr_u	0.13	0.08	—		—		0.14	0.06
OHp_u/Cr_u	0.018	0.002	—		—		0.021	0.003

* gHA, grams of hydroxyapatite

Table 2 Modifications of symptoms during treatment

Symptom	%
Vasomotor symptoms	93
Vaginal dryness	87
Reduced libido	43
Headache	37
Spotting	19

Table 3 Results of therapy with intranasal buserelin

Stage	*Complete recovery*	*Amelioration*	*Non-responders*
I	6 (66.6%)	—	3 (33.4%)
II	14 (40.0%)	8 (22.9%)	13 (37.1%)
III	—	11 (64.7%)	6 (35.3%)

DISCUSSION

In this study buserelin appeared to be an effective drug in the reduction of the total rating of endometriosis (−52.5%). Our data are similar to those reported by other studies[2,3]. Results would be even more convincing (−62%) if the adhesion rating was not considered, as adhesions are scarcely affected by medical treatment[4].

Grouping according to the stage of disease has shown that complete responders are only first and second stage patients, suggesting an inverse correlation between severity of disease and treatment efficacy.

Our data confirm the validity of the therapeutic approach to endometriosis which recommends a combined surgical and medical therapy in moderate and severe forms (III–IV stage) but only hormonal treatment of second stage patients[5,6]. The side-effects are principally the results of the hypoestrogenic state; most of the patients complained of vasomotor symptoms and vaginal dryness (93% and 87% respectively). The fall in libido is a likely consequence of low sexual steroid levels (43%). The side-effects were generally well tolerated and no severe adverse reactions caused any patients to drop out. The mild side-effects reported by the patients disappeared as soon as ovarian endocrine activity recurred.

Buserelin appeared to be safe. It did not influence blood glucose, the hematopoietic system nor liver and kidney functions. Changes in the lipidic pattern were due to drug-induced hormonal variations. The slight modifications of the plasma lipids are probably a result of the reduction in estrogen levels.

Our data have not shown significant bone density variations (−0.7%), in contrast to the results of other authors[7,8]. It should be noted that the bone content loss during the early postmenopausal period is about 4% per year; therefore GnRH analogues might induce, over a 6-month course, a bone content loss of 2%, which would represent the lower limit of detection in relation to the method of quantification used. Incomplete suppression of ovarian function, the amount of adipose tissue, consumption of tobacco and alcohol and the intensity of physical activity are probably further relevant factors.

A slight rise in urine calcium and hydroxyproline and in plasma osteocalcin was found, however. This suggests a mild increase in the mineral turnover of bone tissue. As reported in other studies[9,10], our data imply the pituitary production of α chains during the course of treatment. In fact, monoclonal LH significantly dropped in the 2nd week, while LH, quantified by the polyclonal method, did not fall below the baseline level throughout the course of the treatment. A less noticeable difference was found in the monoclonal and polyclonal assay of FSH: both methods afforded similar results, although values obtained by the polyclonal method were higher. The rise in the LH/FSH ratio detected by polyclonal assay is probably not the result of more elevated plasmatic concentrations of complete molecules of LH (α and β subunits) but the effect of the increase in release of α subunits or LH fragments[11].

In relation to the significant decrease in biologically active LH and FSH, estradiol showed a marked diminution at the end of the 1st month in those patients who began therapy in the early follicular phase and at the 1st week in the patients who commenced therapy in the late luteal phase.

We concluded that the ovarian inhibition induced by GnRH agonist analogs is produced by a hypogonadotropic condition characterized by low FSH levels and an inadequate LH release. Our data show that buserelin is an effective drug in the treatment of endometriosis through the induction of a pseudomenopause and that the drug-related side-effects occurring in a 6-month treatment course are mild and well tolerated, where hyperandrogenic aspects are absent.

REFERENCES

1. Williams, T.J. and Pratt, J.H. (1977). Endometriosis in 1000 consecutive celiotomes: incidence and management. *Am. J. Obstet. Gynecol.*, **120**, 245
2. Dmowski, W.P., Radwanska, E., Binor, Z., Tummon, I. and Pepping, P. (1988). GnRH analogues in the management of endometriosis. *Gynecol. Endocrinol.*, **2**, (suppl. 2), 12
3. Lemay, A., Maheux, R., Jean, C., Faure, N. and Fazekas, A.T.A. (1984). Reversible hypogonadism induced by a luteinizing hormone release hormone (LHRH) agonist (buserelin) as a new therapeutic approach for endometriosis. *Fertil. Steril.*, **41**, 863
4. Brosens, I. and Cornillie, F. (1988). Is there a rationale for GnRH analogue therapy in endometriosis? *Gynecol. Endocrinol.*, **2**, (suppl. 1), 29
5. Donnez, J., Nisolle, M., Clerckx, F. and Casanas, F. (1988). Combined therapy in endometriosis. *Gynecol. Endocrinol.*, **2** (suppl. 1), 81
6. Elstein, M. and Bancroft, K. (1988). Endometriosis: the goals of treatment. *Gynecol. Endocrinol.*, **2** (suppl. 1), 99
7. Comite, F. and Jensen, P. (1988). Bone density changes associated with GnRH analogues. *Gynecol. Endocrinol.*, **2** (suppl. 1), 105
8. Devogelaer, J.P., Donnez, J., Thomas, K. and Nagant De Deuxchaisneis, C. (1988). Differential effects of the GnRH agonist buserelin on the axial and the appendicular skeleton at different scanning sites. Preferential loss of trabecular bone. *Gynecol. Endocrinol.*, **2**, (suppl. 1), 17
9. Hubert, J.F., Simart, J., Labrie, C. and Labrie, F. (1988). Regulation of alfa-subunit and LH-beta mRNA levels by LHRH and (d-Trp^6, des-Gly-$NH_2{}^{10}$)LHRH ethylamide in rat anterior pituitary cells in culture and *in vivo*. *Gynecol. Endocrinol.*, **2**, (suppl. 1), 99
10. Lahlon, N., Roger, M., Chaussain, J.L., Toublaur, J.E., Scholler, R. and Schally, A.V. (1988). Pattern of free gonadotropin alpha-subunit (Gn-alfa) secretion as a function of time in children treated with D-Trp^6-LHRH microcapsules. *Gynecol. Endocrinol.*, **2**, (suppl. 1), 141
11. Meldrum, D.R., Chang, R.G., Lu, J., Vale, W. and Rivier, J. (1982). Medical oophorectomy using a long-acting GnRH agonist: a possible new approach to the treatment of endometriosis. *J. Endocrinol. Metab.*, **54**, 1081

Section 4 continued

Part J

Menopause and osteoporosis

115

Menopause and osteoporosis – the Malmö study

N.-O. Sjöberg, B. Bjerre, S. Jeppsson, O. Johnell, G. Rannevik and L. Svanberg

Malmö is the third town of Sweden and is situated in the south. The town has around 250 000 inhabitants and is a typical trade and commercial city. Malmö has only one hospital and serves only the Malmö town and community. For that reason there are great possibilities to perform prospective studies. The population is well defined and the city files are very complete.

Concerning fractures, Malmö is unique because the department of Radiology has saved all the films since 1950 and all fractures have been registered separately.

Between 1950 until 1987 all types of fractures have increased. As an example the hip fractures in women were 70 in 1950 and 620 in 1987 (Figure 1). One reason for this is, of course, that the mean age of the inhabitants has

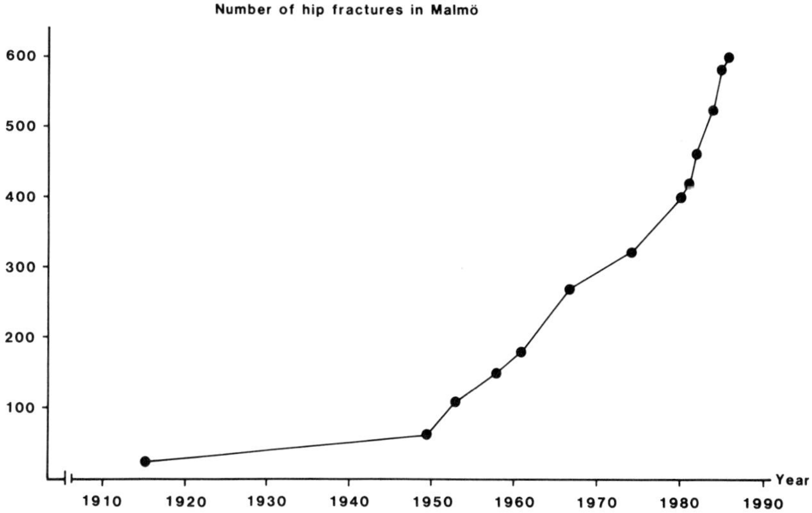

Figure 1 Frequency of hip fractures in women between 1950 and 1987

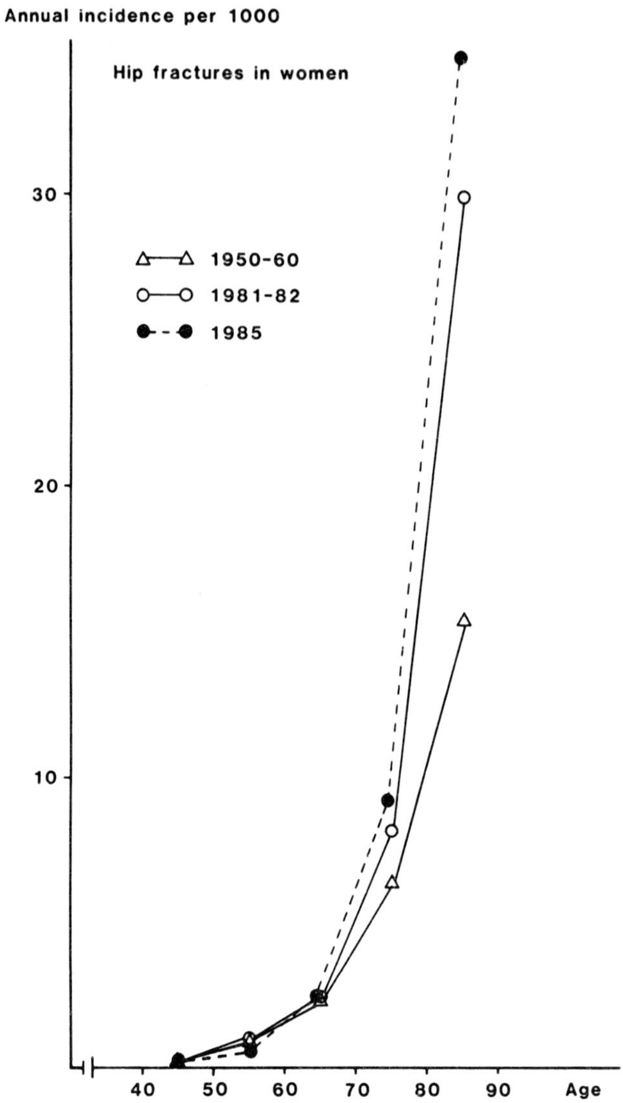

Figure 2 Incidence of hip fractures in women in 1950 and 1985

increased, but other factors must be involved in this increase. The risk for fractures per inhabitant in different age groups has also increased during the last decades (Figure 2). For example the incidence of hip fractures in women was in 1950 15 per 1000 inhabitants. In 1987 this incidence was 40 per 1000 inhabitants. All fragility fractures have the same pattern as the hip fractures with increasing incidence over the last decades.

The risk factors for osteoporosis have been under intensive debate and the factors most frequently listed are menopause, body mass, physical activity,

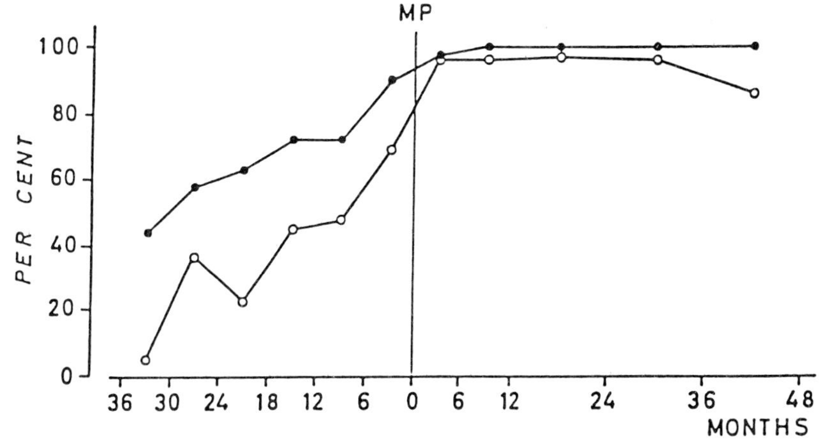

Figure 3 Percentage of women with elevated serum levels > 4 μg/l of FSH (closed cirlces) and LH (open circles) before and after the menopause (MP)

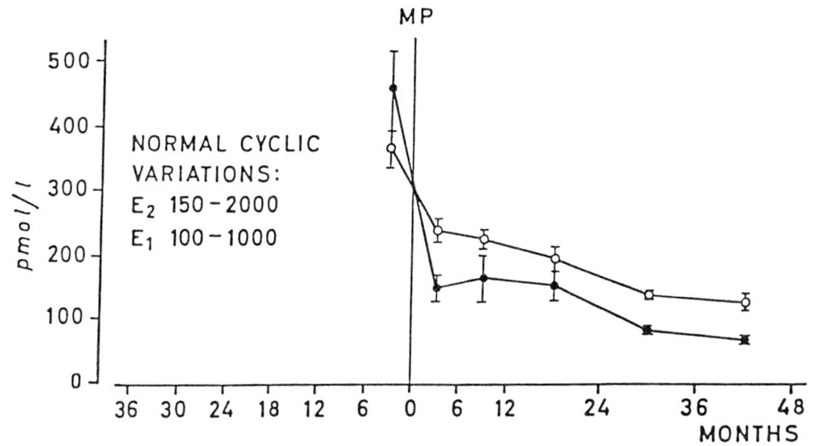

Figure 4 Serum levels of estradiol (closed circles) and estrone (open circles) before and after menopause (MP)

calcium intake, drugs, smoking, diseases, social network and falling tendency.

In Malmö there are many ongoing studies focusing the different risk factors. In this paper we will give you some details from a study concerning the perimenopausal years including measurement of bone mass.

In 1977 this study started and included 192 women born in 1929, i.e. 48 years old. All of them had menstrual periods and normal premenopausal levels of follicle-stimulating hormone (FSH). These women have been followed during 12 years concerning hormonal profile and bone mass (single photon densitometry) and the study will go on for a further 20 years. This means that this study is unique in that it is a prospective longitudinal study.

In the Malmö study the menopause is defined according to WHO: the

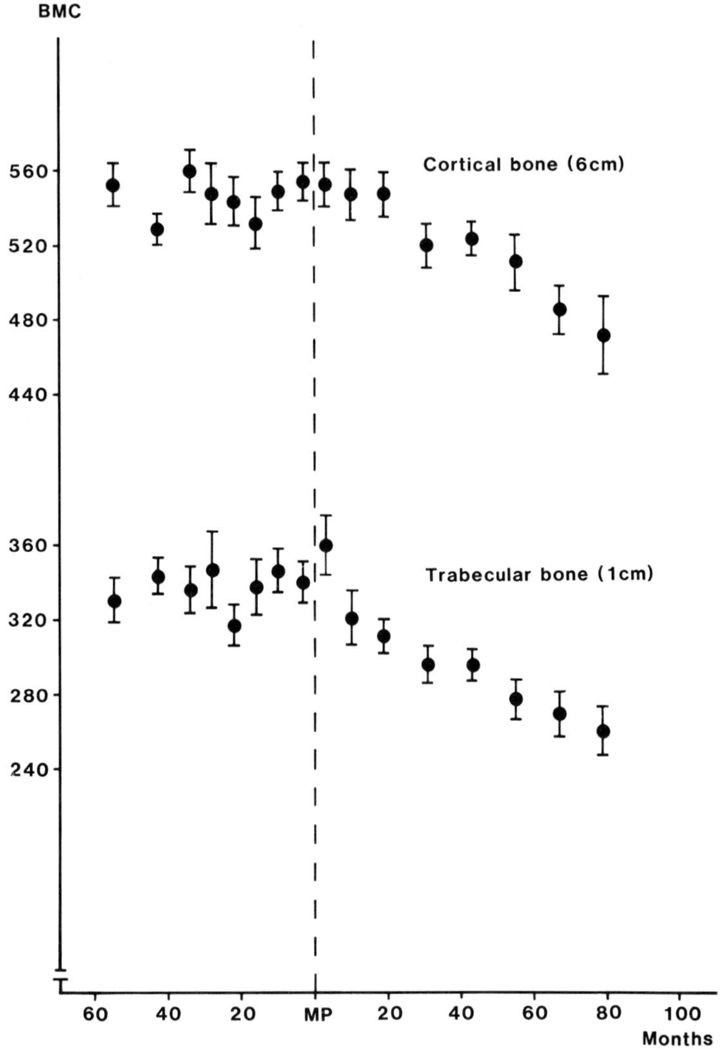

Figure 5 Bone mass content in trabecular and cortical bone before and after menopause

permanent cessation of menstruation (due to the loss of ovarian follicular activity).

In this prospective study the onset of the menopause was established retrospectively after 12 months of spontaneous amenorrhea. Already, at the menopause almost 100% of the women have elevated levels of FSH and luteinizing hormone (LH) and the rise had started a few years previously (Figure 3). Postmenopausally, we can confirm the well-known decrease in estrogen secretion with the typical change in estradiol/estrone ratio (Figure 4). However, it is interesting to note that although there is a certain amount of estradiol (E_2) production during the first few postmenopausal years, no menstrual bleedings occur. It is not until approximately 3 years after the menopause, that E_2 constantly shows low levels with narrow variations.

The single photon densitometry measurements have been performed on the forearm. The trabecular bone has been studied 1 cm from the wrist and the cortical bone 6 cm from the wrist. The densitometry measurements have shown that the bone mineral content decreases continuously after the menopause (Figure 5). In this prospective study bone mineral content is decreasing with 3% per year in the trabecular bone and 1% per year in the cortical bone.

In this prospective study only 10% of the women developed climacteric symptoms. These few women have been given different types of hormonal treatment and the densitometry measurements have shown that the bone mineral content in the women, who received estrogen remained unchanged.

Beside the Malmö study there is another prospective study from Oslo in Norway. Doctor Jan Falk and co-workers have studied the bone turnover with biochemical parameters. They have shown that around the menopause there is an increased bone turnover parallel to advancing osteoporosis. This is caused by an imbalance in the bone turnover where the resorptive factors are dominating.

In Sweden a consensus conference has been held concerning estrogen treatment in the menopause. It has been stated that the bone mass does not reduce after estrogen intake. The frequency of fractures also decreases after estrogen intake. The main problem is, however, the risk for developing uterine and breast carcinoma. Since gestagen has been introduced as a complement to estrogen treatment the risk for uterine adenocarcinoma has been abolished. However, it has been observed in a hitherto unpublished study, that there is an increased risk ratio for breast carcinoma after long treatment with estrogen postmenopausally. This increased risk is not abolished by adding gestagen. For this reason estrogen in Sweden is not approved as general prophylaxis against osteoporosis.

In the Malmö prospective ongoing study there are some tendencies. The first measurement in 1977 showed more bone mass in those women who had an early menarche. It also seems that women with low bone mineral content before menopause have an increased frequency of fractures.

We think, that bone mass before menopause is a good predictor for fractures in the future and the challenge for the twenty-first century is to find risk factors and risk patients in the Malmö study, which is prospective and will last for further 20 years.

At the present time it is impossible to state dogmatic rules regarding the treatment of choice for osteoporosis. It could be estrogen, calcitonine, fluor, calcium and anabolic steroids, but maybe the biggest challenge to prevent osteoporosis after menopause is physical activity.

116

Reliability of quantitative computerized tomography of the lumbar spine in postmenopausal osteoporosis: 2 years of experience

G. Mollica, B. Bagni and F. Pansini

The mineral content of bone is not constant throughout life but undergoes progressive increase up to 30–35 years of age and progressive loss thereafter. This phase of decrease of bone density is characterized by a striking sexual dimorphism: this is manifested as a largely increased rate of bone loss in women at the time of menopause, dependent on the abrupt disappearance of estrogens from circulation.

Any decrease in the density of bone after the bone mass peak is reached, is defined as 'osteopenia', and at least three different types are recognized in women[1]. Physiological osteopenia, as the progressive decrease of bone density normally evident after the 30th–39th year of age; this progresses towards accelerated osteopenia a stage of increased loss of bone mass (greater than 1% per year) which is evident transiently following the time of menopause, because of the lack of ovarian steroids; and finally, in some women an elevated osteopenia is present (which corresponds to high osteoporotic risk) as the decrease in bone density below a fracture threshold limit, defined as the mean density value characteristic of the bone peak age diminished by twice the standard deviation[2,3]. Eventually, within the elevated osteopenia two degrees can be distinguished (A and B) on the hypothesis that the actual decrease in bone density is restricted within two negative standard deviations from the mean of age-matched women or exceeds this value.

In the established osteoporosis syndrome, defined as the association of radiographically recognized fractures in patients with elevated osteopenia, at least two different clinical entities are recognized: the senile osteoporosis, typical of male and female patients above 65 to 70 years of age which involves both compact and spongious bone, and the postmenopausal osteoporosis, mainly involving the trabecular bone in women in a younger age group (below 65 to 70 years of age)[4]. In this respect data on the incidence of fractures after minimal trauma in postmenopausal women at 70 years of age demonstrate that 44% of the subjects suffered from fractures and the large majority of them involved bones which are prevalently composed of trabecular tissue (spine, forearm and wrist)[5].

The severity of postmenopausal osteoporosis and the difficulties of adequate therapeutic measures after the syndrome is established, led researchers to develop diagnostic procedures to select women at risk for appropriate prophylaxis. The diagnostic means actually available are all instrumental and they are recalled in Table 1[6–8].

With the exception of quantitative computed tomography (QCT) all the procedures are based on the relative photonic absorptiometry of radiations produced by radioisotopic sources (^{125}I, ^{241}Am, ^{167}Gd) or of filtered X-rays. In contrast, the QCT technique evaluates the bone trabecular mass at the level of vertebral bodies in comparison with an anthropomorphic phantom which contains in the center of vertebral simulate bodies a figure of hydroxyapatite density.

In both cases therefore the attenuation power of the tissue is expressed as weight equivalent of mineral content but the reference unit differs in both cases: the absorptiometric procedures, and single photon absorptiometry (SPA) represents its most extreme form, refer to the surface projection of the bone scanned, taking therefore into account both the trabecular and the compact bone components, while in QCT the density equivalent is referred to the unit volume of bone analyzed, usually the cubic centimeter (cm^3), and when properly utilized on vertebral bodies or femur neck allows the selective exploration of trabecular bone, the target element of postmenopausal osteoporosis. To summarize the information obtained from absorptiometry methods takes in large account the compact bone, which is irrelevant for the purpose of detecting early changes of postmenopausal osteoporosis; in contrast, the QCT is highly selective for this purpose although it must be interpreted with great caution because its sensitivity allows the determination of false results in the case of a large proportion of bone marrow or blood vessels are occasionally included in the explored volume. In general, both techniques are useful when properly adopted and find differential applications: the easy use of SPA and relatively low dose of radiation make this the selective technique for following-up patients to monitor progressive loss of bone, i.e., for longitudinal purposes, while QCT finds its best application for the immediate diagnostic purposes since it allows the determination of

Table 1 Comparison of bone mineral measurement techniques

Technique	*Precision*	*Accuracy*	*Radiation*
Photon absorptiometry:			
single energy (SPA)	3–5%	1–4%	2–5 mrem
double energy (DPA)	1–3%	4–6%	2–5 mrem
Computerized tomography:			
single energy	1–3%	0–25%	200–250 mrem
dual energy	3–5%	2–4%	500–750 mrem
Quantitative digital radiography (double energy) (QDR)	0.8–1%	1–4%	5–10 mrem

the actual mineral content in trabecular bone.

Quite recently a new technique has been proposed, quantitative double energy digital radiography (QDR), which might be satisfactory applied to both longitudinal and cross-sectional studies: by this technique single surfaces are identified, predominantly composed of either compact or trabecular bone, and serially analyzed by a focused beam of X-rays to achieve information which is highly reproducible to a variation of loss than 1% of the spine phantom values.

The sensitivity of QDR is definitely higher than that of SPA, and of any other technique but QCT, and combines it with a selectivity which approaches that of QCT. The technique however has been introduced too recently for a critical analysis of the data at present (H. W. Wahner, personal communication).

Our further discussion on the limits and benefits of SPA and QCT to detect early signs of osteopenia in menopausal preosteoporotic women is centred on the results we have obtained in our Centre for Menopause and prevention of postmenopausal osteoporosis.

During the period January 1987 to January 1989 we have admitted 666 women with complaints of menopausal related disturbances. All of them were subjected to SPA analysis on the distal radius and to anamnestic selection criteria (physical inactivity, smoking, alcoholism, dietary factors, reproductive history and lactation, heredity, malabsorption of calcium, low body mass index, previous cortisone or FANS therapy) to define a potential risk of osteoporosis. Thus, 185 women were selected and studied further. Fifty-seven patients had undergone ovariectomy and represent a heterogeneous group because a large fraction of them received hormonal replacement therapy (HRT). They were therefore excluded from further study as well as 14 patients in spontaneous menopause who had X-rays demonstrating established osteoporosis as revealed by signs of body vertebral alterations (crush fractures, fish vertebrae, wedge images, etc.). On the residual 114 patients the bone mass density was determined by both SPA and QCT and referred to, as stated above, as g/cm^2 and mg/cm^3.

The data are presented in Figures 1 and 2 and in Table 2 in the function of age. The graphical presentation which is part of a normal distribution with an onset of accelerated decrease of bone mass at apparent age of 52 years for SPA and 48 for QCT. This age difference is presumably due to the ability of QCT, but not of SPA, to detect ongoing physiological osteopenia, while both techniques reveal the beginning of the accelerated osteopenia. For clarity these same results are presented in Table 2. The extreme resolving power of QCT is further demonstrated by the data in Table 3 which summarize our experience on the 185 women we have analyzed by this technique. In particular, the osteopenic condition might be divided, in relation to the risk of developing osteoporosis, into two groups of patients whose bone density is below the fracture threshold limit but within the range of two negative standard deviations for the age-matched mean value (group A), or in the most severe cases, even below the limit of two negative standard deviations from the mean (group B); with this distinction, in the premenopausal women, we detected a limited number of severe osteopenic

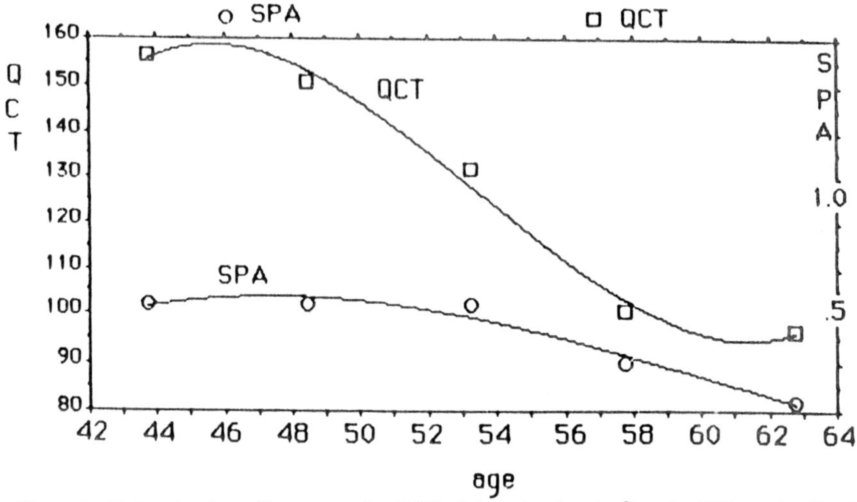

Figure 1 Determination of bone mass by QCT of the spine (mg/cm^3) or by SPA on the distal radius (g/cm^2) on 114 patients without radiographically detectable osteoporosis (premenopause and spontaneous menopause)

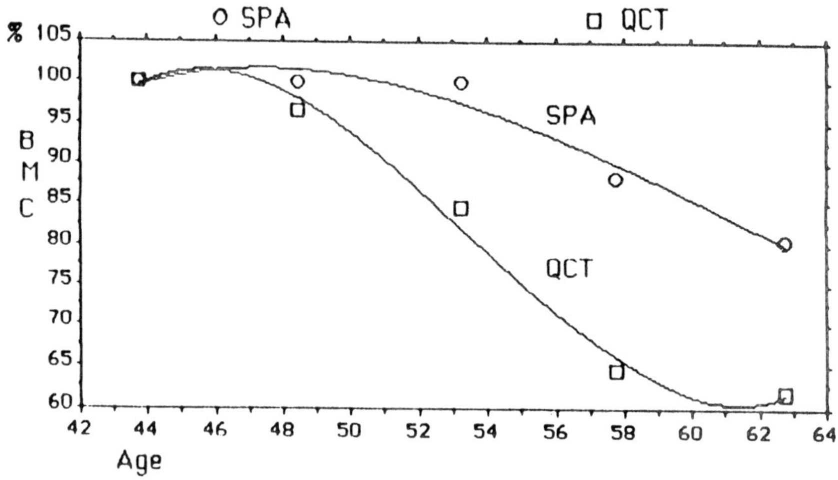

Figure 2 The data of Figure 1 are replotted as per cent decline of bone mineral content (BMC) as a function of age of patients. The 100 per cent value was assigned to the BMC of the first class examined

patients but only at the elevated osteopenia of stage A, while in post-menopausal women both types of defect were detected and accounted together for more than 50% of the patients analyzed.

Curiously, in the surgical menopause group, which should *a priori* be a more severe condition than that produced during spontaneous menopause, the incidence of severe osteopenia is lower than that observed in the spontaneous menopause, possibly because these patients are routinely

Table 2 Bone mineral content in normal women

No.	*Class* (mean age ± SD)	*SPA* (distal radius g/cm^2)	QCT (spine L2–L5 mg/cm^3)
7	44 ± 0.95	0.51 ± 0.09	156 ± 23
27	48 ± 1.34	0.51 ± 0.12	151 ± 25
26	53 ± 1.25	0.51 ± 0.07	132 ± 27
12	58 ± 1.29	0.45 ± 0.08	100 ± 19
8	63 ± 2.50	0.41 ± 0.06	97 ± 21

Table 3 Detection of elevated osteopenia by computerized quantitative tomography (spine L2–L5)

	Premenopause (*n* = *33*)	*Spontaneous menopause* (*n* = *95*)	*Surgical menopause** (*n* = *57*)
Elevated osteopenia (A) <110 mg/cm^3 within −2SD	18%	27%	18%
Elevated osteopenia (B) <110 mg/cm^3 below −2SD	0	26%	16%

* Some of the surgical patients were treated by hormone replacement therapy

admitted to hormonal replacement therapy. This is a further confirmation of the benefit of such therapy in the prophylaxis of postmenopausal osteoporosis by steroid hormones.

In conclusion, this comparative study between the two methods on the same patients demonstrates definitively the superiority of QCT to establish the diagnosis of the osteopenic condition, while maintaining the potential usefulness of SPA in monitoring longitudinally the state of the individual patients within time. Two additional considerations seem worthy, that the sensitivity of QCT allows the early detection of changes at the menopausal phase which easily escape detection by SPA and that it allows the recognition in the advanced osteopenic state of two different populations with increasing osteoporotic risk.

REFERENCES

1. De Deuxchaisnes, C.N. (1987). Plaidoyer pour la prevention de l'osteoporose post menopausique. In Prodim, (ed). *La Menopause – Traitement de la Menopause et Prevention de l'Osteoporose*, pp. 11–34. (Paris: Maloine)
2. Genant, H.K., Cann, C.E., Boyd, D.P., Kolb, F.O., Ettinger, B. and Gordan, G.S. (1983). Quantitative computed tomography for vertebral mineral determination. In Frame, B. and Potts, Y.T. (eds). *Clinical Disorders of Bone and Mineral Metabolism*, (Amsterdam: Excerpta Medica)
3. Cann, C.E., Genant, H.K., Kolb, F.O. and Ettinger, B. (1985). Quantitative computed tomography for prediction of vertebral fracture risk. *Metab. Bone Rel. Res.*, **6**, 1–7
4. Riggs, B.L. and Melton, L.J., III (1983). Evidence for two distinct syndrome of involutional osteoporosis. *Am. J. Med.*, **75**, 899–901
5. Christiansen, C. and Bente, J.R. (1987). Optimal prophylaxis for postmenopausal bone loss. In Genant, H. K. (ed.). *Osteoporosis Update 1987*, pp. 259–65. (University of California Printing Services)
6. Riggs, B.L. and Melton, I.J. (1986). Involutional osteoporosis. *N. Engl. J. Med.*, **314**, 1676–86

7. Mazess, R.B. (1983). The non invasive measurement of skeletal mass. In Peck, W. A. (ed.) *Bone and Mineral Research Annual Journal*, pp. 223–79. (Amsterdam: Excerpta Medica)
8. Laval-Jeantem, A.M., Roger, B. and Bovysse, S. (1986). Influence of vertebral fat content on quantitative CT density. *Radiology*, **159**, 463–6

117

Correlation between biochemical and biophysical indices of bone turnover in postmenopausal osteoporosis

C. Gennari, D. Agnusdei, R. Civitelli, S. Gonnelli and A. Vattimo

INTRODUCTION

The main characteristic of postmenopausal osteoporosis is the reduction of bone mass following natural or surgically induced menopause. Histomorphometric studies, performed to establish bone turnover in untreated osteoporosis, have shown the heterogeneity of this disorder. Some subjects show low bone turnover with formation less than resorption; others show accelerated turnover with resorption greater than formation; and yet other, who perhaps started with a low bone mass, show a normal rate of bone turnover[1-3].

Bone turnover is usually assessed by histomorphometric analysis of bone biopsies, which is probably the most direct way available at present, of assessing the kinetics of formation and resorption. However, transiliac bone biopsy is an invasive technique, and it yields information only at a single time point and on a restricted area of bone, which may not be representative of the entire skeleton and finally it cannot tell us what has happened previously. Kinetic and calcium balance studies have been used to assess bone remodeling and turnover rates[4,5], but these techniques are laborious and not suitable for the study of large numbers of subjects.

Recently, skeletal uptake of bone-seeking radiopharmaceuticals, expressed as whole body retention (WBR) of the tracer, has been proposed as a non-invasive and effective method for measurement of bone turnover[6-10]. More recently, on the basis of an early report of Caniggia and Vattimo[11], a study done in Denmark[12,13] demonstrated that the determination of 24 h urinary excretion of 99m-technetium-methylene diphosphonate (99m-Tc-MDP) is highly correlated to WBR, estimated by whole body counting. This allows a great simplification of the method.

In the present cross-sectional study we used this method to assess bone turnover and remodeling rates in a large number of patients with established postmenopausal osteoporosis. The aim of this investigation was to determine whether the rate of bone remodeling could be correlated with bone mineral content (BMC), as assessed by dual photon absorptiometry of the lumbar spine and whether WBR can be used to predict the severity of postmenopausal bone loss.

PATIENTS AND METHODS

From a large number of patients referred to Institute of Medical Semeiotics, Center for the Diagnosis and Treatment of Osteoporosis at the University of Siena, a cohort of 107 consecutive postmenopausal women (mean age $\pm$ SD, 56.5 $\pm$ 7.3 yr) with radiological evidence of osteoporosis (presence of vertebral wedging or crush fractures) was selected to participate in this study. Besides the presence of osteopenia the patients were in general good health. The dietary calcium intake of our postmenopausal women was 500–800 mg/day. In each patient BMC of the lumbar spine, WBR, urinary excretion of hydroxyproline/creatinine (HOP/Cr) ratio and osteocalcin (OC) were evaluated.

Bone mineral content of the lumbar spine (BMC-LS) was measured by dual photon absorptiometry, using the BMC Lab 22a system (Novo Diagnostic, Bagsvaerd, Denmark), which use ^{153}Gd as radioactive source. Fractured vertebrae were excluded from the measurements. The precision of the method was 3.18% as detailed elsewhere[14].

Whole body retention of 99m-Tc-MDP was assessed according to the method of Hyldstrup *et al.*[12], with the following modification. After voiding, patients received by injection of an intravenous dose of 0.5–1.0 mCi 99m-Tc-MDP (Medrotek, Sorin, Saluggia, Italy), and immediately a 24 h urine collection was started. At the end of the collection period, the activity of 2 ml urine sample counted in a gamma counter (Tri-Carb, Packard Instruments, Downers Grove, IL, USA). A sample taken from the injected solution was counted as standard together with the urine sample. The total injected dose and urinary excretion of 99m-Tc-MDP were extrapolated, and WBR was calculated as $100 \times (1 -$ total urine counts/total injected counts); which represents the fraction, in per cent, of the injected dose retained in the body 24 h after injection.

Serum OC was measured by a radioimmunoassay using the Osteocalcin RIA Kit (Incstar Corp., Stillwater, MN, USA). Urinary hydroxyproline was determined in 24 h urine samples according to the method of Prockop and Udenfriend[15], using the Hypronosticon Kit (Organon, Baxtel, The Netherlands), and expressed as the HOP/Cr ratio in mg/g). Creatinine was assayed using the Creatinine-kine test (Sclavo, Siena, Italy).

Data were analyzed by applying linear regression models (Pearson's correlation coefficient).

RESULTS

The osteoporotic patients were divided into two groups, according to their WBR values. The cut-off value was established at 34%, which corresponds to the upper limit of the 95% confidence interval in the normal population. Forty-two patients (39.2%) had WBR above the cut-off value, and these were considered as having high turnover osteoporosis (HTOP); the other 65 patients (60.8%) were grouped as normal turnover osteoporotics (NTOP).

To investigate whether bone turnover was an important determinant of bone loss in postmenopausal osteoporosis we evaluated the interrelation of WBR with parameters of bone formation and resorption, with bone mass and with the years since menopause (YSM). As shown in Figure 1 a highly significant positive correlation was found between WBR and OC, considered a sensitive marker of bone formation. Figure 2 shows a similar significant positive correlation between WBR and urinary HOP/Cr ratio, a good index of bone resorption. These two positive correlations confirm the validity of WBR as a marker of bone remodeling. As regards the interrelation of WBR with BMC-LS (Figure 3) in our osteoporotic patients, a significant negative correlation ($r = -0.19, p < 0.05$) was found. A significant positive correlation ($r = 0.21$, $p < 0.05$) was evident, as shown in Figure 4, between WBR and years since menopause.

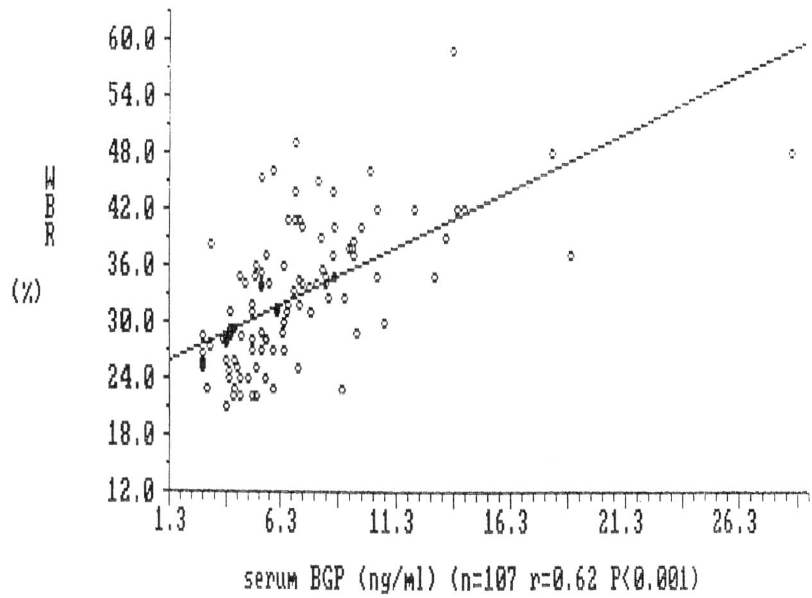

Figure 1 Correlation between whole body retention (WBR) and osteocalcin in 107 patients with postmenopausal osteoporosis

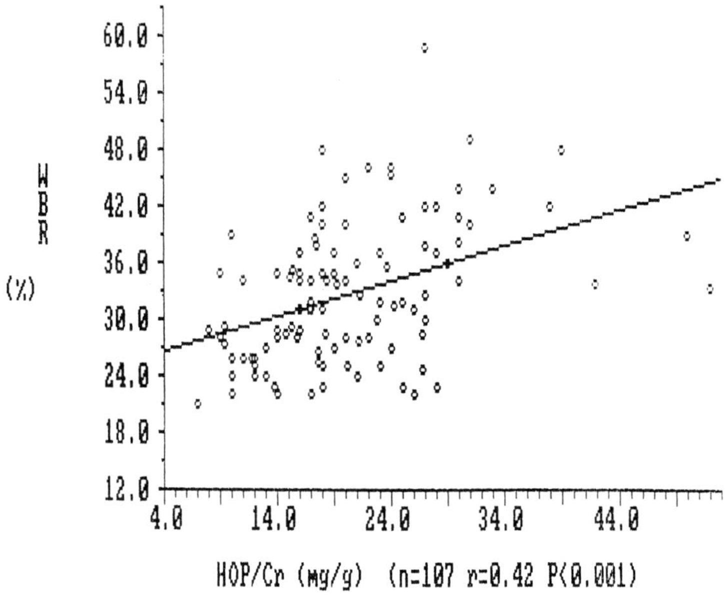

Figure 2 Correlation between whole body retention (WBR) and urinary excretion of hydroxyproline/creatinine (HOP/Cr) ratio in 107 patients with postmenopausal osteoporosis

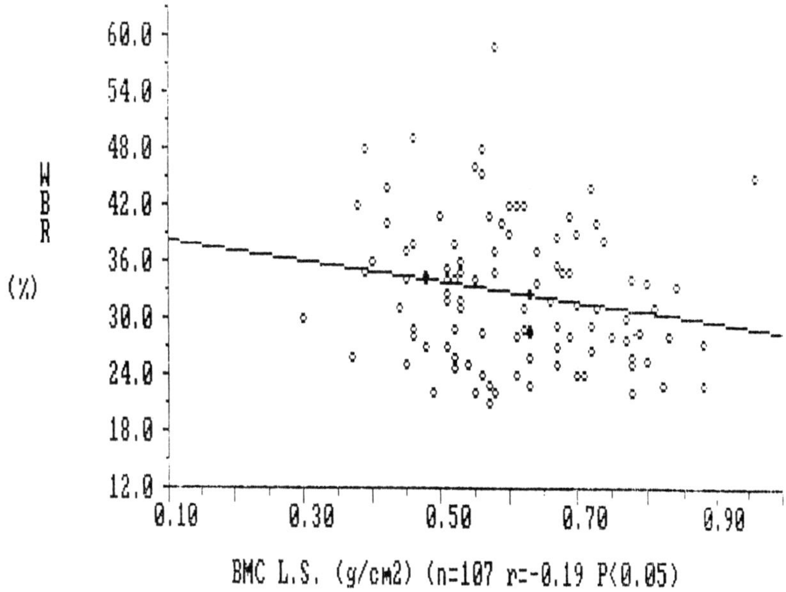

Figure 3 Correlation between whole body retention (WBR) and bone mineral content of the lumbar spine (BMC-LS) in 107 patients with postmenopausal osteoporosis

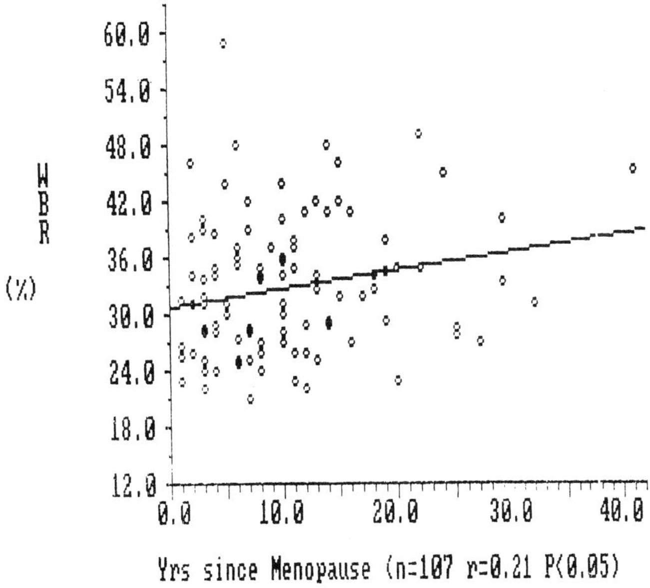

Figure 4 Correlation between whole body retention (WBR) and years elapsed since menopause in 107 patients with postmenopausal osteoporosis

DISCUSSION

This study confirms the heterogeneity of bone remodeling in patients with postmenopausal osteoporosis, and suggests that the severity of bone loss could be related to higher bone turnover rates in these patients. This is supported by the significant negative correlation between WBR and BMC-LS observed in our patients. Skeletal uptake of diphosphonate occurs predominantly at sites of new bone formation[7], and thus it is thought to be dependent upon osteoblastic activity[9]. In fact, significant correlation has been found between WBR and both biochemical[11,12,16-18] and histomorphometric indices of bone formation[18]. Some authors also reported that retention values are closely related to urinary HOP/Cr excretion[8,11,12,17] a marker of bone resorption. Our data are in agreement with these observations, showing high correlation between WBR and both OC and HOP/Cr, this confirming the validity of WBR as estimate of skeletal turnover.

Recent studies[19,20] indicated that although rates of bone remodeling can be related to rates of bone loss, a single determination of biochemical estimates cannot predict the degree of bone loss in a large number of postmenopausal osteoporotic patients. Determination of WBR in our patients revealed that 39.2% of them presented a bone turnover higher than normal women. These data are in agreement with previous studies based on histomorphometric analysis of iliac crest bone biopsies[1-3,21]. Unfortunately, from the data of our cross-sectional study, is not possible to establish whether the enhanced bone remodeling represents a selected population with a particular form of the disease or is suggestive of a longitudinal heterogeneity of the disorder, expressing phases of different bone remodeling rates at different times.

In conclusion, the present study demonstrates that the assessment of bone remodeling rates by a single determination of either biochemical parameters, such as osteocalcin and urinary hydroxyproline, or distribution of bone-seeking radioisotopes, cannot help to predict the degree of bone loss in postmenopausal osteoporosis, but it can be useful as a diagnostic tool in selecting the proper therapeutic approach.

REFERENCES

1. Whyte, M.P., Bergfeld, M.A., Murphy, W.A., Avioli, L.V. and Teitelbaum, S.L. (1982). Postmenopausal osteoporosis. A heterogeneous disorder as assessed by histomorphometric analysis of iliac crest bone from untreated patients. *Am. J. Med.*, **72**, 193–202
2. Meunier, P.J., Sellami, S., Briancon, D. and Edouard, C. (1981). Histological heterogeneity of apparently idiopathic osteoporosis. In De Luca, H.F., Frost, H.M., Jee, W.S.S., Johnson, C.C., Jr and Parfitt, A.M. (eds). *Osteoporosis: Recent Advances in Pathogenesis and Treatment*, pp. 293–301. (Baltimore: University Park Press)
3. Parfitt, A.M., Mathews, L., Rao, D., Frame, B., Kleerekoper, M. and Villanueva, A.R. (1981). Impaired osteoblast function in metabolic bone disease. In De Luca, H.F., Frost, H.M., Jee, W.S.S., Johnson, C.C., Jr and Parfitt, A.M. (eds). *Osteoporosis: Recent Advances in Pathogenesis and Treatment*, pp. 321–30. (Baltimore: University Park Press)
4. Caniggia, A., Gennari, C., Bencini, M., Cesari, L. and Borrello, G. (1970). Calcium metabolism and 47 calcium kinetics before and after long-term thyrocalcitonin treatment in senile osteoporosis. *Clin. Sci.*, **38**, 397–407
5. Heaney, R.P., Recker, R.R. and Saville, P.D. (1978). Menopausal changes in bone remodeling. *J. Lab. Clin. Med.*, **92**, 964–70
6. Fogelman, I., Bessent, R.G., Turner, J.G., Citrin, D.L., Boyle, I.T. and Greig, W.R. (1978). The use of whole body retention of tc-99m diphosphonate in the diagnosis of metabolic bone disease. *J. Nucl. Med.*, **19**, 270–5
7. Fogelman, I. (1980). Skeletal uptake of diphosphonate: a review. *Eur. J. Nucl. Med.*, **5**, 473–6
8. Fogelman, I., Bessent, R.G., Cohen, H.N., Hart, D.M. and Lindsay, R. (1980). Skeletal uptake of diphosphonate. Method for prediction of post-menopausal osteoporosis. *Lancet*, **ii**, 667–70
9. Fogelman, I. and Bessent, R. (1982). Age-related alterations in skeletal metabolism-24 h whole-body retention of diphosphonate in 250 normal subjects: concise communication. *J. Nucl. Med.*, **23**, 296–300
10. Hyldstrup, L., McNair, P., Jensen, G.F., Mogensen, N.B. and Transbol, I. (1984). Measurement of whole body retention of diphosphonate and other indices of bone metabolism in 125 normals: dependency on age, sex and glomerular filtration. *Scand. J. Clin. Lab. Invest.*, **44**, 673–8
11. Caniggia, A. and Vattimo, A. (1980). Kinetics of 99m technetium-tin-methylene-diphosphonate in normal subjects and pathological conditions: a simple index of bone metabolism. *Calcif. Tiss. Int.*, **30**, 5–13
12. Hyldstrup, L., Mogensen, N., Jensen, G.F., McNair, P. and Transbol, I. (1984). Urinary 99m-Tc-diphosphonate excretion as a simple method to quantify bone metabolism. *Scand. J. Clin. Lab. Invest.*, **44**, 105–9
13. Thomsen, K., Nilas, N., Mogensen, T. and Christiansen, C. (1986). Determination of bone turnover by urinary excretion of 99m-Tc-MDP. *Eur. J. Nucl. Med.*, **12**, 342–5
14. Civitelli, R., Agnusdei, D., Nardi, P., Zacchei, F., Avioli, L.V. and Gennari, C. (1988). Effects of one year treatment with estrogens on bone mass, intestinal calcium absorption and 25-hydroxyvitamin D-1 alpha-hydroxylase reserve in postmenopausal osteoporosis. *Calcif. Tiss. Int.*, **42**, 77–86

15. Prockop, D.J. and Udenfriend, S. (1960). A specific method for the analysis of hydroxyproline in tissues and urine. *Anal. Biochem.*, **1**, 228–39
16. Fogelman, I., Bessent, R.G., Beastall, G. and Boyle, I.T. (1980). Estimation of skeletal involvement in primary hyperparathyroidism. *Ann. Intern. Med.*, **92**, 65–7
17. Thomsen, K., Johansen, J., Nilas, L. and Christiansen, C. (1987). Whole body retention of 99m-tc-diphosphonate. Relation to biochemical indices of bone turnover and to total body calcium. *Eur. J. Nucl. Med.*, **13**, 32–5
18. Podenphant, J., Johansen, J.S., Thomsen, K., Riis, B.J., Leth, A. and Christiansen, C. (1987). Bone turnover in spinal osteoporosis. *J. Bone Min. Res.*, **2**, 497–503
19. Thomsen, K., Rodbro, P. and Christiansen, C. (1987). Bone turnover determined by urinary excretion of 99m-Tc-diphosphonate in the prediction of postmenopausal bone loss. *Bone Min.*, **2**, 125–31
20. Civitelli, R., Gonnelli, S., Zacchei, F., Bigazzi, S., Vattimo, A., Avioli, L.V. and Gennari, C. (1988). Bone turnover in postmenopausal osteoporosis. *J. Clin. Invest.*, **82**, 1268–74
21. Marie, P.J. and Caulin, F. (1986). Mechanisms underlying the effects of phosphate and calcitonin on bone histology in postmenopausal osteoporosis. *Bone*, **7**, 17–22

118

Calcitonin and parathyroid hormone in bone metabolism disease

C. Marcocci, E. Schipani, F. Catalano, G. Bruno-Bossio, F. Cetani and A. Pinchera

INTRODUCTION

A highly integrated and complex endocrine system maintains calcium, phosphate and mineral homeostasis. It involves an interplay between the action of two polypeptide hormones, parathyroid hormone (PTH) and calcitonin (CT), and a steroid hormone, 1,25-dihydroxycholecalciferol (1,25-$(OH)_2D_3$). The sites of action of these hormones are the bone, the intestine and the kidney.

The relationships between the multiple components involved in maintaining mineral homeostasis are illustrated in Figure 1. Under physiological conditions, there are small fluctuations in plasma calcium. Decreases in plasma calcium increase PTH secretion and decrease CT secretion. These changes in hormone secretion, and particularly the increase of PTH, lead to

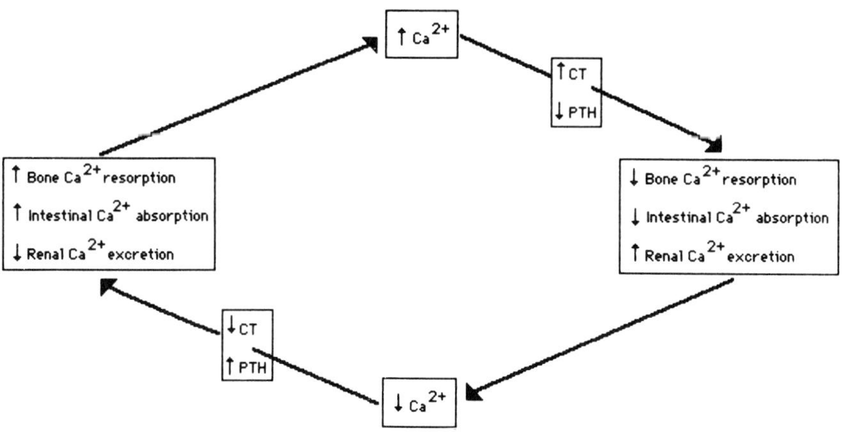

Figure 1 Regulation of calcium homeostasis. Relationships between serum calcium concentration, parathyroid hormone (PTH) and calcitonin (CT), and physiological events which occur in response to a decrease (left side) or an increase (right side) of serum calcium

an increased bone resorption, decreased renal excretion of calcium, and increased intestinal calcium absorption. The latter effect is mediated by 1,25-$(OH)_2D_3$. PTH in fact, either directly or by decreasing serum phosphate, stimulates the renal 1α-hydroxylase enzyme, which converts the inactive 25-OHD_3 to the active form 1,25-$(OH)_2D_3$. Following these events plasma calcium rises slightly above its physiological concentration, inhibiting PTH secretion and stimulating CT secretion. These changes, and particularly the increase of CT, decrease bone resorption, increase the renal excretion of calcium, and decrease the intestinal absorption of calcium, causing plasma calcium to fall below the physiological levels.

In this paper the potential pathogenetic role of abnormalities of CT secretion in the development of postmenopausal osteoporosis, and the clinical usefulness of PTH assay will be briefly discussed.

CALCITONIN AND THE DEVELOPMENT OF POSTMENOPAUSAL OSTEOPOROSIS

Osteoporosis is a common skeletal disorder of heterogeneous etiology, which is characterized by excessive bone resorption particularly in postmenopausal women[1].

The model proposed by Riggs and Melton[1] to explain the pathophysiology of postmenopausal osteoporosis is shown in Figure 2. The concept that osteoporosis was related to estrogen deficiency caused by ovarian failure was originally proposed by Albright *et al.*[2]. However, it is worth noting that only a small proportion of postmenopausal women develop osteoporotic changes, even though all are estrogen deficient. Therefore, other factors, in

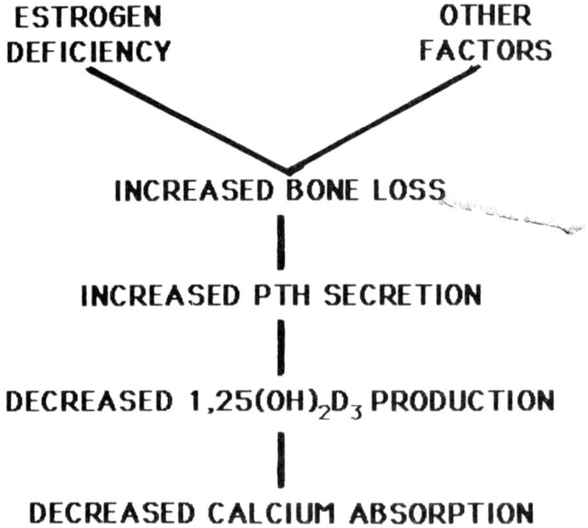

Figure 2 Pathogenesis of postmenopausal osteoporosis (from Riggs and Melton[1])

addition to menopause, must be involved to determine the individual susceptibility. In any case, the final effect responsible for osteoporosis is an accelerated bone loss which decreases PTH secretion[3] and consequently the production of 1,25-$(OH)_2D_3$[4]. The reduced concentration of 1,25-$(OH)_2D_3$ results in an impaired intestinal calcium absorption[5], which may further increase bone resorption in an attempt to maintain calcium homeostasis[6].

The relevant role of estrogen deficiency in the pathogenesis of postmenopausal osteoporosis is demonstrated by the beneficial effect of estrogen administration to these patients[7]. However, the exact nature of this protective effect of estrogen on the skeleton has not yet been defined. It has been suggested that the effectiveness of estrogen in retarding skeletal loss could be mediated by CT and that abnormalities in CT secretion and/or action could be involved in the pathogenesis of postmenopausal osteoporosis[7]. To clarify this possibility, the relationships between age, sex, and osteoporosis itself and both CT secretion and CT levels have been widely examined.

Some studies have shown that circulating levels of CT in normal adult women are lower when compared to those of normal adult men[8–10] although exceptions exist[11,12]. Moreover, a large proportion of women have undetectable CT levels. On the basis of these observations it was proposed that the lower CT levels in women could be responsible for the higher prevalence of osteoporosis in females.

Aging has been reported to be associated with a progressive decrease of basal immunoreactive CT levels both in normal men and women[12]. In addition, in both sexes, there is a progressive decline in CT responses to a 10-min infusion of calcium, that is more dramatic in women[12,13]. However, these CT changes related to sex and aging have not been confirmed by Body and Heath[8], who found no difference in basal whole plasma CT between young and elderly healthy men and women. These authors have also developed a sensitive CT assay, based on silica extraction and concentration of plasma, in order to measure monomeric CT, which is considered to be the active form of the hormone. Using this assay the monomeric CT levels in women were only half those of men, a difference greater than that previously reported by other investigators. By the use of the same assay a reduced CT response in women following calcium infusion was found, but no difference was observed in CT levels between young and elderly men and women.

Based on the observation that CT levels were lower in women than in men, and that at least in some studies aging was associated with a decrease of basal CT and with an impaired responsiveness to secretory stimuli in females, it was suggested that estrogen may have a role in CT secretion and that CT deficiency might be responsible for the development of postmenopausal osteoporosis.

Hillyard and coworkers[9] have reported that both pregnancy and the administration of estrogen–progestogen contraceptive pills to premenopausal women were associated with an increase of plasma CT, up to values similar to those found in normal men.

To evaluate the relationship between CT secretion and postmenopausal osteoporosis better, several investigators have measured CT concentration in osteoporotic patients[14–17].

Although variable findings have been reported, the large majority of investigators have found no difference in basal plasma CT between osteoporotic and normal age-matched women[14–17]. On the other hand, when the calcium-stimulated CT response was evaluated, a decreased response of plasma immunoreactive CT was found by Taggart *et al.*[15], whereas Tiegs and co-workers[16], measuring CT in silica-extracted plasma, found no difference in the monomeric CT response between osteoporotic and normal women. On the basis of these findings these authors concluded that postmenopausal osteoporosis was not associated with, and does not result from, CT deficiency.

Further support for this conclusion derives from studies of Leggate and co-workers[18], who failed to show a relationship between basal CT levels and changes in bone density measured over a period of 10 years. In particular, there was no difference in serum CT levels in women showing an increase, no change, or a decrease of bone density during the study period. The same authors also showed that all women treated with estrogen gained or at least maintained their bone density, whereas the majority of placebo-treated patients showed decreased bone mass. However, when the plasma CT levels were compared, no difference was found between estrogen- and placebo-treated groups, suggesting that the protective effect of estrogen administration on the skeleton did not involve CT.

In an attempt to clarify the role of CT deficiency in the development of osteoporosis, the skeletal effect of iatrogenic CT deficiency and of spontaneous CT excess have been studied. Cross-sectional studies in patients submitted to total thyroidectomy, with well documented CT deficiency, have produced conflicting results, showing normal[19] or reduced bone mineral density in the radius[20] and spine[21]. On the other hand, patients with medullary thyroid carcinoma, a tumor associated with a marked increase of plasma CT concentrations, showed normal radial and reduced spinal density values, despite elevated levels of CT lasting for at least 8 years[19].

In conclusion, the balance of current evidence suggests that CT deficiency, either naturally occurring or iatrogenic, does not play a significant etiological role in the pathogenesis of postmenopausal osteoporosis and, therefore, that CT deficiency cannot be considered as the link between estrogen deficiency and postmenopausal osteoporosis.

Recent studies have provided evidence that bone cells, and particularly osteoblast-like cells, have estrogen receptors[22]. Studies performed in our laboratory have shown that estradiol is able to increase collagen synthesis in UMR cells, a rat osteoblastic cell line, suggesting that estrogen may have a direct effect on bone cell metabolism[23].

CLINICAL USEFULNESS OF PTH ASSAY

The intracellular pathway of PTH biosynthesis and secretion[24,25] is shown in Figure 3. The initial product of synthesis, the preproPTH, is converted to proPTH by removal of the amino-terminal methionine residues on the

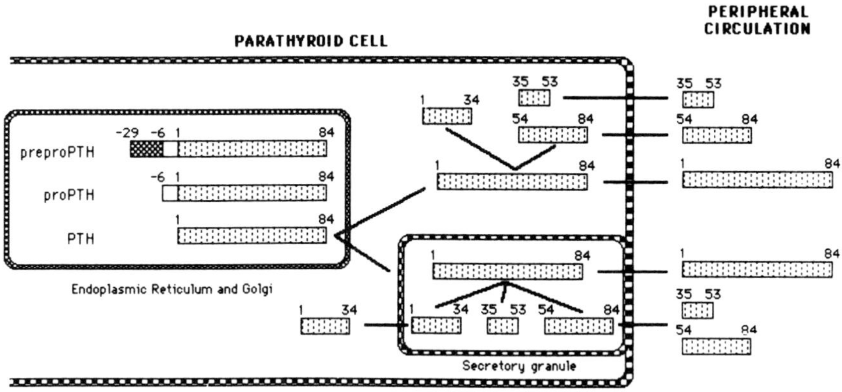

Figure 3 Schematic representation of the intracellular pathways of parathyroid hormone (PTH) biosynthesis (see text)

ribosomes and of the amino-terminal sequence of 23 amino acids in the endoplasmic reticulum. Subsequently, the proPTH reaches the Golgi region where it is converted to PTH by removal of the amino-terminal hexapeptide. Therefore, PTH is either stored in secretory granules or released into the cytoplasm, where it remains until it is secreted into the bloodstream in response to a fall of plasma calcium. The intact PTH, which is composed of 84 amino acids, undergoes at least two cleavages while in the secretory granules, and possibly in the cytoplasm. These cleavages generate the amino-, mid-, and carboxy-region fragments; fragments 1–34, 35–53 and 54–84 respectively. The mid- and carboxy-region fragments are secreted in the circulation along with intact PTH, whereas the amino-region fragment is not released and is degraded within the cell. The intact PTH released into the circulation undergoes metabolic degradation in the liver and kidney. It is important to note that all the biological activity of PTH lies in the first 34 amino acids at the amino-terminal region, and, therefore, that mid- and carboxy-region fragments are biologically inert[12].

Circulating PTH is heterogeneous, consisting of the intact 84-amino acid peptide and multiple degradation fragments[26]. The relative quantities of intact PTH and its fragments in the serum are not precisely known, but there are more circulating fragments than intact hormone. The rate of disappearance of carboxy-region fragments is slower than that of intact PTH or amino-region fragments. This difference in metabolic turnover probably also accounts for the larger pool of carboxy-region fragments and small pool of intact PTH and amino-region fragments in the circulation.

At present all available PTH antisera used in radioimmunoassays are multivalent, and contain antibodies directed at multiple regions of the PTH molecule[27]. As shown in Table 1, antibodies directed against the mid- or carboxy-regions of the PTH molecule recognize the inactive mid- and carboxy-region fragments as well as the intact, biologically active, PTH, whereas antisera directed against the amino-region recognize only the intact

Table 1 Characteristics of the available assays to measure circulating parathyroid hormone (PTH)

	Antibody specificity		
	1–34	*44–68*	*65–84*
Name of assay	N-tact PTH (intact)	PTH-MM	C-terminal
PTH circulating fragment			
1–84	×	×	×
35–65	—	×	—
35–84	—	×	×

active PTH. Nonetheless, mid- and carboxy-region assays have provided surprisingly good diagnostic tools in the evaluation of patients suspected of having primary hyperparathyroidism[28]. In fact, their diagnostic sensitivity was as good as that of amino-terminal PTH assays. This is fortunate because the concentration of intact PTH in the circulation is so low that, with few exceptions, it is beyond the sensitivity of the amino-region assays.

It is important to remember that the absolute PTH values, measured by mid- or carboxy-terminal assays, in patients with surgically proven hyperparathyroidism may be within the normal range, and that the degree of overlapping between control and hyperparathyroid patients may vary from one assay to another[29].

The individual steady-state levels of PTH are dependent on the serum concentration of calcium. In normal humans there is an inverse relationship between the fasting levels of serum calcium and serum immunoreactive PTH. A better discrimination between normal and hyperparathyroid patients may be obtained by evaluating the serum PTH value as a function of the serum calcium concentration[29]. In fact, patients with surgically proven primary hyperparathyroidism and PTH levels at the upper limit of the normal range had values of the hormone inappropriately high when compared with those of normal subjects with similar serum calcium concentration.

Of particular interest is the recently developed immunoradiometric assay of intact PTH. This assay employs two different polyclonal antibodies, prepared by affinity chromatography. These purified antibodies are specific for two different regions of the PTH molecule. The first antibody, specific for the 39–84 carboxy-terminal region, is bound to the solid phase. Thus, the intact PTH molecule as well as all the carboxy-terminal fragments will bind to the coated beads, whereas the other fragments will not stick to the plastic. The second antibody is specific for the 1–34 amino-terminal region of PTH and is labeled with ^{125}I. This antibody will recognize only the intact PTH molecule bound to the solid phase and the radioactivity associated to the plastic beads will be proportional to the concentration of intact PTH in the serum.

Using this assay, a more clear-cut separation of patients with hypercalcemia due to primary hyperparathyroidism from those with hypercalcemia of malignancy may be obtained[30]. However, it should be noted that also using this assay some PTH values of hyperparathyroid patients may occur at the upper limit of normal range.

REFERENCES

1. Riggs, B.L. and Melton, L.J., III (1986). Involutional osteoporosis. *N. Engl. J. Med.*, **314**, 1676–86
2. Albright, F., Smith, P.H. and Richardson, A.M. (1941). Postmenopausal osteoporosis. *J. Am. Med. Assoc.*, **116**, 2465–74
3. Gallagher, J.C., Riggs, B.L., Jerpbak, C.M. and Arnaud, C.D. (1980). The effect of age on serum immunoreactive parathyroid hormone in normal and osteoporotic women. *J. Lab. Clin. Med.*, **95**, 373–85
4. Riggs, B.L., Hamstra, A. and DeLuca, H.F. (1981). Assessment of 25-hydroxyvitamin D 1-alpha-hydroxylase reserve in postmenopausal osteoporosis by administration of parathyroid extract. *J. Clin. Endocrinol. Metab.*, **53**, 833–5
5. Gallagher, J.C., Riggs, B.L., Eisman, J., Hamstra, A., Arnaud, S.B. and DeLuca, H.F. (1979). Intestinal calcium absorption and serum vitamin D metabolites in normal subjects and osteoporotic patients: effect of age and dietary calcium. *J. Clin. Invest.*, **64**, 729–36
6. Gallagher, J.C., Jerpbak, C.M., Jee, W.S.S., Johnson, K.A., DeLuca, H.F. and Riggs, B.L. (1982). 1,25-Dihydroxyvitamin D_3: Short- and long-term effects on bone and calcium metabolism in patients with postmenopausal osteoporosis. *Proc. Natl. Acad. Sci., USA*, **79**, 3325–9
7. Lindsay, R. (1987). Estrogen in prevention and treatment of osteoporosis. In Avioli, L.V. (ed.) *The Osteoporotic Syndrome*, pp. 91–107. (New York and London: Grune & Stratton)
8. Body, J.J. and Heath, H., III (1983). Estimates of circulating monomeric calcitonin: physiological studies in normal and thyroidectomized man. *J. Clin. Endocrinol. Metab.*, **57**, 897–903
9. Hillyard, C.J., Stevenson, J.C. and MacIntyre, I. (1978). Relative deficiency of plasma-calcitonin in normal women. *Lancet*, **i**, 961–4
10. Heath, H., III and Sizemore, G.W. (1977). Plasma calcitonin in normal man: differences between men and women. *J. Clin. Invest.*, **69**, 1135–40
11. Parthemore, J.G. and Deftos, L.J. (1978). Calcitonin secretion in normal human subjects. *J. Clin. Endocrinol. Metab.*, **47**, 184–8
12. Deftos, L.J., Weisman, M.H., Williams, G.W., Karpf, D.B., Drumar, A.M., Davidson, B.J., Pathermore, J.G. and Judd, H.L. (1980). Influence of age and sex on plasma calcitonin in human beings. *N. Engl. J. Med.*, **302**, 1351–3
13. Shamonki, I.M., Frumar, A.M., Tataryn, I.V., Meldrum, D.R., Davidson, B.H., Parthemore, J.G., Judd, H.L. and Deftos, L.J. (1980). Age-related changes of calcitonin secretion in females. *J. Clin. Endocrinol. Metab.*, **50**, 437–9
14. Chesnut, C.H., III Baylink, D.J., Sisom, K., Nelp, W.B. and Roos, B.A. (1980). Basal plasma immunoreactive calcitonin in postmenopausal osteoporosis. *Metabolism*, **29**, 559–62
15. Taggart, H.M., Chesnut, C.H., III Ivey, J.L., Baylink, D.J., Sisom, K., Huber, M.B. and Roos, B.A. (1982). Deficient calcitonin response to calcium stimulation in postmenopausal osteoporosis? *Lancet*, **i**, 475–7
16. Tiegs, R.D., Body, J.J., Wahner, H.W., Barta, J., Riggs, B.L. and Heath, H., III (1985). Calcitonin secretion in postmenopausal osteoporosis. *N. Engl. J. Med.*, **312**, 1097 100
17. Stevenson, J.C., White, M.C., Jopin, G.F. and MacIntyre, I. (1982). Osteoporosis and calcitonin deficiency. *Lancet*, **ii**, 1010–11
18. Leggate, J., Farish, E., Fletcher, C.D., McIntosh, W., Hart, D.M. and Sommerville, J.M. (1984). Calcitonin and postmenopausal osteoporosis. *Clin. Endocrinol.*, **20**, 85–92
19. Hurley, D.L., Tiegs, R.D., Wahner, H.W. and Heath, H., III (1987). Axial and appendicular bone mineral density in patients with long-term deficiency or excess of calcitonin. *N. Engl. J. Med.*, **317**, 537–41
20. McDermott, M.T., Kidd, G.S., Blue, P., Ghaed, V. and Hofeldt, F.D. (1983). Reduced bone mineral content in totally thyroidectomized patients: possible effect of calcitonin deficiency. *J. Clin. Endocrinol. Metab.*, **56**, 936–9
21. Rosenstein, B.D., Awbrey, B.J., Thomas, C.G. and Talmage, R.V. (1985). The effect of thyroid disease and thyroidectomy treatment on calcitonin and bone density in women. *Trans. Orthop. Res. Soc.*, **10**, 261–75
22. Komm, B.S., Terpening, C.M., Benz, D.J., Graeme, K.A., Gallegos, A., Korc, M., Greene, G.L., O'Malley, B.O. and Haussler, M.R. (1988). Estrogen binding receptor mRNA, and

biologic response in osteoblast-like osteosarcoma cells. *Science*, **241**, 81–4

23. Schipani, E., Vitti, P., Ceccarelli, P., Marcocci, C., Cucchi, P., Gryczynska, M. and Pinchera, A. (1988). 17-beta estradiol increases proteins synthesis and collagen synthesis in an osteoblastic cell line. *G. Ital. Metab. Min. Eletr.*, **2**, 137 (Abstract)
24. Cohn, D.V. and MacGregor, R.R. (1981). The biosynthesis, intracellular processing, and secretion of parathormone. *Endocr. Rev.*, **2**, 1–26
25. Habener, J.F., Rosenblatt, M. and Potts, J.T. (1984). Parathyroid hormone: Biochemical aspects of biosynthesis, secretion, action, and metabolism. *Physiol. Rev.*, **64**, 985–1053
26. Martin, K.J., Hruska, K.A., Freitag, J.J., Klahr, S. and Slatopolsky, E. (1979). The peripheral metabolism of parathyroid hormone. *N. Engl. J. Med.*, **301**, 1092–7
27. European PTH Study Group (1978). Interlaboratory comparison of radioimmunological parathyroid hormone determination. *Eur. J. Clin. Invest.*, **8**, 149–55
28. Raisz, L.G., Yajnik, C.H., Bockman, R.S. and Bower, B.F. (1979). Comparison of commercially available parathyroid hormone immunoassay in the differential diagnosis of hypercalcemia due to primary hyperparathyroidism or malignancy. *Ann. Intern. Med.*, **91**, 739–40
29. Insogna, K.L., Mitnick, M.E., Stewart, A.F., Burtis, W.J., Mallette, L.E. and Broadus, A.E. (1985). Sensitivity of the parathyroid hormone–1,25-dihydroxyvitamin D axis to variations in calcium intake in patients with primary hyperparathyroidism. *N. Engl. J. Med.*, **313**, 1126–30
30. Chu, S.Y. and Chu, A.K. (1986). Intact vs C-terminal/Mid-region parathyrin (PTH) assay in diagnosis of hyperparathyroidism. A clinical evaluation. *Clin. Chem.*, **32**, 2206–7

Section 4 continued

Part K

Osteoporosis: pathogenesis, prophylaxis and treatment

119

Eel calcitonin in the prophylaxis of postmenopausal osteoporosis

M. Franchi, A. La Fianza, L. Babilonti, L. Torretta and P. Poggi

Postmenopausal bone loss is persistent and virtually irreversible in the elderly, and it is the reason for the rising incidence of fractures in older women[1]. Prevention is therefore the only therapeutic possibility. Several clinical studies confirmed that premenopausal oophorectomy predisposes to early development of postmenopausal osteoporosis[2]. In the Obstetrics and Gynecology and Semeiotic Departments of Pavia University the possibility of using eel-calcitonin (eCT) as an alternative to estrogen and/or gestagen treatment in the prophylaxis of postmenopausal osteoporosis in women with surgical menopause is under evaluation. In particular the aim of the research is the evaluation of the activity and the side-effects of this new and interesting calcitonin[3–5].

SUBJECTS AND METHODS

The study was performed in 40 premenopausal patients aged between 42 and 54 years, who underwent surgical bilateral oophorectomy for benign gynecological pathology in our Institutions. All the patients were non-smokers, negative for chronic diseases, without previous consumption of drugs affecting mineral metabolism. The subjects were randomized into controls (no prophylaxis: 17 patients) or those given therapy for 12 months with eCT and oral calcium (23 patients). The pharmacological protocol is shown in Table 1.

Bone mineral content (BMC) was evaluated by Quantitative Computed Tomography (QCT) before surgery and at 6 and 12 months at the level of

Table 1 Dosage schedule

100 U s.c. every day for 12 weeks		
100 U s.c. on alternate days for 12 weeks		
100 U s.c.	on alternate days on alternate months	for 24 weeks
Oral calcium 50 mg DIE		

L1–L3 vertebral spongiosa, as previously reported[6,7]. The BMC, expressed in mg/ml of K_2HPO_4, was the mean value of (L1 + L3)/2 density. For the statistical evaluation of the results, Student's t test was employed.

RESULTS

Patients' mean age, weight, height and presurgical vertebral BMC ($\pm$ SD) are shown in Table 2. The randomized groups of patients are comparable save for a slight difference in age. Three patients (7.5%) were lost at follow-up after presurgical QCT (all were controls). Type and incidence of side-effects of the eCT, including the drop-out due to the side-effects, are respectively shown in Tables 3 and 4 and in Figure 1. In Table 5 is shown bone density expressed in mg/ml K_2HPO_4. The variation (%) of vertebral BMC before surgery and during the follow up are shown in Figure 2.

DISCUSSION AND CONCLUSIONS

The two groups of randomized high-risk patients for postmenopausal osteoporosis are comparable, even if a mild difference in age is observed.

Table 2 Characteristics of patients

	*Age**	*Height*	*Weight*	*BMC* (L1 + L3)/2
eCT ($n = 23$)	48.3 ± 2.9	160.7 ± 3.9	48.3 ± 2.9	171.4 ± 28.9
Controls ($n = 17$)	46.3 ± 2	162.3 ± 4.7	59.5 ± 10.9	162.9 ± 23.9

*ecT vs Controls: $p = 0.02$

Table 3 Incidence of side-effects with eCT treatment

	Side-effects	*Drop-out for side-effects*	*No side-effects*
6 months eCT	13/23 (56.5%)	7/23 (30.5%)	3/23 (13%)
12 months eCT	6/12 (50%)	2/12 (16.6%)	4/12 (33%)

Table 4 Side-effects of eCT

	6 months	*12 months*
Gastrointestinal	11/20 (55%)	3/8 (38%)
Vascular	8/20 (40%)	4/8 (50%)
Others	1/20* (5%)	1/8† (12%)

* Pollachiuria, poliuria;
† Hypothermia

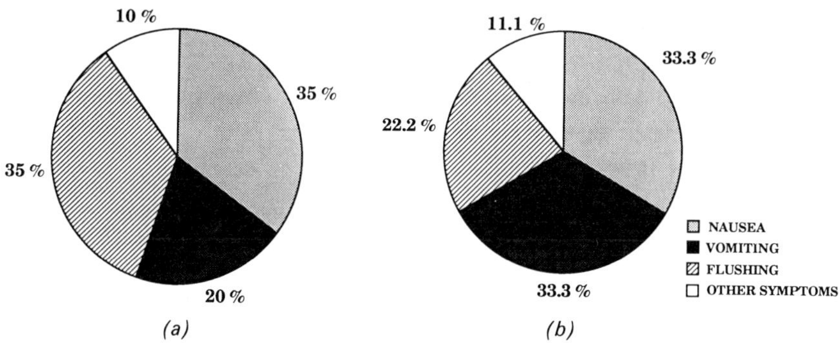

Figure 1 (*a*) Type of side-effects found in 20 patients after 6 months of therapy and (*b*) reasons for drop-out in nine patients

Table 5 Bone mineral content measured as (L1 + L3)/2 and given as mean mg/ml $K_2HPO_4 \pm SD$

	0 months	*6 months*	*12 months*
eCT	171.4 ± 28.9 ($n = 23$)	146.4 ± 24.3 ($n = 16$)	137.9 ± 23.9 ($n = 10$)
Controls	162.9 ± 23.9 ($n = 17$)	134.6 ± 23.3 ($n = 17$)	123.3 ± 25.4 ($n = 14$)

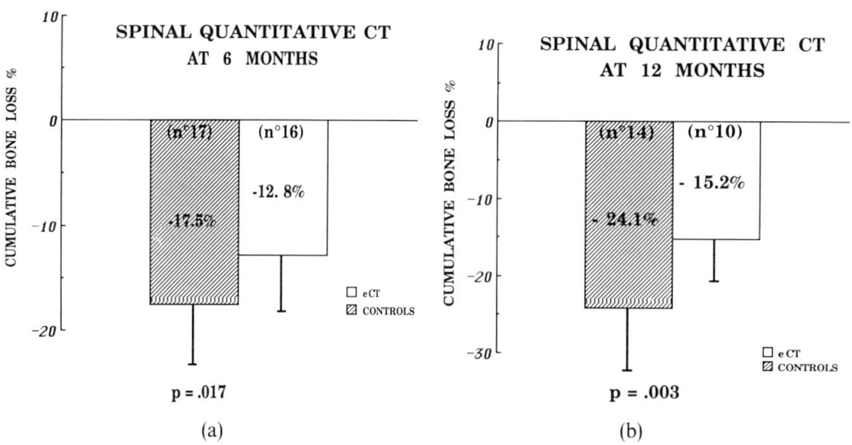

Figure 2 Spinal quantitative CT at (*a*) 6 months and (*b*) 12 months

The study is ongoing but we believe that the number of subjects at 12 months of follow-up is adequate for drawing considerations about side-effects and activity of the drug.

Most of the patients reported side-effects (87%). Of these, 35% (seven of 20) stopped the treatment after 6 months, 25% (two of eight) after 12 months.

Nausea, vomiting and abdominal pain were the most commonly reported gastrointestinal side-effects; amongst vascular symptoms the most common was flushing (Figure 1). The side-effects most commonly implicated in drop-out were gastrointestinal as reported for other calcitonins[8]. It seems that at 12 months vascular side-effects were more frequent than gastrointestinal ones (Table 4).

Our reported incidence of side-effects is higher than the 20% generally reported in patients treated with eCT for postmenopausal osteoporosis. However, there are few data about the incidence of side-effects of eCT employed in normal subjects as a prophylactic drug. As we previously reported, the incidence of side-effects and drug discontinuation in patients with surgical menopause is remarkable also with other calcitonins (55% of side-effects at 6 months and 25% of drop-out for low dose of salmon calcitonin)[8,10]. A good analysis of the data about side-effects and compliance of parenteral eCT is difficult because of the psychological distress of the patients with recent hysterectomy and salpingo-oophorectomy and for the similarity of vascular side-effects of eCT to common symptoms of the climacteric. As shown in Table 4 at 12 months from surgery the side-effects are mainly of vascular type and not gastrointestinal as at 6 months. Therefore we believe that these side-effects are due to the climacteric rather than to eCT. In order to solve the problem we activated a research comparing side-effects of eCT to a placebo.

In concern to the activity of parenteral eCT in preventing the vertebral trabecular bone loss (Figure 2) the presented results are promising. The percentage variation of BMC in treated patients is significantly less than in the controls ($p = 0.017$ at 6 months; $p = 0.003$ at 12 months). Our trabecular bone loss in oophorectomized subjects is of the same order as that of authors that employed a similar measure system by QCT[11,12].

In conclusion, from our data at 12 months, eCT as other calcitonins, seems to have a potential value in preventing axial trabecular bone loss prior to such loss occurring. However, to demonstrate its definitive usefulness in prophylaxis it is necessary to obtain longer term results. The action of calcitonin seems to decrease in long-term therapy[13]. This resistance to the drug's action is possibly due to a down-regulation of receptor sites on osteoclasts as observed in the treatment of Paget's disease[14]; or more likely to the reinstitution of normal coupling mechanisms after a transient uncoupling of bone resorption and formation (CT is an antiresorptive agent)[15,16].

The compliance of the drug administered parenterally in prophylaxis is not satisfactory. At the moment a new mode of administration of eCT by suppositories is under evaluation and preliminary data are extremely promising in respect to the increasing drug compliance for long-term use in prophylaxis.

REFERENCES

1. Heaney, R.P. (1987). Prevention of osteoporotic fracture in women. In Avioli, L.V. (ed.) *The Osteoporotic Syndrome*, pp. 67–90. (New York: Grune and Stratton)

2. Chesnut, C.H. (1987). Report from the NIH Consensus Conference, 1984, and NIH/NOF workshop, 1987. In Genant, H.K. (ed.) *Osteoporosis Update 1987*, pp. 3–6. (San Francisco: Radiology Research and Education Foundation)
3. Lattanzi, F. (1988). Struttura chimica, tecnologia di sintesi, di purificazione, di stabilizzazione. *Presented at the Symposium: Attualità in tema di osteopatie metaboliche*, p. 37, November, Rome
4. Zanelli, J. (1988). Standardizzazione biologica internazionale della calcitonina di anguilla. *Presented at the Symposium: Attualità in tema di osteopatie metaboliche*, p. 38, November, Rome
5. Guidobono, F., Netti, C., Sibilia, V. and Pecile, A. (1988). Aspetti di farmacologia sperimentale. *Presented at the Symposium: Attualità in tema di osteopatie metaboliche*, p. 39, November, Rome
6. Dore, R., La Fianza, A., Franchi, M., Spinillo, A., Cichero, P. and Biazzi, L. (1987). Tomografia computerizzata quantitativa (TCQ) della spongiosa vertebrale. Proposta di una metodica applicabile allo studio dell'osteoporosi postmenopausale (PMO). *Rad. Med.*, **74**, 166–70
7. La Fianza, A., Dore, R., Spinillo, A., Franchi, M. and Danesino, V. (1987). Prediction of fracture risk in patients with postmenopausal osteoporosis (PMO) by quantitative computed tomography (QCT). In Christiansen, C., Johansen, J.S. and Riis, B.J. (eds). *Osteoporosis 1987*, pp. 382–3. (Copenhagen: Osteopress)
8. Franchi, M., Babilonti, L. and La Fianza, A. (1988). Effetti collaterali della calcitonina di salmone (sCT) nella profilassi della osteoporosi postmenopausale (PMO). In Bottiglioni, F. and de Aloysio, D. (eds). *Il Climaterio Femminile: Esperienze Italiane di un Decennio*, pp. 335–42 (Bologna: Monduzzi Editore)
9. Gennari, C. and Avioli, L.V. (1987). Calcitonin therapy in osteoporosis. In Avioli, L.V. (ed.) *The Osteoporotic Syndrome*, pp. 121–42. (New York: Grune and Stratton)
10. Franchi, M. and La Fianza, A. (1988). La calcitonina di anguilla non modificata (eCT) nella profilassi dell'osteoporosi postmenopausale (PMO). *Presented at the Symposium: Attualità in tema di osteopatie metaboliche*, pp. 53–55, November, Rome
11. Genant, H.K., Block, J.E., Steiger, P. and Gluer, C.C. (1987). Quantitative computed tomography in the assessment of osteoporosis. In Genant, H.K. (ed.) *Osteoporosis Update 1987*, pp. 49–71. (San Francisco: Radiology Research and Education Foundation)
12. Genant, H.K., Ettinger, B., Harris, S.T., Block, J.E. and Steiger, P. (1988). Quantitative computed tomography in assessment of osteoporosis. In Riggs, B.L. and Melton, L.J. (eds). *Osteoporosis*, pp. 221–49. (New York: Raven Press)
13. Danesino, V., La Fianza, A. and Franchi, M. (1988). Valutazione dell'efficacia della profilassi con calcitonina nell'osteoporosi postmenopausale (PMO). In Salvadori, B. and Vadora, E. (eds). *Aggiornamenti in Ostetricia e Ginecologia*, pp. 261–72. (Roma: CIC)
14. Chesnut, C.H. (1988). Drug therapy: calcitonin, biphosphonates, anabolic steroids, an hPTH (1-34). In Riggs, B.L. and Melton, L.J. (eds). *Osteoporosis*, pp. 403–14. (New York: Raven Press)
15. Chesnut, C.H. (1984). Synthetic salmon calcitonin, biphosphonates, and anabolic steroids in the treatment of postmenopausal osteoporosis. In Christiansen, C., Arnaud, C.D., Nordin, B.E.C., Parfitt, A.M., Peck, W.A. and Riggs, B.L. (eds). *Osteoporosis. Proceedings of the Copenhagen International Symposium on Osteoporosis*, pp. 549–555. (Aalborg: Stiftbogtrykkeri)
16. Franchi, M., La Fianza, A., Dore, R., Babilonti, L. and Bolis, P.F. (1987). Efficacy of ADFR therapy in prophylaxis of postmenopausal osteoporosis (PMO). In Christiansen, C., Johansen, J.S. and Riis, B.J. (eds). *Osteoporosis 1987*, pp. 586–7. (Copenhagen: Osteopress)

120

Effect of estrogen and eel calcitonin therapy in the early postmenopausal period

V. De Leo, P. Inaudi, D. Lanzetta and N. D'Antona

INTRODUCTION

Postmenopausal bone loss with increased incidence of bone fracture is a serious health problem in postmenopausal women. Estrogen deficiency is considered to be the main factor responsible for postmenopausal bone loss[1] and accelerated bone loss has been observed after surgical menopause due to ovariectomy[2] and after natural menopause[3]. This negative effect can be counteracted by hormonal substitution therapy[4,5]. It is generally assumed that menopause occurs as a result of depletion of follicular reserves and the consequent reduction in plasma estrogen levels. Estrogen replacement is currently the principal therapy for this skeletal disorder. The protective effect of estrogens against postmenopausal bone loss involves the suppression of bone turnover[6], and this has also been demonstrated for estrogen replacement therapy[7]. It has been postulated that estrogens effect calcitonin secretion from the thyroid cells, increasing its reserves[8]. Calcitonin is well known to inhibit bone resorption[9,10]. There are now many calcitonins, the latest of which is unmodified eel calcitonin (eCT), reported to produce marked hypocalcemia in rats and humans[11].

The action of estrogen replacement therapy can be transient if not begun in the first 5 years of menopause or if suspended for some years. The risks and benefits of estrogen treatment have to be evaluated for every individual woman. Estrogen replacement therapy may have certain adverse physiological effects and can increase the incidence of endometrial cancer, however this is thought to be counteracted by the addition of progesterone[12].

The aim of the present study was to examine the effect on bone metabolism of conjugated estrogens and eCT, both singly and in combination in early postmenopausal women and in women with osteoporosis.

MATERIALS AND METHODS

We studied 46 physiological postmenopausal women: 20 healthy subjects (49–52 years) in the 1st year of menopause, and 26 (53–59 years) in established menopause with osteoporosis and bone pain especially of the back and radiological evidence of one or more atraumatic vertebral crush fracture. The wrist BMC was below the first standard deviation in healthy subjects and below the second standard deviation in osteoporotic subjects.

None of the subjects was on drugs known to influence calcium metabolism. All women had a past history of regular menstrual periods and none had received hormonal therapy after menopause. All gave their informed consent to participate in the study. The healthy and osteoporotic subjects were studied as follows:

(1) Healthy 1st year menopause subjects: six women received 10 MRC Units of synthetic unmodified eCT (Sclavo, Siena, Italy) injected every day for 3 months and then on alternate days for a further 3 months; six women received therapy with conjugated estrogens (Premarin, Ayerst, USA) at 1.25 mg/day for 21 days + medroxyprogesterone acetate (MPA) at 10 mg/day for 11 days every month for 6 months; eight women acted as controls and did not receive any treatment.

(2) Osteoporotic subjects in established menopause: eight women received conjugated estrogens at 1.25 mg/day for 63 days followed by 10 mg/day MPA for 10 days plus eCT as above; 10 women received eCT as above plus calcium (1000 mg/day); eight women acted as controls.

In all subjects blood samples were taken three times in 6 months: at the beginning, after 3 months and at the end of the study. Concentrations of gonadotropins, estradiol, prolactin and osteocalcin were measured by radioimmunoassay in all samples. Bone mineral content (BMC) was evaluated every 3 months by dual photon bone densitometry (NIM, Verona, Italy) at the distal radius of the non-dominant arm (1/10 forearm length from wrist) and expressed in mg/cm^2.

Statistical analysis was performed by Student's *t* test. To evaluate time changes in bone mass, the initial value was taken as 100% and the values obtained during and at the end of treatment were expressed as percentage change.

RESULTS

Tables 1 and 2 show the clinical data and hormonal changes in all women during and at the end of therapy. Hormonal patterns, except for osteocalcin, remained unchanged in all patients who received treatment. In the healthy 1st year menopause group wrist BMC progressively increased in the subjects treated with eCT or conjugated estrogens whereas the control subjects showed a slight loss of bone after 6 months (Figure 1). The wrist bone BMC increase was more evident in the estrogen-treated group (+2.1% $\pm$ 0.3); in the eCT-treated group the increase was +1.8% $\pm$ 0.4; in the control group bone loss was about 3% $\pm$ 0.5.

In the women with osteoporosis, BMC progressively increased in both

Table 1 Clinical and hormonal* data (means ± SEM) before and after 6 months of treatment in early postmenopausal women

	Conjugated estrogens		*eCT*		*Control*	
	Before	*After*	*Before*	*After*	*Before*	*After*
Age (years)	47 ± 2		50 ± 2.1		46 ± 1.3	
Menopausal duration (months)	4 ± 1.5		8 ± 3.4		5 ± 2	
Weight (kg)	58 ± 2.7		61 ± 1.4		64 ± 2	
Osteocalcin (ng/ml)	4.2 ± 0.7	4.6 ± 0.9	4.6 ± 0.9	3.9 ± 0.6	4.9 ± 0.7	5.2 ± 1
LH (mU/ml)	50.6 ± 8	26 ± 9	48 ± 12.5	55 ± 10	40 ± 5.9	57 ± 15
FSH (mU/ml)	83 ± 14	35 ± 7	85 ± 6.6	91 ± 9	75 ± 13	87 ± 9
PRL (ng/ml)	9.4 ± 1.7	12 ± 2	12.7 ± 2.4	14 ± 2	15.6 ± 4	13 ± 2
E_2 (pg/ml)	20 ± 4	32 ± 8	18.2 ± 3.0	15 ± 1.8	20 ± 2.8	16 ± 3
E_1 (pg/ml)	25 ± 3	30 ± 4.6	26 ± 4.7	30 ± 7	28 ± 5	25 ± 4

*LH, luteinizing hormone; FSH, follicle-stimulating hormone; PRL, prolactin; E_2, estradiol; E_1, estrone

Table 2 Clinical and hormonal* data before and after 6 months of treatment in osteoporotic women

	Conjugated estrogens		*eCT*		*Control*	
	Before	*After*	*Before*	*After*	*Before*	*After*
Age (years)	56 ± 3.4		57 ± 2		54 ± 3	
Menopausal duration (months)	52 ± 9.3		63 ± 11		59 ± 7	
Weight (kg)	63 ± 2.4		60 ± 3		62 ± 2.4	
Osteocalcin (ng/ml)	6.5 ± 1.7	5.2 ± 0.9	5.7 ± 1.1	4.8 ± 0.7	6.2 ± 0.9	6.0 ± 1
LH (mU/ml)	52 ± 15	40 ± 9	47 ± 9	50 ± 10	62 ± 19	70 ± 15
FSH (mU/ml)	105 ± 22	82 ± 16	71 ± 12	88 ± 7	115 ± 26	90 ± 16
PRL (ng/ml)	10 ± 3	16 ± 4	12 ± 1.8	11 ± 0.9	9 ± 0.7	8.4 ± 0.5
E_2 (pg/ml)	12 ± 4	38 ± 10	18 ± 6	13 ± 2	10 ± 1.4	9 ± 0.7
E_1 (pg/ml)	28 ± 6	43 ± 9	33 ± 7	30 ± 5	25 ± 6	31 ± 7

*LH, luteinizing hormone; FSH, follicle-stimulating hormone; PRL, prolactin; E_2, estradiol; E_1, estrone

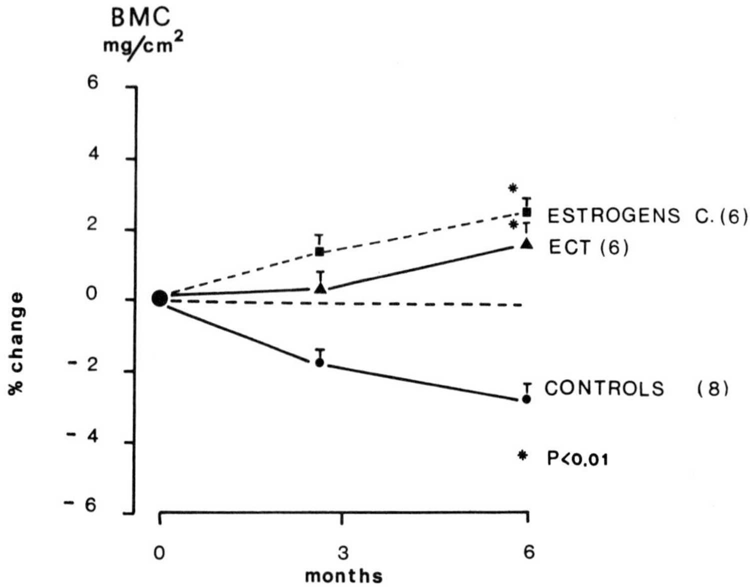

Figure 1 Mean (± SEM) values of bone mass measurements at the distal radius in early postmenopausal women before and after 6 months treatment. ■ = conjugated estrogens group; ▲ = eCT group; ● = control group; $*p < 0.001$ vs basal value

treatment groups, with a more evident rise in eCT plus estrogen treated subjects (+3% ± 0.40 after 6 months) (Figure 2). In the group treated with eCT plus Ca, the rise was 2.7% ± 0.4. The control subjects continued to lose in bone mass, which was −2.1% ± 0.2 at the end of the study. the pattern of osteocalcin, high at the beginning of the study, showed a significant reduction after treatment ($p < 0.01$).

DISCUSSION

After menopause, loss of bone mass exposes many women to the risk of osteoporosis. The present study shows that CT therapy can be considered an alternative to estrogens in preventing bone loss in healthy menopausal women and makes it possible to treat subjects who cannot take estrogens.

In the literature there are many reports of the administration of CT to women after ovariectomy[13,14], because the risk of substantial bone mineral loss is linked to the sudden drop in concentrations of circulating estrogens. This is particularly true in women who undergo ovariectomy before menopause, when estrogens are still at fertility levels. In physiological menopause, estrogen levels are already much lower before the last menstrual bleeding[15], so that certain women only shortly after their last period already have lower than normal BMC. The present study investigated the effect of unmodified eCT in this type of subject and found that treatment either with conjugated

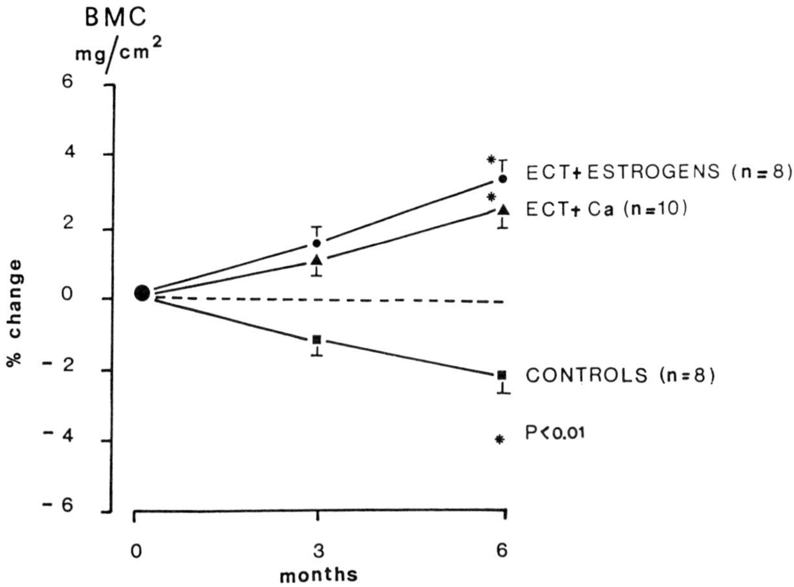

Figure 2 Mean (± SEM) values of bone mass measurements at the distal radius in osteoporotic women before and after 6 months treatment. ● = eCT + conjugated estrogens group; ▲ = eCT + calcium group; ■ = control group; *$p < 0.01$ vs basal value

estrogens or eCT led to an increase in BMC with respect to untreated controls.

The second part of this study concerned the treatment of postmenopausal osteoporosis with eCT + calcium and with eCT + conjugated estrogens. Besides having low BMC these women complained of bone pain particularly of the back and there was radiological evidence of at least one atraumatic vertebral crush fracture. The combination of eCT and estrogens was justified by the need to establish whether bone mass could be recovered more rapidly using the two hormones most implicated in this disease[16]. Since estrogens determine a reduction in bone turnover in rats[17,18] and CT decreases osteoclast activity[19–21] the combined administration of both hormones might potentiate these effects. Our results showed an increase in BMC which was substantially the same with the two types of treatment, whereas controls continued to suffer slow but progressive bone loss. In the treated groups there was a reduction in osteocalcin, a known index of bone turnover. The fact that there was a similar increase with either treatment shows that bone recovery is a very slow process which is not influenced by the contemporaneous administration of eCT and estrogens. Unmodified eCT was well tolerated, episodes of flushing, gastrointestinal disorders and other side-effects were responsible for a drop-out rate of 18% in eCT-treated patients.

In conclusion it is possible to confirm that 6 months treatment with unmodified eCT was effective in preventing bone loss in women immediately after menopause and in increasing bone mass by inhibiting bone resorption in women with postmenopausal osteoporosis.

REFERENCES

1. Richelson, L.S., Wahner, H.W., Melton, L.J. and Riggs, B.L. (1984). Relative contributions of aging and estrogen deficiency to postmenopausal bone loss. *N. Engl. J. Med.*, **311**, 1273
2. Aitken, J.M., Hart, D.M., Anderson, J.B., Lindsay, R., Smith, D.A. and Speirs, C.F. (1973). Osteoporosis after oophorectomy for nonmalignant disease in pre-menopausal women. *Br. Med. J.*, 325
3. Hui, S.L., Wiske, P.S., Norton, J.A. and Johnston, C.C., Jr (1982). A prospective study of change in bone mass with age in postmenopausal women. *J. Chron. Dis.*, **35**, 715
4. Lindsay, R., Hart, D.M., Aitken, J.M., MacDonald, E.B., Anderson, J.B. and Clarke, A.C. (1976). Long-term prevention of postmenopausal osteoporosis by estrogen. *Lancet*, **i**, 1038
5. Nachtigall, L.E., Nachtigall, R.H., Nachtigall, R.D. and Beckman, E.M. (1979). Estrogen replacement therapy I: a 10-year prospective study in the relationship to osteoporosis. *Obstet. Gynecol.*, **53**, 277
6. Frost, H.M. (1973). In Thomas, C. (ed.) *Bone Remodeling and its Relationship to Metabolic Bone Disease.* (Springfield)
7. Christiansen, C., Christensen, M.S., Larsen, N.E. and Transbol, I. (1982). Pathophysiological mechanisms of estrogen effect on bone metabolism. Dose-response relationships in early postmenopausal women. *J. Clin. Endocrinol. Metab.*, **55**, 1124
8. Morimoto, S., Tsiyi, M., Okada, Y., Ouishi, T. and Kumahara, Y. (1980). The effects of oestrogens on human calcitonin secretion after calcium infusion in elderly female subjects. *Clin. Endocrinol.*, **13**, 135
9. Baylink, D.J., Morey, E. and Rich, C. (1969). Effect of calcitonin on the rates of bone formation and resorption in the rat. *Endocrinology*, **84**, 261
10. Austin, L.A. and Heath, H., III (1981). Calcitonin, physiology and pathophysiology. *N. Engl. J. Med.*, **304**, 269
11. Chapui, M.C. and Meunier, P.J. (1982). Comparison of the acute effect of eel and salmon calcitonins in Pagetic patients. *Horm. Metab. Res.*, **14**, 559
12. Geola, F.L., Frumar, A.M. and Tataryn, I.V. (1980). Biological effects of various doses of conjugated equine estrogens in postmenopausal women. *J. Clin. Endocrinol. Metab.*, **51**, 620
13. Zara, C., Perotti, F., Ferraro, R., Lauri, A., Saviotti, C., Montrasio, M.G., Caprotti, M. and Polatti, F. (1988). Trattamento di pazienti ovariectomizzate con calcitonine sintetiche per via intramuscolare e spray nasale. *Minerva Endocrinologica*, **1**, 214
14. Christiansen, C., Riis, B.J., Podenphant, J. and Johansen, J.S. (1987). Intranasal calcitonin in the treatment of postmenopausal osteoporosis. In Christiansen, C., Johansen, J.S. and Riis, B.J. (eds). *Osteoporosis 1987*, Vol. 2, p. 853. *Second International Symposium on Osteoporosis*, Denmark
15. Sherman, B.W. and Korenman, S.G. (1975). Hormonal characteristics of the human menstrual cycle throughout reproductive life. *J. Clin. Invest.*,**55**, 699
16. Sherman, B.W., West, J.H. and Korenman, S.G. (1976). The menopausal transition: Analysis of LH, FSH, estradiol, and progesterone concentrations during menstrual cycles of older women. *J. Clin. Endocrinol. Metab.*, **42**, 629
17. Stevenson, J.C, Abeyasekera, G., Hillyard, C.J., Phang, K.G., MacIntyre, I., Campbell, S., Townsend, P.T., Young, O. and Whitehead, M.I. (1981). Calcitonin and the calcium-regulating hormones in post-menopausal women: effect of oestrogens. *Lancet*, **i**, 693
18. Anderson, J.J.B., Greenfield, J.W., Posada, J.R. and Crackel, W.C. (1970). Effect of estrogen on bone mineral turnover in mature female rats as measured by strontium-85. *Proc. Soc. Exp. Biol. Med.*, **135**, 883
19. Cruess, R.L. and Hong, K.C. (1979). The effect of long term estrogen administration on bone metabolism in the female rat. *Endocrinology*, **104**, 1188

20. Holtrop, M.E., Raisz, L.G. and Simmons, H.A. (1974). The effects of parathyroid hormone, colchicine and calcitonin on the ultrastructure and the activity of osteoclasts in organ culture. *J. Cell. Biol.*, **60**, 346
21. Chambers, T.J. and Moore, A. (1983). The sensitivity of isolated osteoclasts to morphological transformation by calcitonin. *J. Clin. Endocrinol. Metab.*, **57**, 819
22. Nicholson, G.C., Moseley, J.M., Sexton, P.M., Mendelsohn, F.A.O. and Martin, T.J. (1986). Abundant calcitonin receptors in isolated rat osteoclasts. *J. Clin. Invest.*,**78**, 355

Section 4 continued

Part L

Benefits and risks of hormonal treatments in women

121

Benefits and risks of a substitutive therapy in the prevention of osteoporosis

F. Polatti, F. Perotti, A. Lauri, F. Beneventi, R. Ferraro, G. Panese and C. Zara

In women, the physiological process of bone loss is linked to the age of onset of menopause. This phenomenon can be more or less accentuated and from 60 years of age is responsible for vertebral and femoral fractures etc. In the last 20 years, a woman's average life span has increased by about 10–15 years while the average age of menopause onset has not changed[1], causing a great increase in the number of severe cases of osteoporosis.

Almost 50 years ago Albright stated that a substitutive estrogen therapy could impede bone loss[2]; initially this treatment was used only to reduce symptoms of menopause.

Osteoporosis has always been considered a disease of the elderly and has always been treated by the internists or orthopedists, while gynecologists have rarely considered the concept of prevention.

Recently, the possibility of quantifying calcium loss and the demonstration of estrogen receptors in bone tissue have led gynecologists to confront the problem of postmenopausal bone loss[3].

Conjugated estrogens, mestranol, and ethinylestradiol, administered orally and transdermally[4–8], have been used for prolonged periods in postmenopause and have demonstrated a positive effect on calcium phosphate metabolism, cutaneous tropism, the genital urinary system and women's behavior. However, along with these beneficial aspects, various negative side-effects have contraindicated the use of estrogens alone in postmenopause.

The association of a progestin for at least 12 days in every cycle of estrogen treatment has become mandatory to avoid the risk of endometrial cancer[9]. Christiansen[10] and Shaigill[11] have clearly demonstrated how a long-term substitutive estroprogestin therapy can play a role in the prevention of postmenopausal osteoporosis. This new therapeutic strategy, which should be initiated immediately in pre- or postmenopause, should be prolonged for a period equal to the increase in a woman's average life-span (10–15 years).

Today the use of estroprogestins in fertile women still presents contra-indications regarding lipid and carbohydrate metabolism, which clearly increase with age. For many years, research in pharmacology has strived to obtain hormonal preparations which do not alter these parameters.

Medroxyprogesterone acetate (MAP)[13] and cyproterone acetate[14] are progestins which do not induce modifications of the lipid metabolism, proving to be advantageous when associated with estrogens. Jensen and colleagues[14] and Polatti and colleagues[15] have shown that substitutive therapy with estradiol valerate and cyproterone acetate prevents bone loss due to both the estrogen and progestenic activity[16], in addition it does not cause significant variations in lipid and carbohydrate metabolism.

Transdermal estrogen administration[17,18] avoids the hepatic circulation, and therefore significantly reduces liver involvement. At the moment, there are not sufficient data on a widespread basis or for period of administration greater than 5–6 years, which discuss the recently observed advantages of bandage administration of estradiol combined with progestins which have no effect on lipid metabolism.

At present prevention of osteoporosis can be obtained using 'low-risk' estroprogestinic combinations, or transdermal estrogen preparations, combined with cyproterone acetate or MAP, progestins which are metabolically safer.

These two treatments present many well-known benefits yet the extensive duration of therapy should be taken into account when considering administration. A correct evaluation of the patient's general and hormonal condition, along with a detailed examination of the absolute and relative contra-indication associated with the use of estroprogestins is the basis of the approach towards preventive hormonal treatment of osteoporosis.

However, periodic and systematic monitoring during treatment can create a relationship of trust and collaboration between a patient and her gynecologist who is responsible for the artificially extended ovarian activity. In this way, a woman can definitely improve the quality of her life and eventual risks are minimized when compared to the benefits obtained.

Prevention of osteoporosis and estrogen deficiency in women with contra-indications to estroprogestin use still poses a problem.

However, it seems that vaginal administration of estriol (a weak estrogen)[17,18] combined with calcitonin therapy can guarantee a better future to these patients as well.

REFERENCES

1. Bottiglioni, F. and DeAloysio, D. (1988). In Angelini, A. (ed.), *La Menopausa. Aspetti Clinico Terapeutici.* Vol. II (Rome: Ed. Scientifiche Angelini)
2. Albright, F., Bloomberg, E. and Smith, P.H. (1940). Post-menopausal osteoporosis. *Trans. Ass. Am. Physician*, **55**, 298–305
3. Eriksne, E.F. and Riggs, B.L. (1987). In Christiansen, C. *et al.* (eds). *I International Congress of the European Foundation for Osteoporosis and Bone Disease*, Alborg, Denmark
4. Ribot, C., Tremollieres, F., Pouilles, J.M., Louvet, J.P. and Peyron, R. (1987). Transdermal administration of $17\beta E_2$ in postmenopausal women: Preliminary results of a longitudinal study. In Christiansen, C. *et al.* (eds) *Osteoporosis*, **1**, pp. 546–8. *International Symposium on Osteoporosis*, Denmark
5. Ribot, C., Tremollieres, F., Pouilles, J.M. and Louvet, J.P. (1987). Prevention of post-menopausal bone loss by percutaneus $17\beta E_2$. Preliminary results of a two years prospective study. In Christiansen, C. *et al.* (eds) *Osteoporosis*, **1**, pp. 549–50

6. Lindsay, R. *et al.* (1984). *Obstet. Gynecol.*, **3**, 759
7. Lindsay, R. *et al.* (1980). *Lancet*, **ii**, 1151
8. Horsman *et al.* (1983). *N. Engl J. Med.*, **309**, 1405
9. Peterson, H.B., Lee, N.C. and Rubin, G.L. (1987). Genital neoplasia. In Mishell, D.R. (ed.) *Menopause: Physiology and Pharmacology*. (Chicago: Year Book Medical Publisher)
10. Christiansen, C. (1984). Prophylactic treatment for age-related bone loss in women. In Christiansen, C. *et al.* (eds.). *Osteoporosis*, **2**, pp. 587–93. *International Symposium on Osteoporosis*, Denmark
11. Shargil, A.A. (1987). Hormone replacement therapy for prevention of menopausal bone loss: A controlled prospective study for up to 15 years. In Christiansen, C. *et al.* (eds). *Osteoporosis*, **1**, pp. 559–63. *International Symposium on Osteoporosis*, Denmark
12. Council of Scientific Affairs (1983). Estrogen replacement in the menopause. *J. Am. Med. Assoc.*, **3**, 359–61
13. Crona, N., Enk, L., Samsioe, G., Silfverstolpe, G. and Skryten, A. (1983). High dose depot-MAP: effects on lipid and lipoprotein metabolism. *Eur. J. Obstet. Gynecol. Reprod. Biol.* **16**, 97–105
14. Jensen, J., Riis, B.J., Jensen, P.B. and Christiansen, C. (1987). Cyproterone Acetate an alternative progestogen in post-menopausal hormone replacement therapy? In Christiansen, C. *et al.* (eds). *Osteoporosis*, **1**, pp. 551–4. *International Symposium on Osteoporosis*, Denmark
15. Polatti, F., Mandelli, B., Lauri, A., Perotti, F., Ferraro, R. and Zara, C. (1989) Estradiolo Valerato e Ciproterone Acetato nella prevenzione della demineralizzazione ossea post-menopausale. *II Congress Nazionale di scienze Ginecologica Ostetrici*, Isola d'Elba 1988 (in press)
16. Lindsay, R., Hart, D.M., Purdie, D., Ferguson, M.M., Clarke, A.C. and Kraszewsky, A. (1978). *Clin. Sci. Mol. Med.*, **54**, 193–5
17. Englund, D.E. and Heimer, G.M. (1986). The effect of enterohepatic recirculation in oral and vaginal oestriol treatment. In Genazzani, A.R. *et al.* (eds). *Research on Gynecological Endocrinology*, pp. 483–7. *1st International Congress of Gynecological Endocrinology*, Madonna di Campiglio
18. Englund, D.E. and Heimer, G.M. (1986). Pharmacokinetic study on Oestriol: the influence of time, route of administration and food habits. In Genazzani, A.R. *et al.* (eds). *Research on Gynecological Endocrinology*, pp. 475–82 *1st International Congress of Gynecological Endocrinology*, Madonna di Campiglio

122

Estrogen replacement therapy: relationship to osteoporosis in young and old women

T. Motta, L. Santoro, C. Messina, C. Clerici and S. Casazza

INTRODUCTION

Hormone replacement therapy (HRT) has been closely scrutinized and the biological effects of various estrogens have been examined extensively during the past years. Inevitably, the last 50 years have witnessed frenetic swings in the popularity of postmenopausal hormone therapy as potential benefits or potential risks of such treatment were discovered.

Potential risks of HRT include endometrial cancer, hypertension, gall-bladder disease, abnormal uterine bleeding and probably breast cancer. On the other hand, there is no consensus that HRT modifies the risk of developing myocardial infarction, cerebral vascular accident, pulmonary embolism or abnormal glucose metabolism.

Currently, specific benefits of low-dose estrogen therapy in menopausal women include relief of vasomotor symptoms, urogenital atrophy and prevention of osteoporosis.

ESTROGENS AND OSTEOPOROSIS IN OLDER WOMEN

The effect of estrogen on the skeleton is certainly not unique to equine estrogens and probably not to the oral route, or even to estrogens themselves. However, the most effective oral dose of conjugated equine estrogens in the prevention of osteoporosis is 0.625 mg/day; increasing the dose further does not confer added benefits[1]. Estradiol given orally has been shown to prevent bone loss successfully[2] and the most effective oral dose is 2 mg.

Twenty-five μg/day of ethinylestradiol are required to produce any estrogenic effect on mineral homeostasis[3]. The precise mechanism of the action of estrogen on bone metabolism is unknown.

Recently, estrogen receptors have been identified in bone and it is possible that the hormone mechanism of action may be direct[4,5].

Otherwise estrogen acts via an indirect action through marrow-stem cell differentiation or through other calciotropic chemical mediators.

In fact, Stevenson *et al.* have suggested that estrogen stimulates calcitonin (CT) production[6]. The resulting reduction in bone resorption leads to a small reduction in serum calcium and consequently a rise in secretion of parathyroid hormone (PTH).

PTH stimulates 1α-hydroxylation of 25-hydroxycholecalciferol (25-OHD_3), increasing circulating levels of 1,25-hydroxycholecalciferol (1,25$(OH)_2D_3$) and improving calcium absorption from the gut. As a consequence, serum calcium levels tend to rise.

Currently estrogenic drugs, whether natural or synthetic, and irrespective of their route of administration, have been shown to be effective in the prevention of bone loss, if given at sufficient doses. The use of oral estrogens for replacement therapy is well established and actually it is still the preferred route. From the patient's point of view, oral therapy requires daily patient compliance and if given cyclically there may be a return of symptoms in the treatment-free week. Oral estrogens are absorbed through the gut wall and enter the liver via the portal system before continuing on into the general circulation. In the liver a third of the dose of oral estrogen is converted to estrone-3-glucuronide which is excreted in the urine and bile without producing the desired effect. In premenopausal women the physiological ratio of plasma estradiol to estrone is greater than one. When estrogens are administered orally a large proportion are converted to estrone: thus the ratio of estradiol/estrone is reversed. Oral estrogens produce an increase in sex hormone-binding globulin (SHBG), thyroxine-binding globulin (TBG) cortisol-binding globulin (CBG) and renin substrate. This increase is much greater following oral administration of synthetic estrogens (diethylstilbestrol and ethinylestradiol) than with natural estrogens[7]. Finally, synthetic estrogens are also associated with an increased platelet aggregation and reduced anti-thrombin III[8].

For this reason it is essential to use a route of administration which bypasses the liver while maintaining the beneficial effects of the estrogen. Percutaneous estrogen, as a transdermal estradiol patch, is a relatively new method of hormonal administration (TTS).

In fact serum estradiol levels resulting from the transdermal application of 25, 50 or 100 mg of 17β-estradiol (E_2) are both ineffective on renin substrate and on sex hormones.

Relief of hot flushes, irritability, sleep disturbance and vaginal atrophy has been shown to equal oral administration of conjugated equine estrogens[9,10]. The TTS is well tolerated with only infrequent local irritation[9,11].

Since recent studies have suggested that CT is also effective in the prevention of osteoporosis, at least in the short term, this could be an effective alternative to HRT in women unable or unwilling to take estrogens. It is also possible that the combination of CT with estrogen may permit a smaller dose of the latter.

In a 2-year placebo control randomized trial carried out in 70 early postmenopausal women, we have recently shown that both CT and E_2, when administered by TTS, are equally effective in the prevention of bone loss compared with controls ($p < 0.05$).

Further, in women treated with both CT and E_2 there may have been an additive effect ($p < 0.005$)[12]. Thus, optimal protection of both vascular system and skeleton could be obtained.

The disadvantage of the necessity for administration of CT by injection may be overcome with the development of alternative systems such as the recent intranasal spray.

ESTROGEN AND OSTEOPOROSIS IN YOUNGER WOMEN

All the hypogonadal and ovulatory disorders of the adolescent age are associated with a hypoestrogenic state and some of them clearly predispose to bone loss. In fact, exercise-induced amenorrhea, anorexia nervosa, premature ovarian failure, gonadal dysgenesis and hyperprolactinemia are well-documented causes of bone loss[13–20].

In females, bone mineral density (BMD) normally increases in adolescence, reaching a peak by the end of the second decade[16].

It has not been demonstrated whether the reduction in BMD is secondary to bone loss or to arrested skeletal maturation.

On the other hand, hypogonadal individuals and patients with exercise-induced amenorrhea and anorexia nervosa have lower peak bone mineral masses: complete compensation for growth delay may not occur with refeeding or when training is interrupted. It is a reasonable supposition that lower trabecular bone mass in amenorrheic runners[18] is a consequence of estrogen deprivation and reflects increased bone loss. Bone mineral accretion ordinarily continues into the third decade, so we cannot exclude the alternative explanation that lower bone mass is due to arrested skeletal maturation. Cann *et al.* have suggested that treatment of amenorrheic athletes must be initiated early, perhaps within the first 2 or 3 years, to prevent or reverse the bone loss[17]. In fact, estrogen therapy effectively prevented bone loss if started within 2 months of ovarian activity cessation[21]. If started 3–6 years later, the bone loss may be replaced. Beyond 6 years the bone loss was not replaced and further bone loss was not prevented. These effects lasted as long as estrogen was given. On cessation of therapy rapid bone loss resumed[22].

Although it is generally accepted that low estrogen levels in premenopausal women with endocrine dysfunction are related to the osteopenia, the role of estrogen in bone dynamics, as in postmenopausal women, is not fully understood.

As previously indicated, one such indirect route may be the effect of estrogen on calcium balance. Postmenopausal women with osteoporosis may have increased basal urinary calcium excretion.

If the skeletal changes in amenorrheic patients are due to mechanisms similar to those after menopause, alteration of the calcium-related variables measured, would be predicted. On the contrary, in agreement with other authors we found no statistically significant changes in calcium phosphate, PTH, CT, 25-OHD$_3$ levels in women with exercise-induced amenorrhea, anorexia nervosa, gonadal dysgenesis (GD), premature ovarian failure (POF) and hypothalamic primary amenorrhea (HPA)[13–19].

In GD, serum alkaline phosphatase, and 1,25(OH)$_2$D$_3$ levels are elevated and reduced, respectively[13,16].

Thus, the physiological data do not resolve the question of bone loss versus maturation arrest, and further evaluation of both possibilities will require longitudinal assessment of bone mass in cyclic and amenorrheic women. More recently, we have studied a group of young patients with GD, POF and HPA, subjected to an i.v. infusion of calcium (3 mg/kg over a 3-min period) before and after 3 months of HRT. The CT response to provocative test showed a not significant rapid increase of this hormone before therapy and a partially blunted CT response, as in the control group, after therapy[23].

The changes of radial BMD, measured at the distal third of the non-dominant forearm at the start of the trial and after 1 year, are shown in Figure 1. Slight increase in radial BMD was not statistically significant. Further, reduction in both plasma bone-specific alkaline phosphatase and osteocalcin was found in the treatment group (Figures 2 and 3) but only

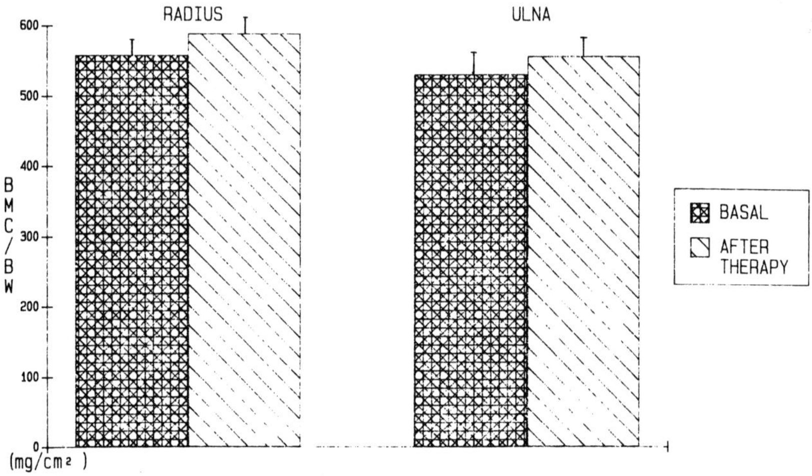

Figure 1 Changes of radial BMC/BW at the start of the trial and after 1 year of substitutive therapy

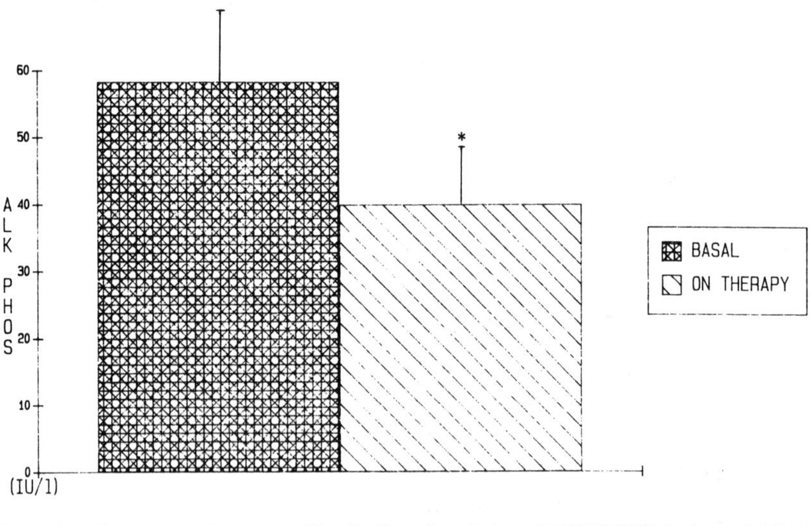

Figure 2 Changes of plasma specific alkaline phosphatase (ALK PHOS) during substitutive therapy; $*p < 0.05$

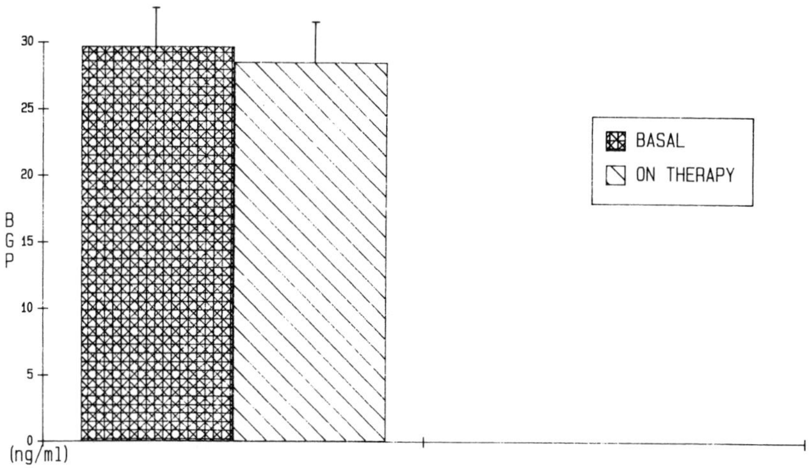

Figure 3 Changes of plasma osteocalcin (BGP) during substitutive therapy

the former was significant (58.3 ± 26.9 IU/ml compared with 40 ± 22.2; mean $\pm$ S.D.; $p < 0.05$). Our data partially support the efficacy of HRT in reducing osteoporosis in primary amenorrhea. In fact the slight increase of BMD is probably due to the few patients examined or to the minimal dose of estrogen used in our study (0.625 mg of conjugated estrogens).

Moreover our data suggest, as demonstrated elsewhere[23], that in GD, estrogen deficiency does not impair CT secretion and that osteoporosis is not associated with an alteration of CT secretion.

The pathogenesis of bone loss in GD, POF and HPA is probably multifactorial. Other hormonal factors, i.e. cortisol, growth hormone, somatomedin C etc., are implicated.

REFERENCES

1. Lindsay, R., Hart, D.M. and Clark, D.M. (1984). The minimum effective dose of estrogen for prevention of postmenopausal bone loss. *Obstet. Gynecol.*, **63**, 759–63
2. Lindsay, R., Hart, D.M., Purdie, P., Ferguson, M.M., Clark, A.C. and Kraszewski, A. (1978). Comparative effects of estrogen and a progestogen on bone loss in postmenopausal women. *Clin. Sci. Mol. Med.*, **54**, 193–5
3. Conference Report Consensus Development Conference: Aalborg, Denmark (1987). Prophylaxis and treatment of osteoporosis. *Br. Med. J.*, **314**, 1676–86
4. Ernst, M., Schmid, Ch. and Froesch, E.R. (1987). 17 beta-estradiol stimulates proliferation and type I procollagen gene expression in primary osteoblasts. In Jensen, J., Riis, B. and Christiansen, C. (eds.) *International Symposium on Osteoporosis*, 27 September–2 October, Denmark
5. Eriksen, E.F., Berg, N.J., Graham, M., Colvard, D.S., Mann, K.G., Spelsberg, T.C. and Riggs, B.L. (1987). Multiple sex steroid receptors in cultured human osteoblast-like cells. In Jensen, J., Riis, B. and Christiansen, C. (eds.) *International Symposium on Osteoporosis*, 27 September–2 October, Denmark
6. Stevenson, J.C., Abeyasekera, G. and Hillyard, C.J. (1983). Regulation of calcium-regulating hormones by exogenous sex steroids in early postmenopause. *Eur. J. Clin. Invest.*, **13**, 481–7

7. Mashchak, C.A., Lobo, R.A., Dozono-Takano, R., Eggena, P., Nakamura, R.M., Brenner, P.F. and Mishell, D.R. (1982). Comparison of pharmacodynamic properties of various estrogen formulations. *Am. J. Obstet. Gynecol.*, **144**, 511–18
8. Gambrell, R.D., Jr. (1982). The menopause: benefits and risks of estrogen–progestogen replacement therapy. *Fertil. Steril.*, **37**, 457–74
9. Padwick, M.L., Endacott, J. and Whitehead, M.I. (1985). Efficacy, acceptability and metabolic effects of transdermal estradiol in the management of postmenopausal women. *Am. J. Obstet. Gynecol.*, **152**, 1085–91
10. Steingold, K.A., Kaufer, L., Chetkowski, R.J. *et al.* (1985). Treatment of hot flashes with transdermal estradiol administration. *J. Clin. Endocrinol. Metab.*, **61**, 627–32
11. Place, V.E., Powers, M., Darley, P.E., Schenkel, L. and Good, W. (1985). A double blind comparative study of estraderm and premarin in amelioration of postmenopausal symptoms. *Am. J. Obstet. Gynecol.*, **152**, 1092–9
12. Motta, T. (1988). Efficacia della terapia sostitutiva con estradiolo transdermico in menopausa. In Fioretti, P. and Melis, G.B. (eds) *Secondo Congresso Nazionale di Scienze Ginecologiche ed Ostetriche*, 12–19 June, Isola d'Elba, pp. 339–45. (Rome: CIC Edizioni Internationali)
13. Brown, D.M., Jowsey, Y. and Bradford, D.S. (1974). Osteoporosis in ovarian dysgenesis. *J. Pediatr.*, **84**, 816–20
14. Shore, R.M., Chesney, R.W., Mazess, R.B., Rose, P.G. and Bargman, G.J. (1982). Skeletal demineralization in Turner's Syndrome. *Calcif. Tissue. Int.*, **34**, 519–22
15. Motta, T., D'Alberton, A., Acaia, B., Conserva, P., Maggi, G., Ortolani, S., Corghi, E. and Caraceni, M.P. (1985). Reduced bone mineral mass in primary amenorrhea. In Flamigni, C., Venturoli, S. and Givens, J.R. (eds). *Adolescence in Females*, pp. 461–2. (Chicago: Year book Publishers, Inc.)
16. Motta, T., Casazza, S., Clerici, C., Giorda, G., Santoro, L., Maggi, G., Benedetti, U. and D'Alberton, A. (1987). Bone mineral content, mineral metabolism and puberal pathology. In Massi, G.B. and Bruni, V. (eds). *III European Symposium on Pediatric and Adolescent Gynaecology*, pp. 555–64. (Roma: C.I.C. Edizioni Internazionali, s.r.l.)
17. Cann, C.E., Martin, M.C., Genant, H.K. and Jaffe, R.B. (1984). Decreased spinal mineral content in amenorrheic women. *J. Am. Med. Assoc.*, **251**, 626–9
18. Drinkwater, B.L., Nilson, K., Chesnut II, C.H., Bremner, W.J., Shainholtz, S. and Southworth, M. (1984). Bone mineral content of amenorrheic and eumenorrheic athletes. *N. Engl. J. Med.*, **311**, 277–81
19. Lindberg, J.S., Fears, W.B., Hunt, M.M., Powell, M.R., Boll, D. and Wade, C.E. (1984). Exercise-induced amenorrhoea and bone density. *Ann. Intern. Med.*, **101**, 647–8
20. Klibanski, A., Neer, R.M., Beitins, I.Z., Ridgway, E.C., Zervas, N.T. and McArthur, J.W. (1980). Decreased bone density hyperprolactinemic women. *N. Engl. J. Med.*, **303**, 1511–14
21. Aitken, J.M., Hart, D.M. and Lindsay, R. (1973). Oestrogen replacement therapy for prevention of osteoporosis after oophorectomy. *Br. Med. J.*, **3**, 515–18
22. Lindsay, K., Hart, D.M., MacLean, A., Clarke, A.C., Kraszewski, A. and Garwood, J. (1978). Bone response to termination of oestrogen treatment. *Lancet*, **i**, 1325–7
23. Saggese, G., Bertelloni, S., Baroncelli, G.I., Buggiani, B. and Papini, A. (1988). La secrezione di calcitonina nell'osteoporosi della sindrome di Turner. *Riv. Ital. Ped.* (*I.J.P.*), **14**, 674–7

123

Estrogen replacement therapy: a theoretical estimation of its effects on mortality in Italy

G.B. Serra, E. Parlati, P. Manna and R. Capocaccia

In Italy there are over 29 000 000 women, of whom more than 30% are older than 50, with a fairly homogeneous distribution between 50 and 75 years old (Table 1)[1]. The fact that almost one third of the female population is older than 50 emphasizes the necessity of an accurate medical care towards this segment of population to obtain, not only longevity, but also a good quality of life.

In order to achieve this goal there has been in several industrialized countries a net increase of estrogen replacement therapy (ERT) to minimize the discomforts related to estrogen deficiency. Different studies report that between 30 and 50% of women over 50 years of age in the USA use ERT[2,3].

In Italy, considering the marketing of all estrogenic compounds used for ERT, and assuming that all blisters have been regularly used once purchased, there is a total use of only 11 000 g of estrogens, equivalent in months of therapy to roughly 650 000 cycles, that is to say 56 000 women years of therapy (Table 2). Based on these calculations it can be assumed that only 3% of women between 50 and 54 have been treated, or less than 0.6 of all postmenopausal women. It seems reasonable to attribute this low consumption of ERT to either the scarce consideration of the beneficial effects, or to an exaggeration of the potential risk of its use. Thus, from a clinical point

Table 1 Estimates of Italy female resident population by age and percentage of total female population

Age (yr)	*No.*	%
All ages	29 112 400	100
50–54	1 829 600	6.2
55–59	1 758 900	6.0
60–64	1 191 600	4.0
65–69	1 495 000	5.1
70–74	1 223 800	4.2
over 75	1 640 200	5.6

Table 2 Estimated consumption of conjugated estrogens and estriol in Italy in 1987. (Farmindustria)

	Blisters sold	*mg*	*Monthly cycle equivalents*
Conjugated estrogens	213 000	5 237 700	323 777
Estriol			
Ovestin	270 000	5 400 000	257 142
Colpogyn	164 000	492 000	98 400
Total	647 000	11 129 700	679 419

of view, the postmenopausal population in Italy represents an interesting model for a quantitative evaluation of estrogen deficiency-related effects in the absence of any ERT. In addition, in the absence of any ongoing prospective cohort study, this medical habit seems to urge a verification of the expected and theoretical mortality if ERT came into use.

Imagining the treatment of 30% of all women between 50 and 54 (540 000 women out of 1 800 000) with adequate dosages (0.625 mg/day) of estrogen for a 10-year period, and applying the specific relative risks for estrogen use, it should be possible to calculate eventual changes in mortality, thus providing an initial evaluation of a benefit/risk balance.

Since ERT prevents postmenopausal accelerated bone loss and osteoporosis it has been calculated that ERT may reduce the mortality risk for hip fractures to 0.4[5]. Applying this protective effect in the ERT group, a decrease of the mortality from the actually observed 71 cases to 28, equivalent to a 40% decrease, should be obtained (Table 3).

In analogy, considering the positive effects on metabolic parameters, such as high-density lipoproteins, ERT seems to decrease the relative cardiovascular mortality risk to 0.8[6]. If this evaluation is correct, even a decrease as little as 20% will produce a reduction of mortality from 537 to 431 (Table 3) in the ERT-treated group.

Therefore, considering mortality from both fractures and cardiovascular diseases, ERT should provide a reduction of 148 out of the 600 deaths now observed for these specific causes in the absence of any estrogen treatment.

The obvious major risk of ERT seems to be of oncogenetic nature, related to the two most prominent estrogen-dependent neoplasis: mammary and endometrial carcinomas.

Table 3 Specific mortality incidences and absolute variations calculated in the 30% of postmenopausal women aged 50–54 (540 000 women) now observed without significant use of ERT, and expected with adequate estrogen doses for a 10-year period

Specific mortality risks	*No. with hip fractures*	*No. with cardiovascular disease*	*No. with breast cancer*	*No. with endometrial cancer*	*Total*
Now observed	71.7	537.1	625.5	127.8	1362.1
Expected under ERT	28.6	431.7	625.5	259.5	1345.3
Variations	−43.1	−105.4	0	+131.7	−16.8

Although both mammary and endometrial tissue are estrogen targets, recent studies have shown differences in the timing of mytotic acme and in the mechanism of cellular depletion, requiring different considerations related to the ERT risks.

Increased risk of mammary carcinoma has been claimed on the basis of the first retrospective studies on estrogen users[7]. Several biases however make those results almost useless. Recent studies, both retrospective and cohort-based, have now produced convincing and unanimous evidence that the relative risk for adequate estrogen use in a 10-year period should not exceed a factor between 0.8 and 1.2[8–10]. Only in particular subgroups, as in patients with familial history positive for breast carcinoma before the age of 40, or with epithelial proliferative breast lesions, may a significant increase of the relative risk occur. On this basis it seems reasonable to conclude that ERT should not increase the expected 625 cases of mortality for mammary carcinoma over a 10-year period (Table 3).

As far as endometrial carcinoma is concerned, data from the literature are unanimous in proving a risk at least double if ERT is given. In Italy the national statistical data do not differentiate between cervical and endometrial carcinoma, so that mortality for uterine cancer may not be further and separately analyzed. However, even considering that as much as 75% of all the mortality in postmenopausal women referred to as due to uterine cancer was of endometrial origin, the doubling of specific deaths as a consequence of ERT, would result in an increase of mortality to not more than 131 cases compared with the actually observed 127 in the absence of any estrogen therapy (Table 3). It may be of interest in the future, if more data are collected suggesting a possible responsiveness of the uterine cervix to estrogen effect, to evaluate eventual modification of the relative risk for cervical carcinoma also.

At present and in conclusion, after a 10-year period of ERT at a dosage of 0.625 mg/day, out of 540 000 women aged 50–54 the mortality should be decreased by 17 cases, corresponding to a 1.5% decrease of the present mortality.

These data indicate that any fear of increased mortality seems to be unjustified. Moreover three considerations deserve attention in this regard: the first is that under ERT a shift seems to occur from more acute and irreversible causes of death, such as those due to hip fractures or cardiovascular pathology, to a slower disease, the endometrial carcinoma. This condition may be easily recognized when the disease is still in an occult state, or even in a precancerous one, thus remaining highly curable, both because it is predictable and for the low malignant histological grading, it is amenable to complete recovery, after treatment with either hormones or surgery.

As a second consideration, since the occurrence of endometrial cancer seems to be the only significant risk, ERT appears to be mandatory in all postmenopausal women previously hysterectomized for non-neoplastic disease.

Finally, it must be considered that even though the mortality balance is the first way to evaluate a risk/benefit ratio, nevertheless, the general improvement in well-being obtained with ERT should be adequately considered and fully appreciated.

REFERENCES

1. Capocaccia, R., Farchi, G., Morietti, S. *et al.* (1984). La mortalita' in Italia nel periodo 70–79. *Rapporti Istisan*, **54**
2. Jones, H.W. and Jones, G.S. (1981). *Novak: Textbook of Gynecology*. Tenth edition, p. 797. (Baltimore: Williams and Williams)
3. Kennedy, D., Baum, C. and Forbes, M. (1985). Non-contraceptive oestrogens and progestins: Use patterns over time. *Obstet. Gynecol.*, **65**, 441–6
4. Capocaccia, R., Farchi, G. and Morietti, S. (1988). La mortalita' in Italia nel 1985, *Rapporti Istisan*, (in press)
5. Lobo, R.A. (1987). Prevention of postmenopausal osteoporosis. In Mishell, D. R. (ed.) *Menopause: Physiology and Pharmacology*, pp. 165–86. (Chicago: Year Book Medical Publishers, Inc.)
6. Ross, R.K., Paganini-Hill, A., Mack. T.M. and Henderson, B.E. (1987). Estrogen use and cardiovascular disease. In Mishell, D. R. (ed.), *Menopause: Physiology and Pharmacology*, pp. 209–23. (Chicago: Year Book Medical Publishers Inc.)
7. Henderson, B.E., Ros, R.K. and Pike, M.C. (1987). Breast neoplasia. In Mishell, D.R. (ed.), *Menopause: Physiology and Pharmacology*, pp. 261–74. (Chicago: Year Book Medical Publishers Inc.)
8. Kaufman, D.W., Miller, D.R. and Rosemberg, L. (1984). Non contraceptive estrogen use and risk of breast cancer. *J. Am. Med. Assoc.*, **252**, 63
9. Wingo, P.A., Layde, P.M. and Lee, N.C. (1987). The risk of breast cancer in postmenopausal women who have used estrogen replacement therapy. *J. Am. Med. Assoc.*, **257**, 209
10. Rohan, T.E. and McMichael, A.J. (1988). Non contraceptive exogenous estrogen therapy and breast cancer. *Med. J. Austr.*, **148**, 7

124

Effects of conjugated estrogens and transdermal estradiol on lipid metabolism and blood clotting during the treatment of menopausal syndrome

G.F. Trossarelli, M. Ardizzoja, E. Chiaudano, A. Defilippi, N. Biglia, M. Musso and M. Massobrio

INTRODUCTION

Estrogens constitute the etiological therapy of menopausal syndrome. The association with a gestagen greatly lowered the oncogenic risk.[1,2] Nevertheless both estrogen and progestogen drugs may exert some effects on lipid and clotting patterns[3–6].

Estrogens seem to reduce the risk of arterial diseases[7–9] and induce the following modifications:

(1) An increase of triglycerides bound to very low density lipoproteins (VLDL) (increase in hepatic synthesis and decrease in lipoprotein lipase (LPL))[10–13];

(2) A decrease of low density lipoprotein (LDL) cholesterol (decrease in peripheral conversion and increase in tissue clearance by an increase of the specific receptors)[10,11,13–15];

(3) A raise of high density lipoprotein (HDL) cholesterol (increase in hepatic synthesis and decrease in hepatic lipase)[7,11,13–21].

The progestogens, by their androgenic power, can induce opposite effects[8,20,22,23].

The known venous thrombophilic action of estrogens may be dose-dependent and is mediated by different mechanisms: vessel endothelium hyperplasia; venous stasis; increase in platelet aggregation (caused by increased thromboxane)[24]; enhanced synthesis and/or activation of clotting factors II, VII, VIII, IX, X, XII and fibrinogen[24–28]; an increased production and a lesser activity of antithrombin III[12,24,25,28–31]; an enhanced fibrinolysis (increase in plasminogen and a release of tissue activators)[5,32,33].

Oral or transdermal delivery, by a different action on hepatocytes, can modify the extent of such effects[11,14,34]. The study goal was to evaluate the lipid metabolism and the clotting system before and during the hormone replacement therapy in menopause.

MATERIAL AND METHODS

We longitudinally studied 40 postmenopausal women (amenorrhea >1 yr, follicle-stimulating hormone (FSH)/luteinizing hormone (LH) ratio >1.5, Kupperman' score >10), aged 44–56 years (mean 50 ± 3.8), without obesity, hypertension, thromboembolic or neoplastic diseases. This group was randomly assigned to receive two different estrogen treatments (21 days every 28 with MAP 10 mg/die from the 10th to the 21st day): oral conjugated estrogens (EC) 0.625 mg/die; or transdermal estradiol (TTS) 50 μg/die.

The following parameters were studied before the start and during the 6th month of therapy: body mass index (BMI, kg/h^2), systolic and diastolic blood pressure in orthostasis (BP, mmHg), FSH, LH (IU/l), prolactin (PRL) (ng/ml), estradiol (E_2) (pg/ml) (radioimmunoassay); triglycerides (TG), total cholesterol (CT), HDL-cholesterol (C-HDL) (mg%, enzymatic method), LDL-cholesterol (C-LDL, mg%, Friedewald' formula)[35], apolipoproteins A1 and B (apoA1, apoB, mg%, nephelometric assay), preβ, β and α-lipoproteins (pre-β, β, α-LP, %, chromatography) and C-HDL/CT, C-HDL/C-LDL, C-HDL/C-nonHDL ratios; PT (ratio)[36], PTT (s)[37], fibrinogen (F, mg%, automatic optical instrument)[38], platelet count (PLT, no. $\times 10^3$/mm^3, focalization hydrodynamic method-TOA Sismex), circulating platelet aggregates (CPA, %)[22], β-thromboglobulin (β-TG) and platelet factor IV (PF_4) (IU/ml, Elisa), VII, VIII and X factors (%, coagulant method with plasma lacking of the measured factor–Instrumental Laboratory), fibrinopeptide A (FPA, ng/ml, ELISA in platelet deprived plasma)[39], antithrombin III (AT III, %, colorimetric method–Chromozym Boehringer)[40], euglobin lysis time (ECLT, min, assay in diluted plasma), plasminogen (PLA)[41] and α-2antiplasmin (α2AP) (%, chromogenic method)[42].

The results are expressed as means $\pm$ SD and statistical evaluations were performed by Student's t test.

RESULTS

Lipid pattern

With TTS no significant variation was observed: CT (250 ± 30 vs 249 ± 44), C-HDL (69 ± 13 vs 62 ± 19), C-LDL (150 ± 6 vs 151 ± 39) and TG (96 ± 27 vs 90 ± 51). With EC we found a significant decrease of CT (250 ± 30 vs 210 ± 24; -16%) and C-LDL (150 ± 6 vs 129 ± 8; -14%), (Figure 1). C-HDL/CT, C-HDL/C-LDL and C-HDL/CnonHDL ratios were unmodified with both treatments, (Table 1). Apolipoproteins trend showed a significant reduction of ApoB in oral treatment group (92 ± 22 vs 72 ± 14; -22%). While EC determined a significant increase of preβ-LP (18 ± 8.25 vs 24 ± 8.28; $+15\%$) and decrease of β-LP (52.9 ± 8.92 vs 46.2 ± 6.21; -13.7%), in TTS group we observed only a significant β-LP reduction (52.9 ± 8.92 vs 45.3 ± 6.27; -14.4%), (Figure 2).

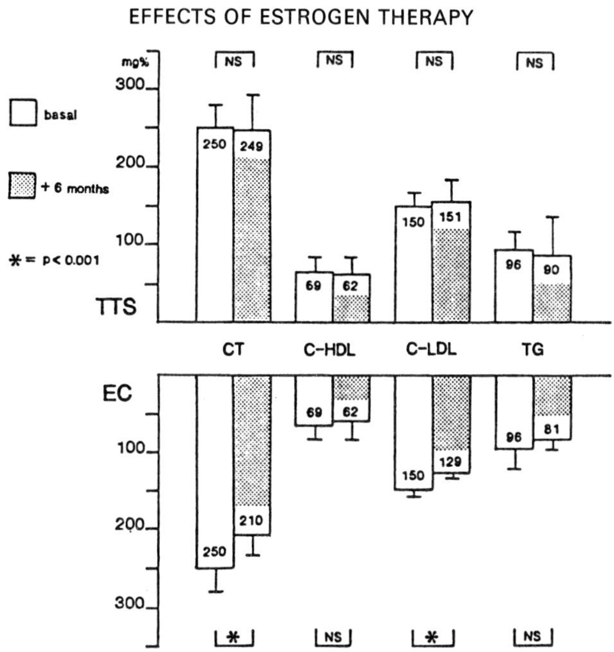

Figure 1 Total cholesterol (CT), HDL-cholesterol (C-HDL), LDL-cholesterol (C-LDL), triglycerides (TG) before and after transdermal estradiol (TTS) or conjugated estrogens (EC) therapy

Blood clotting

Either with TTS or EC PLT, PT and PTT did not significantly change, (Table 1). As regards platelet phase, a significant decrease of PF_4 (3.3 $\pm$ 1.2 vs 1.9 $\pm$ 0.1; -44%) was registered in TTS group; the other parameters did not show any significant variation either with TTS or EC (Figure 3). Factors VII, VIII and X, although unmodified in both therapies, showed a light increase (VII: $+1.2\%$; VIII: $+9.5\%$) with EC (Figure 4). AT III and FPA did not display any significant variation either: however, FPA showed a 28% increase in the TTS group (Figure 5). As expected, F significantly rose with EC (318 $\pm$ 68 vs 381 $\pm$ 66; $+20\%$), (Figure 5). As regards fibrinolysis, ECLT, α-2AP and PLA remained unchanged, (Figure 6).

Hormonal pattern

Both with TTS and with EC a significant decrease of FSH and LH was obtained. Although with a mild estrogen level, we did not obtain a significant increase of PRL, (Table 1). Neither BMI nor BP displayed any significant variation (Table 1).

Table 1

		B.M.I.	BP syst.	BP diast.	FSH	LH	PRL	E_2	PLT	PT	PTT	$\frac{C\text{-}HDL}{CT}$	$\frac{C\text{-}HDL}{C\text{-}LDL}$	$\frac{C\text{-}HDL}{C\text{-}nonHDL}$
Basal	$\bar{x}$	24	130	82	71	38	4.3	11.5	255	1	30	0.27	0.45	0.39
	SD	4.4	18	9.6	27.7	16.5	1.6	7.06	49.5	0.04	3.3	0.06	0.11	0.12
+6 months	$\bar{x}$	22.5	133	82	43.5	29.5	5.7	30	237	1.03	30.3	0.24	0.43	0.35
(TTS)	SD	3.4	27	12.7	18.3	7	2.6	10.8	54.2	0.05	3.3	0.09	0.19	0.17
	%	↓7	↑2.3	—	↓39**	↓23*	↑33	↑160***	↓6.9	↑2.8	↑1	↓12.2	↓4.4	↓10.2
+6 months	$\bar{x}$	24	130	81	45.4	19	4.6	17.6	243	1.01	29.5	0.29	0.5	0.43
(EC)	SD	3.2	14	8.5	19.6	8.1	2	9.7	48	0.04	3.6	0.07	0.12	0.16
	%	—	—	↓1.2	↓36**	↓50***	↑6.9	↑53	↓4.6	↑0.8	↓1.6	↑7.4	↑11.1	↑10.2

*$p < 0.05$; **$p < 0.01$; ***$p < 0.005$

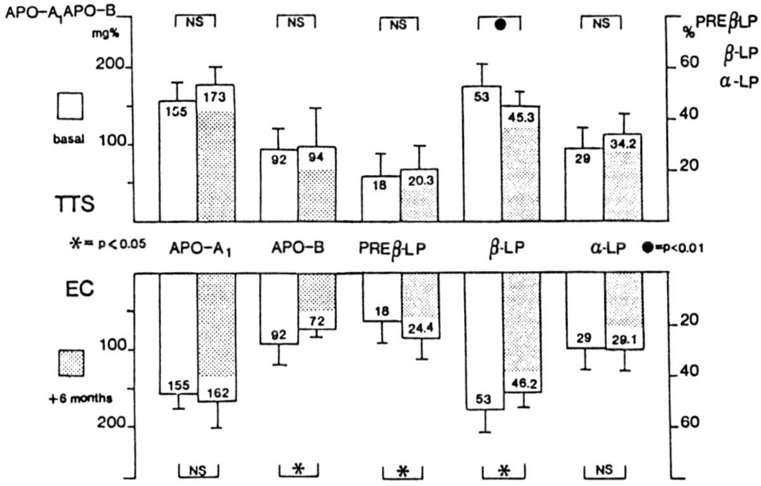

Figure 2 Apolipoprotein A_1 (apo-A_1), apolipoprotein B (apo-B), pre-β, β, and α-lipoproteins (pre-β, β, α-LP) before and after transdermal estradiol (TTS) or conjugated estrogens (EC) therapy

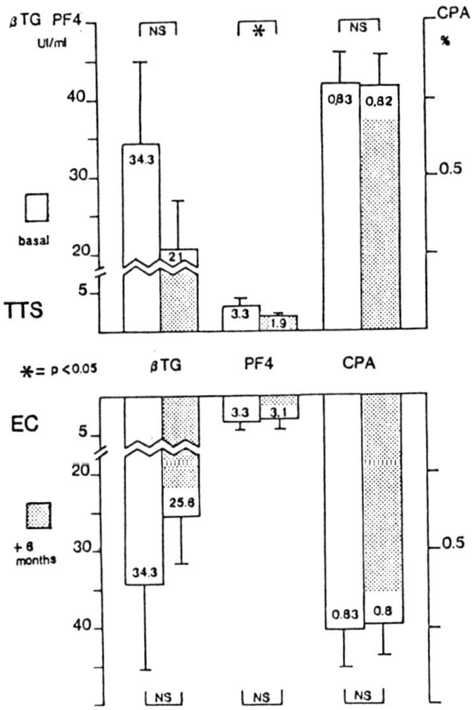

Figure 3 β-thromboglobulin (β-TG), platelet factor IV (PF_4), circulating platelet aggregates (CPA) before and after transdermal estradiol (TTS) or conjugated estrogens (EC) therapy

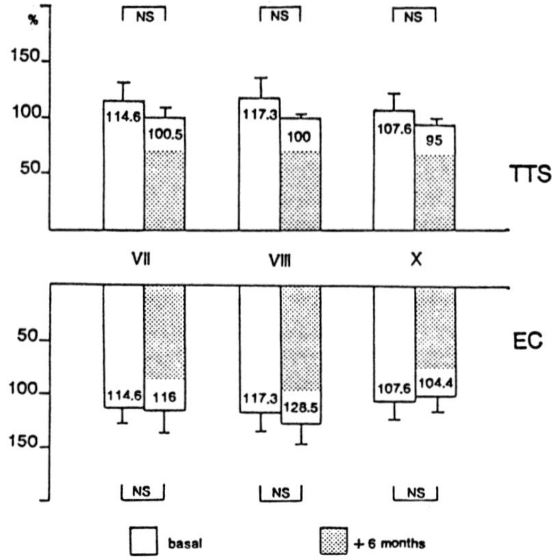

Figure 4 VII, VIII and X factors before and after transdermal estradiol (TTS) or conjugated estrogens (EC) therapy

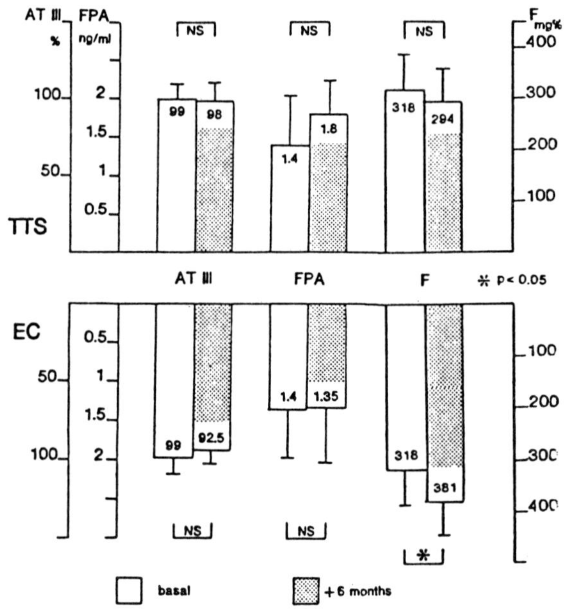

Figure 5 Antithrombin III (AT III), fibrinopeptide A (FPA) and fibrinogen (F) before and after transdermal estradiol (TTS) or conjugated estrogens (EC) therapy

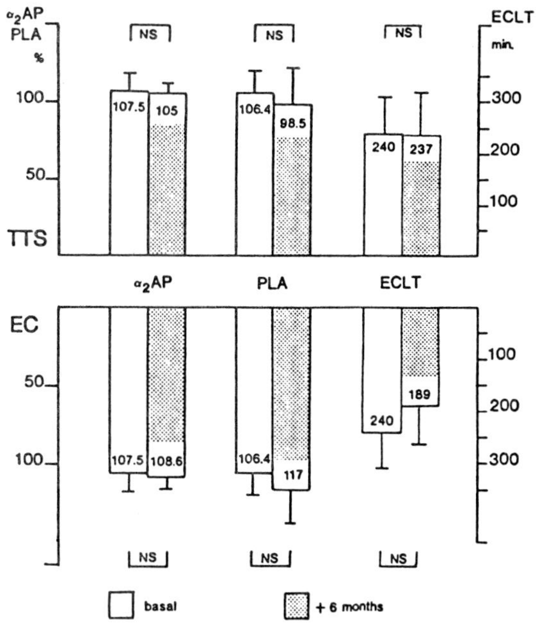

Figure 6 α-2-antiplasmin (α-2-AP), plasminogen (PLA) and euglobulin lysis time (ECLT) before and after transdermal estradiol (TTS) or conjugated estrogens (EC) therapy

DISCUSSION

Lipid pattern

The positive CT and C-LDL trend in EC group is probably due to the greater action of oral therapy on hepatocyte (decrease in HL). It is important to stress that the mild estrogen levels did not determine a TG rise. Whereas our data about EC are according to the literature[11,14], those about TTS are not univocal. Fahraeus[15] and Jensen[18] described a significant decrease of CT and C-LDL; other authors[10,12,14] found unchanged values. According to the CT and C-LDL reduction, apoB and β-LP showed similar behavior with oral treatment. Such a trend is less evident in the TTS group: in fact only β-LP significantly decreased.

Blood clotting

Our data obtained with both therapies suggest a neutrality on platelet activation: CPA and β-TG were similar, while PF_4 significantly decreased with TTS. The last data may be explained only by the few cases and by the assay variability. As regards clotting factors, F was only significantly raised in the EC group: such behavior, obtained by other authors[19,25], is probably due to the estrogen effect on hepatocytes. However, the poor significance of this increase is proved by the steadiness of PT, PTT, VII, VIII, and X factors and especially of FPA, a very sensitive index of thrombinic activation. It is noteworthy that neither treatment induces a significant decrease in AT III activity: this behavior was often observed with synthetic estrogens[19,43]. As regards fibrinolysis, statistically unvaried, we obtained a mild increase of PLA (+10%) with EC, probably due to their greater influence on hepatocyte; ECLT shows with oral therapy an insignificant rise in fibrinolysis, probably due to a lesser inhibition of the endothelial activators. Our data are consistent with the literature[19,25,28,35]

Hormonal pattern

Both treatments seem to be able to inhibit gonadotropins: the lesser reduction of FSH is probably due to the poor ovarian synthesis of inhibin. The low levels of E_2 obtained with EC may be induced by their composition: estrone sulfate (42%), equilin sulfate (26%), dihydroequilin sulfate (18%) and a lower amount of other estrogens. TTS also determined E_2 levels lower than expected: this result may be explained by the employed dosage and/or by a tissue conversion in estrone. The metabolic neutrality of both therapies is confirmed by the unchanged values of BMI and BP.

In conclusion we suggest that both EC and TTS during 6 months do not affect significantly the lipid pattern and the clotting system; the natural conjugated estrogens seem to give some advantages on atherogenic risk.

REFERENCES

1. Gambrell, R.D. (1986). Prevention of endometrial cancer with progestogens. *Maturitas*, **8**, 159
2. Hammond, C.B. and Maxon, W.S. (1986). Estrogen replacement therapy. *Clin. Obstet. Gynecol.*, **29**, 407
3. Gambrell, R.D., Jr (1987). Use of progestogen therapy. *Am. J. Obstet. Gynecol.*, **156**, 1304
4. Hofmann, V. and Straub, P.W. (1977). A radioimmunoassay technique for the rapid measurement of human fibrinopeptide A. *Thromb. Res.*, **11**, 81
5. Krauss, R., Perlman, J.A. and Ray, R. (1988). Effects of estrogen dose and smoking on lipid and lipoprotein levels in postmenopausal women. *Am. J. Obstet. Gynecol.*, **158**, 1606
6. Notelovitz, M., Kitchens, C., Ware, M. *et al.* (1983). Combination estrogen and progestogen replacement therapy does not adversely affect coagulation. *Obstet. Gynecol.*, **62**, 596
7. Barnes, R.B. and Lobo, R.A. (1985). Comparison of lipid and androgen levels after CE or depomedroxyprogesterone acetate treatment in postmenopausal women. *Obstet. Gynecol.*, **66**, 216
8. Bush, T.L. and Miller, V.T. (1987). Effects of pharmagologic agents used during menopause: impact on lipids and lipoproteins. In Mishell, D.R. (ed.). *Menopause: Physiology and Pharmacology.* (Chicago: Year Book Medical Publishers)
9. Bush, T.L., Barret-Connor, E., Cowan, L.D. *et al.* (1987). Cardiovascular mortality and noncontraceptive use of estrogen in women: results from the Lipid Research Clinic's Program Follow-up Study. *Circulation*, **7**, 378
10. Basdevant, A., De Lignieres, B. and Guy-Grand, B. (1983). Differential lipemic and hormonal responses to oral and parenteral 17-βestradiol in postmenopausal women. *Am. J. Obstet. Gynecol.*, **147**, 77
11. Chetkowsky, R.J., Meldrum, D.R., Steingold, K.A. *et al.* (1986). Biological effects of transdermal estradiol. *N. Engl. J. Med*, **314**, 1615
12. Fahraeus, L., Larsson-Cohn, U. and Wallentin, L. (1982). Lipoproteins during oral and cutaneous administration of estradiol-17β to menopausal women. *Acta Endocrinol.*, **101**, 597

13. La Rosa, J.C. (1988). The varying effects of progestins on lipid levels and cardiovascular disease. *Am. J. Obstet. Gynecol.*, **158**, 1621
14. Elkik, F., Gampel, A., Mercier-Boder, D.C. *et al.* (1982). Effects of percutaneous estradiol and conjugated estrogens on the level of plasma proteins and triglycerides in postmenopausal women. *Am. J. Obstet. Gynecol.*, **143**, 888
15. Fahraeus, L. and Wallentin, L. (1983). High density lipoprotein subfraction during oral and cutaneous administration of 17-*β*estradiol to menopausal women. *J. Clin. Endocrinol. Metab.*, **56**, 797
16. Campbell, S. and Whitehead, M.J. (1982). Potency and hepatocellular effects of estrogens after oral, percutaneous and subcutaneous administration. In van Keep, P.A., Utian, W.H. and Vermeulen, A. (eds) *The Controversial Climacteric*, pp. 103–26. (Lancaster: MTP)
17. Friedewald, W.T., Levy, R.I. and Fredrickson, D.S. (1972). Estimation of the concentration of LDL cholesterol in plasma without the use of the preparative ultracentrifuge. *Clin. Chem.*, **18**, 449
18. Judd, H.L. (1989). Estrogen replacement therapy: physiological considerations and new applications. *Bailliere's. Clin. Endocrinol. Metab.*, **1**, 177
19. Ottosson, U.B., Johansson, B.G. and von Schoultz, B. (1985). Subfractions of high density lipoproteins cholesterol during estrogen replacement therapy: a comparison between progestogens and natural progesterone. *Am. J. Obstet. Gynecol.*, **151**, 746
20. Philo, R.D. and Gaffney, P.J. (1982). Comparison of AT III assay using biological and Chromogenic substrates. *Br. J. Med.*, **50**, 147
21. Von Kaulla, E. (1975). Conjugated estrogens and hypercoagulability. *Am. J. Obstet. Gynecol.*, **122**, 688
22. Wu, K.K. and Hoak, J.C. (1974). A new method for the quantitative detection of platelet aggregates. *Lancet*, **ii**, 923
23. Lievertz, R.W. (1987). Pharmacology and pharmacokinetics of estrogen. *Am. J. Obstet. Gynecol.*, **156**, 1289
24. Samama, M., Schleguel, N., Cazenave, B. *et al.* (1980). Synthetic substrates in clinical blood coagulation assays. In Lijnen, H.R. and Collen, D. (eds) p. 93. (La Haye: Martinus Nijhoff)
25. Beller, F.K., Nachtigall, L. and Rosemberg, M. (1972). Coagulation studies of menopausal women taking estrogen replacement. *Obstet. Gynecol.*, **39**, 775
26. Davidsohn, I. and Henry, J.B. (1979). *Clinical Diagnosis by Laboratory Methods*. 16th Edn, (New York: W. B. Saunders Co.)
27. Poller, L., Thompson, J.M. and Coope, J. (1977). Conjugated equine estrogens and blood clotting: a follow-up report. *Br. Med. J.*, **1**, 935
28. Weinstein, L. (1987). Efficacy of a continuous estrogen progestin regimen in the menopausal patient. *Obstet. Gynecol.* **69**, 929
29. Coope, J., Thomson, J.M. and Poller, L. (1975). Effects of natural estrogen replacement therapy on menopausal symptoms and blood clotting. *Br. Med. J.*, **4**, 139
30. Bonnar, J. (1975). Effects of synthetic and natural estrogen on the coagulation system in postmenopausal women. In Campbell, S. (ed.) *The Management of the Menopause and Postmenopausal Years*. (Lancaster: MTP)
31. Volpe, A., Campanini, D., Golinelli, S. *et al.* (1987). Lipid metabolism and menopause. In Genazzani, A.R., Volpe, A. and Fachinetti, F. (eds.) *Gynecological Endocrinology*, pp. 655–666. (Carnforth: Parthenon Publishing)
32. Alkjaersig, N., Fletcher, A.P., De Ziegler, D. *et al.* (1988). Blood coagulation in postmenopausal women given estrogen treatment: comparison of transdermal and oral administration. *J. Lab. Clin. Med.*, **111**, 224
33. Ambrus, J.L. (1976). Estrogen and clotting factors. In van Keep, P.A. and Greenblatt, R.B. (eds) *Consensus on Menopause Research*, pp. 55–8. (Lancaster: MTP)
34. Miale, J.B. (1982). *Laboratory Medicine: Haematology*. 6th Edn. (C. V. Mosby Company)
35. Gambrell, R.D., Jr. (1982). The menopause: benefits and risks of estrogen-progestogen replacement therapy. *Fertil. Steril.*, **37**, 457
36. De Lignieres, B., Basdevant, A., Thomas, G. *et al.* (1986). Biological effects of 17-*β*estradiol in postmenopausal women: oral versus percutaneous administration. *J. Clin. Endocrinol. Metab.*, **62**, 536
37. Notelovitz, M. (1977). Coagulation, estrogen and the menopause. *Clin. Obstet. Gynecol.*, **4**, 107

38. Clauss, A. (1957). Rapid physiological coagulation method for the determination of fibrinogen. *Acta Haemath.*, **17**, 237
39. Jensen, J., Riis, B.J. and Strom, V. (1989). Continuous estrogen-progestogen treatment and serum lipoproteins in postmenopausal women. *Br. J. Obstet. Gynaecol.*, **34**, 130
40. Poller, L. (1975). A double blind cross-over study with conjugated equine estrogens on blood clotting. In Campbell, S. (ed.). *The Management of the Menopause and Postmenopausal Years*, p. 313. (Lancaster: MTP)
41. Stangel, J.J., Innerfield, I., Reyniak, V. *et al.* (1977) The effect of conjugated estrogens on coagulability in menopausal women. *Obstet. Gynecol.*, **49**, 314
42. Soria, C., Soria, J. and Samama, M. (1978). Progress in chemical fibrinolysis and thrombolysis. Davidson, J. F. *et al.* (eds.) (New York: Raven Press) **3**, 337
43. Bruni, B., Abbate, R. and Pinto, S. *et al.* (1987). Effects of gestodene on haemostasis. In Genazzani, A.R., Volpe, A. and Fachinetti, F. (eds.). *Gynecological Endocrinology*, pp. 523–32 (Carnforth: Parthenon Publishing)
44. Campagnoli, C., Prelato-Tousijn, L. *et al.* (1982). Effects of different natural estrogens on clotting factors, plasma lipids and endometrial proliferation in postmenopausal women. In Fioretti, P., Martini, L., Melis, G.B. and Yen, S.S.C. (eds) *The Menopause: Clinical, Endocrinological and Pathophysiological Aspects*, pp. 567–73. (London and New York: Academic Press)

125

Long-term hormonal substitutive therapy with conjugated estrogens in postmenopause

A.R. Genazzani, A. Volpe, A. Maietta Latessa, G. Fabbri, P. Pozzo and A. Grasso

INTRODUCTION

Conjugated estrogens (CE) (Wyeth) are the most widely used drugs for hormonal substitutive therapy in the menopause. The efficacy and safety of the treatment with progestin-associated CE have been documented. However, few studies report long-term effects of this therapy with any entirety. In this chapter we report our experience about this kind of association.

MATERIAL AND METHODS

From 1979 we followed 2132 patients in our Centre, 1270 of them treated with progestin-associated CE. Most of these patients were followed for a short period. Only 72 were followed for a period of 60–84 months (average 58.6). Twenty were in surgical menopause due to ovariectomy, performed in reproductive age. The age of the patients was 39–57 years (average 50.5 years). All the patients had been in the menopause for a period of 1–3 years. We generally used 0.625 mg/die dose of CE for cycles of 21 days and only in those cases in which symptomatology did not completely regress was daily dose of 1.25 mg used. The progestins used in association were medroxin progesterone (MAP), norethisterone (NET) at a 5–10 mg/die dose in the last 12 days of estrogen administration or cyproterone acetate (CA) 12.5 mg/die in the first 10 days. A check-up was performed every 6 months noting subjective symptomatology, side-effects, arterial pressure and with clinical tests on glucidic, lipidic metabolism, blood coagulation, hepatic function. Every year patients underwent a Pap test and an endometrial biopsy, breast checks by palpation, noting subjective symptomatology and eventual mammography. Twelve of these patients underwent a computerized bone mineralometry (CBM) and a dosage of hydroxyprolinuria and calciuria 6 months before and after the treatment.

RESULTS

Efficacy

Vasomotor symptomatology completely regressed in 61 patients (84.7%), and significantly improved in the other 11 patients (15.3%) (Figure 1). CE have been proved effective also on the climacteric symptoms (Figure 2). Only 11 of the patients suffered from vaginal dryness of modest degree. This symptomatology completely regressed with therapy. The efficacy of the treatment in these cases was confirmed by colpocytology, evaluated through maturation volume (Figure 3). CBM was performed in only 12 patients and when checked after 6 months, it did not show significant variation, while a decrease in hydroxyprolinuria, calciuria and phosphaturia was observed.

Side-effects

Bleeding
Forty-three (82.6%) of the patients presented withdrawal bleeding; five (9.6%) had intermenstrual bleeding.

Lipidic metabolism
CE activity on lipidic metabolism appeared different according to associated progestin. A significant increase in apolipoprotein (Apo) A high density lipoprotein cholesterol during the association with NET was observed, while

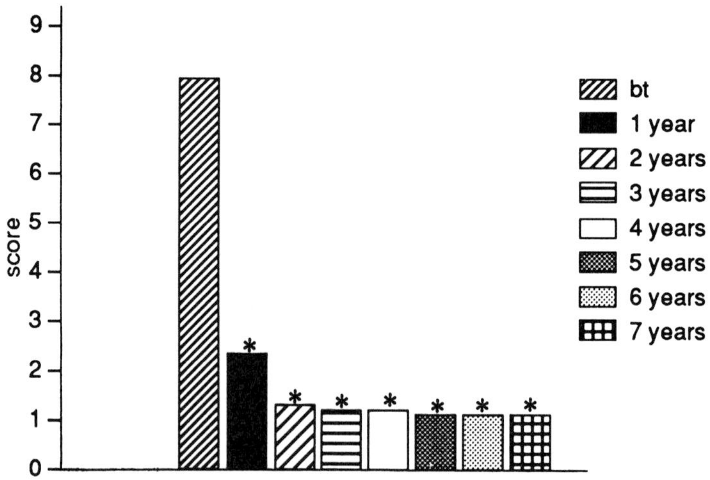

Figure 1 Vasomotor symptomatology before and after hormonal substitutive therapy

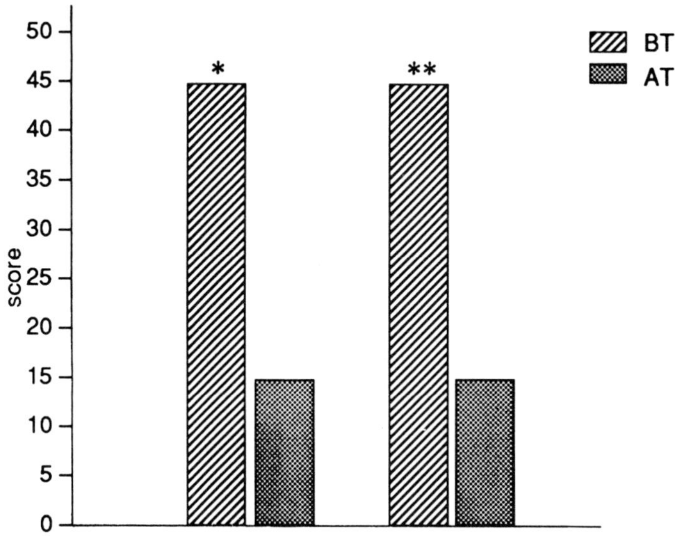

Figure 2 Climacteric symptoms before and after hormonal substitutive therapy: *dizziness, unusual asthenia, back pain and aching muscles; **concentration difficulties, irritability, depression, anxiety and insomnia

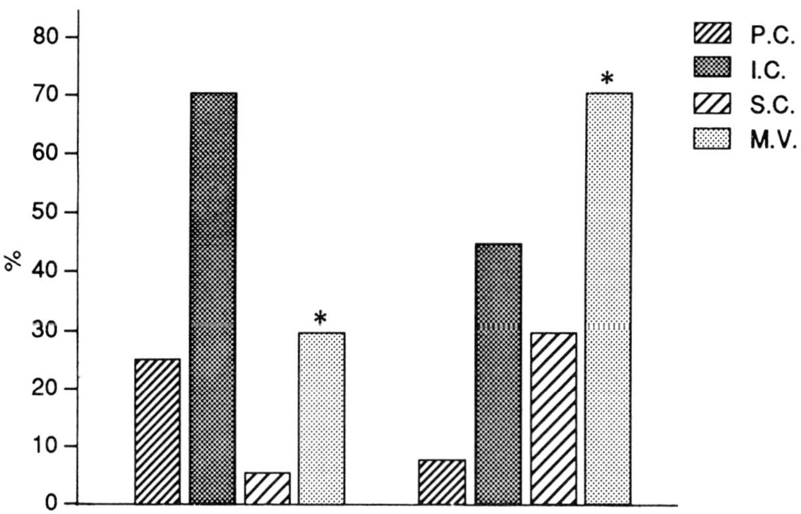

Figure 3 Maturation index and maturation value before and after estro-progestin therapy in postmenopausal women

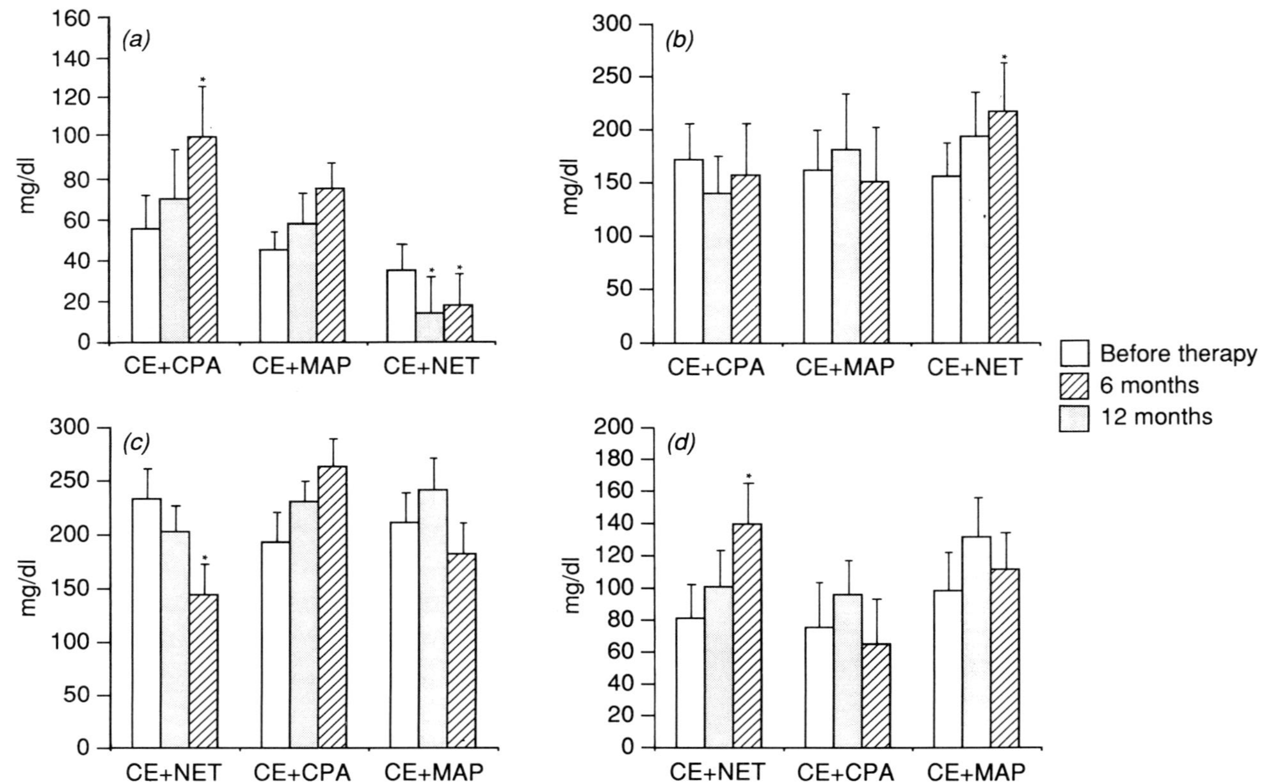

Figure 4 Effects of conjugated equine estrogens and a progestin on lipid metabolism; (*a*) high density lipoprotein, (*b*) low density lipoprotein, (*c*) apolipoprotein A and (*d*) apolipoprotein B

there were no modifications during the association with MAP. Low density lipoprotein and Apo B increased only under CE and NET therapy (Figure 4*a* to *d*).

Coagulation

Fibrinogen, prothrombin time (PT) partial thromboplastin time (PTT), A-fibrinopeptide and antithrombin (AT III) did not significantly change during the therapy (Table 1). Even arterial pressure and parameters of hepatic function did not change during all the years of treatment.

Breast

In 12 out of the 52 patients mastodynia appeared or became worse. In no case was it necessary to stop the treatment. Mammography, performed before and after 3–5 years of treatment in 11 patients showed no changes.

Endometrium

Only in 34 of the 52 patients was comparison of morphology, obtained by biopsy before and after at least 60 months of therapy, possible. Cyclic therapy with CE and progestin did not change endometrial morphology. In some cases this treatment appeared to induce regression of pre-existent hyperplasia.

DISCUSSION

From our data, it appears that CE are effective in the climacteric syndrome and that they are without negative side-effects, if associated with a progestin with weak androgenic activity. According to the results obtained and the analysis of literature we can state that CE, although the first hormones to be used in the treatment of the climacteric syndrome, are today still as effective and safe as the more recently suggested therapies. Hormonal substitutive therapy in the menopause, however, is still used infrequently because of fears of carcinogenic, cardiovascular and thromboembolic risk.

Estroprogestins in postmenopause are actually protective as regards endometrial cancer[1], but they do not seem to modify the risk of breast

Table 1 Changes in coagulation with conjugated estrogen therapy

Clotting system	*Basal values*	*Values after 12 months CE + P therapy*
Fibrinogen (mg/dl)	311.08	358.5
A-fibrinopeptide (mg/dl)	1.5	1.7
(s)	21.2	21.3
PT (%)	97.3	86.0
AT III (mg/dl)	106	100

cancer[2] even though we do not have enough data for a long-term follow-up[3].

As regards cardiovascular and thromboembolic risk, it depends on progestin effects on lipidic metabolism and estrogen effects on the coagulatory system. As our study shows, progestins with weak androgenic activity do not antagonize the positive effect of estrogen on high density lipoprotein[4]. Natural estrogens have a lower activity on the coagulatory systems than synthetic ones.

In conclusion, long-term hormonal substitutive therapy in the postmenopause improves the quality of life[5,6], and reduces the risk of osteoporosis[7], endometrial cancer and systemic cardiac diseases.

REFERENCES

1. Gambrell, R.D. (1977). Estrogens, progestogens and endometrial cancer. *J. Reprod. Med.*, **18**, 31
2. Vessey, M.P. (1987). Cancer of the breast in relation to hormone therapy in the peri-menopause and post-menopause. In Zichella, L., Whitehead, M. and van Keep, P.A. (eds). *The Climacteric and Beyond*, pp. 21–29 (Carnforth: Parthenon Publishiing)
3. Brinton, L.A., Hoover, R. and Fraumeni, J.F. (1986). Menopausal oestrogens and breast cancer risk: an expanded case–control study. *Br. J. Cancer*, **54**, 825
4. Volpe, A., Campanini, D., Golinelli, S., Grasso, A., Baraldi, R. and Genazzani, A.R. (1987). Lipid metabolism and menopause. In Genazzani, A.R., Volpe, A. and Facchinetti, F. (eds). *Gynecological Endocrinology*, p. 655–66. (Carnforth: Parthenon Publishing)
5. Lauritzen, C. (1973). The management of the premenstrual and post-menopausal patient. In van Keep, P.A. and Lauritzen, C. (eds.). *Frontiers of Hormone Research*, vol. 2, *Ageing and Estrogens*, pp. 206–8 (Basel: Karger)
6. Utian, W.H. (1980). *Menopause in Modern Perspective. A Guide to Clinical Practice.* (New York: Appleton-Century-Crofts)
7. Chriastensen, C., Chriastensen, M.S. and Transbol, I. (1981). Bone mass in post-menopausal women after withdrawal of oestrogen-gestagen replacement therapy. *Lancet*, **i**, 459

126

Long-term estrogen–progestogen replacement therapy in healthy postmenopausal women

D. De Aloysio, P. Altieri, A.G. Fabiani, M. Mauloni, L. Miliffi, A. Roncuzzi and F. Bottiglioni

INTRODUCTION

The importance of maintaining complete psychophysical well-being in postmenopausal women has led to an extension in the indications of hormone replacement therapy and its long-term use in order to avoid, not only early climacteric complaints, but also the much more serious postmenopausal degenerative alterations.

In over twenty years of clinical experience answers have been obtained to many of the questions surrounding the replacement estrogen therapy in postmenopause: their efficacy in the treatment of climacteric complaints has been proved to a large extent[1–6], and the evolution undergone by the therapy as regards doses, association with progestogen, type of estrogen and forms of administration, has minimized the risks arising from their use[7–14].

As far as risks are concerned, conjugated equine estrogens have been found to provide the best safety guarantees as they have been used for the longest period of time and have the greatest number of case report histories. However, the question still remains of how long hormone replacement therapy can be prolonged without producing damaging effects.

The aim of this retrospective study is to try to resolve this question by a clinical identikit of the woman who has taken conjugated equine estrogens for more than 5 years.

STUDY GROUP AND METHODS

The study group was composed by 42 women, 23 in natural postmenopause (NPM) and 19 in surgical postmenopause (SPM).

This group was selected from over 1700 outpatients undergoing hormone replacement therapy (HRT) at the Centre for the Physiopathology of the Climacteric and Postmenopause of the University of Bologna from 1976 to 1988.

The selection criteria were as follows:

(1) Replacement therapy with conjugated equine estrogens (CEE) administered for more than 60 months, in different doses (0.625–1.25 mg/day), with the addition of the progestogen (usually medrogestone, 5 mg/day) during the second half of the CEE administration cycle (10th–21st day), in 53% of cycles for the group of women in surgical postmenopause and 76% of cycles for the group in natural postmenopause (ECEP) (see Table 1);
(2) Absence of severe diseases;
(3) Absence of other estrogen replacement therapy previous to ECEP replacement therapy;
(4) Absence of any other drug administration during ECEP replacement therapy.

Table 1 Study group

	No. cases	*Age* (years) $\bar{X} \pm SD$	*Postmenopausal age* (months) $\bar{X} \pm SD$	*Duration of therapy* (months) $\bar{X} \pm SD$	*HRT*
SPM					
K	25	52 ± 4	115 ± 41	—	—
ECEP	19	52 ± 5	115 ± 78	79 ± 35 range: 60–180	[0.625–1.25 mg + P(53%)*]
NPM					
K	25	51 ± 3	95 ± 34	—	—
ECEP	23	50 ± 5	94 ± 34	70 ± 26 range: 60–172	[0.625–1.25 mg + P(76%)*]

* % months of use of progestogen in the second phase of the therapy cycle (10th–21st day)

All personal and medical information collected in the clinical records were studied, including the records of occurrence of complaints supposed to be pertinent to the climacteric syndrome[15] expressed in terms of variations of occurrence in time (attenuation, disappearance, unvariable presence, unvariable absence, accentuation, appearance) and also laboratory screen (hormones, clotting factors, glycolipids, bone metabolism markers, liver and kidney biochemical parameters). All the data were compared to those of two control subgroups (K) comprising women in SPM ($n = 25$) and NPM ($n = 25$), homogeneous according to age and to postmenopausal age. The women in the control subgroups had received no hormone replacement treatment.

The statistical processing of the data used the χ^2 test and analysis of variance.

RESULTS

Laboratory evaluations

Clinical and laboratory monitoring (Tables 2 and 3) showed that the long-term hormone replacement therapy with CEE in association with progestogen does not give rise to damaging effects; on the contrary, it seems to improve

Table 2 Laboratory evaluations showing no statistically significant variations (NPM–SPM) (analysis of variance) in postmenopausal women treated with long-term ECEP replacement therapy

Glycolipid metabolism	Glucose†	Other laboratory evaluations	GOT†
	Triglycerides†		GPT†
	HDL-Cholesterol†		Y-GT†
	Apolipoproteins A†		Alkaline phosphatase†
	Apolipoproteins B†		Uric acid†
	Insuline		Creatinine†
Bone metabolism	Ca†		Creatinine‡
	P†		K‡
	Ca‡		Na‡
	P‡		Quick's time*
	CT*		P.T.T.*
	PTH*		Nitrogen†
	Ca/Cr‡ ratio		
Hormones	HPRL*		
	FSH*		
	LH*		
	TSH*		
	GH*		
	T*		
	ACTH*		
	DHEAS*		
	LH/FSH* ratio		

* Plasma; † serum; ‡ urine

Table 3 Laboratory evaluations (means ± SD) with statistically significant variations in postmenopausal women treated with long-term ECEP replacement therapy

	SPM		*NPM*	
	K	*ECEP*	*K*	*ECEP*
Total cholesterol‡ (mg/100 ml)	NS		234 ± 29*	212 ± 38
Phospholipids‡ (mg/100 ml)	244 ± 45*	286 ± 48	232 ± 20*	254 ± 32
Estradiol† (pg/ml)	7 ± 5*	57 ± 62	12 ± 13*	84 ± 82
Cortisol† (ng/ml)	NS		168 ± 55*	257 ± 88
Triiodothyronine‡ (ng/ml)	1.26 ± 0.15*	1.51 ± 0.31	1.18 ± 0.17**	1.31 ± 0.29
Thyroxine‡ (ng/ml)	83 ± 14*	100 ± 22	81 ± 12*	93 ± 17
K‡ (mEq/l)	NS		4.5 ± 0.3**	4.2 ± 0.3
Na‡ (mEq/l)	141 ± 2**	139 ± 3	141 ± 3**	139 ± 2

* $p < 0.05$; ** $p < 0.01$ (using analysis of variance)
† plasma; ‡serum
NS, not significant

thyroid function (as it induces an increase of mean serum triiodothyronine (T_3) and thyroxine (T_4) levels reduced in premenopause[16]) and it brings about a decrease in the mean serum level of total cholesterol, in spite of the contrasting action of the associated progestogen. Moreover, ECEP therapy induces an increase in the mean serum level of phospholipids and a drop in that of electrolytes Na and K. Finally, with reference only to the NPM subgroup, CEE replacement therapy associated with a progestogen gives rise to an increase in mean cortisol plasma level.

Climacteric syndrome

It is well known that the climacteric syndrome tends to abate as the postmenopausal time proceeds. However, in the women treated with ECEP therapy, this improvement was more evident compared to the control groups (Tables 4 and 5). Moreover, it should also be underlined that the women who underwent ECEP replacement therapy were those suffering from a more accentuated climacteric syndrome.

Table 4 Effects of long-term ECEP replacement therapy on climacteric syndrome (SPM)

		*Effect (%)**			
		Positive (↓↘)	*Negative* (↑↗)	*Nil* (P, A)	*Corrected* χ^2
Arthralgia	K	4.0	8.0	88.0	$p < 0.05$
	ECEP	36.9	10.5	52.6	
Nervousness	K	—	—	—	NS
	ECEP				
Hot flushes	K	36.0	8.0	56.0	$p < 0.01$
	ECEP	63.1	0	36.9	
Sweating	K	32.0	4.0	64.0	$p < 0.01$
	ECEP	63.1	0	36.9	
Paresthesia	K	4.0	0	96.0	$p < 0.01$
	ECEP	36.9	10.5	52.6	
Palpitations	K	0	4.0	96.0	$p < 0.01$
	ECEP	36.8	10.5	52.7	
Fatigue	K	0	4.0	96.0	$p < 0.01$
	ECEP	31.6	21.1	47.3	
Depression	K	0	4.0	96.0	$p < 0.01$
	ECEP	26.3	15.8	57.9	
Headache	K	4.0	0	96.0	$p < 0.01$
	ECEP	26.3	15.8	57.9	
Insomnia	K	—	—	—	NS
	ECEP				
Dizziness	K	4.0	0	96.0	$p < 0.005$
	ECEP	36.8	10.5	52.7	
Chest pains	K	—	—	—	NS
	ECEP				

*(↓) = Disappearance, (↑) = appearance, (P) = unvaried presence, (↘) = reduction, (↗) = increase, and (A) = unvaried absence
NS, not significant

Table 5 Effects of long-term ECEP replacement therapy on climacteric syndrome (NPM)

		*Effect (%)**			
		Positive (↓↘)	*Negative* (↑↗)	*Nil* (P, A)	*Corrected* χ^2
Arthralgia	K	0	8.0	92.0	$p < 0.05$
	ECEP	26.1	26.1	47.8	
Nervousness	K	4.0	4.0	92.0	$p < 0.05$
	ECEP	39.2	13.0	47.8	
Hot flushes	K	32.0	0	68.0	$p < 0.05$
	ECEP	69.6	0	30.4	
Sweating	K	32.0	0	68.0	$p < 0.05$
	ECEP	69.6	0	30.4	
Paresthesia	K	4.0	8.0	88.0	$p < 0.005$
	ECEP	43.6	13.0	43.4	
Palpitations	K	4.0	4.0	92.0	$p < 0.05$
	ECEP	34.8	4.3	60.9	
Fatigue	K	0	4.0	96.0	$p < 0.005$
	ECEP	47.9	8.6	43.5	
Depression	K	4.0	0	96.0	$p < 0.001$
	ECEP	39.2	21.7	39.1	
Headache	K	—	—	—	NS
	ECEP				
Insomnia	K	0	0	100.0	$p < 0.05$
	ECEP	21.8	8.7	69.5	
Dizziness	K	—	—	—	NS
	ECEP				
Chestpains	K	—	—	—	NS
	ECEP				

*(↓) = Disappearance, (↑) = appearance, (P) = unvaried presence, (↘) = reduction, (↗) = increase, (A) = unvaried absence
NS, not significant

Sexual behavior

The benefits of ECEP replacement therapy on the sexual behavior of the postmenopausal women are significant in the SPM subgroup, in which the reduction of sexual activity is most pronounced. This is most evident as regards coital frequency, the parameter least susceptible to the effects of the numerous factors which influence the sexuality of the couple (Table 6).

It seems logical to assume that this benefit is due to both the effects on the climacteric syndrome as well as those on vaginal trophism.

Table 6 Coital frequency (%) in SPM subgroup undergoing longterm ECEP replacement therapy

	*K**	*ECEP**	*Corrected* χ^2
0–1 intercourses per week	36.0	5.3	
2–3 intercourses per week	64.0	89.4	$p < 0.05$
>3 intercourses per week	0	5.3	

* Excluding women who stated an absence of sexual intercourse

Other study parameters

No significant discrepancies emerged between the mean body mass index (BMI) values of the subgroups undergoing ECEP replacement therapy and the control subgroups. The percentage of women subjectively referring weight gain was not significantly different in the subgroups undergoing ECEP replacement therapy compared to the control subgroups.

On the other hand, the mean height (cm) was found to be greater in both subgroups (NPM + SPM) of treated women, compared to both control subgroups (NPM + SPM) (1.57 ± 0.13 compared with 1.55 ± 0.16; $p < 0.05$, using analysis of variance). This appears to suggest an antiosteoporotic effect of ECEP replacement therapy.

The mean values of both systolic and diastolic blood pressure showed no significant differences in the subgroups of treated women compared to the control subgroups.

In the group of women not undergoing therapy (NPM + SPM), there were three cases of vertebral collapse due to postmenopausal osteoporosis (two women in surgical postmenopause and one in natural postmenopause); on the other hand, in the group of treated women (NPM + SPM) there were no cases of fracture.

In the whole group of treated women, gynecological and breast examinations always demonstrated that those women were not affected by any disease. An endometrial biopsy was carried out in 86% of the treated women (NPM + SPM with no hysterectomy): the endometrium was found to be subatrophic in 69% of the cases and in the proliferative phase in 31%. Finally, in the treated women (NPM + SPM), vaginal subatrophy resulted to be considerably less frequent compared to the control subgroups (NPM + SPM) (35% compared with 67%; $p < 0.01$, using χ^2 test).

CONCLUSIONS

The results of this retrospective study allow us to assert that long-term CEE replacement therapy associated with a progestogen leads to an improvement in the quality of life, reduces atrophy of the genital epithelium, prevents bone loss and fractures due to postmenopausal osteoporosis and seems to improve thyroid function. This action takes place without giving rise to damaging metabolic effects, weight gain or increase in endometrial carcinoma risk. Therefore, there is no reason why this hormone replacement therapy should not be prolonged in healthy postmenopausal women, on the condition that clinical and laboratory screen follow-up checks are carefully performed.

REFERENCES

1. Lindsay, R., Aitken, J.M., Anderson, J.B., Hart, D., McDonald, E. and Clarke, A. (1976). Long-term prevention of postmenopausal osteoporosis by oestrogen: evidence for an increased bone mass after delayed onset of oestrogen treatment. *Lancet*, **i**, 1038
2. Hammond, C.B., Jelovsek, F.R., Lee, K.L., Creasman, W.T. and Parker, R.T. (1979). Effects of long-term estrogen replacement therapy. I. Metabolic. *Am. J. Obstet. Gynecol.*, **133**, 525

3. Ettinger, B., Genant, H.K. and Cann, C.R. (1985). Long-term estrogen replacement therapy prevents bone-loss and fractures. *Ann. Int. Med.*, **102**, 319
4. Nachtigall, L.E., Nachtigall, R.H., Nachtigall, R.D. and Beckman, E. (1979). Estrogen replacement therapy. I. A 10-years prospective study in the relationship to osteoporosis. *Obstet. Gynecol.*, **53**, 277
5. Tikkanen, M.J., Nikkita, E.A. and Vartiainen, E. (1978). Natural oestrogen as an effective treatment for type II hyperlipoproteinemia in postmenopausal women. *Lancet*, **ii**, 490.
6. Campbell, S. and Whitehead, M. (1977). Oestrogen therapy and the menopausal syndrome. In Greenblatt, R.B. and Studd, J.W.W. (eds). *Clinics in Obstetrics and Gynaecology*, p. 31. (London, Philadelphia, Toronto: W.B. Saunders)
7. Gambrell, D.R. Jr., Bagnell, C.A. and Greenblatt, R.B. (1983). Role of estrogens and progesterone in the etiology and prevention of endometrial cancer: review. *Am. J. Obstet. Gynecol.*, **146**, 6
8. Hammond, C.B., Jelovsek, F.R., Lee, K.L., Creasman, W.T. and Parker, R.T. (1979). Effects of long-term estrogen replacement therapy. II. Neoplasia. *Am. J. Obstet. Gynecol.*, **133**, 537
9. Nachtigall, L.E., Nachtigall, R.H., Nachtigall, R.B. and Beckman, E.M. (1979). Estrogen replacement. II. A prospective study in the relationship to carcinoma and cardiovascular and metabolic problems. *Obstet. Gynecol.*, **54**, 74
10. Gambrell, D.R., Jr (1982). The menopause: benefits and risks of estrogen replacement therapy. *Fertil. Steril.*, **37**, 4
11. Gambrell, D.R., Jr, Maier, R. and Sanders, B.I. (1983). Decreased incidence of breast cancer in postmenopausal estrogens–progestogen users. *Obstet. Gynecol.*, **62**, 435
12. Kaufman, D.W., Miller, D.R. and Rosenberg, S.D. (1984). Noncontraceptive estrogen use and the risk of breast cancer. *J. Am. Med. Assoc.*, **252**, 63
13. Notelovitz, M., Kitghens, C., Ware, M., Hirschberg, K. and Coone, C. (1983). Combination estrogen and progestogen replacement therapy does not adversely affect coagulation. *Obstet. Gynecol.*, **62**, 5
14. Adams, W.P., Hasegawa, J., Johnson, R. (1979). Conjugated estrogens bioinequivalence: comparison of four products in postmenopausal women. *J. Pharmacol. Sci.*, **68**, 986
15. de Aloysio, D., Bottiglioni, F. and Mauloni, M. (1983). Aspetti sintomatologici del climaterio femminile. In *Atti del LXII Congresso della S.I.G.O.*, p. 21. (Bologna: Monduzzi Editore)
16. de Aloysio, D., Mauloni, M. and Bottiglioni, F. (1988). Transito dal periodo fertile alla premenopausa. In *Atti del III Congresso S.I.M.*, p. 363. (Bologna: Monduzzi Editore)

127

Progestogens, lipid metabolism and cardiovascular disease – a hazardous combination?

G. Samsioe, A. Järnfelt-Samsioe and L.-Å. Mattsson

INTRODUCTION

Several case–control as well as cohort studies have provided evidence of a protective effect by estrogens for cardiovascular disease (CVD) both on morbidity and mortality end points[1–4]. The relative risk (RR) of CVD for estrogen users is in the order of 0.5 and must be regarded as substantial. Considering the overall effects of estrogen-only therapy the RR is 0.8 according to the Leisure world study[4], indicating that benefits outweigh potential hazards. Even if epidemiological evidence is substantial regarding the protective effect on CVD by estrogens little data is available suggesting possible mechanisms.

CVD is multifactorial and several major as well as minor risk factors have been identified as being of importance for a later development of CVD. Estrogen has the potential to influence a number of the risk factors. In an attempt to substantiate this Bush *et al.*[2] applied the Cox proportional hazards model to a number of these factors such as exercise, smoking, alcohol consumption, age and body mass index. None of these significantly altered the protective effect of estrogens. Supported also by other studies these data suggest that the protective effect is virtually the same whether you exercise, smoke or have elevated blood pressure and that the major effect exerted by estrogens would not alter the risk factors mentioned above.

It is also well established that lipids and lipoproteins play a role for the development of arteriosclerosis and later CVD. It has also been repeatedly shown that estrogens influence lipid metabolism as measured by plasma lipid and lipoprotein constituents.

In short, estrogens tend to increase triglycerides and high density lipoproteins (HDL) whereas low density lipoproteins (LDL) are unchanged or reduced. At normal oral doses total cholesterol is virtually unchanged. Although LDL was significantly lower and triglycerides higher in estrogen users neither of these correlated with the adusted death rate by CVD in estrogen users. In contrast HDL was inversely and significantly correlated with CVD mortality in the Bush study but 'only' half of the CVD deaths could be explained this way. In other words at least half of the beneficial effect of estrogens are still unknown. As was recently demonstrated[5], major arteries and the heart itself contain estrogen receptors and a direct effect on the arterial wall would seem intriguing in this respect.

GENERAL ASPECTS OF PROGESTOGENS

A progestogen is defined as any substance that transforms an estrogen stimulated endometrium into secretory phase. This is regardless of the chemical structure of such a compound and thus not necessarily a steroid. In addition the definition does not cover any other qualities such a compound might possess.

In general progestogens counteract the effects induced by estrogens, the so called anti-estrogenic effect mainly by down regulation of estrogen receptors. But non-receptor mediated effects are not affected in the same way. Some effects by estrogens may not be influenced by additional progestogen, others may be augmented even further, such as bone mineral content.

Theoretically progestogenic effects could be subdivided into receptor mediated and non-receptor mediated ones. The receptor mediated effects are usually discussed in terms of anti-estrogenic, androgenic or even progestogenic ones. However effects on lipid metabolism by interaction via the progestogen receptor have been difficult to demonstrate so far. As far as lipids are concerned progestogens tend to reduce the effects induced by estrogens. In other words the addition of a progestogen to an estrogen primed woman woul result in reduced levels of HDL and triglycerides with unchanged or elevation of LDL. A slight increase in total cholesterol is sometimes encountered[6].

The magnitude of these changes of course is dependent on the dose, the time and the choice of progestational agent. As the progestogenic influence on estrogen primed subjects on lipids is regarded unfavourably with respect to CVD the trend to minimize use of progestogens is easily understandable.

This could be achieved by reducing the number of days during which the woman is to take her progestogen. But during the perimenopausal period bleeding problems are likely to occur if progestogens are not given at least bimonthly and for a sufficient number of subsequent days. However, in the postmenopausal period when endogenous fluctuations of estrogen production are scarce the interval between progestogen supplementation could be prolonged. During prolonged usage hepatic clearance of estrogens is often increased leading to altered pharmacokinetics and pharmacodynamics of estrogen with time. This type of hepatic enzyme activation does not influence the metabolism of synthetic progestogens to any major extent and consequently also the oral dose of the progestogen supplementation may be reduced. In other words during the perimenopausal period 2 mg of estradiol may require 1 mg of norethisterone (NET) for 12 days each month but in the postmenopausal period 0.5 mg NET every third month may well be sufficient to control bleeding and endometrial hyperstimulation. A reduction from 150 mg to 25 mg per year is then achieved. It should be remembered that the minipill which corresponds to some 100 mg of NET per annum is not associated with an increased risk of CVD.

Exogenously administered androgens have lipid metabolic effects contrary to estrogens. A reduction in HDL and triglycerides is often accompanied by increased LDL levels during androgen therapy. Indeed, some of the progestogens display androgenic activity and one aim would be to avoid compounds with androgenic qualities. The choice of progestogen is therefore of importance.

CHOICE OF PROGESTOGEN

In 1979 we published some data[7] indicating that progestogens with higher androgenic activity (NET and levonorgestrel) displayed more marked and less desirable effects when given orally in comparison with oral administration of medroxyprogesterone acetate (MPA). It was inferred that the 'negative' lipid metabolic pattern induced by levonorgestrel (LNG) and NET was attributable to androgenicity, the two being derivatives of 19-nortestosterone in contrast to MPA which is derived from 17-alpha-hydroxyprogesterone. Several reports soon followed emphasizing these differences between 17-alphahydroxyprogesterones and 19-nortestosterones. However, almost all reports were based on studies with these three progestogens only.

When desogestrel was introduced it was shown that it was possible to almost abolish androgen activity. In addition this new progestogen also proved itself to have a higher sensitivity and selectivity for the progestogen receptor. Indeed the lipid metabolic pattern induced by the addition of desogestrel showed a much more favorable pattern than did LNG[8]. Another newcomer, gestodene, displayed similar qualities. Despite the fact that desogestrel and gestodene are 19-nortestosterones they have a similar and much more favorable impact on lipid metabolism than NET and LNG.

A closer look at MPA also revealed that non-oral administration and higher doses also induced a decrease in HDL and a slight increase in LDL. Serum triglycerides may further increase with high doses of MPA as some glucocorticoid activity of MPA may be revealed.

During the last decade the oral bioavailability of MPA has been greatly improved and studies with newer formulations of MPA display a similar anti-estrogenic pattern as do other progestogens.

When comparing two clinically relevant doses of another 17-alpha-hydroxyprogesterone derivative, megestrol acetate (MegAc) we were unable to detect any specific quality of MegAc in comparison with two doses of NET. Some of the lipid parameters seemed to be dependent on the dose but no specific pattern emerged[9].

Quite clearly marked differences exist between various progestogens as regards lipid metabolism and the choice of a less deteriorating compound is of importance. But the overall picture is more complex than just a choice between 19-nortestosterone derivatives and 17-alphahydroxyprogestogens.

Minimizing the total progestogen influence and choosing a compound that does not counteract the estrogenic influence are two obvious ways of maintaining the lipid profile as favorably as possible when adding a progestogen in hormonal replacement therapy. It should be remembered however, that a steady state in lipid metabolism is not achieved until some 6–8 months after institution of the hormones. Prior to this, lipid variables fluctuate depending on the prevailing hormonal situation. As estrogens induce formation of progestogen receptors it is evident that the progestogenic influence is at its height during the first few days of progestogen influence. As half-lives of lipoproteins are measured in days the maximal progestational effect is seen about a week after beginning the progestogen period[10]. Short-term studies with sampling 3–10 days into the progestogen period of HRT will ultimately show too high a progestogenic influence and the negative impact might be overemphasized. When giving estrogen–progestogen combinations on a continuous basis a steady state is achieved faster (3–5 months) and receptor amounts are more steady.

It has been a constant finding by us[9,10,11] and others[11,12] that these type of preparations induce reductions in HDL as well as in LDL and triglycerides. No data are available to interpret such a pattern in terms of CVD risk.

As two risk factors are reduced one cannot deduce that these types of regimens would have a negative impact on CVD risk. On the other hand there is no data to support the contrary. Despite the large bulk of data addressing the issues of sex steroids and lipid metabolism some controversies still exist. Some of these are due to variations in methodology. The methods for cholesterol determinations are precise and accurate and have been so for a considerable time. Old and newer data on cholesterol therefore compare well. Methods for triglyceride determinations have improved immensely during the last 10 years or so and the coefficient of variation (CV) has dropped from 20 to 3–5%.

In practical terms this means that the standard deviation of triglyceride determination has dropped substantially being one of the explanations why triglycerides in newer data more often come out at statistically significant levels.

Determinations of lipoproteins is more difficult. A separation can be made by use of ultracentrifugation but this method is laborious, expensive and cannot be used in large population studies, at least not when two or more spins are required.

To avoid ultracentrifugation a precipitation can be made which separates HDL from very low density lipids (VLDL) and LDL. Usually heparin and manganese chloride are being used. By plotting data Friewald *et al.* suggested that VLDL cholesterol could be estimated by using 20% of serum triglycerides. (The constant is 0.45 when values are expressed in mmol/l). Friewald's formula has been extensively used and further developed by DeLong *et al*[12].

The formulation requires that the composition of lipoproteins remain constant, in other words all changes are considered to be changes in the number of particles and not in their composition. Unfortunately alterations occur in both composition and number which limit the use of estimated

LDL. But the formulation often represents the only way to get information on LDL and the precautions using the formulation are sometimes underestimated. The co-existence of several methods and their implications widely contribute to the problems of interpretation of data on sex steroids and lipid metabolism.

To avoid CVD as a result of advancing arteriosclerosis long-term hormone replacement therapy with combinations resulting in an atherogenic lipoprotein pattern should be avoided. After the perimenopausal period progestogens need not be administered more than 3–4 times a year and the dose could often be reduced. There are no data to support the theory that the continuous progestogen–estrogen combination would be hazardous as far as lipids and lipoproteins are concerned. Existing controversies with respect to sex steroids and lipid metabolism can often be ascribed to the designs and methods used.

REFERENCES

1. Stampfer, M.J., Willett, W.C., Colditz, G.A. and Rosner, B. *et al.* (1985). A prospective study of postmenopausal estrogen therapy and coronary heart disease. *N. Engl. J. Med.*, **313**, 1044–9
2. Bush, T.L., Barrett-Connor, E., Cowna, L.D. *et al.* (1987). Cardiovascular mortality and non-contraceptive use of estrogen in women: results from the Lipid Research Clinics Program Follow-up Study. *Circulation*, **75**, 1102–9
3. Paganini-Hill, A., Ross, R.K. and Henderson, B.E. (1988). Postmenopausal oestrogen treatment and stroke: a prospective study. *Br. Med. J.*, **297**, 519–22
4. Henderson, B.E., Paganini-Hill, A. and Ross, R.K. (1988). Estrogen replacement therapy and protection from acute myocardial infarction. *Am. J. Obstet. Gynecol.*, **159**, 312–17
5. Hough, J.L. and Zilversmit, D.B. (1986). Effect of 17 beta estradiol on aortic cholesterol content and metabolism in cholesterol-fed rabbits. *Arterioclerosis*, **6**, 57
6. Crona, N., Enk, L., Mattsson, L.A., Samsioe, G. and Silfverstolpe, G. (1986). Progestogens and lipid metabolism. *Maturitas*, **8**, 141–58
7. Silfverstolpe, G., Gustafson, A., Samsioe, G. and Svanborg, A. (1979). Lipid metabolic studies in oophorectomized women. Effects of three different progestogens. *Acta Obstet. Gynecol. Scand.*, Suppl. **88**, 89–95
8. Crona, N., Silfverstolpe, G. and Samsioe, G. (1985). The effects of two gonadal progestins alone and in combination with ethinylestradiol on serum lipoproteins. *Eur. J. Obstet. Gynecol.*, **19**, 365–74
9. Sporrong, T., Mattson, L.A., Hellgren, M. and Samsioe, G. (1989). Lipid metabolic effects of four progestationally different regimens for climacteric complaints. *Obstet. Gynecol*, **73**, 754–8
10. Mattson, L.A., Silfverstolpe, G. and Samsioe, G. (1984). Lipid composition of serum lipoproteins in relation to gonadal hormones during the normal menstrual cycle. *Eur. J. Obstet. Gynecol.*, **17**, 327–35
11. Mattsson, L.A. and Samsioe, G. (1985). Clinical and metabolic effects of a combined oestrogen/progestogen preparation for climacteric complaints. *Acta Obstet. Gynecol. Scand.*, Suppl. **130**, 58–9
12. Munk-Jensen, N., Pors-Nielsen, S. and Obel, F.R. Personal communication
13. De Long, D.M., De Long, E.R., Wood, P.D. *et al.* (1986). A comparison of methods for the estimation of plasma low- and very low-density lipoprotein cholesterol. *J. Am. Med. Assoc.*, **256**, 2372–7

128

Transdermal 17β-estradiol

R. Sitruk-Ware

INTRODUCTION

The main goal of pharmaceutical research has been to achieve therapeutic improvement by discovering new galenic formulations able to provide sustained, efficient plasma levels of drugs. If we consider conventional galenic preparations (whether administered orally or intravenously), the curve of the plasma levels will first show a peak concentration and then a decrease towards initial pretreatment levels. Plasma concentrations therefore range from the potentially toxic to the ineffective, with considerable interindividual and intraindividual variations. Repeated administration throughout the day could maintain high, efficient plasma values but this is impractical and nocturnal intake is not possible.

Controlled sustained release from long-acting delivery systems would solve the problems of both constancy of plasma levels and acceptability.

Hormonal replacement therapy (HRT) has been recognized to bring benefits to postmenopausal women not only for symptom relief but also and overall, for prevention of osteoporosis and cardiovascular diseases. However, several drawbacks have been ascribed to HRT among which metabolic disturbances and cancer risk were highlighted. The prevention of endometrial carcinoma has been thoroughly investigated and a consensus now exists on the necessity to add to estrogens adequate amounts of progestins for a sufficient period each month in order to avoid endometrial hyperplasia and hence decrease cancer risk[1].

Controversies still exist about the significance of metabolic changes induced by HRT. However in order to avoid any deleterious effect of steroids, alternative galenic formulations have been sought to avoid the so-called first-pass liver effect of oral delivery of HRT.

The alternative delivery systems developed so far include implants, vaginal rings and creams, percutaneous creams and transdermal systems.

PRINCIPLES OF DELIVERING ESTRADIOL THROUGH THE SKIN

Until the turn of this century, scientists generally regarded the skin as totally impermeable to all substances. By the beginning of this century, the skin permeability to lipid-soluble substances and the relative impermeability to water and electrolytes were recognized. Since then the ability of the skin to absorb steroids has been extensively studied[2-4].

While for many decades the skin has been commonly used for topical administration of dermatological drugs to achieve local action, now systemically active drugs and particularly steroids can be applied topically on the skin and distributed into the systemic circulation.

The skin itself can play the role of a rate-controlling membrane and the stratum corneum acts as both a reservoir and a diffusion barrier to drugs. The rate of absorption depends upon the dose that is topically applied and also the surface where the drug is applied[5].

The use of appropriate vehicles represents the key factor to allow the penetration of small molecules unbound to skin proteins through the stratum corneum. The phenomenon of percutaneous or transdermal absorption embraces more than diffusion through the stratum corneum. Different processes occur in sequence. First, the molecules are absorbed within the stratum corneum; then, retention occurs in the stratum corneum (reservoir effect) and third, the molecules diffuse through the epidermis and papillary dermis until they reach the capillary plexus and are transferred to the circulating blood. Each step of these different events is esssential and individual variations at any stage can influence the rate of absorption[2]. Obviously, the thickness of the stratum corneum, and the variations in the degree of hydration of this layer, by occlusion, will affect the permeability of this layer.

In order to achieve a constant sustained release over a long period of time and on a small surface area, several technologies have been developed to provide a control over the rate of release and of the permeation of drugs through the skin. These are called transdermal drug delivery systems (TDDS). For these TDDS, the systemic transdermal delivery rates of the drugs may be the function of the reservoir system itself, the reservoir–skin interface, the drug concentration in the aqueous phase within the skin and the capillary wash-out rate within the skin.

TECHNICAL APPROACH FOR TRANSDERMAL DELIVERY OF ESTRADIOL

An ideal reservoir should hold the drug in a stable condition and have little or no affinity for the drug. It should maintain its structural integrity at high humidity and high body temperature, be self-adhering with a good contact with the skin and non-irritating to the skin. Moreover it should be simple and inexpensive to manufacture.

Transdermal delivery of drugs depends upon the optimization of the reservoir and the barrier membrane that regulates the drug release. Among the polymers that could be used without reacting chemically with the drug, ethylene vinyl acetate (EVA) co-polymer has been used for delivery of estradiol (E_2)[6]. Also, the characteristics of the drug and the use of appropriate enhancers for transcutaneous absorption play an important role in TDDS.

Steroids of low polarity can easily permeate the skin, while addition of further polar groups to the same steroid nucleus considerably lowers the permeability constant[4]. Estradiol answers the requirement for absorption through the skin and the use of ethanol in the system has been used to facilitate the permeation of the drug[6]. Rate-controlled systems for administering 17β-E_2 through intact skin have been designed to be applied twice weekly[7]. They are programmed to release, *in vivo*, 0.025, 0.05 or 0.1 mg E_2 per day, according to patients' needs. Transdermal Therapeutic Systems (TTS) have surface areas of 5, 10 and 20 cm^2 and they contain 2, 4 and 8 mg of E_2, respectively and, 100, 200 and 400 mg of ethanol, respectively. Pharmacokinetic studies in postmenopausal women have shown that following application of the system, therapeutic E_2 levels in serum were achieved in less than 4 h and persisted during the entire wearing of the system. Plasma E_2 rose from a pretreatment level of about 7 pg/ml to approximately 25, 40 or 75 pg/ml respectively, during the use of these systems. The E_2/estrone (E_1) ratio was elevated and maintained close to 1 in the premenopausal range. Within 24 h after removal of the systems, serum concentrations of E_2 and E_1 returned to the pretreatment levels[7,8].

According to further published studies[9–11] the plasma levels of E_2 obtained with these systems approximate 50 to 80 pg/ml with the 10 cm^2 system (ETTS 50) and 80 to 100 pg/ml with the 20 cm^2 system (ETTS 100). Interindividual variations are observed, but very few intraindividual variations occur.

CLINICAL EFFECTS OF TRANSDERMAL E_2

In a placebo-controlled 3-week study, menopausal women experiencing frequent hot flushes (measured by digital thermography) used twice-weekly transdermal systems delivering 0.05 mg of 0.10 mg E_2 per day. Hot flushes decreased from 0.79/h and 0.76/h to 0.35/h and 0.25/h, respectively. E_2/E_1 ratios in both groups increased to those typical of the premenopausal range[12].

Transdermally administered E_2 exerted positive effects on vaginal cytology; the percentage of superficial cells was significantly increased. Follicle-stimulating hormone and luteinizing hormone levels decreased significantly. Blood pressure was not affected during this 3-week period[8,12]. No significant increases in the concentrations of renin substrate or other hepatic proteins (sex hormone-binding globulin, thyroxine-binding globulin, and corticosteroid-binding gobulin) occurred. Thus, transdermal E_2 does not affect the changes in the hepatic function known to occur with oral administration of conjugated and synthetic estrogens.

Transdermal systems have been proved to be as effective as oral conjugated estrogens on menopausal symptoms, without any induction of liver protein production and particularly no modifications of renin substrate or clotting factors[13]. The area of application of transdermal systems should be changed regularly and not always be restricted to the same place. One reason for this is obvious since the occlusive membrane can lead to itching and transient skin irritation. Studies performed to determine the skin tolerability of E_2 transdermal systems compared with BAND-AID at various sites of application have shown that the irritation scores with the two plasters were similar. Moreover this study showed that systems applied on the buttocks, with regular rotation of the application site, gave a very low score of skin irritation, of about 0.9%[14]. It was mostly mild erythema and was always transient. Whether the site of application influences the plasma levels obtained, has been tested and the absorption from various skin areas, like the abdomen, the thighs, the back and the buttocks was shown to be comparable[15].

RESPONSE OF TARGET ORGANS TO E_2 ADMINISTERED TRANSDERMALLY

The endometrium

In women treated with unopposed estrogens, either oral or transdermal, endometrial biopsies performed before and after 18 weeks of therapy showed hyperplasia in five cases out of 238, three cases with transdermal E_2 and two cases with oral conjugated estrogens[16]. More recently Clisham *et al.*[17], studied the endometrial histology of 27 women treated for 1 year either with ESTRADERM 100 only (14 women) or with ESTRADERM 100 and medroxyprogesterone acetate (MPA) 10 mg per day for 12 days per month (13 women). In the group of 14 women treated with unopposed estrogen therapy, eight developed cystic or adenomatous hyperplasia of the endometrium (CAH) but only one of the 13 women who received combined estrogen + progestin therapy exhibited CAH. All abnormalities were reversed to normal after addition of MPA to estrogens for the following 3 months. The authors also noted that the bleeding patterns were not predictive of CAH.

In two other studies[18,19] where respectively nine and eight women received the 50 μg dose of transdermal E_2 for 13 weeks[18] or 6 weeks[19], the predominant aspect of the endometrium was proliferative.

These findings indicate the rapid efficacy of the drug and the absolute need to add sequential progestogen therapy in women with an intact uterus. Among the recommended regimens of therapy, continuous estrogen therapy has been proposed to avoid recurrence of symptoms during a treatment-free interval and the addition of 12 days of progestins has been shown to give a full secretory transformation of the endometrium without hyperplasia[20].

The bone

One of the main beneficial effects expected of HRT is maintenance of bone mass and prevention of osteoporosis. The efficacy of 17β-E_2 delivered through the skin has been demonstrated recently. Ribot *et al.*[21] and Adami *et al.*[22] showed that transdermal E_2 had a preventive effect on bone-loss. Ribot *et al.*[21] studied 29 women for 24 months. Fourteen of them received ESTRADERM 50 and a sequential regimen of progestins and 15 received no treatment. The authors found after 2 years an increase in bone mineral density of 5.9% while the untreated group had a decrease of 1.9% per year. Adami *et al.*[22] followed 39 women for 18 months. Seventeen received ESTRADERM 50 and the 17 others received no treatment. The bone mineral density was increased 5.6 ± 7.7% in the treated group while the untreated group had a decrease of 3.5% ± 4.6%. Further long-term studies with a larger number of women are needed to confirm these preliminary results.

The liver

As stated above, transdermal delivery of E_2 has the main advantage over oral therapy of by-passing the liver, and these systems have been proved to exert no effect on liver proteins, particularly no increase in renin substrate, no change in clotting factors and no modification of lipoprotein profiles[13]. In the study by Chetkowski *et al.*[13] no change in clotting factors was observed either in women who received conjugated equine estrogens or in women using a TDDS of E_2. However, Elkik *et al.*[23] previously showed a significant difference in antithrombin III activity in women receiving either equine estrogens or percutaneous E_2.

The lipid profiles are not modified by parenteral 17β-E_2 to the same extent as after oral E_2 therapy. In a recent randomized trial comparing the effect of non-oral E_2 delivered either by implants or by transdermal systems, Stanczyk *et al.*[11] showed that a significant increase in high density lipoprotein (HDL)-cholesterol and a decrease in total cholesterol/HDL-cholesterol were obvious after 12 weeks of implant therapy and only after 24 weeks of transdermal therapy with ESTRADERM 100. While oral estrogens affect the lipid profiles within the first weeks of administration, indicating their liver impact, the effects of non-oral estrogens on the lipoproteins are delayed and indicate also a beneficial long-term effect on the HDL subfraction of the lipoproteins.

It has been claimed that the increase in HDL_2 fraction observed after oral estrogen therapy was beneficial and could lead to a protective effect against cardiovascular disease[24,25].

It has also been claimed that, a decrease in low density lipoprotein (LDL) would have more relevance to a protective effect than an increase in HDL[26]. In that respect, it was also shown recently in a limited number of patients that hypercholesterolemic postmenopausal women receiving transdermal E_2 at a dose of 200 μg/day had a significant decrease in total cholesterol and in LDL[27]. Further studies would be necessary to confirm these encouraging findings.

Transdermal medication offers many advantages over conventional delivery, namely it bypasses hepatic 'first pass' and avoids gastrointestinal incompatibility, reduces side-effects by optimizing the blood concentration time profile and increases compliance by eliminating the need for multiple-dose schedules.

The therapeutic efficacy is enhanced by constant delivery of effective dosage. This type of medication also minimizes between-patient and within-patient variations due to variable hepatic and renal metabolism, minimizes interaction with other drugs and is easily administered and reversible. The occlusive membrane greatly increases diffusion through the stratum corneum, thus achieving therapeutic efficacy with very low doses of E_2. Also a convenient twice-weekly regimen instead of daily bolus dosing appeared to be highly acceptable by the patients and enhanced compliance to HRT which is a prerequisite for an effective long-term preventive therapy.

REFERENCES

1. Whitehead, M. and Lobo, R. (1988). Progestagen use in postmenopausal women. *The Lancet*, **ii**, 1243–4
2. Scheuplein, R.J., Blank, I.H., Brauner, G.J. and MacFarlane, D.J. (1969). Percutaneous absorption of steroids. *J. Invest. Dermatol.*, **52**, 63–70
3. Vickers, C.F.H. (1980). Reservoir effect of human skin: pharmacological speculation. In Mauvais-Jarvis, P., Vickers, C.F.H. and Wepierre, J. (eds). *Percutaneous Absorption of Steroids*, pp. 19–29. (London: Academic Press)
4. Scheuplein, R.J. (1980). Percutaneous absorption: Theoretical aspects. In Mauvais-Jarvis, P., Vickers, C.F.H. and Wepierre, J. (eds). *Percutaneous Absorption of Steroids* pp. 1–17. (London: Academic Press)
5. Marty, J.P., James, M., Hajo, N. and Wepierre, J. (1980). Percutaneous absorption of oestradiol and progesterone: Pharmacokinetic studies. In Mauvais-Jarvis, P., Vickers, C.F.H. and Wepierre, J. (eds). *Percutaneous Absorption of Steroids*, pp. 205–18. (London: Academic Press)
6. Chien, Y.W. (1987). Development of transdermal controlled release drug delivery systems: an overview. In Kydonieus, A.F. and Berner, B. (eds). *Transdermal Delivery of Drugs*, Vol. **I**, pp. 81–100. (Boca Raton Florida: CRC Press)
7. Powers, M.S., Schenkel, L., Darley, P.E., Good, W.R., Balestra, J.C. and Place, V.A. (1985). Pharmacokinetics and pharmacodynamics of transdermal dosage forms of 17β-estradiol: Comparison with conventional oral estrogen used for hormone replacement. *Am. J. Obstet. Gynecol.*, **152**, 1099–106
8. Laufer, L.R., Defazio, J.L., Lu, J.K.H., Meldrum, D.R., Eggena, M.P., Sambhi, M.S., Hershman, J.M. and Judd, H.L. (1983). Estrogen replacement therapy by transdermal estradiol administration. *Am. J. Obstet. Gynecol.*, **146**, 533–40
9. Simon, J.A., Leal, J.A. and Hodgen, G.D. (1987). Skin and serum pharmacokinetics of percutaneous estradiol absorption in postmenopausal women and nonhuman primates. In Christiansen, C., Johansen, J.S. and Riis, B.J. (eds). *Osteoporosis*, **Vol. II**, pp. 1101–12. (Denmark: Osteopress Aps.)
10. Jasonni, V.M., Bulletti, C., Naldi, S., Ciotti, P., Di Cosmo, D., Lazzaretto, R. and Flamigni, C. (1988). Biological and endocrine aspects of transdermal 17-β oestradiol administration in postmenopausal women. *Maturitas*, **10**, 263–70
11. Stanczyk, F.Z., Shoupe, D., Nunez, V., Macias-Gonzales, P., Vijod, M.A., Lobo, R.A. (1988). A randomized comparison of nonoral estradiol delivery in postmenopausal women. *Am. J. Obstet. Gynecol.*, **159**, 1540–6
12. Steingold, K.A., Laufer, L., Chetkowski, R.J., Defazio, J.D., Matt, D.W., Meldrum, D.R. and Judd, H.L. (1985). Treatment of hot flushes with transdermal estradiol administration. *J. Clin. Endocrinol. Metab.*,**61**, 627–32
13. Chetkowski, R.J., Meldrum, D.R., Steingold, K.A., Randle, D., Lu, J.K. Eggena, P., Hershman, J.M., Alkjaersig, N.K., Fletcher, A.P. and Judd, H.L. (1986). Biologic effects of transdermal estradiol. *N. Engl. J. Med.*, **314**, 1615–20
14. Davis, G.F. and Winter, L. (1987). Cumulative irritation study of placebo transdermal estrogen patches. *Curr. Ther. Res.*, **42**, 712–19
15. Schenkel, L., Barlier, D. and Riera, M. (1986). Transdermal absorption of estradiol from different body sites is comparable. *J. Contr. Rel.*, **4**, 195–201
16. Utian, W.H. (1987). Transdermal estradiol overall safety profile. *Am. J. Obstet. Gynecol.*, **156**, 1335–8

17. Clisham, P., Judd, H., Fu, Y., Lozano, K. and Cedars, M. (1988). Bleeding Patterns and Endometrial Histology (EH) With Long-Term Transdermal Estradiol Therapy (TE). *Fertil. Steril.*, **50** (Suppl.) S24–5, Abstract 070
18. Whitehead, M.I., Padwick, M.L., Endacott, J. and Pryse-Davies, J. (1985). Endometrial responses to transdermal estradiol in postmenopausal women. *Am. J. Obstet. Gynecol.*, **152** 1079–84
19. Johannisson, E., Landgren, B.-M. and Diczfalusy, E. (1988). Endometrial and vaginal response to three different oestrogen preparations administered by the transdermal and oral routes. *Maturitas*, **10**, 181–92
20. Whitehead, M.I., Siddle, N., Lane, G., Padwick, M., Ryder, T.A., Pryse-Davies, J. and King, R.J.B. (1987). The pharmacology of progestogens. In Mishell, D.R., Jr (ed.) *The Menopause* pp. 317–34. (Chicago: Year Book Med. Publ.)
21. Ribot, C., Tremollieres, F., Pouilles, J.M., Louvet, J.P. and Peyron, R. (1987). Transdermal administration of 17β-estradiol in postmenopausal women: Preliminary results of a longitudinal study. In Christiansen, C., Johansen, J.S.L. and Riis, B.J. (eds). *Osteoporosis* 1987, pp. 546–8. (Denmark: Osteopress Aps)
22. Adami, S., Suppi, R., Rossini, M., Maresca, V., Bertoldo, F. and Lo Cascio, V. (1988). Transdermal estradiol in the treatment of postmenopausal bone loss. *XII World Congress of Gynecology and Obstetrics, Rio de Janeiro, Brazil*, Abstracts Book, p. 522
23. Elkik, F., Gompel, A., Mercier-Bodard, C., Kuttenn, F., Guyenne, T.T., Corvol, P. and Mauvais-Jarvis, P. (1982). Effects of percutaneous estradiol and conjugated estrogens on the level of plasma proteins and triglycerides in post-menopausal women. *Am. J. Obstet. Gynecol.*, **143**, 888–92
24. Bush, T.L., Barrett-Connor, E., Cowan, L.D., Criqui, M.H., Wallace, R.B., Suchindran, C.M., Tyroler, H.A. and Rifkind, B.M. (1987). Cardiovascular mortality and noncontraceptive use of estrogen in women: results from the Lipid Research Clinics Program follow-up study. *Circulation*, **75**, 1102–9
25. Fahraeus, L., Larsson-Cohn, U. and Wallentin, L. (1982). Lipoproteins during oral and cutaneous administration of oestradiol-17-beta to menopausal women. *Acta Endocrinol.*, **101**, 597–602
26. Steinberg, D. (1987). Lipoproteins and the pathogenesis of atherosclerosis. *Circulation*, **76**, 508–14
27. Cholst, I.N., Ginsberg, H.N., Bush, T. and Goldberg, I.J. (1988). Lipoprotein and apoprotein levels during treatment of post-menopausal women with transdermal estrogen replacement. *XIIth Congres of Gynecology and Obstetrics, Rio de Janeiro, Brazil.* Abstracts Book, p. 206

Section 4 continued

Part M

Hormonal transvaginal therapy in climacteric women

129

Effect of estrogens on central nervous system

C. Nappi, G. Colace, C. Di Carlo, A. Fatatis, M. Taglialatela and L. Annunziato

INTRODUCTION

It is well known that in mammals steroid hormones of gonadal and adrenal origin influence cerebral functions, sexual differentiation, behavior and neuroendocrine activity. Particularly, it has been demonstrated that these hormones promote neuronal growth in the different stages of development and regulate synaptic function and neurotransmission[1].

Steroid hormones can cross the blood–brain barrier and penetrate into the central nervous system (CNS) acting on different groups of neurons which express receptorial binding sites for different classes of steroids, as demonstrated by autoradiographical and biochemical studies[2].

CNS STEROID RECEPTORS

In particular, neurons sensitive to estrogens are located in the preoptic area, hypothalamus and amygdala and are surrounded by groups of neurons devoid of receptors.

Surprisingly, in the spinal chord of the rat, particularly in those areas which are involved in the estrogen-induced lordosis behavior, it is possible to find neurons which express estrogen receptors. These cells are in small number if compared with those present in the CNS. However, the lack of autoradiographical evidence of steroid receptors in an area of the CNS does not necessarily mean the absence of steroid receptors at that level. Indeed, biochemical methods can demonstrate the presence of steroid receptors which are not visualized by autoradiography[2].

Some estrogen and androgen receptors are present in the fetal rodent hypothalamus during the last trimester of gestation, about the time of final neuronal cell division. However, estrogen receptor levels in the male and female rat brain increase markedly beginning shortly before birth, whereas androgen receptor levels increase markedly around 1 week after birth[2].

Physicochemical and immunological properties of steroid receptors in the brain do not differ from those in peripheral tissues. Neurons which react to steroid hormones are part of complex neuronal circuits connecting sensorial stimuli with response effectors. A typical example of this connection is given by the anatomical basis of the lordosis behavior of the female rat. Sensorial stimuli and circulating estradiol (E_2) influence the neuroendocrine effector (hypothalamus). The hypothalamus releases gonadotropin-releasing hormone (GnRH) in the hypophyseal portal blood. GnRH stimulates luteinizing hormone (LH) production and secretion at the hypophyseal level. Circulating LH stimulates E_2 secretion at the ovarian level and induces ovulation. In turn, E_2 reaches brain and hypophysis and, acting on its specific cellular receptors, modulates neuronal circuits which control GnRH secretion and lordosis behavior[3].

MECHANISM OF ESTROGEN ACTION

Estrogens seem to act on neuronal cells both through effects at genomic level, mediated by intracellular receptors[1] and also through direct actions on the neuronal membrane (non-genomic effects). Both direct (non-genomic) and indirect (genomic) effects of steroid hormones may occur at pre- or postsynaptic level.

Moreover, the effects of steroid hormones can be divided into primary and secondary. Primary effects are those caused by the direct interaction of the steroid hormone with specific neuronal cells. Secondary effects, on the other hand are mediated through the action of other hormones. For example numerous E_2 effects on the turnover of central neurotransmitters are mediated by prolactin (PRL), which is synthesized in response to E_2 stimulation.

Genomic effects

Genomic effects present an indirect mechanism of action. In other words, genomic effects take place at intranuclear level modifying the synthesis of proteins which are then carried (along axon and dendrite) to the synapses interacting with pre- and postsynaptic events.

Genomic activation in steroid target regions of the brain can be demonstrated in different ways. For example, E_2 administration induces a transient activation of RNA polymerase II activity in hypothalamic neurons and actinomycin D, and a well known RNA synthesis inhibitor is able to block estrogen action on female sexual behavior and on preovulatory LH release. Furthermore, very recent studies on the estrogen receptors have shown that they comprise a highly conserved DNA binding domain and an independent, less well conserved domain responsible for hormone binding and transcription activation[4].

Genomic effects are typically of long latency (hours or days) and of prolonged duration. They are responsible for the main estrogen effects on neuronal differentiation and organization processes (which mainly take place during fetal or neonatal life) and on some complex behavioral responses.

Moreover, the interactions between steroid hormones and neurotransmitters are mediated mainly by modifications at the genomic level.

Non-genomic effects

Non-genomic effects are characterized by short latency and brief duration (minutes or hours). They consist of direct actions on cytoplasmic membrane which induce variations in the available neurotransmitter amount, synthesis and metabolism and in changes of membrane permeability and of neurotransmitter receptors function. In more detail, the direct action of estrogens at the presynaptic level can interest all four phases of the neurotransmitters turnover (biosynthesis, release, reuptake and inactivation[1]).

In particular, as far as the effect of estrogens on central neurotransmitter release is concerned, we have been interested in studying the possible interference of estrogens with the processes involving the influx of Ca^{2+} ions into purified presynaptic nerve terminals (synaptosomes) in the rat brain, due to the fundamental role played by this bivalent cation in the process of neurotransmitter release. Among the various Ca^{2+} transporting systems which could mediate Ca^{2+} influx into synaptosomes, our attention has been focused on the study *in vitro* of:

(1) Voltage-dependent Ca^{2+} channels, which are opened by the depolarization of the neuronal membrane.
(2) The Na^{+}–Ca^{2+} antiporter, which could mediate bidirectional Ca^{2+} transport, depending on the direction of the Na^{+} electrochemical gradient.

Ca^{2+} uptake mediated by voltage-operated channels has been investigated by depolarizing the synaptosomal membrane with 55 mM K^{+} ions, whereas Ca^{2+} influx operated by the Na^{+}–Ca^{2+} antiporter has been evaluated by substituting extracellular Na^{+} ions with an equimolar concentration of the impermeant monovalent cation choline, therefore causing a reversal of the resting Na^{+} electrochemical gradient which favors Ca^{2+} entrance mediated by the Na^{+}–Ca^{2+} exchanger.

The results obtained show that both these two Ca^{2+} transporting systems can be inhibited only by elevated estrogen concentrations which are in the pharmacological range. In fact doses of 100 μM of β-estradiol, were able to modify the activity of Ca^{2+} voltage-operated channels and of the Na^{+}–Ca^{2+} exchanger in central synaptosomes.

The *in vitro* inhibitory effect of β-estradiol on the Na^{+}–Ca^{2+} antiporter was also shown by estriol, a 17β-estradiol derivative, even at the lower concentration of 10 μM.

These results appear to suggest that estrogen hormones are able to modulate the activity of the membrane proteins which are responsible for Ca^{2+} translocation across the synaptic membrane; by this means, estrogens could interfere with neurotransmitter release from central neurons, therefore explaining at least some of the neurochemical actions exerted by these ovarian hormones.

The presence of specific receptors for steroid hormones in synaptosomes or isolated membrane fractions has never been demonstrated. Moreover, the short latency of non-genomic effects can hardly coexist with a receptorial mechanism of action.

However, the presence of a binding with a relative specificity but a scarce affinity for E_2 and testosterone has been demonstrated in rat brain synaptic membranes.

At the postsynaptic level, steroid hormones interact with the specific receptors of some neurotransmitters. In isolated membrane E_2 may induce a decrease of serotonin receptors and may compete, if present at high concentrations, with α-adrenergic and dopaminergic receptors.

ACTIONS OF ESTROGENS ON LUTEINIZING HORMONE-RELEASING HORMONE RELEASE

Estrogens have two different effects on luteinizing hormone-releasing hormone (LHRH) release: low estrogen concentrations inhibit (negative feedback) while high estrogen concentrations stimulate (positive feedback) LHRH release.

The negative feedback action is so rapid that it can not be mediated by protein synthesis. Therefore it is likely that estrogens may inhibit LHRH release through a direct action on membranes, ionic channels and enzymes.

On the contrary, the positive feedback action which lasts 26–48 h is believed to happen through the activation of protein synthesis. Indeed, RNA and protein synthesis blockade by means of actinomycin D is able to inhibit estrogen stimulation of LH release.

Immunocytochemical and histoautoradiographical studies demonstrated that only a small part (one out of 435) of hypothalamic LHRH neurons are provided with estrogen receptors.

Therefore, estrogen effects on LHRH release which display a genomic mechanism of action must be mediated through neurons which do not release LHRH but are provided with estrogen receptors and act on LHRH neurons. These are noradrenergic (NA) neurons which stimulate LHRH release and dopaminergic (DA) and opioid neurons which inhibit LHRH release.

Indeed, estrogen receptors have been demonstrated in NA and DA neurons (DA neurons may be also activated by the estrogen-induced hyperprolactinemia).

The role played by serotoninergic neurons has not been well ascertained. They may interfere with circadian regulation of LHRH release. Indeed, a suprachiasmatic nucleus shows an extensive serotoninergic innervation, and serotonin synthesis blockade inhibits diurnal LH surge (in long-term estrogen-treated rats) as well as spontaneous LH surge.

NEUROCHEMICAL ACTIONS OF ESTROGENS

Neurochemical actions of estrogens in the brain include:

(1) Stimulation of neuronal growth and promotion of sexual differentiation;
(2) Induction of progestin receptors in the hypothalamus, preoptic area and pituitary (as well as in all estrogen target tissues). The increase of

progesterone receptor concentration is necessary for the induction of sexual behavior during the estral period;

(3) Modifications of neuronal cell firing;

(4) Modifications of monoaminergic neurons turnover in various hypothalamic and striatal nuclei;

(5) Modifications of the activity of various neuronal enzymes (increase of choline acetyltransferase in the preoptic area, decrease of monoamino-oxidase and tyrosine hydroxylase in the hypothalamus, etc);

(6) effects on cerebral neurotransmitter release and reuptake [DA, NA, γ-aminobutyric acid (GABA), acetylcholine (ACH)];

(7) influence on the receptors for various neurohormones or neuromodulators [thyrotropin-releasing hormone (TRH), LHRH, DA, ACH].

SEXUAL DIFFERENTIATION

It is well known that gonadal hormones contribute to the process of sexual differentiation promoting cellular and biochemical differentiation of specific groups of neurons, during a critical phase of the development. Testosterone secretion is responsible for the sexual differentiation of males while its absence brings about female sexual characteristic development. Two different mechanisms of action are involved in this process. The first is the aromatization of testosterone to E_2 by enzymes present in specific groups of cells of the CNS, followed by the interaction of E_2 with its specific cerebral receptors. The other mechanism is conversion of testosterone to 5α-dihydrotestosterone (5-HT) followed by the interaction of 5-HT with androgen receptors. The first mechanism is responsible for CNS defeminization in the male rats, while the second brings the development of masculine characteristics[5].

It is important to note that in female newborn rats estrogen, being bound to α-fetoprotein, cannot cross the blood–brain barrier[6–9].

EFFECTS ON MONOAMINERGIC SYSTEMS

Among the secondary effects of estrogens, an important role is played by those on cerebral catecholaminergic systems.

In the brain cortex, E_2 administration, *in vivo*, increases the turnover rate and decreases the turnover time of NA and catecholestrogens induce a significant increase of DA turnover rate.

In the hypothalamus, E_2 administration induces, *in vivo*, a significant increase in the turnover rate and a significant decrease in the turnover time of NA, but also a decrease in DA turnover rate. This last effect is due to the fact that while NA is present in the whole hypothalamus, DA is contained only in the median eminence (a very small part of the hypothalamus). It is, therefore, a mistake to consider the turnover rate of DA in the whole hypothalamus. In median eminence, *in vivo*, DA catabolites dihydroxiphenylacetic acid (DOPAC) and homovanillic acid (HVA) increase after E_2 administration.

Among the various catecholaminergic cerebral systems one of the most sensitive to estrogen influence is the tuberoinfundibular dopaminergic (TIDA) system. TIDA neurons are located in the mediobasal hypothalamus. In the rat their cellular bodies are distributed in the arcuate and the rostral parts of the periventricular nuclei and their axons project to the median eminence, in proximity to the perivascular spaces surrounding capillary loops of the portal blood vessels. Dopamine is released at this level and then transported to the anterior pituitary, where, acting on specific receptors located on the lactotropes, tonically inhibits the release of PRL[10,11].

Hyperprolactinemia increases DA turnover in the lateral palisade zone (LPZ) of the median eminence. It has been recently demonstrated that DA turnover and synthesis in the LPZ is reduced in states of high secretion of LH, indicating an inhibitory role of DA in the regulation of LHRH release. Moreover LHRH and DA nerve terminal networks in the LPZ largely overlap, and LHRH injection in hypophysectomized male rat selectively increases DA turnover in the LPZ. Therefore it seems that the ultrashort feedback action of LHRH on its own secretion may involve an activation of DA release from the adjacent DA nerve terminals. Labeled estrogens accumulate in approximately half of the arcuate DA neurons' bodies, indicating the presence of estrogen receptors in these cells. Indeed, exogenous estrogens exert a direct inhibitory feedback action on GnRH release, also through an increase of DA turnover in LPZ[12].

TIDA neurons are not directly regulated by DA receptor-mediated mechanisms but are activated by PRL and LHRH.

The activity of TIDA neurons in the female is higher than in the male. This difference appears to be due, in part, to androgen-induced changes in neuronal differentiation during development. Testosterone administration to female rats on day 5 after birth, induces a reduction of TIDA system activity to values similar to those in the adult male. On the other hand, adult male rats castrated on day 1 after birth present higher rates of DA synthesis, similar to those in female rats. Sexual differences in TIDA neuronal activity also appear to be due to differences in the hormonal milieu in the adult.

Indeed the rates of synthesis and turnover of DA are decreased in the female and increased in the male after castration and testosterone or estrogen replacement restores a normal TIDA neuronal activity[10].

In intact rats, acute estrogen treatment induces an increase of DA synthesis and turnover in the median eminence. These effects are absent in the hypophysectomized animals. Therefore, it is likely that the increase of TIDA neurons activity after estrogen administration is due to the increase of circulating PRL levels induced by estrogens. On the contrary, chronic estrogen treatment induces a decrease of DA synthesis and turnover in the median eminence, even in the presence of high PRL levels. In this condition, cytopathological alterations of the arcuate nucleus and TIDA neurons degeneration are present. These anatomical alterations are a direct effect of estrogen, as chronic pharmacological hyperprolactinemia induces elevated DA levels[10].

Gonadal steroids are also able to modulate cerebral NA turnover. Using autoradiography and immunohistochemistry, E_2 receptors have been demonstrated in central noradrenergic neurons in the lower brainstem of the rat. An increase in hypothalamic NA turnover as well as an increase in tyrosine hydroxylase concentration follow castration in rat[13].

The increase of cerebral NA content and turnover, which takes place after ovariectomy, could explain the alteration in body temperature and peripheral vasodilatation which are present in postmenopausal women during hot flushes.

An important role is also played by opioid activity decrease which follows the castration-induced estrogen decrease. In fact, E_2 plasma levels and opioid inhibitory tone are directly related[14,15]. In fact, naloxone, a receptorial opioid antagonist, is devoid of effects on LH secretion before puberty, after menopause and in hypogonadic subjects. Opioid inhibitory tone could act through the modulation of NA and 5-HT activity as the increase of LH induced by naloxone administration can be antagonized by the administration of NA antagonists or 5-HT agonists. The decreased inhibitory opioid tone on brainstem NA neurons could lead to an increased NA stimulation of the preoptic area, which controls thermoregulation and GnRH release, followed by peripheral vasodilatation and increased LH secretion pulsatility[13].

REFERENCES

1. McEwen, B.S. and Parsons, B. (1982). Gonadal steroid action on the brain: neurochemistry and neuropharmacology. *Ann. Rev. Pharmacol. Toxicol.*, **22**, 555
2. McEwen, B.S., Biegon, A., Davis, P.G., Krey, L.C., Luine, V.N., McGinnis, M.Y., Paden, C.M., Parsons, B. and Rainbow, T.C. (1982). Steroid hormones: humoral signals which alter brain cell properties and functions. *Rec. Prog. Horm. Res.*, **38**, 41
3. McEwen, B.S. (1976). Le interazioni tra ormoni e tessuto nervoso. *Le Scienze*, **99**, 235
4. Metzger, D., White, J.M. and Chambon, P. (1988). The human oestrogen receptor functions in yeast. *Nature*, **334**, 31
5. McEwen, B.S. (1985). Steroids and Brain function. *TIPS*, **6**, 22
6. Arnold, A.P. and Gorski, R.A. (1984). Gonadal steroid induction of structural sex differences in the central nervous system. *Ann. Rev. Neurosci.*, **7**, 413
7. Plapinger, L., McEwen, B.S. and Clemens, L.E. (1973). Ontogeny of estradiol binding sites in rat brain. II. Characteristics of neonatal binding macromolecule. *Endocrinology*, **93**, 1129
8. Nunez, E., Savu, L., Engelman, F., Benassayag, C., Crepy, O. and Jayle, M. E. (1971). Origine embryonnaire de la proteine serique fixant l'oestrone et l'oestradiol chex la Ratte impubere. *C. R. Acad. Sci. Paris*, **273**, 242
9. Raynaud, J.P., Mercier-Bodard, C. and Baulieu, E.E. (1971). Rat estradiol binding plasma protein (EBP). *Steroids*, **18**, 767
10. Moore, K.E., Lookingland, K.J. and Gunnet, J.W. (1988). Effects of gonadal steroids and pituitary hormones on the activity of tuberoinfundibular dopaminergic neurons. In Genazzani, A. R., Montemagno, U., Nappi, C. and Montemagno, U. (eds). *The Brain and Female Reproductive Function*, pp. 117–25. (Carnforth: Parthenon Publishing)
11. Annunziato, L. (1980). Regulatory mechanisms of tuberohypophyseal dopaminergic neurons. In MacLeod, R.M. and Scapagnini, U. (eds). *Central and Peripheral Regulation of Prolactin Function*, pp. 59–67. (New York: Raven Press)
12. Fuxe, K., Agnati, L.F., Kalia, M., Goldstein, M., Andersson, K. and Härfstrand, A. (1985). Dopaminergic systems in the brain and pituitary. In Flückiger, E., Müller, E.E. and Thorner, M.O. (eds). *Basic and Clinical Aspects of Neuroscience*, pp. 11–25. (Berlin–Heidelberg; Springer-Verlag)
13. Casper, R.F. and Yen, S.S.C. (1985). Neuroendocrinology of menopausal flush mechanism. *Clin. Endocrinol.*, **22**, 293
14. Quigley, M.E. and Yen, S.S.C. (1980). The role of endogenous opiates on LH secretion during the menstrual cycle. *J. Clin. Endocrinol. Metab.*, **51**, 179

15. Genazzani, A.R., Petraglia, F., Facchinetti, F. and Volpe, A. (1988). Endogenous opioid peptides and the menstrual cycle. In Genazzani, A.R., Montemagno, U., Nappi, C. and Montemagno, U. (eds.) *The Brain and Female Reproductive Function*, pp. 361–7. (Carnforth: Parthenon Publishing)

Estrogen and progesterone receptors in the cervix during estriol vaginal cream therapy

M. Massobrio, A. Revelli, G. Gregori, P. Cassoni, B. Torchio and M. Migliardi

INTRODUCTION

Several investigators demonstrated the presence of estrogen receptors (ER) and progesterone receptors (PR) in the healthy cervix and in cervical malignancies[1-3]. In the normal cervix the concentration of ER and PR is by far lower than in the endometrium or in the uterine myometrium. The columnar epithelium is particularly rich in ER, producing cervical mucus under estrogen control; the cervical stroma contains a significant amount of receptors, while the lowest ER concentration is associated with the squamous epithelium[5]. Sex steroid receptors in the cervix did not seem to be highly influenced by hormonal fluctuations during the cycle, though PR showed a slight increase during the follicular phase[6]. In contrast postmenopausal women showed a significant rise in ER concentration both in the normal cervix[7] and in cervical carcinomas[8], while PR underwent an important decrease[2,4,9]. The very low circulating progesterone concentration during the menopause was classically considered responsible for the increase in ER number, since progesterone inhibits ER synthesis and consequently the replenishment of cellular cytoplasm by recently synthesized ER[10]. The low PR levels are generally attributed to the postmenopausal hypoestrogenic environment, which is unable to exert the stimulating action that estrogens usually have over PR synthesis. According to the above mentioned hormonal regulation the administration of estrogens enhances ER and PR synthesis, while the treatment with progestins causes a marked reduction in ER and PR concentrations[11].

MATERIALS AND METHODS

The study group consisted of 12 healthy postmenopausal women complaining of moderate dyspareunia, postcoital spotting and recurrent vaginal infections.

The age of the subjects ranged from 51 to 66 years (mean age 58 years) and all had been naturally menopausal for at least 18 months (mean 5 years). None had received any local or systemic hormonal treatment during the 6 months preceding this study. Nobody had a history of endocrine or hepatic diseases. For the entire group the mean weight was 63.1 kg and the mean stature 162 cm.

With written informed consent a therapy with estriol vaginal cream (*Colpogyn*, Angelini, F. Acraf S.p.a., Rome, Italy) one application daily (estriol (E_3) 0.5 mg every single dose) for 21 days was recommended. The following investigations were made before starting the treatment and 24 h after its conclusion: plasma luteinizing hormone (LH), follicle-stimulating hormone (FSH), human prolactin (hPRL), estrone (E_1), estradiol (E_2), sex hormone-binding globulin (SHBG) concentrations were assessed by radioimmunoassay (RIA). Circulating antithrombin III, total cholesterol, high density lipoprotein (HDL), γ-glutamyl transpeptidase (GT), aspartate aminotransferase (AST) and alanine aminotransferase (ALT) were evaluated as indexes of hepatic function. A Papanicolaou (PAP) smear was performed to obtain cyto-hormonal evaluation. A routine colposcopy was made, including 1% acetic acid application and Schiller test. Every woman underwent two cervical biopsies, one of which was processed as usual and sent for histological evaluation. The second one was immediately frozen in liquid nitrogen and carried to the laboratory to perform ER and PR assay by dextran-coated charcoal (DCC) method. This frozen tissue was pulverized, suspended in a balanced solution and then centrifuged at high speed to obtain the cytosol fraction. ^{3}H-labeled estradiol (Amersham) and ^{3}H-labeled progesterone (Amersham) were used as chemical reagents and incubated with the cytosol preparation. Following incubation DCC suspension was added to remove unbound steroids. The preparation was then centrifuged to remove the DCC. A part of the surnatant was then added to the scintillation cocktail and counted by a β-counter. The results were calculated according to the method of Scatchard[12] and the receptor concentrations were expressed as femtomoles per milligram cytosol protein (fmol/mg protein). Statistical elaboration was made using the *t* test for paired data.

RESULTS AND DISCUSSION

Previous studies demonstrated that E_3 acts selectively on the epithelium of the cervix and the vagina without stimulating endometrial proliferation[13]. This selectivity of action is thought to be a consequence of the short (about 6 h) binding time to the estrogen receptor as compared with other estrogens which exhibit long binding time and exert their action even on the endometrium[13]. Moreover estriol is not converted into estradiol or estrone which act on the endometrium and the breast[14]. The vaginal method of administration guarantees a satisfactory absorption of the drug and allows the use of much lower doses in comparison with the oral method, since 0.5 mg E_3 vaginal cream corresponds to 8–12 mg of E_3 orally administered. After the vaginal application, circulating free E_3 rises after 60–90 min and its plasma concentration remains high for about 12 h[15]. A slight cumulative effect after 1–3 weeks of daily applications has been observed by some investigators[16,17], but does not seem to have any consequence.

Our experience substantially confirms the published data about the clinical effectiveness of E_3 vaginal cream treatment. After 1 week of therapy we noticed complete relief from dyspareunia and after 3 weeks the postcoital spotting disappeared. No undesirable side-effects were observed. Colposcopy showed the attenuation of atrophic signs and the improvement of Lugol's iodine positivity. In the cytological smear there was a decrease of basal and parabasal cells, with the reappearance of glycogenic superficial cells. The histological examination showed an increased number of cell layers in the squamous epithelium, with a marked reduction of parabasal cells, a higher percentage of glycogenic cells, a decrease of stromal edema and of stromal leucocyte infiltration. The hormonal evaluations (Table 1) confirmed the absence of E_3 conversion into E_1 and E_2 as well as the lack of a significant negative feedback on gonadotropins and the absence of stimulation on hPRL secretion. The SHBG level was not significantly changed. We could not find any significant difference (Table 2) in serum circulating antithrombin III, total cholesterol, HDL, γ-GT, AST and ALT, according to the minimal hepatic potency of vaginally administered E_3.

As far as ER and PR are concerned, the lowest receptor concentrations which allow consideration of tissue as ER+ and PR+, according to Potish *et al.*[2], are 6 fmol/mg protein and 10 fmol/mg protein respectively. Estrogen receptor concentrations ranged from 4.8 to 172.6 fmol/mg protein and 11 of the 12 women we considered were ER+. Progesterone receptor concentrations ranged from 2.8 to 110.2 fmol/mg protein and nine of 12 women were PR+. The mean $\pm$ SEM ER concentration before starting the treatment was 67.61 ± 7.56 fmol/mg protein, while after the treatment it was

Table 1 Hormonal evaluations (mean $\pm$ SD) before and after the treatment with E_3 vaginal cream

	Pretherapy	*Post-therapy*
FSH (mIU/ml)	64.1 ± 21.6	62.9 ± 19.4
LH (mIU/ml)	44.7 ± 15.7	45.2 ± 13.0
hPRL (ng/ml)	7.8 ± 2.1	8.0 ± 1.9
E_1 (pg/ml)	18.2 ± 12.6	18.9 ± 13.1
E_2 (pg/ml)	15.3 ± 8.8	15.9 ± 7.5
SHBG ($\times 10^{-8}$ M)	2.4 ± 0.9	2.5 ± 0.7

All the differences are not statistically significant

Table 2 Hematochemical evaluations (mean $\pm$ SD) before and after the treatment with E_3 vaginal cream

	Pretherapy	*Post-therapy*
AST (IU)	12.0 ± 4.1	12.6 ± 3.8
ALT (IU)	10.4 ± 3.9	11.7 ± 3.1
γ-GT (mIU/ml)	14.1 ± 6.5	14.9 ± 6.2
Cholesterol (mg/100 ml)	227.8 ± 35.3	216.0 ± 41.3
HDL (mg/100 ml)	39.6 ± 7.2	40.1 ± 7.9
AT III (mg/dl)	104.8 ± 19.8	106.5 ± 21.1

All the differences are not statistically significant

32.48 ± 5.4 fmol/mg protein. Progesterone receptor concentration fell from a mean ± SEM of 38.1 ± 5.4 fmol/mg protein before the E_3 administration to 8.7 ± 3.09 fmol/mg protein after the end of the treatment (Figure 1). After the therapy 10 of 12 women were still ER+ and four of 12 women were PR+.

Why does the ER concentration appear to be markedly reduced after the treatment? In the last few years a new model of steroid–receptor interaction has been proposed and much experimental evidence which supports this hypothesis has been presented[18]. According to the new theory the unoccupied receptor lies in the nucleus, bound to nuclear components by low affinity interactions. The steroid molecules have lipophilic properties and can diffuse through the cell membranes, the cytoplasm and the nuclear membrane, reaching their receptors in the nucleus. After, the steroid–receptor binding conformational changes (transformation) of the occupied receptors are induced. As a result the receptor becomes able to bind with the nuclear components with a high affinity interaction and starts the transcription of the genes. The occupied transformed receptor is so strongly bound to the chromatin proteins that usual tissue preparation procedures, such as low salt extraction or homogenization, cannot break the binding. In our study the homogenization of the tissue specimen provoked the precipitation of the nuclear fractions, where occupied receptors were retained. DCC method dosed cytosol receptors, which were mostly unbound, and probably not occupied and not transformed nuclear receptors, weakly bound to DNA. In this way the lower ER concentration can reflect a higher percentage of transformed receptors tightly bound to E_3 in the nuclear fraction and

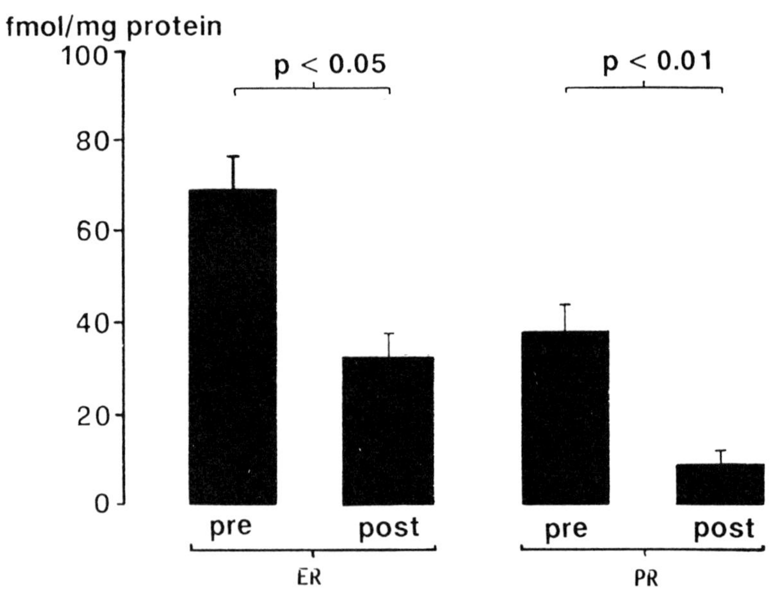

Figure 1 Effect of the treatment with estriol vaginal cream on estrogen receptor and progesterone receptor concentration in the cervix during the menopause ($n = 12$, mean ± SEM)

therefore are undetectable by DCC. A similar effect has been described[19] in rat uterus after parenteral administration of injectable E_3, which determined a marked decrease of cytosol ER concentration due to the increased hormone receptor binding in the nucleus. Moreover the majority of ER is located in the parabasal cells, so the reduction of parabasal cell number after the treatment might contribute to the decrease of ER in the epithelium[20].

It is harder to find a reason for the remarkable decrease of PR after E_3 vaginal cream treatment, since PR are classically considered markers of estrogen activity in the target tissues and they were expected to increase after estrogen therapy. A possible hypothesis to explain this finding is that E_3 could have biological potency sufficient to exert the antiatrophic effect, but not to enhance PR synthesis, which is a late estrogenic effect and perhaps needs a hormone receptor binding time longer than E_3 may guarantee. We think that further evaluations are needed to clarify this finding which is apparently difficult to explain.

REFERENCES

1. Hahnel, R., Martin, J.D., Master, A.M., Ratajaczak, T. and Twaddle, E. (1979). Estrogen receptors and blood hormone levels in cervical carcinoma and other gynecological tumors. *Gynecol. Oncol.*, **8**, 226–33
2. Potish, R.A., Twiggs, L.B., Adcock, L.L., Prem, K.A., Savage, J.E. and Leung, B.S. (1986). Prognostic importance of progesterone and estrogen receptors in cancer of the uterine cervix. *Cancer*, **58**, 1709–13
3. Ford, L.C., Berek, J.S., Lagasse, L.D., Hacker, N.F., Heins, Y.L. and DeLange, R.J. (1981). Estrogen and progesterone receptor sites in malignancies of the uterine cervix, vagina and vulva. *Gynecol. Oncol.*, **15**, 27–31
4. Russo, A., Mondo, F., Francalanci, S., Di Carlo, F., Conti, G., Racca, S. and Reboani, C. (1982). Distribuzione dei recettori per gli estrogeni e dei recettori per il progesterone nell'utero umano ed influenza dei farmaci anestetici. *Min. Ginecol.*, **34**, 755–60
5. Sanborn, B.M., Held, B. and Kuo, H.S. (1975). Specific estrogen binding proteins in human cervix. *J. Steroid. Biochem.*, **6**, 1107–12
6. Sanborn, B.M., Kuo, H.S. and Held, B. (1978). Estrogen and progesterone binding site concentrations in human endometrium and cervix throughout the menstrual cycle and in tissue from women taking oral contraceptives. *J. Steroid. Biochem.*, **9**, 951–5
7. Punnonen, R. and Lukola, A. (1982). High-affinity binding of estrone, estradiol and estriol in human cervical myometrium and cervical and vaginal epithelium. *J. Endocrinol. Invest.*, **5**, 203–7
8. Yajima, A., Yamauchi, R., Wada, Y., Furuhashi, N., Toki, T., Tase, T., Oikawa, N., Sato, S., Takabayashi, T. and Ozawa, N. (1985). Cytoplasmatic estrogen receptors in carcinoma of the uterine cervix. *Gynecol. Obstet. Invest.*, **20**, 103–8
9. Gao, Y.L., Twiggs, L.B., Leung, B.S., Yu, W.C.Y., Potish, R.A., Okagaki, T., Adcock, L.L. and Prem, K.A. (1983). Cytoplasmatic estrogen and progesterone receptors in primary cervical carcinoma: clinical and histopathologic correlates. *Am. J. Obstet. Gynecol.*, **146**, 299–306
10. Hsueh, A.J.W., Peck, E.J. and Clark, J.H. (1976). Control of uterine estrogen receptors levels by progesterone. *Endocrinology*, **98**, 438–44
11. Gorodeski, I.G., Geier, A., Lunefeld, B., Beery, R. and Bahary, C.M. (1987). Progesterone (P) receptor dynamics in estrogen primed normal human cervix following P injection. *Fertil. Steril.*, **47**, 108–13
12. Scatchard, G. (1949). The attraction of proteins for small molecules and ions. *Ann. N.Y. Acad. Sci.*, **51**, 660–7
13. Phillips, A., Hahn, D.W. and McGuire, J.L. (1984). Comparative effects of estriol and equine conjugates estrogens on the uterus and vagina. *Maturitas*, **5**, 147–52

14. Merril, R.C. (1985). Estriol: a review. *Physiol. Rev.*, **38**, 463–79
15. Kikovic, P.M., Cortes Priato, J., Milojevic, S., Haspel, A.A. and Aljinovic, A. (1980). The treatment of post-menopausal vaginal atrophy with ovestin vaginal or suppositories: clinical, endocrinological and safety aspects. *Maturitas*, **2**, 275–81
16. Keller, P.J., Riedman, R., Fisher, M. and Gerber, G. (1981). Oestrogens, gonadotropins and prolactin after intra-vaginal administration of oestriol in post-menopausal women. *Maturitas*, **3**, 47–53
17. Eandi, M., Braggio, N., Andreoli, F. and Andreoli, C. (1986). Hormonal plasma levels following estriol vaginal administration to postmenopausal women. *The Cervix e.i.f.g.t.*, **4**, 91–8
18. Gorski, J., Welshons, W.V., Sakai, D., Hansen, J., Walent, J., Kassis, J., Schull, J., Stack, G. and Campen, C. (1986). Evolution of a Model of Estrogen Action. *Rec. Prog. Horm. Res.*, **42**, 297–329
19. Clark, J.H., Paszko, Z. and Peck, E.J. (1977). Nuclear binding and retention of the receptor estrogen complex: relation to the agonistic and antagonistic properties of estriol. *Endocrinology*, **100**, 91–6
20. Rosner, J.M., Martinez, I.M., Mendizabal, A.F. and Spaltro, N.A. (1971). The in vivo and in vitro uptake of labelled estradiol by different segments of the human uterus. *Steroidologia*, **2**, 283–8

131

Estriol vaginal therapy in the postmenopausal micturitional pathology: evaluation of trigone and urethra receptional population to estrogen and progesterone

G. F. Minini, U. Omodei, C. Simeone, P. Luisi, S. Ghielmi, S. Cosciani Cunico, A. Roggia and A. Gastaldi

INTRODUCTION

Estrogen shortage is commonly known to have an important role in the onset and continuation of typical micturitional disorders in menopause. These are characterized by recurring episodes of frequency, voiding difficulties, urinary infections, sensory urge incontinence and also genuine motor urge incontinence.

Hormone dependency of at least the distal part (trigone and urethra) of the lower urinary tract is also confirmed by the common embryological origin of these structures, that is the same embryonal button which part of the vagina derives from.

From this introduction we have hypothesized the presence of receptor sites to steroids on the trigone and urethra. This hypothesis has prompted researchers to investigate mucosal specimens taken from both samples obtained at operation and cadavers. The main data resulting from this investigation are reported in Table 1.

Table 1 Results of investigations for the presence of estrogen (ER) and progesterone (PR) receptors at various sites

Reference	*Site*	*Cases*	*ER*	*PR*
Saez[1]	Trigone	10	8	4
Iosif and Batra[2]	Urethra	4	4	0
Wilson and Barker[3]	Urethra	5	5	0
Author's cases (1985)	Bladder	20	13	7
Author's cases (1986)	Urethra	20	9	6

MATERIALS AND METHODS

Two objectives have been elected in the present work: first to confirm the presence of steroid receptors in the trigonal and urethral mucosa obtained *in vivo*, i.e. under pretreatment conditions, thus concluding a preliminary phase of research which has been formerly published; second to point out the clinical implications of postmenopausal micturitional pathology in relation to the presence or absence of these receptors, to their density and to their responsiveness to replacement therapy (Table 2).

As regards this aspect, research taking account of the different types of estrogens and different ways of administration is being carried out.

In this work we report some of the results obtained from the topical vaginal administration of estriol. As regards the first aspects, we believe the achieved technique to now be reliable.

Trigonal and urethral mucosa specimens were obtained from biopsies performed during cystoscopy for non-neoplastic pathology. Three samples were taken of the minimum amount needed for receptor determination. While at first we employed a radioimmunoassay technique with dextran-coated charcoal (DCC), at present solid-phase enzyme immunoassays based on the 'sandwich' principle (estrogen receptor, ER-EIA and progesterone receptor, PgR-EIA kits) are believed to be more advantageous and are therefore preferred.

As regards the second objective of this study, we considered 10 patients included in a pre-established research protocol. All of the women were postmenopausal and presented stress incontinence with or without other associated micturitional disorders. The patients were accurately studied by means of anamnestic investigation; objective gynecological examination; biopsy and determination of trigonourethral estrogen and progesterone receptors; urodynamic investigation including cystomanometria, static and dynamic urethral pressure profile, uroflowmetry; endocrine study including the following hormone assays: luteinizing hormone, follicle-stimulating hormone, prolactin, estrone, 17β-estradiol, estriol, sex hormone-binding globulin, thyroxine-binding globulin (TBG), cortisol-binding globulin (CBG), transcortine, testosterone and androstenedione; clinical evaluation for the investigation of the following parameters: urethrovaginal atrophy, dryness and cystourethrocele. Patients with one or more of the conditions reported in Table 3 were ruled out.

TREATMENT

The patients were treated with colpogyn vaginal cream (one application in the evening for 45 days) and re-evaluated at the end of treatment with the

Table 2 Estrogen replacement therapies used in the determination of estrogen and progesterone receptors in menopausal patients

Estriol – vaginal cream
Conjugated estrogens – vaginal cream (low-dosage)
Conjugated estrogens – vaginal cream (high-dosage)
Conjugated estrogens – *per os*
17β-Estradiol – transdermal

Table 3 Criteria of exclusion

Diagnosed or suspicion of estrogen-dependent neoplasm
Endometrial hyperplasia, unexplained genital hemorrhage
Anamnesis or presence of thrombosis, thrombophlebitis, thromboembolic pathology
Anamnesis or presence of cerebrovascular pathology
Anamnesis or presence of coronary ischemic pathology
Chronic or acute hepatic pathology in progress
Clinical diabetes
Uncontrolled arterial hypertension
Positive urine culture
Estrogen replacement therapy in progress or withdrawn for at least 6 months

same pretreatment investigations. Trigonal and urethral biopsies were performed in all of the patients for investigation and determination of the estrogen and progesterone receptors as reported above.

ANALYSIS OF THE RESULTS

In Table 4 we report the clinical parameters evaluated and in Tables 5 and 6 those of laboratory parameters are reported.

Therapy had a positive effect on the subjective symptoms in all cases with especially good results for incontinence and for vulvovaginal burning while no significant change of the cystourethrocele was reported; atrophy and mucosal dryness had a positive response.

The maximum urethral closure pressure increased but not significantly, whereas there was a highly significant increase in the functional length of

Table 4 Clinical results before and after therapy ($n = 10$)

	Before	*After*
Incontinence		
Mild	4	6
Moderate	5	1
Severe	1	0
Absent	0	3
Urethrovaginal atrophy	7	2
Vaginal dryness	9	0
Cystourethrocele	10	10
Maximum urethral closure pressure (mean ± SD)	61.5 ± 9.5	69.9 ± 17.8
Functional length of urethra (mean ± SD)	2.2 ± 0.3*	2.6 ± 0.4*

* $p = 0.003$

Table 5 Modifications of the receptor population (mean ± SD; fmol/mg)

	Before therapy	*After therapy*
Estrogen receptors (bladder)	37.7 ± 42.8	120.1 ± 62.8**
Progesterone receptors (bladder)	27.7 ± 17.3	79.0 ± 55.3*
Estrogen receptors (urethra)	80.9 ± 45.8	85.3 ± 37.2
Progesterone receptors (urethra)	27.6 ± 28.7	44.9 ± 56.3

* $p = 0.03$; ** $p = 0.001$

Table 6 Hormonal modifications (mean ± SD)

	Before therapy	*After therapy*
Luteinizing hormone (mIU/ml)	63.8 ± 20.4	62.7 ± 23.0
Follicle-stimulating hormone (mIU/ml)	111.5 ± 36.9	103.0 ± 35.9
Prolactin (ng/ml)	5.2 ± 1.9	5.2 ± 2.2
Progesterone (pg/ml)	164.6 ± 88.1	128.2 ± 87.9
Estrone (pg/ml)	24.8 ± 10.8	27.7 ± 12.3
Estradiol (pg/ml)	13.3 ± 5.0	13.7 ± 2.9
Estriol (ng/ml)	no det.	no det.
Testosterone (ng/ml)	0.33 ± 0.09	0.38 ± 0.11
Androstenedione (ng/ml)	1.4 ± 0.5	1.4 ± 0.5
Sex hormone-binding globulin (nmol/l)	48.8 ± 20.0	47.5 ± 19.5
TBG (μg/ml)	36.9 ± 7.6	33.9 ± 8.6

the urethra.

All the determined receptor populations increased after therapy: such an increase was highly significant for trigone estrogen and progesterone receptors. The serum hormones and the hepatic transfer proteins were not modified in any way after therapy (Table 6).

CONCLUSIONS

Though our data are limited we may affirm that: the technique adopted is reliable for the determination of estrogen and progesterone receptors in the lower urinary tract *in vivo*; all the receptor populations studied undergo an increase after therapy with a maximum for trigone estrogen receptors; the serum hormones and the transfer proteins are not modified; topical therapy determines a subjective and objective clinical improvement; and there is a significant increase in the urethral functional length.

Finally, it must be remembered that all the above mentioned effects are determined by local action without significant systemic effects.

REFERENCES

1. Saez, P. (1972). Age changes in the female urethra. *Br. J. Urol.*, **44**, 667–76
2. Iosif, S. and Batra, S. (1981). Estrogen receptors in the human female lower urinary tract. *Am. J. Obstet. Gynecol.*, **141**, 817
3. Wilson, P.D. and Barker, G. (1984). Steroid hormone receptors in the female lower urinary tract. *Urol. Intern.*, **39**, 5–8

132

Lipidemic and hemocoagulative changes after treatment with vaginal estriol for climacteric complaints

G.L. Capitanio, A. Ferraiolo, C. Gustavino and M. Leone

INTRODUCTION

Cardiovascular diseases considered in their entirety constitute today the main cause of death for Western populations. During the reproductive age, the woman is somewhat protected, compared to males of the same age, from coronary arteriopathy. Such protection decreases gradually after the menopause until it disappears completely; the disadvantage of males has disappeared by 75 years of age[1]. Cessation of cyclical ovarian activity indeed exposes women to an increased risk of atherosclerosis and all its related pathology.

In developed countries today, 95% of women survive menopause and 65% exceed 75 years of age. Over one-third of the female population is in menopause and a considerable percentage of these women has a high risk potential for atherosclerotic cardiovascular disease[2]: to identify the reasons for the loss of protection from cardiovascular risk is therefore of considerable importance for Public Health.

Maybe the main factor that can be correlated to protection is a correct ratio among the various components of lipoprotein metabolism, and particularly among the low density (LDL) and high density (HDL) lipoprotein subfractions of cholesterol and the ratio between them.

After menopause there is an increase of triglycerides and LDL cholesterol, while the values of HDL cholesterol may diminish or remain the same: the LDL/HDL ratio thus approaches the values found in males and this could explain the sudden increase of cardiovascular risk that occurs after menopause[1,3].

The protecting factor that suddenly vanishes must be correlated to the alterations in hormone balance that occur at this moment of a woman's life, i.e. the more or less abrupt exhaustion of the circulating estrogen fraction.

Indeed, both the estrogens produced by the organism and those administered from the outside have generally positive effects on the metabolism of lipids causing an antiatherogenic lipoproteic response. Indeed they slow down the removal from circulation of LDL by the liver with its consequent decrease while they increase the synthesis and slow the removal of HDL cholesterol[4].

Practically all epidemiological studies published on the subject concur in concluding that the administration of estrogens during postmenopausal years is capable of reducing the risk of mortality and morbidity from cardiovascular diseases[1,5,6]. This administration must however be associated with a progestogen for 12 days: this is necessary in order to decrease the risk of uterine and mammary cancer[7,8]. However, the progestogens derived from 19-nortestosterone possess androgenic characteristics and have a negative influence on the metabolism of lipids, so much so that they suppress the positive effects induced by estrogens[9,10].

Hypercoagulability is another cause of atherosclerosis and of the consequential increased risk of cardiovascular disease. The use of natural estrogens used normally in climacteric complaints seems not to carry with it negative effects on the metabolism of lipids; however, some authors mention modifications of the hemostatic parameters with the use of succinate estriol orally with a daily dosage above at least 4 mg (Table 1)[11–14].

The purpose of our study was to verify the modifications of the lipid metabolism and of the hemostatic parameters in the course of therapy with estriol in cream administered vaginally to a group of 15 women in spontaneous menopause for at least 1 year who complained of problems tied to atrophy of the urogenital tract.

MATERIALS AND METHODS

Fifteen postmenopausal women were admitted to the study in good health, with normal weight, (mean age 64 ± 9.2) who complained of problems due to atrophy of the urogenital tract. None of the patients recruited had undergone substitutive estrogenic therapy of any kind whatsoever during the 6 months before our study.

The means of administration of the drug were as follows: 0.5 mg in cream vaginally (Colpogyn, Angelini Acraf Rome Italy) administered each day for 3 weeks, then 0.5 mg twice a week for a 6-month period.

Before beginning treatment the patients underwent a baseline control of the lipidemic profile (triglycerides, total cholesterol. HDL, HDL_3, LDL, apolipoproteins (Apo)AI and B and the ratio of ApoB/ApoAI) and of the hemostatic parameters (coagulation factors, platelets, platelet aggregation with ADP and collagen, fibrinogen, prothrombin time, partial prothrombin

Table 1 Variations in coagulation factors during oral administration of succinate estriol

Author	*Cases*	*Dosage*	*Variations*
T. Davies *et al.*[11]	10	2 mg/day (1 month)	no variation
	10	4–8 mg/day (3 months)	> factor VII < factor VIII > platelet aggregation
M. McKay-Hart *et al.*[12]	27	2 mg/day (5 weeks)	no variation
	27	6–12 mg/day (4 months)	> factor VII > factor X
J. L. Toy *et al.*[13]	9	12 mg/day (3 months)	> platelet aggregation
C. Campagnoli *et al.*[14]	13	2 mg/day	no variation

time, fibrinopeptide A, Factors VII, VIII, IX and X, fibrinolysis factors: plasminogen, xanthine diphosphate (XDP), antithrombin III). This check-up was repeated after 6 months of therapy.

The blood samples were taken at our Institute always at the same time, 08:00, from the patients who had fasted since the previous evening.

RESULTS AND CONCLUSIONS

The results of our investigation are presented in Tables 2 and 3. From the analysis of these data it can be seen that no statistically significant modification was found for the lipid profile and on the coagulation factors after 6 months of therapy with estriol in cream taken vaginally.

The variations encountered for factors VII, VIII, X and for platelet aggregations that had been reported by some authors after treatment with succinate estriol administered orally at a daily dosage of at leat 4 mg, for a period of time longer than 6 months did not appear in the patients we treated.

Table 2 Modifications of lipidemic metabolism during therapy with vaginal estriol: 15 cases (mean age 64 ± 9.2)

	Baseline values	*6-month therapy*
Total cholesterol (mg/dl)	198.7 (±32.9)	201.5 (±23.3)
Cholesterol-HDL (mg/dl)	64.5 (±9.6)	67.0 (±8.1)
Cholesterol-HDL_2 (mg/dl)	28.6 (±6.6)	28.5 (±6.2)
Cholesterol-HDL_3 (mg/dl)	35.9 (±5.1)	38.5 (±6.0)
Cholesterol-LDL (mg/dl)	155.0 (±30.7)	158.6 (±27.5)
Triglycerides (mg/dl)	130.2 (±40.3)	132.6 (±39.8)
ApoAI (mg/dl)	151.1 (±21.2)	163.4 (±22.1)
ApoB (mg/dl)	94.3 (±17.3)	95.1 (±19.6)
ApoB/ApoAI	0.63 (±0.14)	0.59 (±0.15)

Table 3 Variation of hemostatic parameters during therapy with vaginal estriol: 15 cases (mean age 64 ± 9.2)

	Baseline values	*6-month therapy*
Coagulation factors		
Platelets 10000/mm^3	198	203
Platelet aggregation (ADP)%	50 (±7.0)	52 (±5.0)
Platelet aggregation (coll.)%	75 (±5.0)	75 (±5.0)
Fibrinogen (mg%)	310 (±15)	323 (±10)
Prothrombin time (s)	95 (±3.0)	90 (±5.0)
Partial thromboplastin time (s)	28 (±4.0)	28 (±3.0)
Fibrinopeptide A (ng/ml)	3.9 (±1.8)	4.2 (±1.2)
Factor VII (%)	110 (±8.0)	108 (±10)
Factor VIII (%)	120 (±13)	115 (±9.0)
Factor IX (%)	109 (±12.0)	107 (±8.0)
Factor X (%)	100 (±11)	98 (±10.0)
Fibrinolysis factors		
Plasminogen (mg%)	108 (±10.0)	110 (±9.0)
XDP (ng/ml)	<10	<10
Antithrombin III (mg/dl)	24.4 (±2.3)	23.8 (±2.5)

On the other hand we noticed a certain tendency towards improvement of the lipidemic profile with respect to the baseline situation (it was indeed possible to observe a slight increase of HDL and a decrease of LDL while the ApoB/ApoAI ratio was modified in a positive direction). However, it is necessary to point out that it is only a 'tendency' towards improvement since, as we mentioned previously, these changes were not significant from the statistical point of view and they will have to be confirmed by a study extended to a larger number of patients.

Therefore, based on our results, we can conclude that long-term therapy with estriol in cream taken vaginally can be administered with ease and safety to women with problems due to atrophy of the urogenital tract since, aside from effectiveness, it does not modify atrophic endometria, as we had previously proved, nor the lipidemic or hemocoagulative profile.

REFERENCES

1. Lila, E. and Nachtigall, (19xx). Cardiovascular disease and hypertension in older women. *Obstet. Gynecol. Clin. N. Am.*, **14**, 86–105
2. Keller, P.J. (1987). Estrogen replacement therapy in the postmenopause. In Genazzani, A.R., Volpe, A. and Facchinetti, F. (eds) *Gynecological Endocrinology*, pp. 667–72. (Carnforth: Parthenon Publishing)
3. Carlton, M. and Gibson, L.A. (1980). Vascular disease risk factors in women with premature menopause. *Horm. Metab. Res.*, **12**, 208–11
4. Capitanio, G.L., Bertolini, S., Semino, G., Elicio, N., Croce, S., Montanari, D., Valice, S. and Pistocchi, G. (1983). Considerazioni sulle modificazioni lipoproteiche e conseguente rischio aterogeno indotte dagli estrogeni e dai progestinici. In Cagnazzo, G. (ed.). *Menopausa* (Bologna: Monduzzi Editore)
5. Ross, R.K., Paganini-Hill, A., Mack, T.M., Arthur, N. and Henderson, S.E. (1981). Menopausal oestrogen therapy and protection from death from ischaemic heart disease. *Lancet*, **i**, 858–60
6. Henderson, B.E., Ross, R.K. and Paganini-Hill, A. (1986). Estrogen use and cardiovascular disease. *Am. J. Obstet. Gynecol.*, **154**, 1181–6
7. Gambrell, R.D. Jr. (1986). Role of progestogens in prevention of breast cancer. *Maturitas*, **8**, 169
8. Gambrell, R.D. Jr (1986). Prevention of endometrial cancer with progestogens *Maturitas*, **8**, 159
9. Knopp, R.H., Walden, C.E., Wahl, P.W., Hoover, J.J., Warnick, G.R., Albers, J.J., Ogilvie, J.T. and Hazzard, W.R. (1981). Oral contraceptive and postmenopausal estrogens effects on lipoprotein triglycerides and cholesterol in an adult female population: relationships to estrogen and progestin potency. *J. Clin. Endocrinol. Metab.*, **53**, 1123
10. Ottosson, U.B., Johansson, B.G. and Von Schoultz, B. (1985). Subfractions of high-density lipoprotein cholesterol during estrogen replacement therapy: a comparison between progestogens and the natural progesterone. *Am. J. Obstet. Gynecol.*, **151**, 746–50
11. Davies, T., Fieldhouse, G. and McNicol, G. P. (1976). The effects of therapy with oestriol succinate and etinyloestriol on the hemostatic mechanism in post-menopausal women *Thromb. Haemost.*, **35**, 43
12. McKay Hart, D., Lindsay, R. and Purdie, D. (1978). Vascular complications of long term oestrogen therapy. *Front Horm. Res.*, **5**, 174
13. Toy, J.L., Davies, J.A. and McNicol, G.P. (1978). The comparative effects of a synthetic and "natural" oestrogen on the haemostatic mechanism in patients with primary amenorrhea. *Br. J. Obstet. Gynaecol.*, **85**, 359
14. Campagnoli, C., Prelato Tousion, L., Dolfin, M., Ferruzzi, L., Belforte, P. and Morra, G. (1982). Effects of different natural oestrogens on clotting factors, plasma lipids and endometrial proliferation in post-menopausal women. In Fioretti, P., Martini, L., Melis, G.B. and Yen, S.S.C. (eds). *The Menopause: Clinical Endocrinological and Pathophysiological Aspects*, p. 567. (New York: Academic Press)

133

Estriol in the treatment of postmenopausal osteoporosis

C. Zara, A. Lauri, F. Perotti, F. Beneventi, R. Ferraro, G. Panese and F. Polatti

Bone loss in the postmenopause is related to the lack of ovarian estrogen secretion. Estroprogestinic therapy provides a perfect solution in the prevention of this[1] calcium deficit. However, given the age of these patients the various contraindications of hormonal treatment favor the use of calcitonin[2,3]. The administration of salmon calcitonin (sCT), subcutaneously or more recently in the spray form, inhibits bone loss and in addition can increase bone mineral content (BMC)[4,5].

Nonetheless the symptoms of estrogen deficiency persist in these patients sometimes even to the point of modifying life quality.

Estriol (E_3) is considered to be a weak estrogen, given its insignificant effect on the endometrium when compared to estradiol[6]. This can be easily understood when considering that E_3 is rapidly absorbed, has a brief bonding time (6 h) with the estrogenic receptor, bonds weakly with plasma proteins, is not converted to estrone or estradiol and is rapidly excreted[7].

Data regarding estriol activity in calcium phosphate metabolism are scarce, contradictory and refer only to oral administration. The possibility of vaginal administration[8,9] of estriol has shown, that, by avoiding the hepatic filter, free estriol plasma concentrations are obtained which are more stable in time and about 20 times greater than those obtained *per os*[10]. The absence of collateral effects on lipid and carbohydrate metabolism on coagulation and on the endometrium even in the case of prolonged administration in addition to its efficacy in reducing menopausal symptoms induced us to study the effects of vaginal administration of estriol alone and in association with sCT on calcium phosphate metabolism.

MATERIALS AND METHODS

The first study examined a group of 14 women ovariectomized during menstrual flow. The patients were randomly divided into groups of seven. The first group (A) received 100 IU/dl of sCT spray and 1 g of calcium for 12 months, the second group (B) received 0.5 mg of E_3 administered vaginally three times a week and 100 IU of sCT spray and 1 g/die of calcium for 12 months.

Each patient underwent bone mineralometry with a single ray source of ^{125}I, before the basal administration and this was repeated periodically after 3, 6, 9 and 12 months to evaluate BMC. Alkaline phosphatase and hydroxyprotine levels were determined after 6 and 12 months.

The second study consisted of 24 patients in physiological menopause for 24 years, randomly divided into three groups of eight. The first group received 0.5 mg estradiol administered vaginally three times a week for 12 months and 1 g/die of calcium. The second group received 100 IU of sCT spray/die and 1 g Ca^{2+}. BMC, alkaline phosphate and hydroxyproline levels were also measured in these women following the protocol mentioned above.

Intensity and frequency of hot flushes and sweating were measured in these woman using an arbitrary scale – at basal conditions and after 6 and 12 months of treatment. We excluded patients presenting lipid metabolism alterations or those having recently received prolonged cortisone treatment. Use of drugs interfering with calcium phosphate metabolism was not permitted during the study.

RESULTS

Table 1 shows the percentage variations with respect to the basal (preadministration) values of BMC in the two groups of patients studied. Group A, treated with sCT spray, presented a 0.7% reduction at the third month following treatment which progressively increased to 0.8% at 12 months.

In Group B, treated with sCT spray and E_3, the percentage of increase went from 0.8% at 6 months (Table 1) to 1.8% at 12 months. Table 2 shows the variations in levels of alkaline phosphatase and hydroxyproline. No significant changes were reported for either alkaline phosphatase or hydroxyproline during the 12 months of the study with respect to pretreatment values.

Table 1 Changes (%) of BMC in the ovariectomized women

	n	*0*	*3 months*	*6 months*	*9 months*	*12 months*
Group A (sCT)	7	—	−0.7	+0.2	+0.6	+0.8
Group B (E_3 + sCT)	7	—	−0.2	+0.8	+1.2	+1.8

Table 2 Changes of alkaline phosphatase and hydroxyproline (mean ± SD) in the ovariectomized women

	n	*0*	*6 months*	*12 months*
Group A (sCT)	7			
Alkaline phosphatase		148 ± 9.7	151 ± 11.4	142 ± 6.8
Hydroxyproline		17.7 ± 3.4	15.4 ± 2.6	16.1 ± 3.2
Group B (E_3 + sCT)	7			
Alkaline phosphatase		157 ± 11	152 ± 9.6	158 ± 13
Hydroxyproline		19.4 ± 4.3	17.5 ± 3.9	16.8 ± 4.1

Percentage variations of BMC (with respect to basal values) of the women in physiological menopause in the second study are reported in Table 3.

Group A, treated with E_3 and calcium presented a moderate progressive increase until the eighth month (41.3%) and a successive reduction to 0.8% at the twelfth month.

Group B, (sCT + E_3 + calcium) presented a 3% increase in the third month, increasing to 4.8% at the twelfth month of the treatment.

Group C, (sCT + calcium) showed a progressive percentage increase reaching 12.9% at 12 months. Table 4 reports average values (±SD) of alkaline phosphatase and hydroxyproline in the three groups examined. There were no significant variations in average values of alkaline phosphatase at the sixth and twelfth month with respect to basal values. All three groups presented a significant reduction in hydroxyproline secretion after 12 months of therapy with respect to basal values.

Table 5 reports variations in intensity and frequency of hot flushes and sweating in all three groups. In group A (vaginal E_3) there was a 65% and 68% reduction in intensity after 6 and 12 months respectively while frequency was reduced to 61% (6 months) and 71% (12 months). The per cent reduction

Table 3 Changes (%) of BMC in women with physiological menopause

	n	*0*	*3 months*	*6 months*	*9 months*	*12 months*
Group A (E_3)	8	—	+0.9	+1.2	+1.3	+0.95
Group B (E_3 + sCT)	8	—	+3	+4.4	+4.6	+4.8
Group C (sCT)	8	—	+1.6	+2.3	+2.7	+2.9

Table 4 Changes of alkaline phosphatase and hydroxyproline (mean ± SD) in physiological menopausal women

	n	*0*	*6 months*	*12 months*
Group A (E_3)	8			
Alkaline phosphatase		148 ± 14	157 ± 12	154 ± 11
Hydroxyproline		29.6 ± 4.1	23.2 ± 3.4	18.5 ± 3.1
Group B (E_3 + sCT)	8			
Alkaline phosphatase		163 ± 9	154 ± 13.4	161 ± 11
Hydroxyproline		31.3 ± 4.4	21.0 ± 6.1	15.4 ± 5.3
Group C (sCT)	8			
Alkaline phosphatase		144 ± 11.3	156 ± 14.6	152 ± 12.0
Hydroxyproline		28.5 ± 3.8	20.4 ± 4.3	16.8 ± 3.5

Table 5 Changes (%) of intensity and frequency of sweating and hot flushes in the patients in physiological menopause

	3 months		*6 months*		*12 months*	
	Intensity	*Frequency*	*Intensity*	*Frequency*	*Intensity*	*Frequency*
Group A (E_3)	−46	−55	−61	−65	−71	−68
Group B (E_3 + sCT)	−42	−51	−58	−66	−65	−64
Group C (sCT)	−15	−12	−21	−23	−27	−22

in intensity and frequency of sweating of group B was similar to that observed in group A; In group C (sCT spray) at the end of the treatment there was a slight reduction of the symptoms studied to 27% in frequency and 22% in intensity.

DISCUSSION

These two studies clearly demonstrate the positive role of calcitonin in spray form in calcium phosphate metabolism. However, a particularly interesting notion emerges in the group treated with sCT and estriol. This combination provides a significantly greater increase in BMC with respect to the use of only one or the other drug. This was clearly demonstrated in the ovariectomized women but above all in those in physiological menopause reaching a 4.8% increase at 12 months following treatment. Undoubtedly, estriol has a positive role in calcium phosphate metabolism when examining the data of women in postmenopause.

These results depend on the route of administration which permits an increase of concentration 20 times greater than that obtained with oral administration of the hormone. Our observation of estriol's positive role in calcium phosphate metabolism is justified by the presence of hormone receptors in the bone[11] and the effect of estrogen stimulus on calcitonin secretion[12]. The combined activity of the association of sCT and estriol at various levels on bone metabolism, determine calcium loss and create a more rapid and significant increase in BMC.

In this way we resolve the problem of estrogen deficiency and its repercussions in postmenopausal women who present contraindications to the use of progestinics alone, since estriol presents no contraindications and does not need to be associated with a progestinic.

REFERENCES

1. Gennari, C., Agnusdei, D., Zara, C. and Polatti, F. (1987). Profilassi dell'osteoporosi post-menopausale con Estro-Progestinici. In Fioretti, P. and Melis, G. B. (eds). *Aggiornamenti in Scienze Ginecologici ed Ostetrici*, pp. 253–61 (Milan: CIC)
2. Council of Scientific Affairs (1983). Estrogen replacement in the menopause. *J. Am. Med. Assoc.*, **3**, 359–61
3. Zara, C., Caprotti, M., Mandelli, B., Lauri, A., Perotti, F., Ferraro, R. and Polatti, F. (1988). L'uso della calcitonina spray nasale in ginecologia. *II Cong. Naz:di Scienze Ginec. ed Ost. Isola d'Elba*, 1988 (in press)
4. Zara, C. and Polatti, F. (1987). Analisi retrospettiva dell'efficacia di diversi trattamenti con calcitonina in donne ovariectomizzate. In Genazzani, A. R. *et al.* (eds.). *Ost. e Gin. Seminario invernale di aggiornamento*. pp. 543–7 (Milan: CIC Ed.)
5. Zara, C. and Polatti, F. (1988). Prevenzione della demineralizzazione ossea nella post-menopausa fisologica e chirurgica con sCT spray. In Mazzuoli, G. F. (ed.). *Int. Symp.: Calcitonin '88: New Therapeutic Perspectives. The nasal spray*. pp. 105–9
6. Clark, J.H., Paszko, Z. and Peck, E.J. (1987). Nuclear binding and retention of receptor estrogen complex: relation to the agonistic properties of oestriol. *Endocrinology*, **100**, 335
7. Englund, D.E., Elamsson, K.E. and Johansson, E.D.B. (1982). Bioavailability of Oestriol. *Acta Endocrinol.*, **99**, 136–40
8. Lindsay, R., Hart, D.M., LacLean, A., Garwood, J., Clark, A.C. and Kraszewski, A. (1979). Bone loss during Oestriol therapy in postmenopausal women. *Maturitas*, **1**, 279–85

9. Christiansen, C. and Rodbro, P. (1984). Does Oestriol add to the beneficial effect of combined hormonal prophilaxis agonist early post-menopausal osteoporosis? *Br. J. Obstet. Gynaecol.*, **9**, 489–93
10. Englund, D.E. and Heimer, G.M. (1986). Pharmacokinetic study on Oestriol: the influence of time, route of administration and food habits. In Genazzani, A. R. *et al.* (eds) *Research on Gynecological Endocrinology*, pp. 475–82
11. Eriksne, E.F. and Riggs, B.L. (1987). *I Cong. Int. dell'European Foundation for Osteoporosis and Bone Disease*, Alborg, Denmark
12. Whitehead, M.I., Lance, G., Morsman, J., Myers, C.H. and Stevenson, J.C. (1984). Effect of castration on calcium regulating hormones. In Christiansen, C. *et al.* (eds) *Osteoporosis 1*, pp. 331–2, Copenhagen

134

Effect of estriol on the transport of blood cells

C. Romanini, L. Mazzanti, A.L. Tranquilli, H. Valensise and N. Cester

INTRODUCTION

The present tendency concerning the symptoms and alterations induced by menopause foresee an active treatment aimed not only at therapy but also at prevention.

Among a number of available protections, the use of estrogens is widely supported either as systemic drugs or as topical dressing for the trophic alterations of the vaginal mucosa. The rational basis of the latter use is the fact that such alterations may be due to the estrogenic deficiency present in the menopausal period.

However, the estrogen effects on the structure and functions of the cellular membranes are not completely understood, while the mechanisms of action at the receptorial level are well known.

In the light of these observations we considered it of interest to investigate the action of an estrogen of large clinical use, estriol, on some membrane activities involved in the process of cellular and organic aging. The goals of our study were primarily the transport activities of enzymes such as Na^+/K^+-ATPase and Ca^{2+}-ATPase. In fact, a number of substances exert their biological activities through the activation of these enzymes. The modification of membrane activities determines modifications in the intracellular micro-environment inducing specific biological activities depending on the functional specificity of the cell. Moreover, with regards the action of estrogens on transmembrane transport enzymes contrasting data exist in the literature. In fact, a reduction of the Na^+/K^+-ATPase activity was found in some encephalic areas in ovariectomized rats after estrogen treatment[1] which is not in agreement with the depolarizing activity usually ascribed to these hormones and with the reported increase in calcium influx in rat myometrium referred to an activation of calcium channels[2].

Another problem that we analyzed is based on the finding that the processes of both cellular and organic aging[3] are accompanied by an increase in free radicals, derived from different processes. It is well known that lipid peroxidation at the cellular membrane is a phenomenon probably related with aging and that it may be responsible for negative events, such as a structural modification of the membrane with subsequent functional variations. The increased fluidity and permeability of biological membranes with respect to the artificial ones is due to the higher content in polyunsaturated fatty acid rich phospholipids.

In fact, the presence of double bonds determines a less compact spatial configuration (increased fluidity), with more compatibility with the complex activities of the cellular microenvironment. However, polyethylenic fatty acids are particularly prone to peroxidation, with subsequent reduction of membrane fluidity and parallel decrease of the transport enzymatic activities.

Free radicals produced inside the cell also are able to insert themselves in the membrane, giving rise to a chain of noxious reactions, with alteration of transmembrane gradients, break in disulfide bonds between protein structures (with modifications of specific activities) or formation of new links between proteins and lipids (protein–protein or lipid–lipid crosslinking) causing a deep alteration in cellular microenvironment. Moreover, malondialdehyde is produced resulting from the oxidation of fatty acid[4].

Lipoperoxidation is able by itself to produce a decrease in the activities of the cellular membrane, probably related to the deep modifications of its structure. The activities of transmembrane transport systems might also be involved[5], the accumulation of malondialdehyde being responsible for the decrease of the Na^+/K^+-ATPase activity[6].

Therefore, peroxidative damage is complex and extensive, resulting either in deep modifications of lipid–protein interactions which are regulated by a definite structural and functional balance, either in alterations of polarity, upset by the prominence of peroxidated acyl radicals changed in their polarity and by the deep subversion of the structural composition.

It must be underlined that the cellular alterations related to the production of free radicals are not specific to the aging processes, but can be induced by a number of physical, environmental and pharmacological factors, such as irradiation, tobacco smoking, exposure to high partial tensions of oxygen, some anesthetics and solvents, some pesticides and antibiotics.

Lipid peroxidation is assumed to be the cause of some forms of hemolytic anemias with reduced erythrocyte survival caused by an altered membrane stability[7].

Moreover, it has long been known that the hepatotoxicity of carbon tetrachloride is due to an increase in lipoperoxidation[8].

Therefore, substances stabilizing the cellular membrane are able to exert an antiperoxidative action. Among these substances, vitamin E and cholesterol oppose the diffusion of the peroxidative process inside the lipid bilayer, by means of an isolation effect; a further protective action of cholesterol is due to its opposition to the access of free radicals external to the membrane, and it increases the thickness of the membrane.

Recently, an antiperoxidative action on hepatic microsomes has been attributed to estrogens[9]. This finding suggests the hypothesis that a similar action of estrogens could exist at the level of the plasma membrane, representing the basis of the present research. Moreover, it has been considered interesting to investigate the intracellular calcium content, using platelets as experimental models, measuring its concentration by the probe Fura 2 and determining its response to treatment with thrombin, which causes a calcium influx through specific membrane channels[10].

The relevance of this part of the study is due not only to the above mentioned report[2], but also to the important role that the intracellular concentration of the cation plays in the regulation and functionality of the cellular microenvironment.

MATERIALS AND METHODS

Cytosolic free calcium concentrations

Blood was drawn and immediately mixed with citrate–citric acid–dextrose (CCD: citrate 0.1 mol/l, citric acid 7 mmol/l, dextrose 140 mmol/l pH 6.5) in a ratio of 9:1. Platelet rich plasma (PRP) was obtained after centrifugation of whole blood for 20 min at 140 × *g* at room temperature. The platelet count was adjusted to 300 000/mm^3 by adding platelet poor plasma (PPP).

Ionized calcium in blood platelets was measured according to the method of Rao[11]. Platelets were washed twice in antiaggregating buffer (Tris–HCl 10 mmol/l, NaCl 150 mmol/l, EDTA 1 mmol/l, glucose 5 mmol/l pH 7.3) and subsequently incubated at 37°C for 45 min with Fura-2-acetoxymethylester (Fura-2 AM) 1 μmol/l in a solution containing NaCl 145 mmol/l, KCl 5 mmol/l, $MgSO_4$ 1 mmol/l, HEPES 10 mmol/l, glucose 10 mmol/l pH 7.4 for the loading of the calcium-sensitive probe. Thereafter, cells were washed in the same solution to remove the excess dye.

Intracellular Ca^{2+} levels were measured in a Perkin Elmer MPF-66 fluorescence spectrophotometer at 37°C according to the method of Grynkiewicz *et al.*[12]. The fluorescence intensity was read at a constant emission wavelength (490 nm) with changes in the excitation wavelength (340 and 380 nm). The calibration was carried out as described by Grynkiewicz *et al.*[12] using the following equation:

$$[Ca^{2+}]_i = K_d \times \frac{R - R_{min}}{R_{max} - R} \times \frac{Sf2}{Sb2}$$

where K_d (dissociation constant of Fura 2) = 224 nM; R = ratio of the fluorescence intensities at the excitation wavelengths of 340 and 380 nm; $-R_{min}$ and R_{max} = ratio of the fluorescence intensities in the absence of calcium (R_{min}) and with saturating levels (R_{max}); Sf2 and Sb2 = fluorescence intensities at 380 nm without calcium (Sb2) and with saturating levels of Ca^{2+} (Sb2).

R_{min} and Sf2 were measured after cellular lysis with Triton X100 25% and addition of EGTA 10 mmol/l pH 8.3; R_{max} and Sb2 were measured after lysis and addition of $CaCl_2$ 10 mmol/l.

Thrombin (0.2 U/ml) and ADP (3 μmol/l) were added in the presence of external Ca^{2+} ($CaCl_2$ 1 mmol/l) or in the absence of extracellular Ca^{2+} (EGTA 1 mmol/l).

Ca^{2+}-ATPase assay

Platelets were washed in a buffer containing Na_2HPO_4 8 mmol/l, NaH_2PO_4 2 mmol/l, EDTA 10 mmol/l, KCl 5 mmol/l, NaCl 135 mmol/l pH 7.0 and centrifuged at 3000 × *g* for 30 min to obtain the plasma membranes. Activity of the Ca^{2+}-ATPase was determined according to the method of Davis *et al.*[13] by measuring inorganic phosphate (P_i) hydrolysed from Na_2ATP 1 mmol/l at 37°C in the presence and absence of Ca^{2+} 0.15 mmol/l. The reaction medium contained EGTA 0.1 mmol/l, NaCl 75 mmol/l, KCl 25 mmol/l, $MgCl_2$ 1 mmol/l and Tris–HCl 25 mmol/l pH 7.4. ATPase activity in the absence of Ca^{2+} was subtracted from the total ATPase activity to calculate the activity of Ca^{2+}-ATPase.

Results are expressed as μmolP_i/(mg membrane proteins × 90 min). Inorganic phosphate was measured according to Fiske and Subbarow[14]. Protein concentration was determined by the Lowry method[15], using albumin as standard.

Na^+/K^+-ATPase assay

Na^+/K^+-ATPase activity was determined as previously described[16]. Briefly, the ATPase activity was assayed by incubating membranes at 37°C in 1 ml of medium containing $MgCl_2$ (5 mmol/l), NaCl (140 mmol/l), KCl (14 mmol/l) in Tris–HCl 40 mmol/l pH 7.7 according to the method of Kitao[17]. ATPase reaction was started by the addition of 3 mmol/l Na_2ATP and stopped 20 min later by the addition of 1 ml of 15% trichloroacetic acid, Inorganic phosphate (P_i) hydrolyzed from reaction was measured as previously described[14].

Enzyme activity was expressed as difference in inorganic phosphate released in the presence and absence of 10 mmol/l ouabain. ATPase activity in the presence of ouabain was subtracted from the total Mg^{2+} dependent ATPase activity to calculate the activity of the ouabain-sensitive Na^+/K^+-ATPase. Results are expressed as μmol P_i/(mg membrane proteins × 60 min).

Malondialdehyde determination

The determination of malondialdehyde in serum and membranes was performed according to the method of Yagi[18], that is based on the reaction of malondialdehyde with thiobarbituric acid to give a fluorescent product. The erythrocyte membranes were prepared according to the method of Burton[19].

RESULTS

Na^+/K^+-ATPase

Increasing concentrations of estriol added to the incubation medium of whole platelets demonstrated an activation of Na^+/K^+-ATPase that was manifested at a concentration of 0.5 ng per mg protein, after 24 h of incubation (Figure 1a). At lower concentrations a tendency to increase the activity is present, but the difference relative to the basal value was not statistically significant.

Also on erythrocyte ghosts the addition of estriol demonstrated an activation on the enzyme, already beginning from concentration of 0.2 ng/mg protein (Figure 1b).

Ca^{2+}-ATPase

The experiments performed with increasing concentrations of estrogens and after different incubation times have not given evidence of significant variations of the studied activity, neither on platelets nor on erythrocyte membranes (Figure 2).

Ca^{2+}

The intracellular calcium, detected with the fluorescent probe Fura 2 before and after activation with thrombin, increased as a function of the added, increasing concentrations of estriol relative to the basal values. It does not seem, overall, to exist a quantitative relationship between the increase of estrogen concentration and that of intracellular calcium.

Malondialdehyde

The formation of peroxides, evaluated by the fluorescence of malondialdehyde, was significantly depressed by increasing concentrations of estriol added to the system both with serum and erythrocyte membranes.

COMMENTS AND CONCLUSIONS

The results obtained permit us to have some considerations of the interaction between estriol and the cellular microenvironment.

(1) Addition of estriol induces a specific response at the level of Na^+/K^+-ATPase activity that is increased both in the whole platelets and on erythrocyte membranes, demonstrating the capacity of estrogen to activate the enzyme.

(2) Modification of Ca^{2+}-ATPase activity was not demonstrated, independent of hormone concentration and of the substrate used, hence confirming that the response is specific to Na^+/K^+-ATPase.

(3) The increase of intraplatelet Ca^{2+} detected by using Fura 2 seems overall to refer to the activation of calcium channels, in agreement with the data of Batra[2]. Moreover the ATPase dependent transport system is not involved, as shown above.

(4) The malondialdehyde level demonstrated an antiperoxidant activity of

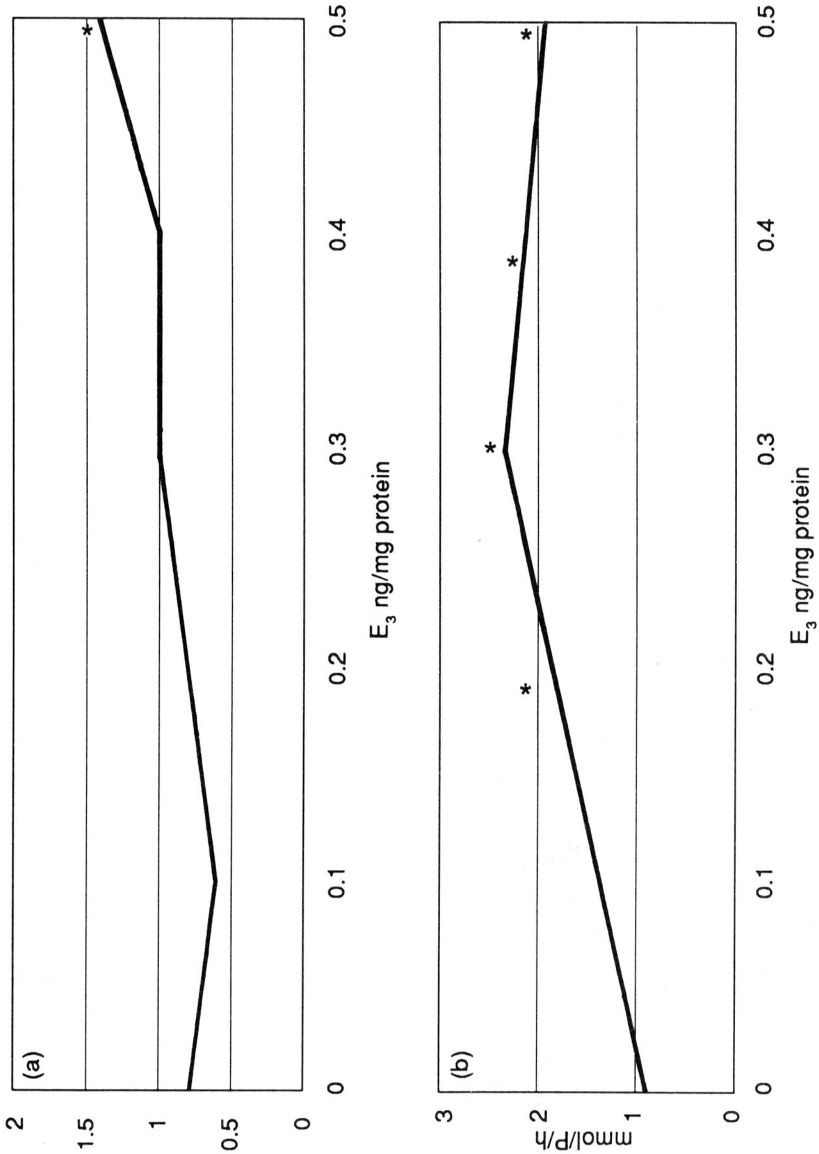

Figure 1 Effect of increasing E_3 concentration on Na^+/K^+-ATPase activity after 24 h incubation: (a) whole platelets and (b) erythrocyte ghosts

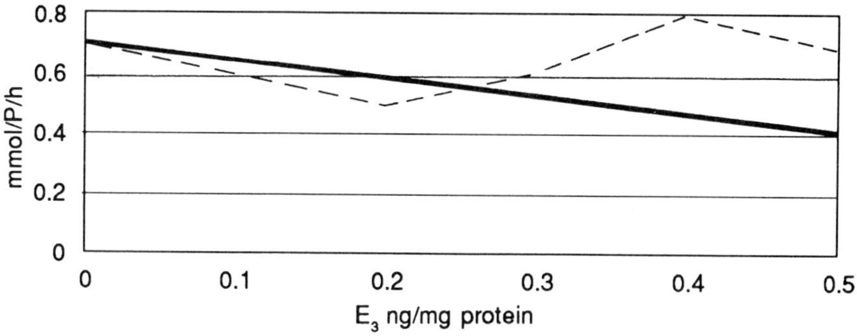

Figure 2 Effect of increasing E_3 on Ca^{2+}-ATPase activity after 24 h incubation

the addition of estriol both to plasma and to cellular membranes. The inrease of Na^+/K^+-ATPase activity may therefore derive from direct action of estriol or from the reduced formation of peroxides that may have inhibitory action on the transport enzymes and specifically Na^+/K^+-ATPase[6].

(5) The reduction of lipoperoxidation shows protective activity toward the cells, against alterations by free radicals, by estriol.

The experimental evidence obtained therefore confirms that estriol expresses an antioxidant activity at the cellular level, accompanied by stabilization of the membrane and increase of active and passive transport activity, that fits into its complex action of cellular protection and activation. Such action, in the specific context of the modifications provoked by menopause, may result in great utility or interest because it seems to contrast specifically the unfavorable effects of the syndrome at the cellular and tissue level.

ACKNOWLEDGEMENTS

The authors wish to thank Drs R. A. Rabini, G. Benedetti and A. M. Cugini for helping during the work.

REFERENCES

1. Rodriguez del Castillo, A., Battaner, E., Guerra, M., Alonso, I. and Mas, M. (1987). Regional changes of brain Na^+/K^+-transporting adenosine triphosphatase related to ovarian function. *Brain Res.*, **416**, 113
2. Batra, S. (1989). Increase by estrogen of calcium entry and calcium channel density in uterine smooth muscle. *Br. J. Pharmacol.*, **92**, 389
3. Rockstein, M., Sussmen, M.L. and Chesky, J. (eds) (1974). *Theoretical Aspects of Aging* (New York: Academic Press)
4. Freeman, B.A. and Crapo, J.D. (1982). Biology of disease-free radicals and tissue injury. *Lab. Invest.*, **47**, 412

5. Kesner, L., Kindya, R.J. and Chan, P.C. (1979). Inhibition of erythrocyte membrane activated ATPase by Ozone-treated phospholipids. *J. Biol. Chem.*, **254**, 2705–9
6. Uysal, M. (1986). Erytrocyte lipid peroxidation and Na^+/K^+-ATPase activity in cholesterol fed rabbits. *Intern. J. Vit. Nutr. Res.*, **56**, 307–10
7. Chiu, D. and Lubin, B. (1979). Vitamin E and glutathione peroxidase levels in sickle cell anemia. Evidence for increased susceptibility to lipid peroxidation *in vivo*. *J. Lab. Clin. Med.*, **94**, 542–8
8. Dianzani, M.U., Gabriel, L., Gravela, E. and Paradisi, L. (1976). Interference of CCL14 metabolites with subcellular structures. *Pammin. Med.*, **18**, 310
9. Sugioka, K., Shimosegawa, Y. and Nakano, M. (1987). Estrogens as natural antioxidants of membrane phospholipid peroxidation. *FEBS Lett.*, **210**, 37–9
10. Zschauer, A., Van Breemen, C., Buhler, F.R. and Nelson, H.T. (1988). Calcium channels in thrombin activated human platelet membrane. *Nature*, **334**, 703–5
11. Rao, G.H.R. (1988). Measurement of ionized calcium in normal human blood platelets. *Anal. Biochem.*, **169**, 400–4
12. Grynkiewicz, G., Poenie, M. and Tsien, R.Y. (1985). A new generation of Ca^{2+} indicators with greatly improved fluorescence properties. *J. Biol. Chem.*, **6**, 3440–50
13. Davis, F.B., Davis, P.J., Nat, G., Blas, S.D., MacGillivray, M., Gutman, S. and Feldman, M.J. (1985). The effect of *in vivo* glucose administration on human erythrocyte Ca^{++}-ATPase activity and on enzyme responsiveness *in vitro* to thyroid hormone and calmodulin. *Diabetes*, **34**, 639–46
14. Fiske, C. and Subbarow, Y. (1925). The colorimetric determination of phosphorus. *J. Biol. Chem.*, **66**, 375–400
15. Lowry, O.H., Rosenburg, M.Y., Farr, A.L. and Randall, R.T. (1951). Protein measurements with the Folin phenol reagent. *J. Biol. Chem.*, **192**, 265–75
16. Testa, I., Rabini, R.A., Danieli, G., Tranquilli, A.L., Cester, N., Romanini, C., Bertoli, E. and Mazzanti, L. (1988). Abnormal membrane cation transport in pregnancy-induced hypertension. *Scand. J. Clin. Lab. Invest.*, **48**, 7–14
17. Kitao, T. and Hattori, K. (1983). Inhibition of erythrocyte ATPase activity by aclacynomycin and reverse effects of ascorbate on ATPase activity. *Experientia*, **39**, 1362–4
18. Yagi, K. (1984). Assay for blood plasma or serum. *Meth. Enzymol.*, **105**, 328–31
19. Burton, J.W., Ingold, K.U.U. and Thompson, K.E. (1981). An improved procedure for the isolation of ghost membranes from human red blood cells. *Lipids*, **16**, 946

Index